Leeds Metropolitan University
17 0212524 8

Hollinshead's

Textbook of Anatomy

Hollinshead's

Textbook of Anatomy

Fifth Edition

Cornelius Rosse, M.D., D. Sc.
Professor

Penelope Gaddum-Rosse, Ph.D.
Associate Professor

Department of Biological Structure
University of Washington School of Medicine
Seattle, Washington

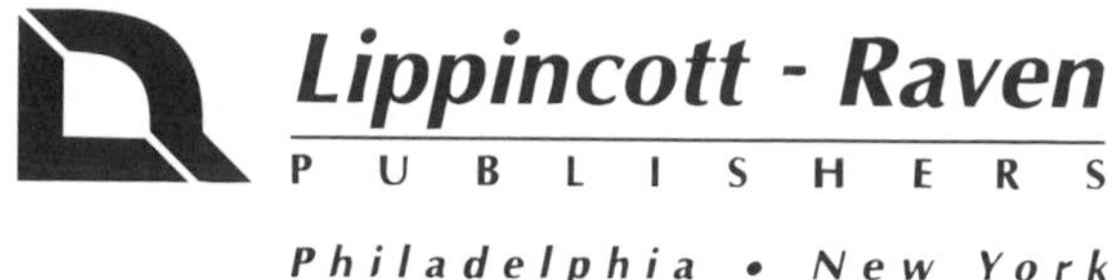

Philadelphia • New York

Acquisitions Editor: Richard Winters
Senior Developmental Editor: Delois Patterson
Project Editor: Bridget H. Meyer
Production Manager: Caren Erlichman
Senior Production Coordinator: Kevin P. Johnson
Design Coordinator: Kathy Kelley-Luedtke
Indexer: Kathi Unger
Compositor: Maryland Composition Company, Inc.
Printer: R.R. Donnelley and Sons Company

5th Edition

Library of Congress Cataloging-in-Publication Data

Rosse, Cornelius.
Hollinshead's textbook of anatomy. — 5th ed. / Cornelius Rosse, Penelope Gaddum-Rosse.
p. cm.
Rev. ed of: Textbook of anatomy. 4th ed. / W. Henry Hollinshead, Cornelius Rosse. c1985.
Includes bibliographical references and index.
ISBN 0–397–51256–2 (alk. paper)
1. Human anatomy. I. Gaddum–Rosse, Penelope. II. Hollinshead, W. Henry (William Henry), 1906– Textbook of anatomy. III. Title.
[DNLM: 1. Anatomy. QS 4 R828h 1997]
QM23.2.H57 1997
611—dc20
DNLM/DLC
for Library of Congress 96–8005
CIP

Care has been taken to confirm the accuracy of the information presented and to describe generally accepted practices. However, the authors, editors, and publisher are not responsible for errors or omissions or for any consequences from application of the information in this book and make no warranty, express or implied, with respect to the contents of the publication.

The authors, editors, and publisher have exerted every effort to ensure that drug selection and dosage set forth in this text are in accordance with current recommendations and practice at the time of publication. However, in view of ongoing research, changes in government regulations, and the constant flow of information relating to drug therapy and drug reactions, the reader is urged to check the package insert for each drug for any change in indications and dosage and for added warnings and precautions. This is particularly important when the recommended agent is a new or infrequently employed drug.

Some drugs and medical devices presented in this publication have Food and Drug Administration (FDA) clearance for limited use in restricted research settings. It is the responsibility of the health care provider to ascertain the FDA status of each drug or device planned for use in their clinical practice.

Preface

The motivation for this fifth edition of *Textbook of Anatomy* remains essentially unchanged from that expressed by its original author, W. Henry Hollinshead, PhD, who first published the book in 1962 and revised it through two successive editions: "to present to the student of medicine and dentistry an account of anatomical facts and concepts that he will need to know, or know where to acquire, during his years of formal study in his chosen profession; to provide a foundation of anatomical knowledge sufficient to build upon when more detailed knowledge becomes necessary; and to help make the study of anatomy more meaningful by emphasizing functional aspects and indicating some of the many ways in which anatomical knowledge influences medical practice." Weakened by protracted illness, Professor Hollinshead lived to voice his approval of the new aspects and directions introduced in the fourth edition, but passed away soon after its publication. His long and distinguished career was dedicated chiefly to graduate medical education in the surgical specialties. His three volume *Anatomy for Surgeons* is without equal in anatomical scholarship. The *Textbook of Anatomy* he prepared for students of medicine and dentistry was steeped in the same spirit. It is our intent to keep that spirit alive for future generations of students in the health-related professions and provide a resource of anatomical information that retains its usefulness and value through the ever changing trends of medical education.

The unprecedented expansion of biomedical knowledge during recent decades has necessitated an evaluation of curricula in the health-related professions. Consequently, the relatively stable period in medical education that prevailed during the middle third of this century has been followed by experimentation with curricular content and the design of new strategies and resources for learning. One of the noteworthy features of this process has been the active involvement of students, not only as experimental material but as critical monitors of the experimental results.

Three main conclusions may be drawn at this stage from the curricular reforms of the recent past: 1) experimentation and evaluation must continue, and flexibility must be built into the health-related professional curricula, anticipating not only the continued expansion of the biomedical sciences but also changes in the educational background of future student populations and in the needs of the health professions; 2) students are capable of, and motivated for, independent learning. Appropriate learning resources must be developed for this purpose, and curricular structure must place the responsibility for much of the learning on the student in order to foster an attitude for continued independent learning beyond graduation; and 3) it is not adequate to define curricular content by the sets of facts and skills on which the everyday practice of the profession relies. Unless the use of such facts and skills is based on a thorough and broad *understanding* of human biology, the practitioner will be restricted to the routine and conventional, degrading health care delivery from the professional to the trade level. Preparation for the practice of a *profession* demands education rather than mere training. *Education* is a protracted developmental process, resulting in a qualitative change in the learner's ability to integrate and use diverse types of information to handle not only routine but also novel and unfamiliar situations. In the process of education, the learner inevitably encounters many facts and concepts that will not surface in the everyday practice of the profession; yet, without such facts and concepts, an understanding of human biology could not be obtained.

Anatomy is basic to education in the health-related professions. ". . .The ultimate purpose of anatomy education is to assist the student in developing an implicit and fully internalized understanding of the 3-dimensional (3-D) dynamic structure of the living human body so that he or she can apply the appropriate cognitive skills when clinical problems call for anatomical reasoning. Anatomical reasoning is the cognitive process that relates manifestations of normal and abnormal function to anatomic entities and seeks to explain these manifestations in terms of the attributes of different anatomic structures. Anatomical reasoning is required for intelligently engaging in such fundamental clinical tasks as performing a physical examination, interpreting symptoms and signs of normalcy and disease, selecting appropriate diagnostic tests, particularly those concerned with imaging the body and interpreting the findings, and administering treatment for problems encountered in primary care and medical emergency settings." (*Rosse, Academic Medicine, 1995; 70:499.*).

Contrary to the opinion of many, the study of anatomy need not consist of the memorization of long lists of names; rather, it should rely on the visualization of parts and regions of the body in three dimensions based on an understanding of how these relationships have come about and why they exist. Such an understanding may be gained through the study of embryology. Therefore, developmental considerations have been included liberally in this text without an attempt to present a comprehensive account of embryology. Many chapters and sections of the book begin with an introductory account of embryology in order to present the organizational plan of an anatomic region or organ. Developmental considerations are also used throughout the chapters to explain anatomical relationships and to introduce relevant congenital abnormalities as well as other concepts. The organization of chapters that deal with the gross anatomy of body regions and parts is such that it facilitates integration of the text with dissection of the cadaver. Many of these chapters, or their major sections, end by summarizing anatomy from the perspective of the physical examination. In our opinion, the physical examination is, in fact, the assessment of functional anatomy. Skills for eliciting physical signs would be most profitably learned in conjunction with the study of anatomy, an approach that would promote anatomical reasoning in clinical practice. Although examples of various clinical conditions are used abundantly to illustrate anatomical principles, the main emphasis is on the anatomical knowledge required for performing and interpreting physical signs in particular regions or parts of the body.

Our motivation for promoting anatomical reasoning requires that a comprehensive account be given of the anatomy of the human body. We have made no attempt to limit the information to so-called essential facts. Defining what is essential, and for what purpose, is an intractable problem. A comprehensive view of anatomy should enable both students and practitioners of medicine and dentistry to put into appropriate context the detailed information that is relevant to the problems they intend to solve. Each chapter and each of its sections usually begin with an overall view that sets the scene for enhancing this basic information in the remaining parts of the chapter or individual section. A different font is used for presenting a third layer of information which provides insights into the material from different viewpoints.

The aim of this three-tiered approach is to make apparent a system according to which anatomical information can be organized. Such a framework should enable both the student and the practitioner of medicine and dentistry to filter anatomical information, and to use detailed information through reasoning rather than by recalling memorized facts.

Through the emphasis placed on anatomical reasoning, this textbook should fill an important need in educational settings that rely increasingly on problem-based learning and on computerized representations of anatomy. Both of these approaches require a resource that, instead of giving concisely packaged answers to discrete questions, provides explanations in the context of relationships and systems that interrelate components of the human body. Although we do not present clinical cases for problem solving, the use of this textbook should be a valuable resource in solving problems in the dissection laboratory and at the bedside.

There are many references in this book to the methods of obtaining anatomical data and also to the knowledge gaps that still exist in certain areas. New information is being published in anatomy at a more rapid rate than ever before. New methods for imaging the body are producing anatomical data on a large scale and the findings are being reported in a number of journals. In fact, new journals have been established for this particular purpose. Such scholarly publications include, for example, *Surgical and Radiologic Anatomy, Clinical Anatomy, Acta Anatomica, Anatomical Record, Anatomy and Embryology, Annals of Anatomy, Journal of Anatomy, Developmental Dynamics, Acta Radiologica, American Journal of Radiology, British Journal of Radiology* and *Investigative Radiology,* as well as journals in the various surgical sub-specialties. Perhaps even more important than these journals is the availability of on-line information sources such as MEDLINE through which information relevant to any anatomical topic can be pursued. We encourage students and practitioners of anatomy to make use of these resources because they will meet their needs better than the limited and selective lists that can be included in publications such as this textbook.

The fifth edition conforms in general to the previous editions. Following an introductory section in Part I, nine brief chapters in Part II give a general account of the tissues and systems of the body. In these chapters the emphasis is on continuities in a particular organ system from one region of the body to another. The function of each system is discussed as a whole. Parts III to VIII encompass the remaining twenty-three chapters, which deal with the regions of the body.

The seven chapters that comprise the back (Part III) and the limbs (Part IV) have been entirely re-written. They now conform in orientation and approach to Parts V, VI, and VII (thorax, abdomen, pelvis and perineum), which were rewritten for the fourth edition. In these parts, developmental considerations and "living anatomy", the basis for the physical examination, are integrated with the description of topographical anatomy.

Over 200 new figures have been added to the fifth edition and a substantial number of existing illustrations have been modified. The new illustrations include many radiological images obtained with different methods. They illustrate normal anatomy as well as lesions, which assist in understanding the appearance of normal structures.

It is our hope that the changes made in the fifth edition of this *Textbook of Anatomy* respond in a constructive manner to the demands of contemporary educational needs in the health-related professions. By aiming to provide the conceptual and functional basis for understanding the human body at the macroscopic level of organization, we hope to stimulate students to acquire the ability to think and reason in anatomical terms. The presentation of the material will, we hope, lend itself to independent study of the subject as well as to use in conjunction with structured courses. The degree of our success in realizing our intentions can be gauged by the feedback that we invite from our students and colleagues who select this book as an aid to learning and teaching anatomy.

Cornelius Rosse, MD, DSC
Penelope Gaddum-Rosse, PhD

Acknowledgments

We wish to record our thanks to a number of our colleagues and associates who have generously contributed to the fifth edition of this book.

Parts III and IV of the fifth edition have benefited extensively from long-standing collaborations with Dr. D. Kay Clawson, formerly Chairman of the Department of Orthopaedics at the University of Washington and, until recently, Executive Vice Chancellor, University of Kansas. Chapters dealing with the back and the limbs draw extensively on *Rosse and Clawson: The Musculoskeletal System in Health and Disease,* Harper & Row Publishers, which has been out of print for some time. Considerations of functional anatomy and its application to clinical conditions owe a great deal to Dr. Clawson's direct and indirect contributions. His generosity in agreeing to the use of material from *The Musculoskeletal System in Health and Disease* in this book is particularly appreciated. Dr. Walter C. Stolov, Professor and Chairman of the Department of Rehabilitation Medicine, University of Washington, has likewise allowed us to base descriptions of the gait cycle in this book on his chapter in *The Musculoskeletal System in Health and Disease.*

The sections in Chapter 21 dealing with the normal and abnormal development of the heart were written in close collaboration with Dr. Lore Tenckhoff, Cardiologist, Clinical Professor of Pediatrics and Radiology at the University of Washington. The section on the breast in Chapter 15 has benefited substantially from the criticism and input provided by Dr. Roger E. Moe, Professor and Director, Breast Cancer Program, Department of Surgery and UWMC BioClinical Breast Cancer Unit, and Dr. Mariann Drucker, Acting Assistant Professor, Director of Mammography, in the Department of Radiology, both at the University of Washington. The radiographs that illustrate the anatomy of the breast were kindly provided by Dr. Drucker.

A large number of the radiographs that enrich the chapters in Parts III and IV were provided by Dr. Rosalind H. Troupin, Professor, Department of Radiology, Hospital of the University of Pennsylvania while she taught musculoskeletal anatomy at the University of Washington as a member of a team that also included Drs. Clawson and Stolov, as well as one of us (CR). We are grateful to her for granting permission to use this extensive material in this book. Dr. Thurman Gillespy, III, Associate Professor, and Dr. Eric Effmann, Professor, both in the Department of Radiology at the University of Washington, have responded generously to our requests to provide MRI scans and x-ray films illustrating normal anatomy and the development of bones, respectively. The numerous radiographs that appear throughout Parts V to VII, without specific credit, have all been provided by members of the faculty of the Department of Radiology, University of Washington. The helpfulness and high professional standards of this department deserve praise and our boundless gratitude. We would like to thank Drs. Melvin M. Figley, Leon A. Phillips, and Charles A. Rohrmann for their generosity and cooperation.

Dr. Raymond F. Gasser, Professor, Department of Anatomy, Louisiana State University, Dr. Adrianne Noe, Director of the Human Developmental Anatomy Center, Armed Forces Institute of Pathology, Dr. William J. Larsen, Professor of Cell Biology, Neurobiology and Anatomy at the University of Cincinnati and Dr. Robert O. Kelley, Professor and Chairman, Department of Anatomy, University of New Mexico, have all responded generously to our requests for assistance with sections of this book that deal with embryology. Dr. John Loeser, Professor, Department of Neurological Surgery, and Director, Multidisciplinary Pain Center at the University of Washington, advised us on developmental defects of the vertebral canal and spinal cord. We are grateful for the detailed suggestions of Dr. Gasser and William J. Swartz for many desirable changes in the fifth edition.

Newly written sections of this book have benefited from the contributions of a number of medical artists. They include Grace von Drasek Ascher, Charlotte P.G. Kaiser, Kate Sweeney, and the late Jessie Phillips. We are grateful for the painstaking work of Brent Dietrich who digitized and enhanced all the new illustrations with the computer, and also generated a number of original figures.

Shelley R. Golard has served as an invaluable resource in the capacity of administrative research assistant. We are grateful for her dedication and the overall support she has provided in all aspects of preparing the fifth edition.

We wish to thank Mr. Mike Belknap of the Visual Information Section, Mayo Clinic, for his cooperation in providing for us, in digitized form, numerous illustrations owned by the Mayo Clinic that have been published either in this textbook or in *Anatomy for Surgeons*. Our publishers have been patient during the protracted preparation of this new edition and we thank them for the support and cooperation they have given us.

Contents

Part V Thorax 419

Part VI Abdomen 513

Part VII Pelvis and Perineum 639

Part VIII Head & Neck 701

Hollinshead's

Textbook of Anatomy

PART I

INTRODUCTION

Hollinshead's Textbook of Anatomy, by Cornelius Rosse and
Penelope Gaddum-Rosse.
Lippincott-Raven Publishers, Philadelphia, © 1997.

CHAPTER 1

The Study of Anatomy

CONTENT AND SUBDIVISIONS OF THE SUBJECT

The word *anatomy* is derived from Greek roots that mean "to cut up" or "to dissect." The study of human anatomy in its early stages was adequately defined by this term, for anatomy dealt only with structures that could be displayed by dissection and that were visible to the naked eye, what we now call *gross anatomy*. Although essentially a morphologic science, anatomy was never purely that. Even in the earliest writings there were speculations concerning the importance of the various parts and how they worked. Thus, a consideration of the use to which a part is put and how it fulfills its functions has always been a part of anatomy. Without considering function, anatomic study would be analogous to learning the names and arrangement of all the parts of an automobile engine and having no concept of what the engine does or how it works. Although there are a few exceptions, all structures have a function associated with them that is quite obvious, even to a lay person. Function is dependent on structure, whether it is gross, microscopic, or molecular.

Physiology, a discipline primarily concerned with the study of function in biologic systems, became separated from anatomy as a science in its own right as methods of investigating structure and function became increasingly complex. The division between anatomy and physiology, however, can never be as sharp as intimated by their separate names and the different academic units concerned with their study.

It is difficult to make a sharp distinction between anatomy and physiology, and it is even more difficult to do so between the various subdivisions of anatomy. These subdivisions fall conveniently into four general spheres: gross anatomy, neuroanatomy, microscopic anatomy or histology, and developmental anatomy or embryology. Such subdivisions are purely arbitrary and are for the convenience of instruction only. Furthermore, it is important to appreciate that none of the subdivisions can be understood without some knowledge of the others.

In short, the study of anatomy is concerned primarily with structure, ranging from the molecular to the macroscopic, and properly includes a consideration of the formation and functional importance of all parts of the organism. Human anatomy, therefore, is a sector of special interest within the field of human biology. Just as it is true in medicine that treatment should be directed at the patient and not at a specific disease, so it is true of anatomy, that it should concern itself with all the aspects of human biology that are necessary for an understanding of the function of the living body. The field of anatomy is an enormous, expanding area that no one ever completely masters. Different specialties in the health professions concern themselves in greater or lesser depth with certain aspects of this large body of knowledge. However, to apply this knowledge, it is necessary to have a basic understanding of the structure of the human body as a whole.

Gross anatomy itself is sometimes divided according to methods of approach. Systemic anatomy attempts to treat the body according to systems: skeletal, vascular, and so forth. Regional anatomy deals with several systems located in a particular region of the body. Practical or surgical anatomy emphasizes certain features that are of particular importance to the practitioners of medicine and surgery. All three of these approaches necessarily deal with the same basic subject matter. The student of gross anatomy needs to combine all three approaches. A general understanding of the systems of the body aids in an appreciation of the more detailed regional anatomy and of the interrelations between parts and regions. The regional approach is commonly used in the dissection room and is also most useful to the physician and surgeon. Consideration of the functional and clinical aspects of anatomy provides a better background on which to build clinical knowledge. This functional approach aids learning by emphasizing the importance of what may seem to be a mass of unrelated minutiae.

CONTENTS OF THIS TEXT

Any one-volume textbook of anatomy necessarily omits many details; there is enough available information to fill volumes. Therefore, this book does not contain enough detail to meet all the possible present and future requirements of the student. Other sources of information will be needed. Fortunately, however, it is possible to recognize a fairly large body of information as being necessary to any thorough study of gross anatomy, and that is what this book attempts to present.

Even though gross anatomy is an old science, interpretations of anatomic facts sometimes change rapidly, and there are some points about which there are long-standing differences of opinion among anatomists. Ideally, the student should be made aware of such differences of opinion. However, divergent views can properly be presented only in detail, and this is not possible in a short text. Occasionally, therefore, views presented in this book will not agree with those of the student's instructors, because some necessarily represent only one opinion.

Certain aspects of gross anatomy are understandable only when there is a background of knowledge in neuroanatomy, histology, and embryology. Yet students are rarely well versed in these fields at the time they are introduced to gross anatomy. For this reason, certain fundamentals that belong more properly to another field, such as a discussion of the histology of a nerve or the explanation of the development of a part, are introduced at appropriate places in the text. The aim is to elucidate the gross anatomy, not to give a well-rounded picture of any other field. It is assumed that the student has texts in those fields and will turn to them, as necessary, for further information.

Although some of the systemic anatomy presented in this text is acquired by many students in courses in comparative anatomy, parts of it will be new to most students. It is suggested, therefore, that the student read pertinent chapters of the systemic anatomy as early as possible in an anatomy course. Chapter 2 (Anatomic Terminology) should be understood from the very beginning. Because one cannot dissect anywhere without encountering skin, fascia, muscles, nerves, and vessels, Chapter 3 (The Skin and Appendages), Chapter 4 (The Connective Tissues), Chapter 5 (The Skeletal System), Chapter 6 (The Muscular System), Chapter 7 (The Nervous System), and Chapter 8 (The Cardiovascular and Lymphatic Systems) contain background information useful from the very first part of the dissection. The parts of Chapter 7 dealing with the autonomic and central nervous systems can be postponed, if desired, until dissection involves some parts of these, and so can Chapters 9 (The Digestive and Respiratory Systems), 10 (The Urogenital System), and 11 (The Endocrine System).

In the discussion of regional parts, some of the material appears in a different font than that used for the main text. This is material that usually cannot be verified in the dissecting laboratory, or it is of an explanatory nature that amplifies the main part of the text. Because it includes discussion of functional and developmental aspects and of clinical applications, it should not be thought of as less important; indeed, much of the material in these sections is necessary for an understanding of the presentation as a whole.

Structures are described, on the whole, in the order in which they can be found during the dissection. Because this type of presentation does not permit complete description of nerves and vessels, only parts of which are usually visible at any one stage of dissection, summaries of the nerves and vessels are provided in introductory sections or in summaries.

HINTS ON STUDYING

Anatomy is a visual science. It is essential for the student to engage the "mind's eye." The time spent on repeated reading of the text will be less effective than the time spent thinking about the subject and visualizing a structure and its relation to other parts or regions. It is well to read the text before going to the dissection room, to become familiar with the region, to learn what to look for, and to gain some understanding of the functional implications of the parts to be dissected. Even at this stage, it is useful to try to visualize what is being read, and it is an added advantage to be able to see it with the book or atlas closed. The text should be consulted again to fill in specific gaps, rather than to reread a complete section. Dissection is usually performed with the aid of special guides, and in performing the dissection, the student should anticipate the structures that are already in the mind's eye. This way, dissection will be a challenging experience, and its reward will be discovery. Knowledge gained from the textbook and atlases will be reinforced and expanded by dissection. Before embarking on the next area of study, the student should again, by way of a summary, recall visually the dissected parts and return to the textbook to reinforce the known concepts and to pick up additional details that may have been overlooked in the first reading.

It is helpful to meet with fellow students periodically to discuss the material and quiz each other on what has been learned. Instead of merely giving answers to isolated questions, being able to explain anatomy is the best proof of its thorough understanding.

RECOMMENDED READINGS

Crisp AH. The relevance of anatomy and morbid anatomy for medical practice and hence for postgraduate and continuing medical education of doctors. Postgrad Med J 1989; 65: 221.

Dalley AF II, Driscoll RE, Settles HE. The uniform anatomical gift act: what every clinical anatomist should know. Clin Anat 1993; 6: 247.

Druce M, Johnson MH. Human dissection and attitudes of preclinical students to death and bereavement. Clin Anat 1994; 7: 42.

Evans EJ, Fitzgibbon GH. The dissecting room: reactions of first year medical students. Clin Anat 1992; 5: 311.

Garrison FH. An introduction to the history of medicine, with medical chronology, suggestions for study and bibliographic data, 4th ed. Philadelphia: WB Saunders, 1929.

Gustavson N. The effect of human dissection on first-year students and implications for the doctor-patient relationship. J Med Educ 1988; 63: 62.

Persaud TVN. Early history of human anatomy from antiquity to the beginning of the modern era. Springfield, IL: Charles C Thomas, 1984.

Singer C, Underwood EA. A short history of medicine, 2nd ed. New York: Oxford University Press, 1962.

Weeks SE, Harris EE, Kinzey WG. Human gross anatomy: a crucial time to encourage respect and compassion in students. Clin Anat 1995; 8: 69.

Hollinshead's Textbook of Anatomy, by Cornelius Rosse and Penelope Gaddum-Rosse.
Lippincott-Raven Publishers, Philadelphia, © 1997.

CHAPTER 2

Anatomic Terminology

Anatomy is a descriptive science. Therefore, its terminology is mainly descriptive; it is also logical. An accurate use of anatomic terms in anatomy is essential to avoid confusion. There is an international nomenclature, the basis of which is Latin. Despite the use of Latin, however, many of the meanings of the words are immediately obvious. For those that are not, the student must learn the meaning. In many instances, it is common and accepted practice to translate the Latin into the vernacular of the particular country concerned, but it is largely a matter of custom as to which terms are so translated and which are rendered in their original Latin form.

Over the history of anatomy, many structures have acquired multiple names. It was estimated in the latter part of the 19th century that there were some 50,000 anatomic terms in use, but that these actually applied only to some 5000 to 6000 structures. The German Anatomical Society studied the question of multiplicity in terms and, in 1895 in Basle, adopted a standard nomenclature that came to be known as the Basle Nomina Anatomica, or the BNA. This was generally adopted in Germany and in the English-speaking countries. In succeeding years, however, as it became obvious that there were some inaccuracies and infelicities in the BNA, several countries undertook to revise it, and synonyms again began to be common. A thorough revision of the BNA was finally undertaken by the International Congress of Anatomists and was approved at a meeting in Paris in 1955. The list of terms there adopted is known as the Nomina Anatomica, or NA, and is now the official terminology.

Nomina Anatomica retains the BNA principles of eliminating synonyms and trying to make terms precisely descriptive. The International Nomenclature Committee from time to time revises NA.

In this text, the 1989 edition of NA is followed, usually in the anglicized form. The original Latin terminology is given where there might be cause for confusion. Although there should no longer be any necessity to learn synonyms, the student cannot avoid hearing and seeing some. Synonyms and alternative terminology will be encountered in the literature and in clinical practice. Consequently, some of the more common synonyms are included in the text. Also, there is appended a short, incomplete glossary of terms frequently encountered in the clinical literature.

Anatomic terms can be divided into two general categories: names of parts of the body and descriptive terms that include adjectives and verbs. Not only the names, but also the adjectives (e.g., proximal, distal) and the verbs (e.g., flex, extend) must be used precisely to avoid misunderstanding.

PARTS OF THE BODY

The body is divided into three parts, or regions: the head and neck, the trunk, and the limbs. The trunk, in turn, is divided into the thorax, abdomen, pelvis and perineum. The limbs, formerly called **appendages,** now are called **membra,** but this is generally translated into **limbs,** rather than members. Names of parts of the limbs are considered in Chapter 14, but it might be noted that "arm" and "leg," although popularly used as synonyms for the upper and lower limbs (superior and inferior members), are not anatomic synonyms for these limbs; the arm (brachium) is that part of the upper limb between shoulder and elbow, and the leg (crus) is that part of the lower limb between knee and ankle.

To understand even introductory anatomy, it is necessary to know the meaning of some Latin terms. The head is the **caput;** hence, the term **capitis** (of the head). The skull is the **cranium;** hence, the adjective **cranial; cephalic** is used in the same sense as cranial, but the prefix **cephalo-** is used as a combining form (e.g., cephalothoracic, relating to the head and chest). There are two words that mean neck, **collum** and **cervix,** and from these terms are derived the possessive forms, **colli** and **cervical.** The back of the neck is the **nucha,** but its derivative, **nuchal,** is more commonly used for structures relating to the neck.

TERMS OF POSITION, PLANES, DIRECTION, AND MOVEMENT

Terms of position, planes, direction, and movement must be used in reference to the anatomic position, and they must be used consistently to avoid confusion. The **anatomic position** is defined as the erect position with the arms at the sides and palms of the hands facing forward.

The **median plane** bisects the body into right and left halves. Any plane parallel with the median plane is a **sagittal plane. Medial** describes a position nearer to the median plane, and **lateral** describes a position farther from it. A **coronal plane** is at right angles to the sagittal plane and bisects the body into **anterior** and **posterior** portions. The position of a structure nearer the front of the body is described as **anterior** and that nearer the back of the body as **posterior.** The terms **ventral** and **dorsal** may be used synonymously with anterior and posterior, but properly should apply only to the embryo. A **transverse plane** is horizontal and bisects the body into upper and lower parts. **Superior** means lying above, and **inferior,** lying below. Terms such as **internal** and **external,** or **superficial** and **deep,** are readily understandable and refer to relations to the surface of the body. **Proximal** and **distal,** meaning closer to and farther from, are general terms, but in reference to the limbs, they are used to designate structures nearer to or farther from the attachment of the limb to the trunk.

In describing the limbs, all of the foregoing terms may be used. However, to avoid confusion, it is customary to describe the limbs in terms of the positions of their paired bones. Thus, in the upper limb, the radius is the lateral bone of the forearm and the ulna is the medial one, so **radial** refers to the thumb side and **ulnar** to the little-finger side. In the leg, the tibia is the medial bone and the fibula is the lateral one, so **tibial** refers to the big-toe side and **fibular** to the little-toe side. Also, the adjective used in describing structures of the anterior surface of the hand is **palmar,** rather than anterior; similarly, **plantar** is used in describing structures of the sole of the foot. The other surface of either the hand or the foot is known as the **dorsum.**

In the embryo, some additional terms are used: Structures close to the head or movements toward the head are described as **cranial** or **rostral** (rostrum meaning beak), rather than superior; structures closer to the tail or movements toward the tail are described as **caudal** (cauda meaning tail, because the embryo possesses a tail), rather than inferior.

Terms describing movement also are a necessary part of anatomic terminology. For purposes of clarity, they sometimes need to be qualified, and at some joints, movements are complex enough to demand special description and definition. Terms generally used are flexion and extension, abduction and adduction, rotation, and circumduction.

Flexion means bending in a direction that approximates the surfaces that in the embryo formed the ventral surface of the body, including the limbs. **Extension** is the reverse of flexion and usually straightens a part by movement toward the surface that was dorsal in the embryo. With the exception of the lower limbs, flexion approximates the anterior surfaces of the body and extension reverses this movement. Because of the developmental rotation of the lower limb explained in Chapter 14, flexion of the knee approximates surfaces of the thigh and leg that face posteriorly, and extension straightens the knee. Also, during development the foot assumes a position that makes a 90° angle with the leg, so that its embryonic ventral surface becomes the sole (*planta* in Latin), which faces downward, and its dorsal surface faces upwards. Therefore, flexion of the foot is often spoken of as **plantarflexion,** a movement that increases the 90° angle; extension of the foot is often referred to as **dorsiflexion,** a movement that decreases the same angle.

Abduction means to draw away from and **adduction,** the reverse, draw toward. These terms are used in reference to the median plane of the body, except when they pertain to movements of the digits. Abduction of the trunk is the same as bending it laterally, and its adduction restores it to the vertical position. Abduction of the limbs lifts them away from the body, and adduction approximates them. The reference line for movement of the digits is the middle finger or the second toe. Spreading the digits is abduction, and drawing them together is adduction.

Rotation is the movement of a part around its long axis. When the anterior surface rotates laterally, the movement is called **lateral rotation,** and rotation of the anterior surface medially is **medial rotation.** Movements that are reminiscent of rotation take place in the forearm and in the foot. These movements receive the names of **supination** and **pronation** of the hand and **inversion** and **eversion** of the foot. In the anatomic position, the forearm and the hand are supinated. When the dorsum of the hand is turned forward without rotation of the upper arm, the hand and the forearm are pronated. With the elbow bent, the palm of the supinated hand faces the ceiling; in the same position at the elbow, the palm of the pronated hand faces the floor. Inversion is the movement that turns the sole of the foot inward or medially, and eversion turns the sole outward or laterally.

Some joints permit several movements to take place. When a part is moved successively through flexion, abduction, extension, and adduction, it circumscribes a cone of space, with its distal point drawing a circle. Such a movement is called **circumduction.**

ABBREVIATIONS

Most abbreviations used in anatomic texts and figures are clear if one knows the words being abbreviated; for instance, "flex. poll. long.," when referring to a muscle, adequately identifies the flexor pollicis longus muscle. There are, however, a few commonly used abbreviations with which the student needs to be familiar: a. for artery or the Latin *arteria*, aa. for arteries or *arteriae*; v. for vein or *vena*, vv. for veins or *venae*; n. for nerve or *nervus*, nn. for nerves or *nervi*; and m. for muscle or *musculus*, mm. for muscles or *musculi*.

In referring to vertebrae or spinal nerves, which are designated both by region and by number within the region (e.g., the sixth cervical or the eighth thoracic), it is often convenient to use shorter forms: **C** for cervical, **T** for thoracic, **L** for lumbar, and **S** for sacral. Thus, the third nerve and vertebra of each of the regions may be identified as C-3, T-3, L-3, and S-3. In older literature, dorsal (D) is synonymous with thoracic; however, since vertebrae in all regions are located dorsally in the body, this use of the term should be abandoned.

RECOMMENDED READINGS

Bergman RA, Thompson SA, Afifi AK, Saadeh FA. Compendium of human anatomic variation: text, atlas, and world literature. Baltimore: Urban & Schwarzenberg, 1988.

Bouchet A. For the love of Greek. Surg Radiol Anat 1994; 16: 217.

Dobson J. Anatomical eponyms. 2nd ed. Edinburgh: E & S Livingstone, 1962.

Grignon B, Roland J, Braun M. Employment of the anatomical terminology of the Nomina Anatomica in the radiologic literature. Surg Radiol Anat 1995; 17: 289.

Moore KL. Anatomical terminology/clinical terminology. Clin Anat 1988; 1: 7.

Nomina Anatomica. 6th ed. Edinburgh: Churchill Livingstone, 1989.

Pepper OHP. Medical etymology. Philadelphia: Saunders, 1949.

Skinner HA. The origin of medical terms. 2nd ed. Baltimore: Williams & Wilkins, 1961.

Squires BP. Basic terms of anatomy and physiology. 2nd ed. Toronto: Saunders, 1986.

Staubesand J, Steel F. A note on degenerative changes in anatomical terminology. Acta Anat 1988; 133:265.

Tobias PV. Some changes in anatomical nomenclature (editorial). Clin Anat 1990; 3: 79.

PART II

Tissues and Systems of the Body

Hollinshead's Textbook of Anatomy, by Cornelius Rosse and Penelope Gaddum-Rosse.
Lippincott-Raven Publishers, Philadelphia, © 1997.

CHAPTER 3

The Skin and its Appendages

The skin is the organ system that covers the surface of the body. Its primary function is to seal off the fluids of the body from the immediate environment of the animal and, thus, to preserve the fluid environment that cells must have if they are to live. In connection with this protective function, the skin has developed certain appendages that increase its effectiveness: nails as a protection against wear, hair as a protection against too much loss of heat. The skin also has excretory glands that discharge directly to the outside. It is the medium through which much information concerning the immediate environment of the body is obtained (that is, it is a particularly important sense organ), and it is important in regulating the loss of heat from the body.

The skin (*integument*) is composed of two fundamental layers: an outer epithelial one, the **epidermis** and an inner one of dense connective tissue, the **dermis** or corium. The term *cutis* sometimes is used to refer to the dermis only, but more properly it refers to the skin as a whole. However, *derma* is regularly employed in all combining words (dermatitis, dermatome) in the sense of the skin as a whole. Some of the confusion here may be that the dermis is frequently defined as the true skin. It is this felted layer of dense connective tissue that is treated by tanning to make leather, the epithelial component being destroyed in the process.

For the most part, the skin is thicker on the posterior aspect of a part than it is on the anterior aspect, but this condition is reversed in the hand and foot. Here the palmar and plantar surfaces, respectively, are provided with much thicker skin than are their dorsal aspects.

The outer surface of the skin presents a series of delicate creases, intercepting in a manner such that they enclose elongated polyangular spaces that vary in prominence. These minute folds help lend elasticity to the skin; hence, they tend to run in the same direction as the tension lines of the skin. They are more prominent in loose skin, especially that close to joints. The outer surface of the skin of the palm and sole differs from skin elsewhere in that it is arranged in a series of alternating ridges and grooves (*cristae* and *sulci cutis*), which may be fairly straight lines, but toward the tips of the digits become elaborated into loops and whorls. It is this pattern that is recorded in fingerprints and footprints. Numerous sweat glands open on the summits of the ridges; hence, fingerprints are left when a smooth object is grasped. The ridges and sulci serve to increase the grip of the hand and foot by increasing friction. The skin of these surfaces is particularly closely bound to deeper structures, this decreased mobility being necessary for a firm grip.

EPIDERMIS

The epidermis is a layer of stratified squamous epithelium derived directly from the surface ectoderm of the body. Its exposed surface is composed of dead cornified cells that offer effective resistance both to passage of fluid and to friction. The thickness of the layer of cornified cells varies markedly. It is thin in such locations as the abdominal wall, but thicker than all other layers of the skin combined on the sole of the foot, especially in the areas most constantly subjected to pressure. Cells from the outermost surface of the cornified layer are constantly being desquamated and replaced by cells that gradually move outward from the deepest layer. The maintenance of the epithelial layer of the skin, therefore, demands a steady mitotic activity on the part of the deepest-lying cells to maintain the necessary rate of regeneration of the epidermis.

DERMIS

The part of the dermis immediately adjacent to the epidermis is less dense in texture than elsewhere and contains the terminal capillaries of the skin and most of its nerve endings (no blood vessels and only a few nerve fibers penetrate the epidermal layer). On its deep surface, this loose layer, the **papillary layer** (*stratum papillare*), blends with the dense and thicker portion of the dermis, the reticular layer. On its outer surface, the papillary layer gives rise to numerous nipplelike projections, dermal papillae, that fit into conical excavations on the deep surface of the epidermis. It is particularly in the papillae that vascular loops and nerve endings are prominent. The reticular layer of the dermis is composed of densely interwoven connective tissue, largely collagenous, but also containing elastic fibers. Its varying thickness is, in most locations, responsible for differences in the thickness of the skin.

Although the fibers of the dermis run in all directions, in most regions of the skin, a greater number of fibers run in one direction than any other, and this predominant direction, in general, tends to parallel the lines along which the skin is folded and stretched during movement. The prevailing direction of these fiber bundles can be determined on the fresh cadaver by inserting a sharp, rounded object, such as an ice pick, into the skin. When this is done, the point separates fiber bundles more than it severs fibers, and the wound left by the instrument becomes slitlike in the direction of the fibers, rather than being round. The lines of the skin determined by this method are known as cleavage or tension lines (Fig. 3-1). Cuts made in the direction of these lines cause less disruption of connective tissue bundles than do cuts made across them, and the skin gapes less widely when incisions follow them. Some surgeons do, some do not, consider the prevailing direction of the tension lines in planning surgical incisions. Cutting across the prominent flexion lines at joints almost always results in excess scar formation. Therefore incisions are made zigzag across the joint. The

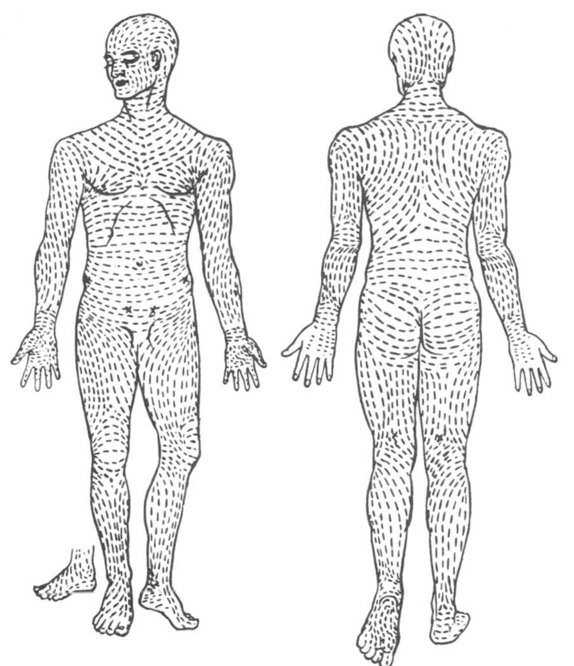

FIGURE 3-1.
Cleavage lines of the skin. (Cox HT. Br J Surg 1941; 29:234.)

incisions above and below the flexion line are connected by an oblique incision almost paralleling the line.

On its deep surface, the dermis is usually connected to the underlying *tela subcutanea,* commonly termed the **superficial fascia.** The loose texture of this layer provides easy movement of the skin over the underlying structures. In some locations, however, the dermis is bound tightly to underlying deep structures, either over a general area, as it is over the tibia in the leg, or over localized areas. The attachment of the skin to the tela subcutanea and deeper structures is through connective tissue bands, the *retinacula cutis.* Where these are locally well developed and are attached to firm, deeper-lying tissue, they produce permanent folds and dimples in the skin. The permanent flexure lines in the skin are such areas of firmer anchorage; the skin on either side of them is moved toward these lines during flexion. Certain muscles of the face and neck also attach into the skin, and dimples on the cheek and chin are produced by the action of these muscles on the skin.

GLANDS

The glands of the skin develop as growths from the epithelial layer; hence, they grow into the dermis with the larger glands growing through the dermis to invade the tela subcutanea. Cutaneous glands fall into two general groups: *sudoriferous* (sweat) and *sebaceous* (oily) glands, but various modifications of these occur in certain regions. The breast is a modified cutaneous gland, of such size that it invades the underlying tela subcutanea. It is described with the pectoral region (see Chap. 15).

The more common type of **sweat gland,** sometimes known as an *epicrine* (eccrine) sweat gland, secretes clear sweat that passes through a duct opening directly onto the surface of the skin. The largest sweat glands, found especially in the axilla but also on the areola of the breast and in the genital and circumanal regions, differ from ordinary sweat glands in that they discharge into hair follicles, rather than directly onto the surface, and in that the material they discharge is not purely a secretion, but consists in part of a portion of the cell cytoplasm. These are called *apocrine glands.* Apocrine glands are primarily responsible for the characteristic odor of sweat. The apocrine sweat glands, like the breast (a modified apocrine sweat gland), enlarge at the time of puberty. The *ceruminous glands,* the secretion of which hardens on exposure to air to form the wax found in the external ear canal, are modified apocrine sweat glands. Stimulation of the sympathetic nervous system provokes a discharge of sweat from sweat glands.

Sebaceous glands secrete an oily material, sebum, that coats the hairs. Each hair follicle is provided with from one to six sebaceous glands opening into it. However, sebaceous glands also open directly on the surface of the skin, particularly on the nose (where the openings of the larger ducts, occluded with debris, appear as "blackheads"), in the genital and circumanal region, on the areola and nipple, and in the eyelids (where they are called "tarsal glands").

HAIRS, NAILS, AND TEETH

Hairs (*pili*) are, like the glands of the skin, derived from ectoderm. A glandlike growth of the epidermis into the dermis gives rise to the hair follicle, and the hair, composed of tightly packed cornified cells, grows upward from the base of the follicle through its central aperture. Hairs are constantly being shed and replaced by the growth of new hairs from the same follicle. The earliest hairs of the fetus and newborn, the lanugo, are particularly fine. In parts of the body, hairs only a little coarser than this, usually referred to as down hairs, persist throughout life. In other regions, notably the scalp, the eyebrows and eyelashes, the axilla, the pubic region, and the beard in the male, most of the finer hairs are replaced by coarser ones of succeeding generations, and there is a tendency for the hairs to grow still more coarse with advancing age.

The hairs in certain regions have special names: those of the eyebrows are the supercilia, those of the eyelashes the cilia, those of the beard the barba, the coarse ones in the outer part of the external ear the tragi, those in the outer part of the nasal cavity the vibrissae, those of the scalp the capilli, those of the axilla the hirci, and those of the pubic region the pubes. Few of these terms are actually used very often. Colloquial or descriptive terms (eyebrows, eyelashes, pubic hair) are more commonly used.

Hair follicles typically have associated with them bundles of smooth muscle, the *arrectores pilorum* muscles, that are attached in such fashion to the hair follicle that they tend to erect the usually obliquely lying hairs. At the same time, they exert pressure on sebaceous glands and provoke the discharge of their secretion into the hair follicle. Contraction of these muscles in many animals serves important functions. For instance, in the cat, contraction of the muscles and raising of the hairs in a cold environment increases the amount of air trapped among the hairs and, thereby, the insulating value of the hair coat. Also, contraction during anger increases the apparent size of the animal and, consequently, the possibility of appearing more frightening to an enemy. In the human, general contraction of these muscles gives rise to "goose flesh."

Nails (*ungues*) are plates of tightly packed, cornified epithelial cells. The thin uncornified epithelium on which the nail plate lies is the *nail bed*. A proximal, thicker part of the nail bed, the *matrix*, is responsible for growth of the nail. The nerves and the blood supply of the nail bed enter it from its deep surface and are derived exclusively from anterior (palmar or plantar) nerves and vessels, never from posterior ones.

Teeth (*dentes*) are derived from both epithelial and connective tissue layers of the oral mucous membrane, itself modified skin, differing from usual skin in that it does not possess a cornified layer. The hard outer **enamel** of teeth is developed from the epithelium and the bonelike **dentin** from the connective tissue. **Cementum,** modified bone softer than dentin, covers most of the dentin of the root of the tooth and attaches the tooth to the **periodontium** or periodontal membrane (the periosteum that lines the dental alveoli—sockets—of the upper and lower jaws). Nerves and blood vessels running in the bony jaws send branches into the teeth through their apical foramina. The gross anatomy of teeth is briefly described later with the oral cavity (see Chap. 31).

FUNCTIONAL ASPECTS

The thin, moist skin of some animals, such as the frog, is permeable to various substances, and it is a rather effective organ of respiration, excreting carbon dioxide and absorbing oxygen. A small amount of carbon dioxide is lost through the skin of humans, apparently partly dissolved in the sweat, but human skin is largely impermeable to gases and to water and other liquids, although oily substances are absorbed somewhat better. In contrast with normal skin, skin in which the epidermal layers have been peeled off by blistering allows the ready passage of substances in either watery or oily solution, as do the thinner, moist mucous surfaces, such as the conjunctiva and the mucous membrane of the nose, that represent modified skin. Most of the **excretion** carried out by the skin is through the sebaceous and the sweat glands. Salt is a prominent component of sweat, and excessive sweating without adequate intake of salt leads to a deficiency of sodium and chloride ions in the body. Sweat also contains small amounts of protein and urea.

The **protective function** of the skin is best illustrated by the effects of the loss of large areas. For instance, in severe burns of the skin, there is not only the clinical problem of minimizing absorption of toxic substances, but also the problems of minimizing infection and loss of fluid, both of which are obvious sequelae to loss of the protective function of the skin.

The **temperature regulatory function** of the skin is controlled in humans by two mechanisms. One depends on dilation and constriction of the blood vessels of the skin, so that more or less blood is allowed to radiate its heat to the outside. The second is through the evaporation of sweat. Sweat secretion is evoked by a rise in temperature of the blood reaching the central nervous system.

The function of the skin as a **sense organ** depends on the abundant innervation sent to it by cranial and spinal nerves. The larger nerve trunks to the skin run in the tela subcutanea, and branches leave these to penetrate the skin, where they at first form coarse networks. Branches from these, in turn, form finer and finer networks as they come closer to the epidermis. Certain specialized endings are found in the skin, especially in the dermal papillae; however, a great deal of evidence indicates that there are relatively few specialized sense organs in the skin of humans and that the common type of nerve ending in the skin is in connection with the finer networks close to the epidermis. This is apparently true not only for fibers concerned with pain, as has been generally agreed for some time, but also for those concerned with heat and cold and even touch. Hairs add to the sensitivity of a region of skin to touch, as hair follicles have about them a complex plexus of nerve fibers. Deeper-lying, encapsulated nerve endings, usually called pacinian corpuscles or Vater-Pacini corpuscles, occur in both the dermis and the tela subcutanea (and also in deep tissues, even within the abdominal cavity) and are generally believed to be associated with sensations of pressure. The concept, once held, that each type of sensation from the skin is mediated by a fiber specific for this type of sensation and also by an anatomically discrete and different nerve ending is no longer widely believed; there are not enough morphologically discrete types of nerve endings to support the concept of *anatomic* specificity of nerve endings.

Gross anatomic aspects of cutaneous innervation, and the concepts of peripheral nerve innervation and segmental innervation or dermatomes are discussed in Chapter 13.

RECOMMENDED READINGS

Ebling FJG, Eady RAJ, Leigh IM. Anatomy and organization of human skin. In: Champion RH, Burton JL, Ebling FJG, eds. Textbook of dermatology. 5th ed, vol 1. Boston: Blackwell Scientific Publications, 1992: 49.

Fawcett DW. Skin. In: Bloom and Fawcett: a textbook of histology. 12th ed. New York: Chapman & Hall, 1994: 525.

Holbrook KA, Wolff K. The structure and development of skin. In: Fitzpatrick TB, Eisen AZ, Wolff K, Freedberg IM, Austen KF, eds. Dermatology in general medicine. 4th ed, vol 1. New York: McGraw-Hill, 1993: 97.

Inoue H. Three dimensional observations of microvasculature of human finger skin. Hand 1978; 10: 144.

List CF, Peet MM. Sweat secretion in man. Arch Neurol Psychiatry 1938; 39: 1228.

Montagna W, Parakkal PF. The structure and function of skin. 3rd ed. New York: Academic Press, 1974.

Taylor GI, Palmer JH. The vascular territories (angiosomes) of the body: experimental study and clinical applications. Br J Plast Surg 1987; 40:113.

Watterson PA, Taylor GI, Crock JG. The venous territories of the human body: anatomical study and clinical implications. Br J Plast Surg 1988; 41: 569.

Hollinshead's Textbook of Anatomy, by Cornelius Rosse and Penelope Gaddum-Rosse.
Lippincott-Raven Publishers, Philadelphia, © 1997.

CHAPTER 4

The Connective Tissues

The term *connective tissue* is used to include a variety of tissues that, despite their common derivation from embryonic mesenchyme, assume distinctive gross and microscopic features and subserve a variety of functions. For example, connective tissues include the dermis and the underlying subcutaneous fat (adipose tissue), ligaments, tendons, as well as bone and cartilage. As the name implies, the universal function of connective tissue is to hold together more specialized tissues, welding them into organs and retaining them in their proper anatomic relations. Connective tissue also circumscribes the various morphologic and functional units of organs and supports nerves and blood vessels as they course between different parts of the body. In its specialized forms, connective tissue supports the entire body and retains the shape of many of its parts.

Connective tissue consists of cells dispersed in extracellular matrix produced by the cells. Derived from embryonic mesenchyme, these cells retain, throughout life, morphologic similarity in the various types of connective tissues. They have, however, differentiated at some point of embryonic development and are able to produce different types of extracellular matrices in different locations of the body. The special properties of the various types of connective tissue are determined by the composition of the extracellular matrix. Consequently, the classification of connective tissues is based on the differences in this matrix.

Extracellular matrix is composed of **fibers** and amorphous **ground substance.** Only two basic types of fibers are admixed in various proportions in all connective tissues: **collagen fibers** and **elastic fibers.** On the other hand, the composition and consistency of ground substance varies considerably between the different connective tissue types. These tissue types include: 1) *ordinary* or **proper connective tissues** (e.g., loose connective tissue, tendon, ligament, or fascia; and 2) **specialized connective tissues** (namely, cartilage and bone).

In connective tissue proper, the ground substance has the physical properties of a thin gel, whereas in cartilage it forms a firm gel of distinct chemical composition. The ground substance specific for bone tissue becomes impregnated by inorganic bone salts that lend rigidity to this tissue.

The density and type of connective tissue fibers determine whether the particular tissue is of primary mechanical importance in musculoskeletal function or whether it forms loose packing material through which nutrients and cells can pass. **Loose connective tissue** consists of an open meshwork of fibers and cells, the interstices of which are filled by ground substance. Loose connective tissue is the prototype of all the more specialized connective tissues and most closely resembles embryonic mesenchyme. When loose connective tissue is extensively infiltrated by fat cells, it is spoken of as **adipose tissue.** Loose connective tissue can also be greatly distended by large amounts of extracellular fluid, which causes swelling (edema) of various parts and organs.

Dense connective tissue is formed by the preponderance of fibers. Tendons and ligaments represent dense connective tissue in which collagen fibers are closely packed in a regular pattern. Although less regular, dense connective tissue also constitutes deep fascia and intermuscular septa. An ordered collagen fiber network is also present in articular cartilage and bone. However, these fibers are masked by the staining properties of cartilage and bone matrix, and special methods are needed for their demonstration.

Densely arranged elastic fibers make up the bulk of the extracellular matrix in **elastic tissue.** Elastic tissue is found in certain ligaments associated with the vertebral column (ligamenta flava) and in the walls of certain arteries.

All connective tissues are dynamic, in that there is a constant turnover of their constituent molecules, and they are readily reorganized in their structure in response to various stimuli and mechanical stresses. Various types of connective tissue may change radically, even in an adult body, and new connective tissue may arise. This is most dramatically demonstrated in the remodeling of bone in healing fractures or the reorganization of scar tissue.

The specialized connective tissues, cartilage and bone, are discussed in Chapter 5, which is concerned with the skeleton and its joints. This chapter deals with gross anatomic forms of connective tissue proper. Ordinary connective tissue is recognized by the naked eye as loose connective tissue, fat, fascia, ligaments, and tendons. This chapter also describes the spaces that develop in connective tissue, including bursae and tendon sheaths.

LOOSE CONNECTIVE TISSUE

Macroscopically, loose connective tissue, or *areolar tissue*, is a fine, cobweblike packing material that fills the interstices between organs and serves as padding. It may be seen, for instance, when the fiber bundles in a muscle such as the biceps, are pulled apart. The same type of tissue is found between the dermis and an underlying structure (muscle or bone) over parts of the body that are devoid of subcutaneous fat (the dorsum of the hand, for example). Areolar tissue creates a plane of cleavage along which tissues or organs may be pulled away from one another, and it also aids the sliding of these structures over each other.

There may be large numbers of fat cells among the connective tissue fibers, in which case the tissue is usually referred to as **fatty (adipose) tissue,** rather than as loose connective tissue. Accumulations of fat in fat-storing cells form the visible depots of fat in the body. Such adipose tissue appears yellow to the naked eye. Body fat under the skin is known to gross anatomists as **superficial fascia.** In Latin terminology, superficial fascia is referred to as *tela subcutanea* or *panniculus adiposus*. Superficial fascia serves as padding to fill out the body contours and to conserve body heat. Over the palms of the hands and soles of the feet, the fat is arranged in rather tight lobules to absorb pressure.

Microscopically, loose connective tissue is a framework of interwoven collagen fibers intermingled with occasional elastic fibers. The large spaces between the fibers are filled with fluid and also contain the cells found in connective tissue (e.g., fibroblasts, phagocytes, migratory elements of the blood). This basic structure also exists in adipose tissue, but most of the spaces are occupied by the distended fat cells. Adipose tissue that is not under the skin is similar in structure to superficial fascia, but is known simply as fat.

FASCIA

The term *fascia* is rather loosely applied in anatomy and in surgery. When used without qualification, it most often denotes a readily visible connective tissue membrane that consists of a thin layer of dense connective tissue without obvious organization of its fibers. The exception to the definition is superficial fascia, which is not a membrane, but a padding. Most fascias are arranged in sheets or tubes and form a more or less obvious connective tissue layer between or around structures. For instance, all muscles, nerves, and blood vessels, as well as most organs, are encased in such connective tissue coverings. Some fascias are dense, rather strong sheets; others are flimsy. No exact division exists between the indistinct, flimsy layer of fascia and loose connective tissue.

Descriptions of fascias tend to be confusing, because fascias are simply more obvious layers of the general connective tissue packing of the body; all connective tissue in the body is continuous with all other connective tissue. Thus, in one sense, a fascia has no beginning and no end, and any description of fascias is necessarily somewhat arbitrary. For instance, custom and convenience usually determine whether a fascia attaching to a bone is considered to continue across the bone or to end there, being replaced beyond the bone by a differently named fascia. Similarly, when a fascia splits into two or more layers, custom and convenience largely determine whether the two layers are separately named.

The description of a fascia as forming a dissectable layer implies that the connective tissue on each side of it, binding it to surrounding structures, is looser in texture and more irregularly arranged. However, there is no standard for how skillful the dissector must be or how sharp the scalpel, and no absolute criterion determines what "looser" and "firmer" mean. Thus, arguments about the existence of a certain fascia may be largely a question of semantics. Surgically useful fascias are those that are strong enough to hold sutures, but the fact that a connective tissue layer is that strong is not an invariable justification for giving it a name of its own.

Fascias may actually be a part of the wall of an organ, as, for instance, the outer connective tissue layer of blood vessels, the *adventitia*. The connective tissue layer that forms the surface of a voluntary muscle, the *epimysium*, is also called the fascia of the muscle. Structures lying in or traversing loose connective tissue tend to have a condensation of fascia on or around them. For example, organs in the neck and pelvis and in the loose connective tissue of the posterior abdominal wall have fascial layers or tubes associated with them.

Microscopically, fascia is distinguished from loose connective tissue by the greater amount of collagen fibers. Most of these fibers may be more organized than in loose connective tissue, but are much more irregular than collagen fibers in tendons or aponeuroses.

In addition to the numerous and variable fascias, there are two rather distinct fascial systems that are of special importance to the anatomist and surgeon. The internal fascia lines the thoracic and abdominal cavities, and the external or investing fascia lies deep to the tela subcutanea and is usually referred to as the deep fascia.

Internal Fascia

The internal fascia that lines the thoracic cavity is called *endothoracic fascia*, and the fascia that lines the abdominal cavity is the *endoabdominal fascia*. These internal fascias form a barely discernible lining of the thoracic and abdominal cavities, and their chief function is to affix the parietal layer of the serous sacs—the pleura in the thorax and the peritoneum in the abdomen—to the inner aspect of the body wall. The terms *endothoracic* and *endoabdominal fascia* do not usually include the loose connective tissue that fills the spaces between the thoracic and abdominal organs. Such loose connective tissue is particularly abundant in the pelvis, and here the packing material is often spoken of as *endopelvic fascia*. The endopelvic fascia is a continuation of the endoabdominal fascia into the pelvic cavity.

Specializations exist in the internal fascias that are named in their own right. For instance, the suprapleural membrane is a thickening in the endothoracic fascia as it roofs over the superior aperture of the thorax and covers the apices of the lungs. Internal fascia may also be named according to the muscles with which it is in contact (e.g., transversalis fascia, diaphragmatic fascia, psoas fascia, or superior fascia of the levator ani). In most instances, these named fascias covering the muscles are not distinguishable from each other and are synonymous with the endoabdominal fascia. This is particularly important to remember in connection with the transversalis fascia, the name most often used when speaking of the endoabdominal fascia. Only over the psoas is the endoabdominal fascia sufficiently thickened to make it anatomically distinct from the rest of the endoabdominal fascia. Likewise, specializations exist in endopelvic fascia. These include membranous condensations of endopelvic fascia over some of the muscles that form the walls of the pelvic cavity (fascia of the obturator internus) and rather poorly defined bands of dense connective tissue that support the pelvic organs and are called ligaments (e.g., pubocervical, uterosacral ligaments).

The inner layers of endoabdominal fascia may become laden with fat, which can be separated from the more membranous layer adjacent to the abdominal wall muscles. In some areas, such adipose tissue is specially named (e.g., around the kidneys, perirenal fat); otherwise, it is spoken of, especially by radiologists, as *preperitoneal fat*.

Deep Fascia

After removal of the superficial fascia (*tela subcutanea*) by blunt dissection, the deep fascia appears in most locations as a thin grayish layer on the surface of the muscles, separable from them only by sharp dissection. Where one muscle overlies another, the deep fascia between them can be split into two layers, one for each muscle. The ease of splitting and the clarity of the two fascial layers depend on the density of the fascia adjacent to the muscles' surfaces and the amount of looser connective tissue between the muscles. Where muscles attach to bone, the deep fascia becomes continuous with the periosteum of the bone.

In the neck and in the limbs, the deep fascia is a tough fibrous layer that surrounds the entire part and from its deep surface sends septa among the muscles. In some locations, such as the back of the arm, the deep fascia is fused to the epimysium of the muscle; in other locations, such as the front of the arm, it forms a loosely fitting envelope around the muscles. In some locations, also, the deep fascia and its septa provide attachment for muscles, so that it is more tendinous than fascial in nature (with most fibers running in one direction, rather than crisscrossed). Where the deep fascia and its septa meet subcutaneous bone (e.g., around the joints of the limbs) they blend with the periosteum.

In the limbs, the chief septa of the deep fascia are medial and lateral ones, which reach the bone and separate the originally ventral (anterior or flexor) muscles from the originally dorsal (posterior or extensor) ones (see, for instance, Figs. 16-10 and 18-10). In the neck, the septa are more complicated and are usually described as forming, in addition to sheaths for various muscles, several distinct layers in the front of the neck (see Fig. 30-3). At the levels of the wrist and ankle joints, the deep fascia is strengthened by special transverse fibers. These thickened portions hold the tendons close to the joints across which they pass, and are known as *retinacula* (see for instance, Fig. 18-45).

The arrangement of fibers in deep fascia forms a more or less regular, widely open, lattice pattern. Although elastic fibers are more numerous than in tendons, deep fascia provides a firm support for muscles; the power of muscle contraction is diminished when its deep fascia is stripped. Because of the limited compliance of deep fascia, pressure rises in the muscle compartment during muscle contraction. The intermittent increase in pressure aids venous return from pendant limbs. Excessive pressure in a compartment, caused by swelling or hematoma, compresses the veins, leading to edema, and eventually will endanger the arterial blood supply of the musculature. The muscle cells will die unless the deep fascia is incised and the pressure released.

LIGAMENTS

The term *ligament* (NA: *ligamentum*; plural, ligamenta; meaning a binding together) is used so loosely in anatomy that it conveys no clear idea of structure. However, there are in general two kinds of ligaments: those that connect viscera to each other or to the body wall, and those that connect one bone to another. The two groups have nothing in common, save that they both "connect" something to something else. Tendons also connect, but they always connect voluntary muscle to something else.

Visceral Ligaments

It is in this group that the greatest diversity lies. Some visceral ligaments, such as those connected to the stomach, are actually only parts of a mesentery (a thin double sheet of connective tissue, with epithelial [mesothelial] surfaces, that conducts blood vessels, lymph vessels, and nerves to a viscus; see Fig. 9-4). Others, such as those between liver and diaphragm, are modified mesenteries in which the connective tissue is much increased and actually holds two parts closely together. Some are fibromuscular remains of structures that had a function in the fetus (for instance, the medial umbilical ligaments are formed from the umbilical arteries). Others, such as some of those in the pelvis, are merely the connective tissue padding about blood vessels and nerves. Still others contain some smooth muscle or are formed largely by it.

Some authorities have insisted that a true visceral ligament must contain smooth muscle and those that do not are false ligaments, but the distinction is not generally followed. In the first place, there is increasing evidence that some of the supposedly "true" ligaments actually contain no smooth muscle other than that of the blood vessels in them. Second, a ligament containing a smooth muscle bundle is often called a muscle, rather than a ligament, or even both. For instance, the rectococcygeus muscle, a band connecting the bowel to the coccyx, is called a ligament only when it is fibrous, rather than muscular, and the suspensory ligament and suspensory muscle of the duodenum are parts of the same structure.

Skeletal Ligaments

Skeletal ligaments are more or less distinct bands of connective tissue that bind together two bones or bony parts. Across joints that have cavities, they usually blend with the fibrous wall (i.e., capsule) of the joint cavity and perhaps, in this instance, are best considered as being special thickenings of the fibrous capsule. Indeed, because of their close association with the capsules of joints, some of them are called capsular ligaments.

Because skeletal ligaments must withstand pull at the joints they cross, the majority of their fibers run in the same direction. Most are composed almost entirely of closely packed collagen fibers and, therefore, allow little stretch. However, some ligaments, notably the ligamenta flava of the vertebral column, are composed almost entirely of elastic fibers. They stretch with movement in one direction, shorten with movement in the opposite direction and, therefore, tend to remain taut rather than to become lax and double up. Ligaments composed of elastic tissue are, in the fresh condition, yellowish. Those composed primarily of collagenous tissue are white, and some of the heavier ones resemble tendons, and a few so-called ligaments really are tendons. For example, the tendon at the front of the knee attaches to the tibia, but is so interrupted by the kneecap (patella) that its lower segment is called the patellar ligament.

TENDONS

Tendons are actually parts of muscles and are best discussed in detail along with other aspects of muscles. However, they deserve mention with fibrous connective tissue because they are one type of very dense collagenous tissue. Even more than in most ligaments, their fibers run in one direction, so that they are able to withstand great pull. Because the densely packed parallel bundles of a tendon are held together by only a few cross fibers, it can be fairly easily shredded. The predominance of parallel collagen fiber bundles gives a tendon its white, shiny appearance.

A *tendon* is defined as the tissue that attaches skeletal muscle to another structure; thus, one end of a tendon is always attached to muscle. At the end away from the muscle, tendon fibers blend with the fibrous connective tissue of the structure to which they attach—usually bone, where they are continuous both with the fibrous outer covering, the periosteum, and with the fibers that form a part of the substance of the bone. In some instances, they blend with the dense connective tissue that forms the deep layer of the skin (the dermis or corium).

Tendons, although thinner than the muscles to which they belong, are usually of the same general form (i.e., broad and flat when they are a part of broad and flat muscles, cordlike when they are a part of long slender muscles). The long, rounded tendons running into the hand and foot are colloquially called "leaders." Very broad, flat tendons are known as **aponeuroses** and because of their breadth and thinness resemble dense fascias. The characteristic difference is that an aponeurosis, like other tendons, is composed of predominantly parallel collagenous bundles, whereas a fascia has interwoven fibers.

Tendons usually have special protection where they work across bone or across other tendons at such angles that friction and fraying may occur. Usually, this protection is simply the special lubrication offered by a bursa or tendon sheath (see the following section). However, in some locations cartilage or bone (sesamoid bones) develops within tendons at points of special friction. The fibroblasts present in the tendon can be induced to form cartilage or bone, even in the adult, although the factors that regulate such a transformation are not completely understood.

Because tendons, fascias, and ligaments all have the same fundamental structure, they tend to blend with each other when they are close together. A fascia may contain tendon fibers, and a ligament may be reinforced by a tendon that blends with it. Indeed, tendons and ligaments are so similar that some ligaments are apparently tendons that have lost their muscle fibers.

Tendons and ligaments have a low vascularity and their capacity for regeneration is limited. A torn tendon or ligament heals by scar tissue formation. The stresses acting on the scar tissue may align some of its fibers with those of the tendon or ligament.

TISSUE SPACES, FASCIAL SPACES, BURSAE, AND TENDON SHEATHS

Tissue spaces filled with interstitial or tissue fluid surround or are adjacent to most living cells. Extracellular fluid serves as the medium for interchange between the cells and the blood and is drained by lymphatics or directly into the venous system. The largest tissue spaces occur in loose connective tissue, where the interstices between fibers are spacious and the cellular elements are few. Consequently, fluid easily collects in the subcutaneous tissue if interference with the lymphatic drainage of a part occurs, if local block or cardiac failure impedes venous drainage, or if excess body fluid collects as a result of inadequate excretion of fluid by the kidneys or because of certain nutritional deficiencies. This excess accumulation of fluid, known as edema (dropsy), may occur in tissue spaces at any site and may interfere with the function of an organ or part through pressure, restriction of mobility, or reduction of nutrients or oxygen reaching the cells.

Fascial spaces are potential spaces filled with loose connective tissue between or among more dense layers of connective tissue. Fascial spaces are usually described as being areas of loose connective tissue that lie between muscles or are bounded by connective tissue layers dense enough to be called fascia. Because of the looseness of their connective tissue and their distensible walls, fluid, such as pus or blood, can accumulate in these crevices and convert them into "spaces" of considerable size.

Fluid or air accumulating in a fascial space may spread into other fascial spaces with which it is continuous. This spread is determined by the arrangement of the loose connective tissue and the surrounding fascial layers. It seems definite that the spread of air and noninfected fluid is determined largely by the arrangement of the looser connective tissue, but clinical opinion differs sharply on the importance of fascial spaces in the spread of infectious processes. One opinion is that infections do so spread, following the path of least resistance. The contrasting opinion is that the swelling and the proliferation of connective tissue produced by infection tend to encapsulate (form a wall around) the process and that this prevents spread through fascial spaces. Since both phenomena have been documented by clinical studies, it may be that the nature of the infection, rather than the anatomy of the fascial spaces, is often the determining factor.

Bursae (*bursa,* meaning purse) are closed connective tissue sacs filled with fluid. The outer surface of these delicate fibrous sacs blends with the surrounding loose connective tissue, whereas their inner surface is smooth and glistening, moistened by synovial fluid in an amount sufficient to lubricate the inside of the bursa. They develop in response to friction between tendon and bone, ligament, or other tendons, or between bone and skin. Most deep-lying bursae develop before birth, but subcutaneous bursae may appear in adult life over prominences exposed to unusual friction (e.g., a bunion). Certain bursae that develop in close relation to joint cavities frequently fuse with these, so that what was once a bursa becomes an extra-articular extension or recess of the joint cavity.

There are some 50 named and fairly constant bursae in the entire human body and many other, usually small, inconstant ones. The majority of both groups are subtendinous or submuscular, but a few are subfascial and several are subcutaneous.

Bursae are typically flattened and essentially collapsed spaces, containing only enough fluid to moisten their walls. When they become infected or are injured, the inflammation (bursitis) causes swelling. Because deep bursae lie between a muscle and a bone or between two muscles, any movement that involves contraction of an adjoining muscle will produce pressure on the inflamed bursa; hence, it will be painful. Subcutaneous bursae, between bony prominences or muscles and tendons and the skin, become visibly swollen and tender to the touch when they are inflamed.

Tendon sheaths are similar to bursae in their fundamental structure, but rather than being simple connective tissue pockets, they are complex tubes wrapped completely around tendons. Tendon sheaths develop like bursae (i.e., the connective tissue splits and forms a cavity), but their structure can be most easily understood if a tendon sheath is thought of as first developing as a bursa on one side of the tendon and then extending around the tendon (Fig. 4-1). One layer of the tendon sheath is closely applied to the surface of the tendon and is usually referred to as the visceral layer. The outer layer, surrounding the cavity, is known as the parietal layer. These two layers, moist and glistening on their apposed surfaces, are for the most part separated from each other by a film of fluid. They are continuous with each other at the ends of the tendon sheath and are often also continuous with each other through a mesotendon (Fig. 4-2). Mesotendons vary greatly, for they may persist throughout the length of a tendon sheath, may partly disappear or become much fenestrated, or may be completely absent. Mesotendons allow blood vessels to reach the tendon as it courses through the sheath, rather than to have to enter only at the ends of the tendon sheath. The small and rather constant remains of mesotendons in connection with the flexor tendons of the fingers and toes are known as vincula.

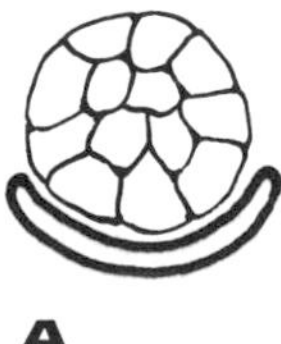

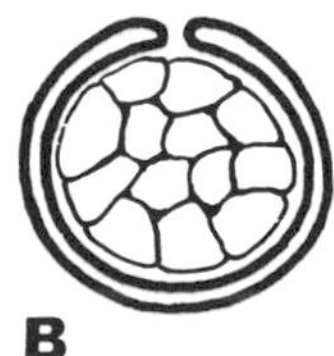

FIGURE 4-1.
Diagram indicating the similarity between bursae and tendon sheaths; (A) a bursa underlying a tendon, can be converted into (B) a tendon sheath, simply by extension around the tendon. Synovial membrane is represented by a *red line.*

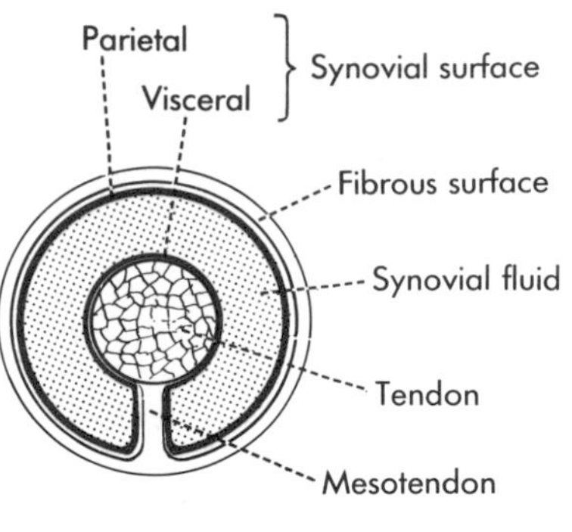

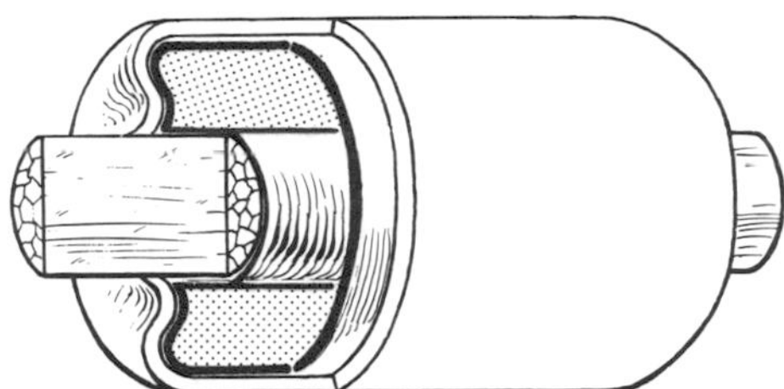

FIGURE 4-2.
Diagrams of a tendon sheath: Cut edges of synovial membrane are represented by *red lines. Above* is a cross section, with a mesotendon also included. *Below* is a view from the side, with a large segment removed and parts cut away at various levels on the *left* side.

RECOMMENDED READINGS

Alexander HG, Dugdale AE. Fascial planes within subcutaneous fat in humans. Eur J Clin Nutr 1992; 46: 903.

Avelar JM. Regional distribution and behavior of the subcutaneous tissue concerning selection and indication for liposuction. Aesthetic Plast Surg 1989; 13: 155.

Fawcett DW. Connective tissue. In: Bloom and Fawcett: a textbook of histology. 12th ed. New York: Chapman & Hall, 1994: 133.

Ger R, Evans JT. Of fat and fascia: clinical conundrum corner. Clin Anat 1995; 8: 66.

Hay ED, ed. Cell biology of extracellular matrix. 2nd ed. New York: Plenum Press, 1991.

Hull D. Distinction of brown from white adipose tissue. Nature 1966; 212: 469.

Hull D. The function and development of adipose tissue. In: Davis JA, Dobbing J, eds. Scientific foundations of paediatrics. London: Heinemann Medical Books, 1974.

Le Gros Clark WE. The tissues of the body: an introduction to the study of anatomy. 4th ed. Oxford: Clarendon Press, 1958.

LeRoy EC. Collagens and human disease. Bull Rheum Dis 1975; 25: 778.

Lockwood TE. Superficial fascial system (SFFS) of the trunk and extremities: a new concept. Plast Reconstr Surg 1991; 87: 1009.

Ross R. Connective tissue cells, cell proliferation and synthesis of extracellular matrix: a review. Philos Trans R Soc Lond B Biol Sci 1975; 271: 247.

Rosse C, Ross R. Tissues of the musculoskeletal system. In: Rosse C, Clawson DK. The musculoskeletal system in health and disease. Hagerstown: Harper & Row, 1980.

Slavin BG. The cytophysiology of mammalian adipose tissue. Int Rev Cytol 1972; 33: 297.

Hollinshead's Textbook of Anatomy, by Cornelius Rosse and Penelope Gaddum-Rosse.
Lippincott-Raven Publishers, Philadelphia, © 1997.

CHAPTER 5

The Skeletal System

The skeletal system provides the structural frame for the body as a whole and also for its regions and most of its parts. In addition to assuring support and retaining shape, the skeletal system, through its close integration with the muscular system, makes possible physical interactions with the environment. The skeletal system is made up of a large number of discrete bones that are secured to one another by various types of joints or articulations. The bones of the body collectively constitute the skeleton. Each bone of the skeleton is a discrete organ composed primarily of bone tissue. It is the association of this bone tissue with other tissues (cartilage, different varieties of proper connective tissue, hemopoietic tissue, or bone marrow) as well as with blood vessels and nerves, that forms a discrete bone (e.g., femur). Joints are also constituted of different types of connective tissue, and like bones, are supplied by blood vessels and nerves.

The first section of this chapter considers the specialized connective tissues of the skeletal system: namely, cartilage and bone; subsequent sections deal with bones as organs and the skeleton, concluding with an account of joints.

SPECIALIZED CONNECTIVE TISSUES

Cartilage

In contrast with fibrous connective tissue, which is adapted particularly well to withstand pull, cartilage (like bone), withstands both pressure and pull. Although its matrix contains connective tissue fibers, the interstices between the fibers are filled with ground substance that gives cartilage its solid feel and appearance. However, the extracellular matrix of cartilage is softer than that of bone, so cartilage possesses a springiness that bone does not. **Chondrocytes,** the cells that make the matrix, occupy small cavities within cartilage. When blood vessels invade cartilage, they destroy it to do so. Normally, this occurs during ossification of the cartilaginous primordia of bones and, abnormally, in varying disease conditions. Otherwise, cartilage is avascular.

General Distribution

Almost all the bones of the body first take form as cartilage. Most of the cartilage is destroyed and replaced by bone in the prenatal or early postnatal period. However, in many bones, growth in length depends on continued growth of cartilage, so regions of cartilage, called epiphyseal cartilages, or growth plates, typically persist in bones until the person has ceased to grow in height. Normally, throughout adult life, cartilage also persists at the ends of bones that articulate in freely movable (synovial) joints. Such cartilage has a smoother surface than bone and is called articular cartilage. It allows the joint to move with less friction than would bony surfaces. In addition, the greater springiness of cartilage presumably allows the articular cartilages to absorb some of the shock delivered to the joints during movement.

Distribution of cartilage in the adult is limited mostly to articular surfaces of bones and to certain locations at which springiness in the skeleton is an advantage and the shape of soft tissues must be retained. The cartilaginous component of the ear, for example, and that of the lower part of the nose, retains the shape of these parts and, at the same time, allows bending, whereas bone in the same location would fracture. In the same way, the persistence of the anterior ends of the ribs as cartilages contributes to the elasticity of the thoracic wall. Cartilaginous, rather than bony, support of the air passages to the lungs is also advantageous because these passages have to remain open while undergoing constant movement with breathing.

Calcification of (deposition of calcium salts in) the matrix occurs regularly in cartilage that is to be replaced by bone. It also may occur, with advancing age, in the permanent cartilages which, as might be expected, reduces their resiliency and renders them brittle.

Types of Cartilage

Although all cartilage contains connective tissue fibers, the fibers may be either collagen or elastic; thus, cartilage is divisible into three types: hyaline cartilage, fibrocartilage, and elastic cartilage.

Hyaline cartilage is glassy in appearance (the meaning of hyaline) because its felted collagen fibers are masked by the homogeneous ground substance deposited about the fibers. **Fibrocartilage** also contains collagen fibers, but the fibers are in heavier bundles, and there is less ground substance. **Elastic cartilage** has elastic, rather than collagen, fibers embedded in its matrix.

Hyaline cartilage in the adult is largely confined to articular cartilages, the cartilages of the ribs, and the rings and plaques that support the trachea and its branches. The greatest concentration of fibrocartilage is in disks that lie between adjacent vertebrae (intervertebral disks). Fibrocartilage is especially capable of absorbing shocks, an important function of the intervertebral disks. Fibrocartilage also exists in some freely movable joints. These fibrocartilages form disks, or C-shaped pads, and completely or partially subdivide the joint cavity (see under joints). Elastic cartilage primarily occurs in the external ear and the lower part of the nose.

Growth and Repair

After its rapid growth during developmental stages, cartilage grows little. Damaged articular cartilage does not regenerate. Grafts of cartilage, whittled to the proper shape and size, are sometimes used in plastic repair of the face. Such grafts of living cartilage, usually obtained from a rib cartilage of the person on whom the plastic operation is being done, typically live, but neither grow nor decrease in size.

Bone as a Tissue

Bone is a mineralized connective tissue; its cells, the **osteocytes,** are enclosed in lacunae of the rigid matrix, and maintain contact with one another by cytoplasmic processes through tiny canals that pervade bone matrix. Osteoblasts and osteocytes secrete all the organic components of bone matrix, 90% of the protein of which is collagen. This collagen is identical with that found in tendon, ligament, fascia, and loose connective tissue, but is distinct from the collagen of cartilage. On the other hand, bone matrix shares with hyaline cartilage the notable property of being calcifiable. The extracellular matrix in either case becomes impregnated with calcium salts, mostly in a complex form of calcium phosphate and calcium hydroxide belonging to the apatite series of minerals. Whereas cartilage is essentially of homogeneous construction and relatively avascular, bone is highly porous and highly vascular.

Unlike chondroblasts and fibroblasts, osteoblasts are polarized cells in that they secrete matrix initially only from the cell surface facing the bone. Subsequently, the matrix is refashioned into thin **lamellae,** the architectural arrangement of which meets precisely the mechanical stresses to which a particular bone is subjected (Fig. 5-1). Such adaptability is wanting in calcified cartilage. Thus, bone is a living tissue—hard, supportive, and protective, yet also plastic, resilient, changeable, and reparable. It also serves as an important store of quickly usable calcium and other electrolytes.

Excluding the water content of some 25% to 30%, adult bone consists of about 30% to 40% collagen and about 60% to 70% mineral deposit. Collagen fibers give the bone tensile strength (resistance to being pulled apart), and calcium salts give it compressive strength (resistance to being compressed or crumbled). In general, bones of children have an excess of collagen compared with mineral matter and, therefore, are more easily bent. In elderly persons, bone becomes less compact, and the calcium salts are often reduced, so that the bones become brittle and fragile. Although there are no constant values for the strength of bone, good adult bone is said to have a tensile strength of about 12,000 to more than 17,000 lb/in^2 (that of copper is 28,000, that of white oak along the grain is about 12,500) and a compressive strength of 18,000 to 25,000 (that of copper is about 42,000, that of granite 15,000, and that of white oak along the grain only 7000).

Bone tissue is organized into discrete units of characteristic shape and form. Such an anatomic unit is called a bone (*os* in Latin).

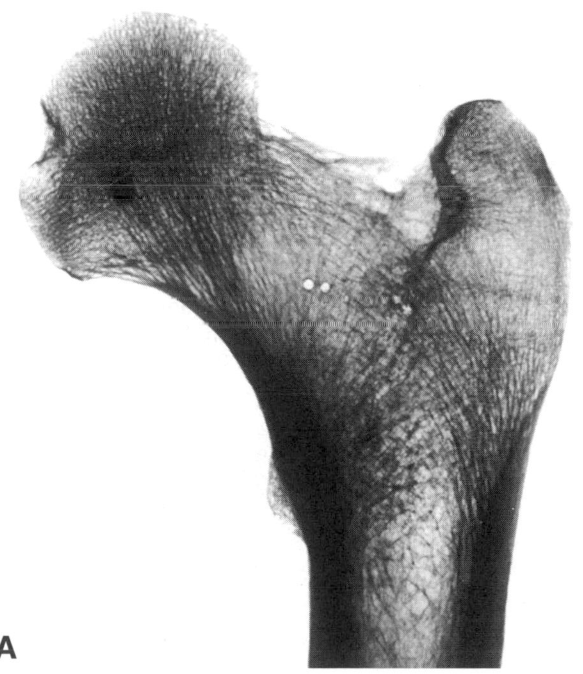

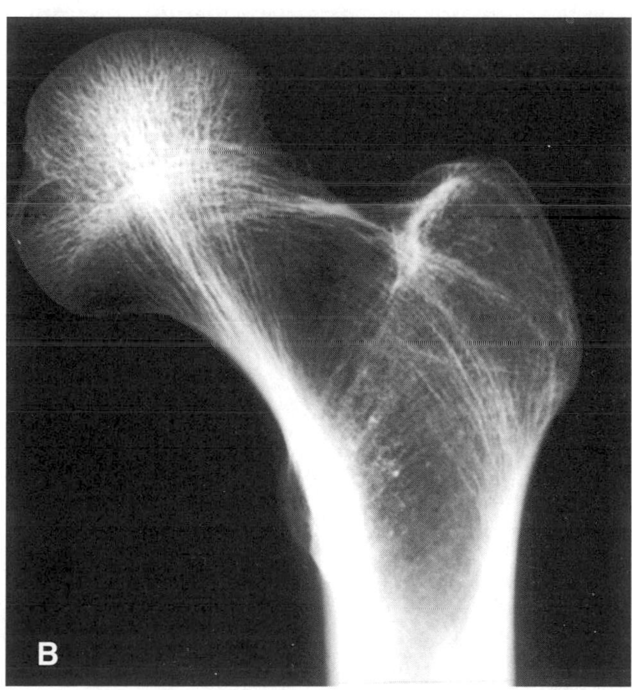

FIGURE *5-1.*
The upper end of the femur showing the arrangement of bony lamellae in cancellous bone: (A) This specimen was prepared by John Hunter, an 18th century anatomist and surgeon. It was decalcified and cut in the coronal plane. Only the fixed bone matrix remains. (B) A radiograph of a femur that exhibits a lamellar architecture. Inorganic bone salts are responsible for generating this image. The deposition of the mineral phase of bone conforms to the orientation of the organic matrix, which is secreted by the osteoblasts (A, courtesy of Huntarian Museum, Royal College of Surgeons, London; B, courtesy of Dr. Rosalind H. Troupin.)

BONES

Shape and Structure of Bones

Bones vary greatly in shape and size. It is possible to learn to distinguish even the smaller bones from each other and to state from which side of the body the bone was taken. Despite their diversity, however, bones can be classified according to their shape. The larger bones of the limbs are **long bones;** those of the wrist and ankle are **short bones;** others, particularly some of those of the skull, can be classified as **flat bones;** and still others, such as the vertebrae, are **irregular bones.**

Regardless of their shape, bones have the same general structure (Fig. 5-2; see also Fig. 12-3). The outer surface, called the **cortex,** is dense and hard, composed of bony layers closely packed together; it may be thick or thin. At the articular surfaces of freely movable joints, the cortex is covered by a layer of hyaline cartilage (articular cartilage). The space enclosed by the cortex of a flat or irregularly shaped bone, and that at the ends of a long bone, is occupied by **trabeculae** (beams) of bone, individually weak, but together forming a strong bracing system. Because the trabeculation gives a spongy appearance, the bone is called **cancellous** or **spongy bone.** The interstices between trabeculae are filled with marrow that is concerned with forming blood cells; from its color is derived the name "red marrow." The major part of a long bone, called the body or shaft, has a particularly heavy cortex that is tubelike and surrounds a large **medullary cavity** that is devoid of bony trabeculae. In the normal adult, the marrow here, although potentially capable of forming blood cells, is a storage place for fat; hence, its name of "yellow marrow."

Except for their articular surfaces, bones are invested by a connective tissue membrane called the **periosteum** (Fig. 5-3). The outer layer of the periosteum is fibrous, like a strong fascia, and contains periosteal blood vessels. The inner layer is looser connective tissue and contains **osteogenic cells** that can, even in the adult, proliferate and change into osteoblasts for the reconstruction of fractured bone. The surface of the bone abutting the marrow cavity is also lined by a layer of connective tissue, the **endosteum.** It is thinner than the periosteum and contains cells capable of forming bone. Thus, both endosteum and periosteum participate in the healing of a fracture.

Periosteum is bound to bone by fibers that continue into the bone to become fibers of the bone itself, but the density of these fibers varies. In many locations, periosteum can be stripped from bone, but it is always firmly bound to the bone at the places of insertion of tendons. Although some tendon fibers blend with the periosteum, most pass through the periosteum to become continuous with the fibers of the bone.

As bones grow, they tend to be modeled by tensile and compressive forces. A well-known example of this occurs in the femur, where the trabeculae of the head and neck (upper end) are arranged in interlocking arches that correspond with the calculated lines of stress evoked by the weight of the upper part of the body (see Fig. 5-1). The tube of cortical bone that forms the body of the femur is more efficient, weight for weight, in withstanding the strain placed on it than is any other structure in the body. A bone subjected to unusual strain as a result of change in the direction of the forces that act on it will gradually un-

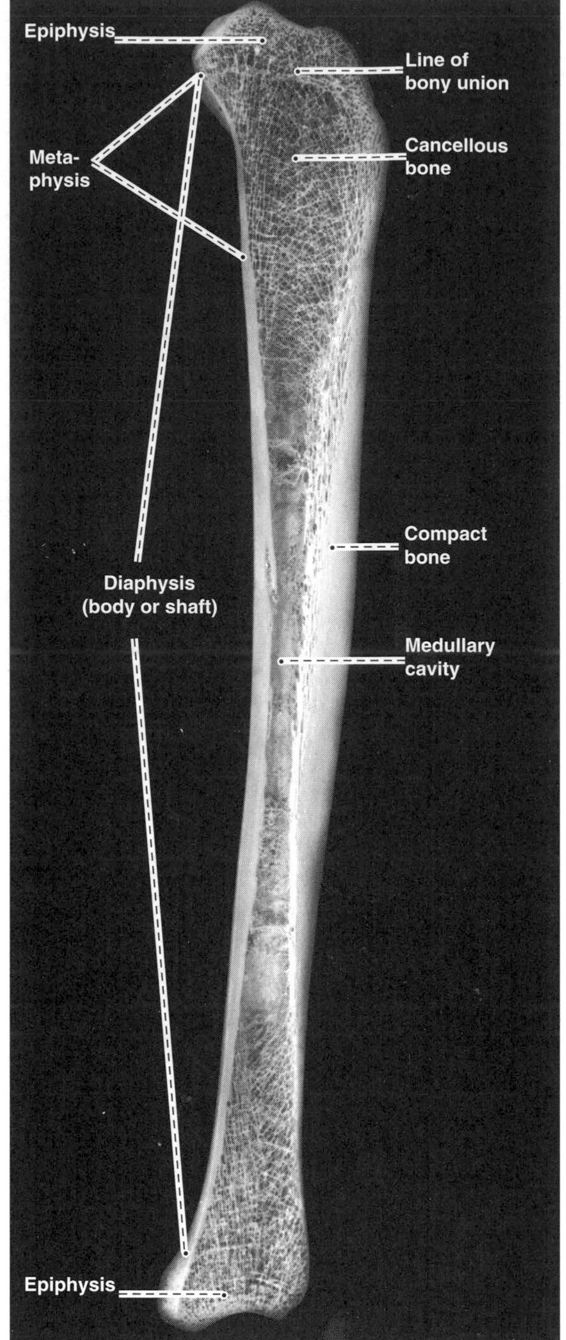

FIGURE 5-2.
Longitudinal section across a long bone of the appendicular skeleton (tibia) to show its different regions. Articular cartilage, covering the ends of the bone, and periosteum, investing the diaphysis, have not been retained in this specimen.

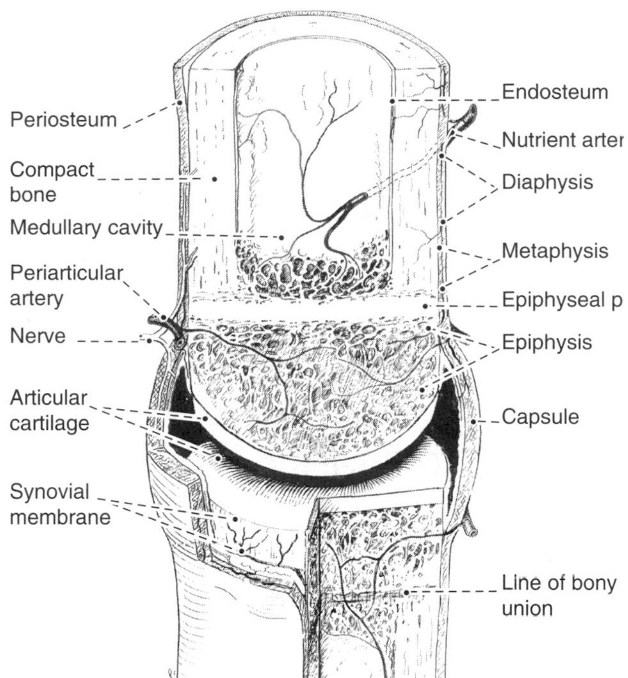

FIGURE 5-3.
Blood and nerve supply to a long bone and to the synovial joint through which it articulates with another bone. The upper bone is shown *before*, and the lower bone *after*, obliteration of the epiphyseal cartilage. The blood vessels that enter the periosteum from the attached muscles have been omitted from the drawing.

dergo resorption and rebuilding of its structure to fit the new pattern of forces acting on it; this occurs, for instance, from weight bearing after an improperly set fracture.

The pull of muscles on a bone also participates in modeling it. Most of the projections of bones, whether called ridges, crests, or tubercles, result from such modeling by muscles. This is why the skeletons of more heavily muscled bodies, regardless of sex, have more clearly marked bones than the skeletons of less muscular individuals.

Regardless of their size, **long bones** have a characteristic anatomy (see Fig. 5-2). A tubular **shaft,** also called the **body,** or **diaphysis,** terminates at either end in an expansion, called the **epiphysis.** Much of the free surface of the epiphysis is covered by articular cartilage. Bone tissue in the diaphysis and epiphyses develops independently (discussed later), and the eventual line of their fusion remains identifiable as the line of bony union, or *epiphyseal line*. The region of the diaphysis adjoining the epiphyseal line is often designated the **metaphysis.** Less significant in fully formed bones, the metaphysis is a particularly active region during the growth of long bones and is a preferential site of bone infection or osteomyelitis (see Fig. 17-15).

Short bones and **flat bones** have a simple structure; flat or curved plates of cortical bone surround cancellous bone in the interior. Much of the surface of short bones is covered by articular cartilage, whereas, as a rule, flat bones lack cartilaginous articular facets, because they are joined together either by fibrous tissue or cartilage (see later under Joints). **Irregular bones** have a variety of anatomic parts. The cancellous bone of vertebrae is filled by red marrow; several irregular bones of the skull contain large spaces filled with air (pneumatic bones).

Blood and Nerve Supply

The **blood supply** to bones varies according to their shape. Small bones may have a single artery entering them (typically accompanied by two or more veins); larger ones may have several, often irregularly spaced; and long bones tend to have a chief artery of the shaft and a variable number of smaller arteries supplying each end.

Because the artery to the shaft, or body, of a long bone is usually the largest, it is known as the **nutrient artery** (see Fig. 5-3). The nutrient artery enters the bone during early development, and as the bone grows, the **nutrient canal** in which it lies usually has its external end carried toward the faster-growing end. In most long bones, growth in length of the bone occurs much more at one end than at the other; thus, the slant of the canal from surface to marrow cavity is commonly toward the end that has grown less rapidly, which allows one to determine the relative growth of the two ends. The nutrient artery or arteries supply most of the marrow and cortex, their branches running in haversian canals of the cortical bone.

The ends of long bones typically have several arteries entering them and several veins leaving, so that numerous vascular foramina are usually visible on the epiphyses of dried bones. These vessels supply both the marrow and the bone.

Lymphatics occur in the periosteum of bone, and it is thought that some accompany blood vessels into the bone.

Nerve fibers to bone are not numerous, but some do accompany blood vessels and some occur in the periosteum. They consist of both afferent (sensory) and sympathetic efferent fibers, the latter representing the motor nerve supply to the blood vessels. This nerve supply apparently does not play any important part in controlling the growth or repair of bone. Afferent fibers within bone are primarily concerned with pain, which may be the first indication of a tumor within the bone. Most of the pain associated with fracture of a bone, however, undoubtedly arises from surrounding soft tissues.

THE SKELETON

The adult bony skeleton (Fig. 5-4) typically consists of 206 bones. This number is subject to some variation, for supernumerary bones are fairly common, especially in the hands and feet. The bony skeleton can conveniently be divided into axial and appendicular skeletons, the latter being the skeleton of the limbs, the former that of the head and the trunk.

Axial Skeleton

The axial skeleton consists of the skull, the vertebral column, the ribs and the sternum. The anatomy of the skull

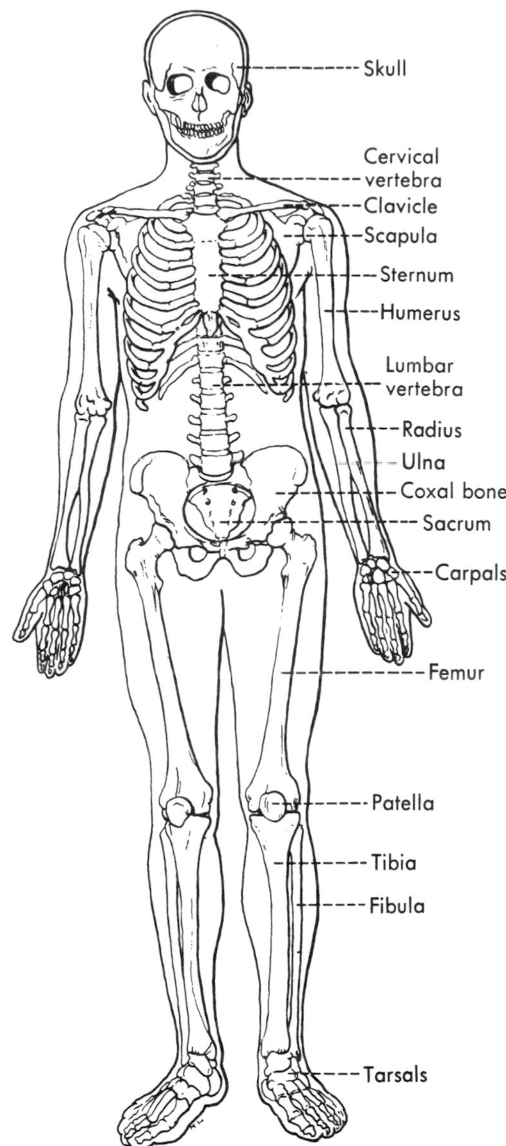

FIGURE **5-4.**
The human skeleton, anterior view.

is described in Chapter 31, that of the vertebral column in Chapter 12, and that of the rib cage in Chapter 19. This section presents these parts chiefly to introduce terminology and general concepts. The bones of the **skull** can be divided into two groups: those that protect and support the brain and the organs of sight, hearing, and balance; and those of the jaws and face. The remainder of the axial skeleton tends to be arranged segmentally (metamerically). The **vertebral column,** or backbone, is composed of 32 or 33 segments that remain as separate **vertebrae** (irregular bones) throughout the neck and most of the trunk, but fuse together inferiorly to form the sacrum. The **ribs,** extending laterally from the vertebral column, are strictly metameric and, together with their cartilages and the sternum, form the rib cage.

Although there are regular differences in the vertebrae in different regions, they are all built on the same fundamental pattern. The 7 vertebrae of the neck are the **cervical vertebrae.** They are followed by 12 **thoracic vertebrae,** which have the ribs articulated with them. These are followed by 5 **lumbar vertebrae** that lie in the small of the back. The next 5 vertebrae fuse together to form the **sacrum,** which transmits the weight of the upper part of the body to the hip bones. Because its original segments (i.e., vertebrae) can still be identified in the adult skeleton, it is customary to refer to, for instance, the second sacral segment or vertebra, even though the vertebrae are not separate. The remaining vertebrae are vestigial and together form the **coccyx.**

Appendicular Skeleton

Of the appendicular skeleton (so termed from the earlier designation of the limbs as "appendages"), the bones of the two upper limbs are essentially mirror images of each other, as are those of the two lower limbs. In addition, the bones of the upper and lower limbs are analogous. Those of each limb can be divided into two chief groups: a **girdle,** closely associated with the trunk, and the skeleton of the **free limb,** the part distal to the shoulder joint or hip joint. The developmental and functional anatomy of the appendicular skeleton is described in Chapter 14.

The upper limb girdle is also called the **pectoral girdle** (*pectus,* meaning chest) and consists of two bones, the **clavicle** or collar bone and the **scapula** or shoulder blade. The lower limb girdle is also called the **pelvic girdle** (*pelvis,* meaning basin), because the right and left girdle, together with the sacrum, form a basin. In contrast with the pectoral girdle, the three bones on each side, the **pubis, ilium,** and **ischium,** are fused together and constitute the **os coxae** or hip bone. They are also firmly united to the sacrum, so that they can better transmit the weight of the trunk to the lower limbs.

The upper and lower limbs are much more similar relative to the **skeleton of the free limb** than they are relative to the girdle. In each limb, a single long bone forms the proximal segment of the skeleton of the limb: the **humerus** in the arm and the **femur** in the thigh. In the next segment of each limb there are two long bones: the **radius** and the **ulna** in the forearm, the **tibia** and the **fibula** in the leg.

The wrist and ankle each consists of several short bones. Those of the wrist are the **carpal bones,** and those of the ankle; the **tarsal bones.** The latter contribute almost half the length of the sole of the foot.

Five bones, the **metacarpals,** form the major part of the palm of the hand; the skeleton of the anterior part of the foot likewise consists of five bones, the **metatarsals.** Each bone that forms a segment of a digit is known as a **phalanx,** whether in the foot or the hand. Although much shorter than the bones in the more proximal segments of the limbs, metacarpals, metatarsals, and phalanges are long bones in that they have a shaft containing a medullary cavity and an epiphysis at one of their ends.

Sesamoid bones (so called because the smallest ones resemble sesame seeds in size) are bones that develop within tendons or ligaments. They develop first as sesamoid cartilages. Sesamoid bones occur regularly in some locations, with varying frequency in others. The patella or kneecap, the largest sesamoid bone of the body, interrupts the great extensor tendon on the front of the knee. There are usually two sesamoid bones at the base of the thumb and two at the base of the big toe, all of which are much larger than implied by the term "sesamoid." Others may occur in ligaments of the toes and fingers, or in certain tendons at points of increased friction.

BONE FORMATION

The first stage in the formation of any bone is a condensation of **mesenchyme,** that is, the loose embryonic connective tissue. The cells in these mesenchymal primordia may then give rise to bone in one of two different ways. A limited number of bones, primarily the bones of the roof of the skull, are formed by the direct transition of mesenchyme into bony tissue. Because the mesenchymal condensation resembles a membrane, this process of bone formation is known as **intramembranous ossification,** and the resulting bones are sometimes called membrane bones. Phylogenetically, bones of this type are believed to be derived from the dermis of the skin (which is also a derivative of mesenchyme) and are often termed "dermal bones." In most bones, however, including most of those of the skull, the entire vertebral column, the ribs and sternum, and virtually all the bones of the limbs, the mesenchymal condensation is first transformed into cartilage. The mesenchymal primordium produces a rough model of the bone in cartilage. As the cartilage grows, it is invaded by blood vessels and accompanying cells that destroy the cartilage and replace it with bone. This process of bone formation is known as **endochondral ossification,** and the resulting bones are known as **cartilage bones.** It should be emphasized that cartilage is never actually transformed into bone; rather, whenever bone replaces cartilage, the cartilage is destroyed and bone is deposited by a new cohort of cells in its place.

Growth of a membrane bone is essentially by a process of accretion on the surfaces and edges of the bone. This is illustrated by the gradual postnatal closure of the fontanels, the soft spots of the child's skull. The fontanels are simply areas of membrane between edges and corners of certain bones; the bones grow into the membrane and close the fontanels by addition of bone along these edges. While bone is being added to the outside of a membrane bone, there is absorption and reorganization on its inner surface. The cancellous bone in the interior is also remodeled along with the bone as a whole, preventing the bone from becoming too thick.

Formation and growth of cartilage bones are somewhat more complicated than those of membrane bones (Fig. 5-5). Briefly, the cartilage representing a bone is invaded, usually at about its center, by blood vessels. Osteoblasts brought in by the mesenchyme along the blood vessels give rise to bone, representing the first or **primary center of ossification.** As this center of bone formation becomes larger, bone is also laid down by the adjacent periosteum. Growth in the diameter of a cartilage bone, therefore, occurs in essentially the same fashion as does that of membrane bone, by the laying down of successive concentric layers by the periosteum. Constant remodeling of the marrow cavity ensures an adequate balance between lightness and strength.

In some cartilage bones, notably the small ones of the wrist (see Fig. 16-8) and most of those of the ankle, the rapidly growing cartilage is eventually replaced entirely by bone spreading from the original center of ossification. The vertebrae and the long bones of the limbs, however, develop more than one center of ossification (see Figs. 12-6, 16-4, 17-7, and 18-5); these additional centers are known as **epiphyses** or **secondary centers of ossification.** Epiphyseal centers of ossification appear for the most part after birth and enlarge rapidly. During the entire growth period they are separated from the primary center of ossification, which forms the **diaphysis,** or body, by a plate of cartilage, known as the **epiphyseal cartilage** (also called **growth plate** or growth plate cartilage).

A large long bone has at least two epiphyses, one at each end. Smaller "long" bones, such as those of the fingers and toes, typically have an epiphysis at only one end. There may be separate epiphyseal centers of ossification for projections of bone developed in connection with the attachments of muscles (e.g., the trochanters of the femur; see Fig. 17-7); these are sometimes known as traction epiphyses.

Growth of the body (shaft) of the bone is responsible for most of the increase in length and occurs entirely from the epiphyseal cartilages. Chondrocytes in the epiphyseal cartilage proliferate, generating progeny that adds new cartilage to the adjacent diaphysis. In this growth region of the diaphysis, called the **metaphysis,** new cartilage is replaced by bone. The epiphyses themselves grow by expansion of the secondary centers of ossification. As growth of the epiphyseal cartilages slows toward the end of puberty, the rate of ossification begins to approach and then exceeds the rate of proliferation of cartilage, so that the entire epiphyseal cartilage is replaced by bone and growth in length ceases. In general, centers of ossification appear earlier in the female than they do in the male, and the disappearance of the epiphyseal cartilages, with cessation of growth, usually occurs about 3 years earlier in the female.

In the long bones that have two epiphyses, growth usually occurs much more rapidly at one epiphyseal cartilage than at the other. In the femur, the faster-growing epiphyseal cartilage is the lower one, whereas in the tibia, it is the upper one.

Interference with the growth of an epiphyseal cartilage may occur as a result of disease, hormonal imbalance, or trauma. If the injury is in one of the long bones of the limbs, an inequality in the length of the limbs will result.

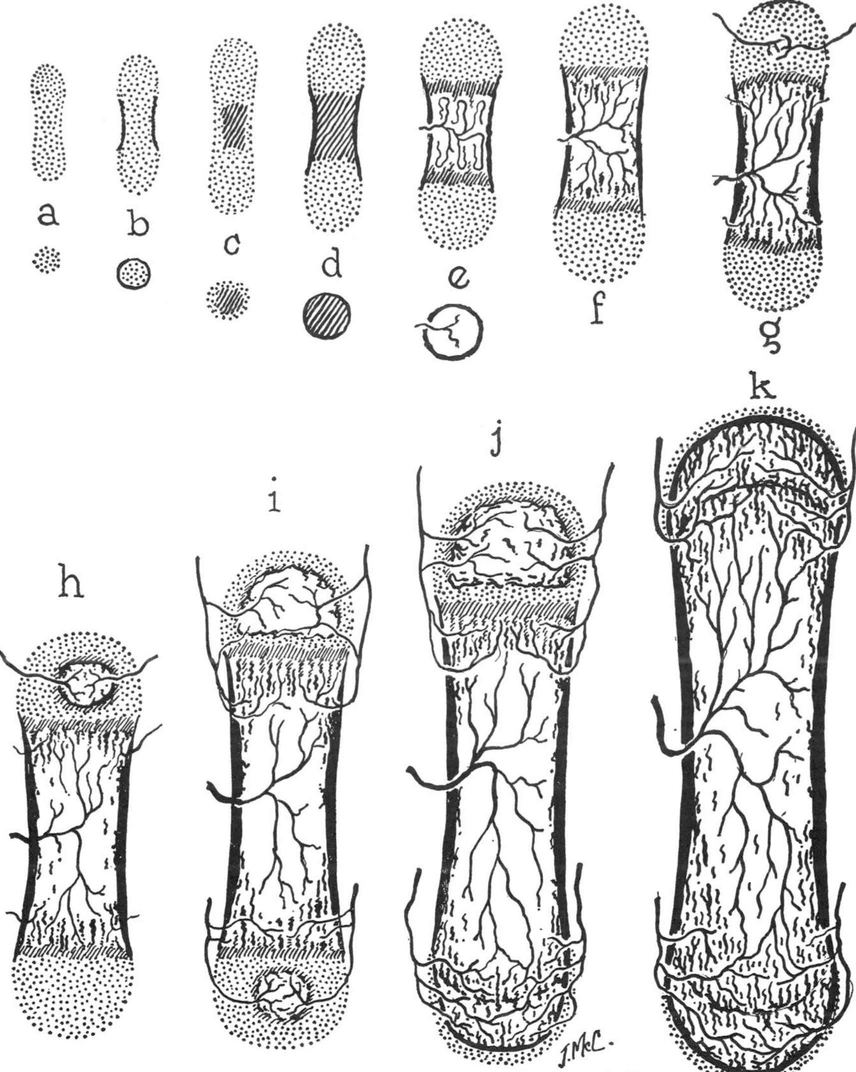

FIGURE 5-5.
Development of a typical long bone. (a) Cartilage model. (b) Periosteal bone collar appears. (c) Center of calcifying cartilage. (d) Further development of calcified cartilage. (e) Vascular mesenchyme enters, resorbs calcified cartilage, and new bone is laid down toward either extremity of the model. (f) Endochondral ossification is further advanced and bone increased in length. (g) Blood vessels and mesenchyme enter upper epiphyseal cartilage. (h) Development of epiphyseal ossification center. (i) Ossification center develops in lower epiphysis. (j and k) The lower and then the upper epiphyseal cartilage plates disappear, bone ceases to grow in length, a continuous bone marrow cavity traverses the entire length of the bone, and blood vessels of diaphysis, metaphysis, and epiphysis intercommunicate. (Adapted from Maximow AA, Bloom W. Textbook of histology. Philadelphia, WB Saunders, 1968)

This has important consequences on body posture and gait if one of the long bones of a lower limb is affected.

Fracture and Repair

Fracture of a bone may result from a crushing injury, but in the long bones it is more often due to an excessive bending force. Because the tensile strength of bone is less than its compressive strength, fracture of a long bone regularly begins on the convex edge of the curve into which it is bent. The heavier fibrous and lower mineral content of young, growing bones leads to irregular splitting fractures resembling those produced when a green stick is broken. For this reason such fractures that break a long bone only on one side are frequently referred to as "greenstick fractures." In old age, the lessened fibrous and mineral content of bones may lead to such fragility that the bone can no longer carry out its usual supporting tasks. Fracture of the neck of the femur, a common fracture of the aged, is thought to result not always from a fall, but sometimes from weakening of the femoral neck to the extent that it can no longer sustain the weight of the body. The sudden fracture then produces the fall, rather than the fall producing the fracture.

A fracture may be merely a crack extending partly into the bone, or it may involve complete interruption of the bone. In the latter event, the ends of the bone fragments may be jammed together (impacted) or widely separated (distracted) from each other. The direction in which the fragments are displaced may depend on the direction of the force causing the fracture, but it is frequently influenced by the actions of muscles that attach to the bone fragments. An overriding of the ends of the fragments of a fractured bone, as a result of the pull of the muscles crossing the fracture line, is common. On the other hand, there may be wide displacement if muscles pull the proximal fragment in one direction and the distal fragment in another (see Figs. 15-8 and 17-8). The sharp, displaced ends of fractured bones sometimes penetrate blood vessels or nerves and may even protrude through the skin (compound fracture). Pain from displacement of the ends of a fractured bone produces reflex or automatic muscular spasm. Knowledge of the anatomy of the involved muscles aids in determining the forces that must be overcome in reducing the fracture.

Repair of a fracture takes place primarily through the combined activity of the periosteum and endosteum, both of which contain osteoblasts capable of forming bone. The best repair of bone occurs when the ends can be put in close apposition and held that way, requiring accurate reduction of the fracture and fixation of the bone fragments through splints or other methods.

Bone grafts are sometimes used in orthopedic surgery. The grafted bone itself will not survive, but it serves as a scaffold on which new bone is laid down, uniting firmly the distracted edges of the fractured bone. Such grafts seem to stimulate the formation of new bone.

JOINTS

A joint, or articulation (*arthrosis*), is a union of two or more skeletal elements. Whether the chief function of a joint is to provide a stable union or a free range of movement is largely determined by the type of tissue of which the joint is constructed. In the great majority, free articular surfaces slide, spin or roll on one another, there being no other tissue interposed between them. Movement in such joints is facilitated by a lubricant called synovial fluid, and they are known as **synovial joints** (*diarthroses*). In the remaining **nonsynovial joints** (*synarthroses*), there are no free surfaces and connective tissue of considerable strength unites the osseous surfaces. Such an arrangement largely precludes movement, although some angulation and distraction are occasionally possible. There are two types of synarthrosis: if the intervening tissue is dense fibrous connective tissue, the joint is called a **fibrous joint** and, if it is cartilage, a **cartilaginous joint.**

All bones and the joints that unite them develop in the embryo from condensations of mesenchyme. As described earlier, some bones develop by direct transformation of the mesenchymal primordia into bone; in others (the majority) ossification is preceded by the development of a cartilage model. In either event the mesenchyme that remains between the developing bones represents the primitive joint (Fig. 5-6). The further development of this

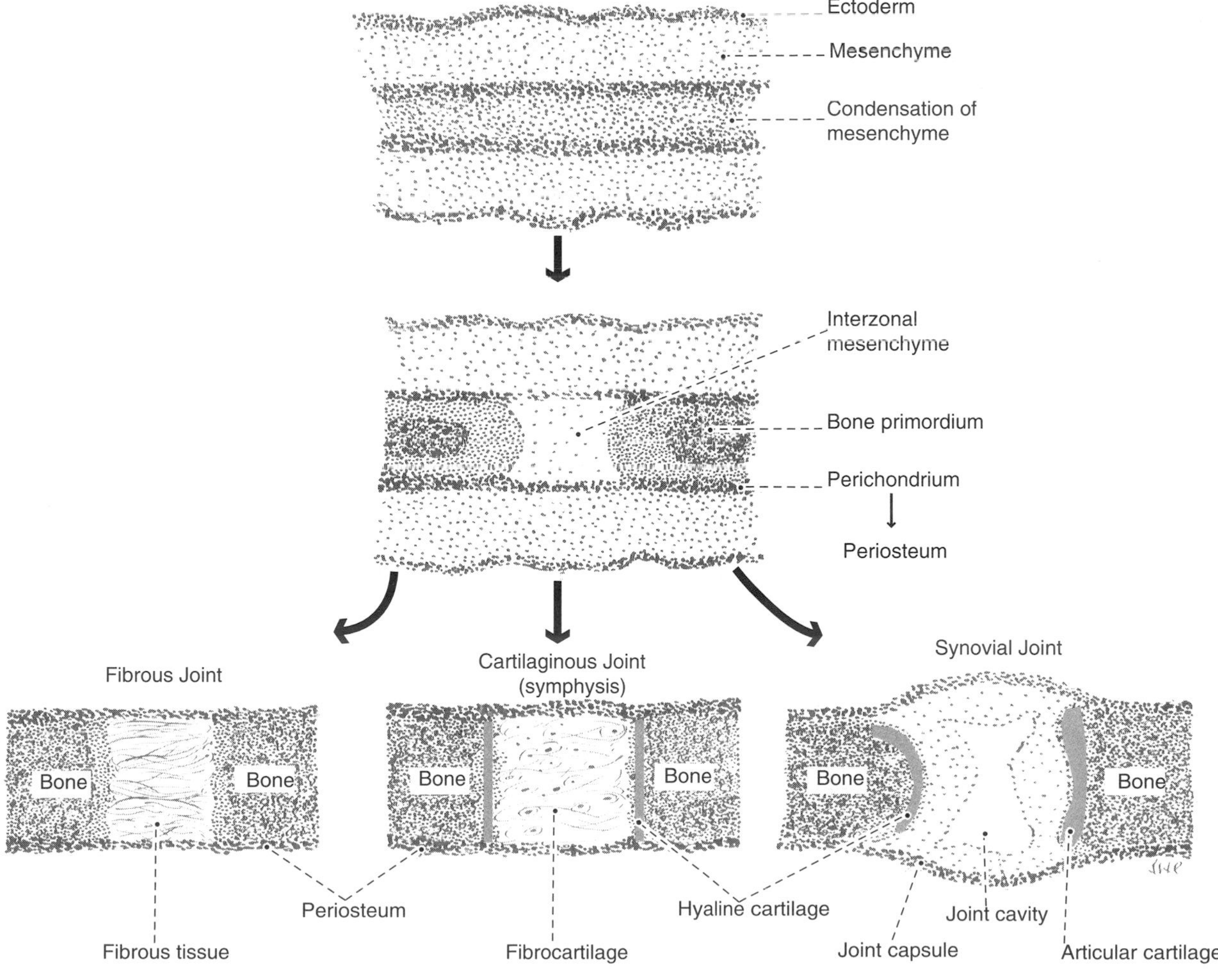

FIGURE 5-6.
Schematic representation of the embryologic development of different types of joints.

tissue, referred to as *interzonal mesenchyme*, determines the type of joint that will form. Where it remains solid, a fibrous or cartilaginous joint develops. Where a synovial joint is to form, the mesenchyme develops a narrow, fluid-containing cavity.

Each of the three categories of joint may be further subdivided, according to a number of different criteria. The classification of joints tends to be somewhat arbitrary and inconsistent: indeed, it is difficult to devise a simple scheme that encompasses all of the varieties of joints found in the body. The classification used here follows the officially recognized one in Nomina Anatomica.

Fibrous and Cartilaginous Joints

Fibrous Joints

There are three types of fibrous joint (Fig. 5-7). In a **suture,** the bones are held together by a very small amount of fibrous tissue. Periosteum is continuous from bone to bone, over the suture. Typically, the osseous surfaces have irregular areas of contact, such as serrations or ridges, which provide resistance to shearing forces or torsion. Sutures are essentially immovable joints. They occur only in the skull. With age, the fibrous tissue is gradually replaced by bone and the suture becomes a completely bony union or *synostosis.*

In a **gomphosis** (*dentoalveolar joint*), like in a suture, essentially a very small amount of fibrous tissue anchors a tooth into its bony socket (alveolus) in the maxilla or mandible.

A **syndesmosis** comprises more fibrous tissue than either a suture or a gomphosis. It may take the form of an interosseous ligament or membrane, or a slender fibrous cord between two bones. Authorities differ in their definition of a syndesmosis; therefore, in the range of structures that they include within this category. Nomina Anatomica lists nine officially recognized syndesmoses. Most of these are named ligaments associated with the vertebral column (e.g., ligamenta flava or interspinous ligaments). In the appendicular skeleton the interosseous membranes of the forearm and the leg (see Figs. 16-2 and 18-2) can be considered syndesmoses. The tibiofibular syndesmosis, which unites the lower ends of the tibia and fibula, is particularly important for the integrity of the ankle region (Fig. 5-7; and see Fig. 18-59). Compared with sutures and gomphoses, syndesmoses do permit a slight degree of movement, but their chief function is to provide a stable union.

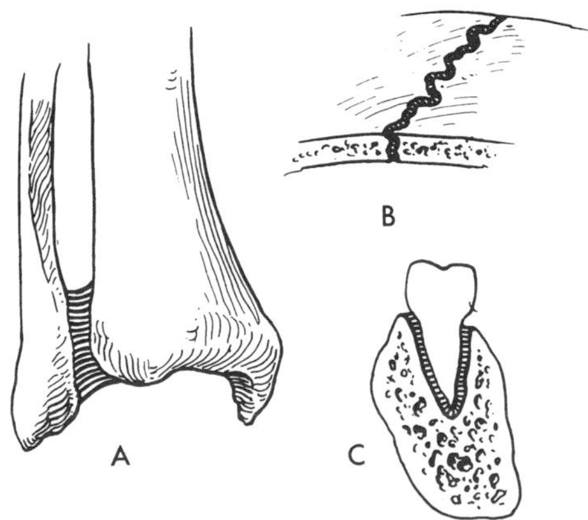

FIGURE 5-7.
Types of fibrous joints: (A) the tibiofibular syndesmosis; (B) a suture of the skull; (C) a gomphosis, the attachment of a tooth.

Cartilaginous Joints

Two categories of cartilaginous joints are recognized. When the uniting tissue is hyaline cartilage, the joint is a *synchondrosis,* and when it is fibrocartilage, a *symphysis.* These two groups have also been called *primary* and *secondary cartilaginous joints*, respectively.

A **synchondrosis** is a plate of hyaline cartilage interposed between two bony elements. Synchondroses occur between adjacent endochondral centers of ossification, permitting growth to take place, yet holding the two bony elements together in a firm union. The epiphyseal plate between the diaphysis and epiphysis of a long bone is an example. Other synchondroses occur in parts of the skull. Yet others are found in the sternum in young individuals: between the growing sternebrae, for example, or at the manubriosternal and xiphisternal junctions. Indeed, synchondroses occur in any postcranial bone that develops from two or more centers of ossification.

All true synchondroses disappear sooner or later. The hyaline cartilage is usually replaced by bone forming a *synostosis;* occasionally, it is transformed into fibrocartilage, forming a *symphysis,* as in the manubriosternal and xiphisternal joints. (Even here, bony union usually occurs eventually). The age at which this transformation occurs varies over a wide range; some synchondroses remain functional into the second or third decade.

In a **symphysis,** the binding material is fibrocartilage. Hyaline cartilage is also present, but only as thin layers covering the apposing bony surfaces; between these layers is a fairly thick, deformable, fibrocartilaginous pad that is well-suited to take compression, tension, shearing forces, or torsion. An important example is the intervertebral disk: these symphyses bind the bodies of adjacent vertebrae together and yet permit the column to bend. The symphysis pubis is another example, as is the manubriosternal joint mentioned earlier.

Other Joints Involving Cartilage. The majority of bones develop by endochondral ossification, from cartilaginous models. Although most of this cartilage is eventually replaced by bone, some relatively large pieces of it remain cartilaginous throughout life. The costal cartilages, for example, are merely the unossified anterior portions of the ribs. Thus, the skeleton must be considered to include cartilaginous, as well as bony, elements. Each cartilaginous element forms junctions with neighboring parts of the skeleton, be they bones or other cartilages. Such junctions do not fit in the most common definition of a joint; namely, a union of two or more bones. Nevertheless, they are unions of skeletal elements and should be included in a general discussion of joints. This category includes, for example, junctions between contiguous cartilages in the cranium and in the larynx. They resemble some of the fibrous joints between bones, described earlier, and perhaps should be included among them. Likewise, the costal cartilages display a variety of junctions—with the sternum, with their own ribs, and with each other—which resemble fibrous or, in some instances, synovial joints between bony elements.

Synovial Joints

General Anatomy

A synovial joint is characterized by the presence of a joint cavity and free articular surfaces: what holds the articulating bones together is a well-developed capsule, together with associated ligaments, rather than solid tissue between the osseous surfaces as in synarthroses. Such a joint is well adapted for movement. The actual range of movement varies greatly, however, depending on the requirements for function and stability.

The basic structure of a synovial joint is shown in Figure 5-8. The **fibrous capsule** (*joint capsule* or *articular capsule*) consists chiefly of interlacing collagen fiber bundles that provide strength, but little elasticity. It is usually reinforced by localized thickenings of parallel fiber bundles, known as **capsular** (*intrinsic*) **ligaments**. Additional or **accessory ligaments** may also be found independent of the capsule, and they may be either inside or outside the joint (intracapsular or extracapsular accessory ligaments). In general, ligaments are found in planes in which the joint requires greater stability, where they restrain motion in an undesirable direction.

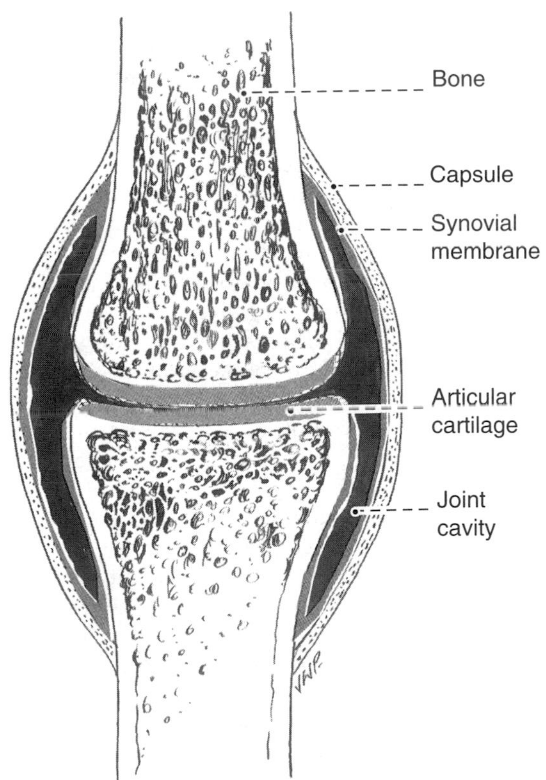

FIGURE 5-8.
Diagrammatic representation of the anatomic features of a typical synovial joint seen in a section cut across the *middle* of the joint. The extent of the joint cavity is exaggerated to show the anatomic arrangement of the synovial membrane more clearly.

The **synovial membrane** lines the capsular sleeve and attaches around the edges of the articular surfaces (see Fig. 5-8). It covers nonarticular bony surfaces in the joint cavity and ensheathes intracapsular ligaments and tendons when present. It also covers fat pads, which sometimes occur between the membrane and the fibrous capsule. Some authorities classify the synovial membrane as an integral part of the articular capsule: the latter is characterized as a structure having two components, an outer *fibrous membrane* (described here as the fibrous capsule) and an inner *synovial membrane*. In the present context, the synovial membrane is treated as a separate structure, as it is not limited to lining the fibrous sleeve, but invests other surfaces within the joint as well.

In appearance, the membrane is delicate, pink, smooth, and shiny. The surface facing the joint cavity is made up of synovial cells (synoviocytes) embedded in an extracellular matrix. Because the cells form a discontinuous layer, and a basement membrane is lacking, matrix is directly exposed to the synovial fluid in places. Beneath the surface is highly vascular loose connective tissue. Some of the synovial cells are thought to be responsible for secreting mucin, chiefly hyaluronic acid, into synovial fluid, whereas others appear to be involved in pinocytosis and phagocytosis.

Articular cartilage covers the articulating surfaces of the bones. In most joints, it is hyaline cartilage, but it differs from hyaline cartilage elsewhere in several respects: it is not covered by perichondrium, its collagen fibers form a three-dimensional network adapted to load bearing and maintaining the integrity of a smooth surface (Fig. 5-9), and it never ossifies. Owing to the capacity of collagen fibrils to bind proteoglycans into a highly resilient, water-filled, structural gel, articular cartilage can resist and distribute into subchondral bone the large compressive forces developed by muscle action and gravity. Articular cartilage is devoid of both nerves and blood vessels, its nourishment being largely dependent on synovial fluid. Its cells rarely divide after the cessation of growth. Once damaged, articular cartilage does not regenerate. Gaps generated in it may become filled by fibrous tissue or, when it is destroyed by inflammatory or degenerative processes, the underlying bone will remain bare.

Some joints contain an **articular disk,** a piece of fibrocartilage interposed like a shelf or pad between the articulating surfaces. Around its circumference the disk is anchored in the fibrous capsule. Where the disks are incomplete and crescent-shaped, as in the knee joint, they are known as *menisci*. Among the functions that have been assigned to disks and menisci are shock absorption, assistance in providing for a more even distribution of weight and synovial fluid, and improvement of the fit of articular surfaces. Like articular cartilage, they are free of synovial membrane.

Synovial fluid moistens and lubricates the articular

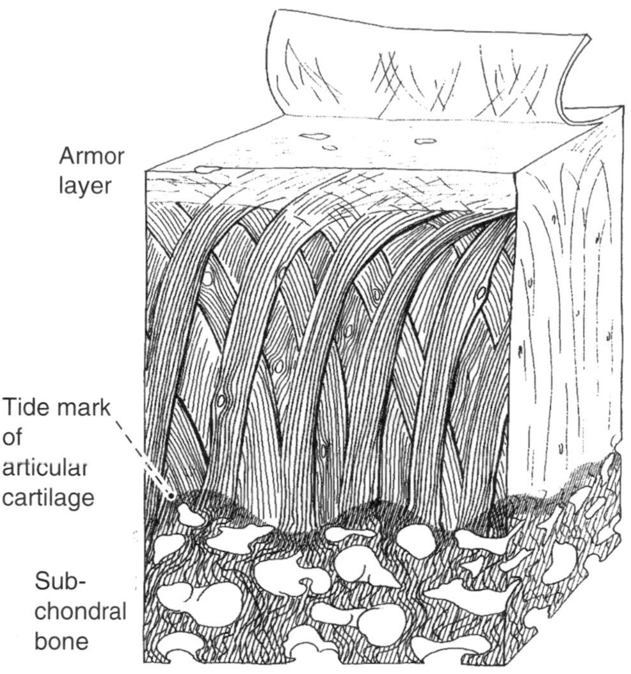

FIGURE 5-9.
Schematic view of the collagen fibrillar organization in human articular cartilage in a full-thickness block from the surface to the deep subchondral bone. The most superficial lamina of the armor layer (lamina splendens) has been incised, peeled off, and reflected. (Redrawn from Minns RJ, Steven FS. J Anat 1977; 123: 437.)

surfaces, the synovial membrane and the articular disks. Primarily a filtrate of plasma, it contains electrolytes and other small molecules at concentrations similar to those in plasma, but with a much lower level of total protein. Its most distinguishing characteristic is the presence of hyaluronic acid. These glycosaminoglycan molecules make the fluid viscous and slimy.

Blood and Nerve Supply

Anastomotic plexuses of blood vessels (*periarticular anastomosis*) and nerves surround the capsule on the exterior, and branches of these plexuses penetrate the capsule as well as the bone (see Fig. 5-3). The periarticular anastomosis is fed by branches of arteries passing the joint and is the source of blood to the capillary bed in the synovial membrane and also to the epiphyses.

Joint pain and the awareness of the precise position of the limbs (proprioception) testify to the rich innervation of joints and associated structures. Articular nerves are composed of **somatic sensory fibers**, which mediate sensations of pain, pressure, vibration, and position sense (proprioception), and of autonomic **vasomotor fibers**. The nerves are distributed to the fibrous capsule, ligaments, synovial membrane, and the periosteum. Articular cartilage is devoid of nerve supply. Practically all nerves in the synovial membrane are thought to serve a vasomotor function. Proprioceptive and pain impulses generated in the capsule and ligaments play a major role not only in informing us of the position of our limbs, but in influencing reflex contraction and inhibition of muscles that act on the joint. As a rule, each joint is supplied by branches of the nerves that innervate the muscles producing movement at that joint. In most joints, the aspect of the capsule stretched by the contraction of one muscle is supplied by the nerve innervating the antagonists of that muscle. This relation is likely to be an important factor in preventing overstretching of the capsule.

The afferent impulses arising in joints are generated by several types of receptors. These nerve endings include lamellated Ruffini and pacinian corpuscles, concerned with proprioception, and free nerve endings sensitive to pain. In addition, tendon organs are present in some ligaments. When the nerve supply is lost, the joint rapidly undergoes degenerative changes, suggesting that the innervation of joints is an important factor in maintaining their normal structure.

Movements in Synovial Joints

The simplest movement possible between two articulating surfaces is *sliding* or gliding—one bone moving bodily across the surface of the other. If the surfaces are fairly flat, gliding may take place in any direction, but angular or rotational displacements are unlikely to occur between the articulating bones. Because of the flatness of the surfaces, such joints are known as **plane joints.** Many articulations between the bones of the carpus and tarsus (intercarpal and intertarsal joints) as well as between neighboring arches of vertebrae are of this type.

The effective use of the limbs and movements of the head rely on joints in which the articular surfaces present pronounced curvatures, which may be considered as segments of spheres, ellipsoids, cones, and cylinders. The lack of complete congruity as well as disproportion in size between the mating surfaces permits some *rolling* (or rocking) and *spinning* of one bone upon the other. In most joints, the movement of greatest amplitude is achieved by one bone sliding on the other, the axis of motion being placed at the center of the arc defining the convex member of the pair. As a consequence, the end of the moving bone distal to the articulation describes arcs. Traditionally, such movements have been explained with reference to the **axes** placed through the center of the curved articular surfaces. The number of such possible axes around which movement may be produced, *independently* and actively, determines the **degrees of freedom** in a joint.

The varieties of synovial joints and their characteristic movements are most satisfactorily explained on an elementary level by retaining this traditional concept of joint axes and classifying the joints accordingly. It is important, however, to carry the analysis of movements a step further and consider the mechanics of joints in the light of concepts developed in kinesiology. A later section will concern itself with such an analysis, but first, synovial joints are discussed according to joint axes and the types of movements their anatomy permits.

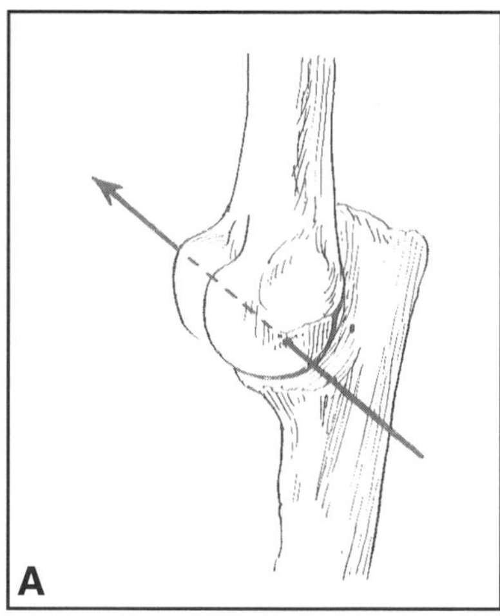

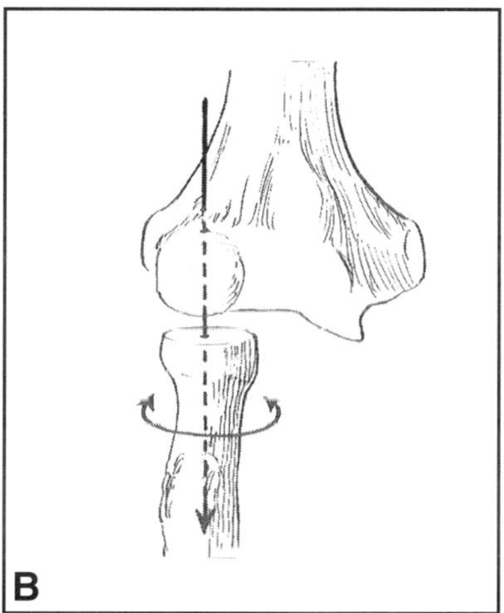

FIGURE *5-10.*
Uniaxial joints: (A) hinge joint (elbow); (B) pivot joint (superior radioulnar joint).

Varieties of Synovial Joints and Their Movements

Those joints in which one or more articular surfaces are perceptibly curved may be classified as uniaxial, biaxial, and polyaxial. These varieties of joints possess one, two, or three degrees of freedom, respectively.

Uniaxial Joints. Movement is possible around only one axis. This axis may be transverse across the articular surfaces, in which case the joint is regarded as a **hinge joint** (Fig. 5-10A); or the axis may lie longitudinally along the shaft of the bone, in which case one speaks of a **pivot joint** (see Fig. 5-10B). The humeroulnar joint at the elbow and the interphalangeal joints of the hand and feet are hinge joints; the radioulnar and the atlantoaxial joints are pivot joints.

The movements permitted in a hinge joint are flexion and extension. **Flexion** occurs when the angle between the adjoining bones is decreased, as when the elbow is bent forward. **Extension** occurs when the angle between the adjoining bones is increased, as when the arm is straightened at the elbow. Both movements take place in one and the same plane.

Only one movement is permitted in a pivot joint, rotation. **Rotation** occurs when a bone spins around a central longitudinal axis without undergoing any displacement from that axis. This is true of the radius which rotates in a stationary osseoligamentous ring (see Chap. 16), and of the atlas which, as a ring, rotates around the stationary dens of the axis vertebra (see Figs. 12-11 and 12-22).

Biaxial Joints. Movement is possible around two axes that lie at approximately 90° to one another. Ellipsoid and saddle joints fall into this category (Fig. 5-11).

In an **ellipsoid joint,** a convex ellipsoid surface is received into a concave ellipsoid surface, like an egg resting in a spoon. One axis is along the long diameter and the other along the short diameter of the articular surfaces

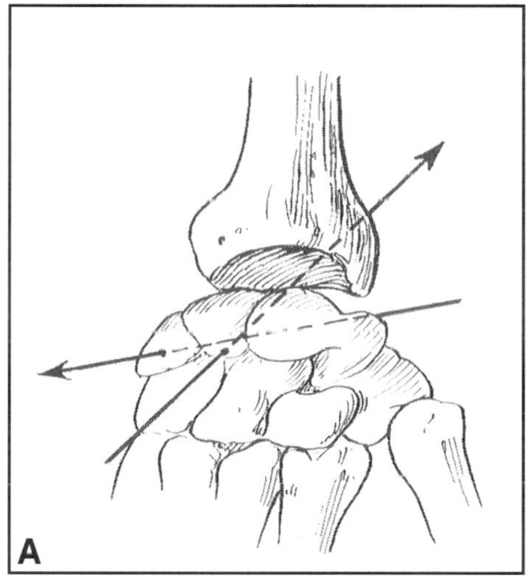

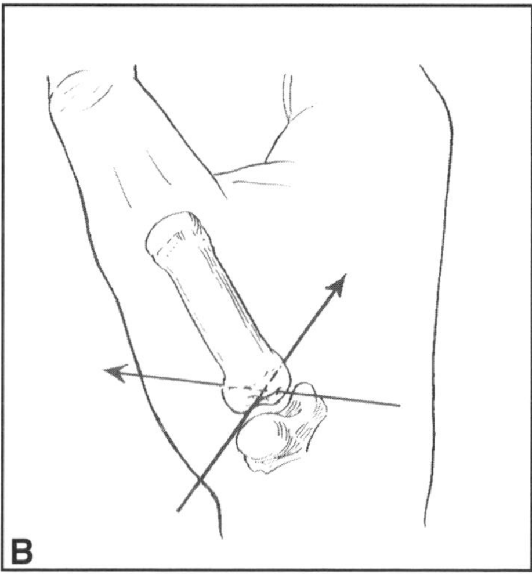

FIGURE *5-11.*
Biaxial joints: (A) ellipsoid joint (radiocarpal joint); (B) saddle joint (carpometacarpal joint of the thumb).

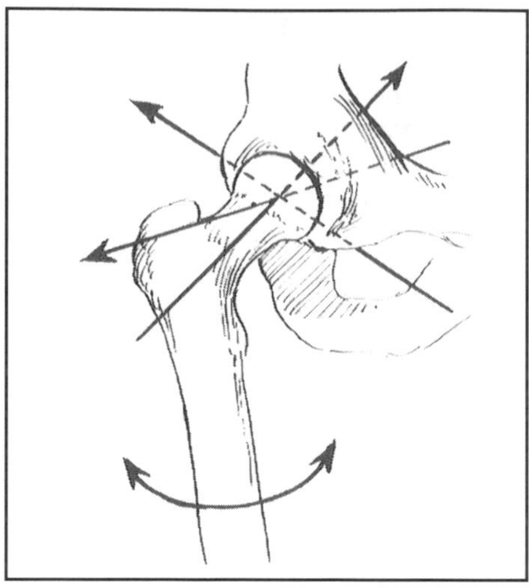

FIGURE *5-12.*
Polyaxial joint: The diagram shows the ball-and-socket joint at the hip; only three of the innumerable axes are shown.

(see Fig. 5-11A). The wrist joint and the metacarpophalangeal joints are shaped in this manner. Movement on the long axis produces **flexion and extension** in one plane, whereas on the short axis, abduction and adduction take place in another plane. **Abduction** is movement away from the median plane and **adduction** is movement toward it.

In a **saddle joint** (see Fig. 5-11B), the articular surfaces are saddle-shaped as, for example, in the carpometacarpal joint of the thumb. The same movements are possible as in an ellipsoid joint. In the anatomic sense, ellipsoid and saddle joints do not permit independent or active rotation of the bones, but **circumduction,** the harmonious combination of flexion–abduction–extension–adduction, gives the impression of rotation as the bone circumscribes a conical space.

Polyaxial Joints. Movement is possible around innumerable axes, exemplified by ball-and-socket joint. In a **ball-and-socket** joint (Fig. 5-12), the articular surfaces are reciprocal segments of a hypothetical sphere, for example, as in the shoulder and hip joints. All the types of movements described so far are possible at a ball-and-socket joint, including rotation and circumduction.

Mechanics of Movement

The foregoing consideration of movements, though helpful, does not reflect the true behavior of joint surfaces. More accurate concepts in the mechanics of joint movement are useful in understanding such complex joints as the shoulder, hip, and knee. The following discussion anticipates the analysis of movement at these joints, and their movements are dealt with in the appropriate chapters.

Nature of Articular Surfaces. As already implied, articular surfaces are geometrically imperfect, and in all varieties of synovial joints, including plane joints, the surfaces are composites of several convex or concave ovoids. In most joints, convex or male ovoid surfaces articulate with concave or female ovoids, and there is considerable disparity in size and curvature between the male and female surfaces in any given joint. In other joints, each surface is composed of ovoids convex in one plane and concave in the other (sellar or saddle-shaped surfaces), and the larger of these is considered the male. In all but one position of a joint, contact between the surfaces is restricted to a small area only, which is due to the incongruity of the mating pair. The male ovoid, as a rule, has a smaller radius than the female. This arrangement is decidedly unstable and greatly enhances the tendency for movement. Movement is further facilitated by the lubricating properties of synovial fluid that fills the wedge-shaped spaces between the divergent surfaces around the restricted area of contact.

Basic Types of Movement. All the types of movements discussed in the previous section are the outcome of three basic displacements. These displacements are: a **spin,** a **roll,** and a **slide.** The definitions of these movements are explicit in Figure 5-13. It should be evident that in view of the unstable relation between the articular surfaces, and because of the composite nature of forces that act on the bones, pure spins and pure rolls are rather un-

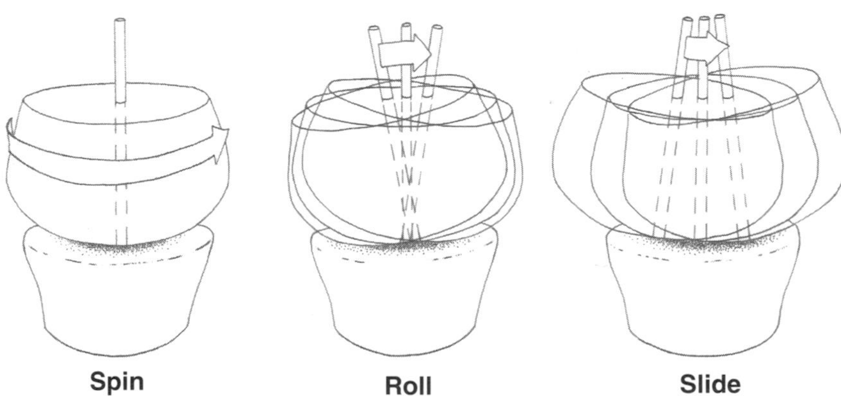

FIGURE *5-13.*
The three basic types of movement possible between a pair of male and female articular surfaces in a synovial joint: In the example illustrated, the male surface moves over a stationary female surface. A moving female surface on a stationary male surface would be likewise free to *spin, roll,* or *slide.* Usually these movements occur in combinations. (Redrawn from Williams PL, Warwick R, Dyson M, Bannister LH eds. Gray's anatomy. 37th ed. New York: Churchill Livingstone 1989.)

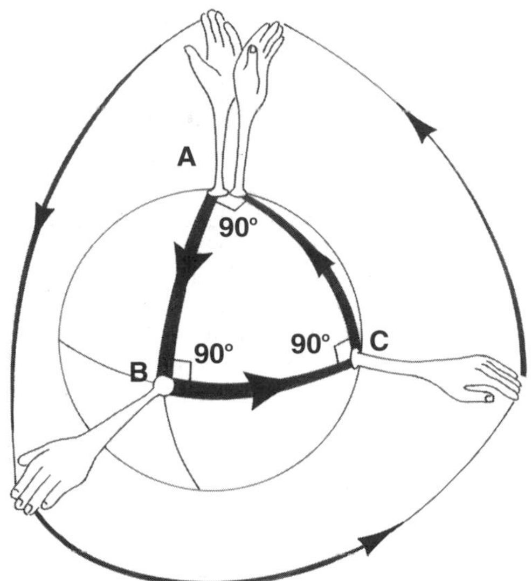

FIGURE 5-14.
Graphic explanation of the spin or *conjunct rotation* that accompanies a succession of slides occurring between two reciprocally curved articular surfaces. A model arm carrying a hand is moved on the surface of a sphere from point A → B → C → A along the shortest possible paths connecting the consecutive points (i.e., along chords). It is clear from the position of the thumb and the plane of the palm that the succession of slides results in 90° rotation of the arm by the time it is returned to position *A*. In this instance each angle of the triangle enclosed by chords *AB*, *BC*, and *CA* measures 90°, giving a total of 270; that is more than 180° because the triangle is on a convex, rather than flat surface. The amount of conjunct rotation or spin is always equal to the sum of the three angles minus 180° namely, 270° = 180° = 90°. For further explanation see text. (Redrawn from Williams PL, Warwick R, Dyson M, Bannister LH, eds. Gray's anatomy. 37th ed. New York: Churchill Livingstone, 1989.)

usual events. As a rule, spins and rolls of a bone in all varieties of joints are accompanied by sliding. At the same time, it must be appreciated, although it is not intuitively obvious, that when a bone is moved on a curved surface by a succession of slides the paths of which make angles with one another, the bone will inevitably undergo a spin. In other words, using anatomic terminology, the bone will be rotated even though an active force required for independent rotation (for pure spin, that is) has not been called into operation. The geometric and mathematic proof of this will not be developed here, but this principle of **conjunct rotation** should become comprehensible with reference to Figure 5-14 and to the description of shoulder abduction discussed in Chapter 15.

Loose Pack and Close Pack Positions. The joint is said to be in **loose pack** when the movements described in the foregoing are permitted. The contact of articular surfaces is assured by atmospheric pressure, surface tension of synovial fluid, and by the tone of the muscles that surround the joint, whereas the joint capsule and ligaments are relatively loose. In loose pack it is possible to distract the surfaces, and it is in these positions that the joint is most prone to dislocation. A position can be reached, however, in all joints where, instead of a limited area, there is extensive contact between the articular surfaces with maximal congruence of their male and female surfaces. Such a situation obtains at one extreme of habitual movements (abduction of the shoulder, extension of the hip, knee, and interphalangeal joints), and the joint is then said to be in **close pack.**

In most joints, the position of close pack is attained by conjunct rotation during the final phase of a slide. This slide may or may not be accompanied by rolling. Because of the twist imparted by this rotation, the capsule and ligaments become maximally spiraled and taut. As a consequence, the articular surfaces will be tightly compressed and cannot be distracted; the two bones in essence become one. Further movement owing to muscle contraction is reflexly inhibited by the activation of mechanoreceptors in the stretched capsule and ligaments. In close pack, the joint is "locked" or "screwed home," and it has to be unlocked or unscrewed by a force vector that reverses the conjunct rotation before the joint can return into loose pack. In close pack the joint is least susceptible to dislocation; however, when excessive force is applied, the joint surfaces are particularly prone to trauma, and the capsule and ligaments to tearing.

From a functional point of view, the close pack position is especially important in those joints that transmit the weight of the body in the standing position. Close pack furnishes stability to these joints with the minimum expenditure of muscular energy. At the hip, knee, and ankle, attainment of close pack is assisted by the force of gravity (see Chap. 17 and 18).

Factors of Joint Stability

There are three main factors that provide stability to a joint: 1) the shape of the articular surfaces, 2) ligaments (including the capsule), and 3) muscles.

The relative importance of these factors varies in different joints. For instance, stability in the hip joint is provided mainly by the deep bony socket into which the head of the femur fits. In the shoulder joint the socket is shallow and, therefore, muscles are the most important factor in joint stability. On the other hand, the knee in the standing position relies primarily on its ligaments for stability. In the treatment of joint injuries the relative importance of these three factors must be considered for each joint.

Atmospheric pressure and surface tension of synovial fluid also contribute significantly to the maintenance of joint stability, especially in loose pack positions. Their importance may be readily demonstrated by the common phenomenon of knuckle cracking. The relaxed, extended middle finger may normally be moved through at least 30° of abduction and adduction at the metacarpophalangeal joint, thus demonstrating that the joint is in loose pack and its ligaments are not taut. The joint, however, cannot be distracted until the traction reaches about a 10-kg force, when the joint cracks. At that time the articular surfaces suddenly separate and a small bubble of gas appears within the joint cavity, which may be demonstrated radiographically. In this phenomenon, the distraction force acting across the joint is opposed both by atmospheric pressure and by the surface tension of the synovial fluid. The latter acts as an adhesive to maintain the apposition of the articulating surfaces. When these forces are overcome, the intraarticular pressure falls suddenly to a level so far below atmospheric pressure that gas is released from the water phase and an audible crack occurs. The instructive message of this example lies in the relatively large force required to distract such a small joint. In larger joints, the stabilizing forces contributed by surface tension and atmospheric pressure must be proportionately greater. However, these forces are exceeded by the forces generated by muscle action, and without ligamentous or muscular support joints cannot perform the functions required of them.

RECOMMENDED READINGS

Barnett CH. Synovial joints: their structure and mechanics. Springfield, IL: Thomas, 1961.

Benjamin M, Evans EJ. Fibrocartilage: a review. J Anat 1990; 171: 1.

Buckwalter JA, Glimcher MJ, Cooper RR, Recker R. Bone biology. Part I: structure, blood supply, cells, matrix, and mineralization. J Bone Joint Surg Am 1995; 77A: 1256.

Buckwalter JA, Glimcher MJ, Cooper RR, Recker R. Bone biology. Part II: formation, form, modeling, remodeling, and regulation of cell function. J Bone Joint Surg Am 1995; 77A: 1276.

Cooper RR, Milgram JW, Robinson RA. Morphology of the osteon: an electron microscopic study. J Bone Joint Surg Am 1966; 48A: 1239.

Fawcett DW. Bone. In: Bloom and Fawcett: a textbook of histology. 12th ed. New York: Chapman & Hall, 1994: 194.

Gardner E. The anatomy of the joints. American Academy of Orthopaedic Surgery, Instructional Course Lectures 1952; 9: 149.

Hancox NM. Biology of bone. Cambridge: Cambridge Univ Press, 1972.

Koch JC. The laws of bone architecture. Am J Anat 1917; 21: 177.

Lawson JP. Clinically significant radiologic anatomic variants of the skeleton. Am J Roentgenol 1995; 163: 249.

Minns RJ, Stevens FS. The collagen fibril organization in human articular cartilage. J Anat 1977; 123: 437.

Noback CR. The developmental anatomy of the human osseous skeleton during the embryonic, fetal and circumnatal periods. Anat Rec 1944; 88: 91.

Norkin CC, Levangie PK. Joint structure and function: a comprehensive analysis. 2nd ed. Philadelphia: F.A. Davis, 1992.

Raisz LG, Kream BE. Hormonal control of skeletal growth. Annu Rev Physiol 1981; 43: 225.

Raisz LG, Kream BE. Regulation of bone formation. N Engl J Med 1983; 309: 29.

Ralphs JR, Benjamin M. The joint capsule: structure, composition, ageing and disease. J Anat 1994; 184: 503.

Rosse C, Clawson DK. The musculoskeletal system in health and disease. Hagerstown: Harper & Row, 1980.

Sokoloff L, editor. The joints and synovial fluid. New York: Academic Press, 1978.

Tavassoli M, Yoffey JM. Bone marrow structure and function. New York: Alan Liss, 1983.

Uhthoff HK. The embryology of the human locomotor system. New York: Springer-Verlag, 1990.

Williams PL, Bannister LH, Berry MM, et al. eds. Gray's anatomy. 38th ed. New York: Churchill Livingstone, 1995.

Wislan NJ, Van Sickle DC. The relationship of cartilage canals to the initial osteogenesis of secondary centers of ossification. Anat Rec 1970; 168: 381.

Zambrano NZ, Montes GS, Shigihara GS, Sanchez KM, Junqueira LC. Collagen arrangement in cartilages. Acta Anat 1982; 113: 26.

Hollinshead's Textbook of Anatomy, by Cornelius Rosse and
Penelope Gaddum-Rosse.
Lippincott-Raven Publishers, Philadelphia, © 1997.

CHAPTER 6

The Muscular System

The muscular system is made of up of all the muscles of the body that are composed of **skeletal muscle,** one of the three types of muscle tissue that exist in the body of vertebrates. The two other types are **cardiac muscle,** confined to the heart, and **smooth muscle,** found predominantly in the walls of blood vessels; in the ducts; in tubes and hollow organs of the digestive, respiratory, urinary, and genital systems; as well as in association with hair follicles (*arrectores pilorum*) in the skin. The fundamental property of all muscle tissue is contractility, and its primary function is to generate mechanical force. Force generated by smooth and cardiac muscle propels or blocks the contents of cavities that the muscle surrounds, whereas force generated by skeletal muscles produces or prevents displacements of bones relative to one another at joints, thereby resulting in movement or stabilization of parts of the body or the body as a whole. Thus, the muscular and skeletal systems are closely integrated, and in many functional contexts, it is useful to think of them together as the *musculoskeletal system*.

The cellular unit of skeletal muscle is the **muscle fiber** (Fig. 6-1), which is a long, multinucleated, cylindrical cell derived during prenatal development from the fusion of many (up to several hundred) myogenic precursor cells. Viewed under the microscope, muscle fibers exhibit striations because of the regular arrangement of *myofilaments* within their cytoplasm (see Fig. 6-1). Therefore, skeletal muscle is sometimes described as *striated muscle.* Striations are also discernible, however, in cardiac muscle. Skeletal muscle tissue is also designated sometimes as *voluntary muscle* because muscles composed of it are innervated by nerve fibers through which voluntary control can be exercised. However, all such muscles contract reflexly (i.e., involuntarily) as often as under volition, and several are difficult to influence voluntarily (e.g., diaphragm). Although there may be reservations about applying the term *skeletal muscle*, it nevertheless seems to be the most appropriate identifier.

In the human, almost half of the body weight is constituted of skeletal muscle tissue. This large tissue mass is divided into several hundred discrete muscles, each of which may be considered a true organ, with a specific function. The function of most individual muscles is to control the movement of specific parts of the skeletal system.

Although some muscles attach to skin and other soft tissues (e.g., the muscles of facial expression, those of the tongue, and the extraocular muscles), most muscles attach to bones by tendons and cross one or more joints. When contraction shortens the muscle, movement is produced at the joint, but when contraction occurs without a change in muscle length, the joint is stabilized and movement by other forces is resisted. In either event, stored chemical energy is converted by the muscle into mechanical energy.

Even when they contract reflexly, skeletal muscles are under the direct control of the somatic or voluntary nervous system. Activation of muscle contraction is achieved by impulses that arise in the central nervous system, proceed along the axons of motor neurons, and are transmitted to the muscle at specialized neuromuscular junctions. Afferent impulses are generated within muscles and tendons by changes in length, tension, and speed of movement, and these impulses are fed back to the central nervous system (see Fig. 7-4). Through the reflex arcs thus established, the voluntary movements are moni-

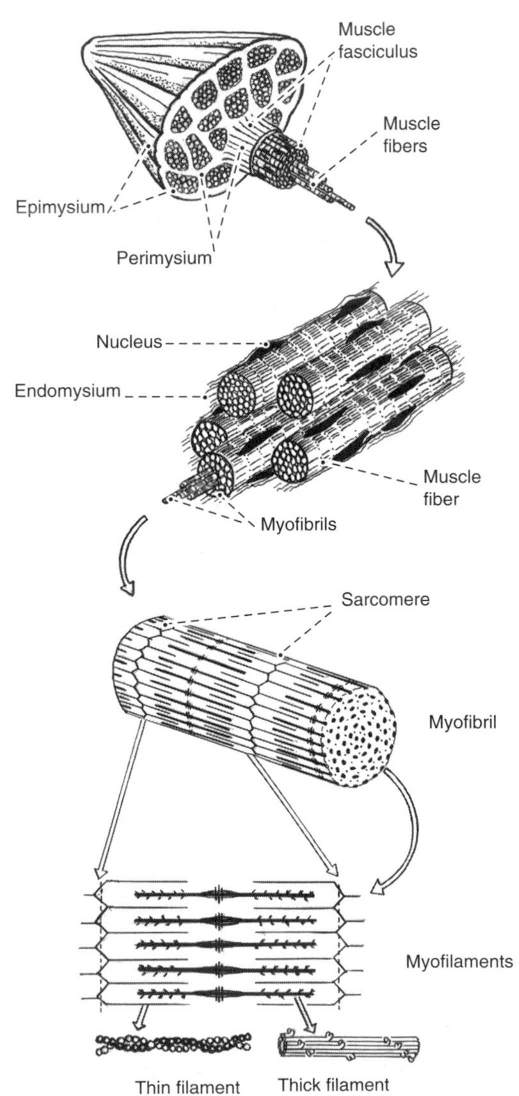

FIGURE *6-1.*
Diagrammatic representation of the organization of skeletal muscle from the gross anatomic to the submicroscopic level. Subunits of a whole muscle are shown with the associated connective tissue elements. (Redrawn from Williams PL, Warwick R, Dyson M, Bannister LH, eds. Gray's anatomy. 37th ed. New York. Churchill Livingstone, 1989.)

tored, and at the same time other muscles that cancel out or prevent unwanted movements are reflexly activated. This chapter deals with the form and structure of muscles as anatomic organs and with the actions they perform in moving parts of the body. The neural control of these actions is discussed with the somatic nervous system in the next chapter (see Chap. 7).

STRUCTURE AND FORM OF MUSCLES

Although some muscles are thin and ribbonlike, some broad and flat, some fan-shaped, and some almost cylindrical with tapering ends, they are all essentially similar in structure. Also, the contractility and the structure of skeletal muscle cells or muscle fibers are similar in all muscles. The forces that different muscles can exert, however, are determined not only by the number and size of these contractile units, but by their three dimensional arrangement within the muscle.

Anatomic Subunits of Muscles

Connective Tissue of Muscles

All muscles are ensheathed by a continuous layer of deep fascia called the **epimysium** (see Fig. 6-1). This connective tissue covering defines the muscle anatomically and facilitates its sliding on surrounding structures. Connective tissue septa extend inward from the muscle's fascia and this **perimysium** subdivides the muscle into macroscopically visible fiber bundles or **fasciculi.** In their finest extensions the septa surround all individual muscle fibers, the cellular units of skeletal muscle, and constitute the **endomysium** (see Fig. 6 1).

This extensive connective tissue stroma subserves three important functions:

1. It largely determines the extent of stretching and deformability in a relaxed muscle, lending it elasticity and a certain degree of stiffness.
2. It constitutes the pathways for nerves, blood vessels, and lymphatics.
3. It transmits the forces generated by the muscle through its tendon to bones and functions as a spring or the *series elastic element.*

The connective tissue of a muscle is largely collagenous, but some elastic fibers occur among the collagen fibers. The endomysium is composed of a delicate network of collagen fibers, usually described as reticular connective tissue. A meshwork of blood capillaries surrounds the individual muscle fibers. Small nerves and individual nerve fibers wind among the muscle fibers and branch to end upon them.

Within a muscle bundle or **fascicle** (*fasciculus*), there may be some muscle fibers that run its entire length. (Fibers as long as 34 cm have been reported, but most muscle fibers in the human are no longer than 10 to 15 cm, and many are much shorter.) Muscle fibers in a fascicle have tapering ends that overlap the tapering ends of neighboring fibers and are bound to them by connective tissue so that several fibers in a row can act as if they were a single fiber. At each end of the muscle, the tapering muscle fibers are affixed to the collagen fibers of the endomysium, forming a complex called the **myotendinal junction.**

Muscle–Tendon Relations

The anchoring of the muscle is accomplished by its connective tissue stroma, which condenses into a tendon at the muscle's site of attachment to bone. At the myotendinal junction, force is transmitted from the muscle fibers to the endomysium, to the tendon, and then to the periosteum and bone. Collagen fibers of the tendon can be traced directly into the bone matrix through the periosteum.

Tendinous tissue is always present at the muscle's attachment to bone, even when macroscopically this attachment appears to be entirely fleshy. On the other hand, in muscles that exert their actions at a distance, the tendon may be longer than the muscle itself.

As noted in Chapter 4, tendons consist of heavy parallel bundles of collagen fibers. However, although the large bundles composing the tendon are parallel to each other, each large bundle is made up of smaller ones that intertwine, so that the muscle fibers' pull on it is spread throughout the whole bundle, rather than being concentrated on individual fibers. Tendons are much stronger than muscles for any given cross-sectional area. The usual ratio is that a tendon can resist at least twice the pull that the muscle can exert on it. In consequence, when a sudden strain is thrown on a muscle, a normal tendon does not rupture. Instead, the muscle itself will rupture across its belly or at the myotendinous junction. Alternatively, the tendon may come loose at its insertion, often pulling out with it a fragment of the bone to which it is attached. Although tendons can rupture through their middle, especially about the shoulder, this seems to be a result of previous pathologic degeneration in the tendon.

The Motor Unit

Each muscle fiber is innervated by one of the terminal branches of an axon. The collection of muscle fibers supplied by the terminal branches of one axon derived from a motor neuron located in the spinal cord or the brain is called a **motor unit.** The motor unit is the unit of contraction in skeletal muscle, and when the motor neuron fires, all muscle fibers in the motor unit contract synchronously. Several motor units are included in a muscle fasciculus and these units are activated in turn during normal muscle action.

The size of the motor unit is determined by the number of muscle fibers innervated by a single motor neuron. Motor unit size is large (several hundred muscle fibers per nerve cell) in the large lower limb muscles, and small (fewer than ten muscle fibers) in muscles concerned with fine movements, such as those of the eye. Powerful muscles have a coarse texture owing to large muscle fasciculi, whereas in muscles concerned with precise movements, the fasciculi are fine.

Under the usual conditions of moving a part or maintaining a position, contraction is automatically rotated among various motor units so that fatigue is minimal; however, the more powerful the movement demanded, the more motor units must be engaged. It is by this mechanism of recruiting more and more motor units that the strength of a movement can be varied voluntarily, although the precise mechanisms employed by the central nervous system to do this are not understood. Because we can use different motor units, we can also voluntarily contract only a specific part of a muscle. This becomes particularly important when a single muscle has two opposing actions, as does, for instance, the deltoid muscle that covers the tip of the shoulder. The anterior part of this muscle can help in flexing the arm, the posterior part in extending the arm. By choosing which movement we want, we automatically activate the nerve circuit that causes contraction of either the anterior or posterior part of the deltoid.

Arrangement of Muscle Fasciculi

The overall size and shape of a muscle and the arrangement of its fasciculi are adapted to the range of movement and strength required at the joint it serves. The range of effective movement is dependent on the length of the muscle fibers. Because muscle fibers can shorten to approximately half their length, long muscles produce a greater range of movement than short ones. This direct relation holds true only if the fasciculi are more or less parallel to the muscle's line of pull, as in so-called **strap muscles** (e.g., rectus abdominis; see Fig. 23-6), or in **fusiform muscles** (e.g., biceps brachii; see Fig. 16-11). When the fasciculi are oblique to the line of pull, represented usually by the tendon of insertion, only a proportion of the force generated is effective in producing movement. However, this arrangement lends itself to increasing the number of muscle fibers without unduly increasing the muscle's diameter or bulk.

Oblique muscle fiber arrangements include forms that resemble a triangle, a half or complete feather form (**unipennate** and **bipennate,** respectively), and composite or **multipennate** forms, for which several tendons receive the obliquely arranged fasciculi. The loss of efficiency in force transmission to the tendon is outweighed in practice by the large number of short fibers of which such muscles are composed. Powerful movements of limited range are executed, as a rule, by muscles composed of obliquely set fibers. Some muscles are twisted or spiralized. Their contraction untwists them, usually resulting in rotation of the bone that they move.

The actual range and type of movement produced by a muscle is modified by factors independent of the muscle's architecture. These factors include 1) the shape of articular surfaces at the joint served by the muscle, 2) leverage, and 3) the action of stabilizing synergistic and antagonistic muscles, described in the next section.

THE ACTIONS OF MUSCLES

Some skeletal muscles move parts of the face, the lips, and the eyelids, and others function as sphincters, closing and opening orifices. Yet others compress the abdominopelvic cavity by pulling on sheetlike tendons as their fibers shorten (diaphragm; see Fig. 25-3), or on an intermuscular ligament or raphe (levator ani; see Fig. 27-4). However, most muscles move bones or cartilages when they contract. This section is concerned with the actions that muscles exert through their attachment to bones or cartilage.

The **action** of a muscle is the effect of its contraction, which is usually stated in terms of the flexion, extension, or other movement of a part. In most instances, the type of movement a muscle can produce by its contraction can be readily deduced from its anatomy. The factors to be considered include the type of joint that the muscle crosses, the axes around which movement can occur at the joint, and the anatomic relations of the muscle's line of pull relative to the joint axes. For instance, both the biceps and triceps muscles cross the elbow joint, which functions as a hinge (see Fig. 5-10A). The line of pull exerted by the biceps is anterior to the joint axis; therefore, the biceps flexes the elbow, whereas the triceps extends it because its line of pull falls posterior to the joint axis. This deduction is reached from taking into account the muscle's attachments, the location of its tendon in relation to the joint axis, and the anatomy of the joint itself.

In many instances, however, because of the more complex fascicular structure of the muscle and the multiple axes around which movement may occur at the joint, such reasoning can lead to simplistic or even erroneous conclusions. The actions that muscles exert, therefore, must be investigated by several methods. This may be done by physical examination. Palpation of a contracting muscle or its tendon during a particular movement can confirm the muscle's participation in that movement. Likewise, testing the muscle's strength, while the movement it produces is opposed by an examiner, is a valuable and informative clinical method. Both these methods, however, are also prone to errors of interpretation when several muscles participate in producing the movement that is being tested.

Individual muscles can be stimulated by electric current applied to them through an electrode placed on the overlying skin or inserted into the muscle. The resulting movement can be observed and the muscle's action deduced. The electrical activity of a muscle can also be recorded through needle electrodes while the muscle is contracting as it participates in a particular movement. This latter technique of *electromyography* can yield detailed and reliable information, and it is in clinical use for assessing the integrity of muscles and of the nerves that supply them. Nevertheless, electromyography will not reveal the precise role the muscle has in the movement. Is the muscle primarily responsible for the movement, or does it cancel out unwanted action by other muscles that also cross the joint? To answer such questions, attention must be paid to the precise attachment of muscles and to the types of actions they can exert at a particular joint.

Fixed and Moving Points of Muscle Attachment

Movement of one bone in relation to another takes place at a synovial joint, and it is produced actively by the isotonic contraction of muscles that cross the joint. As the contracting muscle shortens, it approximates one of its sites of attachment to the other one. When the muscle is twisted or spiralized, its shortening also brings the line of its insertion into one and the same plane with the line of its other attachment, imparting a spin to the moving bone. The attachment site that remains fixed during a movement is considered the **origin,** whereas the attachment site that describes an arc in a given movement, whether or not there is an element of spin, is considered the muscle's **insertion.**

The fixed and moving points may be reversed in some instances, owing to the stabilizing action of a different set of muscles, or to external forces. For instance, the *usual* action of the pectoralis major is to adduct the arm against the rib cage. In this movement the muscle's attachment to the sternum and the ribs represents its origin, and its attachment to the humerus its insertion. However, when a patient in respiratory distress leans on both elbows, the two humeri become stabilized, serving now as the site of origin for the pectoralis major muscles; the contracting muscles will now lift the ribs, assisting in respiratory movements by expanding the rib cage. In this instance, origin and insertion have been reversed. This principle is important when normal and deranged movements are analyzed. However, in anatomic terminology, the attachment site that remains fixed during a muscle's *usual* or *habitual* action is spoken of as its origin, and the attachment site that moves under the same circumstances is considered its insertion. Accordingly, the pectoralis major is said to originate on the sternum and ribs and insert on the humerus.

Prime Movers and Antagonists

Many muscles cross more than one joint. When such a muscle contracts, movement will occur at all the joints crossed by the muscle or its tendon. At each joint the resulting movement depends on the shape of the articular surfaces and on the relation of the muscle's line of pull to the axes of the joints. To produce the desired result, movement at some of the joints may have to be prevented. Therefore, when a movement is carried out, a combination of muscles is called into action. The muscle or muscles in this combination responsible for initiating and maintaining the desired movement are known as the **prime movers.** The muscle or muscles capable of directly opposing this movement, or initiating the converse movement, are known as the **antagonists.** For instance, if flexion of the fingers (interphalangeal joints) is desired, the prime movers will be the flexor digitorum superficialis and flexor digitorum profundus muscles, and the antagonists, the digital extensors (extensor digitorum and interossei; see Fig. 16-20).

It has been established by electromyography that the antagonists remain inactive while the prime movers do their work, and the resistance offered by the antagonists to prime mover force is due to their viscosity and elasticity. The relaxed antagonists are stretched by the contracting prime movers and, during the active phase of the movement, contraction of the antagonists in response to the stretch is reflexly inhibited.

Gravity as the Prime Moving Force

When the prime moving force is generated not by muscle action, but by **gravity,** the movement will be controlled paradoxically by muscles capable of producing the converse movement, that is, by the antagonists. For instance, if the forearm resting on the elbow is allowed to fall passively to the table, the prime moving force responsible for this elbow extension is provided by gravity. Control over this movement is exerted by the antagonists, that is, by the elbow flexors. The weight of the forearm subjects the elbow flexors to a sustained stretch, in response to which tension is generated in these muscles. Under voluntary control the flexors will elongate while contracting, the elbow will extend, and the forearm will come to the table at the desired rate.

This mechanism is particularly important in the maintenance of upright posture. All antigravity muscles function in response to the stretches to which they are subjected by the force of gravity. Gravity must be taken into consideration in the clinical assessment of all normal and abnormal movements.

Stabilizers and Synergists

The site of a muscle's origin has to be immobilized; in the limbs, which consist of a series of joints, this is accomplished, as a rule, by muscle action. Prime movers and antagonists contract in unison functioning as **fixation** or **stabilizer muscles.** For instance, during push-ups the scapula and the shoulder joint are stabilized by the contraction of surrounding muscles to provide a firm base for the contracting elbow flexors and extensors, which work against gravity at a controlled rate. The stabilizers are called into action as part of the total movement, without any specific command.

Not only does the muscle's origin need to be stabilized, but the unwanted components of its action have to be cancelled out if the muscle crosses more than one joint, or if its unrestrained pull produces more than one type of movement at a single joint. The elimination of unwanted movements is done by **synergists.** As their name implies, synergists assist the prime movers in exerting an action in such a manner that, by working together, a movement is produced that neither muscle could bring about by itself. The example of finger fiexors, quoted previously, illustrates the principle. The digital flexors originate in the forearm, and when they contract, flexion of the wrist as well as of the interphalangeal joints will occur, unless wrist movement is eliminated by synergists. Extensor muscles of the wrist contract reflexly when finger flexion is attempted, and the wrist will be noticeably extended to facilitate a powerful grip by the flexing fingers.

Spurt and Shunt Action of Muscles

The force generated by prime mover contraction can be resolved into two vectors (Fig. 6-2). One vector acts *across* the moving bone and causes the point of insertion to swing through an arc, whereas the other vector, acting *along* the moving bone, forces the two articulating bones against each other. The two force components have been called the **spurt** and **shunt action** of a muscle, respectively. If a muscle originates far from a joint and inserts near it, its pull across the moving bone will be greater than along it, and such a muscle is considered a **spurt muscle.** On the other hand, if a muscle originates close to a joint and inserts far from it, its pull along the moving bone will be greater than across it, and such a muscle is considered a **shunt muscle.** Among flexors of the elbow, for example, the brachialis and biceps are spurt muscles, whereas the brachioradialis is a shunt muscle.

The importance of spurt muscles is self-evident, and they are primarily recruited to execute the desired movement. The need for shunt muscles can be appreciated by considering that 1) spurt muscles impart a centrifugal force to the bone that moves on a curved articular surface, causing it to tend to fly off at a tangent to the articular surface, and 2) spurt muscles may move the bone into such a position that their force vector acting along the bone will tend to dislocate the joint (see Fig. 6-2). The brachioradialis, functioning as a shunt muscle at the elbow, can be expected to be active during rapid movements whatever the direction of the swing. It has, indeed, been confirmed by electromyography that the muscle contracts during rapid elbow flexion and extension. Thus, during movement, the shunt action of muscles contributes to maintaining joint integrity. In those positions of the joint where the ligaments are lax, shunt muscles guard against dislocation.

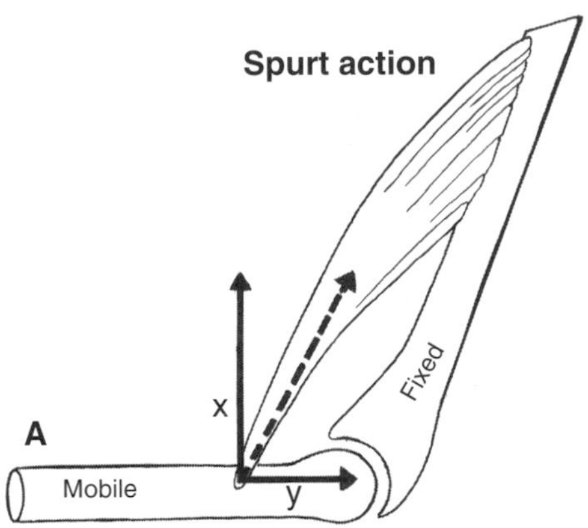

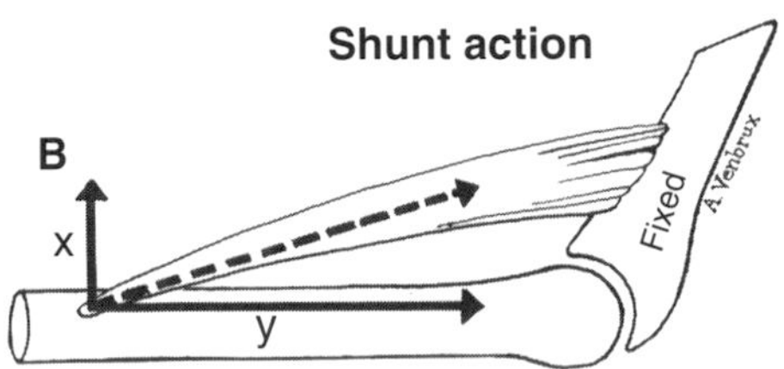

FIGURE 6-2.
Spurt and shunt action of muscles: The force generated by contraction of the muscle (*dashed arrow*) can be broken down into two vectors, *x* and *y*. *Spurt action* is due to vector *x* acting across the mobile bone, whereas *shunt action* is due to vector *y* acting along the mobile bone. The muscle shown in panel A is a spurt muscle ($x > y$), the muscle in panel B is a shunt muscle ($y > x$). (Modified from Williams PL, Warwick R, Dyson M, Bannister LH, eds. Gray's anatomy. 37th ed. New York: Churchill Livingstone, 1989.)

Versatility of Muscle Action

It will be appreciated that a single muscle can act in a variety of ways. As a prime mover, a muscle may flex one joint and extend another, as the hamstrings, for instance, flex the knee and extend the hip. In converse movements the same muscle functions as an antagonist, and in other circumstances it will participate in a movement as a fixator or synergist. The same muscle may function as a spurt or shunt muscle at the same joint, depending on which of its attachments is stabilized to serve as its origin. With the foot off the ground, the hamstrings flex the knee by their spurt action, acting at the same time as shunt extensors at the hip. On the other hand, when a foot is planted, the same muscles become shunt flexors at the knee and spurt extensors at the hip. In some instances, a muscle contracts isometrically; in others, isotonically. In the latter, it may shorten or lengthen as it counteracts the load.

For a muscle to perform in such a versatile way it must be endowed with a sophisticated sensory apparatus and with mechanisms for feedback to the motor neurons and to higher centers of coordination to be able to contribute appropriately to the execution of a voluntary act.

INNERVATION AND BLOOD SUPPLY

Nerves and blood vessels enter a muscle at one or two well-defined points (neurovascular hila) by piercing the muscle's fascia and then arborizing in the perimysium and endomysium. The capillaries embedded in endomysium surround individual muscle fibers, and the terminal branching of nerve fibers also takes place in this tissue.

Motor and Sensory Innervation

Muscles are supplied by branches of nerves that invariably contain nerve fibers that stimulate the muscle to contract, as well as sensory nerve fibers that relay information from the muscle to the central nervous system (see Figs. 7-4 and 7-5).

Peripheral Innervation

The innervation of a muscle is not haphazard, with the muscle receiving nerve fibers from any nerve in its neighborhood; rather, it is fixed early in development. It is easy to see, in the course of a series of dissections, that a muscle tends to be innervated constantly by branches from a certain major nerve, regardless of which other nerves may be close by. For instance, either of the two major nerves on the anterior side of the forearm could supply all the muscles there, yet each supplies only certain muscles. Furthermore, although the two nerves are of approximately equal size, one supplies almost all the muscles and the other supplies only a few.

Only a small number of muscles are regularly innervated by two named nerves, rather than one, or sometimes by one nerve and sometimes by another. Some muscles, however, particularly those of the hand, may receive a truly anomalous innervation; that is, an innervation from a nerve that normally does not supply them. Such a situation sometimes arises when two nerves originate and run close together: nerve fibers may grow down the connective tissue sheath of the wrong nerve.

Segmental Innervation

Only a few muscles in the trunk retain a truly segmental arrangement corresponding to the original segments of the body. These extend from one vertebra to the next or one rib to the next. As expected, each of these muscles is supplied by the single spinal nerve belonging to the corresponding segment of the spinal cord.

Other muscles (the larger muscles of the back and the abdominal muscles) extend over several vertebral segments and, therefore, lie on level with several the segmental spinal nerves. As expected, these muscles are supplied by branches of a series of spinal nerves. In general, a muscle is innervated by the nerves of the segments over which it extends, and the longer the muscle, the more extensive its segmental nerve supply.

Thus, the muscles of the trunk are innervated by the segmental spinal nerve or nerves associated with the segment (or segments) from which the muscle arose. As explained in Chapter 14, although such segmentation is not evident in the limbs and their muscles, a segmental pattern of spinal nerve distribution can be defined to limb muscles as well.

Distribution of Nerves Within Muscles

The distribution of a nerve within a muscle typically follows a fixed pattern: the nerve branches and rebranches in the connective tissue of the muscle, and the branches follow such courses as to bring them into contact with all the muscle fibers within a muscle. The pattern of distribution of a nerve within a muscle, therefore, partly depends on the shape of the muscle. For instance, in a long, fusiform muscle, the major nerve branches run longitudinally with the muscle bundles to reach all of them, whereas in a short, wide muscle, the branches run transverse to the muscle fibers, only the smaller ones becoming longitudinal to reach muscle fibers at the ends of the muscle.

Motor Fibers

Every individual muscle fiber eventually receives input from a nerve fiber, for skeletal muscle contracts only when it is stimulated to do so by means of nerve impulses reaching it. The nerve fiber forms, with the substance of the muscle, a structure known as the **neuromuscular junction,** at which the impulses delivered by the nerve are transformed into the trigger mechanism that induces contraction of the muscle fiber. Acetylcholine, released by the nerve fiber, is an essential part of this mechanism; therefore, nerve fibers to skeletal muscle are known as **cholinergic fibers.** Substances that interfere with the action of acetylcholine necessarily produce paralysis (lack of contraction) of the muscle. This is the basis on which curare, the South American poison, has been adapted to clinical use and employed when complete quiescence of muscle is desired, as during some surgical procedures.

Not all the nerve fibers entering a voluntary muscle are motor ones destined for the muscle fibers. Some are derived from the sympathetic system and innervate blood vessels, although these are markedly smaller in diameter than are the motor fibers to the muscle itself.

Sensory Fibers

In addition to motor or efferent fibers, a nerve to a muscle also contains a large proportion of afferent, or sensory fibers, constituting as much as 40% to 50% of the total number of fibers in the nerve. Therefore, it is incorrect to consider a nerve to skeletal muscle as being a purely motor nerve.

Some of the afferent fibers have to do with the reception of stimuli that give rise to the sensation of pain. Others end in the muscle and its tendons and form endings that are stimulated by the contraction of, or the passive tension on, the muscle and tendon. These endings, being activated by happenings in their immediate environment, rather than by stimuli from the outside, are among the types known as **proprioceptive endings.** The best known example is the **muscle spindle,** a collection of specialized, slender muscle fibers enclosed within a delicate connective tissue sheath. Afferent nerve fibers are intertwined among the muscle fibers of the spindle. Proprioceptive endings and fibers in muscle are probably not concerned with conscious appreciation of movement of a part, but rather with reflexes that help maintain the desired or necessary degree of contraction (tone) in a muscle. If, for instance, the sensory roots of the nerves contributing to a given muscle are cut, not only are the obvious muscle reflexes lost (e.g., knee jerk), but the resting muscle also undergoes a diminution in tone (the relatively small amount of contraction demonstrable in muscles that are not completely relaxed). Similarly, deafferentation of an entire limb leads to clumsy and poorly coordinated movements of that limb, which cannot be attributed entirely to loss of conscious sensation in the limb; instead, they seem to be due to incoordination among the muscles as a result of the lack of information delivered to the central nervous system concerning the state of contraction of the various muscles. Other receptors, particularly those associated with tendons, do provide information that informs us of the position of our limbs and the posture of our joints.

Denervation, Degeneration, and Regeneration. When the nerve to a muscle is interrupted, the muscle not only ceases to contract, but the muscle fibers composing it begin to degenerate. This is a slow process in which the muscle fibers gradually become smaller and are eventually largely replaced by connective tissue. Because it is partly brought on by the lack of contraction of the muscle, electrical stimulation and massage of the muscle are valuable in increasing the blood supply and slowing the degeneration of a denervated muscle. It is generally agreed that the process of degeneration in a muscle as a result of denervation is largely reversible for a period of at least 12 months; if nerve fibers succeed in reaching the muscle fibers within this time, the muscle can begin to function again and will eventually recover most of its former structure and strength. For a time, the amount of recovery in a denervated muscle probably depends more on the condition of the nerve than on the extent of degeneration of the muscle fibers. However, a permanently denervated muscle is eventually transformed into a fibrous mass in which no muscle fibers are evident.

It is often stated that skeletal muscle does not regenerate. This erroneous belief comes from clinical studies of muscle injuries in which the scar tissue formed was very extensive and seriously limited any possibility of proliferation by cells other than fibroblasts. It has been known for many years that skeletal muscle does regenerate under experimental conditions (limb amputations in amphibia, crush and cold injuries in mammals), some of which mimic quite closely the types of injuries seen in clinical practice. Presumably, if scar tissue formation could be controlled, some regeneration of muscle could also be anticipated in human muscle.

It has now been established that some primitive mesenchymal cells, known as **satellite cells,** persist in skeletal muscle and retain their potential for generating muscle cells. Following injury, these reserve muscle precursors respond to specific regulatory molecules by dividing and giving rise to new myoblasts, which then fuse to form muscle fibers. Experiments using cell-labeling techniques in vivo espouse the idea that satellite cells are indeed reserve cells for muscle regeneration.

Blood Supply

As a general rule, an artery and one or two veins accompany the nerve into the muscle, and their larger branches accompany the nerve branches in the connective tissue within the muscle. However, blood vessels do not have the early and permanent connection with developing muscle that nerves do, and muscles that spread over a considerable distance or area frequently gain additional blood supply from blood vessels in several areas. Thus, the blood supply of a muscle is not as specific as its nerve supply; nevertheless each muscle typically has its characteristic pattern of blood supply. A general rule is that the one or several blood vessels that should supply the muscle, because of the close spatial relations between it and the vessels, usually do so.

Muscular tissue depends on its blood supply to deliver the oxygen and glucose necessary for its contraction and to dispose of its metabolic wastes. Death of the muscle results from interruption of its blood supply. Any drastic lowering of the blood supply, even if insufficient to bring about death of the muscle fibers, interferes with the action of the muscle. Clinically, muscle ischemia (reduced blood supply) is marked by pain in the muscles and easy fatigability and, hence, by rapid loss of the strength of contraction. Ischemia may be chronic, resulting from permanent narrowing of the vessel supplying the muscle or muscle group, or it may be intermittent or spasmodic, appearing and disappearing with the activity and rest of the muscle, which demand increased and reduced amount of blood flowing through the muscle, respectively.

Whatever the pattern of distribution of the blood vessels to and within a voluntary muscle, the capillaries uniting the arteries and veins are so arranged among the muscle fibers that each fiber is in intimate contact with one or more capillaries. Muscle is highly vascular, and much oozing of blood can be expected to occur at the cut surface of a living muscle, even when no blood vessel of appreciable size is severed by the cut.

Tendon, in contrast to muscle tissue, has a sparse blood supply consonant with its low metabolic activity. The vessels of tendons are typically continued into them from the muscle substance, but long tendons receive additional twigs from vessels in their vicinity as well as close to their termination.

To what degree changes in the blood supply of a tendon contribute to pathologic weakening of the tendon is unknown, but blood supply is of particular importance in the healing of a severed tendon. The increased metabolic processes associated with healing demand an adequate blood supply, and tendons that have such a supply heal more quickly, and generally with better end results, than tendons that must depend on particularly long vessels to supply them.

NAMING OF MUSCLES

The attributes by which muscles are named include their shapes and sizes, as well as their positions, attachments, and actions. The trapezius, rhomboid, and deltoid muscles (of the shoulder) are named from their shapes; the latissimus dorsi is named from its size and position (broadest muscle of the back); the interossei of the hand and foot attain their names because of their positions between bones of the hand and foot; and the supraspinatus and infraspinatus are named from their positions above and below the spine of the scapula, respectively. The biceps brachii and the quadriceps femoris are named in accordance with their shape and position: the biceps brachii has two heads of origin and lies in the arm, and the quadriceps femoris has four heads of origin and lies in the thigh. The coracobrachialis is named from its attachments to the coracoid process and the arm (brachium). The levator scapulae and supinator muscles are named from their actions, lifting the scapula and supinating the forearm, respectively. The two pronator muscles of the forearm are named according to a combination of their actions and shapes: the pronator teres is a rounded muscle that pronates, and the pronator quadratus is a quadrilateral one that pronates. The flexor digitorum superficialis and flexor digitorum profundus are named from their actions and positions, both being flexors of the fingers, but one lying superficial and the other deep. Thus, for the most part, the names of muscles are descriptive of some particular feature of the muscle. The student will find it advantageous to attempt to understand why a muscle is named as it is, because such an understanding will minimize what would otherwise be a task of rote memory.

RECOMMENDED READINGS

Basmajian JV, DeLuca CJ. Muscle interactions. In: Muscles alive: their functions revealed by electromyography. 5th ed. Baltimore: Williams & Wilkins, 1985.

Cooper S, Daniel PM. Muscle spindles in man: their morphology in lumbricals and the deep muscles of the neck. Brain 1963; 86: 563.

Cronkite AE. The tensile strength of human tendons. Anat Rec 1936; 64: 173.

Desaki J, Uehara Y. The overall morphology of neuromuscular junctions as revealed by scanning electron microscopy. J Neurocytol 1981; 10: 101.

Edwards DAW. The blood supply and lymphatic drainage of tendons. J Anat 1946; 80: 147.

Fawcett DW. Muscular tissue. In: Bloom and Fawcett: a textbook of histology. 12th ed. New York: Chapman & Hall, 1994: 260.

Goss CM. The attachment of skeletal muscle fibers. Am J Anat 1944; 7: 259.

Huber GC. On the form and arrangement in fasciculi of striated voluntary muscle fibers. Anat Rec 1916; 11: 149.

Lockhard, RD. Anatomy of muscles and their relation to movement and posture. In: Bourne GH, ed. The structure and function of muscle. Vol 1 (Pt 1). 2nd ed. New York: Academic Press, 1972: 1.

MacConaill MA. The movements of bones and joints. 2. Function of the musculature. J Bone Joint Surg Br 1949; 31B: 100.

MacConaill MA, Basmajian JV. Muscles and movements: a basis for human kinesiology. Baltimore: Williams & Wilkins, 1969.

Patton NJ, Mortensen OA. An electromyographic study of reciprocal activity of muscles. Anat Rec 1971; 170: 255.

Rosse C, Clawson DK. The musculoskeletal system in health and disease. Hagerstown: Harper & Row, 1980.

Uhthoff HK. The embryology of the human locomotor system. New York: Springer-Verlag, 1990.

Hollinshead's Textbook of Anatomy, by Cornelius Rosse and Penelope Gaddum-Rosse.
Lippincott-Raven Publishers, Philadelphia, © 1997.

CHAPTER 7

The Nervous System

The nervous system of vertebrates consists of the brain, the spinal cord, and the nerves that issue from those organs and pervade all parts of the body. Although a detailed discussion of the structure and function of the nervous system is beyond the scope of this book, a general understanding of these topics is necessary to fully appreciate the gross anatomy of the system.

THE NEURON

The anatomic unit of the nervous system is the nerve cell or **neuron.** Although neurons vary widely in both shape and size, each has a region known as the *cell body* where the nucleus is located; in addition, there are usually several processes extending away from the cell body, one of which is the *axon* and the remainder, the *dendrites.*

Dendrites (from *dendron,* meaning tree) are characterized structurally by a branching, treelike form. In most instances their function seems to be to increase the surface area available for the reception of signals from other neurons. As such, their surfaces are usually covered by the specialized endings of other neurons, the points of contact being known as *synapses.*

In contrast to the dendrites, the **axon** (one per neuron) is relatively unbranched over most of its length. Usually, however, it branches repeatedly close to its termination. In typical neurons its function is to conduct impulses away from the cell body and transmit signals to other cells. Whereas some axons are relatively short, others may be very long and, therefore, capable of conducting impulses over large distances. In some motor neurons, for example, the axon may be up to 1 m in length. Almost all information concerning the conduction of nerve impulses has been derived from the study of axons, and the term *nerve fibers* refers to axons, not dendrites.

Basically, neurons simply link a **receptor** and an **effector,** but only in certain primitive invertebrates does a single nerve cell form such a direct link. In higher animals, neurons are linked into chains or units of varying complexity, so that even the simplest reaction resulting from a stimulus must be mediated through two or more neurons, and most reactions involve great numbers of such cells. Some neurons are in the direct line of transmission from receptor organ to effector organ, but others are parts of circuits that interlock with this direct line of transmission and, through their activity, vary the response resulting from the stimulus.

Some Basic Groupings of Neurons

There are relatively few tissues into which nerve fibers do not penetrate. Nerve cell bodies, by contrast, are not scattered at random through all tissues. The greatest accumulation of cell bodies, as well as of nerve fibers, is represented by the brain and spinal cord, together known as the **central nervous system;** nerve fibers and cell bodies outside the brain and spinal cord constitute the **peripheral nervous system.** In the latter system, nerve fibers may convey impulses either toward, or away from, the central nervous system; these two types of fibers are known as *afferent* or *efferent fibers,* respectively. In like manner the neurons of which they are parts are known as *afferent* or *efferent neurons.* Because afferent neurons frequently convey signals that, after reaching the central nervous system, give rise to sensations (touch or pain, for example), they are also referred to as *sensory neurons.* The designations "afferent" and "sensory" are not truly synonymous, however; indeed, there are many afferent neurons that, when stimulated, convey signals to the central nervous system that do not result in conscious sensations. Nonetheless, the terms afferent neuron and sensory neuron tend to be used interchangeably. Efferent neurons, on the other hand, carry impulses to effector organs, where they cause some change in activity (muscle contraction, for example) and therefore, are often referred to as *motor neurons.*

The distinction between central and peripheral nervous systems is a gross anatomic one only. The former is dependent on the latter both for reception of stimuli and for transmission of impulses to the effector organs. Moreover, the connections between the afferent and efferent parts of the peripheral nervous system occur in the central nervous system. Furthermore, many of the cell bodies, the fibers of which form the peripheral nervous system, are themselves housed within the central nervous system.

Within the central nervous system, accumulations of cell bodies are known as **gray matter** because of their color in the fresh condition. Accumulations of axons are known as **white matter** because the fatty sheath (myelin) that covers many axons appears white in the fresh condition. Accumulations of nerve cell bodies outside the central nervous system are known as **ganglia** (*ganglion,* meaning swelling), and bundles of nerve fibers outside the central nervous system form the nerves. There are two types of ganglia: sensory and autonomic. Sensory ganglia lie close to the central nervous system and house the cell bodies of afferent (sensory) neurons. Autonomic ganglia may also lie close to the central nervous system, or they may be scattered more peripherally. They contain the cell bodies of some of the efferent (motor) neurons of the autonomic nervous system, to be described later.

Cell bodies and nerve fibers in the central nervous system are enmeshed in **neuroglia,** which can be considered the connective tissue peculiar to the central nervous system. Neuroglia differs from connective tissue elsewhere, not only in its form, but also in its origin, for it is derived from ectoderm, rather than mesoderm. However, a certain amount of ordinary mesodermal connective tissue is brought into the central nervous system, along with the blood vessels that penetrate it. The cells and fibers of the ganglia and nerves of the peripheral nervous system are bound together by the usual type of fibrous connective tissue, although some cellular elements within ganglia and nerves are apparently derived, as are the neuroglia, from ectoderm.

DEVELOPMENT OF THE NERVOUS SYSTEM

The first evidence of the nervous system appears in the trilaminar embryo as a longitudinal thickening of the ectoderm along the dorsal midline, called the **neural plate.** This structure then forms the **neural tube** (see Fig. 13-7), the enlarged cephalic end of which becomes the brain, and the narrow caudal portion the spinal cord. Some cells of the neural plate that are excluded from the neural tube form the **neural crest.** The neural crest gives rise to all the neurons that are located outside the brain and spinal cord. The cell bodies of such neurons are located in ganglia, either sensory or autonomic. The neural crest also gives rise to a variety of other cell types that become incorporated into such structures as the heart and the skin.

Central Nervous System

Many of the cells of the neural tube, after a period of proliferation, become transformed into *neuroblasts.* Neuroblasts, in turn, are transformed into true nerve cells. Aggregates of neurons in the central nervous system form its gray matter, and their processes, most of which become ensheathed by myelin, form its white matter. Other cells in the neural tube are transformed into neuroglia (supporting) cells, and a limited number remain as rather primitive epithelial cells—ependymal cells—that line the cavity of the neural tube.

The cell bodies of the neurons of the central nervous system tend to remain grouped close to the central canal, but they send their longer processes into the periphery of the tube; here the processes grow up or down the tube, or across it, as nerve fibers to form **tracts.** Thus, the gray matter of the central nervous system tends to be centrally located and the white matter, peripherally located. Exceptions to the central location of gray matter are the thin layers (cortices) on the surfaces of the cerebellum and cerebrum (parts of the brain). Here, although masses of gray matter remain centrally located, many neurons migrate to the surface and cover the white matter.

Neurons in the cerebral and cerebellar cortex form layers, whereas in the central gray matter they tend to form groups called **nuclei.** Neurons in a nucleus tend to share similar functions. Those concerned with motor functions (causing muscle cells to contract and glands to secrete) extend their axons through the surface of the brain and spinal cord and contribute motor fibers to the nerves that issue from the central nervous system. The sensory component of nerves is made up of processes of neurons that develop from the neural crest.

Peripheral Nervous System

Neural crest cells in the ganglia of the peripheral nervous system, whether they be sensory or autonomic ganglia, form *neuroblasts.* In sensory ganglia, the neuroblasts destined to become **sensory neurons** initially develop two processes. Later on these combine into a single short stem that divides into two branches: one grows out to the periphery (to the skin, for example), as a sensory (afferent) fiber of a nerve; the other grows into the neural tube, making connections with cells there. With other similar fibers, the latter forms the **sensory** (afferent) **root** of the nerve. Thus, a single nerve cell conducts from a peripheral sense organ to the central nervous system. Neuroblasts in autonomic ganglia also differentiate into neurons; their anatomy and function, however, are best described later.

The fibers that form the **motor** (efferent) **root** of a nerve arise as processes of neuroblasts that lie within the central nervous system. These become multipolar cells (that is, cells with many processes), but their numerous dendrites remain within the central nervous system, whereas their single axons grow out to join the sensory part of the nerve peripheral to the sensory ganglion. Once they have mingled with the sensory fibers, some motor fibers grow out to skeletal muscle, to end there, whereas others leave the main nerve and end in autonomic ganglia. Here they relay their impulses to other neurons, the cell bodies of which lie in the ganglia.

Myelin, a fatty layer formed around many nerve fibers, is laid down by **Schwann cells,** one of the nonneuronal cell types that are derived from neural crest and become associated with growing nerve fibers. The presence of myelin increases the conduction velocity in nerve fibers, and all of the larger fibers in the peripheral nervous system become myelinated. Even the smaller, so-called unmyelinated fibers, however, are encased by Schwann cells. (Myelination is also a requirement for many fibers in the central nervous system, but here it is carried out by oligodendroglia, one of the neuroglial cell types, rather than by Schwann cells.)

The neural crest cells that give rise to **autonomic ganglia** assume various positions in the body, but most accumulate either along the anterolateral aspect of the vertebral column, to form the *paravertebral ganglia* of the paired sympathetic trunks, or around large vessels that supply viscera and form the *collateral* or *prevertebral ganglia* of the sympathetic system. Others form relatively small and irregularly placed autonomic ganglia of the head, and still others migrate into the walls of the digestive tract to form tiny autonomic ganglia or intramural nerve plexuses. Each neuroblast in an autonomic ganglion develops short dendrites and a single axon that grows out to smooth muscle, cardiac muscle, or glands. These neurons are essentially similar in appearance to many of the multipolar cells in the central nervous system.

THE BRAIN, SPINAL CORD, AND MENINGES

The spinal cord and the brain compose the central nervous system (Fig. 7-1). Between them, they give rise to all the motor fibers in the spinal and cranial nerves and receive all the sensory ones. They consist of enormous numbers of neurons. One cerebral cortex, only a part of one side of the brain, has been estimated to contain about 7 billion nerve cells. As mentioned earlier, the nerve cell bodies are usually grouped together into masses that are collectively called gray matter, whereas the longer fibers tend to be grouped as the white matter. The white matter of the central nervous system, composed of axons, serves to connect various groups of gray matter and, therefore, consists of fibers running in many different directions.

Spinal Cord

The spinal cord (*medulla spinalis,* or "marrow of the spine") is the simplest part of the central nervous system and can be thought of as a modified tube with enormously thickened walls. The lumen of the tube is called the central canal. The gray matter in its thick walls is arranged around the central canal, and the white matter largely surrounds the gray matter.

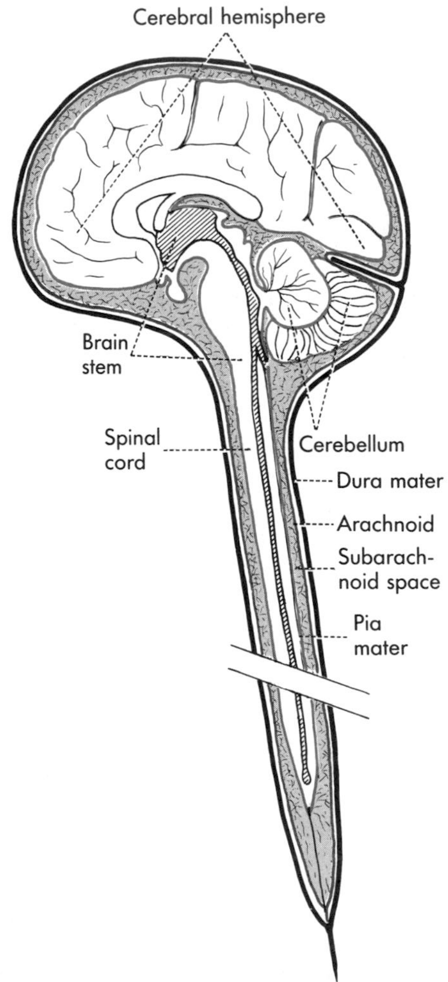

FIGURE *7-1.*
Diagram of the central nervous system and its meninges in a sagittal section. The spinal cord is much foreshortened.

The anatomy of the spinal cord is discussed in some detail in Chapter 13; only a few general aspects are mentioned here. In cross section (see Figs. 13-10 and 13-11), the uneven distribution of the gray matter around the central canal is obvious. The projections on each side of the midline are known as the **posterior** and **anterior horns.** In general, the posterior horns receive the incoming sensory fibers and disperse their nerve impulses to other parts of the cord and to the brain. In the anterior horns are large cells that give rise to the fibers that go to skeletal muscle. In some parts of the cord, there is a small **lateral horn** that contains the cell bodies that ultimately innervate smooth muscle, cardiac muscle, and glands.

The white matter of the spinal cord is composed of fibers that run between parts of the spinal cord, from the spinal cord to parts of the brain, or from parts of the brain to the gray matter of the cord (see Figs. 13-9, 13-12, and 13-13). Through it, therefore, impulses entering the spinal cord are disseminated and also forwarded to higher levels in the brain. In addition, various parts of the brain can influence, through the white matter of the cord, the voluntary and reflex activities that are mediated by cells located in the spinal cord. Fibers that have the same function tend to be grouped together in the spinal cord, and such groupings, although not necessarily visible, constitute the tracts of the cord (see Fig. 13-12). Some of the major tracts are sensory, ascending toward the brain, whereas others are motor, descending from the brain to various levels of the spinal cord.

Brain

The brain (*encephalon,* meaning in the head), the enlarged upper end of the central nervous system lodged within the skull, is much more complicated than the spinal cord and is properly studied in the neuroanatomy laboratory. General features of its gross anatomy are presented in Chapter 32; only a brief summary is given here.

The **brain stem** is a direct upward continuation of the spinal cord, but is somewhat more complex. Here the gray and the white matter are more intermixed than they are in the spinal cord. Furthermore, in some places the surface is formed of white matter as it is in the cord, whereas, in others, gray matter comes to the surface. The gray matter that corresponds most closely to the horns of the spinal cord tends to be close to the modified central canal of the brain stem. Much of this gray matter sends motor fibers into, or receives sensory fibers from, cranial nerves through cell groups that are called the nuclei of the cranial nerves. The white matter of the brain stem, like that of the cord, is largely collected into tracts; some of these are continuous with sensory and motor tracts in the spinal cord, whereas others originate from (or end in) gray matter at the brain stem level.

Surmounting the brain stem, and originating as outgrowths from it, are the **cerebellum** (little brain) and the **cerebrum** (brain). The cerebrum is composed of paired cerebral hemispheres. Both the cerebrum and the cerebellum are distinguished from the brain stem by their size and structure. Although both contain deep-lying masses of gray matter, called nuclei, each also has an extensive convoluted surface composed of gray matter, known as **pallium** (cloak or mantle) or **cortex** (bark, therefore, outer layer). Here nerve cells are spread out in layers. Through the white matter, the cortices of both the cerebellum and the cerebrum are connected to lower-lying centers of the brain stem and spinal cord, and to each other. Various areas of the cerebral cortex of the same and opposite hemispheres also have extensive connections with each other.

The cerebellum is concerned mainly with helping guide, through lower centers, the activity of skeletal muscle. The cerebrum is literally "the brain" in the colloquial sense and is concerned not only with initiating voluntary movements, but also with sensations, judgments, interpretations, emotions, and all those activities grouped together as mental. Most sensory impulses to the cerebrum cross to the opposite side before they reach it, and most impulses to skeletal muscle cross after they leave it, so that each cerebral cortex mediates, for the most part, sensation and movement on the opposite side of the body.

Meninges and Cerebrospinal Fluid

The *meninges* are connective tissue wrappings of the central nervous system that intervene between it and the surrounding bone. Together with the fluid that they enclose, they cushion the nervous system. There are three layers, each continuous from brain to spinal cord.

The **dura mater,** the tough outermost layer of the meninges, lines the skull as it surrounds the brain and forms a simple tube around the spinal cord. Immediately internal to the dura mater, and forming a similarly shaped sac, is the thin **arachnoid membrane** (arachnoidea). The arachnoid membrane is separated from the innermost meninx, the **pia mater,** by a fluid-filled space. The pia mater is also a thin layer but, unlike the arachnoid, it is closely applied to the brain and spinal cord. The space between the arachnoid and pia is the **subarachnoid space,** and the fluid that fills the space is called cerebrospinal fluid.

The colorless **cerebrospinal fluid** is formed largely in the cavities (ventricles) of the brain and escapes from them to fill the subarachnoid space. From here, it eventually drains into the venous system.

NERVES

Nerves are bundles of nerve fibers that lie outside the central nervous system. Most nerves contain both motor (efferent) and sensory (afferent) fibers. The nerves that make their exit through the skull are known as **cranial nerves.** Twelve pairs of these are described and named as being typical of all mammals. They are all attached to the brain.

Those nerves that make their exit below the skull and between vertebrae are **spinal nerves.** There are 31 pairs of these; they arise from the spinal cord throughout its length.

Structure of Peripheral Nerves

Connective Tissue

All peripheral nerves, whether spinal or cranial, are similar in structure. The nerve fibers or axons that make up a nerve become bound together, somewhat like the individual wires in a cable, by connective tissue. The connective tissue of a large nerve makes up what are called the epineurium, perineurium, and endoneurium (Fig. 7-2). The **epineurium** surrounds the entire nerve and holds it loosely to the connective tissue through which it runs. It also sends septa into the nerve that divide the nerve fibers into bundles (*fasciculi* or *funiculi*) of varying size. The **perineurium** surrounds each fasciculus and splits with it at each branching point. The **endoneurium** is a delicate

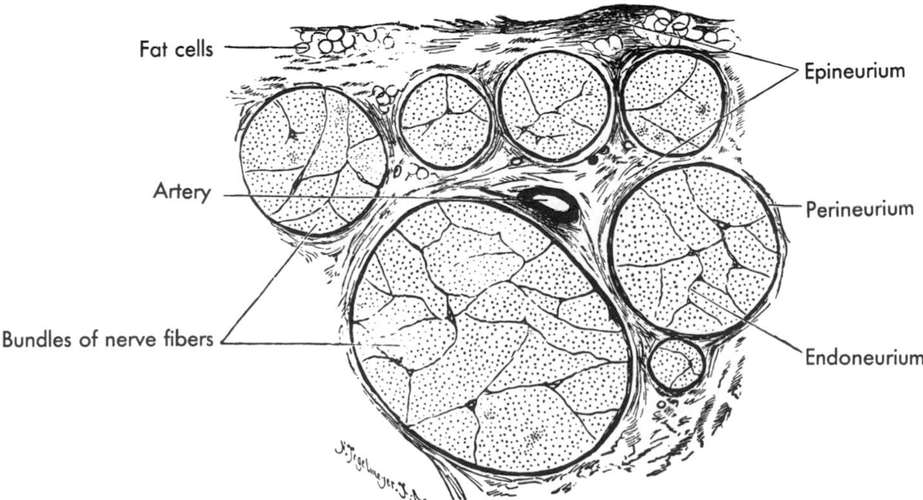

FIGURE 7-2.
Cross section of part of the human median nerve to show its connective tissue components. (Bremer JL, Weatherford HL. A textbook of histology. Philadelphia: Blakiston & Son, 1944.)

layer of connective tissue around each nerve fiber (and lies, therefore, within the perineurium).

The connective tissue of a nerve permits a certain amount of stretch without damage to the nerve fibers. The latter tend to be "wavy," and by the time the slack in them is taken up, the connective tissue fibers are also under tension and resist further stretch. The maximal stretch that can be imposed on any given length of nerve without appreciable damage is approximately 10%, although nerves that contain fat allow a little more. Nerves that are most likely to be stretched during normal movements typically contain more fat than do other nerves.

Anastomoses and Branches. When a nerve branches, the branching is a separation of nerve bundles, not a branching of axons. Similarly, when two nerves join, their fibers do not unite, but simply intermingle and become surrounded by a common epineurium.

The connective tissue of a nerve is so tough, compared with the nerve fibers themselves, that it generally cannot be removed without tearing the fibers. However, when two nerves join, it is sometimes possible to separate them for a little distance beyond their point of juncture, because they may not interchange fibers immediately, and their epineuria may fuse only superficially instead of blending decisively. Thus, nerves may seem to join higher or lower than usual, depending on the density of the connective tissue first connecting them. The fasciculi of such nerves do not remain separate long, however, but divide and rejoin each other repeatedly; therefore, a little beyond the junction there is no fasciculus that contains fibers from only one nerve.

The same type of branching and regrouping of nerve fiber bundles occurs throughout the length of all the larger nerves, whether or not they are formed by the union of other nerves. Thus, there is a sorting and resorting of sensory and motor fibers, or fibers from different segments, leading finally to the isolation of a particular bundle of nerve fibers. This bundle then leaves the main nerve as a branch. The fibers destined for a given branch are grouped together a variable distance above the level at which they leave the nerve and are merely held to the remainder of the nerve by enveloping connective tissue. Accordingly, depending on the development of the surrounding connective tissue, a branch may leave a nerve either higher or lower than its usual level of exit. Variations in the level of origin of nerve branches, largely the result of variations in the surrounding connective tissue, are very commonly seen.

Blood Supply

Nerves receive twigs from adjacent blood vessels along their course. The twigs to large nerves are of macroscopic size, somewhat irregularly placed, and their branches tend to join together (anastomose) to form a longitudinally running vessel that supplies the nerve, giving off subsidiary branches. Opinions differ about whether damage to a nerve from pressure or stretch is due to interference with its vascular supply or direct trauma to nerve fibers.

Degeneration and Regeneration of Nerves

Regeneration of neuron cell bodies, whether inside or outside the central nervous system, is not possible, for once a neuroblast differentiates into a nerve cell it loses its capacity to divide. Loss of nerve cells, whether in the brain or in the peripheral nervous system, therefore, is irreparable. Clinical recovery from an apparent loss results from one of two processes: either the nerve cells concerned were not actually destroyed, but merely injured sufficiently to produce temporary arrest of their function; or, alternatively, uninjured cells were capable of taking over, to some extent, the functions of the destroyed cells.

In contrast with nerve cell bodies, nerve fibers do regenerate after injury, but only in the peripheral nervous system. Nerve fibers within the central nervous system do not appear to regenerate to form functional connections. Similarly, interruption of the sensory roots of spinal and cranial nerves is not followed by functional regeneration, for the fibers must enter and grow within the central nervous system to make functional connections. Consequently, sectioning of sensory nerve roots, sometimes carried out for relief of intractable pain, can be expected to produce permanent results.

Presumably, the absence of Schwann cells and endoneurium are among the factors responsible for the lack of regeneration in the central nervous system, for regeneration of nerve fibers seems to follow the same general principles that govern and guide the early outgrowth of the fibers in the embryo. The most important principle is that the outgrowing fiber must have a structure that it can grow along if it is to reach an end organ. Regenerating peripheral nerve fibers, but not fibers in the central nervous system, have a "guiding thread" in the form of cells and connective tissue fibers immediately around the exon (see following).

Degeneration. When an axon in a peripheral nerve is interrupted, all of that axon distal to the level of interruption (that is, the part that is no longer connected to the cell body) degenerates. If the axon is myelinated, its myelin sheath also degenerates. The Schwann cells, however, appear to survive. So do the delicate "tubes" of connective tissue (endoneurium) that encase the axons. Thus, a freshly degenerated peripheral nerve, although devoid of functioning axons distal to the lesion, still has the same connective tissue framework that it had before the lesion occurred.

Regeneration. After complete interruption of a peripheral nerve fiber, its proximal end, still connected to the cell body, passes through a period of relative inactivity. During this period, the Schwann cells multiply and, by their apposition, form tiny threads within the endoneurial tubes.

Actual regeneration begins with the sprouting of several very fine fibrils from the distal end of the intact part of each axon. The growing tip of each fibril seeks out or encounters the ends of nearby endoneurial tubes and attempts to grow down them (as the ameboid tip of a nerve fiber in tissue culture will grow along a fine matrix). Of the regenerating axon tips that enter a single endoneurial tube, some are quickly outstripped in their growth by others and tend to degenerate. Of the others, the one that first reaches the end organ and establishes a functional connection with it persists as the single nerve fiber within the endoneurial tube, whereas the others degenerate.

Because regenerating nerve fibers must reach endoneurial tubes if they are to grow any distance, it is important that tubes and ameboid tips be close together when regeneration begins. If there has been no break in the continuity of the nerve as a whole, but only in the nerve fibers within it, the endoneurial tubes distal to the level of interruption are still continuous with those surrounding the regenerating axon. Each nerve fiber then tends to regenerate along the same pathway that it originally followed; therefore, it reaches the same end organ with which it was originally connected. Obviously, a lesion of a nerve that does not interrupt the continuity of its connective tissue offers favorable conditions for regeneration, and regeneration may be expected to occur.

If the nerve as a whole has been interrupted, bringing the cut ends together and holding them in that position is the nearest approximation to continuity that can be achieved. The most important problem is to prevent scar tissue from forming between the adjacent ends, which would block the growth of axons into the peripheral part of the nerve. When the nerve ends are so far separated that they cannot be approximated without too much tension, a nerve graft, employing appropriate lengths of a cutaneous nerve from the same person, must be used as a bridge to connect the two ends if regeneration is to be obtained.

For perfect regeneration, every regenerating axon would seemingly have to make connection with exactly the same end organ with which it was once connected. This may be reasonably well achieved where there has been no interruption in the continuity of the connective tissue framework of the nerve. In any other circumstance, it seems inevitable that some growing axons would regenerate down the wrong endoneurial tubes and, hence, terminate in contact with end organs with which they were not previously associated. If the end organ is of the same type as that originally reached by the fiber, functional regeneration can be expected. For example, recovery is probable if an axon that once supplied muscle regenerates to muscle. The fiber is capable of forming functional connections with muscle cells that it did not originally supply, and the central nervous system is capable of readjusting its output and sending signals to a given muscle by a nerve different from the one that previously conducted impulses to that muscle. This ability to readjust is sometimes purposely used by surgeons. For instance, in a case of irreparable damage to a proximal part of the facial nerve, with resulting paralysis of the face, the accessory nerve (to muscles of the shoulder) can be sectioned and its proximal end sutured to the distal part of the facial nerve. After the regenerating accessory fibers have reached the facial muscles, the patient obtains fairly adequate control over these muscles, although it requires, at first, thinking of shrugging the shoulder when intending to move the face.

However, if a sensory fiber regenerates down an endoneurial tube that brings it in contact with muscle fibers, it cannot form motor endings on those muscles as would a motor nerve fiber. Neither can a fiber originally connecting with muscle form functional sensory endings in the skin. Regeneration of fibers down the wrong pathways may be disastrous, leading to no functional regeneration at all. Because of this danger, the surgeon, in suturing a nerve, takes particular care not to twist either end, hoping to bring together nerve bundles that were originally in continuity with each other.

Although nerve fibers grow very rapidly (some of them at the rate of more than 3 mm/day), the great distances over which they sometimes must regenerate, which may be measurable in feet when the injury is close to the spinal cord, make the functional regeneration of nerve fibers a slow process. As a general rule, the farther a regenerating axon tip gets from the nerve cell body, the more slowly it grows. For example, an axon that starts regenerating at the rate of 3 mm/day may drop its rate to 0.5 mm/day or less as it reaches a more peripheral location. Additional time at the beginning and the end of the process must be allowed for in clinical practice. The first period is necessary for reorganization of the cell body and the axon before regeneration begins and the second, for functional maturation of the fiber after it has reached the end organ. The complete process may occupy periods of from several months to a year or more.

THE SOMATIC AND AUTONOMIC NERVOUS SYSTEMS

Components of both the central and the peripheral nervous system may be classified, from a nontopographical perspective, according to the target organs or tissues they serve. On the one hand, components that innervate structures derived from the somites can be classified as forming the **somatic nervous system.** Such structures include skeletal muscle and the dermis, as well as the skeletal system and its joints. On the other hand, those components of the nervous system that serve viscera can be classified as constituting the **visceral** or **autonomic nervous system.** Such structures include the heart and blood vessels; hollow and parenchymatous organs of the digestive, respiratory, urinary, and genital systems; and all glands and smooth muscle located throughout the body, including the skin.

Both the somatic and visceral (autonomic) nervous systems incorporate both motor and sensory neural elements, including nerve fibers, ganglia, and masses of gray matter within the central nervous system (nuclei). Thus, it is customary to speak of *somatic efferents* and *somatic afferents,* or *visceral efferents* and *visceral afferents,* when describing nerve fibers. Likewise, somatic and visceral *efferent nuclei* (nuclei of origin) or somatic and visceral *afferent nuclei* (nuclei of termination) can be distinguished with reference to appropriate groups of neurons within the brain and spinal cord.

The sole target tissue of somatic efferents is skeletal muscle: they do not innervate any other type of tissue. Visceral efferents, on the other hand, terminate on smooth muscle, cardiac muscle, or glands. Somatic efferents deliver impulses to skeletal muscle from somatic efferent nuclei, and their only effect is to cause the muscle cells to contract. Visceral efferents, by contrast, may have a stimulatory effect on their target tissues (causing smooth muscle or cardiac muscle to contract, for example, or glands to secrete), or they may inhibit such activities. Somatic afferents transmit impulses from receptors in skin, skeletal muscle, tendons, joints, bones, and ligaments to afferent nuclei in the central nervous system. Ultimately, these impulses are perceived as pain, temperature, touch, vibration, or position sense (proprioception). Visceral afferents transmit impulses from receptors in blood vessels and viscera to visceral afferent nuclei in the central nervous system. These impulses are ultimately interpreted as pain, or as such visceral sensations as hunger, nausea, or distension. Many visceral afferent impulses do not reach the level of consciousness and are concerned with reflexes that regulate the subconscious activity of viscera. The somatic nervous system also mediates reflex activities, but we become aware of most of these reflexes, despite the fact that we do not initiate them voluntarily.

There is a third component of the nervous system, called the **branchial nervous system,** that may be included in the somatic nervous system. The branchial nervous system is concerned with the innervation of the *branchial apparatus*, which in fishes forms the gills and in mammals gives rise to structures that are incorporated into the head and neck, particularly the larynx and pharynx. Branchial efferents innervate branchial muscles which, although not of somite origin, closely resemble skeletal muscle. Branchial afferents have lost their independent identity in higher vertebrates and have merged with somatic afferents that serve the head and neck regions.

The parts of the brain and the cranial nerves that are concerned with the special senses of sight, smell, hearing, balance, and taste do not readily fit into this classification. They are best thought of in the current context as making up a category of their own. The receptors for the special senses, as well as some of the neural elements of the nerves, are developmentally related to regions of ectoderm that are located outside the neural plate. To emphasize the difference from "ordinary" somatic afferents, the nerve fibers and nuclei concerned with the special senses are, with one exception, designated *special somatic afferents.* The exception involves the sense of taste: neural elements mediating this sense are known as *special visceral afferents.* In contrast, all other visceral afferents are often referred to as *general visceral afferents.*

Nuclei concerned with specific functions are topographically segregated in the gray matter of the central nervous system. For instance, the location in the spinal cord of somatic and visceral efferent nuclei, as well as of somatic afferent nuclei, is illustrated in Figure 13-7 and their development is explained in Chapter 13. A similar topographic segregation holds true in the brain as well, although here, there is a tendency for nuclei belonging to one functional group to fuse with nuclei belonging to a different functional group (e.g., visceral efferent and branchial efferent nuclei). Such fusion is reflected in the coexistence of nerve fibers from these nuclei in the corresponding cranial nerves. Mixing of somatic and visceral efferent and afferent nerve fibers is more the rule than the exception in spinal nerves and most of their branches. In fact, very few nerves are composed of only one type of nerve fiber; they include, for instance, the optic, olfactory, cochlear, and vestibular nerves, all of which belong to the category of special somatic afferents.

Following a brief summary of cranial nerves and spinal nerves, the remainder of this section provides simple descriptions and examples of the organization and fiber pathways in the somatic and autonomic nervous systems. Subsequent chapters dealing with different body regions present relevant aspects of the cranial nerves and of the somatic and autonomic systems in appropriate and greater detail.

Cranial Nerves

Described more fully in Chapter 32, the 12 pairs of cranial nerves are discussed here briefly, summarizing the functional types of nerve fibers that predominate in each pair. The 12 nerves are referred to equally commonly by name or by number. The numbers of individual cranial nerves are usually written in Roman numerals to distinguish them from spinal nerves, the numbers of which are usually written in Arabic numerals. The cranial nerves are

I Olfactory
II Optic
III Oculomotor
IV Trochlear
V Trigeminal
VI Abducens
VII Facial
VIII Vestibulocochlear
IX Glossopharyngeal
X Vagus
XI Cranial accessory
XII Hypoglossal

As explained earlier, the optic and olfactory nerves are special somatic afferents; neither has a sensory ganglion. The oculomotor, trochlear, and abducens nerves are composed predominantly of somatic efferent fibers that serve the extrinsic muscles of the eyeball. The hypoglossal (XII) nerve belongs in the same functional class: it innervates the tongue musculature. The extraocular and tongue muscles are derived from cranial myotomes. Associated with the oculomotor nerve are visceral efferent fibers that innervate the smooth muscle within the eyeball (iris, ciliary muscle). The trigeminal nerve is the chief somatic afferent nerve of the head, and a large sensory ganglion is associated with it. The nerve, however, incorporates a significant motor component, composed of branchial efferents that serve chiefly the muscles of mastication. The facial nerve is chiefly concerned with supplying the facial muscles with branchial efferents. Associated with it, however, are visceral efferents concerned with salivation and special visceral afferents that convey taste sensation. The latter have their cell bodies in a ganglion. The glossopharyngeal nerve is also a mixed cranial nerve: it contains branchial efferents and afferents, mainly for the pharynx, as well as special visceral afferents (taste) and visceral efferents concerned with salivation. The vagus nerve is also complex; its chief components are visceral efferents and afferents (serving extensive parts of the gastrointestinal, respiratory, and cardiovascular systems), as well as branchial efferents and afferents to the larynx. The cranial accessory nerve is a motor nerve and boosts the vagus by contributing predominantly branchial efferent fibers to it.

Two types of ganglia are associated with cranial nerves: 1) sensory ganglia, appearing as relatively large swellings on the nerves (e.g., trigeminal ganglion and superior and inferior ganglia of the vagus); and 2) autonomic ganglia in which visceral efferents synapse (e.g., otic ganglion and ciliary ganglion).

Spinal Nerves

Described more fully in Chapter 13, the 31 pairs of spinal nerves are discussed here briefly, with the object of summarizing the functional types of nerve fibers that predominate in them and the anatomic parts that make up each spinal nerve. The composition of the spinal nerves is considerably less complicated than that of cranial nerves. All 31 pairs of spinal nerves are preponderantly composed of somatic efferents and afferents; admixed among these, however, are some visceral efferents and afferents.

There are 8 pairs of cervical, 12 pairs of thoracic, 5 pairs of lumbar, 5 pairs of sacral, and 1 pair of coccygeal nerves associated in series with the spinal cord. The origin, course, and branches of these nerves are illustrated in Figures 13-9 and 13-22. They are segmentally distributed to skeletal muscle and the skin of the trunk and limbs (see Chaps. 13 and 14).

The parts of a spinal nerve are shown in Figure 7-3. These are the relatively short **spinal nerve** itself, and its **anterior root** and **posterior root,** which connect the spinal nerve to the spinal cord.*

In a more extended sense, the branches of the spinal nerve should also be considered as forming a part of it. The first two branches into which the spinal nerve splits are called the **anterior** and **posterior rami.** Each ramus proceeds in the direction implied by its name and gives off rather well-defined sets of branches (see Fig. 7-3). A sensory ganglion, called the **spinal ganglion,** is associated with the posterior root. (Previous terminology designated the spinal ganglion as the dorsal root ganglion.)

Those anterior rami that supply the limbs form plexuses in a manner explained in Chapter 14 (see Fig. 14-6). Notwithstanding the formation of plexuses, the types of nerve fibers distributed to the limbs are the same as those that are distributed to the anterior and lateral parts

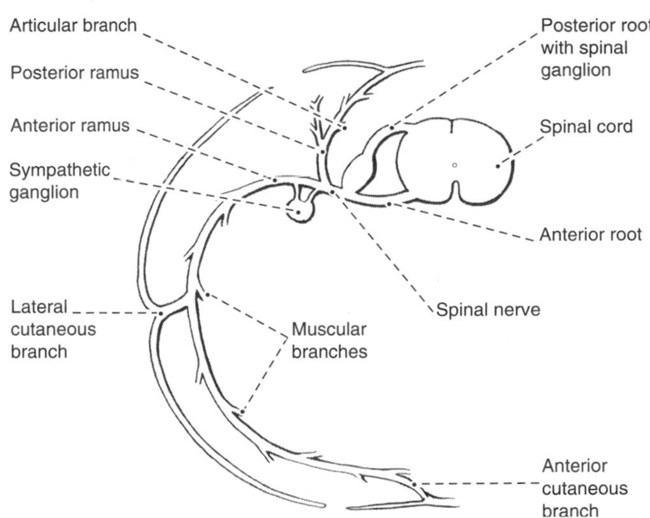

FIGURE *7-3.*
A "typical" spinal nerve, its roots and branches. The outline of the spinal cord is also shown.

of the trunk by the other anterior rami, and to the back by the posterior rami.

Somatic Nervous System

The somatic nervous system is composed of somatic efferent and somatic afferent nuclei in the central nervous system, and of somatic efferent and somatic afferent nerve fibers, as well as sensory ganglia, in the peripheral nervous system. Although such somatic nuclei and nerve fibers are associated with certain cranial nerves as well, it is the spinal cord and the spinal nerves that supply the entire body inferior to the head with somatic innervation.

Disregarding topographic details of the named parts and branches of individual nerves, Figures 7-4 and 7-5 illustrate the anatomic units involved in the functioning of the somatic nervous system.

Figure 7-4 illustrates the pathway for one of the basic reflexes involving the somatic nervous system, the stretch reflex. It has been chosen because it represents the simplest example of the cooperative action of some of the anatomic units of the somatic nervous system. In the example shown, the examiner is passively extending the subject's elbow. The subject is not resisting the maneuver, and the flexor muscle is put on stretch. The stretch stimulates the peripheral endings of somatic afferent fibers within the flexor muscle. These endings, known as sensory receptors because of their ability to detect a stimulus, are housed within specialized units in the muscle, known as muscle spindles. Impulses thus generated in the receptors are transmitted along the peripheral processes of somatic afferent (sensory) neurons, the cell bodies of which are located in spinal ganglia just outside the spinal cord. The central processes of these neurons transmit the impulses to two nuclei in the gray matter of the spinal cord. One of these is a somatic afferent nucleus, from which the message gets transmitted to the brain and may reach consciousness. The other is a somatic efferent nucleus, which

* The roots and rami of spinal nerves have been designated as dorsal and ventral, or posterior and anterior. Previous editions of this text used dorsal and ventral designations for the roots, and posterior and anterior designations for the rami. In conformity with Nomina Anatomica (1989), the terms posterior and anterior are being used here for both the rami and the roots.

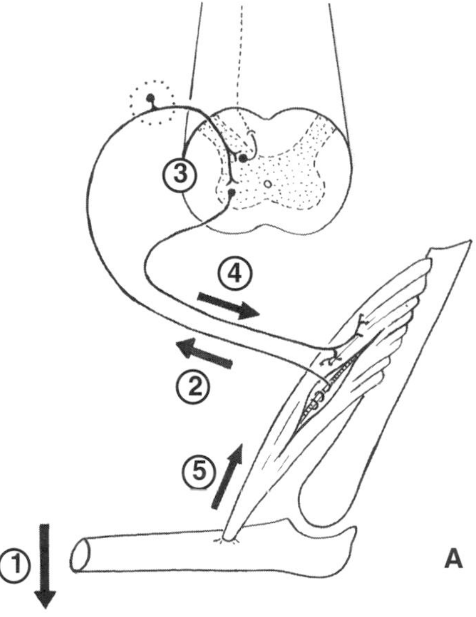

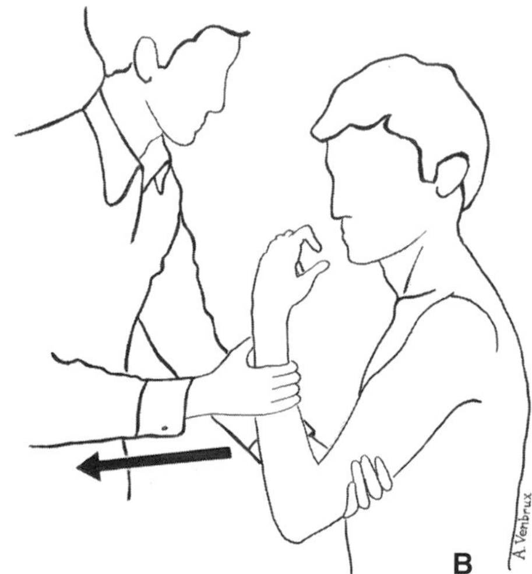

FIGURE 7-4.
An example of the activation of somatic afferent and somatic efferent fibers, as it occurs in the stretch reflex: (A) the pathways involved when the reflex is (B) elicited in an elbow flexor muscle. The events that occur in sequence are (*1*) Passive extension of the elbow by the examiner stretches the flexor muscle; (*2*) some of the spindle afferents are excited; (*3*) excitatory postsynaptic potentials are generated, and some of the somatic efferent neurons are depolarized; (*4*) efferent impulses induce contraction of skeletal muscle; (*5*) resistance is offered to the stretching force (force exerted by the examiner) caused by contraction of the muscle.

responds by firing impulses along somatic efferent nerve fibers, causing reflex contraction of the skeletal muscle fibers in the elbow flexor. As a consequence, the flexor muscle will resist the stretch applied by the examiner, whether the subject wishes it or not. The stretch reflex is the basis of all tendon reflexes (tendon jerks) that are commonly elicited clinically. Testing the reflex tests the integrity of the anatomic components of the somatic nervous system, as well as of the sensory and effector mechanisms within skeletal muscle.

Figure 7-5 illustrates a further example of the function of somatic afferents and efferents; namely, the inhibition of antagonists for a movement coincidental with the contraction of the prime movers. A somatic afferent nerve fiber is activated by a pain stimulus applied to the skin (e.g., the sole of the foot). Impulses are relayed to a somatic afferent nucleus in the spinal cord. So-called interneurons transmit these impulses to the brain and to a somatic efferent nucleus on the same side of the spinal cord (just as in the previous example); in addition, however, impulses are transmitted to a somatic efferent nucleus on the contralateral side of the cord. In this instance, as a consequence of differential synaptic transmission between the incoming somatic afferent neurons and the interneurons, some of the somatic efferent neurons will be excited, whereas others will be inhibited. The response of the subject is reflex withdrawal, that is, flexion of the limb

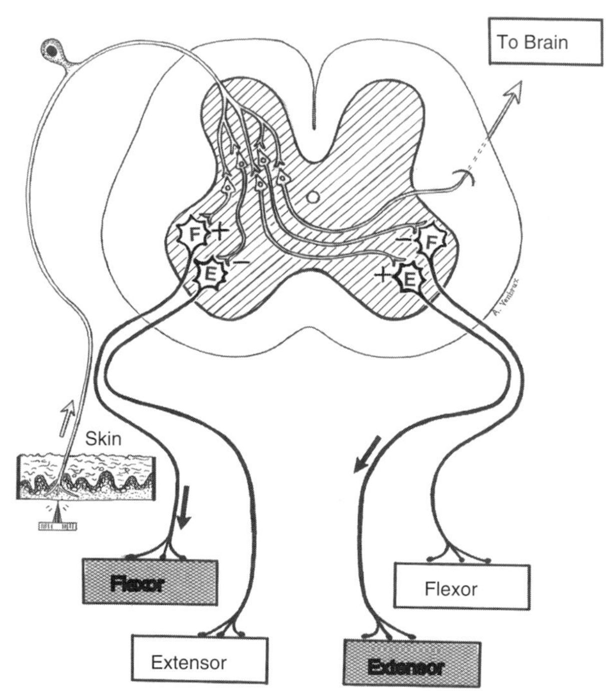

FIGURE 7-5.
A highly schematic representation of reciprocal innervation: Only one interneuron is shown between a terminal branch of the somatic afferent nerve fiber and a somatic efferent neuron, but in reality multiple such interneurons exist. (*E*, extensor motor neuron; *F*, flexor motor neuron; +, excitatory postsynaptic potential; –, inhibitory postsynaptic potential). In the instance illustrated, the afferent impulse is provoked by a pain stimulus applied to the skin. Such a stimulus results in a flexion or withdrawal reflex (excitation of flexor and inhibition of extensor motor neurons) and also in a crossed extension reflex.

that received the pain stimulus. To stabilize the body, however, the opposite limb needs to extend (perhaps even before the pain stimulus is registered by the brain). The arrangement of the circuitry of interneurons within the gray matter of the spinal cord assures that: 1) the extensors of the injured limb are inhibited while its flexors are induced to contract, and 2) the extensors are activated in the opposite limb (to stabilize the body) and the flexors are inhibited. The example illustrates reciprocal innervation within the somatic nervous system: a volley of impulses that generates contraction in one muscle by exciting somatic efferent (motor) neurons, as a rule, turns off motor neurons that supply the opposing muscles. Thus, the possible conflict between prime movers and antagonists is avoided.

Both of the scenarios illustrated in Figures 7-4 and 7-5 involve activation of somatic efferents and contraction or relaxation of skeletal muscle reflexively, without any intent or volition on the part of the subject. An important feature of the somatic nervous system is, however, that it provides the pathways for voluntary control of motor activities.

The motor neurons responsible for causing contraction of elbow flexors or flexors in the lower limb (to use the examples already discussed) can be made to fire by a conscious intent. Impulses descend from a particular region of the cerebral cortex (motor cortex) along tracts in the brain and spinal cord, and are relayed through interneurons to excite the motor neurons of the flexor and, at the same time, inhibit the motor neurons of its antagonist, the extensor. For this reason the somatic nervous system is often, but perhaps not quite justifiably, called the **voluntary nervous system.** It certainly can function voluntarily, but many of its activities do not reach consciousness and, instead, result in involuntary muscle action. Similar reasoning pertains to the somatic afferents. Whereas we are keenly aware of many different kinds of stimuli to which our skin, joints, and bones may be subjected (pain, touch, tactile discrimination of textures, or various postures, for example), a large number of similar somatic afferent impulses are blocked from reaching consciousness. For instance, in the normal course of events, we are unaware of the tactile stimuli on our skin generated by the clothes we wear, unless we choose to be.

The cell bodies of somatic afferent neurons are located in sensory ganglia; there are 31 pairs of spinal ganglia, one pair associated with each pair of spinal nerves. The central process of a ganglion cell in a spinal ganglion enters the spinal cord through the **posterior** (dorsal) **root** of the spinal nerve; its peripheral process passes laterally and helps form the spinal nerve itself by joining the **anterior** (ventral) **root.** Somatic efferents leave the spinal cord through the anterior root. Thus, the anterior and posterior roots of a spinal nerve are composed of purely motor or sensory fibers, respectively, whereas the spinal nerve itself, as well as its **anterior** (ventral) and **posterior** (dorsal) **rami,** are mixed nerves. Somatic afferent fibers segregate in the subsidiary branches of these rami when they supply the skin (cutaneous branches) and joints. Although muscular branches of these rami transmit somatic efferents to the muscles (see Fig. 7-3), they also contain somatic afferent fibers that mediate sensations of stretch, proprioception, and pain from the muscles and their tendons.

Branchial efferents and branchial afferents function in ways similar to their somatic counterparts. We use muscles of the larynx reflexively in a gag, voluntarily in emitting a particular sound of a defined pitch, and without thinking about it, during normal speech. Although relevant pathways involve the brain, rather than the spinal cord, the neural mechanisms are similar in the somatic and branchial systems. The situation is quite different, however, for the visceral (autonomic) nervous system that functions predominantly through reflexes, that is, autonomously, and is largely independent of voluntary control.

Autonomic Nervous System

The visceral (autonomic) nervous system, like the somatic nervous system, is composed of both central and peripheral elements. Centrally, it comprises visceral efferent (motor) and visceral afferent (sensory) nuclei in the brain and spinal cord. Its peripheral division is made up of visceral efferent and afferent nerve fibers as well as autonomic and sensory ganglia.

The anatomic organization of these functional components is complicated by several special features. First, the reciprocal innervation of target tissues (smooth muscle, cardiac muscle, and glands) is accomplished by two separate components of the autonomic nervous system, known as the *sympathetic system* and the *parasympathetic system.* Second, a large proportion of visceral efferents and afferents in both the sympathetic and parasympathetic systems are topographically associated for much of their course with somatic efferents and afferents of spinal nerves or, for a large proportion of parasympathetic fibers, with the vagus and other cranial nerves within the head. The subdivision of the autonomic nervous system into sympathetic and parasympathetic systems requires that qualifiers be added to the terms "visceral afferent" and "visceral efferent." Thus, we speak of *sympathetic* (visceral) *efferents* and *parasympathetic* (visceral) *efferents;* as well as *sympathetic* (visceral) *afferents* and *parasympathetic* (visceral) *afferents.** Furthermore, each visceral efferent pathway is interrupted by a synapse located in an autonomic ganglion. In both the sympathetic and parasympathetic systems, the visceral efferent neuron which is located in a visceral efferent nucleus of the central nervous system is designated a *preganglionic neuron,* and its axon is a preganglionic efferent fiber. The autonomic ganglion cell on which the preganglionic efferent fiber terminates is designated a *postganglionic neuron,* and its fiber is a postganglionic (postsynaptic) efferent fiber.

* The autonomic nervous system was arbitrarily defined early in the century by some authors as a purely motor system. Such a definition is inappropriate from both the anatomic and physiologic viewpoints. It is not unusual, however, to encounter individuals in both clinical and basic science disciplines who continue to adhere to such a definition.

The Sympathetic System

The sympathetic system consists of two columns of gray matter in the spinal cord (intermediolateral cell columns, one on each side) that contain preganglionic neurons; a pair of sympathetic trunks, each comprising a chain of paravertebral ganglia; a number of so-called collateral or prevertebral ganglia associated with blood vessels that supply viscera; and nerves and nerve plexuses that interconnect the spinal cord, the ganglia, and the target organs of the sympathetic nervous system. The effects of sympathetic stimulation include constriction of blood vessels (vasoconstriction); sweating; contraction of the arrectores pilorum, causing "gooseflesh" of the skin; increases in the rate and force of the heartbeat; constriction of the sphincters of hollow viscera and relaxation of the muscle in their wall (including that of the bronchi); dilation of the pupil of the eye; and inhibition of secretions by the glands of the respiratory and digestive systems. It may be deduced from these effects that sympathetic efferents pervade the entire body, including all structures in the head and neck, the limbs, the trunk, and all the viscera. The nerve impulses that attain such widespread distribution, however, all originate from a visceral efferent nucleus of relatively limited extent within the spinal cord. The nucleus is confined to the intermediolateral cell column (also known as the lateral gray column or lateral horn; see Fig. 13-9) in the thoracic and upper lumbar segments of the spinal cord, specifically T-1 to L-2. The restricted origin and widespread distribution of sympathetic pathways are largely responsible for the anatomic complexity of the peripheral component of the sympathetic system (Fig. 7-6).

An understanding of sympathetic pathways is perhaps facilitated by considering separately the following: 1) those that are concerned with the innervation of blood vessels or glands associated with somite-derived structures, whether these be in the body wall, the limbs, or the head and neck; and 2) those that innervate cardiac muscle, glands, and smooth muscle of viscera, including the blood vessels that serve them. The first group of sympathetic efferents can be thought of as having a *somatic distribution* and the second, a *visceral distribution*. Although such a distinction is helpful for achieving an overall view of sympathetic pathways, it should be remembered that fibers in

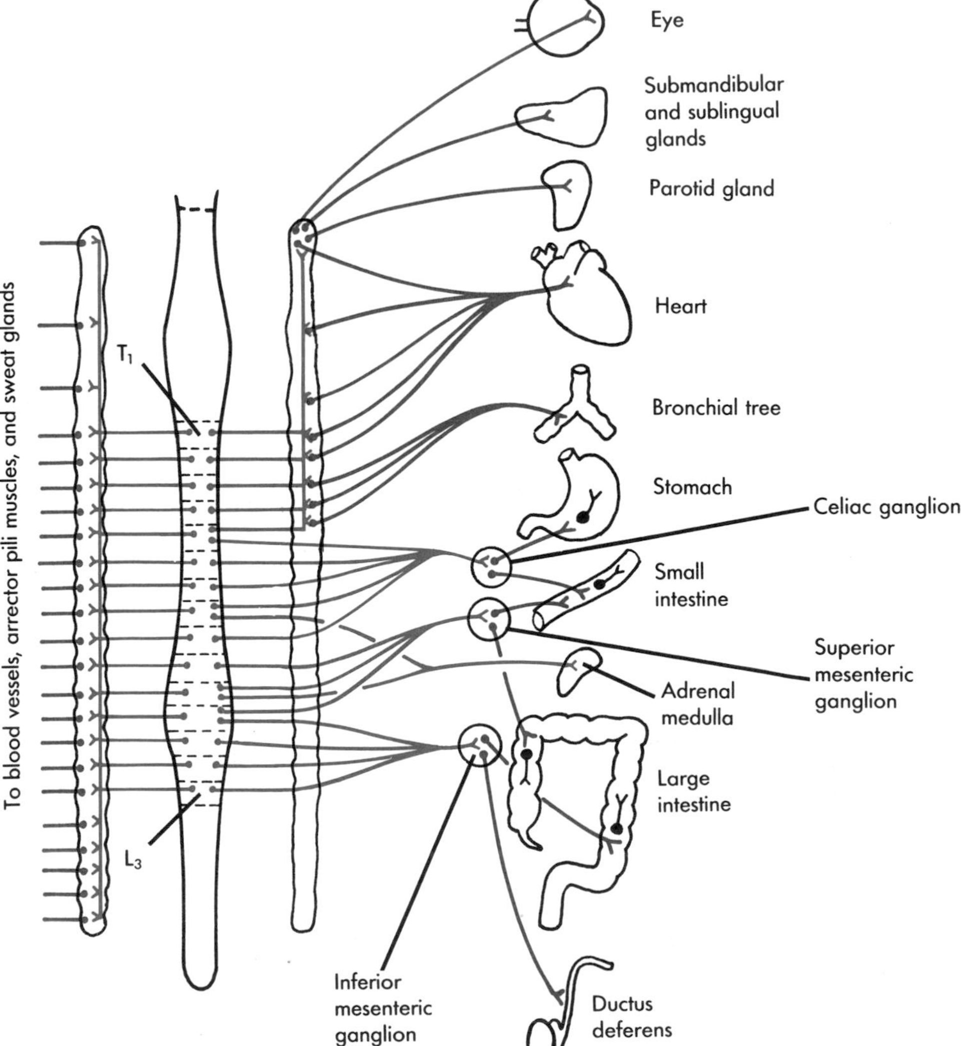

FIGURE *7-6.*
The motor components of the sympathetic nervous system: Preganglionic fibers are *red*; postganglionic fibers *blue*. The left half of the figure shows the spinal cord between the right and left sympathetic trunks. Sympathetic efferents destined for smooth muscles and glands associated with semite-derived structures are shown emerging from one trunk, and sympathetic efferents destined for viscera (shown in the right half of the figure) are emerging from the other trunk. In reality both types of fibers arise from both sympathetic trunks. (Barr ML, Kiernan JA. The human nervous system: an anatomical viewpoint. 4th ed. Philadelphia: Harper & Row, 1983.)

the first group are not, in fact, innervating somatic structures, but rather, smooth muscle and glands associated with such structures (the smooth muscle in the walls of blood vessels within skeletal muscles or the dermis, for example). In reality all the fibers are visceral efferent fibers, regardless of their ultimate distribution.

Sympathetic Efferents with Somatic Distribution. Sympathetic innervation reaches the limbs and the body wall by means of sympathetic efferents that join all 31 pairs of spinal nerves and become intermingled with the somatic efferent and afferent fibers of which these nerves are chiefly composed. By contrast, sympathetic efferents reach structures in the head by passing along blood vessels. The sympathetic trunks provide the synaptic relay stations that distribute the limited preganglionic output from T-1 to L-2 spinal cord segments to this wide distribution territory.

The **sympathetic trunks** are composed of 31 pairs of autonomic ganglia and their interganglionic branches. The ganglia and their interconnections give each trunk a superficial resemblance to a string of beads or a chain. Like the sensory spinal ganglia, the sympathetic trunk ganglia are derived from neural crest cells that accumulate along the ventrolateral aspects of the developing vertebrae, which accounts for their designation as *paravertebral ganglia.* Although there is eventual fusion among a number of neighboring ganglia, especially in the cervical region, there is, in principle, a paravertebral ganglion associated with each spinal nerve.

In addition to its two interganglionic branches, each paravertebral ganglion has two or three other types of branches, the number depending on the spinal nerve with which it is associated. In the ganglia associated with T-1 through L-2 spinal nerves, one of these branches serves to bring preganglionic fibers into the ganglion. (Ganglia at other levels, above T-1 or below L-2, do not have such a branch, but rather, receive preganglionic fibers through interganglionic branches in a manner described in the following.) A second type of branch, common to all paravertebral ganglia, allows postganglionic fibers to leave the ganglion and join the spinal nerve with which the ganglion is associated. A third type of branch transmits fibers from the ganglion to certain viscera and is called its *visceral branch.*

The preganglionic fibers that enter ganglia located at T-1 through L-2 levels are myelinated; the branch that transmits them to a given ganglion at one of these levels, therefore, is called the *white communicating ramus* (**white ramus communicans**). These fibers are the axons of preganglionic neurons located in the intermediolateral cell column of cord segments T-1 to L-2. They reach the white ramus communicans by passing through the anterior root of the spinal nerve (intermingled with somatic efferent fibers), into the spinal nerve itself and, thence, into the nerve's anterior ramus. There is a white ramus communicans linking a paravertebral ganglion to the anterior ramus of each spinal nerve in the T-1 to L-2 range, but they are lacking for all other paravertebral ganglia and spinal nerves. Instead, preganglionic fibers reach paravertebral ganglia in the cervical region by ascending in the sympathetic trunk, from the upper thoracic ganglia; likewise, they reach paravertebral ganglia below the L-2 ganglion by descending in the trunk from lower thoracic and upper lumbar ganglia.

Whereas white rami communicantes carrying *preganglionic* fibers are confined to the thoracic and upper lumbar regions, every ganglion throughout the trunk has a branch carrying *postganglionic* fibers to the anterior ramus of its corresponding spinal nerve. Because these fibers are unmyelinated, the branch is called the *gray communicating ramus* (**gray ramus communicans**).

The preganglionic fibers involved in sympathetic pathways of somatic distribution synapse on postganglionic neurons within the paravertebral ganglia. The synapse may occur at the same level at which the preganglionic fiber enters the trunk, or at a different level if the fiber ascends or descends through interganglionic branches before terminating. In either event, the axons of postganglionic neurons generally enter the corresponding spinal nerve immediately, through the gray ramus (Fig. 7-7). At all levels, most of the postganglionic fibers

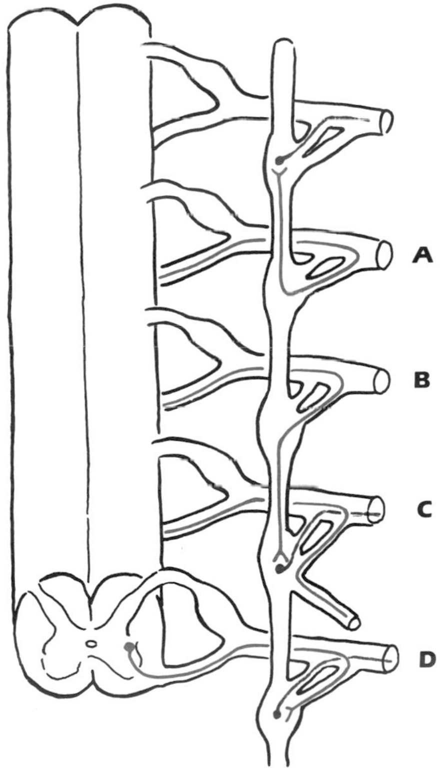

FIGURE 7-7.
Various courses that preganglionic fibers (*solid red lines*) may take through the thoracic sympathetic trunks: *Blue lines* represent postganglionic fibers. (A) The preganglionic fiber ascends to synapse at a higher level in the trunk; (B) it descends to a lower level; (C) it traverses the trunk and the ganglion, leaving as a visceral (splanchnic) branch; and (D) it ends in the ganglion at its own segmental level. The preganglionic fibers in any one nerve may do all of these.

then continue along the anterior ramus and are distributed to smooth muscle and glands by its branches. Some, however, turn medially in the anterior ramus and, at its junction with the posterior ramus, join that ramus to distribute through its branches to smooth muscle and glands in the back. Postganglionic fibers destined for smooth muscle and glands located in the head arise in the uppermost cervical paravertebral ganglia; branches of these ganglia then join the major blood vessels that ascend to the head.

Sympathetic Efferents Destined for Viscera. The preganglionic fibers destined for viscera, like those destined for somatic distribution, enter paravertebral ganglia T-1 to L-2 through their white rami communicantes. Since visceral branches are given off by paravertebral ganglia at all levels, those ganglia above or below T-1 to L-2 levels receive their input through the sympathetic trunk. The location of the synapse in the pathway depends on the location of the viscus within the body cavity. Preganglionic fibers destined for thoracic viscera (e.g., heart or lungs) synapse within paravertebral ganglia, whereas those destined for viscera in the abdominal and pelvic cavities leave the paravertebral ganglia through their visceral branches as preganglionic fibers and synapse in collateral ganglia (see Fig. 7-7C).

During development, at the time when the thoracic viscera are acquiring their innervation, they are located opposite cervical and upper thoracic vertebrae. Their nerves, therefore, are derived from paravertebral ganglia at these levels. Because the synapses occur in these paravertebral ganglia, visceral branches of cervical and upper thoracic (T-1 to T-5 or T-6) ganglia contain postganglionic sympathetic visceral efferents. Proceeding into the thoracic cavity, the visceral branches give rise to *autonomic nerve plexuses* (e.g., cardiac plexus or pulmonary plexus) that reach the respective organs along blood vessels.

In contrast, the visceral branches of paravertebral ganglia in lower thoracic, lumbar, and sacral regions transmit preganglionic, rather than postganglionic, fibers. These fibers initially enter paravertebral ganglia T-7 to L-2 through their white rami communicantes. Some then leave the ganglion at the same level, through its visceral branch, whereas others descend in the sympathetic trunk to exit through visceral branches of lower lumbar and sacral ganglia. The visceral branches of all these ganglia, therefore, contain preganglionic fibers and are usually called **splanchnic nerves.** Depending on the ganglia from which they arise, they are called *thoracic splanchnic nerves, lumbar splanchnic nerves*, or *sacral splanchnic nerves*. They proceed to the anterior aspect of the aorta and enter **collateral** (prevertebral) **ganglia,** in which they synapse. The postganglionic fibers arising from a collateral ganglion pass along the blood vessel that originates from the aorta where the ganglion is located. Pairs of collateral ganglia take their names from these blood vessels: the *celiac, superior mesenteric*, or *inferior mesenteric ganglia*, for example (see Fig. 7-6). Inferior to the bifurcation of the aorta, collateral ganglia in the pelvis are associated with the internal iliac arteries and are called *pelvic* (inferior hypogastric) *ganglia*.

The collateral ganglia are interconnected in front of the aorta by a delicate nerve plexus composed of autonomic fibers. This *aortic plexus* contains both preganglionic and postganglionic efferents (as well as visceral afferents and fibers belonging to the parasympathetic nervous system; see following section). Below the bifurcation of the aorta, the aortic plexus descends into the pelvis and links up with the pelvic ganglia. Passing from the collateral ganglia toward the viscera, postganglionic fibers also form plexuses along the arteries that convey them. These plexuses, like the collateral ganglia from which they arise, are named according to the corresponding artery (e.g., the superior mesenteric plexus along the superior mesenteric artery).

Like the paravertebral ganglia, collateral ganglia are derived from the neural crest. Their arrangement, however, is not segmental; rather it conforms to the organization of the blood vessels that supply the gut and its derivatives.

Sympathetic Visceral Afferents. Although visceral afferents associated with the sympathetic nervous system participate in visceral reflexes, their chief clinical significance is the mediation of pain sensation from most of the thoracic and abdominal viscera. The cell bodies of such visceral afferents are located in the spinal ganglia of those spinal nerves that are linked to paravertebral ganglia by white rami communicantes: namely, T-1 to L-2. The peripheral processes of these cells terminate as receptors within the walls of viscera. Impulses generated by the receptors pass along the afferent fibers that, in general, follow the same path as the corresponding sympathetic visceral efferents. For instance, afferent fibers from the heart pass along the cardiac plexus, the visceral branches of upper thoracic and cervical ganglia, the sympathetic trunk, and through the white rami communicantes of upper thoracic ganglia, into the corresponding anterior rami of spinal nerves. From here, they turn medially along the rami to reach the nerves' posterior roots, on which the spinal ganglia containing the sensory neurons are located. The central processes of the sensory ganglion cells enter the spinal cord along the posterior roots and terminate in a visceral afferent nucleus of the gray matter. From abdominal and pelvic organs, the afferent fibers follow the appropriate nerve plexus along the artery that serves the viscus. They pass through collateral ganglia and splanchnic nerves before ascending in the sympathetic trunk. They eventually leave the trunk through white rami communicantes of T-7 to L-2 ganglia and reach the spinal ganglia on the posterior roots as described earlier. (More detailed accounts of the distribution of pain afferents to different viscera are found in the appropriate chapters.)

Visceral afferents also serve blood vessels in the limbs, body wall, and the head and neck. Presumably they mediate pain sensation. These visceral afferent fibers, however, pursue exactly the same course as somatic afferents and, once they have joined a branch of a spinal nerve, they cannot be distinguished from somatic afferents.

The Parasympathetic System

Concerned primarily with the viscera, the parasympathetic system has a more limited distribution than the sympathetic system. Smooth muscle and glands associated with somatic structures are not innervated by the parasympathetic system. Parasympathetic stimulation in many respects reverses the effects of sympathetic stimulation. For instance, it slows the heart, relaxes the sphincters of hollow viscera, and stimulates the contraction of smooth muscle in their walls; it also induces glands to secrete in the gastrointestinal and respiratory systems. Unlike its sympathetic counterpart, the parasympathetic system has little to do with controlling the degree of vasoconstriction or vasodilation in tissues. In fact, with one notable exception, parasympathetic stimulation has no known effect on the tone of smooth muscle in the wall of blood vessels. (The exception concerns the erectile tissues in the genitalia, where the parasympathetic system causes vasodilation.) It does apparently induce contraction of muscles in the bronchi. The afferent limb of the system is primarily concerned with visceral reflexes, although it may mediate pain sensation from certain viscera (such as the lung).

Like the sympathetic system, the parasympathetic system consists of visceral efferent and afferent nuclei, preganglionic and postganglionic visceral efferents, visceral afferents, and autonomic as well as sensory ganglia. The visceral efferent nuclei of the parasympathetic system are located in two distant regions of the central nervous system: in the brain stem, associated with cranial nerves III, VII, IX, and X; and in the intermediolateral cell column of S-2, S-3, and S-4 spinal cord segments (Fig. 7-8). The anatomy of the parasympathetic system can be sufficiently illustrated by describing the parts of the system associated with the sacral spinal cord and with the vagus nerve. The other cranial nerves are rather specialized and are discussed in chapters dealing with the head.

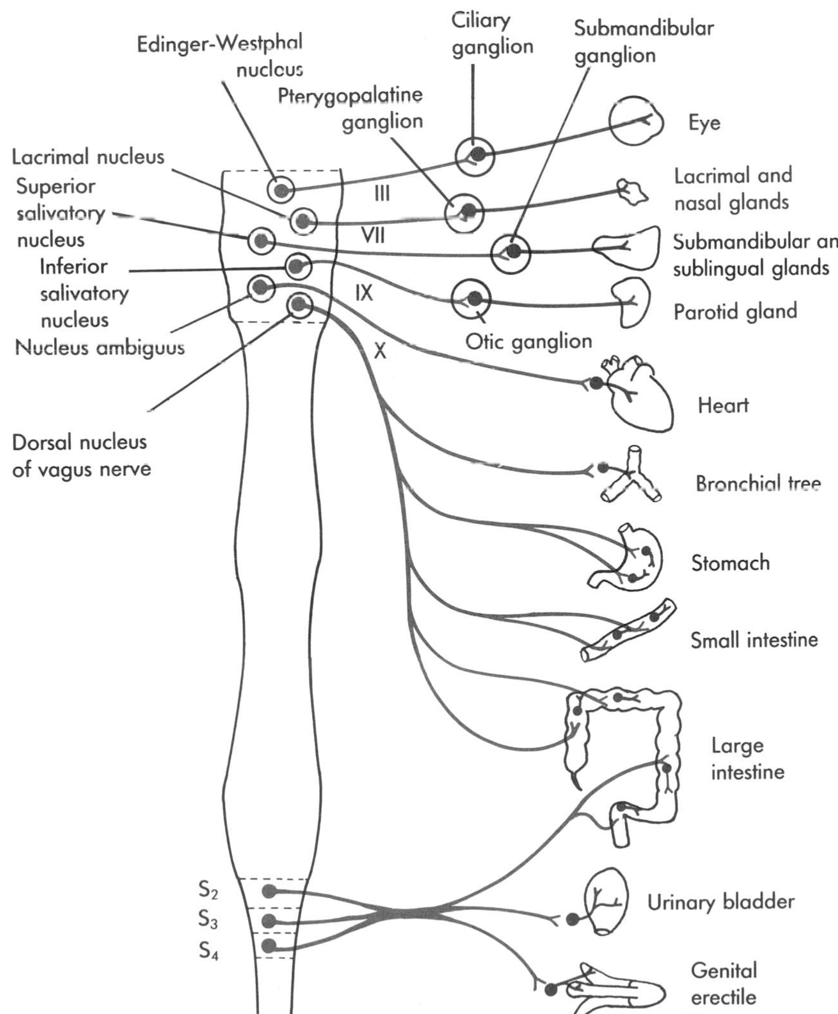

FIGURE 7-8.
The motor components of the parasympathetic nervous system: Preganglionic fibers are *red*: postganglionic fibers *blue*. (Barr ML, Kiernan JA. The human nervous system: an anatomical viewpoint. 4th ed. Philadelphia: Harper & Row, 1983.)

Parasympathetic Visceral Efferents. In S-2 to S-4 segments of the spinal cord, the cell bodies of preganglionic parasympathetic neurons are located in the intermediolateral cell column. Their axons leave the cord along with somatic efferents through the anterior roots of the spinal nerves and, thence, into the anterior rami. Up to this point, the pathway corresponds with that of sympathetic preganglionic fibers, which leave the cord at higher levels (T-1 to L-2). After reaching the spinal nerves' anterior rami, however, the parasympathetic fibers do not enter the sympathetic trunk through white rami communicantes (which, in any event, do not exist in the sacral region), but rather, leave the anterior rami lateral to the sympathetic trunks as independent nerves, called the **pelvic splanchnic nerves.** These nerves, branching directly from the anterior rami and carrying *parasympathetic* preganglionic fibers, are to be distinguished from the sacral splanchnic nerves mentioned earlier, which are the visceral branches of paravertebral ganglia in the sacral region and carry *sympathetic* preganglionic fibers.

The pelvic splanchnic nerves pass medially toward the pelvic viscera. The ganglion cells on which these fibers synapse do not form discrete ganglia; instead, they are spread out in plexuses within the walls of the viscera served by these nerves. Therefore, the postganglionic fibers are of microscopic dimensions and are "intramural." When associated with the gut, these ganglia are called **enteric ganglia,** and the intramural nerve plexus, of which they are part, is described as the **enteric nervous system.**

The viscera that are innervated by pelvic splanchnic nerves include the bladder, the rectum, and the descending and sigmoid colon (parts of the embryonic hindgut; see Fig. 7-8). They also innervate the erectile tissue of the external genitalia in both sexes.

Thoracic viscera and most of the abdominal viscera (those derived from the foregut and the midgut) receive their parasympathetic innervation through preganglionic neurons of the **vagus nerve.** These neurons are located in the vagal visceral efferent nucleus in the brain stem (medulla oblongata) and their axons descend within the vagus, along with other types of vagal nerve fibers, through the neck and thorax and into the abdomen (see Fig. 7-8). The vagus gives off a number of branches for the supply of thoracic viscera as it passes through the neck and the thorax. These fibers join the plexuses that transmit the sympathetic innervation of these viscera (e.g., cardiac plexus or pulmonary plexus). Entering the abdomen, the vagus breaks up into branches and disperses its fibers along the aortic plexus and subsidiary plexuses that accompany arteries to the viscera. After joining a plexus, whether in the thorax or the abdomen, the vagal preganglionic fibers become admixed with postganglionic sympathetic fibers; they terminate on ganglion cells that form plexuses within the walls of the viscera innervated by the vagus.

Preganglionic parasympathetic efferents that leave the brain stem through cranial nerves III, VII, and IX, in contrast with those in the vagus, terminate in discrete autonomic ganglia before they actually reach their target organs (see Fig. 7-8). These are the ciliary, pterygopalatine, submandibular, and otic ganglia, which contain autonomic ganglion cells. The postganglionic fibers are longer than those in the efferent pathways, described in the foregoing, that involve the pelvic splanchnic nerves and the vagus. They terminate on smooth muscle that alters the size of the pupil and the curvature of the lens in the eye, as well as on the lacrimal (tear) glands and salivary glands.

Parasympathetic Visceral Afferents. Visceral afferents are carried in the pelvic splanchnic nerves and the vagus. The cell bodies for visceral afferents in pelvic splanchnic nerves are located in sacral spinal ganglia and correspond to those described for sympathetic visceral afferents. The cell bodies for vagal visceral afferents are located in the sensory ganglia of the vagus, which are swellings on the nerve just before it enters the skull. The types of sensations conveyed by these afferents from different viscera are described in the appropriate chapters.

RECOMMENDED READINGS

Adams WE. The blood supply of nerves: historical review. J Anat 1942; 76: 323.

Angevine JB. The nervous tissue. In: Fawcett DW, ed. Bloom and Fawcett: a textbook of histology. 12th ed. New York: Chapman & Hall, 1994: 309.

Barr ML, Kiernan JA. The human nervous system: an anatomical viewpoint. 6th ed. Philadelphia: Lippincott, 1993.

Collins JD, Shaver ML, Batra P, Brown K. Nerves on magnetic resonance imaging. J Natl Med Assoc 1989; 81: 129.

Devinsky O, Feldmann E. Examination of the cranial and peripheral nerves. New York: Churchill Livingstone, 1988.

Gershon MD. The enteric nervous system. Annu Rev Neurosci 1981; 4: 227.

Granit R. The basis of motor control. New York: Academic Press, 1970.

Haines DE. Neuroanatomy: an atlas of structures, sections, and systems. 4th ed. Baltimore: Urban & Schwarzenberg, 1995.

O'Connell JEA. The intraneural plexus and its significance. J Anat 1936; 70: 468.

Pearson AA, Eckhardt AL. Observations on the gray and white rami communicantes in human embryos. Anat Rec 1960; 138: 115.

Pick J. The autonomic nervous system: morphological, comparative, clinical and surgical aspects. Philadelphia: JB Lippincott, 1970.

Shanthaveerappa TR, Bourne GH. The effects of transection of the nerve trunk on the perineural epithelium with special reference to its role in nerve degeneration and regeneration. Anat Rec 1964; 150: 35.

Sunderland S. The connective tissues of peripheral nerves. Brain 1966; 88: 841.

Triplett B, Ochoa JL. Contemporary techniques in assessing peripheral nervous system function. Am J EEG Technol 1990; 30: 29.

Vallbo AB, Hagbarth K-E, Torebjörk HE, Wallin BG. Somatosensory, proprioceptive and sympathetic activity in human peripheral nerves. Physiol Rev 1979; 59: 919.

Williams PL, Bannister LH, Berry MM, et al, eds. Gray's anatomy. 38th ed. New York: Churchill Livingstone, 1995.

Hollinshead's Textbook of Anatomy, by Cornelius Rosse and Penelope Gaddum-Rosse.
Lippincott-Raven Publishers, Philadelphia, © 1997.

CHAPTER 8

The Cardiovascular and Lymphatic Systems

The *cardiovascular system* is composed of the heart and all the vessels through which blood passes. The heart pumps blood into the arteries; these terminate in capillaries, from which blood is returned to the heart by veins. The lymphatic system consists of lymphatic capillaries that begin blindly in the tissues and collect tissue fluid. The **lymphatic vessels** convey this fluid, called lymph, toward the base of the neck, where they empty it into veins. The lymphatic system also includes collections of lymphatic tissue that have to do with the immune responses of the body.

Radiological examination of various parts of these systems in the living person has become a useful diagnostic tool. The technique, known generally as angiography, consists of injecting a small amount of radiopaque material into an appropriate vessel and taking radiographs that will show the passage of the material through the region to be examined. It has been used to study the heart and great vessels (cardioangiography), various arteries (arteriography), veins (venography), and lymphatics and lymph nodes (lymphangiography or lymphography).

GENERAL STRUCTURE

Vessels

Because blood vessels and lymphatics are built on the same fundamental plan, their essential structure can be discussed together. The blood vessels are classified into **arteries,** vessels that conduct blood away from the heart; **veins,** vessels that conduct blood toward the heart; and **capillaries,** very small vessels distributed through the tissues of the body to bring the blood into close contact with the cells of the tissues and connect the arteries to the veins. **Lymphatics** are divisible into lymphatic capillaries and larger lymphatic vessels.

Because an artery conducts blood from the heart, its wall must be sufficiently strong to withstand the sudden thrust imposed on it with every heart beat. The walls of arteries are, therefore, thicker and stronger than those of veins of similar diameter. Lymphatics have the thinnest walls of all and are particularly difficult to recognize in dissection because of their generally small size and because their contents are colorless.

All blood vessels and lymphatics have a lining of flattened cells, known as **endothelial cells.** The integrity of this layer is essential to normal blood flow. If it is injured, blood cells begin to stick at the point of injury and build up a blood clot. In vessels larger than capillaries, the endothelial cells are supported by a thin layer of connective tissue. The endothelium plus its supporting connective tissue constitutes the **intima** (tunica intima). In blood vessels of the size seen at dissection, the next layer wrapped around the intima is the **media** (tunica media), which consists of a layer of smooth muscle and elastic tissue. The third and outer coat of such a blood vessel is composed primarily of loose connective tissue, the **adventitia** (tunica adventitia). The adventitia binds vessels loosely to the connective tissue in which they run and contains nerves and small blood vessels that supply the wall of the vessel. Larger lymphatics have a similar structure.

The structural differences among arteries, veins, and lymphatics are primarily the degree of development of the media and adventitia, especially the former. For any given size, arteries tend to have a much stronger and thicker media, veins a more poorly developed one, and lymphatics the most poorly developed of all. In both veins and lymphatics, the smooth muscle of the media may be so poorly developed that the connective tissue of the typical three layers blends together with no clear distinction between the layers. Also, the walls of arteries contain fairly prominent elastic tissue, whereas those of veins and lymphatics do not.

Arteries

Arteries are generally divisible into **elastic** and **muscular types,** although the media of most arteries contains some of both types of tissue. Elastic tissue allows the wall of an artery to be distended by the sudden thrust of blood from the heart and then to contract again, which helps force the blood forward, with no initiation of energy by the wall of the vessel. To move the same amount of blood, the thrust—the work of the heart—would have to be much greater if the arteries were inelastic. The large arteries near the heart typically contain a great deal more elastic tissue than do the smaller, more distal ones; in general, the greater the pressure in an artery, the more elastic tissue there is. For example, the pressure in the great trunk (pulmonary trunk) going to the lungs is much less than that in the great trunk (aorta) carrying blood to the body as a whole; therefore, the wall of the aorta contains far more elastic tissue than the pulmonary trunk. Elastic tissue serves the double purpose of cushioning the sudden rise of pressure induced by the heart beat and of smoothing, by its automatic recoil, what would, in an inelastic system, be a sudden drop in pressure. In hardening of the arteries (arteriosclerosis), in which the elasticity is interfered with by the deposition of fatty and, eventually, calcified material in the intima and sometimes the media, the blood pressure undergoes abnormally great fluctuation with each cardiac cycle (beginning of one heart beat to beginning of the next).

In the larger arteries, particularly the aorta, most of the strength of the wall is provided by elastic tissue. If this undergoes degenerative changes, or is destroyed by disease, the arterial wall may bulge, either in one spot or all around. Such a widening of the arterial lumen is an *aneurysm* and always involves the danger that the weakened wall may burst which may be life-threatening

As branches of the aorta are traced distally, the relative amount of elastic tissue becomes less and the relative amount of smooth muscle more. The elastic tissue of the peripheral arteries tends to smooth the pressure and lessen the velocity of the blood. The smooth muscle, controlled by the autonomic nervous system, can contract or relax to vary the caliber of the vessel and, thereby, the blood flow through it. Even rather large vessels, for instance, the chief arteries of the arm and thigh, contain sufficient smooth muscle to reduce to a dangerous level the blood flow through them if they are incited to maximal contraction. The smallest arteries, **arterioles,** have a media composed almost entirely of smooth muscle and are particularly contractile. It is through the activity of the arterioles that blood is shunted from one place to another, and they are the most important governors of the peripheral resistance to blood flow. If too many arterioles are simultaneously relaxed, blood pressure drops drastically; if too many are contracted, or so diseased that they cannot relax, high blood pressure ensues.

Anastomoses and End Arteries. Most parts of the body receive branches from more than one artery, and where two or more arteries supply the same territory, they usually connect with each other (anastomose). The number and size of anastomoses vary considerably with the region or organ (and often with the individual). In many locations, there are one or more macroscopic (dissectible) anastomoses and numerous finer ones. An anastomosis between vessels may be by small terminal branches that result from repeated divisions, or two vessels of considerable size may simply join end to end (inosculate) with such little diminution in caliber that it is impossible to tell at what point the two vessels meet.

Anastomoses between arteries provide alternative ways in which blood can reach a given tissue or organ; therefore, their number and size (ability to conduct blood) are critical when the blood supply from one or more sources is cut off. Usually, a region is supplied more particularly by one artery than by others, and the anastomotic alternative paths by which blood can reach the field of distribution of the chief artery are known as the **collateral circulation.** Since blood vessels enlarge as more and more blood tries to go through them, collateral circulation is best developed by slow occlusion of the main artery. This ability to gradually enlarge is of no help in instances of sudden occlusion unless the collateral circulation is capable of dilating rapidly enough to carry sufficient blood to keep the tissue alive. In general, this depends on the total caliber of the collateral circulation. (Collateral circulation can sometimes, but not always, be effectively increased by a sympathectomy that paralyzes the smooth muscle.) Knowledge of the anatomy of the collateral circulation to a part is essential if the reasons for death or survival of a part (and of a patient) following an arterial occlusion are to be understood. During surgical procedures, the anatomy of the collateral circulation may also be of critical importance; some vessels can be ligated at any level with impunity, others can never be ligated without damage because there is insufficient collateral circulation, and still others must be ligated at a level calculated to spare the greatest possible amount of collateral circulation if further injury is not to be done.

Until the latter half of the 20th century, there was no method of averting gangrene (massive death of tissue), or sometimes death of the patient, when an artery without adequate collateral circulation was occluded by a disease process or by ligation. With various techniques of suturing and grafting (arteries, veins, and synthetic tubes, have all been used as grafts), continuity of the vessel after removing the injured segment can often be restored, thereby preventing or minimizing the damage that would otherwise ensue.

Just as anastomotic channels occur between arteries to a region, so may they also occur between arteries that supply an organ. This is true, for instance, of the vessels in the wall of the stomach, which anastomose so freely with each other that the surgeon does not hesitate to ligate any of the supplying vessels. However, other organs, among them the most vital—the brain, the heart, the liver, and the kidneys—are supplied by arteries that, beyond a certain point, within the organ, have no anastomoses with each other, or such small ones as to be totally inadequate. Arteries that do not anastomose are known as **end arteries.** Occlusion of an end artery interrupts the blood supply to a whole segment of the organ, producing necrosis (death) of that segment; the area of necrosis is known as an **infarct.** Results of infarction necessarily vary according to its size and location. True end arteries occur in the brain, kidney, and liver, but infarctions in the brain are more injurious for a given size because uninjured tissue of the kidney and liver is usually functionally adequate, whereas there are many parts of the brain for which no other part can substitute. The heart does not have true end arteries in its wall, but anastomoses are normally so small that most of the vessels are functional end arteries. The results of ischemia (decreased blood supply) to the heart vary from very mild to fatal heart attacks, the final outcome depending largely on the size of the infarct.

Capillaries, Sinusoids, and Arteriovenous Anastomoses

Most arterioles empty into capillaries, tiny channels (little larger than the diameter of a red blood cell) with endothelial walls through which the blood is in close contact with the tissues. Because of the pressure of the blood, a certain amount of its fluid escapes through the endothelial wall of capillaries to become tissue fluid, thereby providing the liquid environment in which all living cells need to be suspended. Through interchange between the blood plasma and the tissue fluid, oxygen, carbon dioxide, and nutrients, carried by the bloodstream, and metabolic wastes, produced by the cells, can pass back and forth between the bloodstream and the cells.

Although capillary walls apparently contain contractile elements, circulation through any given capillary bed is determined primarily by the arterioles that feed it. In many tissues, capillaries form a dense interconnecting network, fed by several arterioles, but bone and tendon have a relatively poor blood supply, cartilage has no capillary network, and stratified epithelium contains no blood vessels at all. The density of the capillary bed seems to be primarily related to the functional activity of the organ. In some organs, as was intimated in the discussion of end arteries, a large capillary bed receives its blood entirely from arterioles that are all branches of the same artery.

Sinusoids, found in a few locations (for instance, the liver and spleen) are specialized capillaries of unusually large diameter. Instead of the usual lining of endothelial cells, however, the walls of sinusoids are largely composed of special phagocytic cells (in the liver, Kupffer cells).

Although capillaries are the usual connection between arteries and veins, there also are sometimes larger connections, arteriovenous anastomoses. **Arteriovenous anastomoses** are essentially arterioles with especially contractile walls that open directly into venules. Through their contraction and relaxation, they can play an important part in the circulation to the tissues, because their relaxation diverts blood that would otherwise pass through the capillary network, directly into the venous system. Arteriovenous anastomoses have been found in many locations, but the exact way in which they fit into the physiology of the bloodstream is not yet understood. Arteriovenous anastomoses that are normal structures are not to be confused with abnormal communications between arteries and veins. These are properly known as arteriovenous aneurysms or fistulae. In certain locations, arteriovenous anastomoses sometimes give rise to painful tumors, known as "glomus tumors."

Veins and Sinuses

The smallest veins, **venules,** are formed by the junction of capillaries and consist only of an intima and a thin layer of connective tissue, the adventitia. Larger and larger veins are formed by the junction of smaller veins, and in veins of medium size, a media appears, containing smooth muscle in variable amounts, but never to the degree that arteries of comparable diameter do. In the larger veins close to the heart (where the blood pressure is very low), there may be no media, and the adventitia often has longitudinally arranged smooth muscle.

Veins anastomose much more freely than do arteries; therefore, they afford more abundant collateral circulation on the venous side. Consequently, occlusion of veins is rarely a cause of necrosis, although it may be if the occluded vein is large and there are only small anastomotic channels, or if a considerable length of vein is occluded (e.g., by a thrombus) and many collateral channels are shut off. Occlusion of even large veins commonly leads to only temporary edema (accumulation of fluid in the tissues), which disappears as the collateral circulation enlarges.

Sinuses (vascular sinuses; there are also air sinuses, and certain pathologic openings are likewise called sinuses) are veins with very thin walls for their diameter. In the best example, the intracranial sinuses, the true wall of the vein is nothing but endothelium. The endothelium is supported by the heavy connective tissue surrounding the brain (the dura mater) in which the sinuses lie, so this actually replaces the usual media and adventitia of the venous channel.

Valves. The two chief factors in directing the flow of blood in veins toward the heart are the slight positive or even the negative pressure obtaining in the thorax and the massaging action of muscles on veins. In the limbs, the effectiveness of the massage, which might, under certain circumstances, drive blood toward the periphery rather than toward the heart, is ensured by the presence of valves in the veins. Venous valves are infoldings of the intima, so arranged that they allow free passage of blood toward the heart but impede or prevent passage of blood in the reverse direction. Venous valves are often bicuspid, the elements of a pair meeting along their edges in the middle of the vessel, but sometimes they have only one cusp, or they may have three. Inefficiency of the valves in the veins connecting the deep and superficial veins of the lower limb allows the pumping action of the muscles to force blood from the deep venous system into the superficial veins, thus overloading and dilating them. Dilated, tortuous veins are known as varicose veins.

There are few or no functionally efficient valves in the veins of the abdomen, but under the squeezing action of the abdominal muscles and the diaphragm, blood flow into the region of lesser pressure provided by the thorax is far easier than backflow into the valved veins of the lower limb, so valves are not really needed here. In the same way, the veins of the head and neck do not, for the most part, need valves to resist backflow, since flow toward the heart is assisted both by the decreased pressure and by gravity; there are few valves in this part of the venous system.

Lymphatics and Lymph Nodes

Lymphatic capillaries are essentially similar to blood capillaries in that they have only an endothelial wall, through which water and certain larger molecules can pass freely. They differ in that they begin blindly. Lymph, derived from tissue fluid, enters the lymphatic capillaries by passing through the capillary wall. In some tissues, lymphatic capillaries are sparse. In some, such as the central nervous system, they apparently do not exist at all. In still other locations, for instance the dermis of the skin, they may form plexuses so dense that it is almost impossible to inject substances into the tissue without filling the lymphatic plexus. The rapid spread obtained through the lymphatics is used when intradermal, rather than subcutaneous, injections are given, as, for instance, for immunization against typhoid fever.

Larger lymphatics are formed by the union of smaller ones, and these lymphatics resemble veins in structure except that they have an even more poorly developed media than a vein of corresponding size. Lymphatics are regularly provided with valves, like those of the veins of the limbs, to ensure flow of lymph away from the tissues and toward the venous system. They tend to anastomose freely.

In their course toward the venous system, many lymphatics empty into lymph nodes, instead of joining others directly. **Lymph nodes** are collections of lymphocytes (one type of white blood cell) held together by connective tissue and permeated by lymphatic channels. Each lymph node typically receives several lymphatic vessels (termed "afferent," since they are carrying lymph to the node), and the lymph from all these circulates through the lymph channels of the node, leaving it usually by a single efferent vessel. Lymph may pass for some distance through larger and larger lymphatic channels without passing through a lymph node, or it may pass successively through several nodes. Typically, all lymph has passed through several lymph nodes before it is returned to the venous system.

If a lymphatic vessel bears cancer cells that have invaded it and are floating in its stream, the filtering action of the lymph node tends to retain these cells within the node; hence, those cancers that spread through the lymphatic system tend to migrate (metastasize) first to lymph nodes, where they typically grow at the expense of the node, gradually destroying it. Because they do not migrate farther until they are well established in the first node that they reach, cancer that has begun to spread can sometimes be eradicated entirely by removing, in addition to the original lesion, the lymph nodes that first receive the drainage from the region of the lesion (called "primary lymph nodes") or by exposing the nodes to radiation that can inhibit or destroy that type of cancer. Thus, detailed knowledge of the usual lymphatic drainage of an organ and of the lymph nodes into which this drainage passes may be of great importance.

The filtering action of lymph nodes, particularly dramatic when it involves cancer cells, is also apparent when the lymph nodes about the lung of a city dweller are examined. The carbon particles breathed in from the smoke in city air are deposited not only in the connective tissue of the lung (taken there by phagocytes), but also in the lymph nodes draining the lung, so that these nodes' may be black and gritty.

Another function of lymph nodes is to produce lymphocytes, the second most common type of white blood cell. Lymph nodes also participate in the production of antibodies.

The lymphatic vessels act with blood capillaries and veins to remove tissue fluid that leaks out from the arterial side of the capillaries; therefore, obstruction of either the venous or the lymphatic drainage of a part may produce excessive accumulation of tissue fluid, **edema.** In the digestive tract, lymphatics also carry out a function that the blood capillaries apparently cannot perform: They receive almost all of the fat absorbed by the digestive system. In addition to the lymphocytes and the fat that lymphatics return to the venous system, lymph has a high protein content. Loss of large amounts of lymph through rupture of a major lymphatic vessel produces serious deficiencies in the protein and salt content of the blood.

Blood Supply and Innervation of Vessels

Because larger blood vessels and lymphatics have relatively thick walls, the tissue of these walls cannot receive adequate nutrition from the blood contained within the vessel itself; thus, blood vessels that are approximately a millimeter or more in diameter receive vessels, *vasa vasorum,* from adjacent small blood vessels. These lie in the adventitia and form a capillary network there, but do not pass very far into the media in arteries; in veins they are said to go sometimes as far as the intima. Lymphatics even smaller than a millimeter in diameter have a blood supply.

Little is known concerning the innervation of lymphatics. As might be expected, the more muscular arteries have a better innervation than do the less muscular arteries and veins. The motor innervation of the blood vessels is entirely by the sympathetic nervous system, and the usual effect of activity of this system is to cause contraction of the circular smooth muscle of the vessel; hence, constriction of its diameter. The arterioles, with their almost entirely muscular walls, have a particularly rich innervation, and it is primarily through these vessels that peripheral blood flow is regulated by the sympathetic system.

Arteries and veins also receive afferent fibers. Many of these fibers are concerned with pain. In certain locations also, especially on the great veins and arteries close to the heart and on the chief arteries to the brain (internal carotids), there are areas of afferent endings that react to changes of the blood pressure within the vessel and that reflexly affect the autonomic system to raise or lower this pressure. The rate and strength of the heart beat is controlled in part, for example, by impulses originating within the walls of the vascular system, as is the constriction and relaxation of arterioles.

Source of Nerve Fibers. It is common for blood vessels to be accompanied by a nerve plexus, sometimes macroscopic, sometimes microscopic and embedded in the adventitia; but apparently only in the blood vessels to the thoracic and abdominal viscera and to the head does a plexus beginning at the base of a vessel extend throughout the length of that vessel. By contrast, in the limbs, the nerve plexus along a chief artery and its branches is not one continuous plexus, but is a series of interlocking plexuses that are fed at more or less regular intervals by nerve branches derived directly from neighboring peripheral nerves. Interruption of the nerve plexus along the chief artery to the lower limb, for instance, the external iliac, will not abolish the nerve plexus on the femoral or popliteal arteries (the direct continuation of the external iliac into the limb) nor those on their branches. In consequence, a periarterial sympathectomy (stripping the plexus from around a part of an artery), or separation of a length of artery from all neighboring nerves by severing the branches of the nerves to the artery, produces only a local denervation of the vessel. If sympathetic denervation of an entire limb is desired, this can be accomplished only by interrupting the sympathetic nervous system before it has joined the major nerves of the limb. Although the sympathetic fibers travel in these major nerves, it is obviously impractical to interrupt them by sectioning the nerves, since these are also the source of the voluntary motor activity and sensation in the limb.

Heart

The heart (*cor;* cardia) begins its embryologic development as a contractile tube. In spite of the fact that it departs markedly from its original size and shape and, in the adult, is completely divided into right and left sides, it can still be likened to a double-barreled tube, receiving blood at one end (the **atria**) from veins and pumping it out at the other end (the **ventricles**) into the arteries. Because the heart must pump blood in only one direction, it is provided with valves to ensure against backflow from a region of higher to one of lower pressure.

The intimal lining of the heart, continuous with the intima of the vessels connecting to it, is known as the **endocardium** and does not differ essentially from the intima of blood vessels. Reinforced by connective tissue, it also forms the valves that lie between atria and ventricles and at the bases of the two great arterial trunks leaving the heart.

The muscular part of the heart, **myocardium,** is equivalent to the media of a blood vessel. It is a special type of muscle (cardiac muscle) found only in the heart and the great vessels as they attach to it. Although cardiac muscle is striated like skeletal muscle, it differs in all other respects.

The musculature of the atria is thin, because the atria work at a low pressure and have only to drive blood into the relaxed ventricles. The musculature of both ventricles is much thicker than that of the atria, and the musculature of the left ventricle is much thicker than that of the right, as the former must pump blood all over the body, whereas the latter must pump only to the lungs.

The outermost layer of the heart is the **epicardium** (visceral layer of the serous pericardium).

The **pericardium** is a closed sac surrounding the heart. Its outer wall, the fibrous pericardium, is a tough, fibrous, loose-fitting sac. It is lined with the parietal layer of serous pericardium that is reflected onto the heart around the great vessels that are leaving it and along the posterior aspect of the heart where that organ is fused to the pericardium. In these locations the parietal layer of the serous pericardium continues onto the heart as the epicardium or visceral layer of the serous pericardium. Between parietal and visceral layers of the serous pericardium is the **pericardial cavity,** containing a small amount of serous fluid.

The gross morphology of the heart is described later (see chap. 21). This hollow, muscular organ, roughly the size of one's fist, is, in the adult, normally completely divided into sides, through which the blood circulates separately, entering and leaving one side and then returning to the heart to enter and leave the other side (Fig. 8-1). The great veins carrying blood to the heart enter the thin-walled atria; the veins from all of the body except the lungs enter the right atrium, and those from the lungs enter the left atrium. Each atrium opens into the ventricle of its side. The opening is protected by a valve (atrioventricular valve) so arranged that whereas blood can flow freely from atrium to ventricle, the valve closes as blood starts to flow in the reverse direction. Each ventricle gives rise to a large arterial trunk, the right ventricle giving rise to the pulmonary trunk (to the lungs), the left ventricle to the aorta (distributing blood to the rest of the body).

The musculature of the heart is highly vascular and is fed by two arteries, the **coronary arteries,** that arise from the aorta just after it leaves the heart. Obstruction of a ma-

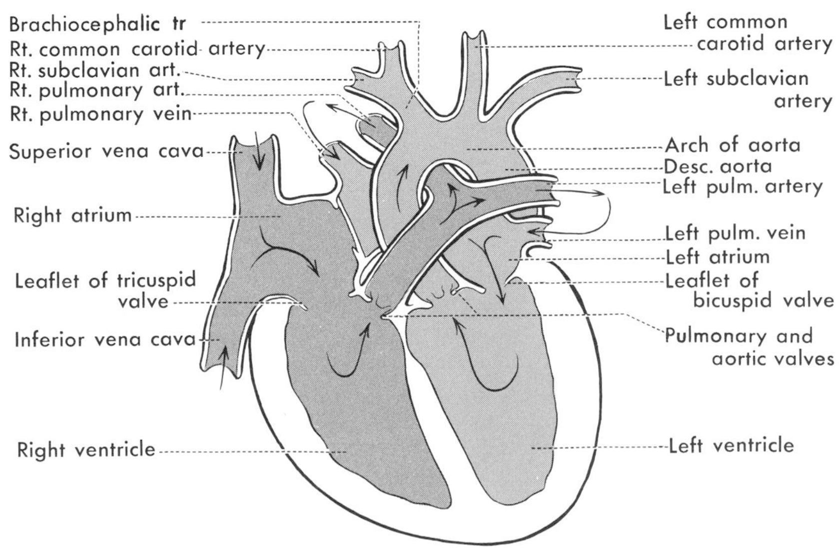

FIGURE *8-1.*
The heart and the great vessels connected to it: The right side of the heart and its connecting vessels are *blue;* the left side of the heart and its connecting vessels are *pink. Arrows* indicate the direction of blood flow.

jor branch of a coronary artery, especially one to a ventricle, is the common cause of a heart attack (myocardial infarct) or sudden heart failure. Too great a narrowing of a major branch of an artery, or occlusion of minor branches, produces ischemia of the cardiac muscle. The pain produced by this is known as *angina pectoris*. For the most part, the cardiac veins that collect the blood delivered to the myocardium by the coronary arteries parallel these arteries, but all the larger ones empty into a single vein, the coronary sinus, that returns the blood to the right atrium.

The heart also has a nerve supply that contains both afferent fibers (including ones of pain) and motor fibers (see Chap. 21). The motor nerve supply acts on the heart to modify (i.e., increase or decrease) the rate and strength of the heart beat according to the needs of the body.

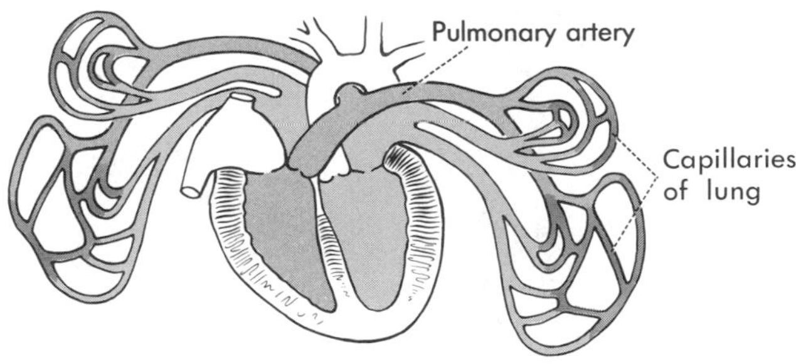

FIGURE 8-2.
The pulmonary circulation: The right ventricle and the pulmonary arterial system are *blue*; the pulmonary veins and the left atrium are *pink*.

CIRCULATION OF THE BLOOD

The anatomy of the circulation of the blood through the heart is very simple. In contrast, the factors governing the peripheral circulation are very complicated and even now not completely understood. An understanding of a few basic phenomena will, however, serve as an introduction to the subject.

Circulation Through the Heart

Because the heart is divided into right and left sides, there are two circulations through it (Figs. 8-2 and 8-3). Both occur simultaneously and are equal in volume, but it is convenient to trace a given quantity of blood from the time it enters one side of the heart until it returns again to that side.

Blood from the head and neck, the upper limbs, and the thoracic wall enters the right atrium by the superior vena cava; blood from the abdomen, pelvis, and lower limbs enters this atrium by the inferior vena cava; and blood that has circulated to the cardiac muscle enters the right atrium through the coronary sinus. The right atrium thus receives blood that has passed through capillaries in the tissues of the body, lost much of its oxygen, and picked up much of the carbon dioxide in the tissues. As the blood runs into the right atrium, some of it continues on into the relaxed right ventricle. Contraction of the right atrium injects more blood into this ventricle. At this moment, the right ventricle begins to contract and to force blood out through the pulmonary trunk to the lungs. Backward passage into the relaxing atrium is normally prevented by the right atrioventricular valve, which is closed by the rising intraventricular pressure. Similarly, the blood forced by the right ventricle into the pulmonary trunk (so called because it is a common trunk for the paired pulmonary arteries) is prevented from returning to the relaxing ventricle by the pulmonary valve at the level of origin of the pulmonary trunk from the ventricle.

After passing through the pulmonary trunk and its branches, and through the capillaries and smaller veins of the lungs, the blood sent to the lungs by the right ventricle is returned to the left atrium by pulmonary veins. As occurs in the right side of the heart, contraction of the left atrium injects additional blood into the left ventricle. Contraction of the ventricle closes the left atrioventricular valve and forces blood out through the aorta. Closure of the aortic valve at the base of the aorta prevents regurgitation of blood into the relaxing left ventricle. The blood is then delivered through the branches of the aorta to the tissues of the body, where it loses oxygen, picks up carbon dioxide, and returns to the right side of the heart to begin its double cycle all over again.

Because the blood is constantly circulating, both to the lungs and to the tissues of the body, it is obviously important that both sides of the heart handle the same amount of blood. If, for instance, the right side fails to send to the lungs all the blood it has received from the left side, it will be overfilled by the next inflow of blood and will have to dilate slightly to receive it. If it then does not beat strongly enough to expel all the blood it has just received plus the residue from the previous beat, it must remain dilated or dilate still more. Normally, dilation of the heart produces a stronger beat, so at some stage of dilation, the beat usually becomes strong enough to restore the balance of circulation (*compensation*). If the heart muscle of the dilated side finally begins to fail (*decompensation*), rapid dilation and more serious or fatal interference with the circulation ensues. Digitalis is useful in minimizing decompensation because it increases the strength of the heart beat and, therefore, the cardiac output. Epinephrine, which mimics the effects of sympathetic stimulation, has the same effect, but acts more powerfully, more quickly, and over a shorter period than does digitalis; it is, therefore, most useful in emergency situations, whereas digitalis is used in chronic cases of incipient cardiac failure.

Cardiac Cycle

The cardiac cycle is the series of events occurring during one beat of the heart as it fills and empties. The period of

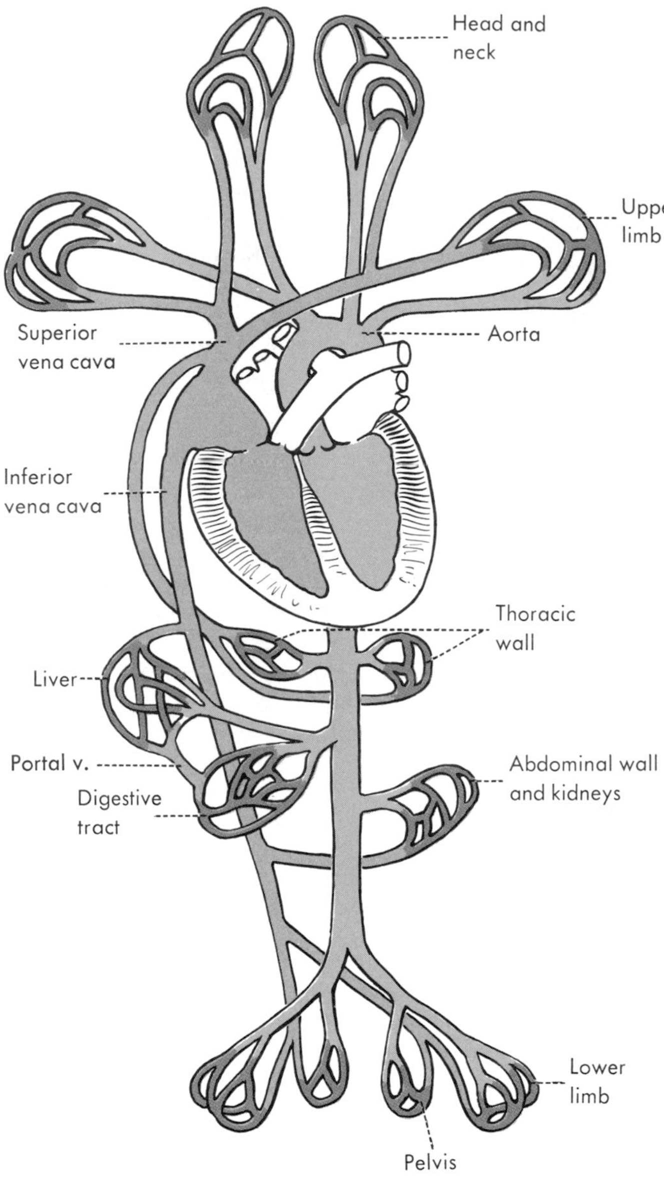

FIGURE *8-3.*
The systemic circulation: The left ventricle, the aorta, and the other arteries are *pink*; the veins, including the portal, are *blue*; the *purple* connections between vessels represent the circulatory pathways in the various parts and organs indicated.

contraction of the heart is **systole,** that of relaxation, **diastole.** Since atria and ventricles contract separately, there is actually an atrial systole and a ventricular systole. Atrial and ventricular diastole overlap. Pressure changes in atrial systole can be measured only by instruments lying within the heart, but ventricular systole can be roughly measured simply by the rapidity and strength of the arterial pulse. Clinically, therefore, the term "systole" usually refers to ventricular systole only, and atrial systole, occurring during ventricular diastole, is usually called a presystolic phenomenon.

The electrocardiogram, based on the principle that contraction of muscle always involves an electrical change, allows the cardiac cycle to be analyzed in detail and thus aids in diagnosis of minor irregularities and local defects in contraction resulting from injury to the musculature. Normal heart sounds are caused by closing of the valves and contraction of the ventricles. A heart murmur is the sound heard when blood under high pressure runs through an abnormal or irregular opening It is often a sign of leakage of blood from ventricle to atrium, or from pulmonary trunk or aorta to ventricle, as a result of imperfect valvular closure.

Contraction of the two atria typically occurs simultaneously and is closely followed by contraction of the ventricles. Although the heart muscle works more continuously than does any other muscle in the body, its periods of rest are greater than its periods of contraction: in a cycle lasting about 0.8 second, atrial contraction lasts for only about 0.1 second, so that the atrial muscle is resting seven-eighths of the time. Ventricular systole lasts only about 0.3 second, so that even the ventricular musculature rests for a longer period than it contracts, and all the cardiac muscle is relaxed at the same time for about half the length of the cardiac cycle.

Peripheral Circulation

The force of the heart beat and the pulsatile contraction of the elastic arteries carry the blood into the capillaries, but because there is a steady increase in the extensiveness of the vascular bed (the total area of channels through which the blood can flow) between the heart and the capillaries, there is also a steady decrease in blood pressure. Blood that leaves the heart through the aorta at a pressure of about 120 mm Hg falls in the capillaries to only 10 mm to 20 mm. Furthermore, the elastic recoil of the arteries gradually converts the pulsatile flow from the heart into a steady flow through the capillaries, and the expansion of the vascular bed slows the velocity of blood from an average of about 0.5 m/sec near the heart to about 0.5 mm/sec in the capillaries. These changes in the blood flow allow a better interchange between the capillaries' contents and the tissues and result in delivery of a steady stream of blood into the venous side of the circulation. The flow into the veins is delivered at very low pressure; therefore, in dependent parts of the body, most notably the lower limbs, the venous return of blood to the heart is made difficult by the effect of gravity. The effect of the valves and of the massage by muscles has already been noted. Blood pressure falls steadily in the veins as they near the heart, often to subatmospheric levels, so that some of the blood is literally sucked into the heart.

The physiology of blood flow and of the factors that affect it and the blood pressure are too complicated to be discussed here, but a few basic principles can be noted. The source of the arterial blood pressure is the thrust given the blood at ventricular systole, but the pressure and rapidity of flow are determined by this and the peripheral resistance together, for the heart must beat more strongly to move blood against greater peripheral resistance. If the arterioles, the chief governors of peripheral resistance, are tonically contracted beyond normal, the heart must work harder to maintain an adequate flow against the increased resistance, and blood pressure rises. In such cases the work on the heart can be lightened and the blood pressure lowered by the administration of appropriate drugs; if, however, the cause of the increased resistance is an arteriosclerotic aorta or irreversible changes in the caliber of the arterioles, such treatment will be useless. The reverse effect occurs in vascular shock, in which, as a result of loss of blood or of pooling of blood in the tissues in consequence of general vasodilation, not enough blood returns to the heart to enable it to maintain normal pressure.

Normally, as blood spreads through the branching arterial system, it encounters some vascular beds that are at the moment more constricted and others that are less constricted; therefore, it flows more freely through the latter, as they are pathways of less resistance. Local vasoconstriction and vasodilation can, therefore, bring about decreased or increased blood flow to an organ or part and shifts in rate of blood flow among parts on the basis of their activity and resultant needs, with no alterations of blood pressure. The volume of blood flow through an artery does not follow the rules that hold for an inelastic system of pipes, in which rate can be calculated from fluid pressure and size of the pipe. Rather, in arteries, the rate of flow drops off far more rapidly with vasoconstriction and with decreases in blood pressure than mathematical calculations would indicate. A general lowering of blood pressure, combined with vasoconstriction in a given part, or even partial block of a large artery, can result in markedly reduced or even total cessation of flow to a part.

Much of the venous blood pressure is hydrostatic; therefore, venous return to the heart is expedited by elevating a part above the level of the heart, a procedure commonly followed in alleviating any swelling caused or contributed to by venous congestion.

BASIC GROSS ANATOMY

A general comprehension of the gross anatomy of the cardiovascular and lymphatic systems is necessary if the parts studied regionally are to be fitted into their proper places in these systems. For the cardiovascular system, it has already been noted that because arteries conduct blood away from the heart, the largest arteries are those that leave the heart. The large arteries branch and rebranch until finally they end in capillaries. In the same fashion, small veins are formed from capillaries, and larger veins are formed by the union of these. The largest veins are those that empty blood back into the heart.

Many branches of the expanding vascular tree, as one follows the arteries, and many tributaries of the contracting vascular tree, as one follows the veins, are named. Generally speaking, although not always, arteries and veins run together and, therefore, have the same name. There is no rule for how small an artery must be to be considered unworthy of a name, but usually the named arteries are those that one can readily dissect. Even in vital organs where the detailed blood supply is of particular interest, named arteries are, for the most part, at least a millimeter in diameter. In locations (such as the limbs) where the finer pattern of branching is not particularly important, the named vessels are generally much larger.

Both arteries and veins vary somewhat in pattern from one person to another, as might be expected from their method of development. As a rule, variations in the arterial pattern are less common than those in the venous pattern. Indeed, many variations in the venous pattern are so common that little attention is paid to them. For instance, the detailed pattern of the superficial veins on the back of the hand is so varied that probably no two patterns exactly coincide, even though all usually correspond to the same general plan. Variations in superficial veins for precise pattern, size, and termination or connections are particularly numerous. The deep veins that accompany arteries tend to vary in the same manner as do the arteries they accompany. Major variations in those veins of the abdomen and thorax that do not quite parallel arteries can usually be explained on the basis of their complex embryologic development.

Because arterial variations are less common than venous ones, they tend to be more striking. Also, because arteries tend to anastomose less freely than veins, and a misplaced artery is often potentially more dangerous (anomalous superficial arteries have been mistaken for veins, and misplaced deep arteries may exert pressure on a vital structure), variations in the arteries tend to be of more anatomic and clinical interest than variations in veins. The common types of arterial variation are those of size and distribution of branches, origin of a vessel at a higher or lower level than usual, combined origin of vessels that usually arise separately, and origin of a usual branch of a vessel either independently from a parent trunk or from another neighboring vessel. More important and less commonly encountered variations (anomalies) are usually combinations of abnormal origin and course; many of these can be understood by knowledge of the normal developmental history of the artery concerned.

Subdivisions of the Blood Vascular System

The peripheral vascular system is divided into two parts: the pulmonary circulation, to the lungs, and the systemic circulation, to the rest of the body. Pulmonary arteries and pulmonary veins go to and from the lungs, and systemic arteries and veins go to and from all the tissues, organs, and organ systems of the body (see Figs. 8-2 and 8-3). In addition, a system of veins drains most of the digestive tract and ends in the sinusoids of the liver, rather than joining veins going to the heart. This system of veins differs from almost all other veins in that it both begins and ends in capillaries. Because it carries blood to the liver, it is known as the portal system. In some lower animals, there is also a renal portal system, through which blood beginning in venous capillaries is filtered through capillaries in the kidney before returning to the heart, but in humans and other mammals the "hepatic" portal system is the only major portal system; hence, the qualifying word "hepatic" is not used.

Pulmonary Vessels

The two **pulmonary arteries,** one to each lung, arise from a single **pulmonary trunk** that, in turn, arises from the right ventricle. At its base, the pulmonary trunk is provided with a pulmonary valve, consisting of three cusps. The trunk is a short stem lying within (i.e., surrounded by) the pericardial cavity, branching at the uppermost part of this cavity into right and left pulmonary arteries. These go to the right and left lungs.

Within the substance of the lung, the pulmonary arteries branch and rebranch, as do systemic vessels elsewhere, but in general they follow the air passages. The arterioles of the pulmonary arteries are, in turn, continuous with capillaries that form a very close network in intimate contact with the air sacs (alveoli) within the lung and, hence, are particularly adapted to easy interchange of gases between the air sacs and the bloodstream.

The pulmonary veins, draining the capillary plexus of the lung, are formed by the confluence of smaller veins. Instead of all the veins from the right lung going together to form a single vein, and those of the left lung doing likewise, however, there usually are two right and two left pulmonary veins. Both sets of pulmonary veins empty into the left atrium, so that this atrium normally receives four veins.

Bearing in mind that the right atrium and ventricle receive blood returned from the general tissues of the body, it should be obvious that the pulmonary arteries carry to the lungs blood poor in oxygen, but rich in carbon dioxide, and the pulmonary veins return to the heart blood low in carbon dioxide, but rich in oxygen.

Systemic Arteries

The left ventricle, receiving oxygenated blood from the lungs by way of the pulmonary veins and left atrium, gives rise to the *aorta* which, in turn, gives rise, directly or indirectly, to all the systemic arteries (Fig. 8-4). As the aorta leaves the ventricle, it is directed upward, but it soon arches to the left and backward to attain a position on the left side of the vertebral column. Because of this arrangement, the aorta is conveniently divided into **ascending aorta, arch** (both of which are short), and **descending aorta.** The descending aorta is, in turn, conveniently described as being thoracic or abdominal, the continuity of the two parts being at the level at which the aorta passes through the diaphragm.

Close to its base and the cusps of the aortic valve, the ascending aorta gives off paired coronary arteries that supply the musculature of the heart. The arch of the aorta normally gives off three arterial trunks, the first being the **brachiocephalic trunk;** the second, the **left common carotid artery;** and the third, the **left subclavian artery.** After a short course upward, the brachiocephalic trunk divides in the base of the neck into a **right subclavian artery** and a **right common carotid.** The left common carotid and left subclavian parallel each other into the base of the neck.

Head and Neck. The two common carotid arteries, left and right, are similar. Each runs upward in the neck, lateral to the trachea or windpipe (where it can be palpated) and divides at about the upper border of the larynx (Adam's apple) into external and internal carotid arteries. Normally, there are no branches of the common carotid except these terminal ones. The **external carotid** gives off a series of branches to structures in the neck (the neck also obtains a blood supply from branches of the subclavian artery), and both superficial and deep branches to the face and jaws. The **internal carotid** artery, in contrast, gives off no branches in the neck. It runs upward and enters the skull and ends by dividing into several important branches to the brain.

Upper Limb. Although differing slightly in origin, the two **subclavian arteries** are essentially similar. At the base of the neck each gives off branches to the neck, the shoulder, and the thorax; one, the vertebral, runs the length of the neck to enter the skull and add to the blood supply of the brain. The subclavian artery leaves the neck by passing across the first rib, between this and the overlying clavicle, into the axilla (armpit), where its name is changed to **axillary artery.**

The axillary artery gives off a number of branches to the shoulder, the uppermost part of the arm, and the thoracic wall. As it leaves the axilla to run down the medial side of the arm, it becomes the **brachial artery.** The brachial artery ends in front of the elbow by dividing into **radial** and **ulnar arteries,** which course downward on the anterior aspect of the forearm in the positions indicated by their names; they end by supplying the hand and digits.

Thorax. Because the lungs and heart, the large organs in the thorax, receive their blood supplies from the pulmonary and coronary arteries, respectively, the chief branches of the **thoracic aorta** (thoracic part of the descending aorta) are small, supplying the thoracic wall (intercostal arteries) and the esophagus.

Abdomen. The **abdominal aorta** (abdominal part of the descending aorta) is the direct continuation of the thoracic aorta. The name of the vessel simply is changed as it passes through the diaphragm from the thorax into the abdomen. The abdominal aorta gives rise to several small paired branches, including ones to the abdominal wall, but its major branches are to the digestive tract and to the

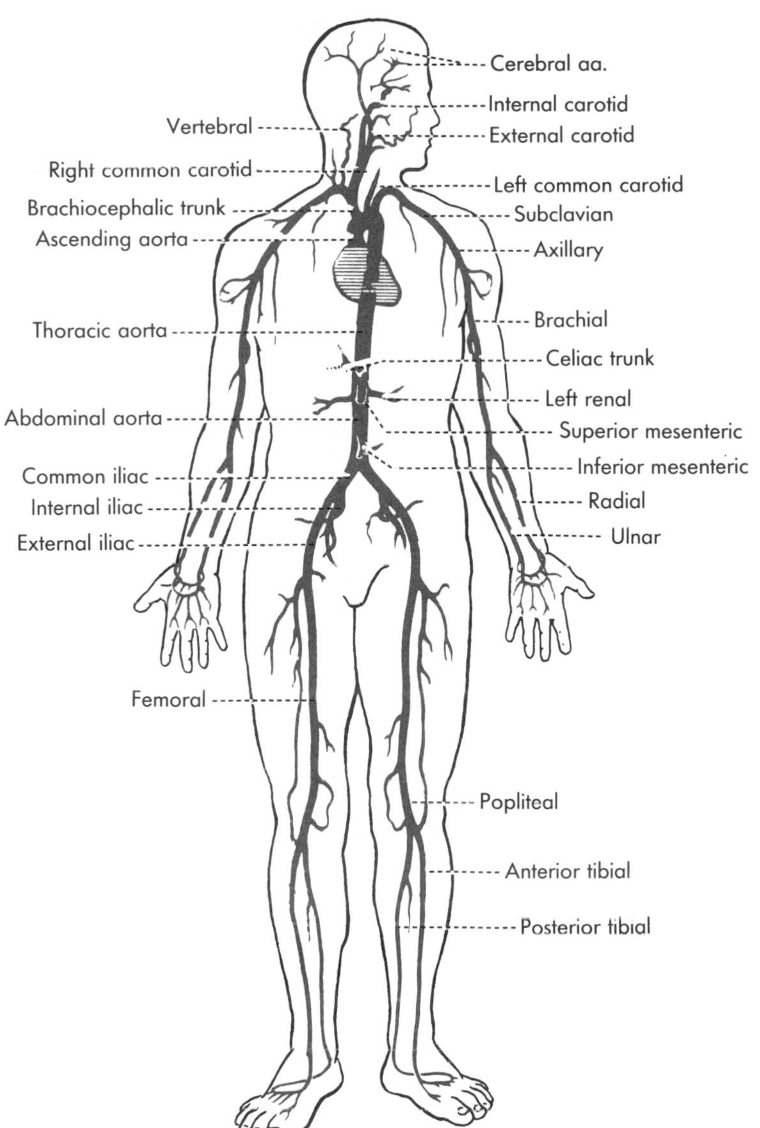

FIGURE *8-4.*
The chief systemic arteries.

kidneys. The three unpaired branches to the digestive tract arise from the front of the aorta. The first is the **celiac trunk,** which, through three major branches, supplies upper abdominal organs (stomach, liver, duodenum, pancreas, and spleen); next is the **superior mesenteric artery,** which partly overlaps the distribution of the celiac trunk, but supplies especially most of the small intestine and much of the large intestine; last is the **inferior mesenteric artery,** supplying the more caudal part of the large intestine.

The arteries to the kidneys (**renal arteries**) arise from the sides of the aorta and are therefore paired, typically one to each kidney. The aorta ends in the lower part of the abdomen by bifurcating into paired **common iliac arteries.**

Pelvis and Lower Limb. The right and left common iliac arteries, the terminal branches of the aorta are essentially similar. Each runs downward and laterally and ends by dividing into internal and external iliac arteries.

The **internal iliac artery** descends into the pelvis and supplies the pelvic viscera (bladder, uterus and vagina in the female, and rectum), sends branches into the buttock to supply muscles there, and sends one branch to the perineum to supply the anal and genital regions.

The **external iliac** continues into the thigh. As it enters the thigh, its name becomes the **femoral artery.** As the femoral artery passes down the thigh, it comes to lie deep to certain muscles, giving off several named branches to muscles in the thigh. The femoral artery eventually appears behind the knee (in the space known as the popliteal fossa), and the name of the artery here changes to **popliteal artery.** The popliteal artery, in turn, ends a little below the knee by dividing into **anterior** and **posterior tibial arteries,** the former passing to and running down the anterior aspect of the leg and into the dorsum of the foot, and the latter running down the posterior aspect of the leg and into the plantar surface of the foot.

Systemic Veins

With a few exceptions (the most notable of which are the veins of the brain, the subcutaneous veins of the limbs, and to some extent, the portal vein draining the digestive tract), the veins largely parallel the arteries and are named as they are, or are called the *venae comitantes* (accompanying veins) of the arteries. Arteries of moderate size, such as the brachial, radial, and ulnar arteries, typically have a pair of veins accompanying them. The two elements of a pair usually unite by numerous cross channels.

The superficial veins of the limbs form a special system of their own, but unite with the deep veins accompanying the arteries. These veins and their tributaries lie in the subcutaneous tissue and are often visible through the skin. Those in front of the elbow are particularly easy to find and are frequently used for withdrawing blood or giving intravenous medication or feeding. The superficial veins are so valved that blood normally can pass only toward the proximal part of the limb, and their connections with the deep veins are so valved that blood normally can pass only from the superficial into the deep veins.

Finally, the veins draining the major part of the intestinal tract, although in part paralleling the arteries supplying this tract, do not empty into the venous equivalent

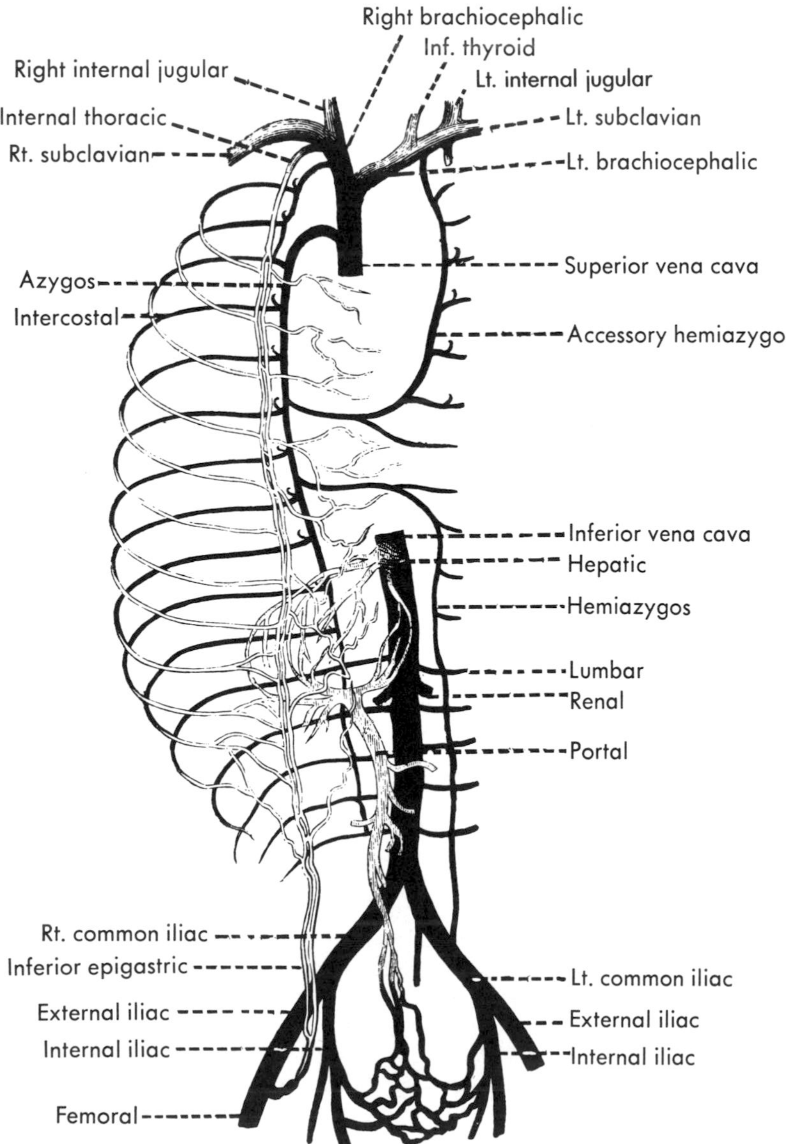

FIGURE *8-5.*
The systemic venous system: Veins of the anterior wall of the trunk are shown in *outline* only, and the portal system is *lightly shaded.* (Henle J. Handbuch der systematischen Anatomie, Bd 3. Braunschweig: Vieweg und Sohn, 1868.)

of the aorta (the inferior vena cava) but carry their blood to the liver; they constitute a separate system, the **portal system** of veins. Although the portal system is systemic in comparison with the pulmonary system, for it does carry blood that has lost oxygen by passing through the tissues, it is sometimes not included among the systemic veins; instead, "systemic" is sometimes used in a restricted sense in comparing the two sets of veins in the abdomen. A general diagram of the veins of the trunk and base of the neck is shown in Figure 8-5.

Head and Neck. The chief veins draining the head and neck are the **internal jugular veins.** Each begins at the base of the skull, where it receives blood brought to the brain by both the internal carotid and vertebral arteries, and is a large vessel that runs straight down the neck alongside the internal and common carotid arteries. It receives tributaries from the face, jaws, tongue, and structures of the upper part of the neck, and it ends at the base of the neck by joining the **subclavian vein** (from the upper limb). Also, a smaller, superficial **external jugular vein** (*jugular,* meaning neck) helps to drain the scalp and usually connects with the upper part of the internal jugular. Just before it ends in the subclavian vein, the external jugular receives some tributaries from the shoulder.

Upper Limb. The deep veins of the upper limb originate in the hand and form paired veins accompanying the radial and ulnar arteries. At the elbow, they unite to form paired **brachial veins** that end above by joining the **axillary vein.** The axillary vein is the upper end of the **basilic vein,** one of the two large superficial veins of the upper limb. As the basilic enters the axilla (armpit), its name changes to axillary. The axillary vein receives the other superficial vein of the upper limb, the **cephalic,** and veins corresponding to branches of the axillary artery. As the axillary vein leaves the arm and enters the neck, its name changes to **subclavian vein.**

The subclavian vein, at the base of the neck, receives the **external jugular** and then joins the **internal jugular.** This union forms the **brachiocephalic vein**. In contrast with the brachiocephalic arterial trunk, normally found only on the right side, the union of subclavian and internal jugular veins to form a brachiocephalic vein occurs on both sides of the body. After its formation, the right brachiocephalic continues the downward course of the right internal jugular, passing down into the thorax. The left brachiocephalic passes to the right side to join the right brachiocephalic vein. The single trunk thus formed, the **superior vena cava,** passes straight downward to enter the upper end of the right atrium, receiving, just before it does so, the **azygos vein** (the chief venous drainage of the thoracic wall). A number of small veins from the neck and the thorax empty into the brachiocephalic veins.

Thorax. Small veins, mostly from the thoracic wall (intercostal veins) and corresponding in general to the thoracic branches of the aorta, empty into a pair of vessels that approximately parallel the thoracic aorta. This pair is the **azygos** ("unpaired") **system,** so named because it is asymmetric. The veins of the left side empty mostly into the larger vein on the right. The largest vein of the system on the left is called the **hemiazygos vein.** The larger vein on the right is the **azygos vein.** It joins the lowermost part of the superior vena cava.

Lower Limb and Abdomen. The deep veins of the lower limb accompany the arteries and bear similar names. The **femoral vein,** paralleling the femoral artery, enters the abdomen, whereupon its name is changed to **external iliac vein.** The external iliac vein is joined by the **internal iliac** from the pelvis and buttock to form the **common iliac vein.** Right and left common iliac veins unite to form the **inferior vena cava.** In its course upward, the inferior vena cava and its tributaries receive vessels corresponding to the branches of the abdominal aorta, except those going to the digestive tract. Finally, just before it leaves the abdomen, the inferior vena cava receives the hepatic veins from the liver, which contain not only the blood from the arteries of the liver, but also the blood from the digestive tract brought there by the portal vein. The inferior vena cava ends in the inferior part of the right atrium, immediately after passing through the diaphragm.

Portal System

The portal system of veins drains the gastrointestinal (digestive) tract from the stomach to the upper part of the rectum. The tributaries of this system unite to form the **portal vein,** which instead of returning blood directly to the heart, as do the venae cavae, delivers it to the sinusoids (essentially dilated capillaries) in the liver.

The tributaries of the portal vein generally parallel the arteries going to the digestive tract (and the artery to the spleen) and are similarly named; however, there is no single trunk corresponding to the celiac trunk of the aorta, and the portal vein itself parallels the artery to the liver (**hepatic artery**). The portal vein ends by dividing into branches that enter the substance of the liver and divide repeatedly. Eventually, they empty into the sinusoids of the liver, as do the branches of hepatic artery. The small veins opening into the sinusoids thus constitute the termination of the portal system of veins.

Blood from the sinusoids, whether brought in by the hepatic artery or the portal vein, is drained by the **hepatic veins.** These, as already noted, empty into the upper end of the inferior vena cava immediately below the diaphragm.

Lymphatic System

The lymphatic system begins in capillaries that begin blindly and drain tissue spaces. Deep lymphatics that drain the muscles and other tissue of the limbs and the body wall are relatively few, but accompany the arteries and veins supplying these parts. Deep lymph nodes are correspondingly scarce in the limbs, but typically do occur in a few locations. The chief lymphatic drainage from

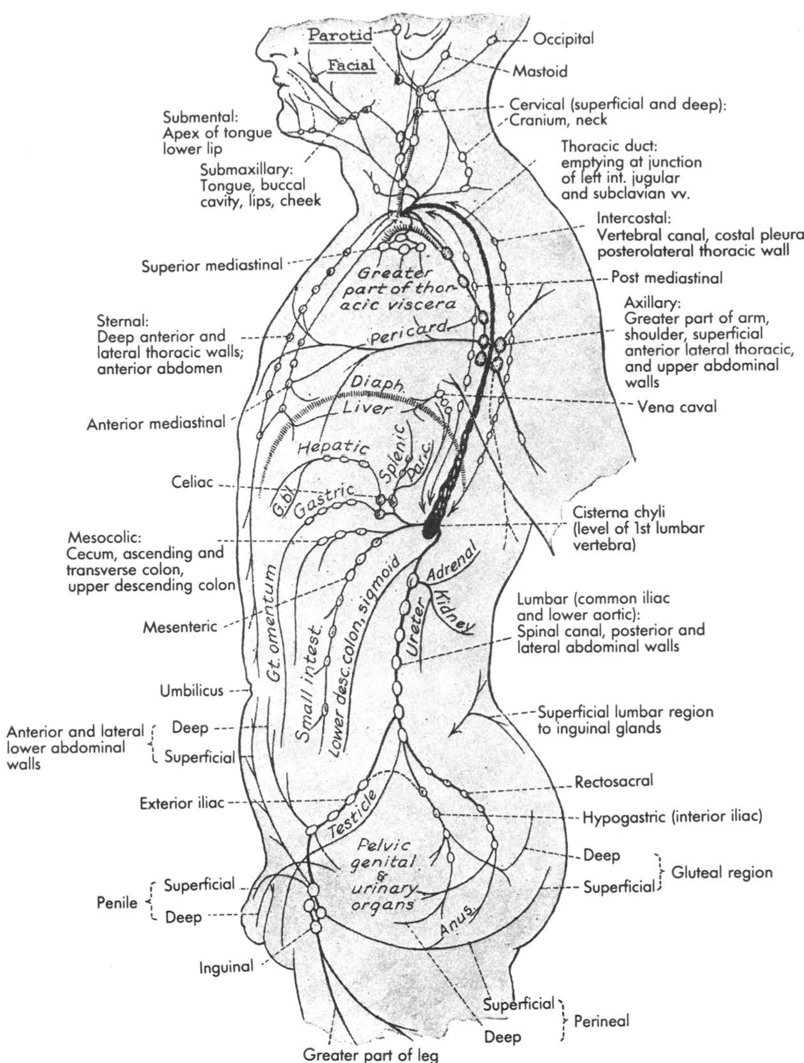

FIGURE *8-6.*
Schema of the lymphatic drainage of the body. (Jones T. Shepard WC. Manual of surgical anatomy. Philadelphia: WB Saunders, 1945.)

the limbs and from the body wall, therefore, is by superficial lymphatics.

In synopsis, most of the lymphatics of the lower limb converge on lymph nodes located anteriorly and superficially in the uppermost part of the thigh (Fig. 8-6). These then drain upward into the abdomen, where many of the lymphatics and lymph nodes are closely associated with the aorta. The abdominal nodes also receive the lymphatic drainage from the pelvic and abdominal viscera. In the uppermost part of the abdomen, the major lymphatics unite to form the largest lymphatic vessel in the body, the **thoracic duct.** This runs upward along the posterior thoracic wall, receiving lymphatics from that, and ends at the base of the neck on the left side by emptying into the venous system at approximately the angle of junction of the internal jugular and subclavian veins.

The lymphatics of the upper limb converge on lymph nodes situated around the axillary vessels, and those of the head and neck converge on lymph nodes grouped especially around the internal jugular veins. Lymphatic trunks from the upper limb and from the head and neck join each other and a trunk from the thorax and empty together, or remain separate and, therefore, empty separately, into veins at the base of the neck on the right side. On the left side they join the thoracic duct, or empty into the venous system close to the ending of that duct.

In addition to the lymphatic vessels and nodes, the lymphatic system includes collections of lymphocytes located under the epithelium of the digestive tract (tonsils and Peyer's patches), the spleen, the thymus, and the bone marrow. Apart from returning tissue fluid from essentially all parts of the body to the venous circulation, the significance of the lymphatic system lies largely in its contribution to the immune responses of the body. The organs of the lymphatic system that are concerned with the production of lymphocytes, the chief immunocompetent cells of the body, are called **primary lymphoid organs.** These include the thymus and the bone marrow. Those lymphoid organs in which the immune response is initiated against antigens are called **secondary lymphoid organs.** These include the lymph nodes, the subepithelial collections of lymphocytes, and the spleen.

The **thymus** is distinct from other lymphoid organs in that instead of being entirely mesodermal in origin, it is derived, in part, from an outgrowth of the embryonic gut (pharyngeal pouch). Its lymphoid elements develop in association with the endodermal epithelium. The **bone marrow** produces all types of blood cells (hematopoietic cells) in addition to lymphocytes.

Antigens that are picked up in the tissues by the afferent lymph stimulate an immune response first in the lymph nodes; those that are picked up by the blood initiate a response first in the spleen.

The **spleen** is enclosed in a part of the mesentery of the stomach, and its parenchyma resembles that of lymph nodes. Lymphatics within the spleen are confined to its capsule and to large trabeculae, so that the lymphatic nodules of the spleen add lymphocytes directly to the bloodstream instead of delivering them first into lymphatic vessels, as the lymph nodes do. Instead of capillaries, the spleen has large sinusoids lined by highly phagocytic cells. The size of the sinusoids allows the spleen to act as a reservoir for red blood cells, which accumulate in it when the splenic circulation is sluggish. The phagocytic walls of the sinusoids are the chief elements concerned with the destruction of red blood cells and the removal of the iron component from them so that this can be used again to form new cells. If the spleen is removed, these functions are carried out by the bone marrow, lymph nodes, and liver. Under abnormal conditions, the spleen may also begin to produce red cells and myelocytes, normally produced only in the bone marrow.

SOME DEVELOPMENTAL CONSIDERATIONS

Details of development necessary to an understanding of the variations and anomalies of specific vessels are best noted in connection with those vessels, and only general comment upon the development of the vascular system is needed here. The heart and all vessels of the vascular and lymphatic systems develop from embryonic mesenchyme. Mesenchyme is the versatile, multipotent, embryonic connective tissue formed from *mesoderm* (see Fig. 9-2), the middle germ layer of the embryonic disk. The vasculature of those organs that are primarily derived from *ectoderm* or *endoderm* (the other two germ layers) is also of mesenchymal origin.

Blood Vessels

All blood vessels develop from capillaries, which grow by sprouting and by coalescing with other capillary spaces to form networks in which certain channels enlarge as a result of a greater amount of blood coursing through them, while others disappear completely, or remain as capillaries. This method of development offers opportunity for much variation in the anatomy of the vascular system, and vascular variations are not so much to be wondered at as is the fact that developmental conditions are so relatively constant from one person to another that a basic and prevailing vascular pattern can be recognized in all. Because from the beginning of the developing circulation, the blood leaving the heart is under greater pressure and flows faster than does blood returning to the heart, it might be expected (in analogy with a river at flood as compared with a slow and winding one) that blood leaving the heart would have the greater tendency to take the shortest and most constant route to a part and that arteries would, therefore, be less variable than veins; indeed, as already noted, this is generally true.

Abdomen and Thorax

The first circulations to develop are to the yolk sac and the placenta. Because the yolk sac is nonfunctional in humans, this circulation is short-lived, and only the proximal parts of the yolk-sac (*vitelline and omphalomesenteric*) vessels persist as the blood supply to the gut (celiac and mesenteric arteries, portal vein). The numerous, originally paired, yolk-sac arteries become single, unpaired ones, apparently by fusion, and are reduced to three. The veins become reduced to a single pair that are interrupted in their course to the heart by the developing liver and become converted into portal veins; parts of both portal veins contribute to the single definitive portal vein.

Unlike the yolk-sac circulation, that to the placenta enlarges steadily and persists up to the time of birth, as the umbilical vessels (the paired vein is reduced to a single one). After birth, the useless parts of the umbilical vessels lose their lumen, but remain throughout life as fibrous cords ("ligaments").

The paired lateral branches of the abdominal aorta to the kidneys are remains of much more numerous paired vessels that originally supplied the nephrogenic ridge, especially the evanescent mesonephros, or "middle kidney." Besides the arteries to the kidneys, other vessels of this group persist as paired arteries to the gonads, the suprarenal glands, and the diaphragm.

The inferior vena cava has a particularly complicated developmental history, for all three pairs of veins formed caudal to the heart—the postcardinals (posterior cardinals), subcardinals, and supracardinals—contribute to the development of this unpaired vessel (see Chap. 25). In consequence of this complicated development, major variations of the inferior vena cava are more common than are variations in any other large vein.

The pulmonary veins are a derivative of the venous plexus on the gut, just as the lungs are an outgrowth from the gut. Anomalous openings of one or more pulmonary veins into the systemic venous system are believed to result from improper separation of the two systems.

The pulmonary arteries are derivatives of the aortic

arch system, as are the arch of the aorta and the great vessels that originate from it (see Chap. 22).

Limbs

The main arterial stems in both upper and lower limbs have a complicated history. In each instance, the first definitive stem is formed by enlargement of one of several vessels feeding the developing limb bud, but in neither one does this stem persist throughout the length of the limb. Rather, a series of branches appear, and first one, then another, takes over the duty of supplying the distal part of the limb, so that the definitive main channels of the adult are composed of portions of several different arteries in series.

The earliest veins of the limbs are superficial and lie especially on the borders of the limb. Most of the channels along the preaxial (radial and tibial) borders of the limbs atrophy, but those along the postaxial borders tend to persist as the proximal parts of the great veins of the limbs, receiving both superficial veins and the definitive deep veins that develop distally along the arteries.

Head and Neck

The veins of the head and neck develop from the paired precardinal (anterior cardinal) veins, which receive the veins from the head and neck and upper limbs just as the posterior cardinal veins originally receive those from the lower limbs and the trunk. The left precardinal vein shunts its blood to the right precardinal and helps form the superior vena cava.

The arteries of the head and neck have a particularly complicated developmental history. Most of them develop from the aortic arch system, which is similar to the system that supplies the gills in fishes and thus aerates the blood.

Heart

The heart, in an early stage, is a single tube like the heart of a fish, receiving blood at one end and propelling it from the other into the aortic arch system. Subsequently, it becomes twisted upon itself and some of its original subdivisions disappear. Partitions that appear and separate the heart into right and left sides then produce a four-chambered heart. This differs drastically from the four-chambered heart of a fish: Instead of four chambers in series, there are two right and two left chambers, and, as noted, the blood must circulate twice through the heart to become aerated and be returned to the body in general.

Lymphatics

Lymphatic capillaries originate either by outgrowth from the venous system in certain locations or by the coalescence of blind lymphatic spaces, or both. Like blood vessels, they increase in size according to the flow of lymph through them. In an early stage of development, enlarged lymphatics or lymph sacs are found at the junction of the chief veins of each of the upper and lower limbs with the cardinal veins into which they empty, and two others are found on the posterior abdominal wall. From these sacs, lymphatics grow along blood vessels: those connected with the limbs grow distally into those parts; those connected with the lower limbs also grow centrally and connect with the upper abdominal lymph sac, which gives rise, in turn, to the thoracic duct, that grows to join the sac connected with the left upper limb; the lower abdominal sac grows peripherally to the intestines and centrally to join the thoracic duct; and the sacs connected with the upper limbs either retain their connections to the venous system here (at the base of the neck) or establish new ones, so that all lymph must return to the bloodstream here.

Anomalous openings of the lymphatic system into the venous system (in locations other than the base of the neck), although rare, indicate the close developmental relation between veins and lymphatics.

RECOMMENDED READINGS

Abramson DI, Dobrin PB, eds. Blood vessels and lymphatics in organ systems. New York: Academic Press, 1984.

Barnhart MI, Lusher JM. The human spleen as revealed by scanning electron microscopy. Am J Hematol 1976; 1: 243.

Castellino RA, Marglin MI. Imaging of abdominal and pelvic lymph nodes: lymphography or computed tomography? Invest Radiol 1982; 17: 433.

Fawcett DW. Blood and lymph vascular systems. In: Bloom and Fawcett: a textbook of histology. 12th ed. New York: Chapman & Hall, 1994: 368.

Franklin KJ. A monograph on veins. Springfield, Il: Charles C Thomas, 1937.

Haagensen CD. General anatomy of the lymphatic system. In: Haagensen CD, Feind CR, Herter FP, Slantez CA, Weinberg JA. The lymphatics in cancer. Philadelphia: WB Sanders, 1972.

Harvey W. Movement of the heart and blood in animals: an anatomical essay. Franklin KJ (trans). Springfield, Il: Charles C Thomas, 1957.

Kendall MD. Functional anatomy of the thymic microenvironment. J Anat 1991; 177: 1.

Lippert H, Pabst R. Arterial variations in man: classification and frequency. New York: Springer-Verlag, 1985.

Maros T. Data regarding the typology and functional significance of the venous valves. Morphol Embryol 1981; 27: 195.

Maximenkov AN. Structural and functional peculiarities in some parts of the venous system. Anat Rec 1960; 136: 239.

Quiring DP. Collateral circulation: anatomical aspects. Philadelphia: Lea & Febiger, 1949.

Ross R, Glomset JA. The pathogenesis of atherosclerosis. Parts I and II. N Engl J Med 1976; 259: 369, 420.

Rouviere H. Anatomie des lymphatiques de l'homme. Paris: Masson et Cie, 1932.

Schlant RC, Alexander RW, eds. The heart, 8th ed. New York: McGraw-Hill, 1994.

Tavassoli M, Yoffey JM. Bone marrow structure and function. New York: Alan Liss, 1983.

Taylor GI, Palmer JH. The vascular territories (angiosomes) of the body; experimental study and clinical applications. Br J Plast Surg 1987; 40: 113.

von Gaudecker B. Functional histology of the human thymus. Anat Embryol 1991; 183: 1.

Watterson PA, Taylor GI, Crock JG. The venous territories of the human body: anatomical study and clinical implications. Br J Plast Surg 1988; 41: 569.

Weiss L. The cells and tissues of the immune system: structure, function, interactions. Englewood Cliffs, NJ: Prentice-Hall, 1972.

Weissleder R, Thrall JH. The lymphatic system: diagnostic imaging studies. Radiology 1989; 172: 315.

Willius FA, Keys TE, eds. Classics of cardiology: a collection of classic works on the heart and circulation with comprehensive biographical accounts of the authors. New York: H. Schuman, 1961.

Yoffey JM, Courtice FC. Lymphatics, lymph, and the lymphomyeloid complex. New York: Academic Press, 1970.

Hollinshead's Textbook of Anatomy, by Cornelius Rosse and Penelope Gaddum-Rosse.
Lippincott-Raven Publishers, Philadelphia, © 1997.

CHAPTER 9

The Digestive and Respiratory Systems

The digestive and respiratory systems of mammals are closely connected, for the respiratory system is largely an outgrowth from the digestive system. Even when fully developed, the two systems share in part a common passageway, the pharynx (Fig. 9-1). Interestingly, the respiratory organs of humans, the lungs, arise from the region of the pharynx that in fishes is provided with gill slits and gills and, thus, has both respiratory and ingestive functions.

The **digestive system** (*apparatus digestorius*) is essentially a long tube with muscular walls and a glandular epithelial lining. Its upper end is the mouth, and its lower end is the anus; most of it lies coiled within the abdomen. Certain glands of the digestive system have become specialized and are too large to be included in the walls of the tube. These glands have grown out of the tube, assuming the status of independent organs, although still retaining ducts that connect them to the tube. These are the three pairs of salivary glands, the ducts of which open into the mouth, and the liver and pancreas, which lie within the abdomen and connect with the small intestine through a ductal system.

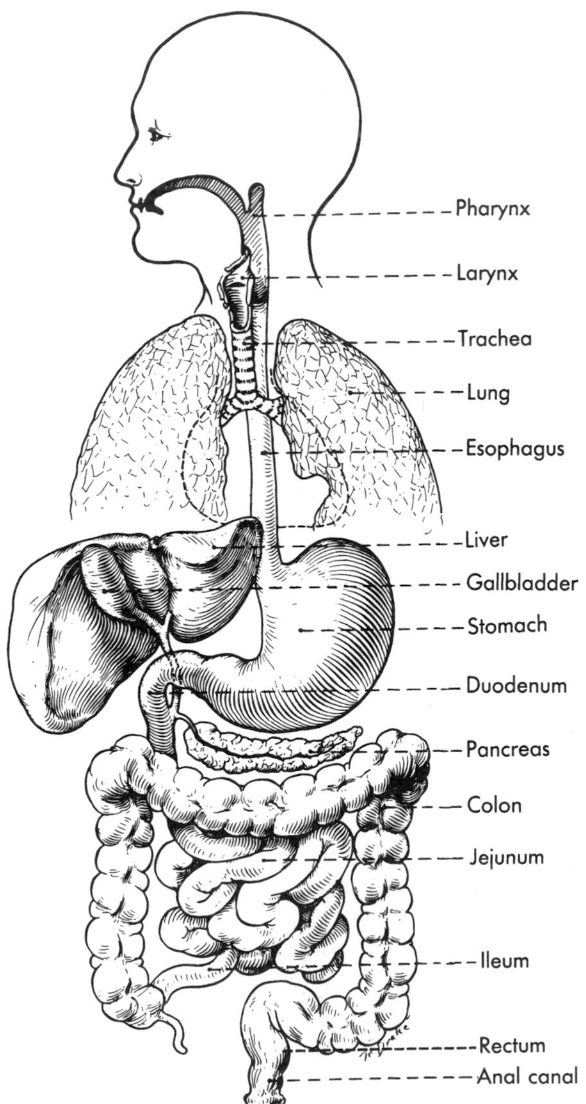

FIGURE *9-1.*
The digestive and respiratory systems: The nasal cavity, here omitted, opens into the uppermost part of the pharynx.

The parts of the tubular digestive system are, in order, the mouth, pharynx, esophagus, stomach, small intestine or small bowel (with three subdivisions, the duodenum, jejunum, and ileum), and large intestine or large bowel (including cecum and vermiform appendix, colon, rectum, and anal canal). All these parts between mouth and anus are referred to collectively as the *alimentary canal.*

The **respiratory system** consists of the nose and nasal passages, part of the pharynx, the larynx (voice box), the trachea (windpipe), the bronchi, and the lungs.

The lungs and most of the digestive tract are surrounded by serous sacs, which line the body cavity and, owing to the small amount of serous fluid the sacs contain, facilitate the movements of the lungs and the intestines. In the thoracic cavity, each lung is surrounded by a *pleural sac,* which encloses a pleural cavity; the *peritoneal sac,* with the peritoneal cavity enclosed in it, is associated with the part of the digestive tract located in the abdominal cavity. All these serous sacs, including the one around the heart, which encloses the pericardial cavity, develop from the primitive body cavity of the embryo called the *intraembryonic celom.*

In addition to introducing the digestive and respiratory systems, this chapter also discusses the development of the intraembryonic celom in the three-layered embryo. Much reference will be made in the remainder of this book to both the intraembryonic celom and the tissues that compose the three-layered embryo.

THE DIGESTIVE SYSTEM

General Functional Anatomy

Mouth and Pharynx

The mouth (*oral or buccal cavity*) is separated from the nasal cavity by the palate. The back end of the palate is movable and capable of coming in contact with the posterior pharyngeal wall to cut off the upper (nasal) part of the pharynx from communication with the oral part of the pharynx. The highly mobile tongue largely fills the oral cavity. In addition to its function in speech, the tongue is used for positioning food between the teeth so that it can be properly masticated. A number of small glands of the cheeks, lips, tongue, and palate empty their secretion into the oral cavity, as do three large pairs of glands; because they secrete most of the saliva, they are known as *salivary glands.*

The mouth opens into the pharynx through a narrow space, on the lateral walls of which are the tonsils (palatine tonsils). The larynx, the beginning of the respiratory pathway to the lungs, leaves the lower part of the pharynx anteriorly. A little below this, the pharynx narrows and is continued as the tubelike esophagus.

The musculature of the walls of the pharynx is voluntary, bronchial muscle and promotes the function of swallowing. The movements of the tongue, which tend to pass food back into the pharynx, initiate the act of swallowing and, together with the constriction of the pharyngeal muscles, increase the pressure within the pharynx. During swallowing, the oral and nasal pharynx are temporarily separated by the palate, preventing liquids in the pharynx from flowing into the nose.

Esophagus and Stomach

The esophagus is the continuation of the pharynx. It runs down through the neck and thorax and, as soon as it reaches the abdomen, enters the stomach.

The **stomach** (*ventriculus* or *gaster,* hence, the adjective "gastric") is a saccular organ, flattened anteroposteriorly and curved along both its upper right and its lower left borders. The esophagus enters the stomach at the left upper end, and the duodenum, the first part of the small intestine, leaves it at its right lower end.

Within the stomach, the digestion of starches, initiated by saliva during mastication, is gradually halted by the effect of the hydrochloric acid secreted there. Excess acid secretion by the stomach is believed to be an important factor in the formation of gastric and duodenal ulcers. Acid-secreting (parietal) cells of the stomach are especially numerous toward its duodenal end. The stomach gradually churns the swallowed food until it becomes liquefied through mixture with the secretions. This liquid material, called *chyme,* is then passed little by little into the duodenum.

Duodenum, Pancreas, and Liver

In spite of its short length, the **duodenum** is particularly important because it receives the ducts from the pancreas, liver, and gallbladder. The pancreatic secretions, containing protein-splitting, fat-splitting, and carbohydrate-splitting enzymes, first begin their digestive action on the chyme within the duodenum. The common bile duct delivers bile from the liver and gallbladder to the intestinal contents; this is essential for adequate emulsification of fats, a necessary step in their proper digestion.

The **pancreas** is largely exocrine: pancreatic juice is secreted by the acini (groups of glandular cells that form the secretion) into a duct system that empties into the duodenum. These acini constitute the exocrine portion of the pancreas, which is concerned with digestion. Among the acini are scattered groups of cells that are so isolated from each other that they appear as islands. These pancreatic islets, also known as islets of Langerhans, are the endocrine part of the pancreas (see Chap. 11).

The **liver** (*hepar,* hence, the adjective "hepatic") is the largest organ of the body, constituting in the average adult about 1/36 of the entire body weight.

The liver is an extremely vascular structure and differs from other glands in that blood flows into it from both the hepatic artery and the portal vein. The **portal vein** is formed by its tributaries, which arise within the walls of the intestinal tract. This large vein, after entering the liver, breaks up into branches that terminate in sinusoids (dilated capillaries) within the liver. Thus, through this **portal system** of veins, blood containing freshly absorbed products of digestion is brought into intimate contact with liver cells before being returned to the general circulation through the hepatic veins. The detoxifying action of the liver on this blood is essential to life. Although mammals, including humans, can survive when only a part of the liver is active, complete removal or destruction of the liver results in death within a few days. In fact, the liver is one of the major centers of chemical activity in the body; the secretion of bile is only one of a number of functions of this organ. Bile pigment, produced from the breakdown of hemoglobin during destruction of red blood cells, is removed from the blood by the liver and secreted as a component of the bile.

Jejunum and Ileum

Succeeding the duodenum is the jejunum, followed by the ileum, with no sharp line of division between them. Digestive activity initiated by the pancreatic enzymes in the duodenum is continued in the jejunum and ileum, which are the longest segments of the digestive tract. The small glands in the walls of these organs add their secretion to the chyme. The small intestine, with an enormous mucosal surface provided by folds of its lining and by the villi that project from these folds, is especially adapted for absorption, and most absorption of food from the alimentary tract occurs in the jejunum and ileum.

Large Intestine

Rather than opening end to end into the large intestine, the ileum opens into its side a little above a blind lower end; this blind lower end is the **cecum,** and the **appendix** (vermiform appendix) is a slender projection from it. The ileum joins the large intestine in the lower right side of the abdominal cavity.

The first part of the large intestine above the cecum is the **ascending colon,** which passes up toward the liver, where it bends to the left to pass across the abdominal cavity to become the **transverse colon.** In the left side of the abdominal cavity, close to the stomach and spleen, the large intestine bends again; turning downward, it forms the **descending colon.** Finally, in the lower left part of the abdominal cavity, the colon becomes somewhat tortuous, forming the **sigmoid colon,** which descends into the pelvis. In the pelvis, the colon becomes the **rectum,** which leads to the anus by way of the **anal canal.**

The large intestine absorbs about four-fifths of the water in the intestinal contents that reach it, thereby being largely responsible for the dehydration necessary to allow formed stools. It is also an excretory organ for almost all the iron, most of the calcium, and usually about half of the magnesium eliminated by the body; the remaining excretion of these substances is through the urine.

General Structure

Below the pharynx, the alimentary canal, or digestive tract, remains essentially the same in structure throughout its length. However, there are certain structural variations along the length of the canal that endow particular parts of the tract with specific functions. Basically, the wall of the digestive tract has four layers. There is a thin, outermost layer of mesothelium and connective tissue, the **serosa;** next are the muscular layers (**tunica muscularis**); following is another layer of connective tissue, the **submucosa;** and finally, there is an innermost layer of more delicate connective tissue with an epithelial surface, called the **mucosa.** These layers are discussed from within outward.

The surface epithelium of the **mucosa** (*tunica mucosa*) gives rise to numerous glands that lie in the connective tissue of the mucosa and, in some locations, also invade the submucosa. In the esophagus, subject to possible damage from hot or cold food and from solid particles, the epithelium is stratified squamous and contains few glands; this is also true of the last part of the gut, the anal canal. Elsewhere, the epithelium is columnar and differs in detail from one region to another. In the small intestine, the mucosa forms innumerable tiny, fingerlike processes that project into the lumen and give a mossy appearance and velvety texture to the lining. Each of these tiny processes is a *villus.* Within each villus are blood vessels and a central, blindly ending lymphatic capillary, called the *lacteal* (so named because fat, which gives the otherwise clear lymph a milky appearance, is absorbed by these lymphatic capillaries). The villi enormously increase the absorptive surface of the small intestine. Since neither the stomach nor the large intestine contains villi, they are not particularly efficient organs in the process of absorption.

The most important glands of the stomach are those that secrete hydrochloric acid and pepsin, a protein-splitting enzyme. Glands of the small intestine are generally small. Some of them apparently secrete some digestive enzymes. There are also mucus-secreting glands, the mucus serving for lubrication. These become more numerous in the lower part of the small intestine and, in the large intestine, constitute the chief type of gland.

The **submucosa** (*tela submucosa*) is a layer of connective tissue between the mucosal and muscular layers. It is particularly vascular and also contains nerve fibers and postganglionic parasympathetic nerve cells that form a *submucous plexus.* Throughout much of the small intestine, the submucosa and the mucosa together form a series of permanent circular folds. Otherwise, the submucosa acts as padding between the mucosa and the muscular layers, allowing the mucosa to be thrown into temporary folds when the musculature contracts.

Throughout most of the digestive tract, the **musculature** consists of an inner circular and an outer longitudinal layer of smooth muscle. Smooth muscle is composed of tapering, overlapping cells or fibers bound together by delicate connective tissue. It is called smooth because it shows none of the striations characteristic of cardiac and skeletal muscle. Smooth muscle possesses the ability to contract in the absence of nerve stimuli, although this varies according to the location of the muscle. This autonomous contractility is especially well developed in the muscle of the digestive tract, where peristaltic (rhythmic) movements occur, even after complete denervation of the tract. *Peristalsis* is responsible for emptying the stomach and moving the contents of the digestive tract along the length of the intestine. This activity is influenced by the autonomic nervous system. Plexuses of autonomic nerve fibers that contain parasympathetic ganglion cells lie between the longitudinal and circular layers of the muscle (the *myenteric,* or intermuscular, *plexus*), which is similar to the submucous plexus. The parts of the digestive tract that have voluntary, rather than involuntary, musculature in their wall are the pharynx and the upper part of the esophagus; the muscle here is striated (bronchial) rather than smooth.

Serosa covers the outer surface of the abdominal part of the esophagus, the stomach, the small intestine, and most of the outer surface of the large intestine. The serosa of these organs is, in fact, their *visceral peritoneum.* This layer is present only on those surfaces of organs that are directly adjacent to the peritoneal cavity; for instance, serosa essentially surrounds the muscular layer of most of the small intestine, but on parts of the large intestine occurs only on the anterior surface. The outer surface of the serosa is a mesothelium, whereas its deeper layer, uniting it to the muscular layer, consists of connective tissue. On nonperitonealized surfaces, such as the thoracic part of the esophagus, there is connective tissue only; when this is substantial, it is called the *tunica adventitia.*

THE RESPIRATORY SYSTEM

The **external nose** and the nasal septum between the two nasal cavities are supported partly by cartilage and partly by bone. The lateral walls of the **nasal cavities** are largely thin bone, on which are prominent ridges, the *conchae* (turbinates), that project medially and downward into the cavity. They are covered by mucous membrane and help warm and moisten the inspired air. They occupy so much space in the nasal cavity that when they become swollen they may block the air passage completely.

The paired nasal cavities are separated by a median septum, and each opens through a narrow posterior aperture into the nasal part of the pharynx, separated from the mouth by the palate. From the nasal part of the pharynx, inspired air passes into the oral part of the pharynx and then enters the **larynx,** the entrance of which is kept permanently open by supporting cartilages. A little below the entrance, projecting folds in the larynx allow the passageway to be closed for swallowing or holding the breath, or to be narrowed to allow a thin column of air to escape between them for phonation. The vocal cords are one pair of laryngeal folds. The prominent anterior cartilage of the larynx (Adam's apple) is the thyroid cartilage, "thyroid" referring to its shape, which is somewhat like that of a shield.

The **trachea,** the continuation of the larynx, is a musculofibrous tube supported by a series of rings of cartilage (*trachea,* meaning "rough") that are incomplete posteriorly. The trachea is thus held permanently open and normally allows easy passage of air. It is palpable in the front of the neck below the larynx; at the base of the neck it disappears into the thorax, where it ends by bifurcating into right and left **bronchi.** Repeated branchings of the bronchi and associated vessels of the lung form the substance of that organ, and the final bronchial branchings, the *alveoli,* provide for intimate contact between the air and blood vessels. (Although *pulmo,* from which the adjective "pulmonary" is derived, is the proper name for the lung, common combining forms referring to the lung are *pneumo* and *pneumato,* which actually mean gas or air.)

The pulmonary arteries that deliver deoxygenated blood to the lung enter it through its hilum, along with the bronchi. The pulmonary veins leave the lung through its hilum and return the oxygenated blood to the left atrium.

DEVELOPMENT OF THE CELOM AND THE DIGESTIVE AND RESPIRATORY SYSTEMS

The Embryonic Disk

At the time the body cavity makes its first appearance, the embryo consists of a flat disk located between two other cavities: above the disk is the **amniotic cavity;** below it the **yolk sac** (Fig. 9-2A). The amniotic cavity and the yolk sac, with the disk between them, are suspended by the **connecting stalk** in yet another larger cavity called the **extraembryonic celom,** enclosed by the chorion. The orientation of the embryo is indicated by the attachment of the connecting stalk to the caudal region of the disk; the rostral, or cranial, region of the disk is opposite the attachment of the connecting stalk.

The surface of the embryonic disk facing into the amniotic cavity is covered by **ectoderm;** the surface facing into the yolk sac is covered by **endoderm.** On each side of the median axis of the disk, two longitudinal ridges of ectoderm are raised up to form the *neural folds,* (see Fig. 9-2B); their contribution to the nervous system is described in Chapter 13. Ectoderm and endoderm are separated from one another everywhere by the third germ layer, the *intraembryonic mesoderm,* except in two small areas: the *oropharyngeal membrane* in the rostral region in front of the neural folds, and the *cloacal membrane,* caudal to the neural folds. These membranes, composed of endoderm and ectoderm, will break down, providing two openings through which the amniotic cavity communicates with the interior of the yolk sac. The gut will be formed from part of the yolk sac, and the openings will become the mouth and the anus.

Intraembryonic Mesoderm

The exterior of the amnion, yolk sac, and connecting stalk are covered by *extraembryonic mesoderm;* only intraembryonic mesoderm sandwiched between ectoderm and endoderm contributes to the formation of the body of the embryo. This mesoderm is organized in distinct structures and regions (see Fig. 9-2B): 1) Along the central axis of the disk, the mesoderm forms the rodlike **notochord,** around which the vertebral column will be organized. 2) Along each side of the notochord, the so-called *paraxial mesoderm* becomes segmented into discrete units called **somites,** from which the axial skeleton and its musculature are derived (see Chaps. 12 and 13). 3) **Lateral plate mesoderm,** spreads as a continuous sheet along the lateral portions of the disk and also extends rostral to the oropharyngeal membrane. 4) On each side, a bar of mesoderm that lies between lateral plate mesoderm and the somites is called **intermediate mesoderm.**

Formation of the Intraembryonic Celom

The body cavity of the embryo, that is, the intraembryonic celom, is formed by a process of cavitation in lateral plate mesoderm (see Fig. 9-2C). The intraembryonic celom splits the lateral plate mesoderm into two laminae: splanchnic mesoderm and somatic mesoderm. The mesodermal lamina adjacent to endoderm is designated as **splanchnic mesoderm** and gives rise to all smooth muscle, connective tissue, and vasculature of the gut and its derivatives, whereas the epithelial lining of the gut and the parenchymal cells of the organs derived from the gut (liver and pancreas) are formed by endoderm. The mesodermal lamina associated with ectoderm is designated **somatic mesoderm** and, together with the ectoderm, forms most of the tissues of the body wall (see Chaps. 19 and 23). The serous pericardial, pleural, and peritoneal sacs develop from those cell layers of these two mesodermal laminae that face into the intraembryonic celom.

The intraembryonic celom extends along each side of the embryonic disk, and these two celomic ducts are connected with each other rostrally, but not caudally: a horseshoe-shaped or an inverted U-shaped cavity is thus created (see Fig. 9-2C). The caudally pointing limbs of the celom, called the *pleuroperitoneal canals,* eventually fuse and give rise to the peritoneal cavity (see Chap. 23); the future pleural cavities are situated at the rostral end of the pleuroperitoneal canals, whereas the transverse portion of the celom will become the pericardial cavity (see Chaps. 19 and 21).

The medial wall of the pleuroperitoneal canals is formed by intermediate mesoderm; along their lateral wall, somatic and splanchnic laminae of lateral plate

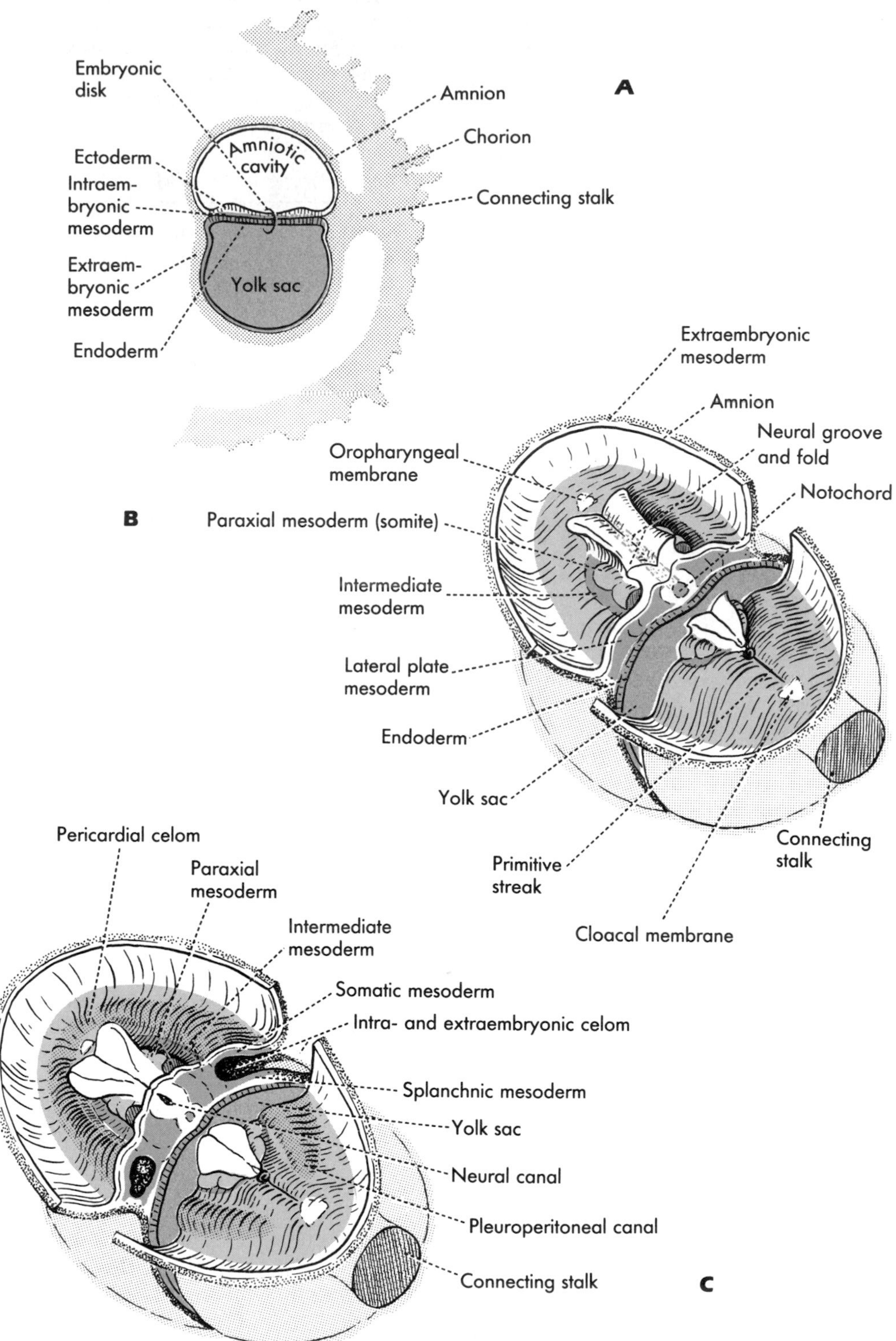

FIGURE *9-2.*
Schematic representation of the trilaminar embryonic disk. (A) The chorion has been sliced open to show the relation of the disk to the amniotic cavity, the yolk sac, and the extraembryonic celom. *(B)* A view of the ectodermal surface of the embryo seen from the amniotic cavity. A transverse section across the disk and the yolk sac below reveals the components of the intraembryonic mesoderm. (C) The location of the intraembryonic celom (black) in the lateral plate mesoderm. The *left* pleuroperitoneal canal is as yet closed; the *right* one has opened and is in communication with the extraembryonic celom.

mesoderm fuse with each other and with extraembryonic mesoderm (see Fig. 9-2C). Thus, at the time of its formation, the intraembryonic celom is a closed cavity; it will, however, soon be breached by the dissolution of a streak of mesoderm in the lateral wall of the pleuroperitoneal canals (see Fig. 9-2C). The communication established with the extraembryonic celom admits into the body of the embryo nutrient-rich fluid from the extraembryonic celom needed before the development of the circulation.

During the folding of the embryonic disk, this communication will be closed and the celom partitioned into the pericardial, pleural, and peritoneal cavities. The division of the celom is discussed in Chapters 19, 23, and 25; the folding of the embryonic disk is dealt with in the next section, because it contributes to the definition of the main subdivisions of the primitive gut.

Formation of the Foregut, Midgut, and Hindgut

The folding of the flat embryonic disk, which rests on the yolk sac, creates a more or less cylindrical organism. This process entraps portions of the yolk sac within the embryo, which become its alimentary canal or gut and also displaces parts of the celom into a plane that is ventral to the central nervous system and the developing vertebral column of the embryo. There are three components to the folding, which progress more or less simultaneously: the head fold, tail fold, and lateral folds.

Concomitant with the rapid growth of the head process, the **head fold** carries the pericardial portion of the celom ventrally and thereby the crescentic ridge of lateral plate mesoderm that formed the rostral wall of the peri-

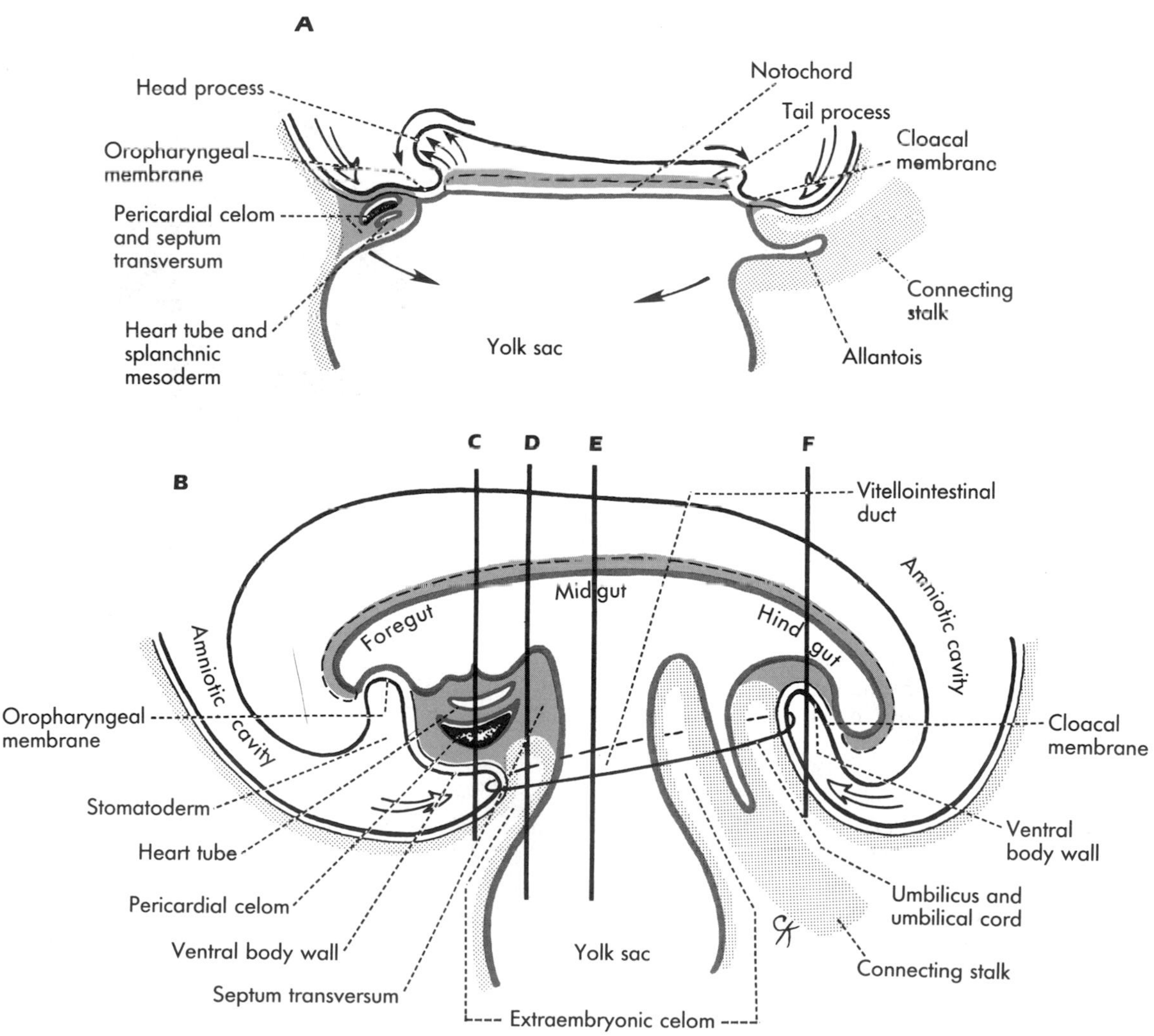

FIGURE 9-3.
Folding of the embryonic disk: (A and B) Two successive stages of the folding in sagittal section illustrate the head fold and tail fold. The positions of transverse sections (C through F) are identified in B.

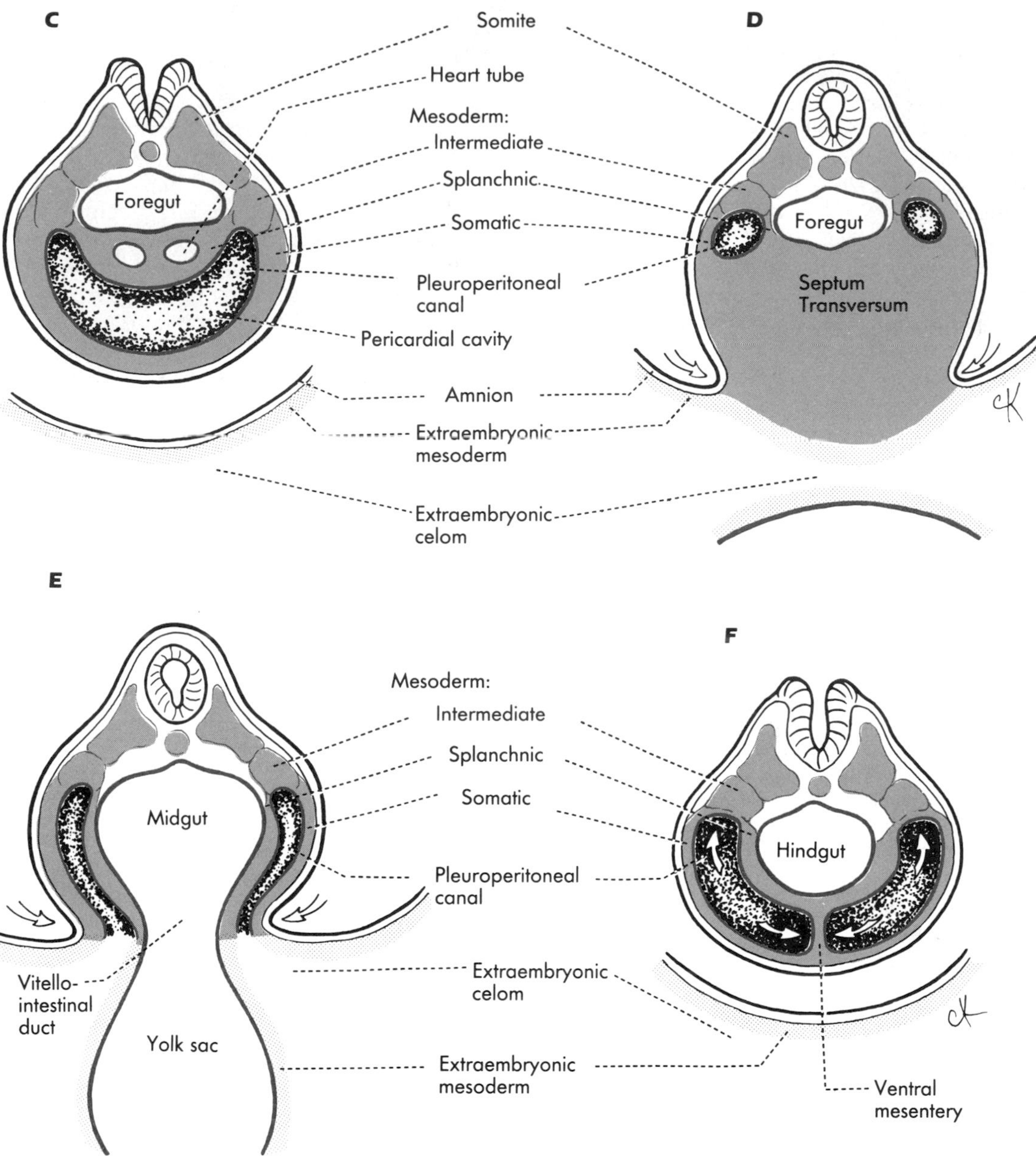

FIGURE *9-3 (Continued).*
(C) a section through the pericardial portion of the celom; *(D)* through the septum transversum; (E) through the vitellointestinal duct; and (F) through the hindgut just anterior to the cloacal membrane.

cardial cavity sharply indents the yolk sac (Fig. 9-3A, and B). The consequences of this head fold are that 1) part of the yolk sac becomes entrapped within the embryo and can henceforth be called the **foregut** (*proenteron*); 2) the pericardial cavity is placed ventral to the foregut (see Fig. 9-3C), 3) a ridge of mesoderm is placed transversely across the ventral aspect of the embryo interposed between the pericardial cavity and the yolk sac—this mesoderm is the **septum transversum** (see Fig. 9-3D); 4) a ventral body wall covered in ectoderm is created in the ventromedian area of the rostral part of the embryo.

At the caudal end, the **tail fold** likewise indents the yolk sac, entrapping the **hindgut** (*metenteron*) in the embryo, and creates a ventromedian body wall (see Fig. 9-3B and F). However, no septum transversum is formed caudal to the yolk sac because a transverse portion of the celom is lacking caudally.

The lateral edges of the embryonic disk also move ventrally as the **lateral folds** indent the lateral wall of the yolk sac and enclose the **midgut** (*mesenteron*) in the now somewhat cylindrical body of the embryo (see Fig. 9-3E). In this manner, the ventrally curved perimeter of the once disk-shaped embryo constricts around the yolk sac from all directions like a purse string, stopping short around an opening that becomes the umbilicus (see Fig. 9-3A and E). A narrow connection persists between the midgut and the

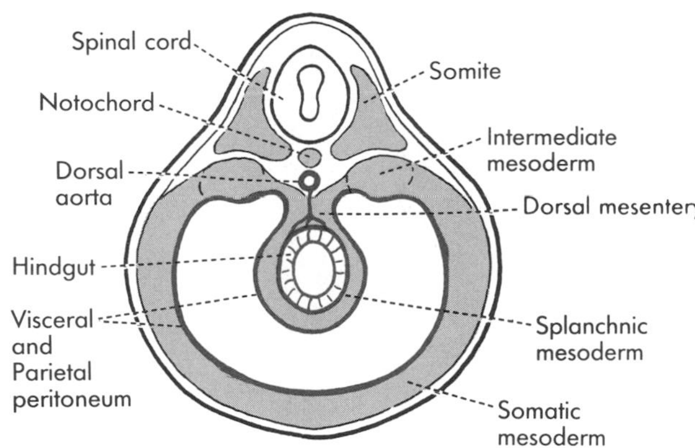

FIGURE *9-4.*
The scheme of the peritoneal cavity, derived from developmental stages shown in Figure 9-3.

extraembryonic yolk sac and is called the *vitellointestinal duct*. Because the amnion remains attached around the embryonic disk during this folding, the amnion will be attached around the umbilicus and will invest the vitellointestinal duct and the connecting stalk, which contains the umbilical veins and the umbilical arteries as these structures enter or leave the body of the embryo, in what can now be called the *umbilical cord*.

The fusion of the edges of the lateral folds with the extraembryonic and splanchnic mesoderm on the exterior of the vitellointestinal duct and with the tail fold, closes the communication between the extraembryonic celom and the pleuroperitoneal canals (see Fig. 9-3E and F). The definitive anatomy of the **serous sacs** is attained by 1) the separation of the pericardial sac from the pleuroperitoneal canals by the *pleuropericardial membranes* (see Fig. 19-12); 2) expansion of the portion of the pleuroperitoneal canals rostral to the septum transversum to form the bilateral pleural sacs (see Fig. 19-12); and separation of the sacs from the distal portion of the pleuroperitoneal canals by the bilateral *pleuroperitoneal membranes*, which complete the septum transversum dorsally (see Fig. 25-4); 3) formation of the peritoneal sac by expansion of the pleuroperitoneal canals distal to the septum transversum and the fusion of the two canals ventral to the midgut and hindgut so that the gut comes to be suspended by a dorsal mesentery (Fig. 9-4).

Differentiation of the Primitive Gut

By the breakdown of the oropharyngeal membrane, the foregut establishes communication with the *stomatodeum*, a depression lined by ectoderm from which part of the oral cavity develops (see Fig. 9-3B). Similarly, by the breakdown of the cloacal membrane, the hindgut establishes communication with the *proctodeum*, a depression or pit lined by ectoderm from which part of the anal canal develops. The cranial part of the foregut forms the pharynx, in the lateral wall and floor of which a number of ridges and epithelial pouches make their appearance. From the epithelial outgrowths develop a number of glands located in the neck, which lose connection with the pharynx. From one of the ventral diverticula of the pharynx develops the trachea and the lung buds (see Chap. 20). This diverticulum retains communication with the pharynx and, at their junction, develops a specialized sphincter, the larynx, which is also adapted for voice production. The lung buds invaginate the pleural sacs (see Fig. 19-12). The remainder of the foregut becomes the esophagus, the stomach, and part of the duodenum. The liver, gallbladder, and pancreas bud off from the distal end of the foregut and will be joined to the duodenum by their excretory ducts (see Fig. 24-21). From the midgut develop the rest of the small intestine and part of the colon; from the hindgut is formed the rest of the large intestine (see Fig. 23-24).

RECOMMENDED READINGS

Anson BJ, Lyman RY, Lander HH. The abdominal viscera in situ: a study of 125 consecutive cadavers. Anat Rec 1936; 67: 17.

Barclay AE. The digestive tract. London: Cambridge University Press, 1933.

Batson OV. Anatomic variations in the abdomen. Surg Clin North Am 1955; 35: 1527.

Boyden EA. Segmental anatomy of the lungs: a study of the patterns of the segmental bronchi and related pulmonary vessels. New York: McGraw-Hill, 1955.

Moody RO. The position of the abdominal viscera in healthy, young British and American adults. J Anat 1927; 61: 223.

Murray JF. The normal lung. 2nd ed. Philadelphia: WB Saunders, 1986.

Thurlbeck WM. Structure of the lungs. Int Rev Cytol 1977; 14: 1.

Williams PL, Bannister LH, Berry MM, et al eds. Gray's anatomy. 38th ed. New York: Churchill Livingstone, 1995.

Hollinshead's Textbook of Anatomy, by Cornelius Rosse and Penelope Gaddum-Rosse.
Lippincott-Raven Publishers, Philadelphia, © 1997.

CHAPTER 10

The Urogenital System

Urinary and genital organs are closely related both anatomically and developmentally and, therefore, are grouped together as the urogenital system. In both sexes, the urinary system consists of the paired kidneys, the duct (ureter) leading from each kidney to the urinary bladder situated in the pelvis, the bladder itself, and the channel (the urethra) by which the bladder opens to the outside. The genital or reproductive system in both sexes consists of paired gonads (ovary or testis), a duct system by which the products of the gonads escape to the outside, and the external genitalia that are associated with these ducts. In the male, the ducts from the testis discharge to the outside by way of the urethra, which the genital and urinary systems share. In the female, the duct system is largely separate from that of the urinary system, and the paired ducts are partly fused together to form the uterus. Genital and urinary systems in the female share a shallow opening (the vestibule) to the outside.

URINARY SYSTEM

Kidney and Ureter

There is no essential difference in the urinary system of the two sexes (Fig. 10-1). Urine is formed in the **kidney** (*ren;* hence, the adjective "renal") by a process of filtration from the blood vessels. This filtrate is modified as it passes down a long and convoluted tubule. Beyond their convoluted portions, adjacent tubules join each other to form collecting tubules.

The *cortex,* or outer part of the kidney, is largely concerned with the formation of urine, whereas the *medulla,* or inner part, consists primarily of collecting tubules that serve for transport (cortex and medulla mean bark and marrow, respectively). The urine in the collecting tubules is delivered into a single large chamber that is drained by the **ureter,** a thick-walled tube that by peristaltic action conducts urine to the urinary bladder.

Because the kidneys are situated in the upper part of the abdominal cavity, against the posterior abdominal wall, and the urinary bladder is situated in the lowest part of the pelvic cavity, the ureters are some 25 cm to 35 cm long. Any interference with the flow of urine through them endangers the life of the kidney. When a ureter is obstructed, the kidney continues to produce urine and the pressure of this gradually destroys the renal substance, so that eventually the kidney loses its excretory power entirely.

Humans readily survive removal of one kidney, but destruction of both kidneys is incompatible with life, for other excretory organs—the skin, the lungs, the colon—cannot take over the functions of the kidney. Visualization of the urinary passages by radiography offers excellent means of determining not only the condition of the urinary tract and the positions of the kidneys, but also the state of function of these important organs.

A more detailed description of the kidneys and the ureters will be found in Chapter 25.

Urinary Bladder and Urethra

The **urinary bladder** (*vesica urinaria*) is a distensible sac located primarily in the pelvic cavity, but rising more or less into the abdomen as it becomes filled with urine. It lies anterior to the rectum in the male and anterior to the uterus and vagina in the female. It receives the two ureters and by the contraction of its smooth muscle discharges the urine to the outside through the urethra.

The **urethra** in the female is short and embedded in the anterior wall of the vagina. Both it and the vagina open between prominent folds, the labia, that are a part of the external genitalia. In the male, the urethra, as it leaves the bladder, is surrounded by the prostate (Fig. 10-2). Enlargement of this gland is a common cause of difficulty in emptying the bladder in the male. After leaving the prostate, the male urethra enters the penis, continuing to the end of this organ. The ducts of the genital system join the prostatic part of the urethra, so that both urinary and genital systems share the major length of the urethra.

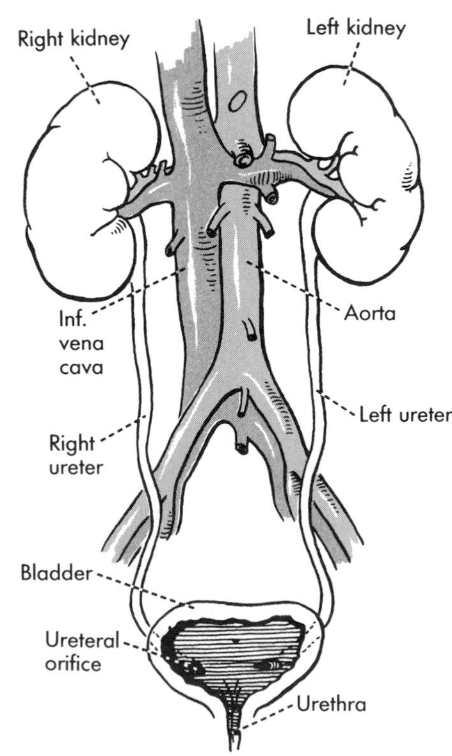

FIGURE *10-1.*
Diagram of the urinary system.

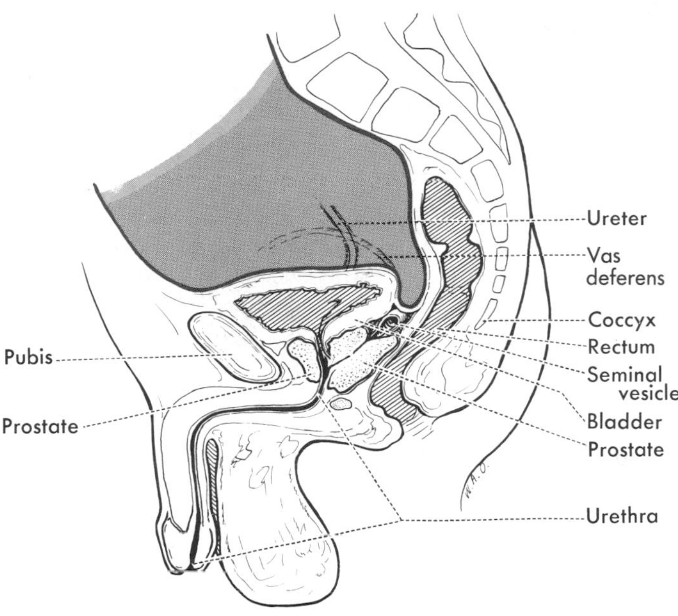

FIGURE *10-2.*
Male pelvis in sagittal section, showing a part of the urogenital system: The cut edge of the peritoneum is shown as a *red* line, and the peritoneal cavity is shaded *pink*.

GENITAL SYSTEM

Male Genital System

The genital system of the male consists of the two **testes** and their ducts, most of the **urethra,** the **prostate** and **seminal vesicles,** and the **external genitalia,** of which the **penis** houses the urethra and the **scrotal sac** houses the testes.

Development of Testis and Ducts

In their early development, the testes originate very close to a primitive kidney, the *mesonephros,* and they make use of the duct system provided by this evanescent kidney. The testis develops a series of *seminiferous tubules* in which, after sexual maturity, male germ cells, or *spermatozoa* are produced. These tubules, at an early stage of development, become connected to tubules of the mesonephros, which then drain the seminiferous tubules. The mesonephric tubules open into the mesonephric duct, but after this duct becomes connected to the testis by the mesonephric tubules, its name is changed to **ductus deferens.** With further development, the lower ends of the two deferent ducts open into the urethra.

Close to their lower ends, the deferent ducts give off blind diverticula that become the **seminal vesicles** (*vesicle,* meaning little bladder), so called because they were once thought to store spermatozoa. They are actually glands that contribute to the *seminal fluid* (ejaculate). The other major gland that contributes to the seminal fluid is the **prostate,** which develops as multiple outgrowths from the urethra and largely surrounds a part of it. The **penis** develops from a swelling just above the opening of the urethra to the outside and by its growth comes to surround the urethra as it elongates.

Although the testis originates in the abdomen, it migrates caudally, passes through the anterior abdominal wall, and descends into the scrotum, a diverticulum of this wall.

Female Genital System

There are many parallels in the development of the male and female genital systems, and homologies of parts of the two systems are easily apparent.

Development

The **ovary** begins its development, as does the testis, at the level of the mesonephric kidneys; however, unlike the testis, it separate completely from the celomic epithelium from which it develops. The mesonephric tubules and mesonephric duct do not become connected with the ovary, and they largely degenerate. Instead of the ovum's being discharged directly into a tube, the mature ovum is therefore discharged from the surface of the ovary into the peritoneal cavity and is picked up by a tube that opens into this cavity. The primitive tube is the paramesonephric duct, which parallels the mesonephric duct, and it is developed in close relation to it. Unlike the mesonephric duct, the paramesonephric duct opens directly into the peritoneal cavity. As they descend toward the pelvis, the two ducts fuse to form the unpaired uterovaginal canal, and the paired upper parts of the ducts remain as the **uterine tubes.**

The ovaries undergo a descent, for a time paralleling that of the testis, but they and the uterine tubes normally end by taking up a position in the pelvis.

Anatomy

In the adult female, each **ovary** lies on the lateral wall of the pelvis, close to that end of the uterine tube that opens into the peritoneal cavity. The other ends of the uterine tubes empty into the **uterus** (Fig. 10-3).The uterus is thick walled because its musculature must be heavy to accommodate and then expel the fetus and because its mucosa (*endometrium*) must accommodate numerous glands, the secretion of which nourishes the developing embryo. The endometrium undergoes a cyclic thickening in preparation for the expected monthly release of the ovum from the ovary. This endometrial hyperplasia occurs as a result of hormones acting on the uterus. Failure of an egg to be fertilized produces a shift in hormonal balances that leads to rapid endometrial degeneration and its discharge during menstruation.

The uterus empties into the much thinner-walled **vagina** through a narrow lower segment known as the **cervix,** which protrudes into the upper part of the vagina. Because carcinoma of the uterus most often starts at the

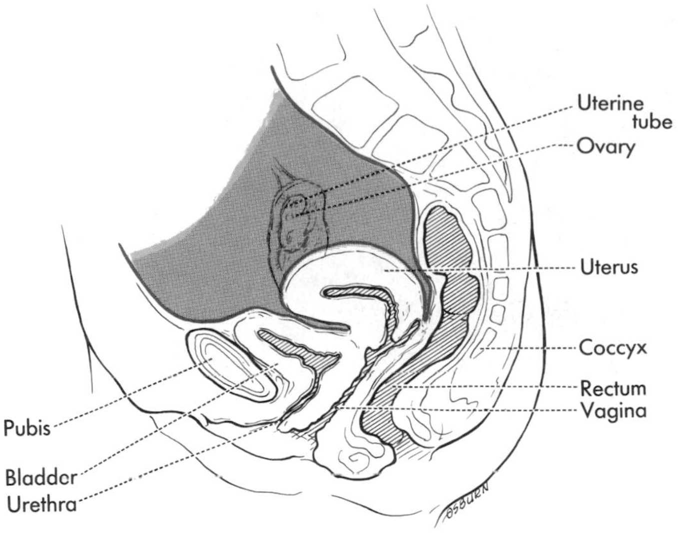

FIGURE *10-3.*
Sagittal section of the female pelvis, showing the chief reproductive organs: The cut edge of the peritoneum is shown as a *red line,* and the peritoneal cavity is shaded *pink.*

cervix, examination of the cervix and of material obtained from the vagina by vaginal smear is often useful in its early detection.

The vagina opens through the pelvic floor into the **vestibule,** into which the urethra also opens. The walls of the vestibule, the **labia minora,** are homologues of part of the penis of the male, and the larger folds outside the labia minora, the **labia majora,** are homologues of the scrotal sac of the male. Another part of the penis is represented by the **clitoris,** the tip or glans of which lies anteriorly where the labia minora come together.

Hermaphroditism

The early development of the male external genitalia is identical with that of the female; therefore, the sex of the fetus cannot at first be determined by examination of the external genitalia. Cessation in development of male genitalia results in their closely resembling those of the female. Overdevelopment of female genitalia produces a condition resembling that of an underdeveloped male. The condition in which testes occur in an individual with apparently female genitalia, or ovaries in a person with apparently male genitalia, is known as *psuedohermaphroditism.* It is more common in males than in females. *True hermaphroditism,* in which an individual has both a testis and an ovary, or a gonad that is a combination of both, is very rare in humans.

RECOMMENDED READINGS

Beeuwkes R. The vascular organization of the kidney. Annu Rev Physiol 1980; 42: 531.

Gosling JA, Dixon JS, Humpherson JR. Functional anatomy of the urinary tract. London: Churchill Livingstone, 1983.

Gray SW, Skandalakis JE. Embryology for surgeons. Philadelphia: WB Saunders, 1972.

Hacker NF, Moore JG. Essentials of obstetrics and gynecology. 2nd ed. Philadelphia: WB Saunders, 1992.

Potter EL. The normal and abnormal development of the kidney. Chicago: Mosby-Year Book, 1974.

Redman JF. Anatomy of the genitourinary system. In: Gillenwater JY, ed. Adult and pediatric urology, 2nd edition. Chicago: Year Book Medical Publishers, 1991.

Smith HW. The kidney. New York: Oxford University Press, 1969.

Walsh PC, Gittes RF, Perlmutter AD, Stamey TA, eds. Campbell's Urology. 6th ed. Philadelphia: WB Saunders, 1992.

Williams PL, Bannister LH, Berry MM, et al eds. Gray's anatomy. 38th ed. New York: Churchill Livingstone, 1995.

Hollinshead's Textbook of Anatomy, by Cornelius Rosse and Penelope Gaddum-Rosse.
Lippincott-Raven Publishers, Philadelphia, © 1997.

CHAPTER 11

The Endocrine System

The endocrine system consists of a few widely separated glands that form discrete anatomic organs and of other smaller groups of cells that are located in organs that belong to other systems. From the anatomic perspective, the endocrine glands are united by one fundamental characteristic: they are glands that do not have ducts, but instead, discharge their secretions (hormones) directly into the bloodstream. A synonym is "ductless glands". The cells of most endocrine glands are epithelial, as are the cells of exocrine glands. Because of the necessary close relation with the bloodstream, endocrine tissue is particularly vascular. For instance, the thyroid gland, one of the endocrine glands, has been said to have the greatest blood supply per unit of tissue of any organ in the body.

Although the endocrine glands differ markedly from each other in many anatomic features, and the hormones that they produce differ widely in chemical composition and in physiologic action, nevertheless, they form a physiologic system: they all produce hormones that act on other tissues of the body; some of these hormones also act on other endocrine glands. Many of the fundamental metabolic activities of the body are governed by the endocrine system.

The recognized endocrine glands are the unpaired hypophysis, four parathyroid glands, the unpaired thyroid gland, and the paired suprarenal glands. In addition to these, the ovaries and the testes have endocrine functions; the pancreatic islets are composed of endocrine cells; certain parts of the digestive tract also liberate hormones; and the liver, has some endocrine functions. Finally, the pineal body, an outgrowth of the thalamus of the brain, is also sometimes described as an endocrine organ. Because the various endocrine organs and tissues are described later in this text, according to their regional anatomy, remarks concerning them here will be limited primarily to physiologic considerations.

HYPOPHYSIS

The hypophysis (pituitary gland) is actually two closely associated endocrine organs. The posterior part of the hypophysis (**posterior lobe** or *neurohypophysis*) is an outgrowth from the floor of the hypothalamus of the brain. A larger part is derived from surface ectoderm that during the growth of the mouth is carried back into the roof of the pharynx. When this part separates from the pharyngeal wall, it becomes closely associated with the posterior lobe and forms the important **anterior lobe** and a part, rudimentary in humans, known as the pars intermedia.

The hypophysis lies immediately beneath the brain and is connected to it by the hypophyseal stalk, representing the stem by which the posterior lobe grew out from the brain. Blood vessels surround the stalk that arise in the hypothalamus and end in the hypophysis, especially the anterior lobe. The *hypophyseal stalk* consists primarily of nerve fibers that end in the posterior lobe. It is generally accepted that the posterior lobe does not itself produce the hormones that it secretes into the bloodstream, but merely releases them into capillaries after they have been formed by nerve cells in the brain and have migrated along the nerve fibers to the posterior lobe.

The **posterior lobe** apparently secretes two recognized hormones, an antidiuretic hormone (also known as vasopressin) and oxytocin. Antidiuretic hormone, or vasopressin, has to do with controlling the amount of water excreted by the kidney and also produces constriction of arterioles and, therefore, a rise in blood pressure. Oxytocin produces contraction of the smooth muscle in the uterus and also has a lactogenic effect, causing expulsion of milk from the lactating breast.

The **anterior lobe** of the hypophysis is glandular, rather than neural, in appearance (hence, also called *adenohypophysis*), and the several types of epithelial cells composing it are believed to secrete several different hormones. Although the secretory activity of the anterior lobe is controlled in part by the nervous system, this control is not through nerve fibers, but through substances released into the blood vessels about the hypophyseal stalk. These begin in the central nervous system and end in the hypophysis (the hypophyseal portal system).

There is no agreement on exactly how many hormones are secreted by the anterior lobe. The most important active principles of this lobe have to do with growth of the body as a whole, with the development and maintenance of the gonads, and with the maintenance of secretory activity by the thyroid gland and the suprarenal (adrenal) cortex. At least six hormones of the anterior lobe are usually named: a growth hormone, a thyrotropic hormone, corticotropin (adrenocorticotropic hormone; rather generally known, even to laymen, as ACTH), and two gonadotropic hormones. Because of its effects on the endocrine activity of the gonads, the thyroid, and the suprarenal cortex, the anterior lobe of the hypophysis is sometimes known as the master endocrine gland.

Loss of growth hormone, or the fraction of the hormone that has to do with growth, in young animals leads to cessation of growth in body size. Similarly, oversecretion of this hormone produces increased skeletal growth, which may be general and lead to gigantism or, if it occurs at a somewhat later time as a result of a tumor of the gland, produces *acromegaly* (characterized by abnormal enlargement of the lower jaw and of the hands and feet). Lack of secretion of the gonadotropic hormones results in failure of secretion by the endocrine portions of the testis and ovary and failure of production of ova or spermatozoa. In young animals, because the development of sexual characteristics is dependent on these secretions, the secondary sex characteristics fail to develop. A similar lack in the adult female leads to cessation of the reproductive cycle, and in adults of both sexes to disappearance of sexual activity and gradual regression of the sex organs. Lack of thyrotropic hormone greatly diminishes the secretory activity of the thyroid gland and, therefore, produces a marked drop in metabolic activity. Lack of secretion of adrenocorticotropic hormone lowers the secretory activity of the adrenal cortex and may produce symptoms of adrenal cortical insufficiency.

The *pars intermedia* in lower animals secretes a hormone that acts on melanophores (pigment cells). Its function in humans is unknown.

SOME HORMONAL INTERRELATIONS

Although the anterior lobe of the hypophysis has been referred to as the master endocrine gland, it must not be supposed that the secretions of the other endocrine glands have no effect on each other's activities or on the activity of the anterior lobe. Interrelations among the endocrine glands and their hormones are extremely complex, and many facts about them remain to be determined.

One of the more obvious interrelations between endocrine glands can be seen in the thyroid gland. Although largely governed in its secretory activity by secretion of thyrotropic hormone from the anterior hypophysis, the secretion of the thyroid gland itself affects the metabolic activity of all tissues of the body and, therefore, the activity of the anterior lobe of the hypophysis and of all the other endocrine glands.

Another interendocrine relation, particularly well known, is the cycle of secretion of the hormone corticotropin by the anterior lobe of the hypophysis and the secretion of certain adrenal cortical hormones by the adrenal cortex. Stated in its simplest form, the anterior lobe secretes corticotropin in sufficient amounts to cause secretion by the adrenal cortex. However, in turn, the amount of adrenal hormones in the bloodstream determines the rate of corticotropin secretion by the anterior lobe. Adrenocortical hormones, circulating to the anterior lobe, depress the activity of the lobe in secreting corticotropin; therefore, when the adrenal hormones have reached an adequate level, the anterior lobe ceases to secrete. Then, as the secretion of adrenocortical hormones drops off in consequence of lack of stimulation through the anterior lobe's hormone, less circulating hormone reaches the anterior lobe and it begins to secrete once again. Accordingly, the adrenal cortex, although governed by the anterior lobe, in turn regulates the activity of the anterior lobe in governing it. Exactly similar "feedback" relations seem to exist between the thyroid gland and the anterior lobe, and the gonads and this lobe.

A clear example of the effect of at least two different hormones on a single organ is seen relative to skeletal growth. The growth hormone apparently produces its effects by increasing the rate of proliferation of cartilage cells which, in turn, under normal conditions (thyroid hormone probably being essential for this), increase the rate of ossification and, therefore, the rate of growth of the bones. However, certain sex hormones have a different effect on the epiphyses; they decrease the rate of proliferation and maturation of the cartilage, so that the process of ossification overtakes the growth of new cartilage and the epiphyseal cartilages are totally eliminated. When this occurs, growth ceases. The earlier secretion of larger amounts of sex hormones by the developing female than by the male, evidenced in the earlier sexual maturity of the female, is responsible for the fact that bone growth in females regularly ceases some 1 to 3 years earlier than it does in males. Another feature of this relation that is of clinical importance is that, because sex hormones tend to interfere with growth, they cannot be given indiscriminately to growing children. For instance, certain hormones that may produce descent of an undescended testis before the age of puberty can have a stunting effect on growth.

THYROID GLAND

The thyroid gland lies in the neck across and lateral to the trachea. Rather than being arranged in irregular cords permeated by blood vessels, as are the epithelial cells of many endocrine glands, the epithelial cells of the thyroid form vesicles. The outer wall of each vesicle is adjacent to an abundant capillary network, and the hollow within the vesicle serves as a storehouse for thyroid hormone until it is needed by the rest of the body.

The nerves to the thyroid gland are probably purely vasomotor and have nothing directly to do with its secretory activity. This apparently is controlled primarily by the activity of the anterior lobe of the hypophysis.

The hormone of the thyroid gland contains iodine, and a supply of iodine in the diet is necessary for its formation. In the absence of an adequate intake of iodine, the thyroid gland attempts to produce a larger amount of hormone, as if to make up for its deficiency in iodine, and the gland becomes markedly larger. This enlargement of the gland is *simple goiter*, once fairly common in certain areas of Switzerland and the United States, where soil and water are deficient in iodine compounds. The availability of radioactive iodine has allowed rather precise study of the ability of a thyroid gland to handle iodine.

The chief effects of thyroid hormone are well known. It is essential to normal metabolism, and marked destruction of the thyroid gland in an adult depresses basal metabolism to such an extent that mental activity is interfered with, and the pulse rate and temperature of the body fall below normal. For reasons not clearly understood, there is also a deposition of subcutaneous connective tissue, which causes the face and hands to appear edematous. This condition is known as myxedema and is readily treated with desiccated thyroid. Absence of adequate secretion by the thyroid gland in infants affects both intelligence and physical growth and, if prolonged, produces idiocy and dwarfism (cretinism). However, treatment with desiccated thyroid, when begun during the infantile period, will usually prevent the otherwise inevitable arrest of physical and mental development.

Quite different from the enlargement of the thyroid gland produced by lack of thyroid hormone is the enlargement occurring, for unknown reasons, in association with markedly increased activity on the part of the gland. In this instance, the enlarged gland secretes more than a normal amount of hormone, with the result that there is an increased metabolic rate, nervousness, and loss of weight (these being symptoms of hyperthyroidism). In connection with this type of enlargement, the eyeballs typically become prominent, so this is known as *exophthalmic* (toxic) *goiter*. Removal of a part of the thyroid gland, thus leaving less glandular tissue to secrete, has been effective in relieving the symptoms of this type of goiter. Removal of more gland than is necessary to achieve the desired results is not serious, because the metabolic activity of the patient can be restored to normal levels by the administration of desiccated thyroid.

PARATHYROIDS

The parathyroid glands, usually four of them, are closely associated with the thyroid gland (typically lying on its posterior surface); but are different from it both in origin and in physiology. They derive from the walls of the third and fourth branchial pouches and only secondarily become associated with the thyroid gland. Although they are small bodies, the presence of one or more is necessary to health. Surgeons, therefore, so plan their operations on the thyroid that they can be rather confident of not removing all parathyroid tissue.

The hormone of the parathyroid glands exerts control over the calcium content of the blood. The normal constant interchange between blood and bone is only partly independent of parathyroid hormone, and lack of the hormone produces a marked fall in the calcium content of the blood. This, in turn, produces nervous and muscular disturbances and tetany. The opposite effect is produced by oversecretion of parathyroid hormone, typically resulting from a parathyroid tumor; here the blood-calcium level is markedly raised, and because the diet of the individual relative to calcium usually has not been changed, the calcium is typically withdrawn in abnormal amounts from the bones, with resulting fragility of those elements. A person with an untreated severe parathyroid tumor may break an arm or a rib by simply turning over in bed. Furthermore, the increased blood calcium level leads to increased excretion of calcium in the urine, and renal stones are not infrequent accompaniments of a parathyroid tumor. Too much parathyroid secretion produces weakness, diarrhea, and vomiting, and, if severe enough, circulatory collapse and death.

SUPRARENAL GLANDS

The suprarenal glands lie behind the peritoneum of the abdominal wall, closely associated with the upper poles of the kidneys; hence their name of suprarenal or adrenal glands. (In humans, they are properly called suprarenal glands, whereas in most animals they are called adrenal glands; however, the latter term is commonly applied to the glands of humans.) A suprarenal gland is composed of cords of epithelial cells with abundant capillaries between these cords. Even on casual examination, it is obvious that there are two distinct types of cells and cell arrangements here. One type of cell forms the outer part of the gland, hence, the **cortex,** whereas the other type forms the center of the gland, the **medulla.**

The cortex and the medulla of the suprarenal gland are really two separate endocrine glands that have become closely associated. Similar to the anterior and posterior lobes of the hypophysis, the two parts of the suprarenal have distinct functions and different developmental histories. The **medulla** arises from some of the neural crest cells, that give rise to the prevertebral sympathetic ganglia, such as the celiac. The **cortex,** however, arises directly by proliferation of the celomic epithelium. In many lower animals, there is no close relation between the cortex and medulla, each occurring, rather, as a series of isolated bodies. Even in humans, there are a few isolated collections of cells identical with those of the adrenal medulla, known as *chromaffin tissue* (a term that also includes the medulla), and there may be small nodes of cortical tissue outside the gland that are not associated with medullary tissue.

The functions of the **suprarenal medulla** are believed to be much simpler than those of the cortex. The medulla secretes into the bloodstream a hormone, usually referred to as epinephrine or adrenaline, but known to consist of two forms, *epinephrine* and *norepinephrine.* Both forms act primarily on smooth muscle, producing the same effects that stimulation of the sympathetic nervous system does. Epinephrine, for instance, increases both the rate and strength of the heart beat and produces constriction of arterioles and, thus, a rise in the blood pressure. Hence, like activity of the sympathetic nervous system, epinephrine prepares the body for an emergency. Epinephrine dilates the pupil, as does the sympathetic nervous system. As a part of a preparation for an emergency, it also promotes the conversion of glycogen into glucose and the latter's discharge from the liver, so that a greater amount of blood sugar is available to the other tissues of the body. It is because of the hyperglycemia (increased sugar in the blood) produced by the liberation of epinephrine that glycosuria (a spilling over of sugar into the urine) may be found during times of stress and tension in persons who are otherwise normal. The finding of sugar in the urine of a student taking examinations, for instance, is usually attributable to oversecretion by the suprarenal medulla, not to the hypoinsulinism of diabetes.

The suprarenal medulla seems to be the only endocrine gland for which activity is controlled entirely by nervous impulses. The medullary cells have an abundant innervation, derived from the sympathetic nervous system. These fibers, preganglionic ones, end directly on the medullary cells without the interposition of the usual postganglionic cells and fibers—an apparent exception to the rule that in the autonomic system, the preganglionic fibers always end on postganglionic neurons. This is, however, easily reconciled when it is remembered that the medullary cells themselves represent postganglionic nerve cells (having the same origin) and produce the same effects as do postganglionic cells (but over the body in general, through the discharge of epinephrine, rather than in specific locations by sending nerve fibers to these locations). The chromaffin system of the body, of which the suprarenal medulla is the largest component, therefore seems to be an adjunct of the sympathetic nervous system. As with the sympathetic system, there is no evidence that the chromaffin system is essential to life. Destruction of all or almost all of this system in experimental animals is entirely compatible with normal existence in the laboratory, although an animal that had to defend itself or flee to save its life would be at a disadvantage.

Chromaffin cell tumors, usually of the suprarenal medulla, but sometimes developing from small chromaffin cell groups found associated with the sympathetic trunks in the thorax or abdomen, are one, but not the most common, cause of high blood pressure (hypertension). The hypertension tends to be spasmodic and to reach levels that endanger the life of the patient, so that when the diagnosis is made, the tumor is sought by surgical exploration and removed.

In contrast with the medulla, the **suprarenal cortex** is necessary to life. Degeneration of the suprarenal glands (Addison's disease) as a result of tuberculosis or other disease process, typically leads to bronzing of the skin, vomiting, and muscular weakness so severe that the individual is incapacitated. The disease typically resulted in death before replacement therapy was available. Several complex steroids have been isolated from the cortex. Some of these, among which cortisone is the most widely known, are particularly active physiologically. Cortisone and its related compounds have been used in the treatment of various diseases, and it is now possible to treat and maintain in good health persons afflicted with Addison's disease. The importance of the suprarenal cortex in reactions to mental and physical stress has been studied in great detail, increased cortical secretion being apparently the most important element in the "alarm reaction."

Hyperplasia of the cortex or functioning tumors (some tumors apparently do not secrete) lead to an excess of cortical hormones, with resultant overaction on other tissues, including other endocrine organs. Clinical findings in hyperplasia and functioning tumors of the cortex vary greatly, for the secretion may be largely cortisonelike material, sex hormones, or a mixture of both, and the effects of sex hormones vary with the sex of the individual. However, symptoms often include premature puberty in children, sexual changes in adults, hirsutism (abnormal growth of hair) in women, and diabetes mellitus (sugar diabetes); mental changes are not uncommon. Certain of these changes apparently depend on simple hypersecretion by the gland and, therefore, are amenable to treatment by operative removal of an appropriate amount of a gland. Others are apparently a result of secretion of estrogens or androgens, as a result of malfunction of the cortex, and are usually treated by the administration of cortisone. Tumors of the gland are removed surgically.

OTHER ENDOCRINE TISSUE

The **endocrine tissue of the pancreas,** the *pancreatic islets* (islets of Langerhans), consists of small groups of cells scattered among the more numerous acini (the exocrine part of the pancreas). The islets, very vascular, consist of two or more types of epitheloid cells, of which one is apparently concerned with the secretion of insulin. *Insulin* is concerned primarily with sugar (glucose) metabolism and is necessary not only for the proper oxidation of sugar, but also for its conversion into glycogen, in which it is stored, particularly in the muscles and the liver. (A substance known as glucagon, also produced by the islets, has an opposite effect—it provokes the liver to convert glycogen into glucose.) Too little secretion of insulin leads to accumulation of glucose in the blood with consequent excretion of it by the kidneys, a part of the syndrome of diabetes mellitus. Improper oxidation of sugar also leads to improper metabolism of fats. In contrast, too much secretion of insulin, which may result from a tumor of one or more pancreatic islets, leads to a dangerous decrease in blood sugar. This can be treated temporarily by supplying more sugar in the diet and can be cured by removing the tumor.

The **endocrine cells of the gonads** include several cell types. The most important are, in the testis, the **Leydig (interstitial) cells,** located between the seminiferous tubules and, in the ovary, the cells of the **ovarian follicles.** After the egg is liberated, they proliferate, change their character, and become cells of the *corpus luteum*. It is the hormones produced by these cells that can be grouped together as **sex hormones,** which (with sex hormones liberated by the suprarenals) are responsible for the development of secondary sex characteristics and, in the female, the institution of the menstrual cycle or its cessation with pregnancy.

Hormones from the digestive tract include a substance released by the duodenal mucosa that causes the gallbladder to discharge bile into the duodenum and another substance that provokes the secretion of enzymes from the exocrine part of the pancreas. One part of the stomach also releases a hormone that provokes the secretion of acid by the stomach.

Whether the **liver** should be classed as an endocrine organ is debatable, but its activity does affect the endocrine balance. Among the activities of the liver is that of inactivating sex hormones (generally classed as *estrogens*, or female sex hormones, and *androgens*, or male sex hormones, both of which are produced in both sexes). With increasing failure of hepatic function, for instance, potent estrogens (which are normally less readily inactivated than androgens) may come to predominate in the bloodstream of a male and produce testicular atrophy, gynecomastia (enlargement of the male breast), and disturbance of the gonadal–hypophyseal relation.

RECOMMENDED READINGS

Bergland RM, Page RB. Pituitary-brain vascular relations: a new paradigm. Science 1979; 204: 18.

Crowder RE. The development of the adrenal gland in man, with special reference to origin and ultimate location of cell types, and evidence in favor of the "cell migration" theory. Contrib Embryol 1957; 36: 193.

Fawcett DW, Long JA, Jones AL. The ultrastructure of the endocrine glands. Recent Prog Horm Res 1969; 25: 315.

Fawcett DW. Bloom and Fawcett: a textbook of histology. 12th ed. New York: Chapman & Hall, 1994.

Hollinshead WH. Anatomy of the endocrine glands. Surg Clin North Am 1952; 32: 1115.

Schalley AU, Kastin AJ, Arimura A. Hypothalamic hormones: the links between brain and body. Am Scientist 1977; 65: 712.

Swinyard CA. Growth of the human suprarenal glands. Anat Rec 1941; 87: 141.

Tixier-Vidal A, Farquhar MG, eds. The anterior pituitary. New York: Academic Press 1975.

Weller GL Jr. Development of the thyroid, parathyroid, and thymus glands in man. Contrib Embryol 1933; 24: 93.

Wilson JD, Foster DW, eds: Williams textbook of endocrinology. 8th ed. Philadelphia: WB Saunders, 1992.

PART III

BACK

Hollinshead's Textbook of Anatomy, by Cornelius Rosse and Penelope Gaddum-Rosse.
Lippincott-Raven Publishers, Philadelphia, © 1997.

CHAPTER 12

The Vertebral Column

The body of all vertebrate animals is built on a central axis known as the vertebral column. This *backbone* or *spine* consists of a series of bones, the **vertebrae** (Fig. 12-1). Reflecting their embryonic origin from segmented paraxial mesoderm, the vertebrae are metamerically arranged bones, firmly connected to one another by joints and ligaments. This arrangement lends a considerable degree of springiness and flexibility, as well as strength, to the entire vertebral column.

Although all parts of the column contribute to its overall role as a robust, yet flexible, axis, five specific **regions** are recognized on the basis of differences in curvature and other functionally important features. They are the **cervical, thoracic, lumbar, sacral,** and **coccygeal** regions (see Fig. 12-1). Typically, there are 7 cervical, 12 thoracic, and 5 lumbar vertebrae; these are succeeded by the **sacrum,** formed by the fusion of 5 vertebrae, and by the **coccyx,** formed of rudimentary vertebrae. The first coccygeal vertebra is commonly separate, whereas the succeeding 3 are fused together. Thus, there are typically 33 vertebrae in the column.

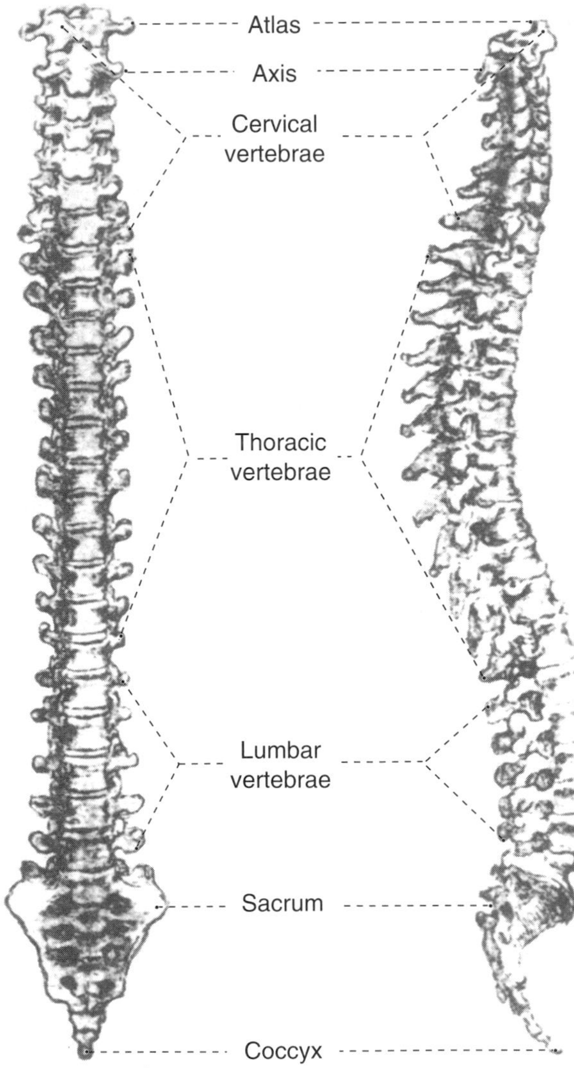

In the human, the vertebral column supports the head and the trunk in the erect position and, through the pelvic girdle, transmits the weight of the body to the lower limbs. From the lower limbs it receives the propulsive impetus during locomotion. Thus, the vertebral column is continually subjected to a variety of forces. The rib cage is suspended on the vertebral column and the articulations between ribs and vertebrae permit the movements necessary for respiration. The vertebral column protects the spinal cord by enclosing it in the **vertebral canal.** From this canal issue all spinal nerves for the supply of the limbs, the neck, and the trunk. The contents of the vertebral canal and the anatomic relations between the spinal cord segments, spinal nerves, and the vertebrae are discussed in Chapter 13. This chapter deals with the bony elements, joints, muscles, and movements of the vertebral column.

FIGURE *12-1.*
The vertebral column, drawn by Leonardo da Vinci, as seen from the *front* and the *side.*

Developmental Considerations

In the trilaminar embryonic disk, the intraembryonic mesoderm is organized into the notochord, which forms the first axis of the early embryo, and three distinct mesodermal regions, the paraxial, intermediate, and lateral plate mesoderm (see Fig. 9-2). Of particular relevance for the development of the vertebral column is the paraxial mesoderm that, as its name implies, comprises a column of tissue on either side of the notochord. It becomes subdivided into brick-shaped, segmentally arranged masses of cells, the somites. The latter give rise to the sclerotomes, myotomes, and dermatomes; these three groups of cells, in turn, are the precursors of the axial skeleton, skeletal muscle, and the dermis of the skin, respectively. The spinal nerves, growing out of the developing spinal cord, and the intersegmental branches of the aorta, become closely associated with these somite derivatives and serve as useful landmarks during the establishment of the definitive segmental anatomy (Fig. 12-2). This anatomy is determined by two major factors: expression of homeobox-containing (*Hox*) genes and local cell interactions. An understanding of these factors and the mechanisms that regulate them is beginning to emerge from experiments in the chick embryo and in transgenic mice. Some of these experiments replicate congenital anomalies of vertebral segmentation that are well recognized in the human.

Sclerotomal cells, induced by the notochord and the ventral portion of the neural tube, proliferate and detach themselves from the ventromedial portions of the somites, and regroup around the notochord; their

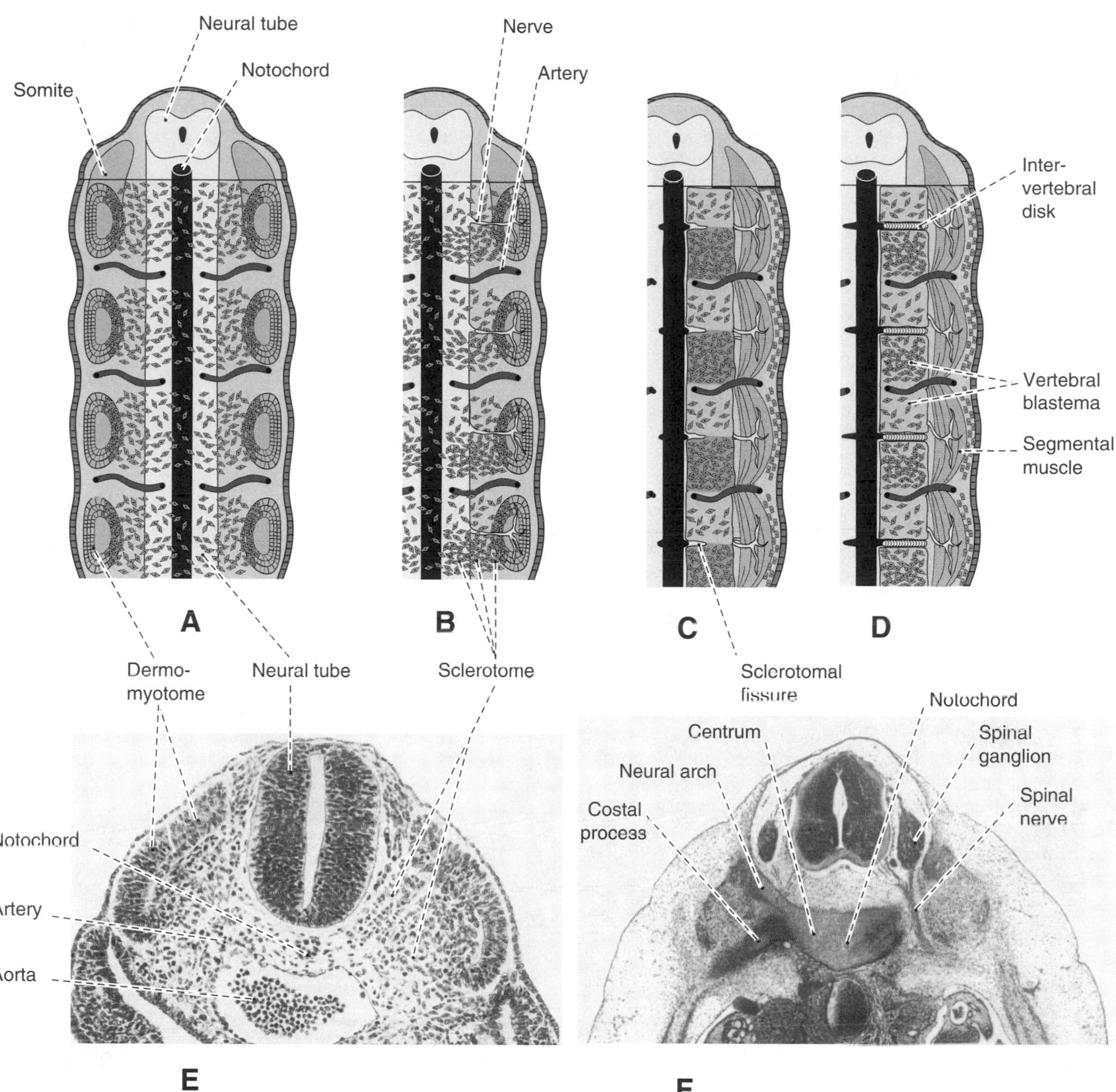

FIGURE *12-2.*
Stages in the differentiation of the somites, sclerotomes, and the vertebral blastema: (A through D) coronal sections cut along the axis of the notochord. Sclerotomal cells are shown migrating medially from the somites to surround the notochord. Note the relation of the intersegmental arteries (*red*) and spinal nerves (*white*) to the somites, myotomes, sclerotomes, and the blastema of the vertebra. The latter is generated by fusion of the dense caudal half of one sclerotome with the loose cranial half of the next sclerotome. (E) Transverse section of a 5-week-old human embryo, which corresponds to stages shown in panels A and B. (F) Two halves of successive transverse sections of a 10-week-old human embryo juxtaposed; the half on the *left* cuts through the centrum and the neural arch of a mesenchymatous vertebra, the half on the *right* through a segmental nerve. (A–D adapted from Hamilton WJ, Boyd JD, Mossman HW. Human embryology. 4th ed. Cambridge: Heffer and Sons, 1972; E, Fitzgerald MJT. Human embryology. New York: Harper & Row, 1978; F, Gasser RF. Atlas of human embryos. New York: Harper & Row, 1975.)

segmental pattern is made evident by the intersegmental arteries (see Fig. 12-2A and B). Within each sclerotome, the mesenchymal cells become loosely arranged cranially and more densely packed caudally. Between these two sclerotomal regions there appears a dense band, and later a fissure, which separates the cranial and caudal halves of the sclerotome. The caudal half of one sclerotome fuses with the cranial half of the next, and it is this aggregate that forms the primordium of the vertebral body (vertebral blastema), whereas the fissure defines the position of the future intervertebral disk. The notochord is soon lost in regions where it is enveloped by developing vertebral bodies, but between the vertebrae, some cells remain and will form the centers of the intervertebral disks. If notochordal remnants persist within vertebral bodies, they may give rise to cartilage tumors later in life (*chordomas*).

Between the developing spinal nerves, cells extend dorsolaterally from the cranial portion of each vertebral primordium to surround the neural tube (see Fig. 12-2F). This extension forms the **neural arch,** whereas the more bulky, ventral portion enclosing the notochord is the **centrum** of the mesenchymal vertebra. Sclerotomal cells also migrate ventrolaterally to form the **costal elements.** Only in the thoracic region, however, do costal elements normally develop into discrete bones, such as the ribs; in other regions they fuse with the vertebra.

Rearrangement of the sclerotomes establishes a number of important relations (see Fig. 12-2D): Each myotome is positioned opposite two vertebrae, and segmental muscles derived from it can produce movement between the two vertebrae. Spinal nerves leave the spinal cord between neural arches to make contact with adjacent myotomes. The relations established with the neural arch will be retained, and the nerve associated with a vertebra will innervate that vertebra, its joints, and ligaments as well as the corresponding myotome and dermatome. Branches of the aorta skirt the ventral surface of the centrum as they pass to the body wall and will also furnish the blood supply to the corresponding segment of the spine.

Chondrification converts the mesenchymal vertebrae into hyaline cartilage, in which ossification centers will appear. The mesenchyme that persists between the cartilaginous vertebrae develops into intervertebral disks between the centra and into ligaments and synovial joints between the neural arches. Growth and ossification of the cartilaginous vertebrae continue well past puberty and are discussed in a subsequent section.

Variation in the Number of Vertebrae. There is evidence that the segmental rearrangement of the sclerotomal mesenchyme is influenced by local cellular interactions. In the chick embryo, removal of the notochord results in unsegmented centra (resembling *block vertebra;* see following), and removal of spinal ganglia results in unsegmented neural arches. In mice, six specific patterns of *Hox* gene expression define the six regions in which vertebrae share morphologic features. These are the occipital, cervical, thoracic, lumbar, sacral, and caudal regions. The occipital vertebrae become incorporated into the base of the skull, and caudal segments in the human are represented only by the rudimentary coccyx. Shifts in the boundaries of *Hox* gene expression, caused by the introduction of transgenes into germline mice or by exposure of the embryo to chemical agents (e.g., retinoic acid), alter the normal constitution of these regions. Some of these induced mutations, for instance, transform the base of the occipital bone into a discrete *proatlas* vertebra, and others resemble some of the spontaneous regional variations in vertebral numbers of the human column (e.g., Klippel-File syndrome, characterized by a short neck owing to a reduced number of cervical vertebrae).

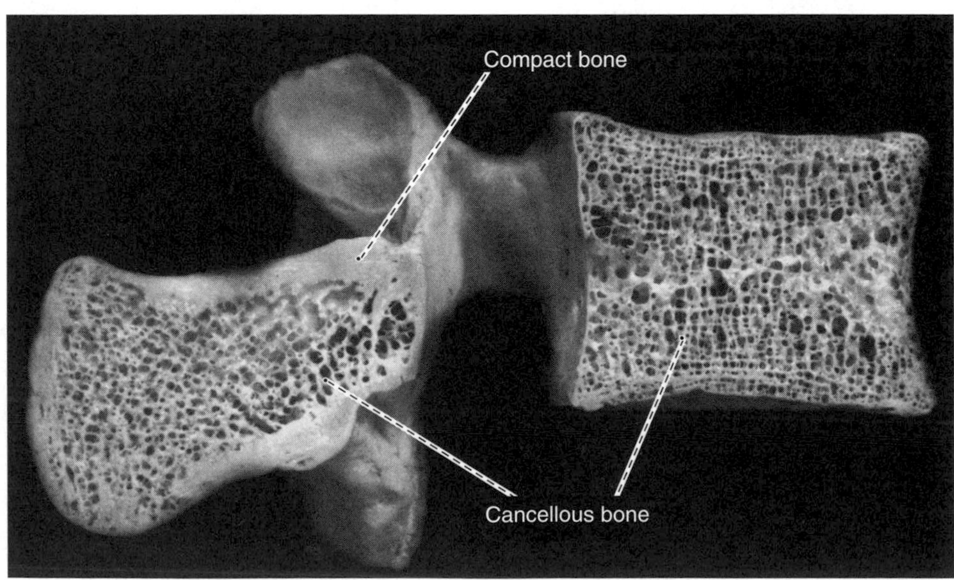

FIGURE *12-3.*
Sagittal section of a vertebra: Cancellous bone is invested by compact bone or cortex, which is very thin over the body of the vertebra and thicker over the spinous process.

Occasionally, a vertebral column may consist of 32 or 34 vertebrae instead of the typical 33. More commonly, however, numerical variations occur within specific regions, rather than in the column as a whole. The lumbar region, for example, may comprise six vertebrae instead of five if the first sacral vertebra fails to fuse with the sacrum. The thoracolumbar portion of the column is thus lengthened in such individuals (6% of cases). In others, there is some degree of fusion, partial or complete, between the fifth lumbar vertebra and the sacrum, thereby shortening the thoracolumbar portion of the spine (5% to 6% of cases, see Fig. 12-7).

THE VERTEBRAE

The Typical Vertebra

Composition and Parts

Vertebrae are made of cancellous (spongy) bone encased in a shell of compact bone (Fig. 12-3). In all regions of the spine, vertebrae have two basic components: the **body** and the **vertebral arch** (Fig. 12-4). The arch projects posteriorly from the body, and the two enclose the **vertebral foramen.** Successive vertebral foramina form the vertebral canal within which lies the spinal cord, enveloped in its meninges.

The **vertebral body** is the bulky, anterior part of the vertebra, shaped like a squat, somewhat irregular, cylinder or truncated cone. It has superior and inferior surfaces; each is flat and covered by hyaline cartilage. Abutting surfaces of two vertebral bodies are held together securely by an **intervertebral disk** composed of fibrocartilage. On the convex anterolateral surface of the body, there are numerous small foramina for nutrient vessels; on the posterior surface, one or two large foramina transmit the large basivertebral veins. The height and circumference of the vertebral bodies and the intervening disks increase progressively in a downward direction until the sacrum is reached (see Fig. 12-1); such an arrangement is consistent with the lower vertebrae having a greater role in weight bearing.

The **vertebral arch** consists of a right and left **pedicle** and **lamina.** On each side, the pedicle projects posteriorly and continues into the lamina. The two laminae fuse in the midline (see Fig. 12-4). The vertebral arch thus formed bears several bony processes, some for articulation with adjacent vertebral arches and others for attachment of muscles and ligaments. On each side, three processes arise from the junction of the pedicle and the lamina: a **transverse process,** which projects laterally, and a **superior** and an **inferior articular process** (*superior* and *inferior zygapophyses*) that project upward and downward, respectively. A **spinous process** extends posteriorly at the union of the two laminae (see Fig. 12-4).

The laminae are flat and broad; their vertical extent is about the same as that of the vertebral bodies. Consequently, in the erect or extended position, virtually no space exists between successive pairs of laminae, and they provide a flat posterior wall, or roof, for the vertebral canal. The pedicles, on the other hand, are rounded bars of bone; as their vertical extent is considerably shorter than that of the vertebral bodies and laminae, the vertebral canal is open laterally between successive vertebrae (see Fig. 12-4). These **intervertebral foramina** are

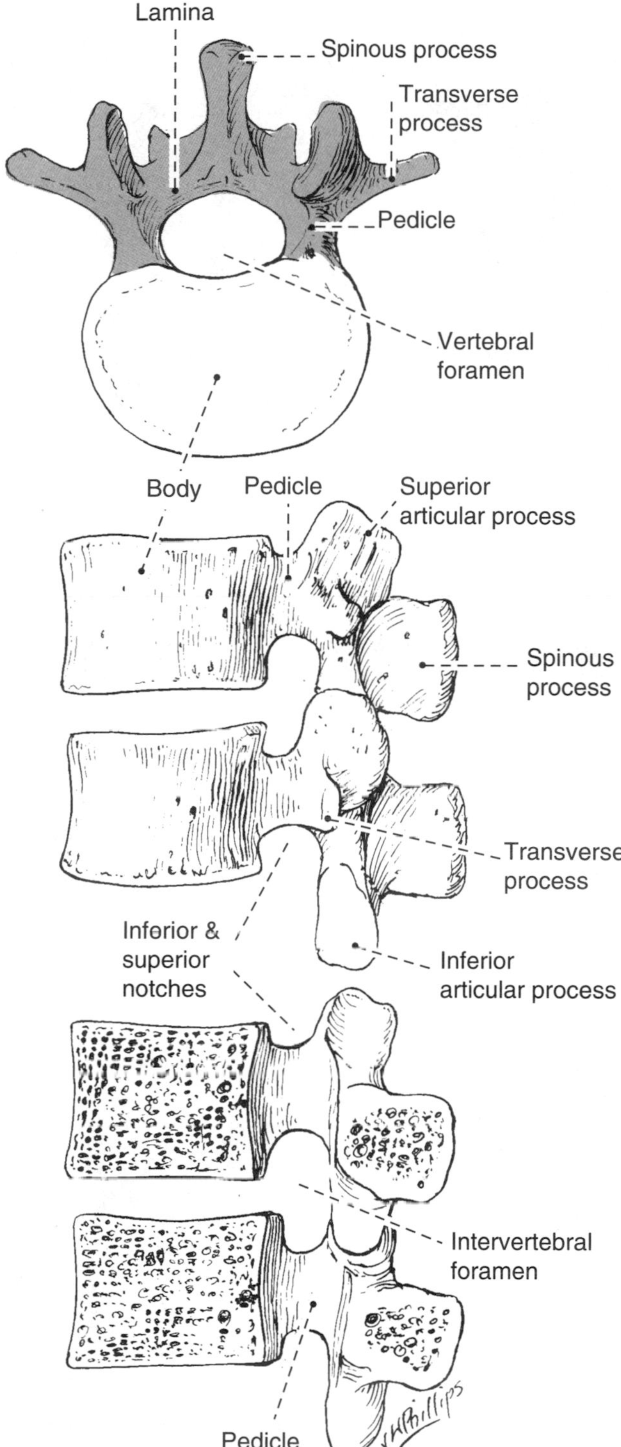

FIGURE 12-4.
Parts of a typical vertebra as seen from *above*, from a *lateral view* and on a *sagittal section*. In the *uppermost* figure, the vertebral arch is shaded.

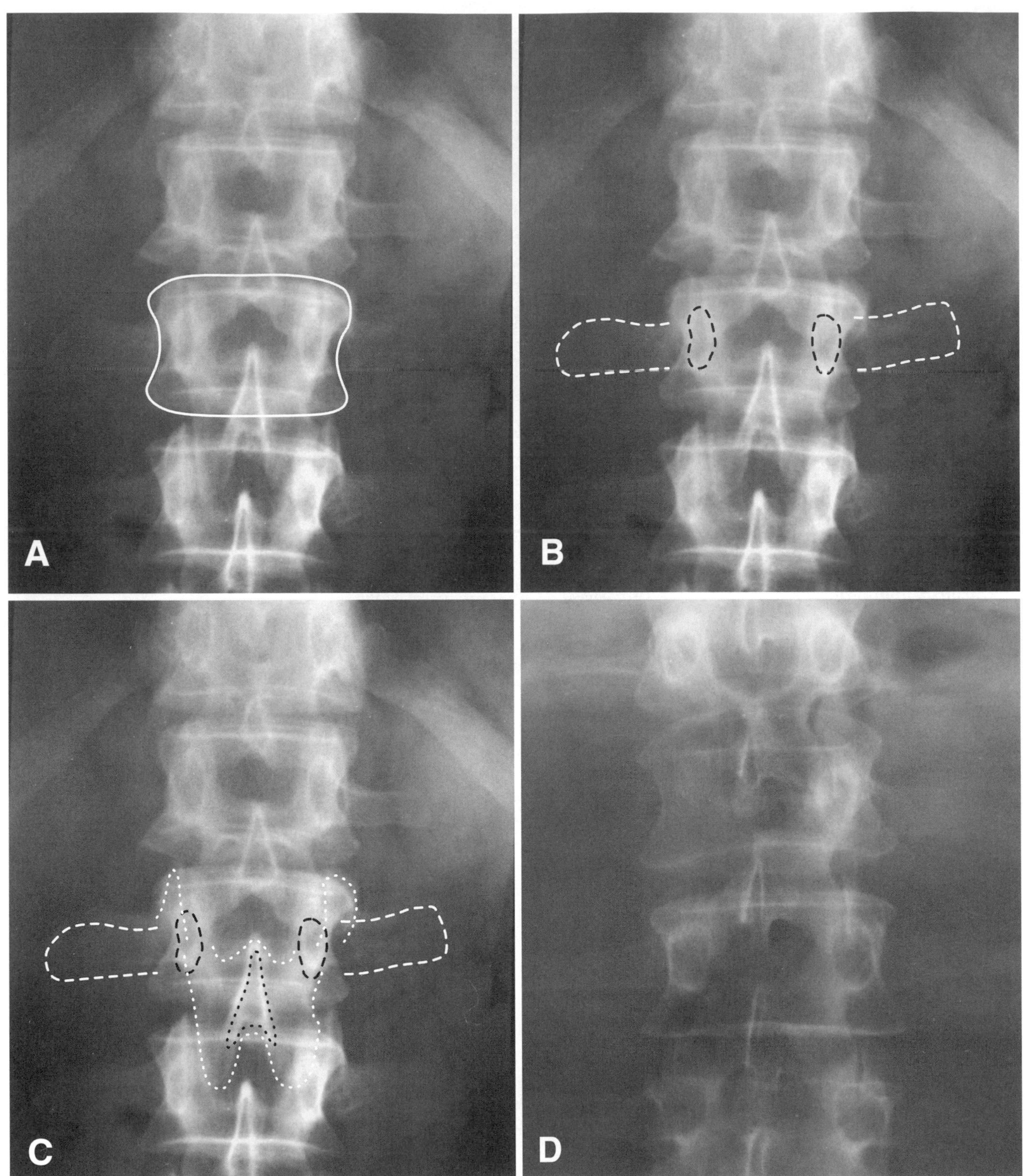

FIGURE *12-5.*
A stepwise approach for identifying the anatomic parts of a vertebra on an anteroposterior radiograph: (A) The contour of the vertebral body; (B), *interrupted lines* define the roots of the pedicles (*black*) and the transverse processes (*white*); (C) *dotted lines* are superimposed on the profile of the laminae, superior and inferior articular processes (*white*), plus the spinous process (*black*), which together resemble a butterfly. (D) Several defects are present in the second of the lumbar vertebrae from the top of the picture. The pedicle, the transverse process, and the superior and inferior articular processes are missing on the *right side* of the patient. They have been eroded by a malignant neoplasm situated in the intervertebral foramen. (Courtesy of Dr. Rosalind H. Troupin.)

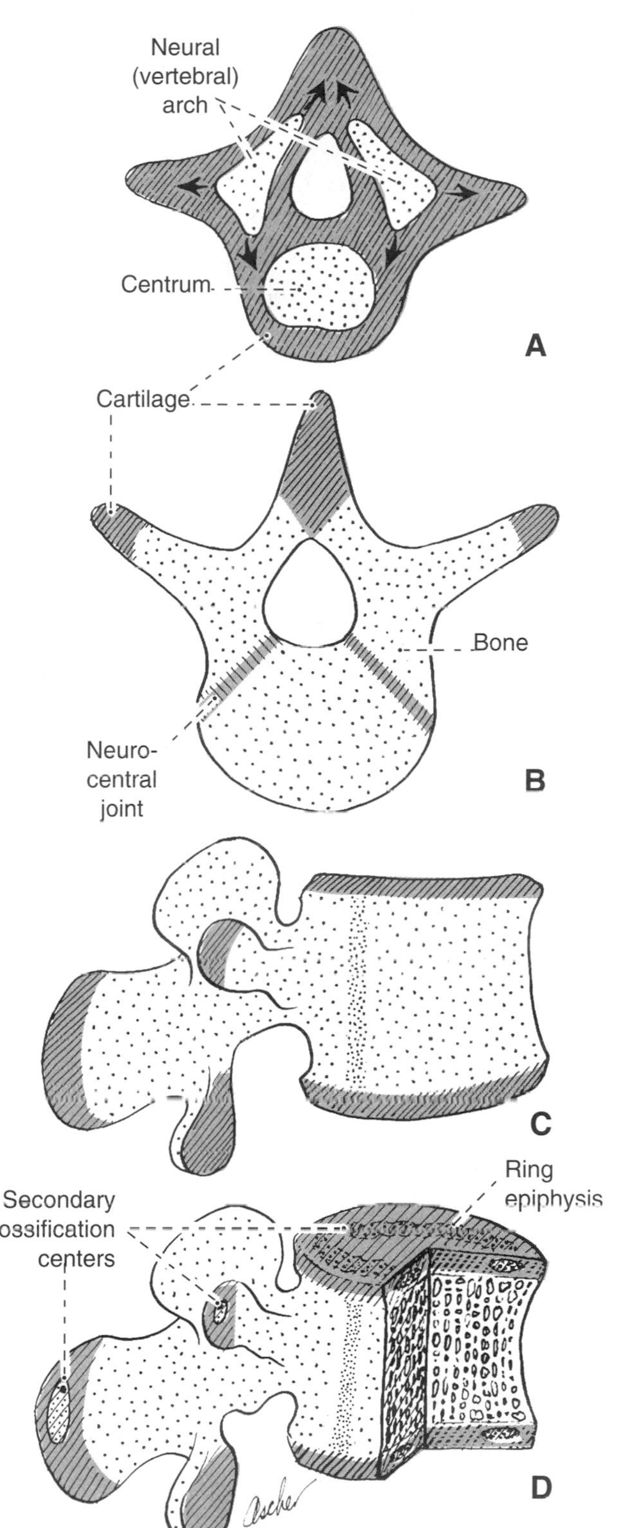

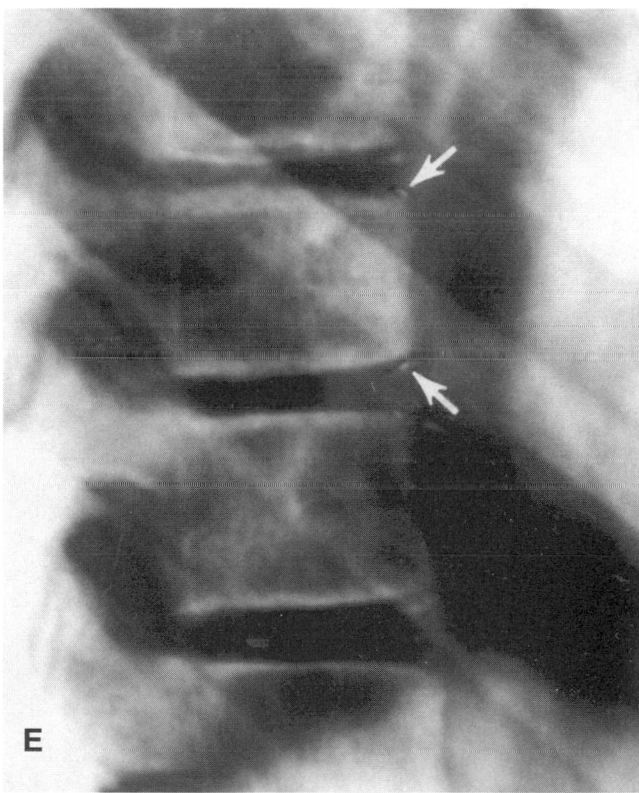

FIGURE *12-6.*
Ossification of a typical vertebra: Cartilage is shown in *blue*, bone in *white*. (A) Primary ossification centers for the centrum and neural arch during the fetal stage; (B) at birth; (C) shortly before puberty. *Dense shading* on the vertebral body indicates the position of the neurocentral junction. (D) secondary ossification centers at puberty; (E) lateral radiograph of the lumbar spine at the age of 13 years. The ring epiphyses are visible anteriorly at the superior and inferior margins of the vertebrae (*arrows*). (E, courtesy of Dr. Rosalind H. Troupin.)

bounded above and below by the pedicles, anteriorly by the vertebral bodies and the intervening intervertebral disk, and posteriorly by the articular processes and the joint capsules that connect them (see Fig. 12-16). The concavities that form the upper and lower boundaries of an intervertebral foramen are the **vertebral notches** (*incisures*), the inferior notch being deeper, as a rule, than the superior one.

Radiographs of Vertebrae

Despite the superimposition of several profiles, all parts of a vertebra can be identified on radiographs by following a simple, disciplined approach. The approach is illustrated in Figure 12-5.

Development and Growth of a Typical Vertebra

Before the growth of the cartilaginous vertebra is completed (see foregoing), three *primary ossification centers* appear within it; one in the **centrum** and one in each half of the **neural arch** (Fig 12-6A). From the centrum develops most of the vertebral body, whereas the neural arch becomes the vertebral arch of the mature vertebra. Overall growth of the cartilage enlarges the vertebra, while at the same time ossification spreads from the primary centers in several directions (see Fig. 12-6A). By the time of birth, the centrum and the two half arches are primarily bony; the apex of the arch is still cartilaginous, however, as is the spinous process. Cartilage also caps the transverse processes, covers the upper and lower surfaces of the vertebral body, and unites the neural arch with the centrum at the **neurocentral joints** (see Fig 12-6B). Since the ossification center of each half arch adds bone to the posterolateral part of the vertebral body, the neurocentral joint is actually within the vertebral body.

During the early postnatal years, the ossifying fronts of the two half arches meet and unite with each other at the back. The neural arch also unites with the centrum, eliminating the neurocentral joints (see Fig 12-6C). At puberty, *secondary ossification centers* (epiphyses) appear within the remaining cartilage in five places: at the tips of the spinous and transverse processes, and as two **ring epiphyses** on the upper and lower surfaces of the vertebral bodies (see Fig. 12-6D and E). Growth at all these epiphyses ensures continued enlargement of the vertebra until they unite with the rest of the bone at 18 to 25 years. As a rule, epiphyseal fusion begins in the cervical region and proceeds toward the sacrum.

Congenital Abnormalities

Malformations of the Vertebral Body. The right and left sclerotomes normally fuse in the midline, obliterating the notochord; if they fail to fuse and the notochordal canal persists, a **cleft** or **butterfly vertebra** is formed (Fig. 12-7). A further malformation may occur later on, after the mesenchymal centrum has formed and chondrification is about to begin. There are normally two chondrification centers (right and left) that develop and soon fuse; if one does not appear, chondrification and subsequent ossification occur only on the contralateral side of the vertebra. The resultant **hemivertebra** predisposes to lateral curvatures or scoliosis of the spine. A third malformation involves

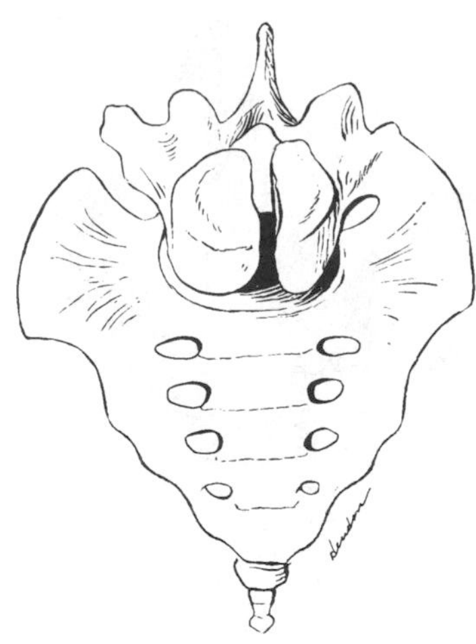

FIGURE *12-7.*
Cleft fifth lumbar vertebra, the transverse process of which has fused with the sacrum on the *left side*, thus sharing the fate of the sacral transverse processes.

the persistence of cartilage in the neurocentral joint, causing defects in the posterolateral parts of the vertebral body.

Malformations of the Vertebral Arch. The most common congenital anomalies of the spine affect the vertebral arch. Defects in midline union exist in different degrees. The simplest is failure of fusion between the ossification centers in the right and left half of the vertebral arch. The condition, called **spina bifida occulta,** is usually asymptomatic (see Fig. 13-20). More serious degrees of nonunion are associated with meningeal and spinal cord abnormalities that are most commonly seen in the lumbosacral region. These are discussed in the next chapter.

Malformations of the Costal Elements. Except in the thoracic region, where they form the ribs, the costal elements normally fuse with the vertebra. They may, however, develop into supernumerary ribs. The cervical rib of the 7th cervical vertebra, and the "gorilla" rib below the 12th thoracic vertebra are the most frequent examples.

Vertebral Fusion. Fusion of all vertebral elements is a normal process in the sacral region, and results in the formation of the sacrum (see later discussion). The centrum of the first cervical vertebra normally fuses with the centrum of the second and is represented by the dens of the axis (discussed in the following). These fusions are influenced by homeobox-containing genes, and it seems likely that mutations of these genes are responsible for abnormal fusions in other regions, which result in so-called **block vertebrae.** The most common site of such fusion is between the fifth lumbar vertebra and the sacrum.

Regional Characteristics of Vertebrae

The similarities and differences between cervical, thoracic, and lumbar vertebrae are illustrated in Figure 12-8.

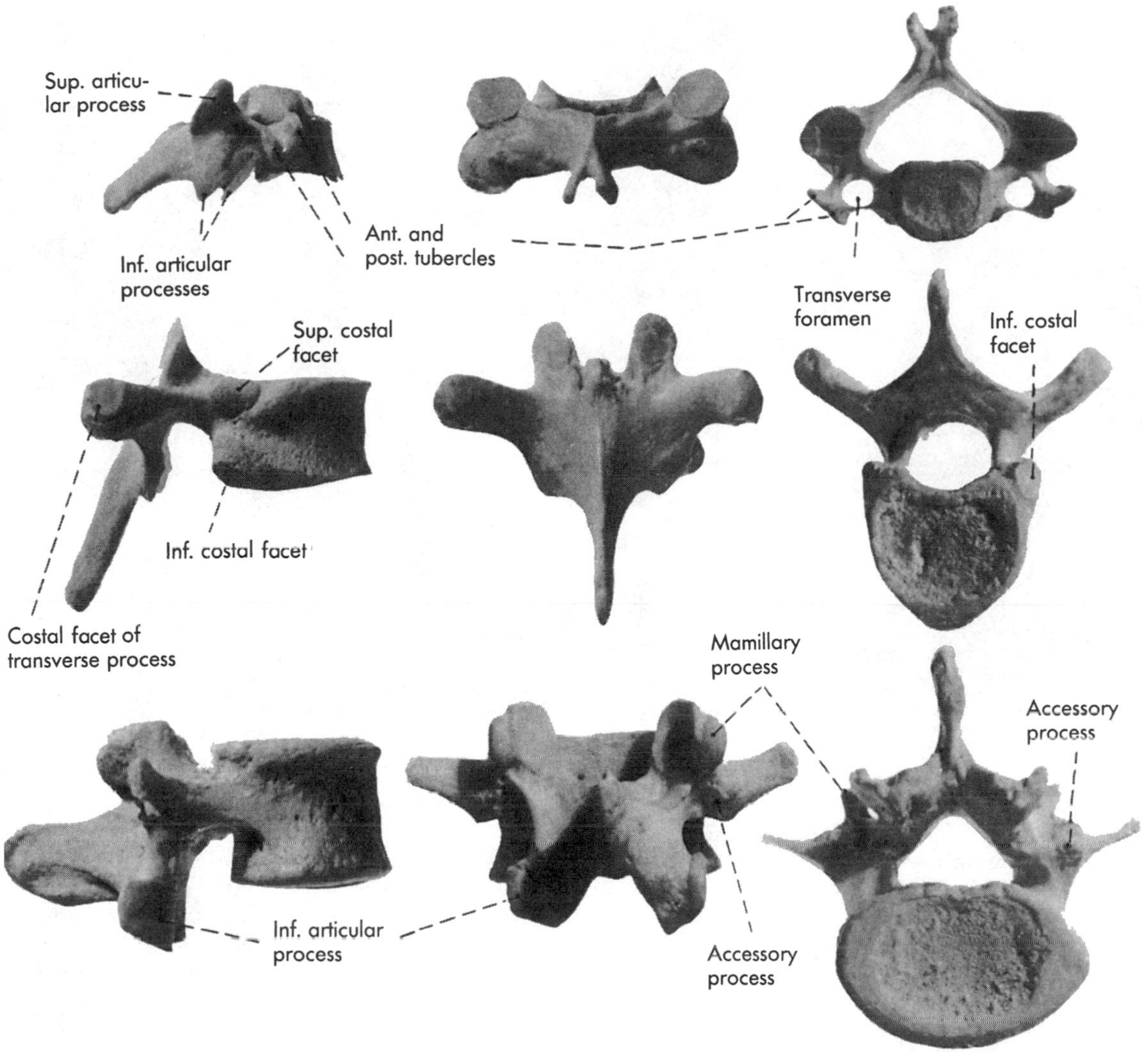

FIGURE *12-8.*
Lateral, posterior, and inferior views of the fourth cervical, seventh thoracic, and fourth lumbar vertebrae.

Cervical Vertebrae

All seven cervical vertebrae (C-1 through C-7) are easily distinguished from other vertebrae by the presence of a **transverse foramen** in each transverse process; these foramina transmit the vertebral vessels and associated sympathetic nerve plexuses. C-1, the **atlas,** and C-2, the **axis,** are highly specialized, and will be described after C-3 through C-7 vertebrae, which share common features. Many of these features are evident on radiographs of the cervical spine (Fig. 12-9).

Each vertebra in the **C-3** through **C-7** range has a relatively small, kidney-shaped body. On the other hand, the *vertebral foramen* is large by comparison with its size in other regions. It provides room for the spinal cord, which is of its greatest diameter in this region. Posterolaterally, the superior margin of the body (derived from the neural arch, rather than the centrum) curves upward as a lip or *uncus* (see Figs. 12-8 and 12-9). The lips articulate with beveled reciprocal facets on the inferior surface of the vertebra above, and form the so-called joints of Luschka (discussed later).

The *pedicles* are short and largely obscured by the broad transverse processes (see Fig. 12-8). Unlike those in other regions, they attach to most of the vertical extent of the body. Consequently, the inferior vertebral notches are shallow and the *intervertebral foramina* narrow. Therefore, the cervical spinal nerves that emerge through these foramina are particularly susceptible to compression. Flexion of the neck tends to open up the foramina, whereas extension, lateral bending, and rotation tend to crowd these spaces. Symptoms caused by nerve compression will be exaggerated by these latter movements and somewhat

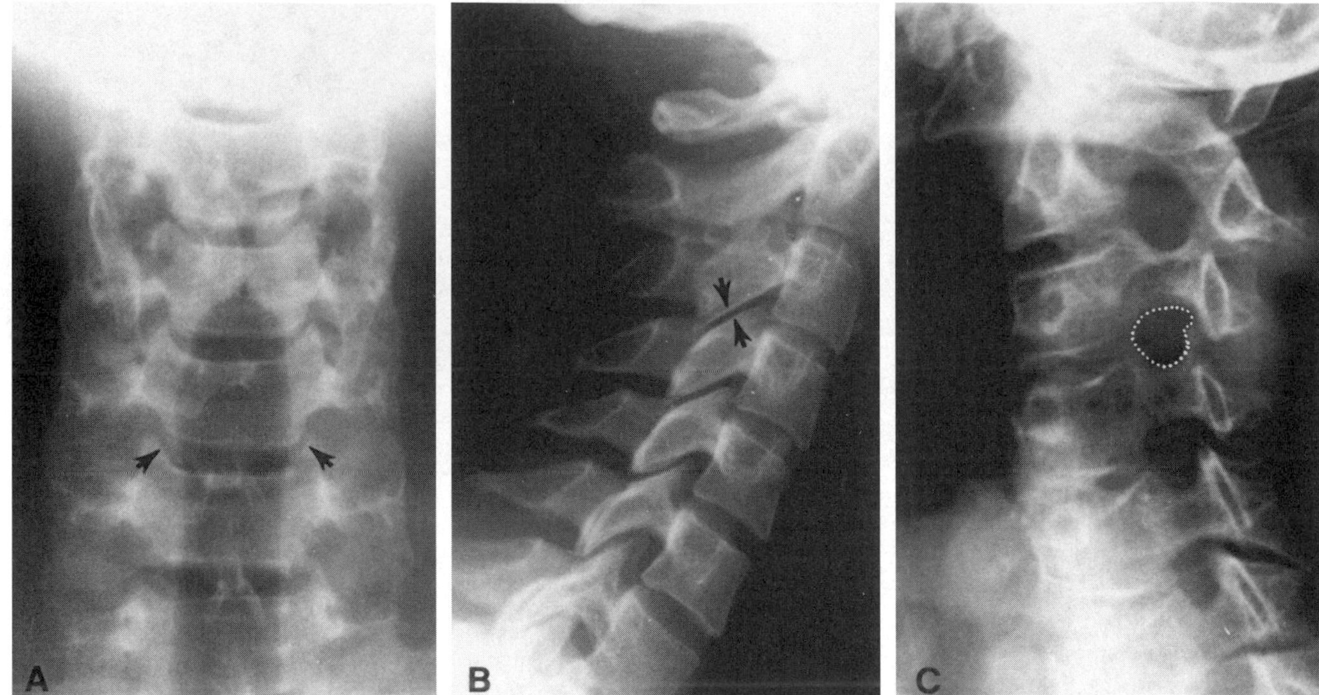

FIGURE *12-9.*
Radiologic anatomy of the cervical spine: (A) in the anteroposterior view, the most superior vertebra is C-3; C-1 and C-2 are obscured by the jaw. The lateral lip of the superior surface of the vertebral body (uncus) projects upward (*arrows*). The so-called joints of Luschka are situated here, replacing the posterolateral part of the intervertebral disk. The central radiolucent shadow is the trachea, which tapers into the larynx superiorly. (B) In the left lateral projection, the vertebral bodies and disks are well outlined, spinous processes are visible, and the joint space is clearly seen between superior and inferior articular processes (*arrows*). (C) A right oblique projection demonstrates the intervertebral foramina to best advantage (one of them outlined). The circular or C-shaped profile in the vertebral bodies anteriorly is the outline of the transverse process on the opposite side. (Courtesy of Dr. Rosalind H. Troupin.)

relieved by flexion. This may be appreciated by studying the radiologic anatomy of the cervical spine, particularly in the oblique projection (see Fig. 12-9).

The *articular processes* are bulky, and together form a column of bone that is interrupted by the *vertebral arch (zygapophyseal) joints* (see Fig. 12-9B). The facets of these joints influence the range of movements in the cervical spine. Those of the superior articular processes are turned backward and slightly upward to face the reciprocally oriented facets on the inferior articular processes (see Fig. 12-8). Sliding of the superior and inferior facets on one another permits flexion and extension of the neck. Because the facets on the right and left side lie more or less in the same coronal plane (see Fig. 12-19), these joints cannot contribute much to rotation of the neck.

The *spinous processes* on C-2 to C-6 vertebrae may or may not be bifid, depending on racial origin: they are bifid in white persons, for example, but usually not so in black people. The long and prominent spinous process of C-7 accounts for the name of this bone, the **vertebra prominens,** even though in a living person the spine of T-1 may be more prominent than that of C-7. The *transverse processes* of cervical vertebrae are complex structures (Fig. 12-10). The parts of the process that surround the transverse foramen have different homologues in other vertebrates. Knowledge of these homologues explains some congenital abnormalities.

The true transverse process is represented by a small bar of bone located posterior to the foramen. All other

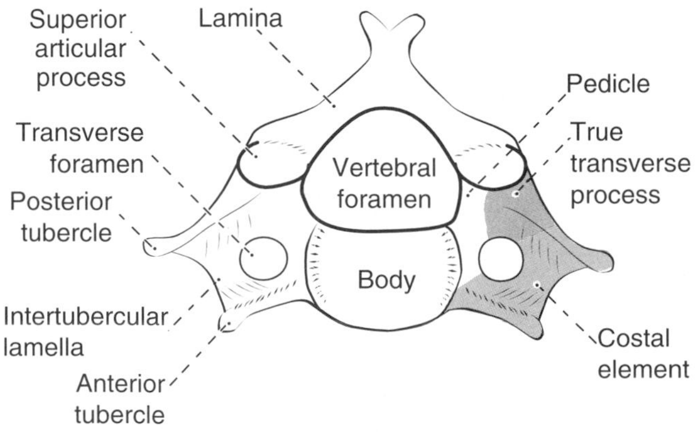

FIGURE *12-10.*
Parts of the transverse process of a cervical vertebra. (Adapted from Cave AGE. J. Zool 1975; 177: 377.)

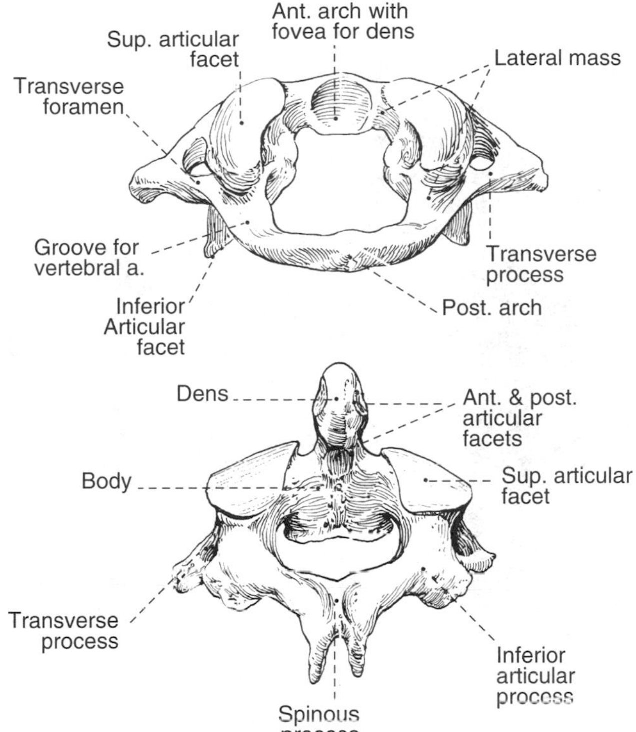

FIGURE *12-11.*
The atlas and axis seen from behind.

parts of the process are components of the **costal element** and correspond to the head, neck, and tubercle of a rib (see Fig. 12-10). These include the bar of bone anterior to the foramen together with the **anterior tubercle** of the transverse process, the **intertubercular lamella** closing the foramen laterally, and the **posterior tubercle** of the process. The costal element may not fuse with the transverse process, in which event it persists as a **cervical rib.** Therefore, the vertebra associated with a cervical rib will lack a transverse foramen. Spinal nerves emerging from the intervertebral foramen pass between the anterior and posterior tubercles, in the sulcus floored by the intertubercular lamella.

As the **vertebral artery** passes through the transverse foramina, it is susceptible to compression by abnormalities of the cervical spine. Because the artery is the main source of blood supply to the hind brain and the cervical spinal cord, a complex set of symptoms and signs may result when the artery becomes occluded.

The Atlas and Axis

The first two cervical vertebrae are especially adapted for the free movements of the head. C-1, the atlas, is the bearer of the "globe." C-2 is called the axis because it provides the axis upon which the atlas, bearing the head, can rotate. In actuality, it is only its toothlike (odontoid) process, the **dens,** that subserves this function.

The **atlas** is the most slender vertebra, and is peculiar in that it lacks a body and consists of an anterior and a posterior arch (Fig. 12-11). The **posterior arch** corresponds to the vertebral arch, but the **anterior arch** (which embraces the dens) has only ligamentous equivalents in other vertebrae. The dens represents the centrum of C-1, which has fused to the axis. The atlas has neither superior nor inferior articular processes; instead the facets for articulation with the skull and the axis are borne on paired **lateral masses,** situated at the junctions of the anterior and posterior arches. The skull rests with its occipital condyles on the **superior articular facets,** thereby forming the *atlantooccipital joints*. The **inferior articular facets** meet the corresponding facets of the axis in the *lateral atlantoaxial joints*. The anterior arch has a small **fovea** or facet for articulation with the dens. Instead of a spinous process, a small **posterior tubercle** projects from the posterior arch. Muscles attach to the **anterior tubercle** on the anterior arch. The transverse processes are prominent and palpable behind the angle of the jaw. As the vertebral artery emerges from the transverse foramen, it turns medially in a groove (*sulcus*) on the upper edge of the posterior arch before ascending into the skull.

Although the **axis** has a body, it is atypical because it is extended into the **dens** (see Fig. 12-11). The dens presents anterior and posterior articular facets that participate in the *median atlantoaxial joint* by articulating with the fovea and the transverse ligament of the atlas. The axis has no real superior articular processes; its **superior articular facets** are placed on the body like shoulder pads. The inferior articular processes, as well as its transverse processes, resemble those of other cervical vertebrae.

Ossification of the Atlas and Axis. As may be predicted from their unusual morphology, the

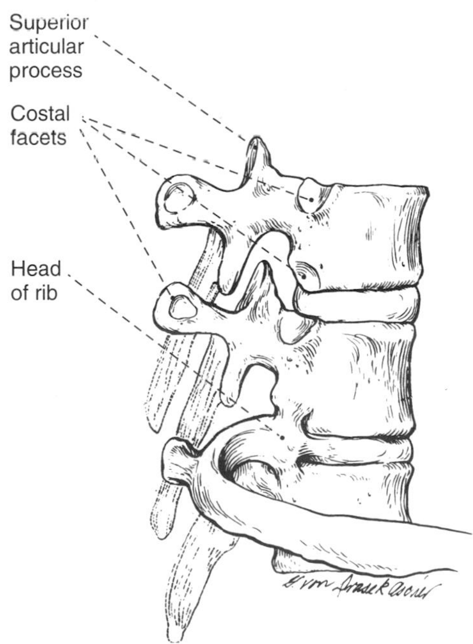

FIGURE *12-12.*
Thoracic vertebrae and one of the associated ribs.

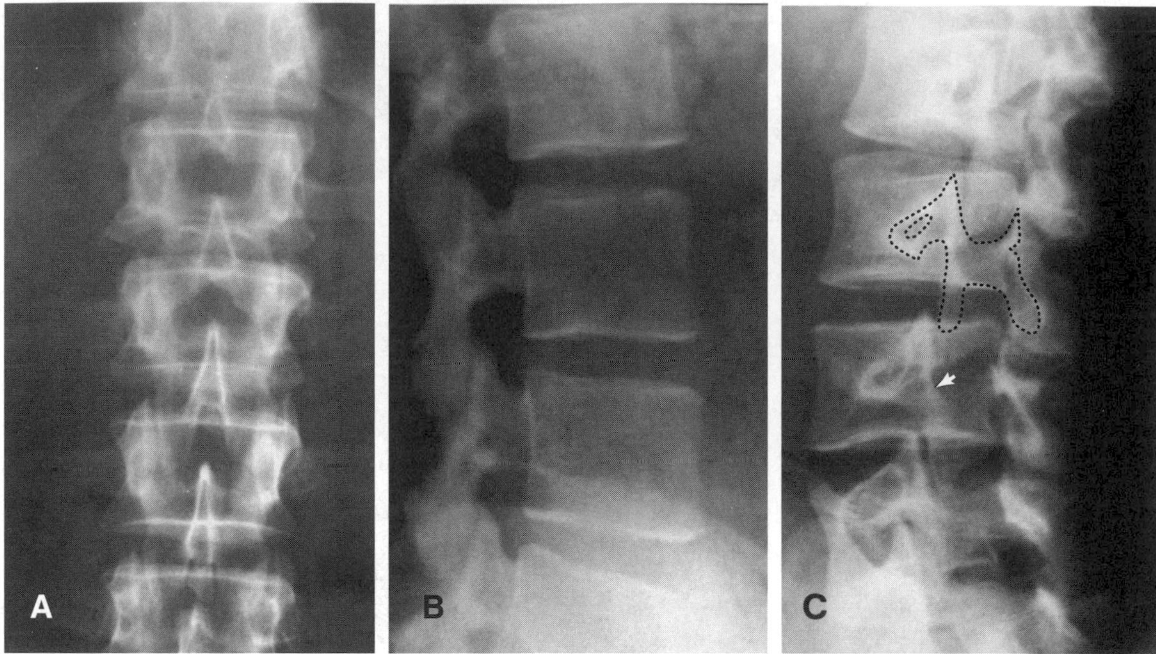

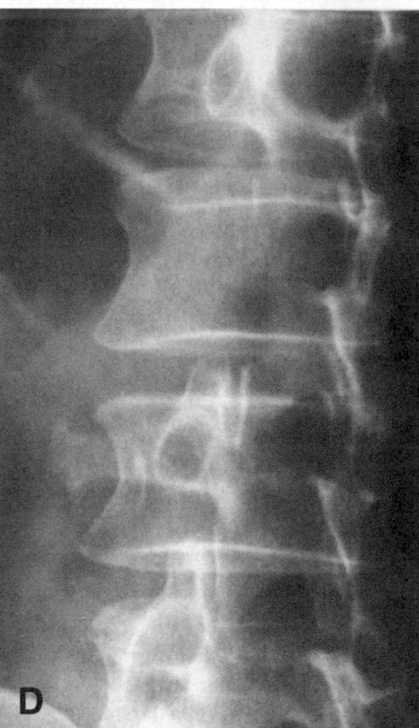

FIGURE *12-13.*
Radiologic anatomy of the lumbar spine: (A) in the anteroposterior view, clearly identifiable are (1) the vertebral body; (2) the space occupied by the intervertebral disk; (3) the roots of the pedicles; (4) transverse and spinous processes; (5) the superior margin of the lamina; (6) superior and inferior articular processes with the joint space between their facets (see Fig. 12-5). (B) The lateral projection gives a good view of the space occupied by the intervertebral disk and the intervertebral foramina with the structures that form their boundaries. (C) The oblique projection in the lumbar region provides a good view of the superior and inferior articular processes and the bridge of bone that unites their bases, which is known as the *pars interarticularis.* Though somewhat fanciful, it helps orientation to recognize the outline of a Scottie dog over the posterior half of the vertebra (*dotted outline*). The dog's head is the root of the pedicle, its large eye the base of the transverse process, its ear the superior articular process, and the front legs the inferior articular process. The neck of the dog (*arrow*) is the pars interarticularis. (D) An oblique view of the lumbar spine of the same patient shown in Figure 12-5D. The Scottie dog is missing in one of the vertebrae. (Courtesy of Dr. Rosalind H. Troupin.)

ossification of these two vertebrae does not conform to the typical pattern described in the foregoing. Although the **atlas** lacks a body, there is a single ossification center for its anterior arch (not analogous to the centrum), and one center for each half of the posterior arch, including the lateral masses that bear the articular surfaces. In the **axis,** the lower part of the body initially has two ossification centers, which soon fuse together. The dens, representing the body of the atlas, shows a similar pattern. There are bilateral ossification centers in the vertebral arch (as in all vertebrae). Thus, at birth, the axis consists of four bony parts embedded in cartilage: the two halves of the vertebral arch soon fuse and join the body; the dens usually becomes united to the fused centers of the body by the age of 6 years. This fusion begins superficially, but a disk of cartilage may persist deeply for many years. Finally, the cartilaginous tip of the dens develops a bony center that fuses with the rest of the dens about age 12.

Thoracic Vertebrae

The distinguishing feature of a thoracic vertebra is the development of its costal elements into a pair of separate bones. Consequently, all thoracic vertebrae (T-1 through T-12) articulate with at least one pair of ribs. In fact, typical thoracic vertebrae (T-2 to T-9) articulate with two pairs

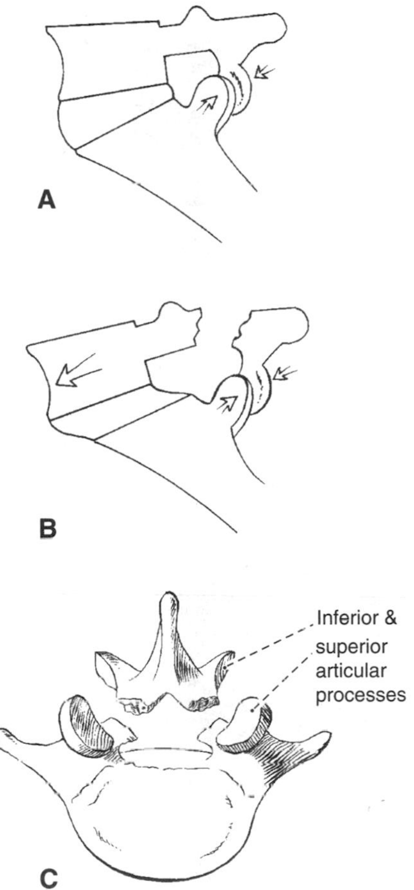

FIGURE *12-11.*
The lumbosacral angle and the role of the articular processes in supporting the vertebral column on the sacrum; (A) normal; (B) disruption of the pars interarticularis (spondylolysis) leading to spondylolisthesis; (C) superior view of L-5 with pars interarticularis defect. (Modified from Mitchell GAG. J Bone Joint Surg 1934;16:233.)

of ribs; the head of a rib contacts a **costal facet** (*fovea*), or demifacet, on the superior margin of one vertebral body and a similar facet on the inferior margin of the vertebral body above (Fig. 12-12). In addition, there is a costal facet on the transverse process of the upper ten thoracic vertebrae.

The **bodies** of the thoracic vertebrae increase in size from the 1st to the 12th (see Fig. 12-1). Their anterior surfaces are highly convex (see Fig. 12-8) and, therefore, the vertebrae protrude deeply into the thoracic cavity. This is exaggerated by the direction of the transverse processes, which point backward and upward, as well as laterally. The *pedicles* are placed toward the upper ends of the bodies; therefore, the inferior vertebral notches, which accommodate the spinal nerves as they leave the vertebral canal, are deep. The *laminae* of an upper vertebra overlap those of the one below. The long and slender *spinous processes* point downward and overlap the succeeding vertebra, a point to be remembered when counting vertebrae and identifying vertebral levels. The spinous processes of lower thoracic vertebrae resemble those of lumbar vertebrae; they are shorter, stouter, and point more posteriorly than those at higher levels. The *superior and inferior articular processes* project away from the root of the transverse process, and bear reciprocal articular facets that lie at an angle to the coronal plane (see Fig. 12-19). The superior facets face posteriorly as well as laterally, thus permitting rotation at the synovial (*zygapophyseal*) joints between neighboring vertebrae. There is an abrupt transition in the orientation of these articular processes at the level of the 11 or 12 thoracic vertebra: although the superior processes retain the characteristics of thoracic vertebrae, the inferior processes are oriented to match those of lumbar vertebrae, eliminating the potential for rotatory movement.

Atypical Thoracic Vertebrae. In addition to the orientation of facets on articular processes described earlier, the 1st and the 9th to 12th thoracic vertebrae present deviations from the typical pattern of costal articular facets (foveae) on the vertebral body or transverse process. The body of the 1st thoracic vertebra has a complete superior fovea for articulation with the head of the first rib and a small inferior fovea along its lower margin for articulation with the head of the second rib. The 9th through the 12th vertebral bodies have single foveae on their upper parts for articulation with the heads of the ribs of corresponding number. The costal facet is absent from the transverse processes of the 12th thoracic vertebra, a condition that may also be true for the 11th, or even the 10th thoracic vertebra.

Lumbar Vertebrae

The characteristic radiologic features of the lumbar spine are illustrated in Figure 12-13. The **body** of a lumbar vertebra is large in comparison with those of other vertebrae, and in proportion to its own vertebral foramen (see Fig. 12-8). The short and heavy *pedicles* arise from the upper part of the body, leaving a very deep inferior vertebral notch and a roomy intervertebral foramen (see Fig. 12-13B). The lumbar *laminae* are stout and broad. There is a distinct gap between one pair of laminae and the next, exposing the ligaments that connect them. (In cervical and thoracic regions, by contrast, adjacent pairs of laminae tend to overlap slightly, and the connecting ligaments cannot be seen.) The gap between lumbar laminae is exaggerated when the spine is flexed. In this position, a needle can be inserted through the gap into the vertebral canal and a sample of cerebrospinal fluid obtained, a clinical procedure known as a *lumbar puncture*.

Seen from the side, the *spinous process* is broad and quadrangular, with thick posterior and inferior margins. The long and slender *transverse process* is a composite structure, much of it actually made up of the costal element. Two small tubercles are homologous with the morphologic transverse process: the **accessory process** at the root of the transverse process, and the **mamillary process** on the posterior margin of the superior articular process.

The *articular processes* are substantial and are oriented predominantly in the sagittal plane. The slightly concave articular facet of the superior process faces medially and meets the reciprocally shaped facet of the inferior process,

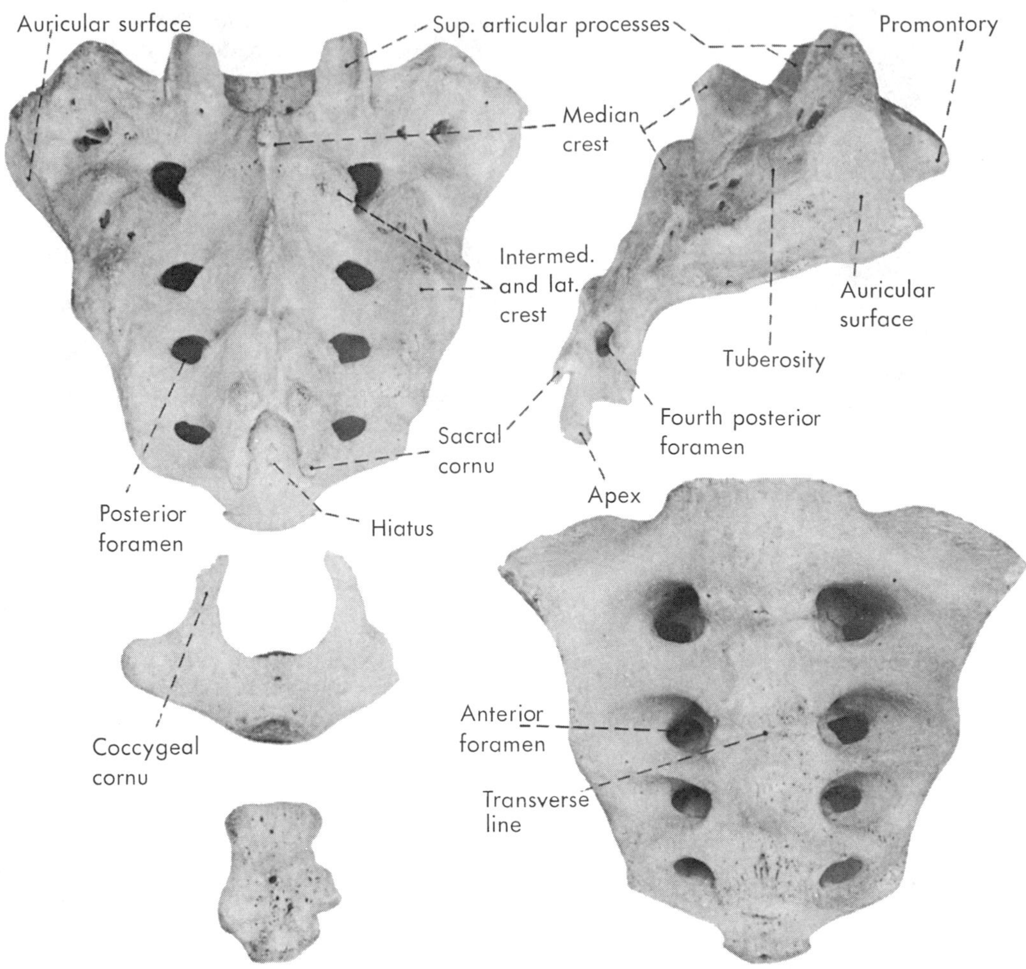

FIGURE *12-15.*
Dorsal, lateral, and pelvic surfaces of the sacrum and a posterior view of the coccyx.

which faces laterally (see Figs. 12-4 and 12-19). These facets slide effectively on one another in flexion, extension, and lateral bending, but there is hardly any freedom for the rotation of one lumbar vertebra on another.

The **fifth lumbar vertebra** (L-5) exhibits some notable features consistent with its role in transmitting weight to the sacrum. It is the largest and heaviest of all vertebrae. The height of its body is greater anteriorly than posteriorly, which contributes to the presence of the **lumbosacral** (sacrovertebral) **angle,** or junction (see Fig. 12-34). This angle is created by the change in spinal curvature between the lumbar and sacral regions of the spine (see Fig. 12-1) and by the angulation of the superior articular surface of the sacrum (Fig. 12-14A). The inferior articular processes of L-5 take a large share in supporting the lumbar spine on the sacrum. Although there is variation, these processes (and the joint facets on them) tend to change from the sagittal to a nearly transverse orientation. Such reorientation allows the processes to minimize the shearing stress imposed on the last intervertebral disk, a stress that is greater at this joint than at any other in the vertebral column (see following discussion).

The bone of the vertebral arch of L-5 that intervenes between superior and inferior articular processes, called the **pars interarticularis**, plays a key role in this weight-supporting mechanism (see Fig. 12-14). When the pars interarticularis is disrupted (spondylolysis) the fifth lumbar vertebra, and the rest of the spine with it, slip forward on the sacrum. The condition is known as **spondylolisthesis.** The ossification center of the developing vertebral arch is uninterrupted across the bases of the articular processes and pars interarticularis defects arise postnatally. Such defects and spondylolisthesis may occur at other vertebrae, but are most common between L-5 and the sacrum. In addition to nerve root compression in the intervertebral foramen, the cauda equina also may be damaged.

The Sacrum

The sacrum is formed by the complete fusion of all elements of five sacral vertebrae, but its five **segments** are still discernible (Fig. 12-15). Wedged in between the two hip bones, the sacrum transmits the weight of the body to these bones by the sacroiliac joints. The irregular, interlocking joint surfaces and the strong ligaments that unite the three bones permit little movement, converting the sacrum and the two hip bones into the rigidly constructed pelvis.

The wide upper end, or *base,* of the sacrum articulates with the body of the fifth lumbar vertebra, and its inferior *apex* with the coccyx. Its concave *pelvic surface* forms the posterior wall of the pelvic cavity, whereas the *posterior surface* is essentially subcutaneous. The two irregular *lateral surfaces* articulate with the hip bones. Enclosed within the bone is the *sacral canal,* the continuation of the lumbar vertebral canal, which terminates at the *sacral hiatus* near the apex.

The center of the **base of the sacrum** is occupied by the upper surface of the *body of the first sacral segment,* which presents a prominent anterior lip called the **sacral promontory.** The lateral, winglike parts of the base are the **alae of the sacrum** (*ala* is wing in Latin). Each ala consists anteriorly of the costal element, and posteriorly of the transverse process. Both components are fused to the side of the S-1 body and to its pedicle, the part of the bone forming the lateral boundary of the sacral canal.

The **pelvic surface** of the sacrum is relatively smooth. Four **transverse lines** (ridges) in its central portion indicate the regions of fusion between the bodies of the five sacral vertebrae. Lateral to these lines are four pairs of **anterior** (*pelvic*) **sacral foramina** through which the anterior (ventral) rami of S-1 through S-4 spinal nerves enter the pelvis. On each side the bars of bone separating successive foramina are in series with the medial portion of the ala and correspond to costal elements. Lateral to the foramina, the costal elements have fused with one another and with the transverse processes, forming the **lateral mass** (*pars lateralis*) of the sacrum.

The slightly convex **dorsal surface** is a rather irregular sheet of bone. The irregularities are mainly due to ridges that indicate the fusion of various vertebral components. The dorsal surface is interrupted by four **posterior** (*dorsal*) **sacral foramina,** from which issue the posterior (dorsal) rami of the upper four sacral spinal nerves.

Fusion of the spinous processes results in the **median sacral crest.** On each side of the crest are the fused laminae. The laminae of S-5 vertebra do not develop, leaving the **sacral hiatus** as an opening into the sacral canal. (The hiatus is roofed over by ligaments and provides a route for introducing anesthetics into the sacral canal.) Lateral to the fused laminae, the **intermediate sacral crest** represents the remnants of the articular processes. The superior articular process of S-1 segment is distinct and well developed for articulation with the fifth lumbar vertebra. The inferior articular processes of the S-5 segment form the **sacral cornua,** which are connected to the coccyx. On the dorsal surface, the lateral mass of the sacrum is formed by the fused transverse processes, the tips of which make up the **lateral sacral crest.**

The **lateral surface** of the sacrum, formed by the *pars lateralis,* presents a smooth **auricular** (ear-shaped) **facet,** which articulates with the ilium through the sacroiliac joint, and the rough **sacral tuberosity** posterior to the auricular surface, which receives the massive sacroiliac ligaments. The **intervertebral foramina,** readily visible from the side in other regions of the spine, are obscured from view by the lateral mass of the sacrum. The sacral spinal nerves, after emerging from the sacral canal through the intervertebral foramina, divide immediately and send their anterior and posterior rami through the anterior and posterior sacral foramina, respectively. The sacral **pedicles** (also obscured from lateral view) are unfused and separate successive intervertebral foramina from one another.

Ossification. Each sacral vertebra conforms in its ossification pattern to that of a typical vertebra. In each sacral segment, primary ossification centers appear before birth in the centrum, in each half neural arch, and in the costal elements just above the anterior sacral foramina. Between the ages of 2 and 8, these centers unite with one another, but bony fusion between adjacent segments begins only at about puberty, proceeds from below upward, and is completed during the third or fourth decade. The growth of the sacrum is assisted by secondary ossification centers, which appear near puberty in locations analogous to the epiphyses of typical vertebrae (see Fig. 12-6).

Variations. The sacrum is one of the bones that shows well-marked sexual dimorphism. In the female, the alae occupy a larger proportion of the base of the sacrum than they do in the male; each ala is roughly equal in length to the transverse diameter of the first sacral body. In the male, by contrast, the first sacral body is relatively wide: its diameter exceeds the length of an ala.

The fifth lumbar vertebra may fuse completely or partially with the sacrum (*sacralization;* see Fig. 12-7), and the same may be true for the first coccygeal vertebra. More rarely, the first sacral segment may persist as a separate vertebra (*lumbarization*), thus increasing the length of the vertebral column above the sacrum. Such a condition increases the strain on the lower part of the lumbar column because of increased leverage. If sacralization or lumbarization are unilateral, rather than bilateral, the vertebral column is more susceptible to damage, apparently because the articulations between the vertebrae at that level are asymmetric; both these conditions predispose to backache.

The Coccyx

Of the four vertebrae that usually make up the coccyx, the last three are regularly fused together (see Fig. 12-15). The first segment articulates with the apex of the sacrum through a rudimentary intervertebral disk. It has short transverse processes and two *cornua,* which represent pedicles and superior articular processes. The last three coccygeal segments hardly resemble vertebrae, but are in fact the remains of vertebral bodies.

Palpation and Percussion of Vertebrae

Only a vague impression can be gained of the vertebral bodies in the cervical and lumbar regions. At the risk of some discomfort, the larynx may be pushed aside when the neck is flexed and the front of the cervical vertebral bodies palpated. In a spare individual, the lumbar vertebral bodies can be felt through the relaxed abdominal wall. The bodies of thoracic vertebrae are inaccessible inside the rib cage. In truth, bony points of the vertebrae accessible for palpation are essentially limited to the tips of the spinous processes. The atlas has no true spinous process but, as already noted, its transverse process can be felt in the gap between the mastoid process and the angle of the jaw. It is sensitive to pressure.

The cervical spine is best palpated by sliding the hands behind the neck of the subject while the latter is lying supine. Alternatively, slight passive extension of the head relieves tension in the ligament connecting the tips of cervical spinous processes (*ligamentum nuchae*) and provides access to the processes of C-2 to C-6. That of C-7 is the most prominent one. Slightly lateral to the spinous processes, ill-defined bony masses can be discerned that represent the articular processes. These may be tender when the cervical spine is affected by arthritis.

For palpating the spinous processes below C-7, the subject has to be sitting, standing, or lying prone. In the thoracic region, the spinous processes overlap the body of the first or even the second vertebra below. In the lumbar region, by contrast, the spinous processes are on level with their own bodies. The posterior surface of the sacrum with its rudimentary spinous processes is quite superficial. The coccyx and the anterior aspect of the sacrum are best palpated through the rectum.

Regardless of any overlap between spinous processes, the cause of the pain elicited by palpating a

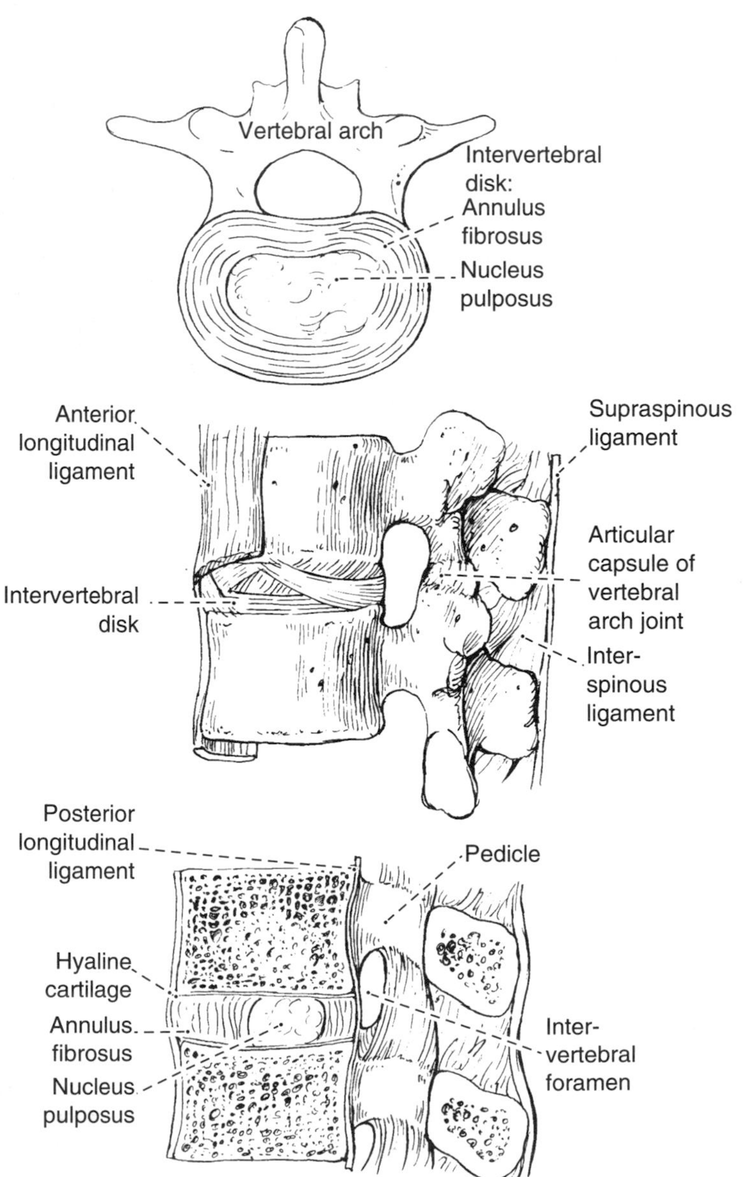

FIGURE *12-16.*
Joints and ligaments of the vertebrae.

spinous process is localized to its own vertebra. Gentle percussion of a spinous process that elicits pain confirms some pathologic process in that vertebra. When it is judged safe, to exclude pathology, the examiner may also use quite forceful percussion by banging along the length of the spine with his or her fist.

Counting Vertebrae. Knowledge of vertebral levels has clinical significance. Counting vertebrae is accomplished with the aid of some landmarks. The anterior arch of the atlas is on level with the hard palate. Cervical and upper thoracic vertebrae can be counted with reference to the prominent processes of C-7 and T-1. Lower thoracic and upper lumbar spines can be identified by locating the 12th rib. The inferior angle of the scapula is usually on level with the spine of T-7, and L-4 vertebra is on level with the highest point along the iliac crest.

ARTICULATIONS OF THE VERTEBRAL COLUMN

Vertebrae articulate with one another by two types of joints: 1) a fibrocartilaginous joint or symphysis between adjacent vertebral bodies, the **intervertebral disk,** and 2) synovial joints between adjacent vertebral arches, the zygapophyseal or **vertebral arch joints.** A set of ligaments is associated with each type of joint (Fig. 12-16). Specialized **craniovertebral joints** exist between the skull, atlas, and axis; they will be discussed after the more typical articulations have been described.

Joints of the Vertebral Bodies

The chief union between adjacent vertebral bodies is secured by the intervertebral disks. This union is reinforced by the anterior and posterior longitudinal ligaments.

The Intervertebral Disk

The intervertebral disk is a symphysis between vertebral bodies (see Fig. 12-16). On radiographs, the disk appears as a translucent space (see Figs. 12-13 and 12-18). It is sandwiched between the plates of hyaline cartilage that cover the superior and inferior surfaces of adjacent vertebral bodies. Each disk is named and numbered according to the vertebra below which it lies. There being no disk between the atlas and axis, the uppermost one is that between the axis and the third cervical vertebra; it is the C-2 disk. The L-5 disk is between the fifth lumbar vertebra and the sacrum. The disk between the sacrum and the first coccygeal segment is rudimentary.

Each intervertebral disk conforms in shape to the apposing surfaces of the vertebral bodies between which it lies (see Fig. 12-16), and together the disks account for one-quarter of the height of the vertebral column above the sacrum. The disks are thickest in the lumbar region, more so anteriorly than posteriorly. The structure of the disk is admirably suited for resisting displacement of vertebrae on one another, while allowing some movement; they withstand and dissipate the forces that are transmitted along the vertebral column. In fact, they are so strong that unless there is disk degeneration, it is impossible to wrench one vertebra from the other; the bone will break before the disk tears. An intervertebral disk consists of a tough, peripheral fibrocartilaginous ring called the **annulus fibrosus** and a more pliable, inner, gelatinous mass, the **nucleus pulposus** (see Fig. 12-16).

The **annulus** is composed of densely packed collagen fibers in the outer, and fibrocartilage in the more central, part of the ring. The fiber bundles run obliquely in concentric lamellae and are anchored in the hyaline cartilage covering the bone surfaces. Their attachment is secured by calcification in the cartilage. Only the superficial fiber bundles attach directly to bone. In alternate lamellae the fibers slant at right angles to one another (see Fig. 12-16), an arrangement that permits, and also limits, rotation between vertebrae. This arrangement also lends a certain degree of elasticity to the fibrous ring. When the nucleus pulposus is compressed, it changes its shape and distends the annulus by slightly altering the angle between the collagen fiber bundles (Fig. 12-17). Fiber orientation is different in the posterior part of the annulus, where the lamellae interdigitate. Because of the eccentric location of the nucleus pulposus, closer to the back than the front, the annulus is also thinner posteriorly. All these factors may predispose to posterior rupture of the ring.

The **nucleus pulposus** can be demonstrated radiographically (Fig. 12-18). Its white, glistening, amorphous substance consists predominantly of semisolid matrix, within which are embedded some collagen fibers, with no specific orientation. Matrix and fibers are produced by the sparse cells found in the nucleus. Many of the cells originate in the notochord, but become replaced by chondrocytes during childhood. The nucleus pulposus has the capacity to absorb water, which it loses when it is compressed. This accounts for the gain in body height of 1 to 2 cm during the night, and a corresponding loss during the day. The water content of the nucleus pulposus is some 70% to 88%, the percentage decreasing with age.

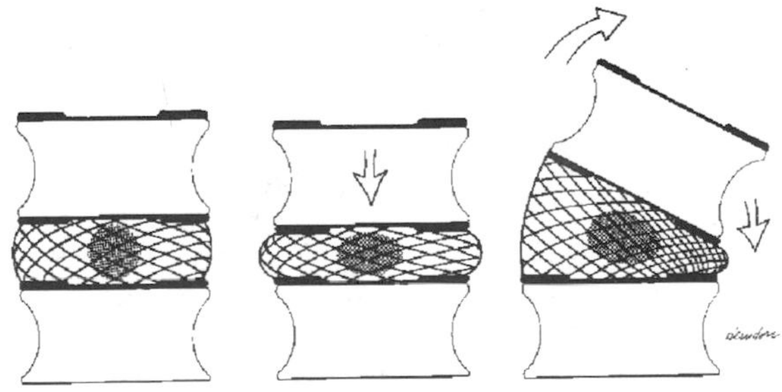

FIGURE *12-17.*
A highly simplified and schematic representation of the structure of the intervertebral disk: The criss-cross arrangement of collagen fiber bundles in the laminae of the annulus fibrosus permits rotation between the vertebrae and also allows for bulging when the nucleus pulposus is compressed.

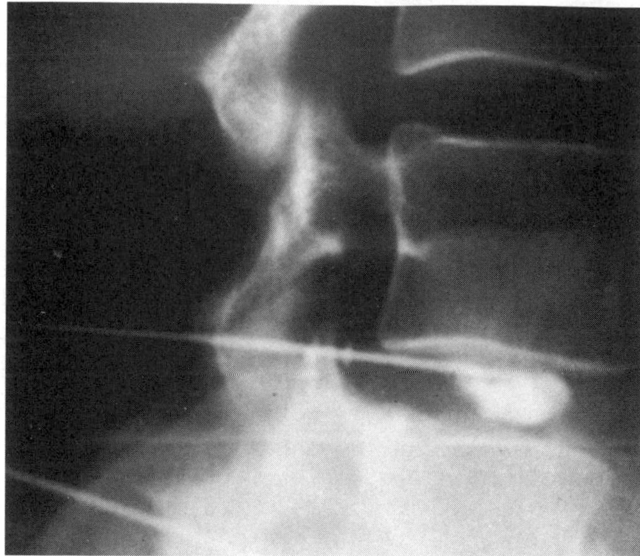

FIGURE *12-18.*
A discogram: A radiopaque, water-soluble substance is injected into the center of the intervertebral disk, and it outlines the extent of the nucleus pulposus which, in this patient, is normal. (Courtesy of Dr. Rosalind A. Troupin.)

With advancing age the disks become thinner, mainly due to changes in the nucleus pulposus. After the first decade, the nucleus is gradually replaced by fibrocartilage, its matrix composition changes, and its capacity for absorbing water diminishes. Nevertheless, the nucleus will still herniate if the annulus fibrosus is ruptured, resulting in intervertebral disk prolapse (see Chap. 13).

Nutrition and Degenerative Changes. Apart from the most superficial layers of the annulus fibrosus, the intervertebral disk in adult life is avascular. Its nutrition is dependent on diffusion across the hyaline cartilage from the spongy bone of the vertebra. During the growth period, however, radial vascular channels are present in the hyaline cartilage. They may leave defects in the cartilage, predisposing to herniation of a portion of the nucleus pulposus into the cancellous bone of the vertebral body. The herniation, known as a **Schmorl's node**, or body, forces its way through the hyaline cartilage and the thin lamella of bone in the center of the upper surface of the vertebral body. Schmorl's bodies, which may arise from other causes as well, usually remain asymptomatic.

Degenerative changes begin in the intervertebral disk during the third decade. Caused by mechanical stresses, they are most marked and common in the last two lumbar disks. They consist of thinning of the hyaline cartilage plate, dehydration, and loss of pliability in the nucleus pulposus, with accompanying cell death, and fragmentation of fibers in the annulus fibrosus. The latter phenomenon is particularly marked posteriorly. These factors contribute to a decrease in disk thickness and predispose to rupture of the annulus with consequent herniation of the disk into the vertebral canal or intervertebral foramina (see Chap. 13).

Joints of Luschka. At about the age of 10, small cavities appear in the posterolateral parts of the cervical intervertebral disks. These cavities have been considered by some as discrete synovial joints (joints of Luschka). They are absent at birth and most likely represent degenerative changes in the disks, although opinion on this point is divided.

Joints of the Vertebral Arches

Consecutive vertebral arches articulate with one another by their articular processes, which form synovial joints (see Fig. 12-16). The correct anatomic name of these joints is the **zygapophyseal joints.** Often referred to by clinicians as the *facet joints*, and by anatomists as the *synovial joints of the spine*, the term *vertebral arch joints* has the advantage of being specific and also refers to function, as it distinguishes these joints from those of the vertebral body. The movements permitted by the intervertebral disk between two vertebral bodies are amplified at the vertebral arch, a finding that is consonant with the synovial nature of vertebral arch joints and the presence of a symphysis between the bodies. Because the intervertebral disk permits movement in any direction, the types of motion possible between a pair of vertebrae are determined by the synovial joints of the arch. All these joints are of the plane or ellipsoid variety, and it is the orientation of the articular processes, rather than the shape of the joint facets themselves, that influences the degrees of freedom for joint motion.

The articular facets on the superior and inferior processes slide on one another in flexion and extension of the spine and also in lateral bending. As described with the regional characteristics of vertebrae, rotation is limited in cervical and lumbar regions because the facets are oriented in a plane that is more or less coronal (cervical region), or sagittal (lumbar region). In the thoracic region the articular facets are positioned roughly along the arc of a circle whose center is in the vertebral body (Fig. 12-19). This orientation is well suited for rotation of vertebrae on one another around this imaginary center.

The facets on the articular processes are covered by articular cartilage and a thin, sleevelike, capsule, lined by synovial membrane, attaches to their margins (Fig. 12-20; see also 12-16). The capsule is relatively easily strained, which can give rise to back pain. It receives its **innervation** from twigs of the *posterior rami* of spinal nerves that are associated with the two vertebral arches participating in the articulation.

When the intervertebral disks become thinner and less pliable, the vertebral arch joints tend to settle; weight-bearing by these joints then increases. The slackened articular capsule and synovial membrane may become pinched between the articular processes, causing pain. These changes often set the stage for joint disease that leads, in turn, to reactive bone formation: bony spurs (osteophytes) are produced at the margins of the articular facets. Because the vertebral arch joints form the posterior boundaries of intervertebral foramina, the

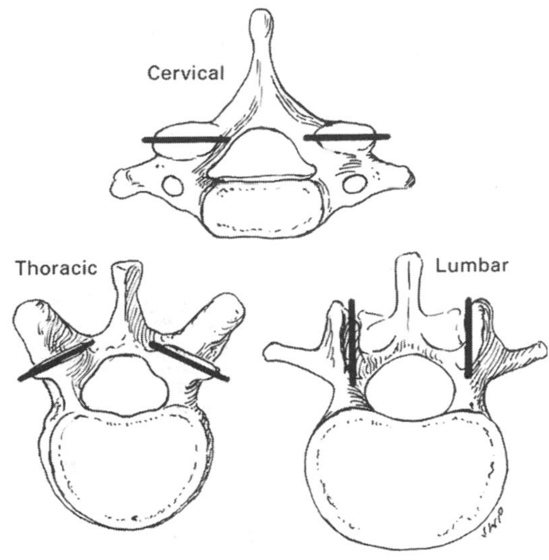

FIGURE 12-19.
Superior view of a cervical, a thoracic, and a lumbar vertebra: *Solid lines* have been placed across the articular surfaces of the vertebral arch joints to illustrate the different planes in which the facets of these joints lie. Only in the thoracic region does the positioning of these facets permit an appreciable amount of rotation between consecutive vertebrae.

swollen joints and osteophytes may compress the spinal nerves exiting through the foramina (radiculopathy). This may cause not only back pain, but pain and other clinical findings in the distribution territory of the nerve.

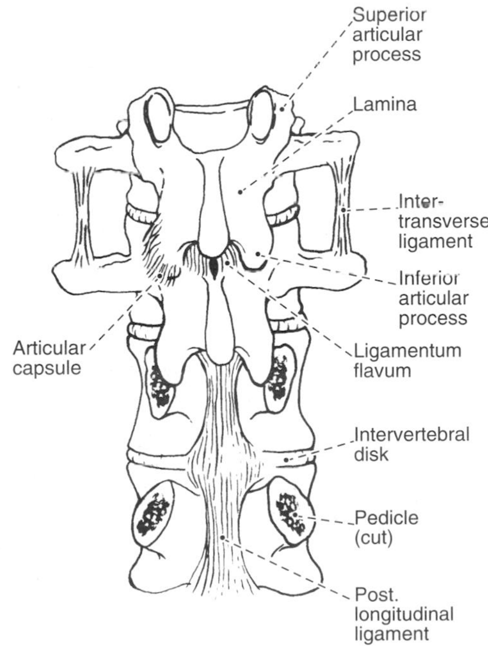

FIGURE 12-20.
Ligaments of the vertebral column seen from the back. The vertebral arches of the lower two vertebrae have been removed.

Ligaments

The ligaments that reinforce the intervertebral symphysis are tough and inelastic, whereas the ligaments associated with the vertebral arch contain many elastic fibers and are stretchable, allowing separation of the arches and the vertebral processes during flexion and rotation of the spine.

Ligaments Associated With the Intervertebral Disk

Between the skull and the sacrum, the **anterior** and **posterior longitudinal ligaments** run uninterruptedly on respective surfaces of the vertebral bodies (see Fig. 12-16). The ligaments resist anterior and posterior displacement of vertebrae on one another. Both ligaments are firmly attached to each intervertebral disk, as well as to bone, but allow some blood vessels to pass deep to them to supply the vertebral bodies.

The *anterior longitudinal ligament* is a broad band, covering much of the anterior and anterolateral surfaces of the vertebral bodies. It is thick anteriorly and much thinner laterally. It limits extension of the vertebral column and is especially important in the lumbar region, where the weight of the body tends to increase the normal posture of extension of the lumbar spine. The *posterior longitudinal ligament* tends to check flexion of the vertebral column. It runs within the vertebral canal and covers the posterior surfaces of the vertebral bodies and disks (see Fig. 12-20). In the thoracic and lumbar regions the ligament narrows over the middle of each vertebral body, where it is separated from the bone by loose connective tissue, and expands over the margins of the vertebral bodies and the intervening disks, gaining firm attachment to them. Blood vessels pass from one side to the other in the loose connective tissue, and enter or leave the bone under cover of the ligament.

Ligaments Associated With the Vertebral Arch

Ligaments run between the laminae, the spinous processes, and the transverse processes of consecutive vertebrae. There are no ligaments between pedicles where the intervertebral foramina are located. On each side, the **ligamentum flavum** connects the laminae of adjacent vertebrae (see Fig. 12-20); the rather thin **interspinous ligament** fills the space between spinous processes (see Fig. 12-16). The **supraspinous ligament** runs over the tips of the spinous processes and blends with the interspinous ligaments. The **intertransverse ligaments** connect succeeding transverse processes and are functionally insignificant (see Fig. 12-20).

The strongest and most important ligaments are the *ligamenta flava* (yellow ligaments). They are composed almost entirely of elastic tissue, which is yellowish. Each ligamentum flavum is a flattened band that stretches from the anterior surface of the lower edge of one lamina to the upper part of the posterior surface of the succeeding lamina. The paired ligaments fill the space between two adjacent laminae except for a narrow slit in the midline (see Fig. 12-20). Laterally, the ligamenta flava tend to blend with the fibrous capsule of the vertebral arch joints.

Flexion separates the laminae and stretches the ligamenta flava, affording more room between laminae for the procedure of lumbar puncture. Conversely, violent extension (hyperextension) of the neck may carry the cervical laminae so close together that the ligamenta flava bulge forward and may impinge on the spinal cord.

The *supraspinous ligament* is a continuous cordlike band, running from the spinous process of the seventh cervical vertebra to the sacrum. Its superficial fibers span several vertebral spines; the deepest ones blend with the interspinous ligaments and attach to neighboring spines. The ligament limits flexion of the spine: violent flexion may tear it. The site of injury may be localized by point tenderness between the spines. The ligament is thin in the lumbar region and may be absent between L-5 and the sacrum.

In the cervical region, the supraspinous ligament is replaced by the **ligamentum nuchae** (ligament of the neck; Fig. 12-21), a sickle-shaped membrane that separates the muscles on the two sides of the neck and provides attachment for them. Its deep fibers, like those of the supraspinous ligament in other regions, attach directly to the spinous processes of cervical vertebrae. Superiorly, the ligamentum nuchae is attached to the external crest and protuberance of the occipital bone. Its posterior margin spans the distance between the external occipital protuberance and the spine of the seventh cervical vertebra. The ligamentum nuchae helps to support the weight of the head when it is inclined forward, as in reading and writing, for instance. The ligament is much stronger in quadrupeds that graze, and in these species it is rich in elastic tissue.

In the coccygeal region, there are no synovial joints, and small **sacrococcygeal ligaments** unite the coccyx to the sacrum. Similar ligaments join the coccygeal segments. These ligaments permit some movement and are painful when they become torn, as may happen, for example, during delivery, owing to displacement of the coccyx by the advancing fetal head.

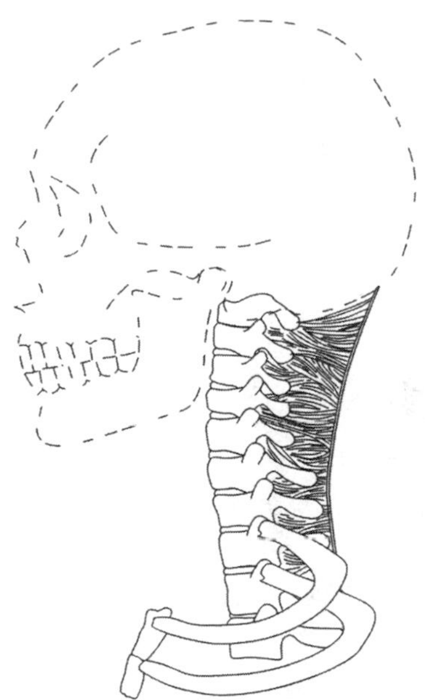

FIGURE *12-21.*
The ligamentum nuchae.

The Craniovertebral Joints

Just as the atlas and axis are specially adapted for movements of the head, so the joints associated with them are also specialized. Although the base of the skull incorporates occipital sclerotomes, there is no intervertebral disk between the atlas and the occipital bone, or between the atlas and the axis. The craniovertebral joints, responsible for the greatest range of head movements, are all synovial. They include a pair of atlantooccipital joints and three atlantoaxial joints (Fig. 12-22).

FIGURE *12-22.*
The anatomy of the craniovertebral joints: (A) Anterior and (B) posterior views of the atlantooccipital and atlantoaxial joints. On one side the articular capsules have been removed to show the apposing articular surfaces. (C) The atlas and axis viewed from *above* and *behind*. All the ligaments associated with the dens (D through F) have been removed except the transverse ligament of the atlas, to illustrate its function. The atlas is depicted as having rotated around the dens (*arrows*). In panel D and E, the occipital bone and the posterior arches of the atlas and axis have been transected and the contents of the vertebral canal removed to reveal the anterior wall of the canal. The layering of the ligaments associated with the dens is shown in a sagittal section in panel F. In panel D, the posterior longitudinal ligament and the tectorial membrane have been removed to show the cruciform ligament, formed by the blending of the transverse ligament and longitudinal fasciculi. Panel E shows the deepest set of ligaments, revealed by removal of most of the cruciform ligament, leaving the transverse ligament of the atlas in place.

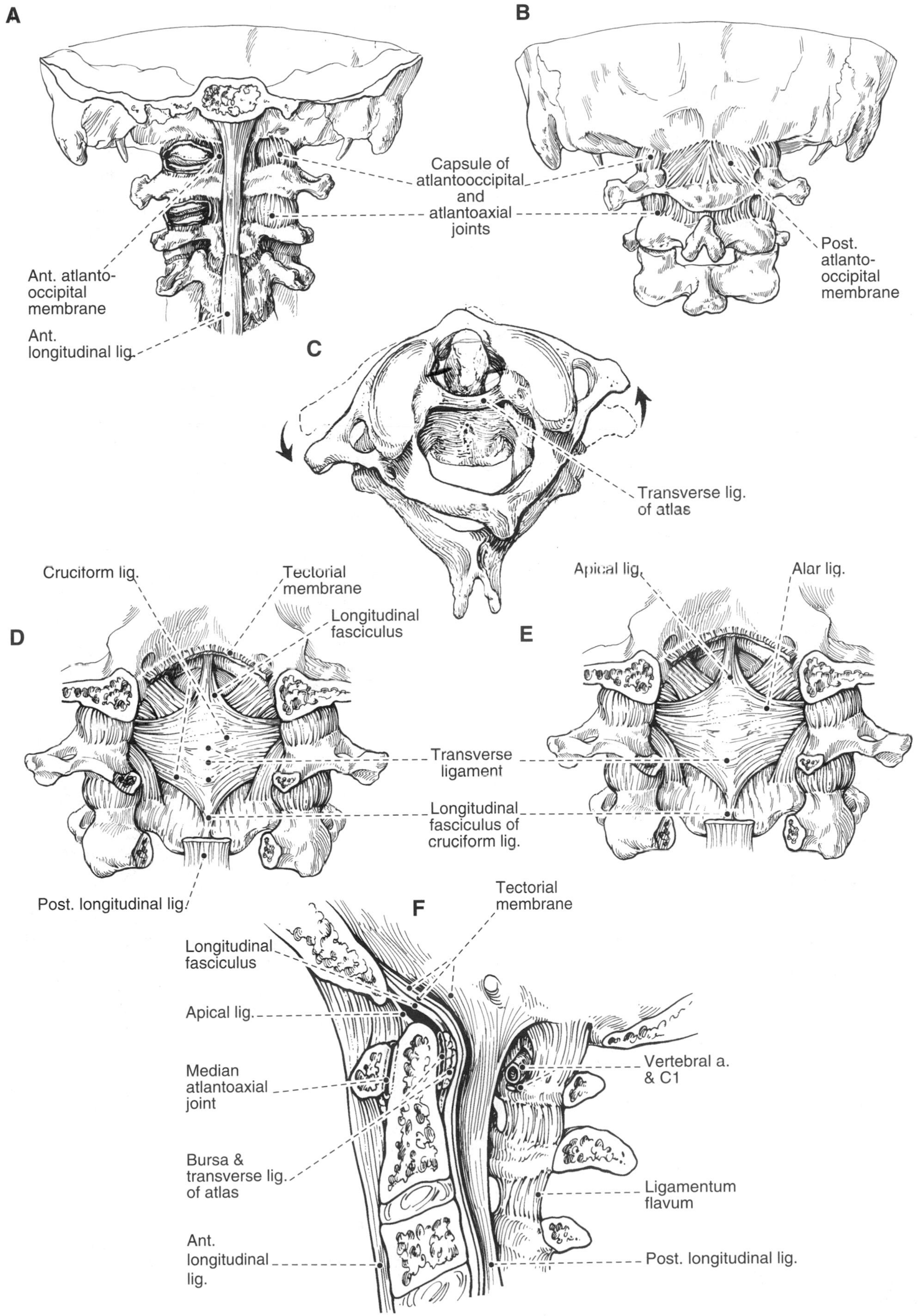
A
B
Capsule of atlantooccipital and atlantoaxial joints
Ant. atlanto-occipital membrane
Ant. longitudinal lig.
Post. atlanto-occipital membrane
C
Transverse lig. of atlas
Cruciform lig.
Tectorial membrane
Longitudinal fasciculus
D
E
Apical lig.
Alar lig.
Transverse ligament
Longitudinal fasciculus of cruciform lig.
Post. longitudinal lig.
F
Tectorial membrane
Longitudinal fasciculus
Apical lig.
Median atlantoaxial joint
Bursa & transverse lig. of atlas
Ant. longitudinal lig.
Vertebral a. & C1
Ligamentum flavum
Post. longitudinal lig.

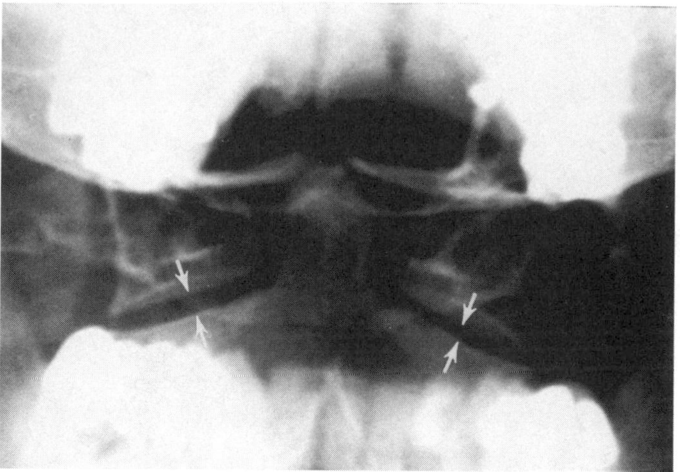

FIGURE 12-23.
The lateral atlantoaxial joints: The dens of the axis projects above the two lateral atlantoaxial joints (*arrows*), the articular surfaces of which permit gliding as the atlas, bearing the head, pivots around the dens. This radiograph is taken in a frontal view through the open mouth, and the tip of the dens can be seen to be on level with the hard palate. (Courtesy of Dr. Rosalind H. Troupin.)

The Atlantooccipital Joints

The articulation is formed on each side by the concave, superior articular facet of the atlas (see Fig. 12-11) and the convex condyle of the occipital bone, both covered with articular cartilage. The oblong, rather bean-shaped facets are obliquely positioned; their long axes would intersect anteriorly. The geometry of these facets permits nodding (flexion and extension) of the head and some lateral bending, but practically no rotation. The two joints act in unison. Each joint, however, is enclosed by a separate fibrous capsule (see Fig. 12-22A and B), though each synovial cavity may communicate with the median atlantoaxial joint.

The Atlantoaxial Joints

Three joints between the atlas and the axis are specialized for head rotation: a **lateral atlantoaxial joint** on each side, formed by the lateral mass of the atlas and the superior articular facet of the axis, and a **median atlantoaxial joint** between the dens and the anterior arch of the atlas (see Fig. 12-11). The inferior articular facets of the atlas are almost plane and match the corresponding, gently curved facets of the axis, permitting free sliding at the lateral atlantoaxial joints during head rotation (Fig. 12-23). The median atlantoaxial joint is a pivot: the atlas pivots around the dens, carrying the head with it (see Fig. 12-22C). The transverse ligament of the atlas is critical to the integrity of the median atlantoaxial joint (see following).

Ligaments

The stability of the craniovertebral joints is enhanced by the presence of several strong ligaments. Most important of these is the **transverse ligament of the atlas,** which converts the anterior arch of the atlas into an osseoligamentous ring (see Fig. 12-22C). A bursa lubricates the movement of the dens against the ligament.

> The transverse ligament of the atlas retains the dens in position, preventing its impingement on the spinal cord. However, when rheumatoid arthritis affects this joint, the ligament may become eroded and may rupture, endangering the spinal cord even in minor whiplash injuries (Fig. 12-24). Normally, the ligament is so strong that when subjected to trauma, as in judicial hanging or in other cases of violent trauma (automobile accidents), it will often not give way; rather, the bone will fracture (hangman's fracture).

The **anterior and posterior atlantooccipital membranes** close the space between the margins of the foramen mag-

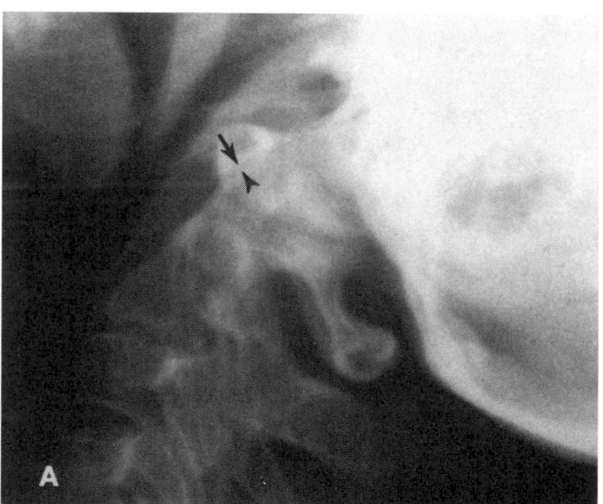

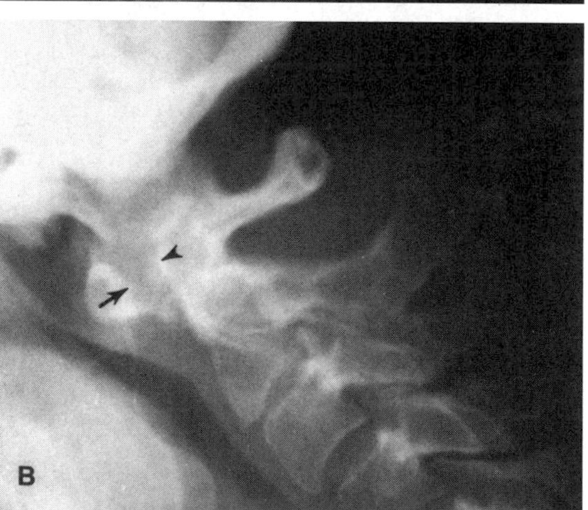

FIGURE 12-24.
The median atlantoaxial joint as seen in lateral radiographs of the cervical spine in a patient suffering from rheumatoid arthritis. (A) The head is extended and the anterior arch of the atlas (*stemmed arrow*) is closely apposed to the dens (*arrowhead*). The hardly perceptible radiolucency separating them represents the articular cartilage of the median atlantoaxial joint. (B) in flexion, the dens moves away from the anterior arch of the atlas, indicating that the transverse ligament, which normally retains it in position, has been eroded by the disease. (Courtesy of Dr. Rosalind H. Troupin.)

num above and the anterior and posterior arches of the atlas below (see Fig 12-22A, B and F). Several ligaments attach the dens to the occipital bone (see Fig. 12-22D through F): the **alar ligaments,** which limit flexion and rotation, the more slender **apical ligament of the dens** (believed to be a vestige of the notochord), and a *longitudinal fasciculus* that extends upward from the transverse ligament of the atlas. This last fasciculus, together with the transverse ligament itself and a similar fasciculus extending downward from the transverse ligament, form a complex called the **cruciform ligament.** All these ligaments are beneath the upward continuation of the *posterior longitudinal ligament*, which forms a distinct, bilaminar structure here, called the **tectorial membrane** (see Fig. 12-22B and F). The *anterior longitudinal ligament* blends with the anterior atlantooccipital membrane, and limits extension of the craniovertebral joints (see Fig. 12-22 A and F).

BLOOD AND NERVE SUPPLY

The vasculature and innervation of the vertebrae and their associated joints and ligaments are discussed in Chapter 13, because the same vessels and nerves supply much of the contents of the vertebral canal as well. Moreover, the topographic relations of these vessels and nerves in the vertebral canal have considerable clinical relevance.

MUSCLES OF THE VERTEBRAL COLUMN

The range and types of movements possible in each region of the spine are determined by the vertebral arch joints, but the control and strength of those movements depend on muscles. Muscles are also essential for the stability of the spine, and for cancelling out or controlling the effects of gravity. They fall into two major functional groups: extensors and flexors. Each group is also capable of rotating and laterally bending the column. The anatomic arrangement that evolves from the simple embryonic pattern of sclerotomes and myotomes, however, is very much more complex than this functional grouping implies.

Developmental Considerations

Differentiation of the sclerotomes, as described earlier, results in a particular segmental arrangement whereby each myotome is positioned opposite two developing vertebrae (see Fig. 12-2). This primitive arrangement, however, becomes greatly complicated by regional specializations in each myotome, and by the subsequent migration and fusion of myogenic cell masses. **Epimeric myosites** migrate from the dorsomedial portion of each myotome to the dorsolateral aspect of the neural arches. Here they will form the extensors of the vertebral column and will be innervated by the posterior rami of spinal nerves (Fig. 12-25). The migration of **hypomeric myosites** from the

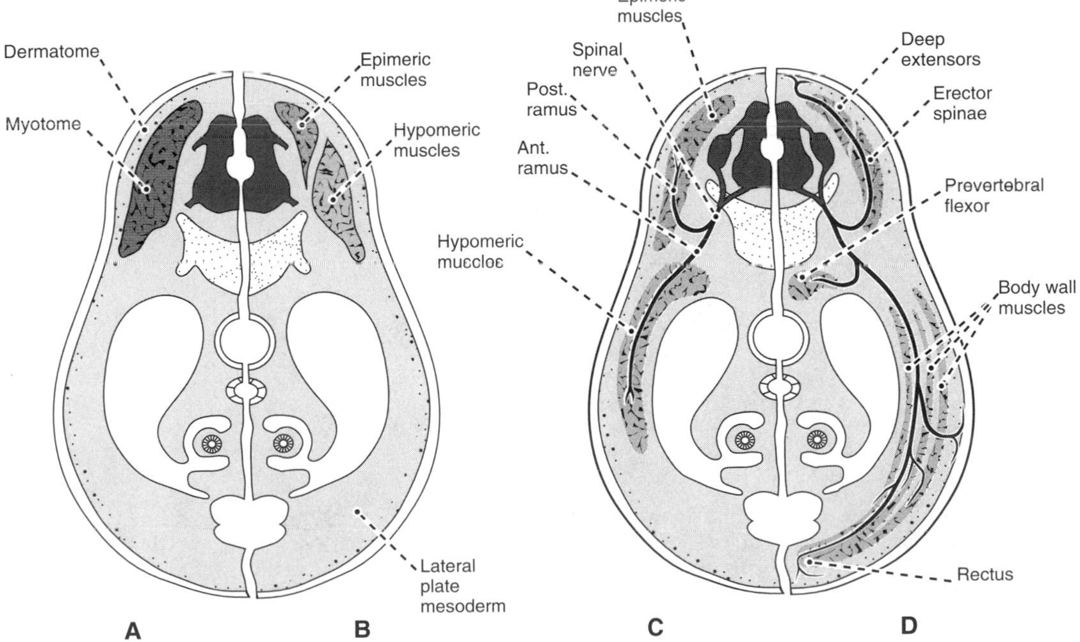

FIGURE 12-25.
Development of the muscles capable of moving the vertebral column and of the nerves that supply them: Successive embryonic stages are shown in *right* and *left halves* of schematic transverse sections. (A) Undifferentiated myotome; (B) separation of epimeric and hypomeric muscle primordia; (C) innervation of the blastemas of epimeric and hypomeric muscle masses; (D) segregation of epimeric and hypomeric myocytes into discrete muscle groups and their association with branches of a spinal nerve.

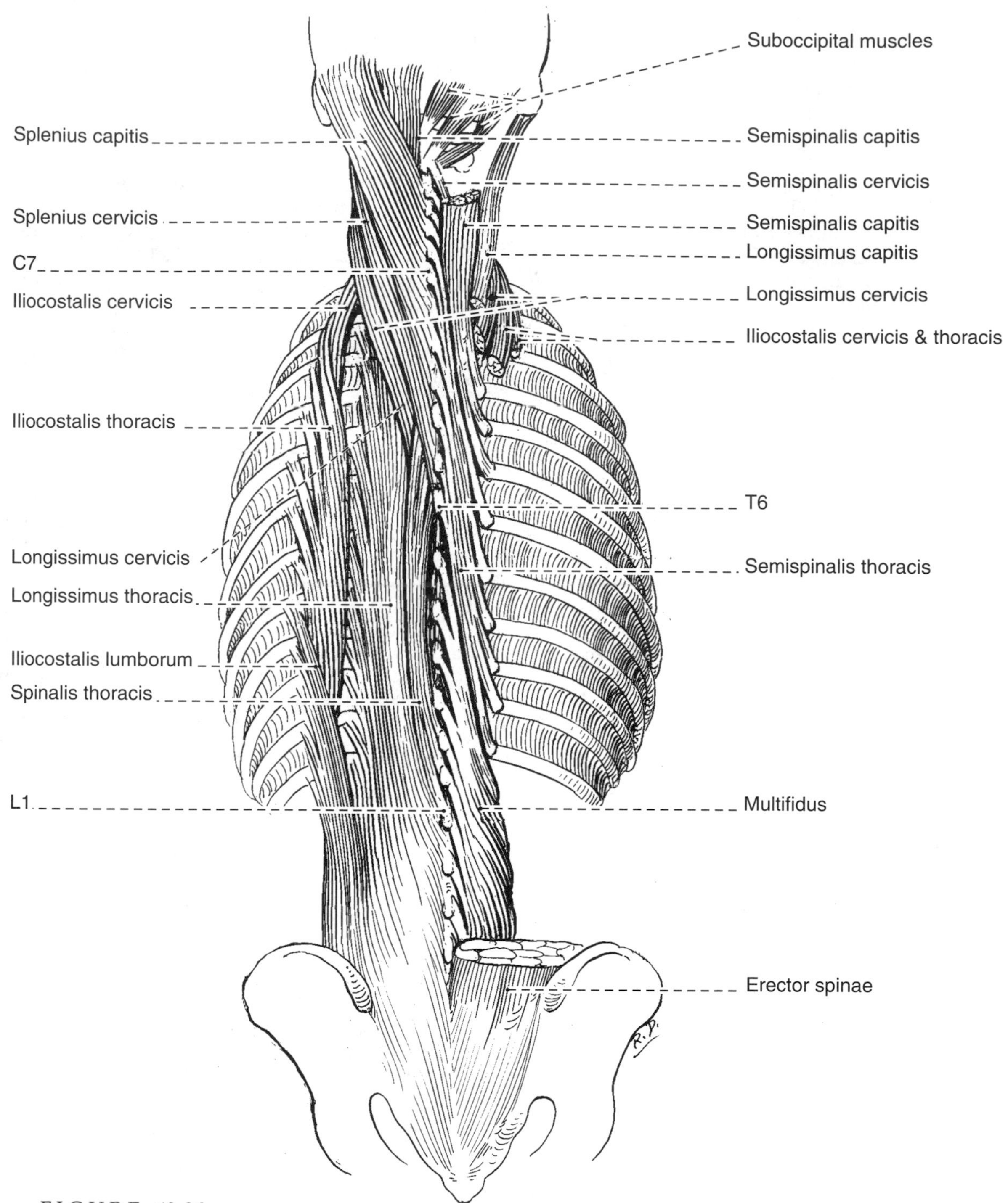

FIGURE *12-26.*
General view of the extensor muscle mass of the vertebral column: Many superficial muscles have been removed on the *right side* to show members of the intermediate layer. Of the deep layer, only the suboccipital muscles are shown.

ventromedial portions of the somites is much more extensive. Although all the hypomeric muscles that arise from them will be innervated by the anterior rami of spinal nerves, only a few will actually attach to vertebrae and, therefore, flex the column directly. The others will contribute to the formation of the body wall and the anterior musculature of the neck. Many of these muscles, however, will flex and rotate the vertebral column in an indirect manner, owing to the pull they exert on the rib cage or the skull.

Morphogenesis of definitive muscles is most likely determined by the regrouping of both epimeric and hypomeric muscle primordia by local factors in embryonic connective tissue. Myotubes derived from one myotome fuse with several successive neighbors, forming muscles that span many vertebrae. Longitudinal and tangential regrouping of these fused myogenic masses permit individual myotomes to contribute to several discrete muscles, and individual muscles to incorporate portions of several myotomes. Only a few muscles retain a truly segmental arrangement: the deepest muscles in the epimeric group, and the intercostal muscles in the hypomeric group. The original segmental pattern of nerve supply, however, will be retained, regardless of the regrouping.

Extensors

The extensors of the spine are placed posterior to the laminae and transverse processes and span the entire back between the occiput and sacrum. They are the only muscles in the body supplied by posterior rami of spinal nerves. For descriptive purposes, they fall into four groups: the **splenius muscles,** the **suboccipital muscles,** the **erector spinae,** and the **transversospinalis.** The first two groups are found in the back of the neck and assist mainly in head movements. The last two, by contrast, span the whole length of the vertebral column and constitute the bulk of the spinal extensor musculature (Fig. 12-26).

The entire back musculature is often referred to as "the erector spinae," or "the back muscles." This seems justified in a clinical context, for individual anatomic units are difficult to evaluate clinically. Two points should be noted, however. First, the erector spinae is not responsible for holding the spine erect during standing, but, as its name implies, restores it to the erect position. In addition to producing extension, it controls flexion of the spine by "paying out rope" against gravity. It contracts just as powerfully during flexion as it does during extension; it may be palpated during both bending over and straightening up from the bent position. Second, these back muscles are covered by various other muscles that do not belong to the spinal extensors and are not supplied by posterior rami of spinal nerves. One such group attaches the upper limb to the vertebral column (trapezius, latissimus dorsi, and rhomboids; see Fig. 12-32). They are important muscles, can be clinically evaluated independently, and are described in a later chapter. Beneath them is a second group, the superior and inferior serratus posterior muscles (see Fig. 12-32); these do not perform a critical function and their action cannot be demonstrated clinically. The concern of this section is the spinal extensors situated deep to these two muscle groups.

Structure and General Grouping

Knowledge of the individual muscles and muscle groups in the spinal extensor musculature is less important than an appreciation of the general arrangement. The deepest muscles are the shortest and extend no farther than the next vertebra, whereas more superficial muscles span many vertebrae. Individual muscles arise and insert by multiple tendinous slips. They cross each other in different layers, establishing a system of guy ropes or trusses. Such an arrangement is ideal for providing stability to the vertebral column. When this mechanism is defective on one side, a pathologic lateral spinal curvature or scoliosis will result.

The subdivision of this large muscle mass by innumerable connective tissue planes, and the multiple attachments of tendons over small areas of periosteum on vertebral processes, may suggest why pain or spasm is so common in the extensor musculature of the spine, and why it is so difficult to offer a specific anatomic explanation for it. Segmental spasm and pain will also be induced in a muscle if a single nerve root is irritated. Conversely, segments of a muscle may go into spasm to guard against movement when a painful lesion is present.

The following section describes the individual components of the spinal extensors with emphasis on their layering and grouping, rather than on their detailed anatomy (Fig. 12-27).

Specific Grouping and Individual Muscles

The *erectors spinae* and *transversospinalis*, the largest of the four muscle groups, are each composed of three subgroups. With one exception each of these subgroups, in turn, is composed of three individual muscles (see Fig. 12-27). The muscles in a given subgroup typically have the same name, but are distinguished from one another by regional designations (semispinalis thoracis, cervicis, and capitis, for example). The other two muscle groups are rather simpler in their composition: the *splenius group* comprises only two muscles and the *suboccipital group,* four muscles.

The muscles are arranged in three fairly well-defined layers (see Fig. 12-27). The superficial layer contains all three subgroups of the erector spinae and, in the neck, the splenius muscles as well. The intermediate layer is made up of two of the transversospinalis subgroups, the semispinalis and multifidus. Deep to these lie the third subgroup of the transversospinalis (the segmental muscles) and, in the neck, the suboccipital muscles. In the following account of the four muscle groups and their subdivisions, the muscles of the superficial layer are described first, then those of the intermediate layer and lastly, those of the deepest layer.

Splenius Muscles. The two muscles of this group are the broad **splenius capitis** and the narrow **splenius cervicis** (see Fig. 12-26). They arise in continuity from

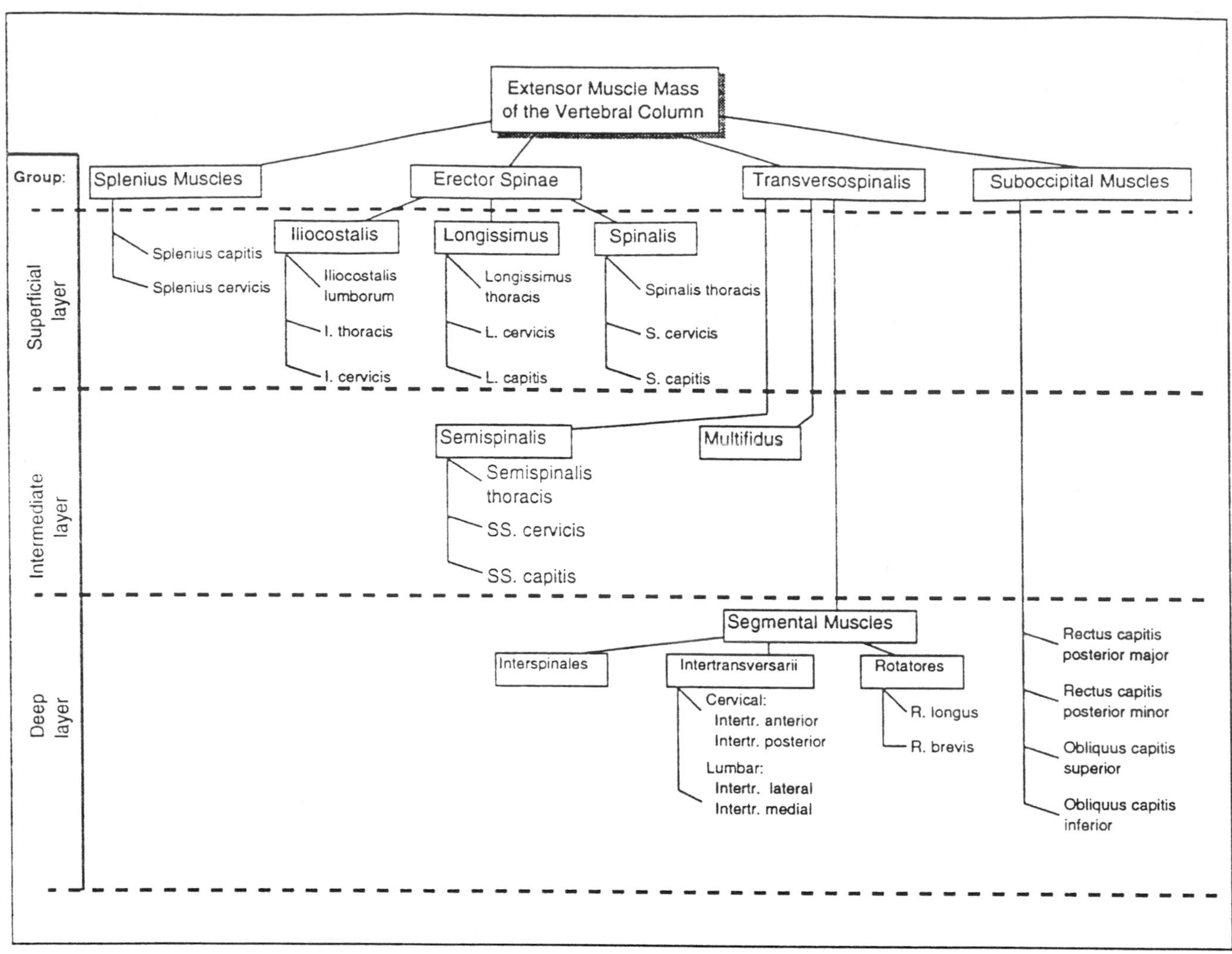

FIGURE *12-27.*
Layers and groups in the extensor muscle mass of the vertebral column.

approximately the lower half of the ligamentum nuchae and the spinous processes of the seventh cervical and upper six thoracic vertebrae. From here they run upward and laterally. The splenius capitis inserts onto the occipital bone (lateral part of the superior nuchal line) and the mastoid process of the temporal bone; the splenius cervicis inserts onto the transverse processes of the upper two to four cervical vertebrae.

Erector Spinae. This large muscular mass has a heavily tendinous and extensive origin from the sacrum, the iliac crest, and the spinous processes of most of the lumbar and last two thoracic vertebrae (see Fig. 12-26). As it becomes muscular in the upper lumbar region, the erector spinae divides into three subgroups that form vertical columns (see Fig. 12-26): The most lateral column is the **iliocostalis,** the intermediate column the **longissimus,** and the medial subgroup, the **spinalis.** Each has regional subdivisions (see Fig. 12-27).

As its name implies, the *iliocostalis* is associated with costal elements. The **iliocostalis lumborum** arises from the lilac crest; its fibers run upward to insert on the angles of the lower six ribs. Here they overlap with the slips of origin of the **iliocostalis thoracis** which, in turn, runs upward to insert on the angles of the upper six ribs. The third muscle in the subgroup, the **iliocostalis cervicis,** takes origin from the upper six ribs, just medial to the insertion slips of the iliocostalis thoracis, and inserts onto the transverse processes of the 4th, 5th, and 6th cervical vertebrae.

The **longissimus** blends with the iliocostalis in the lumbar region, but separates above into three overlapping muscles that are associated with the transverse processes. The largest, the **longissimus thoracis,** forms most of the intermediate column of the erector spinae and inserts into T-3 to T-12 transverse processes and the adjacent ribs. The **longissimus cervicis** arises medial to the upper insertions of the longissimus thoracis and inserts into the transverse processes of the C-2 to C-6 cervical vertebrae. The origin of the **longissimus capitis** overlaps the upper insertions of the longissimus cervicis; it inserts, under cover of the splenius capitis, into the posterior margin of the mastoid process.

The **spinalis** forms the smallest and most medial column of the erector spinae. As implied by its name, it is primarily associated with spinous processes. When it is well developed, there are three muscles in this group: the spinalis thoracis, cervicis, and capitis, respectively. However, the spinalis thoracis is the only constant and relatively independent member of the group. The **spinalis thoracis** arises from the spinous processes of T-10 to L-2 vertebrae, and inserts into the spinous processes of the upper four to eight thoracic vertebrae. The **spinalis cervicis** is frequently absent or represented by only a few muscle fibers attached to the ligamentum nuchae. When well developed, however, it arises from the lower part of the ligamentum nuchae and the spinous process of C-7 vertebra and inserts into the spinous process of the axis. The **spinalis capitis** is not a separate muscle, it being blended laterally with the larger *semispinalis capitis.* It arises with that muscle and inserts with it into the occipital bone.

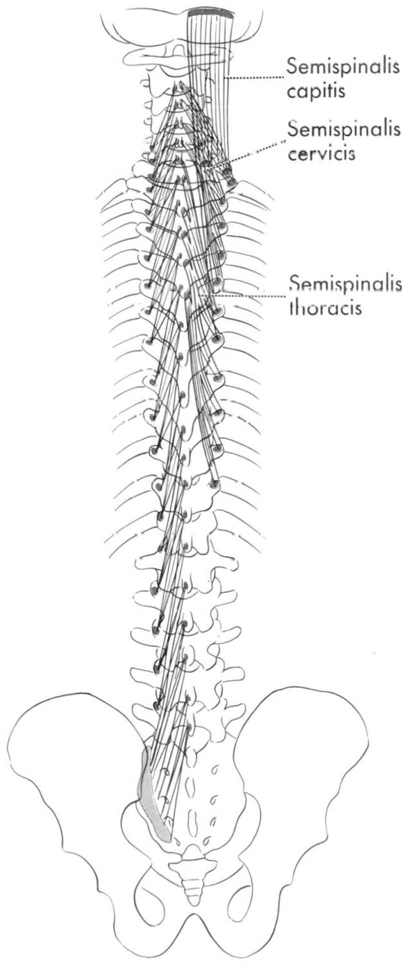

FIGURE *12-28.*
Origins (*red*) and insertions (*blue*) of the semispinalis muscles (*right*) and the multifidi (*left*).

Transversospinalis. The three subgroups of this system are the **semispinalis,** the **multifidus,** and the **segmental muscles** (see Figs. 12-26 and 12-27). They lie deep to the erector spinae. Their fibers are often shorter, those of the last group attaching to neighboring vertebrae. The semispinalis is lacking in the lumbar region, and has *thoracis, cervicis,* and *capitis* portions. No such designations exist for the multifidus, which is present throughout the spine. Among the segmental muscles, one set connects the spinous processes of adjacent vertebrae (*interspinales*), another the transverse processes (*intertransversarii*), and the third set, the *rotators,* connect a transverse process of one vertebra to the spinous process of another one or two segments higher. The segmental muscles are present in all regions.

The **semispinalis** is superficial to the multifidus, and its longest bundles pass over as many as six vertebrae between their origin and insertion; the shortest slips pass over about four (Fig. 12-28, also see Fig. 12-26). The **semispinalis thoracis** arises by long slender tendons from the transverse processes of approximately the lower six thoracic vertebrae, and inserts by similar slender tendons into the spinous processes of upper thoracic and lower cervical vertebrae. The **semispinalis cervicis** arises from the transverse processes of the upper six thoracic vertebrae and inserts into the bifid spinous process of the axis and the three or four spinous processes below it. The **semispinalis capitis** is a large muscle. It arises by tendons from the tips of T-1 to T-6 transverse processes and from the articular processes of the lower three or four cervical vertebrae. Under cover of the splenius capitis, the muscle sweeps upward as a broad band and inserts into the occipital bone between the superior and inferior nuchal lines. The most medial part of this muscle is in fact the *spinalis capitis;* both parts contain a partial tendinous intersection.

The muscle bundles of the **multifidus** are shorter than those of the semispinalis, spanning two to four vertebrae. In the sacral and lumbar regions, the multifidus is covered by the erector spinae, and in the thoracic and cervical regions by the semispinalis. The fibers of the lumbar part arise from the dorsal surface of the sacrum, the posterior superior iliac spine, the deep surface of the erector spinae tendon, and the mamillary processes of lumbar vertebrae (see Figs. 12-26 and 12-28). Farther up, the muscle bundles are thinner and take origin from the transverse processes of T-1 to T-12 vertebrae and the articular processes of the lower four cervical vertebrae. Slanting upward and medially, the fibers of this slender, continuous muscle mass insert into the sides of the spinous processes of all the vertebrae from L-5 to the axis.

The *segmental muscles,* made up of the interspinous, intertransverse, and rotator groups, are the deepest members of the transversospinalis system and lie deep to the multifidus (Fig. 12-29). All groups are better developed in the cervical and lumbar regions than in the thoracic region. In both the intertransverse and the rotator group, two sets of muscles are distinguished by different adjectives.

The **interspinales** stretch between adjacent spinous processes, members of a pair at each segment being

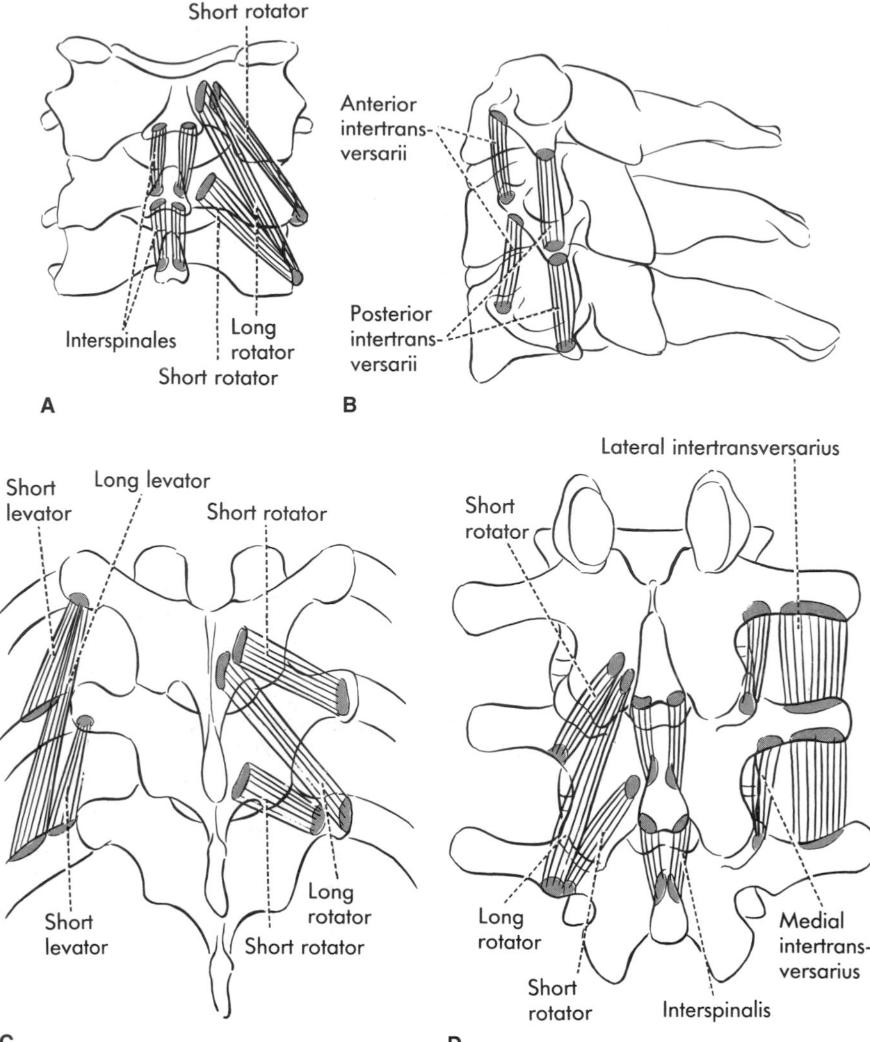

FIGURE *12-29.*
Segmental muscles of the back: (A and B) Cervical region; (C) thoracic region; (D) lumbar region. *Origins* and *insertions* are shown in *red* and *blue*, respectively.

separated from each other by the interspinous ligaments (see Fig. 12-29A and D). The **intertransversarii** run vertically between adjacent transverse processes (see Fig. 12-29B and D). In the cervical and lumbar regions the intertransversarii are divided into two sets. Although these muscles are small, their subdivisions exhibit interesting homologies and provide the dividing line between the territories of muscular distribution of the anterior and posterior rami of spinal nerves.

One set of intertransverse muscles connects the true transverse processes of vertebrae and, the other, the costal elements. The latter set are innervated by anterior rami and, strictly speaking, should not be counted among the extensor muscles of the spine. In the cervical region, these muscles run between the anterior tubercles (costal element) of the transverse processes, and are called *anterior intertransversarii* (see Fig. 12-29B). In the lumbar region, the corresponding muscles, called the *lateral intertransversarii*, connect the prominent, lateral part (costal element) of the transverse processes (see Fig. 12-29D). The equivalent muscles in the thoracic region, called the **levatores costarum** (elevators of the ribs), run between the transverse processes and the ribs (see Fig. 12-29C). The second set of intertransversarii are called the *posterior intertransverse muscles* in the cervical region and *medial intertransversarii* in the lumbar region (see Fig. 12-29B and D). They connect the posterior tubercles of cervical transverse processes and, in the lumbar region, they run between the accessory process of one vertebra and the mamillary process of the next. In the lumbar region the posterior ramus actually passes between the lateral and medial intertransverse muscles. As it does so, it supplies the medial muscle; the lateral muscle, by contrast, receives its innervation from the anterior ramus. In the cervical region, the anterior intertransverse muscles are innervated by anterior rami whereas the posterior muscles actually receive innervation from both posterior and anterior rami. Except for the lower two segments, the equivalents of these muscles are absent from the thoracic region.

The **rotatores** arise on the transverse processes and slope upward and medially to insert on the bases of spinous processes at higher levels. Some insert on the vertebra immediately above and thus, are strictly

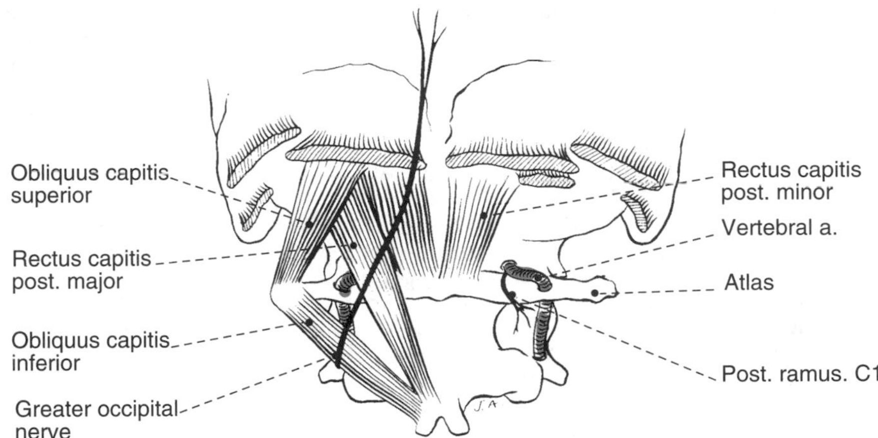

FIGURE **12-30.**
Suboccipital muscles and the suboccipital triangle.

segmental (short rotators), whereas others skip one vertebra and insert on the next one (long rotators; see Fig. 12-29C and D).

Suboccipital Muscles. The group of muscles in the deepest layer that connects the atlas and axis to each other and to the skull is specialized for rotating and extending the head. This suboccipital group is composed of four muscles: a major and minor rectus muscle, and a superior and inferior oblique muscle (Fig. 12-30). Their names imply not only the direction of their fibers, but also their actions: the recti mainly produce extension at the atlantooccipital joints, whereas the obliques rotate the atlas and skull on the axis. The rectus muscles are also designated as posterior because they have flexor anterior counterparts. All suboccipital muscles are supplied by the posterior ramus of the first cervical nerve.

The **rectus capitis posterior major** arises from the spinous process of the axis and inserts into the occipital bone a little lateral to the midline. The **rectus capitis posterior minor** arises from the posterior tubercle of the atlas and inserts just medially to the major. The **obliquus capitis inferior** arises from the spinous process of the axis and extends laterally to insert on the transverse process of the atlas. The **obliquus capitis superior** arises from the transverse process of the atlas and passes upward to insert into the occipital bone deep to the insertions of the splenius and semispinalis capitis.

The obliques and the major recti enclose between them the **suboccipital triangle**, which contains important structures (see Fig. 12-30). The *vertebral artery* emerges from the transverse foramen of the atlas and crosses the triangle, running medially along the posterior arch of the atlas before entering the foramen magnum to supply the brain. The posterior ramus of the first cervical nerve (**suboccipital nerve**) enters the triangle close to the vertebral artery. It supplies all four of the posterior suboccipital muscles and usually helps supply overlying muscles. The **greater occipital nerve**, representing primarily the posterior ramus of the second cervical nerve, appears at the lower border of the obliquus capitis inferior and, after giving off a few muscular branches, crosses over the triangle to reach the scalp.

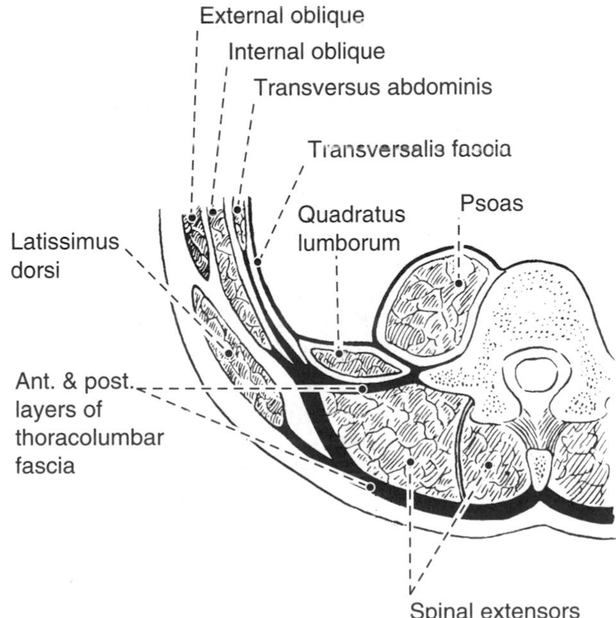

FIGURE **12-31.**
The thoracolumbar fascia (*black*) in a transverse section at the lumbar level.

Associated Fascia

A strong fascia envelops the spinal extensors; it is best developed in the lumbar region, where it is reinforced by aponeuroses, from which the fleshy parts of the latissimus dorsi and some of the abdominal muscles arise (Fig. 12-31). It is known as the **thoracolumbar fascia** and, in the lumbar region, consists of two distinct layers. The *anterior layer* is anchored to the transverse processes; it meets the *posterior layer* along the lateral edge of the erector spinae. Numerous muscle fibers of the erector spinae take origin from both laminae. In the thoracic region, the much thinner fascia blends laterally with the periosteum of the ribs.

In the cervical region, the fascia helps encircle the deep muscles of the neck by blending laterally with the prevertebral fascia.

Associated Muscles

Immediately superficial to the thoracolumbar fascia are the two pairs of rather insignificant and thin **serratus posterior muscles** (Fig. 12-32). The **serratus posterior superior** arises from the lower part of the ligamentum nuchae and the spinous processes of C-7 to T-2 vertebrae (and the intervening supraspinous ligaments). It runs laterally and downward to insert into the second to fourth or fifth ribs. The **serratus posterior inferior** arises from the spinous processes of about T-6 to L-2 vertebrae (and the intervening supraspinous ligaments), and runs laterally and upward to insert into the last three or four ribs. The aponeuroses of origin of both these muscles are fused to the underlying thoracolumbar fascia.

The two serratus posterior muscles assist inspiration. The superior serratus elevates the upper ribs and the inferior serratus stabilizes the lower ribs to prevent them from being pulled upward by the contraction of the diaphragm. Both muscles are innervated by branches of *intercostal nerves* that are associated with two to four of the ribs to which the muscles attach.

The posterior serratus muscles as well as the extensor muscle mass of the spine are covered by muscles of the upper limb, which attach to the midline in continuity from the occiput to the sacrum. The overlapping musculotendinous sheets of the trapezius and latissimus dorsi hide from view not only the spinal extensors and serrati, but the rhomboids as well (see Fig. 12-32). The aponeurosis of the latissimus dorsi blends with the thoracolumbar fascia, but all other muscles are superficial to the fascia.

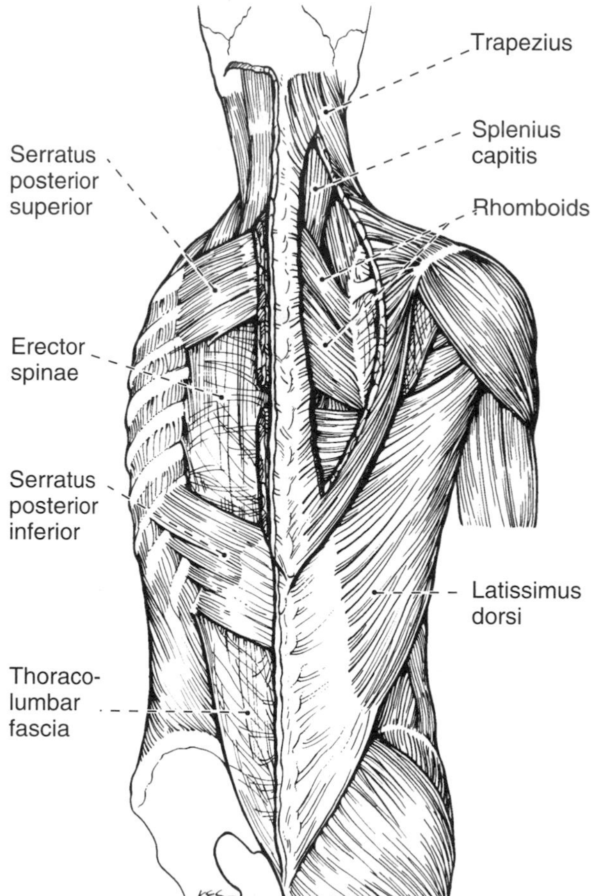

FIGURE *12-32.*
Muscles associated with the spinal extensors: On the *right* are shown the posterior muscles that move the shoulder girdle: the trapezius, cut to show the deeply lying rhomboids, and below, the extensive latissimus dorsi. On the *left side* of the figure, the latissimus dorsi, trapezius; and rhomboids have been removed with the scapula to reveal the superior and inferior serratus posterior muscles. The spinal extensor musculature is deep to the serrati and the thoracolumbar fascia.

Flexors

The flexor musculature is virtually confined to the cervical and lumbar regions of the spine, these being the most mobile regions of the vertebral column. Because gravity plays a major part in flexion, the flexor muscles of the spine are best demonstrated when they are made to work against gravity, as happens, for example, during raising of the head or trunk from the supine position.

The **prevertebral musculature** is the flexor counterpart of the spinal extensors. Attaching directly to vertebrae, these muscles produce movement at intervertebral joints. Owing to their close apposition to the vertebral column anteriorly, they have poor mechanical advantage and, therefore, are ineffectual as a flexor unit; they retain their original function only in the cervical region where they are chiefly represented by the **longus colli** and the **scalene** muscles (Fig. 12-33A). In the thoracic region this muscle group is absent; in front of the lumbar spine it is chiefly represented by the **psoas major** (see Fig. 12-33B). However, the psoas muscle does not function as a flexor of the spine. The distal attachment of the psoas has migrated to the lower limb; when the muscle contracts, it flexes the entire trunk on the lower limb at the hip; it cannot produce flexion at intervertebral joints. When the right and left psoas contract together, they extend, rather than flex, the lumbar spine, owing to their attachment to the posterolateral parts of the vertebrae. The **quadratus lumborum** muscles (see Fig. 12-33B) have a similar action on the spine when they contract together, exerting a pull on the last pair of ribs.

More powerful are the muscles that flex the spine indirectly. They are placed more anteriorly and, therefore, operate at a better advantage than the prevertebral muscles. The **sternocleidomastoid muscles** attach superiorly to the skull and inferiorly to the manubrium and clavicles (see Fig. 12-33A). They not only draw the head forward, but flex the cervical spine. This composite movement anticipates food being placed into the mouth.

The flexors of the lumbar spine are the anterior abdominal wall muscles (see Fig. 12-33C). The two **rectus**

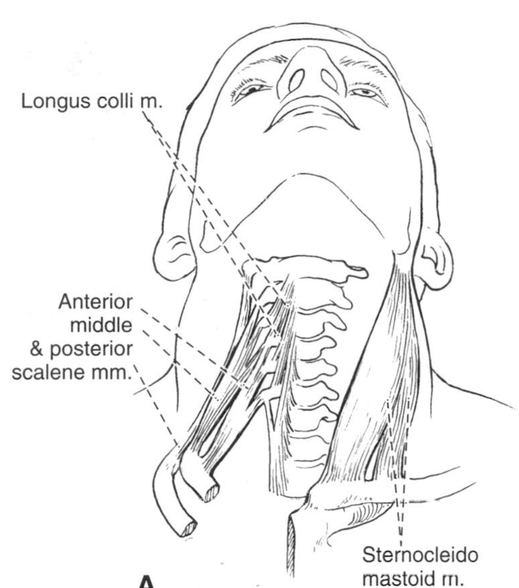

FIGURE 12-33.
(A) Muscles of the neck and (B and C) abdomen involved in flexion and lateral bending of the vertebral column: The psoas major flexes the trunk by producing movement at the hip joint, but it cannot flex intervertebral joints. On the *right side* of (C) the upper portion of the rectus sheath has been cut open to expose the rectus abdominis. On the *left*, the inferolateral part of the external oblique has been removed to expose the internal oblique.

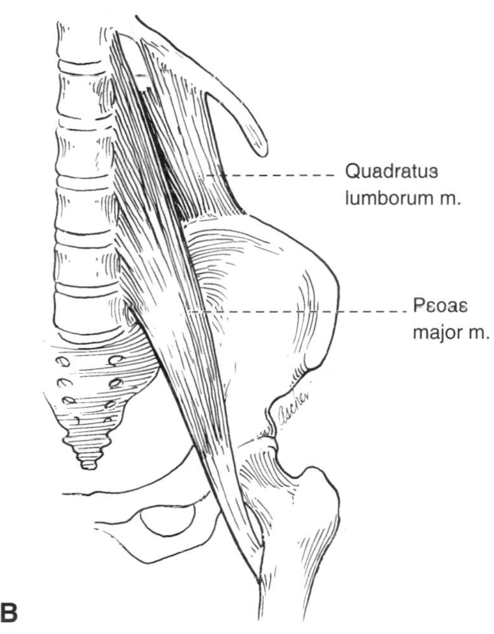

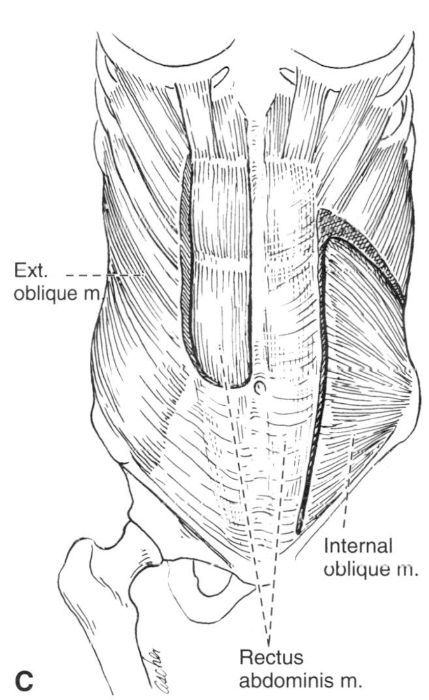

abdominis muscles are attached to the rib cage and the pubis. They are assisted by the **external** and **internal obliques.** These muscles approximate the rib cage to the pelvis. The muscles are put to work during sit-ups, especially when the hips and knees are flexed. With extended hips, sit-ups mainly exercise the psoas.

The prevertebral and the anterior abdominal wall muscles are derived from the hypomeric component of myotomes and are all supplied segmentally by the anterior rami of spinal nerves. The sternocleidomastoid muscle is an exception; it is supplied from cervical spinal cord segments by the spinal accessory nerve whose relation to spinal nerves is not clearly understood.

Lateral Bending

Unilateral contraction of spinal flexors and extensors produces lateral bending. The rotational element that some of these muscles produce must be cancelled out by appropriate antagonists. A muscle that functions chiefly in lateral bending of the lumbar spine is the **quadratus lumborum** (see Fig. 12-33B).

Rotation

Rotation is possible in the cervical and thoracic regions but, for all practical purposes, it is nonexistent in the lumbar spine. When the head is turned fully to one side, 70% of the movement occurs at the **atlantoaxial** and **atlantooccipital joints** and only 30% at joints between the remaining cervical vertebrae.

The sternocleidomastoid is the most powerful rotator, but a combination of muscles is called into action. Although parts of the spinal extensors running between the transverse process of one vertebra and the spinous process of the vertebra above do exert a rotatory action (see Figs. 12-26 through 12-29), the most powerful rotators of the thoracic spine are the abdominal flank muscles, namely the external and internal obliques (see Fig. 12-33C). These muscles run obliquely, at right angles to one another, between the pelvis and the thoracic cage. The right external oblique acts in union with the left internal oblique and together they rotate the costal margin toward the left side.

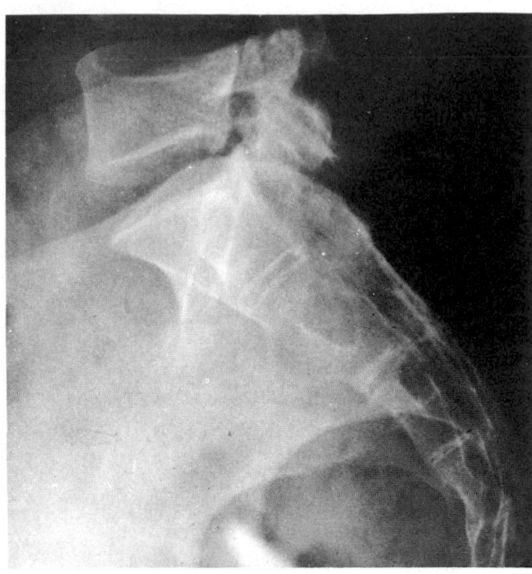

FIGURE *12-34.*
Lateral view of the lumbosacral junction and sacrum: Note the wedge shape of the body of the fifth lumbar vertebra and of L-5 disk. (Courtesy of Dr DG Pugh.)

THE VERTEBRAL COLUMN AS A WHOLE

The vertebral column performs most of its functions as an integrated unit. Clinical evaluation of the vertebral column as a whole is an important part of the physical examination. The evaluation described in this chapter is concerned mainly with the assessment of the spinal curvatures, the ranges of movement and stability, and the strength of the spinal musculature.

Curvatures

Normally, a plumbline, held to the external occipital protuberance of the skull, falls into the cleft between the buttocks and lies over the spinous processes in all regions of the vertebral column. Apart from a minor deviation from the vertical toward the side of handedness in the thoracic region, there are no lateral curvatures in the spine of a normal individual. When viewed from the side, however, the vertebral column shows marked curvatures in the sagittal plane (see Figs. 12-1, 12-9 and 12-13). In the early embryo the column is curved like a C, its concavity facing ventrally. This **primary curvature** persists throughout life in the thoracic and sacral regions. The **secondary curves,** which develop later in the cervical and lumbar regions, are convex anteriorly. Exaggeration of a normal thoracic curve is known as **kyphosis** and an exaggerated lumbar curve is a **lordosis** (see later discussion). These Greek words mean convexity and concavity, and were originally used to describe the curves as seen by the examiner standing behind, rather than in front of, the subject. Although these terms denote abnormal conditions of the spine, it has become customary in clinical contexts to speak of a "normal" kyphotic or lordotic curve when describing the normal spine. The primary and secondary curvatures impart an undulating lateral profile to the whole vertebral column and greatly increase its springiness. The freedom of movement is greater in regions that are convex anteriorly.

The curvatures are determined by the disparate shapes of the vertebral bodies and intervertebral disks in the various regions. The disks are responsible for the cervical curve, because the vertebral bodies in this region actually measure slightly less anteriorly than posteriorly. The shape of vertebral bodies is primarily responsible for the thoracic curve, whereas in the upper lumbar region, the wedge-shaped disks, thicker anteriorly than posteriorly, account for the forward convexity. The convexity is further exaggerated in the lower lumbar region by the wedge shape of both the disks and the vertebral bodies (Fig. 12-34).

> **Development of the Curvatures.** Probably as a result of fetal movements, the original anterior concavity of both the cervical and lumbar regions is abolished before birth, and convexities begin to form in each region. Further development of the cervical curvature is believed to be associated with the ability of the infant to raise and balance its head, whereas the lumbar curve develops when the infant begins to sit up and walk.

Curvatures and Posture

The cervical and lumbar curves are compensatory to the upright habitus of humans. The cervical curve acts as a buttress to the weight of the head, thereby relieving the posterior muscles of the neck of undue strain. Although the thoracic curve tends to put the body at a disadvantage, the lumbar curve, in its turn, buttresses the weight of the trunk and upper limbs.

In the erect stance, the vertical line of gravity of the body tends to maintain the spinal curvatures: it passes behind the bodies of C-2 to C-6 vertebrae, through those of C-7 and T-1, in front of most thoracic vertebrae, through the vertebral bodies at the thoracolumbar junction, behind the

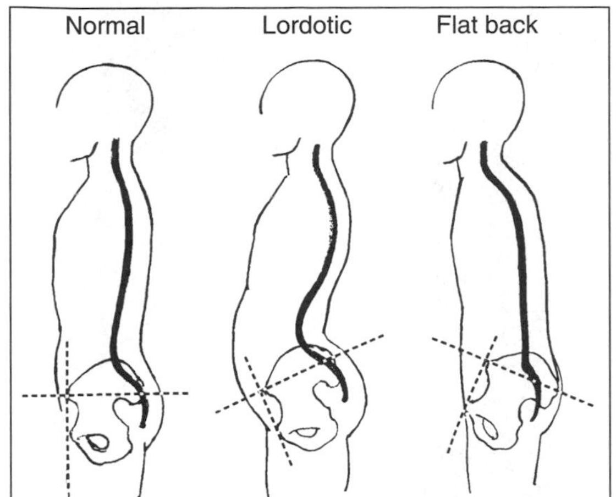

FIGURE *12-35.*
Variations in posture: Tilting of the pelvis is associated with changes in the spinal curvatures. In the normal stance, the *line drawn* across the anterior and posterior superior iliac spines is horizontal and the pubic tubercle and the anterior superior iliac spine lie in the same vertical plane. Forward tilting of the pelvis produces lordosis, and its backward tilt flattens the normal lumbar curve.

center of upper lumbar bodies, and near the center of L-4 and L-5. The least expenditure of muscular energy is required when the center of gravity is so situated. If one curve becomes exaggerated, thereby displacing this center of gravity, reciprocal changes occur in another curve to restore the alignment and conserve muscular energy.

Abnormal Curvatures

Abnormal curves may develop in the vertebral column during the growth period, or as a consequence of disease in the vertebrae or intervertebral joints. Pathologic curves may also result from interference with the normal function of the spinal musculature. Any condition that produces a change in one of the spinal curvatures will cause compensatory changes in the other curves to maintain balance. Abnormal curvatures of the vertebral column are designated as kyphosis (hunchback), lordosis (swayback), and scoliosis (a lateral curvature).

Kyphosis, an exaggeration of the thoracic curvature, can result from defective development of the vertebral bodies. During the rapid phase of spinal growth in the preadolescent- and adolescent-aged group, the ring epiphysis of vertebral bodies may suffer damage anteriorly, where it is less protected (see Fig. 12-6). The result will be wedge-shaped vertebrae because growth proceeds posteriorly at a normal pace, whereas anteriorly it is retarded. The condition should be detected as early as possible, because deformity can be prevented by wearing an appropriate brace during the growth phase. In the older-age-group, the most common cause of kyphosis is osteoporosis of the spine, which is frequently complicated by the collapse of vertebral bodies.

Lordosis, an exaggerated lumbar curve, is usually a compensation for increased obliquity of the sacrum, or for thoracic kyphosis. It is an adjustment toward maintaining the body's center of mass over the feet. The degree of tilting of the pelvis, even in normal individuals, causes recognizable variations in posture that are reflected in the spinal curvatures (Fig. 12-35). Lordosis is seen in obese people and in the later months of pregnancy. It also occurs when, as a result of joint disease, the hip becomes fixed in a flexed position (flexion contracture), a condition that throws the weight of the body forward.

Lateral curves (curvatures in the coronal plane) are always abnormal curves. It is a mechanical principle that one cannot bend a bent column again in a second plane without a concomitant rotation. Hence, a lateral bending deformity of the spine must be accompanied by rotation of the vertebrae, and this complex deformity is termed **scoliosis** (Fig. 12-36). One or more compensatory curves usually develop following establishment of the primary curve, to reestablish a vertical line of gravity between the head and the pelvis.

Scoliosis may be due to a congenital abnormality of the vertebrae, such as a hemivertebra or block vertebra; more frequently, however, it is an acquired condition. For instance, a short leg produces scoliosis because the pelvis must dip to that side for both feet to remain on the ground (see Chap. 17). Scoliosis may also result from unilateral muscle spasm provoked by pressure on a nerve caused, in turn, by a prolapsed intervertebral disk (see Chap. 13). Unilateral paralysis of spinal musculature caused, for example, by poliomyelitis will also result in scoliosis. In each case the imbalance of forces acting on the spine is responsible for the condition. The most common type of scoliosis, however, is idiopathic; that is, the cause or causes cannot be determined. Idiopathic scoliosis is usually associated with rapid growth and is most prevalent in the preadolescent- and the adolescent-aged group. Once scoliosis has started, it will usually progress during the growth period. In the thoracic spine, the deformity includes not only malalignment of the vertebrae but also of the ribs, because of the obligatory rotation associated with the lateral bend (see Fig. 12-36). The ribs are crowded together on the concave side of the curve, and produce the so-called *rib hump* on the convex side. Severe scoliosis will alter respiratory function by diminishing the capacity of the thorax and shifting the mediastinum. As other curvatures, it will also compromise the height of the individual.

Stability and Mobility

The vertebrae may be thought of as a series of levers held together by joints and ligaments and kept in alignment, as well as operated, by muscles and the force of gravity. Considering the number of levers that constitute the column, the forces to which its sinuous architecture is subjected, and the range of movements that are permitted without violating its integrity, the degree of stability that is obtained in the column is indeed remarkable. Perhaps even more remarkable is that many of the anatomic structures that assure stability are also the ones that permit the column to move as freely as it does. As previous sections of this chapter have already suggested, these factors are the intervertebral disks, the ligaments, the articular facets of the vertebral arch joints, and the spinal musculature.

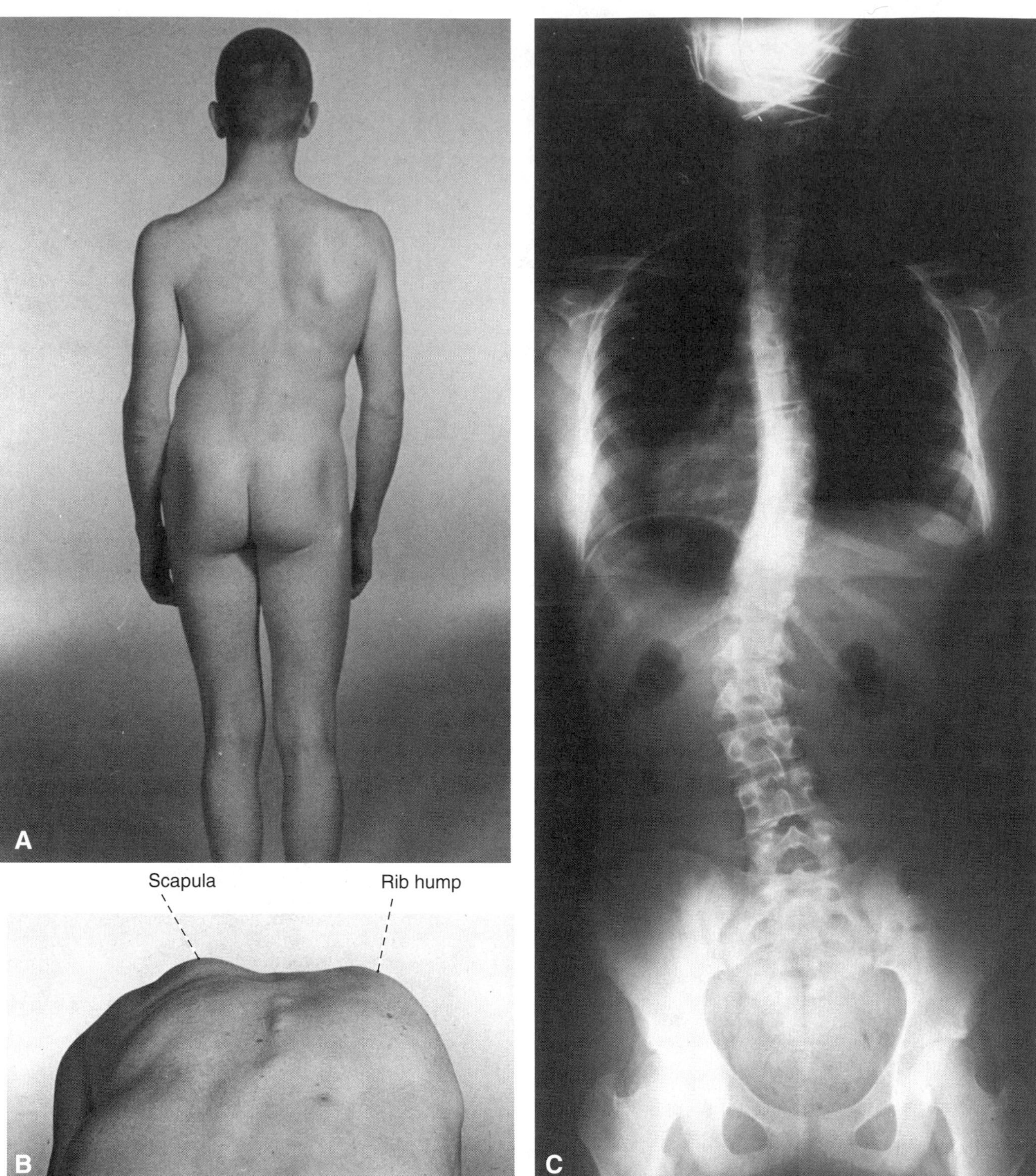

FIGURE *12-36.*
Scoliosis: (A) a scoliotic curve of the thoracic spine is evident. The curve is convex to the right. A secondary curve of the lumbar spine is also present. It is convex to the left. The pelvis and gluteal folds appear symmetric; the right shoulder is higher than the left and the gap between the arm and flank is greater on the right than on the left side; all suggestive of lateral curvatures of the spine. An imaginary plumb line dropped from the occiput aligns with T-1, but not with the gluteal cleft. (B) when the subject bends forward, the lateral curves of the spine remain visible, but the asymmetry of the contour of the rib cage becomes exaggerated. The rib hump on the right obscures the scapula from view at this angle; on the left the scapula is still visible, the curve of the rib cage being much lower than on the right. (C) composite radiograph of a patient with idiopathic scoliosis. In addition to the primary curve in the thoracic spine, there is a secondary compensatory curve in the lumbar region. On close examination the rotatory element of the deformity may be appreciated from the changes in the alignment of the spinous processes and of the bases of the pedicles from vertebra to vertebra.

Stability

As already explained, the structure of the *annulus fibrosus* provides both a strong bond and a certain degree of mobility between the vertebral bodies.

Among the *ligaments,* the anterior longitudinal ligament is the strongest; it checks both anterior and posterior displacement of vertebrae. When the spine is fully flexed, all muscles are silent electromyographically, and the column is supported entirely by its ligaments. The supraspinous and interspinous ligaments, the ligamenta flava, the posterior longitudinal ligament, and the fibrous capsules of the vertebral arch joints provide the support and set the limit of the movement.

The placement and shape of the *articular facets* of the vertebral arch joints (see Fig. 12-19) help resist displacement of vertebrae upon one another. The ribs and the ligaments of the costovertebral joints furnish additional elements of stability to the thoracic part of the vertebral column.

Movements and adjustments in body posture shift the line of force of gravity through the curvatures of the vertebral column and require constant adjustments in the positions of individual vertebrae. These adjustments are made chiefly by the deepest muscles of the extensor musculature which, to a large extent, function as *postural muscles.* The stabilizing influence of the trusses and guy ropes provided by the spinal extensors is illustrated by the scoliotic curves that develop after complete resection of one or more ribs. This undesirable side complication can usually be prevented if the medial portion of the rib, to which these muscles attach, is retained. Once these postural muscles stabilize vertebrae, other muscles can effectively move regions of the column, or the column as a whole. The strength of the muscles that stabilize and move the column is an important factor in relieving the joints and ligaments of the strain imposed by gravity. Assessment of muscle strength, therefore, is as important in the physical examination of the spine as assessment of the ranges of movement.

Ranges of Movement

Familiarity with normal ranges of movement in regions of the spine is particularly important when progressive disability, or its treatment, are being assessed. It is not possible clinically to measure movement between individual vertebrae, nor is it feasible to measure movement in any one region of the spine in actual degrees, although this may be done radiographically. Therefore, assessment is usually limited to comparison of movements in opposite directions and to visual estimates of the range.

Cervical Spine. Full flexion of the cervical spine and the atlantooccipital joints should put the chin on the chest with the mouth closed. Full extension of the same joints catches the examiner's finger between the occiput and C-7, but does not trap it. In lateral bending, when the shoulders are steadied, approximating the ear toward the shoulder should provide a total range of movement between the right and left sides that is somewhat less than 90°. As in scoliosis, lateral flexion is always accompanied by some rotation. These ranges are the sums of the movements taking place at the atlantooccipital, lateral atlantoaxial, and other cervical intervertebral joints.

When the shoulders are steadied, rotation of the head and neck normally brings the chin level with the shoulders. As noted earlier, two-thirds of this range are obtained at the atlantoaxial joints. Combined extension and rotation compresses intervertebral foramina (see Fig. 12-9) and provokes or exaggerates the symptoms caused by nerve compression in these foramina (see Chap. 13).

Thoracolumbar Spine. Mobility of the thoracic spine, particularly in its upper and middle regions, is limited mainly by the rib cage, but also by the narrowness of the intervertebral disks. Flexion, extension, and lateral bending occur mainly in the lumbar region, whereas rotation of the trunk takes place primarily in the thoracic spine. Limitation of flexion, extension, and rotation can be camouflaged by movement at the hip joints, and this must be excluded by stabilizing the pelvis.

Even in the erect, neutral position, the normal lumbar curve holds the lumbosacral angle in extension (see Figs. 12-34 and 12 35). The range of extension is only about 15° to 30°, if movement at the hips is precluded. Extension exaggerates the normal "lordotic" curvature.

The range of flexion can be assessed by bending forward as far as possible with the knees extended. The range of motion is best recorded by placing a tape measure between C-7 and a fixed point on the sacrum in the upright position, and recording the increase in the distance between these two points as full flexion is attained. This measurement is preferable to the distance between the finger tips and the floor because the contribution by hip flexion is excluded.

Lateral bending can be measured by sliding the hand down the side of the thigh as far as possible. Normally, the head of the fibula can be reached without flexing the hip or knee. The distance from the finger tips to the fibula is a reliable measure of the range of the lateral bend. If, during this movement, pain is experienced on the concave side, nerve root compression should be suspected. Pain on the convex side is usually related to muscle, tendon, or ligament abnormalities.

To assess rotation of the thoracolumbar spine, pelvic rotation at the hips must be excluded. The examiner, standing behind the subject, should hold the pelvis firmly at the iliac crests while the subject twists the trunk to look back at the examiner. Alternatively, the subject should be seated while the trunk is rotated. The range of movement is assessed by the change in the position of the shoulders.

Estimation of Muscle Strength

The spinal extensors can be evaluated only as a group. Lying prone, the subject is asked to raise the head and shoulders from the examining table. The examiner may apply resistance to the head or shoulders, testing the strength of the muscles in the cervical and thoracolumbar regions. Contraction of the lumbar part of the musculature can be observed and palpated during this maneuver.

Unless there is regional paralysis, generalized weakness of the spinal extensors is rarely associated with back problems. More commonly, back symptoms are related to weakness of the flexor muscles, particularly the rectus abdominis and the flank muscles. Evaluation of the muscles that move the spine should include attempted sit-ups, while the knees are kept in the flexed position. Inability to do sit-ups in this position signifies marked weakness of the abdominal musculature. Strengthening the abdominal muscles can relieve symptoms caused by strains on the vertebral column.

RECOMMENDED READINGS

Amonoo-Kuofi HS. Changes in the lumbosacral angle, sacral inclination and the curvature of the lumbar spine during aging. Acta Anat 1992; 145: 373.

Amonoo-Kuofi H, El Badwi M, Fatani J. Ligaments associated with lumbar intervertebral foramina. 1. L1 to LA. J Anat 1988; 156: 177.

Asmussen E. The weight carrying function of the human spine. Acta Orthop Scand 1960; 29: 276.

Babic MS. Development of the notochord in normal and malformed human embryos and fetuses. Int J Dev Biol 1991; 35: 345.

Bailey RW, Sherk HH, Dunn EJ, et al. The cervical spine. Philadelphia: Lippincott, 1983.

Bareggi R, Grill V, Sandrucci MA, et al. Developmental pathways of vertebral centra and neural arches in human embryos and fetuses. Anat Embryol 1993; 187: 139.

Basmajian JV, DeLuca CJ. Posture. In: Muscles alive: their functions revealed by electromyography. 5th ed. Baltimore: Williams & Wilkins, 1985.

Bowden REM. Anatomy of the human spine. In: Findlay GF, Owen R, eds. Surgery of the spine. Oxford: Blackwell, 1992.

Brown RC, Evans ET. What causes the "eye in the Scotty dog" in the oblique projection of the lumbar spine? Am J Roentgenol 1973; 118: 435.

Carlson BM. Human embryology and developmental biology. St. Louis: Mosby-Year Book, 1994.

Cotten A, Sakka M, Drizenko A, Clarisse J, Francke JP. Antenatal differentiation of the human intervertebral disc. Surg Radiol Anat 1994; 16: 53.

Coventry MB. Anatomy of the intervertebral disk. Clin Orthop 1969; 67: 9.

Danforth CH. Numerical variation and homologies in vertebrae. Am J Phys Anthropol 1930; 14: 463.

Dumas J-L, Thoreux P, Attali P, Goldlust D, Chevrel JP. Three-dimensional CT analysis of atlantoaxial rotation: results in the normal subject. Surg Radiol Anat 1994; 16: 199.

Dumas JL, Sainte Rose M, Dreyfus P, Goldlust D, Chevrel JP. Rotation of the cervical spinal column: a computed tomography in vivo study. Surg Radiol Anat 1993; 15: 333.

Floyd WF, Silver PHS. Function of the erectores spinae in the flexion of the trunk. Lancet 1951; 260: 133.

Fon GT, Pitt MJ, Thies Jr AC. Thoracic kyphosis: range in normal subjects. Am J Roentgenol 1980; 134: 979.

Gunzberg R, Hutton WC, Fraser RD. Role of the capsulo-ligamentous structures in rotation and combined flexion-rotation of the lumbar spine. J Spinal Disord 1992; 5: 1.

Hollinshead WH. Anatomy for surgeons. Vol 3, the back and limbs. 3rd ed. Philadelphia: Harper & Row, 1982.

Hoppenfeld S. Physical examination of the spine and extremities. New York: Appleton-Century-Crofts, 1976.

Knutsson F. Growth and differentiation of postnatal vertebrae. Acta Radiol 1961; 55: 401.

Kramer J. Intervertebral disk diseases - causes, diagnosis, treatment and prophylaxis. Stuttgart: Thieme Verlag, 1981.

Louis R. Spinal stability as defined by the three-column spine concept. Anat Clin 1985; 7: 33.

MacConaill MA, Basmajian JV. Vertebral column. In: Muscles and movements: a basis for human kinesiology. Baltimore: Williams & Wilkins, 1969.

Morris JM. Biomechanics of the spine. Arch Surg 1973; 107: 48.

Müller F, O'Rahilly R. Occipitocervical segmentation in staged human embryos. J Anat 1994; 185: 251.

Nachemson A. Electromyographic studies on the vertebral portion of the psoas muscle. Acta Orthop Scand 1966; 37: 177.

Nathan H. Osteophytes of the vertebral column, an anatomical study of their development according to age, race, and sex with considerations as to their etiology and significance. J Bone Joint Surg 1962; 44A: 243.

O'Rahilly R, Müller F. Human embryology and teratology. New York: Wiley-Liss, 1992.

Olsen GA, Hamilton A. The lateral stability of the spine. Clin Orthop 1969; 65: 143.

Parke WW. Development of the spine. In: Rothman RH, Simeone FA, eds. The spine. Philadelphia: WB Saunders, 1975.

Rauschning W. Clinical and imaging anatomy of the lumbar spine and sacrum (videodisc). LaserAnatomy Videodisc Series. Uppsala, Sweden: Uppsala University, 1990.

Roberts S, Menage J, Urban JPG. Biomechanical and structural properties of the cartilage end-plate and its relation to the IV disc. Spine 1989; 14: 166.

Scoles PV, Linton AE, Latimer B, Levy ME, Digiovanni BF. Vertebral body and posterior element morphology: the normal spine in middle life. Spine 1988; 13: 1082.

Stephens MM, Evans JH, O'Brien JP. Lumbar intervertebral foramens: an in vitro study of their shape in relation to intervertebral disc pathology. Spine 1991; 16: 525.

Taylor JR. Growth of the human intervertebral disc and vertebral bodies. J Anat 1975; 120: 49.

Verbout AJ. The development of the vertebral column. New York: Springer-Verlag, 1985.

Hollinshead's Textbook of Anatomy, by Cornelius Rosse and Penelope Gaddum-Rosse.
Lippincott-Raven Publishers, Philadelphia, © 1997.

CHAPTER 13
The Vertebral Canal, Spinal Cord, Spinal Nerves, and Segmental Innervation

The vertebral canal contains the spinal cord invested in its meninges. The roots of 32 pairs of spinal nerves issue from the cord, traverse the canal and exit through the intervertebral foramina (Fig. 13-1). The vertebral canal also contains blood vessels that contribute to the supply of the spinal cord, the vertebrae, and the intervertebral joints. Nerves enter the vertebral canal to supply the meninges and blood vessels, as well as ligaments and bones. Potential and real spaces intervene between the spinal cord, the meninges, and the osseoligamentous walls of the vertebral canal. One of these spaces is filled with cerebrospinal fluid. The chief concern of this chapter is the anatomy of the vertebral canal, its contents, and its defined spaces. However, it also deals with the segmental distribution of spinal nerves, because the functional evaluation of these nerves provides information about the anatomic integrity of major structures within the canal: namely, the spinal cord and the nerve roots that proceed from it.

It is important to understand the anatomy of the vertebral canal because function will be seriously impaired by even minor lesions if they compromise available space within the inexpansible canal or within its portals of exit: the intervertebral foramina. The resultant functional losses may be complex and may manifest themselves in structures anatomically removed from the spine. A diagnosis of the causative lesions will be possible only if the anatomy of the vertebral canal and its contents is fully understood. In subsequent sections, two examples will illus-

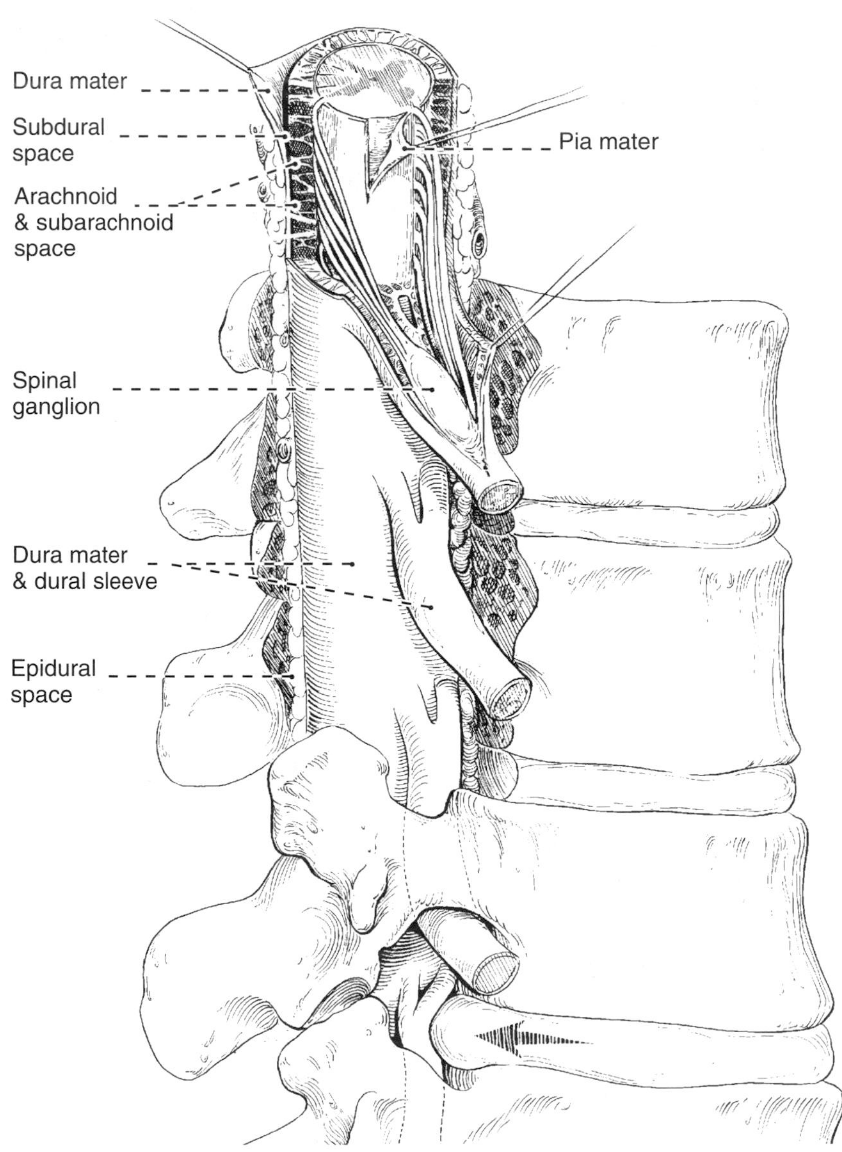

FIGURE *13-1.*
The contents of the vertebral canal: The spinal cord is illustrated with its meninges and associated spaces. Note the rootlets of spinal nerves as they form anterior and posterior roots per segment. The fusiform spinal ganglion is present on the posterior root. A dural sleeve invests the roots and the ganglion as far as the intervertebral foramen. The subarachnoid space is interlaced by delicate strands of the arachnoid and is filled by cerebrospinal fluid (CSF). The disk between the lower two vertebrae is prolapsed and compresses the roots of the exiting nerve.

trate the applied anatomy of the vertebral canal: lumbar puncture and the intervertebral disk syndrome.

THE VERTEBRAL CANAL

The vertebral canal is a sinuous, tubular cavity enclosed within the vertebral column. It is formed by the juxtaposition of the vertebral foramina, which are lined up with one another in series. The canal commences at the **foramen magnum** and terminates at the **sacral hiatus** just above the coccyx (see Fig. 13-3). Its anterior wall is made up of the vertebral bodies and intervertebral disks, over the surfaces of which the posterior longitudinal ligament is draped (see Figs. 12-16 and 12-20). Posteriorly, the laminae and ligamenta flava close the canal. Laterally, nerves and blood vessels leave and enter the canal through the **intervertebral foramina**, which are separated from one another by the pedicles (see Fig. 12-4). Defects in the formation of the posterior wall of the canal are discussed in the section on the spinal cord, because these defects are often associated with maldevelopment of the cord.

The vertebral canal is most spacious in the cervical and lumbar regions. Its terminal portion is rather narrow and is called the **sacral canal.** Notwithstanding these regional variations, the entire canal is roomy enough to accommodate the meningeal spaces; these enhance the protection afforded by the bony canal itself to the spinal cord and its nerve roots.

The vertebral canal is most easily approached, both anatomically and surgically, from the back. After the muscles are stripped away, the laminae of neighboring vertebrae are transected on one or both sides, making it possible to lift away a part of the canal's posterior wall. This procedure, called *laminectomy* (removal of laminae), is usually limited to one side, and to one or several vertebrae, when lesions in the canal are approached surgically. For studying the contents of the canal in a cadaver, however, laminectomy should be done along the entire length of the vertebral column.

THE MENINGES AND RELATED SPACES

The spinal cord is suspended in the vertebral canal within a triple envelope of meninges (*meninx;* Greek for membrane) made up of the **pia**, **arachnoid**, and **dura mater** (see Figs. 13-1 and Fig. 13-2). The outermost meninx, the dura, is a tough membrane (*dura;* Latin for hard), whereas the pia and arachnoid, together known as the **leptomeninges** (*leptos;* Greek for slender, thin) are quite delicate. The spinal cord and the roots and rootlets of the spinal nerves are closely invested by the pia, whereas the dura and arachnoid together form a rather loose sheath around these neural structures. This sheath, known both as the **thecal** or **dural sac** (*theke;* Greek for enclosing case or sheath), is separated from the walls of the vertebral canal by the **epidural space.** Only a potential space exists between the dura and arachnoid (subdural space); the much more extensive **subarachnoid space,** between the arachnoid and pia is filled by cerebrospinal fluid (CSF).

Development. The space between the mesenchymal vertebra and the neural tube becomes filled with loose mesenchyme, sometimes designated *meninx primitiva.* The more central region of this mesenchyme becomes populated by neural crest cells and gives rise to the leptomeninges. Accumulation of fluid in the spaces of this tissue defines the subarachnoid space and distinguishes the pia and arachnoid.

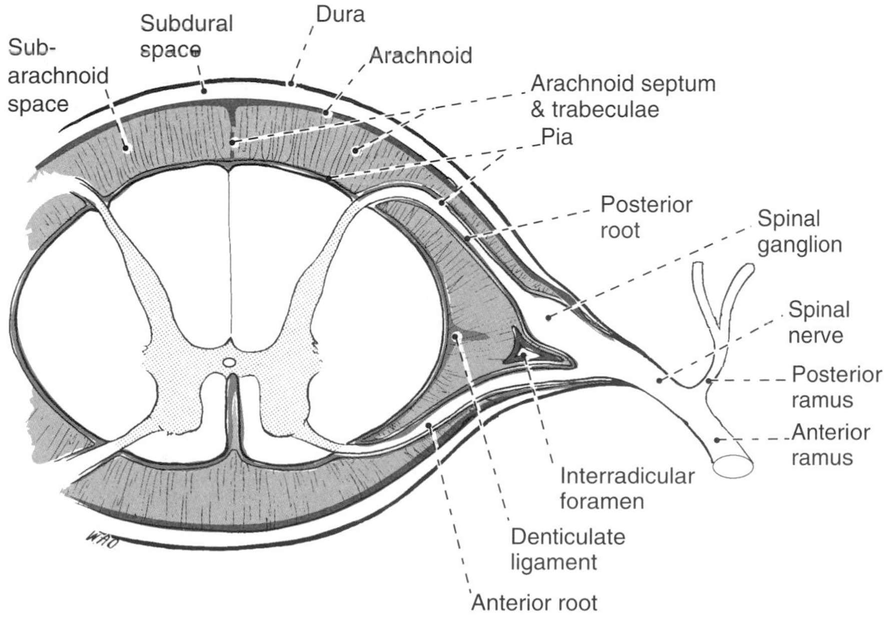

FIGURE 13-2.
Diagram of the meninges and the subarachnoid space in a transverse section of the cord. Note the extensions of the meninges and the spaces around the nerve roots.

The role of neural crest cells is less clear relative to the outer layer of the *meninx primitiva*, which forms the *pachymeninx* (*packy*; Greek for thick) or dura mater. Observations in lower vertebrate embryos suggest that the pachymeninx may be entirely derived from sclerotomal mesenchyme.

The Dura Mater and Associated Spaces

The Spinal Dura Mater

All three meninges invest both the brain and the spinal cord; consequently, they have cranial (or cerebral) and spinal regions. The spinal dura mater is composed of tough longitudinal collagen fiber bundles interwoven with circular elastic fibers. The outer surface of the dura is rough and blends loosely with connective tissue in the epidural space; the inner surface, facing into the subdural space, is smooth and moist, and is covered by a layer of mesothelium.

The rather loose bag of the spinal dura is attached superiorly to the rim of the foramen magnum, where it is continuous with the cranial dura mater (Fig. 13-3). Inferiorly, the thecal sac ends blindly in the sacral canal, most often at the level of the second or third sacral vertebra, but sometimes as high as S-1. Beyond this point, the dura continues as a slender fibrous thread—the dural (external) **filum terminale**—which ends by blending with the posterior longitudinal ligament over the coccyx.

The dural or thecal sac sends sleevelike projections into the intervertebral foramina (see Figs. 13-1 and 13-2), where the dura blends with the epineurium of the spinal nerves. Connective tissue slips in the foramina anchor the dural sleeves so that they can protect the spinal nerve roots from being stretched during movements of the spine. In addition to these tetherings, the dura is attached in places to the posterior longitudinal ligament.

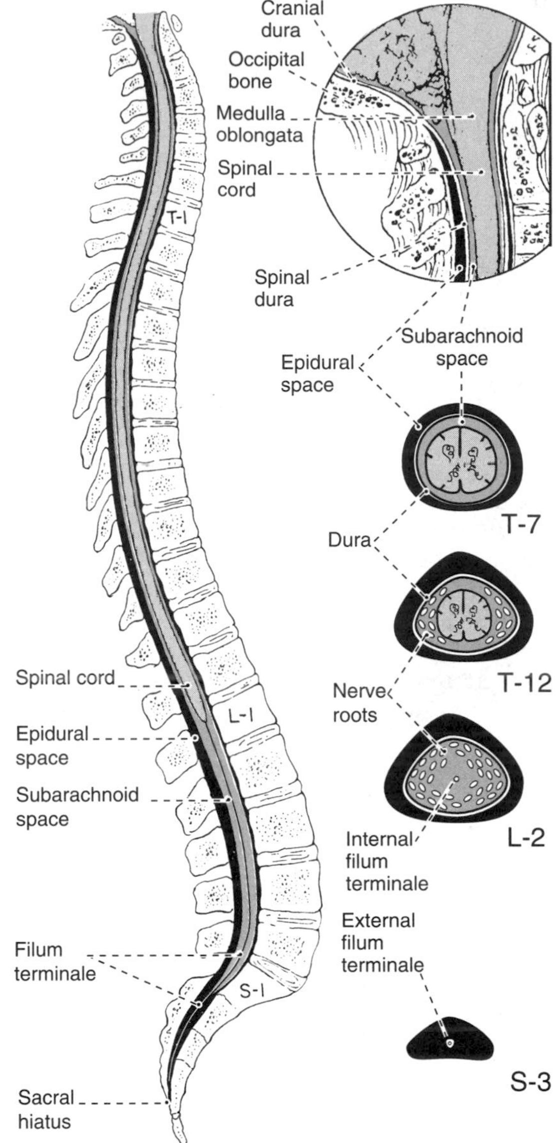

FIGURE *13-3.*
The epidural space: *Left,* sagittal section of the vertebral column with the contents of the vertebral canal. *Right, upper drawing,* Enlarged view of the upper cervical region showing the termination of the epidural space at the margins of the foramen magnum. *Right lower drawings,* Transverse sections of the vertebral canal at various levels. The subarachnoid space is *blue.* (Adapted from Bonica JJ. Principles and practice of obstetric analgesia and anesthesia. Philadelphia: FA, Davis, 1969.)

The Epidural Space

The epidural space (also called the *peridural* or *extradural space*) is limited above by the fusion of the spinal dura to the foramen magnum. Below, it terminates at the sacral hiatus (see Fig. 13-3), where it is sealed by the posterior sacrococcygeal ligaments. The dural sleeves (or cuffs), with the enclosed nerve roots, traverse the space as they extend into the intervertebral foramina (see Fig. 13-1). The entire space is occupied by loose connective tissue laden with variable amounts of fat, thereby providing an effective padding around the thecal sac, with its enclosed spinal cord.

Embedded in the epidural connective tissue is a rich plexus of veins (vertebral venous plexus) that, under certain circumstances, is called on to transmit quite large amounts of blood (see later discussion). The compression and expansion of the loose and fatty epidural connective tissue accommodates to these changing volumes and also permits infiltration by, and spread of, anesthetics introduced into the epidural space.

Epidural block entails the delivery of local anesthetics around the dural sac and its sleeves, selectively blocking the roots of certain spinal nerves, without blocking segments of the spinal cord itself. Such blocks are usually introduced in the lumbar region (spinal, or lumbar epidural block) or through the sacral hiatus (caudal block). For a lumbar block, a needle, or fine trocar and cannula designed for the purpose, is inserted between the vertebral spines, through the ligamenta flava, and into the epidural space. Avoiding puncture of the thecal sac, the epidural connective tissue is infiltrated with the anesthetic. A catheter may also be introduced through the needle and guided to the desired vertebral level in the epidural space, at which anesthetic may be delivered over a time period. The injected substances spread rather well and rapidly in the epidural space, and they also diffuse through the intervertebral foramina into the paravertebral tissues.

The Subdural Space. The potential space between the inner surface of the dura and the adjacent arachnoid contains only enough tissue fluid to moisten the apposed surfaces. Thus, it is virtually impossible to pierce the dura without also piercing the arachnoid. The subdural space communicates with neither the epidural nor the subarachnoid space.

Arachnoid, Pia, and Subarachnoid Space

The Leptomeninges

The two leptomeninges are delicate membranes separated from one another by the rather voluminous subarachnoid space filled with cerebrospinal fluid. All surfaces of the arachnoid and pia that are bathed by CSF are covered by a layer of mesothelium. The substance of the membranes themselves is loose connective tissue.

The **arachnoid mater** lines the entire dural sac and extends into the dural sleeves. In addition, it sends cobweb-like strands or trabeculae (*arachnion;* Greek for cobweb), across the subarachnoid space to the pia. They probably facilitate the mixing of CSF as it percolates through the space (Fig. 13-4, also see Fig. 13-2). Along the posterior midline, the trabeculae form a more or less well-defined subarachnoid septum. Superiorly the spinal arachnoid is continuous with the cranial arachnoid, and inferiorly, it terminates as it lines the blind dural sac within the sacral canal.

The **pia mater** (*pia;* Latin for tender) provides support for the delicate blood vessels that nourish the spinal cord and the nerves that traverse the subarachnoid space. It adheres intimately to the spinal cord, dipping into the long sulci along its surface. The pia forms a separate sheath for each nerve rootlet and root as far laterally as the intervertebral foramen, where it blends with the epineurium (see Fig. 13-2). At the lower end of the cord, the pia continues as a thin thread, the pial (internal) **filum terminale** (see Fig. 13-3). After reaching the lower end of the dural sac, the filum becomes invested by the dural (external) filum terminale and continues to the coccyx.

On each side a fibrous septum, the **denticulate ligament**, helps stabilize the spinal cord within the thecal sac (see Fig. 13-4). Although considered an extension of the spinal pia mater, this "ligament" is actually tougher (being made of dense connective tissue) and less vascular than the pia. From its continuous attachment along the sides of the cord, it extends across the subarachnoid space and is tethered to the dura by a series of 20 to 21 processes or denticulations ("toothlike" projections) that penetrate

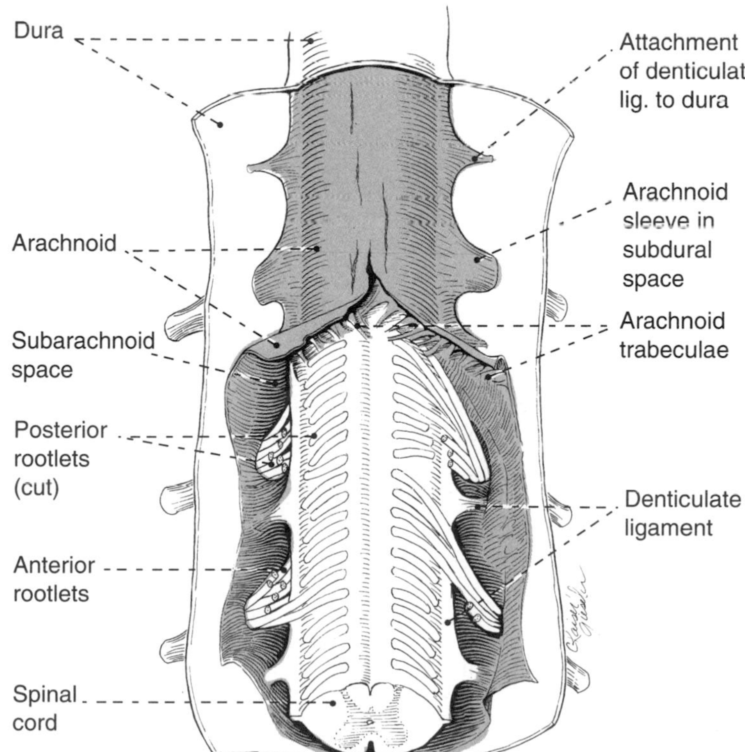

FIGURE *13-4.*
Meninges about the cord seen from *behind.* The dura is intact *above* and reflected *below,* opening up the subdural space between the arachnoid and the dura. The arachnoid has also been opened *below* to show the arachnoid trabeculae in the subarachnoid space, the denticulate ligament and, anterior and posterior to it, the slanting anterior and posterior nerve rootlets, respectively, as they enter their dural sleeves.

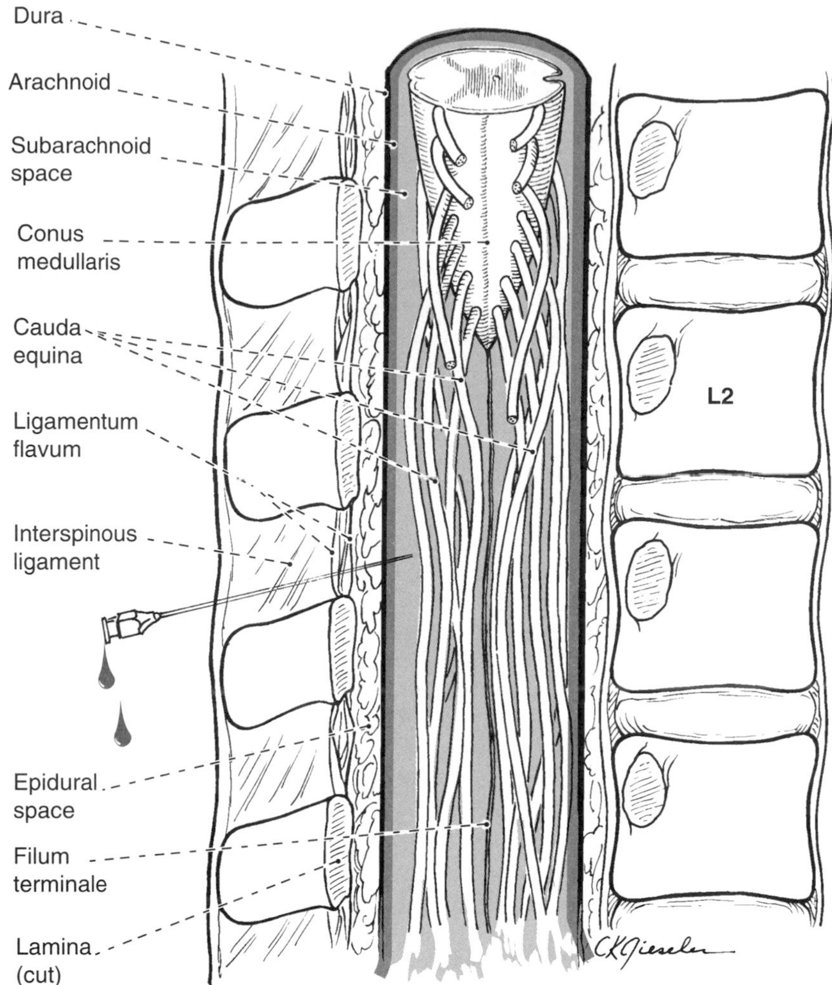

FIGURE 13-5.
Lumbar puncture: The needle has been inserted through the supraspinous and interspinous ligaments and the ligamentum flavum. Lordosis of the lumbar spine has been eliminated by its flexion.

the arachnoid. The uppermost of these is attached to the dura in the foramen magnum, and succeeding ones are attached between the dural sleeves. The last denticulation is above or below the sleeve of the last thoracic nerve.

The Subarachnoid Space

The spinal subarachnoid space communicates freely with the cranial subarachnoid space through the foramen magnum. Its content of CSF, 20 mL to 35 mL, is only a fraction of the total volume of CSF (120 to 150 mL). Somewhat limited in the thoracic region, the space becomes commodious in the lumbar region. The spinal cord tapers to a point above the second lumbar vertebra; the lower third of the arachnoid sac, therefore, contains only the filum terminale and the roots of those spinal nerves that leave the vertebral canal below this level. These roots hang like a horse's tail, or **cauda equina**, from the lower part of the spinal cord (Fig. 13-5; see also Fig. 13-3). The subarachnoid space, with its content of CSF, fills the whole thecal sac, the lower extent of which within the sacral canal has been described in the foregoing.

Cerebrospinal fluid is secreted by the choroid plexuses of the cerebral ventricles. After entering the subarachnoid space directly, or from the ventricles, it is absorbed into the venous system, chiefly through villi specialized for this purpose in the cerebral arachnoid (see Chap. 7). Some absorption also occurs from the spinal subarachnoid space into the vertebral venous plexuses. The presence of CSF allows the arachnoid sac to act similarly to a water jacket, protecting the spinal cord and brain by equalizing pressures around them.

The composition and pressure of CSF is of great diagnostic significance. Although some circumstances may call for directly entering the cranial subarachnoid space or the ventricles of the brain, the fluid is usually sampled in the spinal subarachnoid space by a procedure known as lumbar puncture.

Lumbar Puncture. The success of this procedure, known also as *spinal tap*, depends on applying anatomic knowledge of the bones and soft tissues of the spine (Fig. 13-5). The thecal sac is usually penetrated between the third and fourth, or the fourth and fifth, lumbar vertebrae. Puncture at these levels avoids possible injury to the spinal cord, the latter having terminated at a higher level (see Fig. 13-3). After flexing the vertebral column either in the sitting or lateral recumbent position (to spread apart the spinous processes and laminae), the spinous processes are identified (see Chap. 12), and the level of puncture

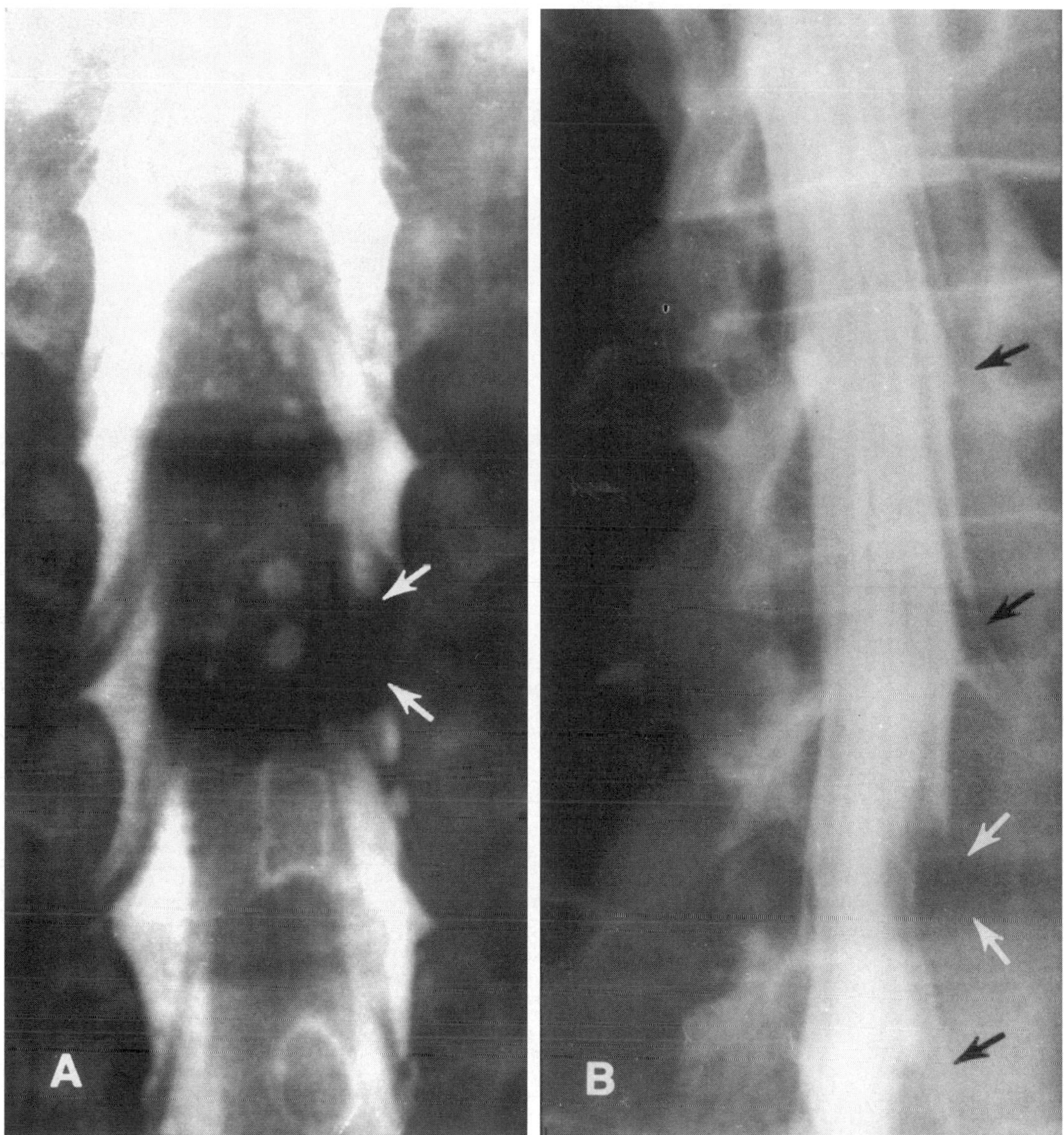

FIGURE *13-6.*
Myelograms of (A) the cervical and (B) lumbar spine. Radiopaque contrast medium has been injected into the subarachnoid space through a lumbar puncture needle. The table was then tilted allowing the contrast medium to flow to the area of diagnostic interest before x-ray films were taken. (A) contrast medium fills the subarachnoid space on each side of the cervical spinal cord (which is radiolucent) and some drops of medium are superimposed over the cord. The anterior and posterior roots are discernible as radiolucent strands as they pass toward the intervertebral foramina within the lateral extensions of the subarachnoid space in the dural sleeves. The regularity of the scalloped pattern along the lateral edge of the thecal sac is distorted by a radiolucent lesion (*arrows*) situated between C-4, and C-5 vertebrae. The patient, a 19-year-old college student, injured his neck rupturing the C-4 disk during wrestling. In addition to neck pain, he had symptoms and signs in his upper limb attributable to the compression of C-5 nerve. (B) A slightly oblique view of the lumbar spine of a 35-year-old man. The thecal sac is filled by contrast medium in which the spinal nerve roots of the cauda equina can be discerned. L-3, L-4, and S-1 dural sleeves are clearly identifiable (*black arrows*), but the sleeve around L-5 is obliterated by a radiolucent lesion (*white arrows*), which represents herniation of the L-5 disk. (Courtesy of Dr. Rosalind H. Troupin.)

decided. The skin and the supra- and interspinous ligaments are infiltrated with local anesthetic. A "spinal needle" containing a stylet is then advanced through, or along one side of, the interspinous ligament. The vertebral canal is entered either through the small midline gap between the ligamenta flava or, preferably, to one side, through the ligamentum flavum (see Fig. 12-20). Overcoming the resistance offered by this ligament is a useful indication of having entered the epidural space (see foregoing section: Epidural Block).

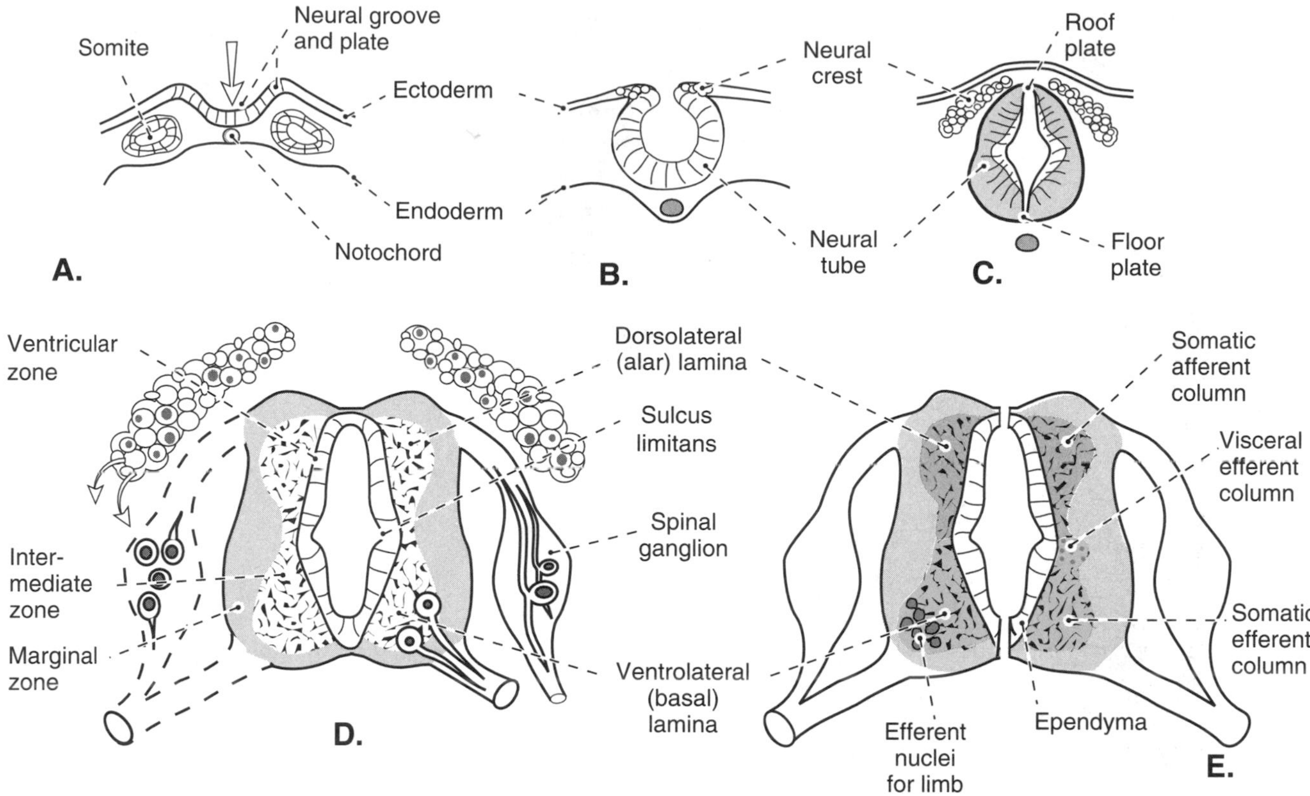

FIGURE *13-7.*
Development of the spinal cord: (A through C) formation of the neural tube and neural crest in early somite embryos; (D) cellular differentiation within the cord; (E) development of cell columns in the alar and basal laminae shown on one side for a segment that innervates the limbs and on the other, for a segment that contains the visceral efferent column.

After turning the bevel of the needle into a vertical position to avoid cutting the vertical collagen fiber bundles of the dura and, thereby, minimize the risk of subsequent CSF leakage, the needle is advanced into the subarachnoid space. Clad in their pial sheaths, the roots of the cauda equina move out of the needle's way and should not be injured. A few seconds after withdrawing the stylet, drops of CSF emerge from the needle. Lumbar puncture is performed for measuring intrathecal pressure, sampling the CSF, or delivering drugs or a radiologic contrast medium into the subarachnoid space (Fig. 13-6).

A manometer attached to the spinal needle can readily register the changes in **intrathecal pressure** caused by physiologic and pathologic processes. For instance, an increase in intrathoracic or intra-abdominal pressure is freely transmitted through the intervertebral foramina into the vertebral canal and to the thecal sac by the communication of veins in the thoracic and abdominal cavities with the vertebral venous plexuses (see later discussion). Forceful expiration against a closed glottis (Valsalva maneuver), as occurs during straining or coughing, causes a rise in CSF pressure and may induce or exaggerate pain owing to lesions that increase tension in the vertebral canal. Free communication between the cranial and spinal subarachnoid space can also be readily assessed. If there is no obstruction in the foramen magnum or in the vertebral canal, CSF pressure registered through a spinal needle should rise when the jugular veins are temporarily compressed by an examiner because the resulting increase in intracranial pressure (caused by venous distension within the skull) is transmitted to CSF in the spinal subarachnoid space (Queckenstedt maneuver).

Spinal anesthesia or *subarachnoid block* entails the introduction of anesthetic solutions into the subarachnoid space through a spinal needle. It is an alternative to epidural block and is frequently used for alleviating the pain of labor and delivery. The spinal cord and the nerve roots are blocked at selected levels. By regulating the specific gravity and volume of the solution, but especially the tilt of the patient, the effect of the anesthetic can be localized to defined regions of the spinal cord.

Myelography is a radiologic procedure for examining the subarachnoid space (see Fig. 13-6). Radiopaque contrast medium is injected through a lumbar puncture needle, and the patient is then tilted on a table, allowing the contrast medium to flow to the area of diagnostic interest before radiographs are taken.

THE SPINAL CORD

The spinal cord (*medulla spinalis; medulla*, Latin for innermost part) is one of the two anatomic components of the central nervous system, the other being the brain. The spinal medulla becomes continuous with the medulla oblongata between the atlas and the foramen magnum. Consonant with its development from the neural tube, the spinal cord contains a cavity, the narrow **central canal.** Around this canal are grouped the cell bodies of neurons concerned with the innervation of the neck, trunk, limbs, and viscera. The bulk of the spinal cord, however, is made up of the nerve fiber fasciculi that transmit impulses between the brain and different segments of the cord. Therefore, lesions that affect discrete regions or segments of the cord usually result in complex clinical syndromes. These include dysfunction, not only in the regions of the body innervated by the injured segments of the cord, but also in regions innervated by other segments that, although undamaged themselves, can no longer function properly if their normal input from higher levels has been compromised.

Developmental Considerations

The tubular central nervous system is formed by the longitudinal folding of the **neural plate,** a region of thickened ectoderm that becomes defined along the length of the embryo under the inducing influence of the notochord (Fig. 13-7). The neural plate invaginates, its lateral edges approximates each other, and fuse along the dorsal midline. This fusion results in the formation of the **neural tube** and, at the same time, separates the tube from the overlying ectoderm. A population of neuroectodermal cells, located in the junctional zone between the neural plate and the somatic ectoderm, are excluded from the neural tube. These cells segregate along the dorsolateral aspect of the tube and form the **neural crest** (see Fig. 13-7C).

All the neuronal cell bodies located within the brain and spinal cord develop from the cell layer that lines the neural tube. The processes of many will extend into tissues and organs of the embryo, establishing the motor innervation of skeletal muscle. All neurons for which cell bodies are located outside the brain and spinal cord develop from cells of the neural crest, and most will aggregate into several discrete ganglia. All neurons concerned with receiving sensory information from tissues and organs throughout the body are of neural crest origin and transmit this information (by their processes) to the brain or spinal cord. Other neurons derived from the neural crest provide motor innervation to smooth and cardiac muscle and glands; their activity is governed by those neurons for which cell bodies lie within the brain or spinal cord.

The closure of the neural tube commences midway along the neural plate, in the region where the first somites appear. Closure proceeds rostrally and caudally, progressively reducing the size of, and ultimately eliminating, the **rostral** and **caudal neuropores** (see Fig. 13-21). Arrest of this process at the caudal or cranial end results in serious birth defects (see later discussion). The cavity of the neural tube expands at the cranial end to form the **cerebral ventricles;** within the spinal cord it persists as the **central canal**; a slight dilation at its caudal end is called the *terminal ventricle.*

Proliferating groups of neurons produce signs of segmentation (neuromeres or rhombomeres) on the surface of the medulla oblongata and neighboring regions of the brain. Although many functions of the spinal cord suggest a segmental organization of its neurons (see later discussion), neuromeres have not been observed on the developing cord. The segmental arrangement of the nerves that enter and leave the cord, as well as of the ganglia associated with them, is determined by the somites and will be discussed later.

External Anatomy

The slender cord, somewhat cylindric in shape, extends from the vertebral foramen of the atlas to the upper lumbar region of the vertebral canal, where it tapers into a cone, the **conus medullaris** (see Figs. 13-5 and 13-8). There is some variability in the level at which the cord actually terminates, but usually, it does not extend beyond the lower margin of the L-2 vertebral body (Fig. 13-8). This disparity between the length of the spinal cord and that of the vertebral canal results from their differential growth rates.

Up to the end of the first trimester the various segments of the spinal cord are aligned with the

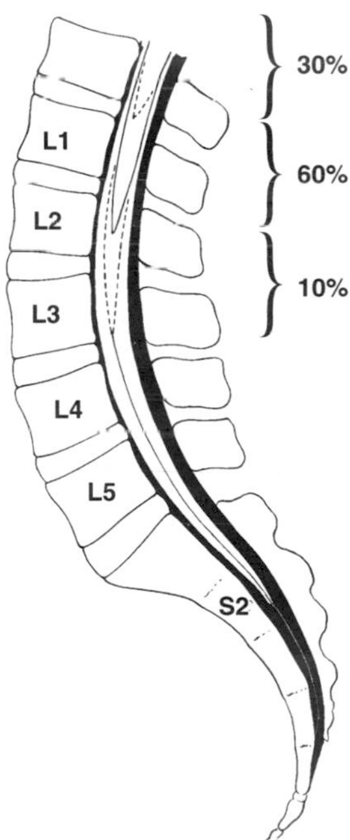

FIGURE *13-8.*
Variations in the level of termination of the spinal cord: The percentages indicate the incidence for each level at which the spinal cord terminated in 129 specimens. The epidural space is shown in *black*, the subarachnoid space in *white*. (Adapted from Bonica JJ. Principles and practice of obstetric analgesia and anesthesia. Philadelphia: FA Davis, 1969.)

corresponding vertebrae. Thereafter, however, the cord grows more slowly than the vertebral column, and the conus medullaris recedes from the coccygeal and sacral regions: at 25 weeks of gestation, the tip of the conus is on level with L-3 vertebra, the approximate level it retains until birth. In some infants the level characteristic of adulthood may be reached by 2 months of age, but variation is considerable up to 15 years of age.

The division of the cord into symmetric right and left halves is suggested on its surface by two longitudinal grooves, the **anterior median fissure** and the **posterior median sulcus** (Figs. 13-9 and 13-10). The deep invagination of the anterior median fissure, lined by pia mater, nearly reaches the central canal and contains a rich plexus of blood vessels that penetrate the cord. The shallow posterior median sulcus marks the position of the *posterior median septum* that, being composed of glia, demarcates the two halves of the cord posteriorly. It prevents nerve fibers from crossing in the posterior half of the cord from one side to the other.

The posterior **rootlets of spinal nerves** enter the cord in an uninterrupted longitudinal row in the shallow *posterolateral sulcus,* and the anterior rootlets emerge from the cord in a similar fashion along the *anterolateral sulcus*. On each side, the rootlets are gathered into posterior and anterior roots. There is one posterior and one anterior root for each segment; their subsequent union forms a spinal nerve (see Fig. 13-9). A **segment of the cord,** therefore, is defined as a portion of the cord to which is attached a set of posterior and anterior rootlets which, in turn, form a single pair of spinal nerves.

The circumference of the spinal cord is preferentially enlarged in two regions, from which the upper and lower limbs are supplied. These are the **cervical** and **lumbosacral enlargements** (see Fig. 13-14). The cervical enlargement extends from the fifth cervical to the first thoracic segment and is widest opposite the sixth cervical vertebra; the lumbosacral enlargement includes L-1 to S-3 segments and is widest opposite T-12 vertebra.

An attempt to correlate spinal segments to vertebral levels, as in the foregoing, shows that the discrepancy between spinal segments and vertebrae of corresponding number increases in a downward direction (see Fig. 13-14). This is an important point to appreciate in cases of cord compression associated with spinal lesions and injuries. As a general rule, the tip of the spine of a cervical vertebra corresponds to the succeeding cord segment (the tip of C-6 spine is on level with C-7 segment, for example); the difference is two segments in the upper thoracic region and three segments in the lower thoracic region (e.g., the tip of T-10 spine is opposite L-1 segment). Lumbar and sacral segments are telescoped within the vertebral canal at the level of T-11, T-12, and L-1 vertebrae. The T-12 spine is opposite the S-1 segment. Variations in the level of termination of the spinal cord displace these landmarks.

Internal Structure

The **central canal**, barely visible to the naked eye, is filled with cerebrospinal fluid (see Fig. 13-9). Around the canal are aggregated, in somewhat-defined groups, the cell bodies of all neurons of the spinal cord. More peripherally, the substance of the cord is made up of myelinated

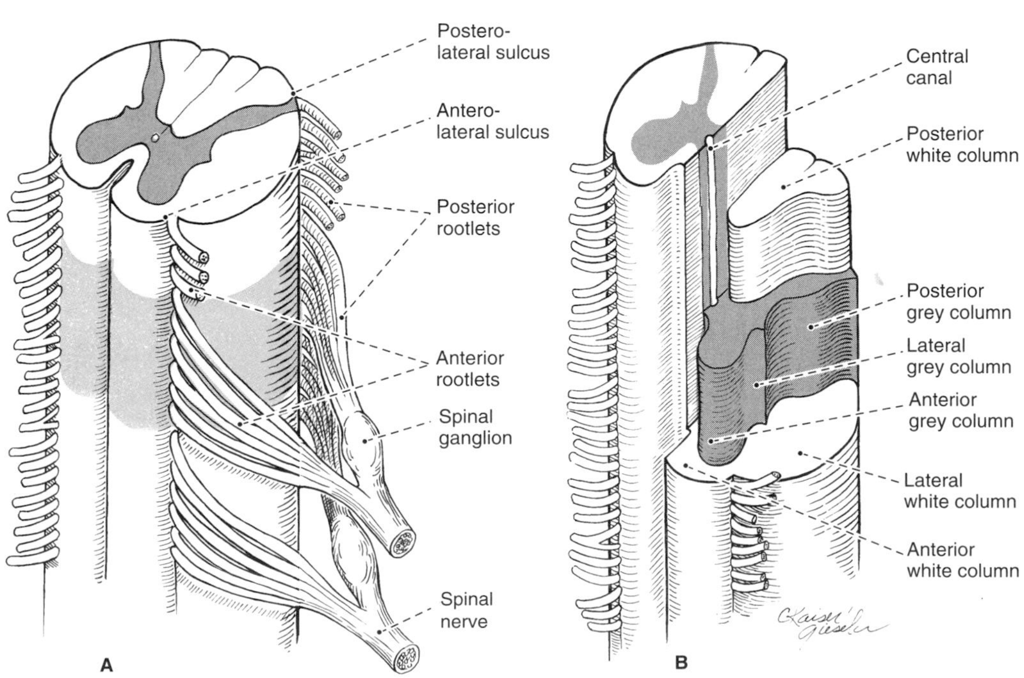

FIGURE *13-9.*
External and internal anatomy of the spinal cord: (A) an anterolateral view; a cord segment is shaded *red*; (B) a dissection of the *white* and *gray* columns of the spinal cord.

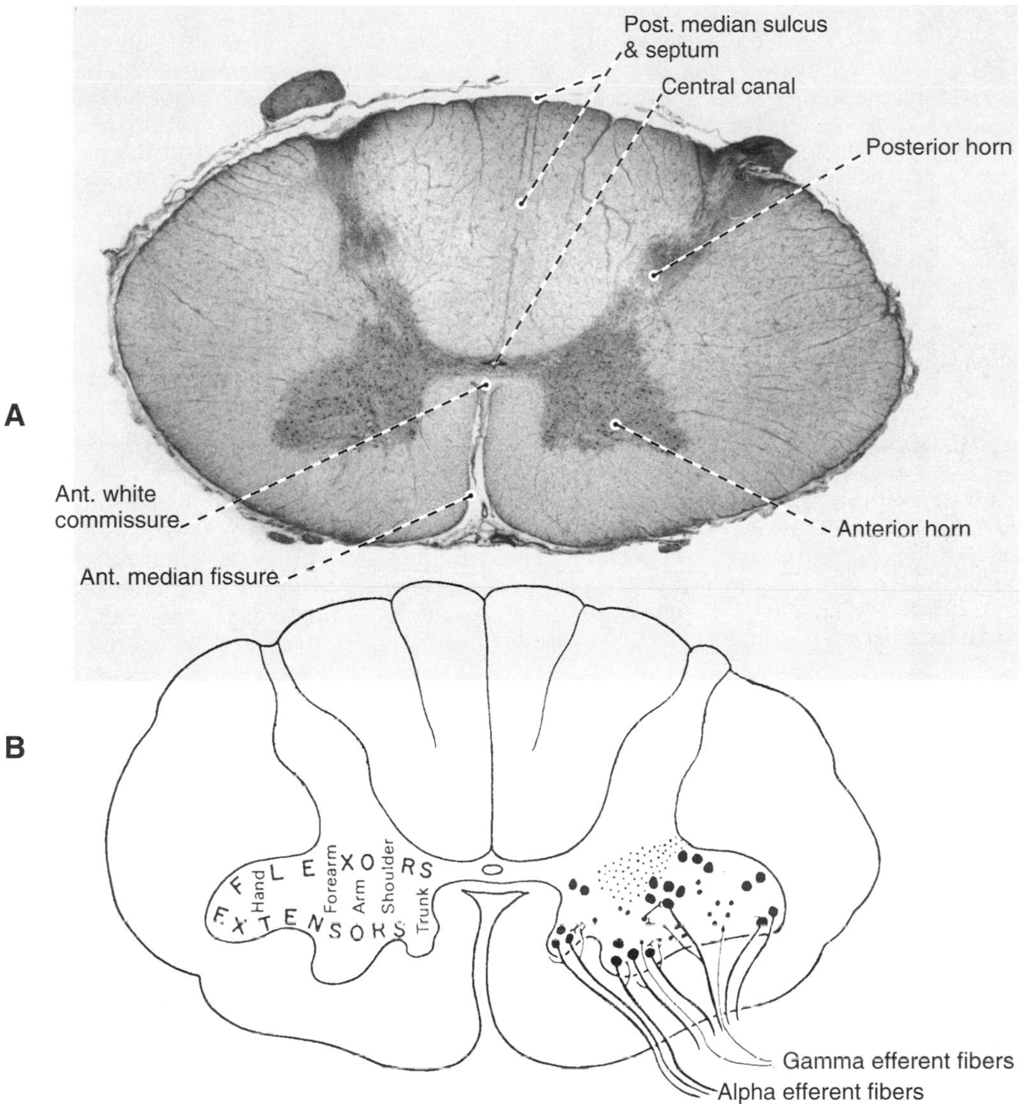

FIGURE *13-10.*
Internal structure of the spinal cord: (A) Photomicrograph of a transverse section of the spinal cord at the cervical enlargement stained with cresyl violet (×10) At this magnification, groups of neurons are visible as black dots. (B) a diagram of the groups of motor neurons in the anterior gray column of the cervical enlargement. On the *left side* is shown the general location of anterior horn cells that send motor axons to specific muscle groups of the upper limb. Individual motor nuclei are shown on the *right*; neurons and axons of gamma efferents are smaller than those of alpha efferents. (A, Everett NB. Functional neuroanatomy. 6th ed. Philadelphia. Lea Febiger, 1971; B, Adapted from Truex RC, Carpenter MB. Strong and Elwyn's, human neuroanatomy. 5th ed. Baltimore. Williams & Wilkins, 1964.)

nerve fibers. On a transverse section, therefore, **white matter**, containing the myelinated fibers, surrounds a central core of **gray matter**, comprising the neuron cell bodies and unmyelinated fibers. Both the gray and the white matter form anterior, posterior, and lateral columns.

A detailed description of the internal structure of the spinal cord is beyond the purpose of this section. Only those concepts are presented that have direct relevance to the anatomy of the spinal cord and to the general plan of innervation of the body. For further details, treatises on neuroanatomy should be consulted. The internal organization of the spinal cord is perhaps best appreciated from its developmental perspective.

Development

The internal anatomy of the spinal cord is established by the descendants of the cells that line the neural tube. Daughter cells of this proliferating **ventricular zone** migrate peripherally and populate the **intermediate zone** (*mantle layer*), which develops into the gray matter of the cord (see Fig. 13-7D). Processes of the neuroblasts in the intermediate zone extend into the peripheral **marginal zone**, where they become myelinated and form the white matter of the cord. The marginal zone is also invaded by the processes of neuroblasts from neighboring or distant cord segments and the brain. Once the proliferative potential of the ventricular zone is exhausted, its cells become the *ependyma* that lines the central canal.

The proliferation and the accumulation of neuroblasts occur chiefly in the lateral walls of the developing spinal cord, leaving relatively thin layers dorsally and ventrally. These thin areas are the *dorsal lamina* (roof plate) and *ventral lamina* (floor plate), respectively (see Fig. 13-7C). As each lateral wall thickens a longitudinal furrow, the *sulcus limitans*, appears on its inner surface. The part of the lateral wall above the sulcus is the **dorsolateral** (*alar*) **lamina**, and that below it is the **ventrolateral** (*basal*) **lamina.** Neurons developing in the ventrolateral lamina will fulfill motor functions exclusively, whereas those in the dorsolateral lamina will form interneurons, many of which will process incoming (afferent) impulses from spinal nerves or from nerve fiber tracts from other segments and the brain.

The groups of neurons developing in the ventrolateral lamina form the **anterior column of gray matter**, and those developing in the dorsolateral lamina form the **posterior column of gray matter**. Nuclei within these columns span regions or segments of the cord. Detailed description of these nuclei is beyond our purpose, but the following broad (and rather simplified) classification will be informative.

Nuclei adjacent to the sulcus limitans in the ventrolateral lamina are concerned with the innervation of smooth and cardiac muscle and glands and are designated as the **visceral efferent column**, for the tissues they innervate constitute viscera (see Fig. 13-7E). In the spinal cord, the development of this gray column is restricted to two regions: segments T-1 to L-2 and S-2 to S-4, where they form the lateral gray column (or lateral horn; see later discussion). Nuclei concerned with the innervation of skeletal muscle derived from the somites develop as the **somatic efferent column** in the remaining ventral part of the ventrolateral lamina. The medial group of these nuclei, which innervate the muscles of the vertebral column and trunk, develops throughout all segments. In the segments concerned with the innervation of the limbs, additional nuclei develop in the lateral part of the somatic efferent column; their presence increases the bulk of the spinal cord and accounts for the cervical and lumbosacral enlargements.

Gray Matter

In a transverse section of the spinal cord the gray matter is shaped like a distorted H or a butterfly, presenting on each side an **anterior horn** and a **posterior horn** (see Fig. 13-10A). These horns are simply the cut surfaces of the **anterior** and **posterior columns** of gray matter (see Fig. 13-9). Somatic motor neurons giving rise to both alpha and gamma efferents (for the innervation of skeletal muscle and muscle spindles, respectively) are located in the anterior gray column. Some degree of functional localization has been demonstrated among these nuclei (see Fig. 13-10B). In both the cervical and the lumbosacral enlargements, the anterior horn is augmented laterally by groups of neurons concerned with the supply of the limbs (compare Figs. 13-10 and 13-11). Groups of neurons of the posterior gray column receive and relay incoming impulses from the posterior roots, other segments, and the brain. The posterior horn is relatively slender in all regions of the cord.

In segments T-1 to L-2, visceral efferent neurons form the **lateral column** of gray matter, known also as the intermediolateral cell column, which is evident on a transverse section as the **lateral horn** (see Fig. 13-11). It contains preganglionic sympathetic neurons that furnish the sympathetic nerve supply to the entire body. A similar cell column in segments S-2 to S-4 contains preganglionic parasympathetic neurons that, as far as is known, are concerned exclusively with the innervation of viscera.

Gray matter in the central region of the spinal cord connects the gray columns in each half and is called the **gray commissure.** The central canal runs through it and

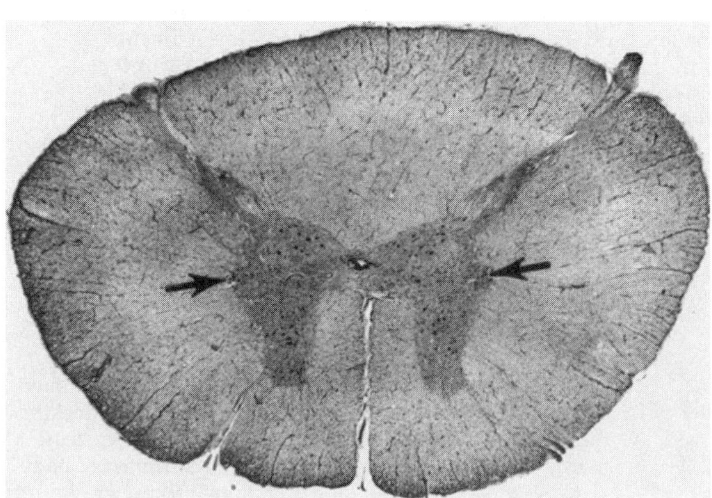

FIGURE *13-11.*
Photomicrograph of a transverse section of the spinal cord in the thoracic region stained with cresyl violet. Compare the size of the anterior horn with that in Figure 13-10A. The lateral horn is indicated by *arrows*. (Everett NB. Functional neuroanatomy. 6th ed. Philadelphia: Lea & Febiger, 1971.)

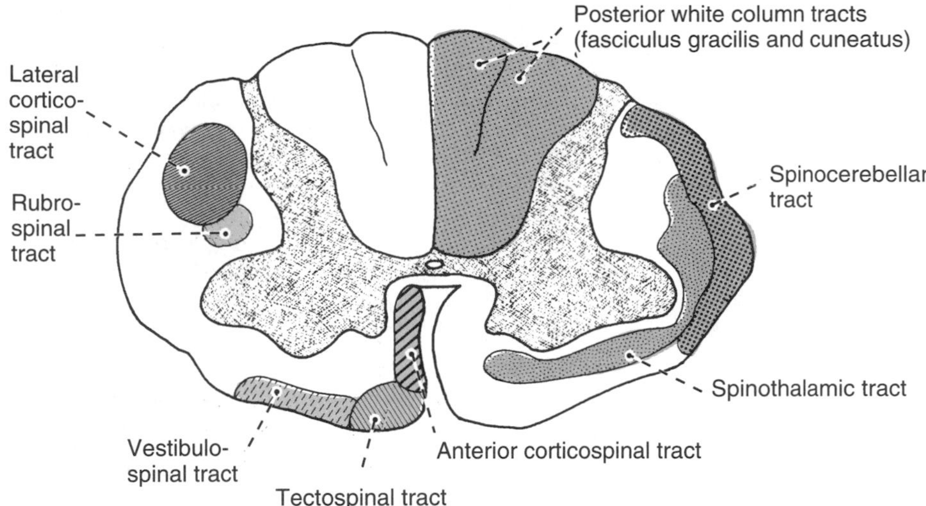

FIGURE 13-12.
A simplified diagram of the main tracts in the white matter in the spinal cord. The ascending tracts are shown on one side in *blue*, and the descending tracts on the other side of the cord in *red*.

marks its division into anterior and posterior components.

White Matter

Anterior, posterior, and lateral **columns** (*funiculi*) of white matter are more or less completely demarcated in the spinal cord by the anterior and posterior horns of gray matter, the posterior median septum, and the anterior median fissure (see Figs. 13-9 and 13-10). In each of these white columns somewhat well-defined **tracts**, composed of nerve fiber bundles, transmit information up or down the cord and are accordingly designated as ascending or descending tracts (Fig. 13-12). In many of these tracts, the fibers are arranged in a roughly somatotopic pattern, laminated according to the segments and regions of the body they serve (Fig. 13-13). The naming of a tract usually designates its origin and termination (e.g., the corticospinal tract begins in the cortex and ends in the spinal cord). Some fibers cross from one side of the cord to the other in the **white commissure**, a narrow strip of white matter between the anterior gray commissure and the anterior median fissure (see Fig. 13-10A). The following description of the white columns gives only a synoptic account of the tracts and their functions.*

The **posterior white column** (*funiculus*) consists of long ascending fibers that convey proprioceptive impulses from joints, ligaments, and tendons, as well as sensations of fine touch, two-point discrimination, vibration, and pressure from the same side of the body, except the head (see Fig. 13-12). Most, but not all, the fibers are the central processes of pseudounipolar neurons in the spinal (posterior root) ganglia and terminate in the medulla oblongata. In the upper thoracic and cervical regions the posterior white column is divided by a partial septum into the *fasciculus gracilis,* conveying fibers from the lower part of the body, and the *fasciculus cuneatus*, made up of fibers from upper thoracic and cervical segments (see Fig. 13-13).

The **lateral white column** (*funiculus*) contains both ascending and descending tracts (see Fig. 13-12). Most important is the **lateral corticospinal tract**, which

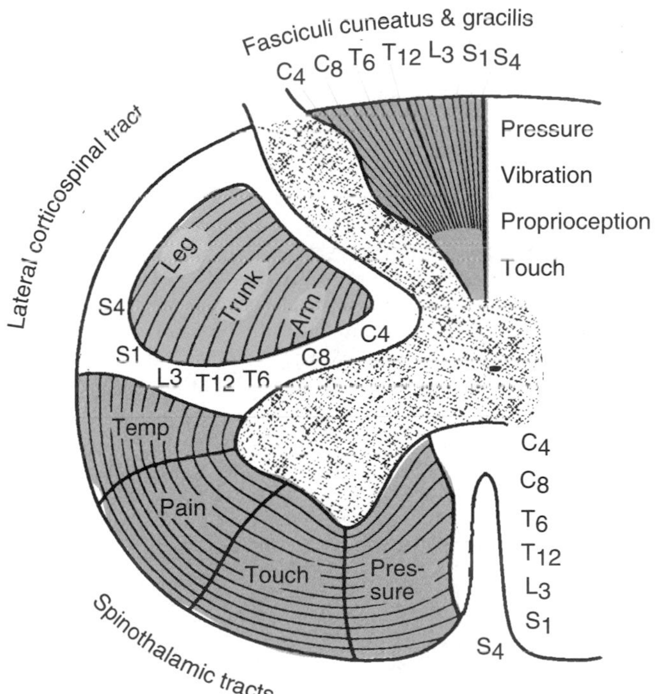

FIGURE 13-13.
The general plan of segmental organization of the fibers in the tracts of the posterior, lateral, and anterior white columns. The probable cross-sectional areas of the tracts shown are arbitrarily enlarged to provide adequate space for illustrating their lamination. (Adapted from Williams PL, Warnick R, eds. Gray's anatomy. 38th ed.; after Foerster, 1936.)

* The terms *column* and *funiculus* are used interchangeably in describing the major constituents of the white matter.

descends from the motor cortex, crosses to the opposite side in the medulla oblongata, and is concerned with the voluntary initiation of movements. Its input is relayed to somatic efferent nuclei for muscles and muscle groups in the anterior gray column. The **rubrospinal tract** descends from the red nucleus in the midbrain (which receives input from the motor cortex and the cerebellum), crosses to the opposite side, and is closely associated with the lateral corticospinal tract. It relays to the same motor neuron pools and is concerned with the regulation of movements.

Two ascending tracts occupy the peripheral region of the lateral white column. The **spinocerebellar tract** originates in nuclei of the posterior gray column of the same side and conveys chiefly proprioceptive information to the cerebellum. The **spinothalamic tract** is the predominant pathway for pain and temperature sensation. It also mediates sensations of crude touch and pressure. Its fibers cross in the white commissure from nuclei in the posterior gray column of the opposite side and ascend to the thalamus, whence they are relayed to the cortex. The tract extends into the anterior white column and, like the spinocerebellar tract, is usually described as having two named components. Because spinothalamic fibers originate in the gray matter, those that are added to the tract in higher segments are adjacent to the gray matter, whereas those conveying sensations from lower body segments are superficially situated in the tract (see Fig. 13-13). A neurosurgical procedure called *chordotomy* can be used to relieve intractable pain in the lower part of the body, on one side, by selectively interrupting the superficial fibers of the tract on the opposite side.

The **anterior white column** (*funiculus*) contains tracts that are similar to those in the lateral white column (see Fig. 13-12). In addition to the anterior portion of the spinothalamic tract, there are three descending tracts concerned with the initiation and regulation of movement. The **anterior corticospinal tract** is similar in all respects to the lateral corticospinal tract, except that its fibers decussate in the anterior commissure, rather than in the medulla oblongata. Although the **vestibulospinal** and **tectospinal tracts** originate in different nuclei of the brain stem than the rubrospinal tract, they likewise provide additional input to the somatic motor neurons, and contribute to the modulation of their activity.

Several well-recognized tracts are omitted from the foregoing account. Mention should perhaps be made of the **intersegmental tract**, in which fibers ascend and descend between spinal cord segments around the fluted surface of the spinal gray matter.

NERVE ROOTS

Descriptions of the external anatomy of the spinal cord, its meninges, and associated spaces in earlier sections of this chapter have made reference to the roots of spinal nerves. This section is concerned chiefly with the course and relations of the nerve roots and spinal nerves in the vertebral canal and intervertebral foramina.

It may be useful to reiterate that the roots of a spinal nerve arise from a segment of the spinal cord as posterior and anterior rows of **rootlets**. Those in each row blend together to form a **posterior** and an **anterior root** that proceed independently toward their respective intervertebral foramen, traversing the subarachnoid space within the dural sac and dural sleeves. The **spinal nerve** is formed by the union of the posterior and anterior root in the intervertebral foramen (see Figs. 13-1 and 13-22). Typically, the spinal nerve emerges through the intervertebral foramen below the pedicle of its corresponding vertebra, an association that is established early in development.

Developmental Considerations

Axons of neuroblasts in the ventrolateral lamina grow ventrolaterally and exit the neural tube along a restricted longitudinal line (the future anterolateral sulcus) that establishes the position of the **anterior rootlets**. They continue their growth laterally, being attracted by the somites. The notochord evidently exerts a regulatory influence, by the ventral lamina (floor plate) of the neural tube, on this pattern of growth. Experiments in chick and quail embryos have shown that interference with notochordal regulation results in ectopic nerve fibers exiting at multiple sites around the circumference of the tube.

Neuronal processes also extend from neuroblasts derived from the neural crest. These neuroblasts aggregate along each side of the neural tube. One process from each enters the dorsolateral surface of the neural tube, helping establish the position of the **posterior rootlets**; the other, attracted by the somites, proceeds ventrolaterally.

Concurrent with these events, sclerotomal cell migration and fusion establishes the centra and neural arches of the mesenchymal vertebrae (see Fig. 12-2). The remaining portions of the somites (dermomyotomes) are invaded by the advancing nerve fibers. It is the gathering of sets of nerve fibers by the dermomyotomes that establishes the segmental pattern of **spinal nerves** and, as a consequence, defines the segments of the spinal cord. At the same time the longitudinal column of neural crest cells that remains associated with the spinal cord becomes segmented into discrete ganglia. The cell bodies of neurons, the central processes of which are in the posterior root of a given spinal nerve, become enclosed in a single **spinal** (*sensory*) **ganglion** (see Fig. 13-7D).

The dorsal extension of the neural arches between the successive bundles of nerve fibers establishes the relation of individual spinal nerves with the pedicles of corresponding vertebrae (see Fig. 12-25). Although, initially, nerve roots proceed horizontally from each spinal cord segment to its corresponding dermomyotome, the relative cranial displacement of the spinal cord within the vertebral canal during later stages of development (described earlier) leads to the elongation of all nerve roots, except those in the upper cervical region. This elongation involves not only the roots themselves, but the meningeal sleeves that develop around them.

Course of Spinal Nerve Roots

Invested in their sleeves of pia mater, posterior and anterior roots pursue independent courses of variable length in the subarachnoid space. They pierce the dura separately before they blend with each other at the intervertebral foramen. The first cervical roots are only 3 mm long but those at lower levels are progressively longer. The roots for T-1 spinal nerve, for example, are close to 30 mm long. Root length increases to 90 mm for L-1, 185 mm for S-1, and over 260 mm for coccygeal nerves. It is not only the length, but the obliquity, that increases greatly from cervical to coccygeal segments. The cauda equina, formed by lumbar, sacral, and coccygeal nerve roots, has already been described.

Each root pursues much of its course within the thecal sac, and only its lateral portion is in the dural sleeve. There may be separate dural sleeves around the posterior and anterior roots for a given spinal nerve, or the two sleeves may be fused; in either event, there is a separate arachnoid sheath around each root, bathing it in cerebrospinal fluid. The dural sleeves in the cervical and thoracic regions project almost horizontally from the thecal sac (see Fig. 13-4); in the lower lumbar region, they are longer and run downward as well as laterally to reach the appropriate level of exit for the spinal nerve (see Fig. 13-1).

Each posterior root presents a fusiform enlargement just proximal to the point of union with the anterior root (see Figs. 13-1 and 13-2). This is the **spinal** (*sensory*) **ganglion**, known also as the posterior or dorsal root ganglion. In it are located the cell bodies of all sensory nerve fibers conveyed by a spinal nerve, including those from viscera. The ganglia are situated in the intervertebral foramina for the most part; there being no intervertebral foramina above the level of the axis, C-1 and C-2 ganglia lie on the vertebral arches of the atlas and axis, respectively. The sacral ganglia lie within the sacral canal.

Exit Levels of Spinal Nerves

As a general rule, spinal nerves leave the vertebral canal by passing *below* the pedicles of corresponding vertebrae (T-6, for example, below the T-6 pedicle). This rule applies to all thoracic, lumbar, sacral, and coccygeal nerves (Fig. 13-14). It does not, however, apply in the cervical region. Here, there are eight spinal nerves and only seven vertebrae; all but the last cervical nerve exit *above* the corresponding vertebra. The C-8 nerve exits between C-7 and T-1 vertebra. This seeming discrepancy between the cervical nerves and all others is understandable in light of the appearance during development of a transient occipitocervical vertebra, the proatlas, at the top of the vertebral column. Although it normally becomes incorporated into the occipital bone, only rarely forming an independent vertebra (see Chap. 12), its presence during development accounts for the observed relation between cervical nerves and their vertebrae. If the C-1 cord segment is assumed to lie on level with the proatlas and sends its nerves out *below* it, in accordance with the general rule for all cord segments below the cervical level, then the C-1 nerve will actually emerge above the C-1 vertebra (atlas). The C-2 through C-7 nerves will likewise exit above the vertebra of the corresponding number. From the T-1 level downward, however, each nerve comes out *below* its corresponding pedicle.

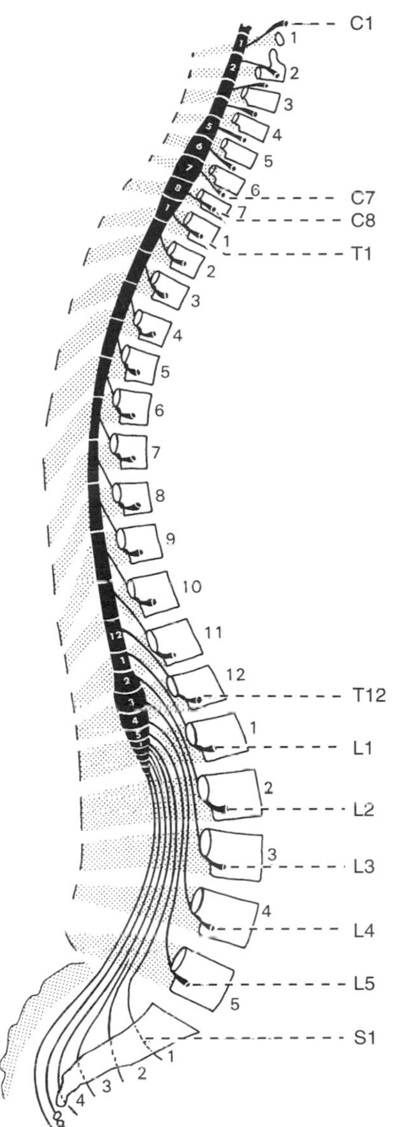

FIGURE *13-14.*
A schematic representation of the relation of spinal cord segments and spinal nerves to the vertebrae. (Based on Haymaker W. Woodhall B. Peripheral nerve injuries. Philadelphia: WB Saunders, 1967.)

In all presacral regions, the first division of the spinal nerve takes place within the intervertebral foramen. The resulting branches are the **posterior** and **anterior rami** (see Fig. 13-22). Sacral spinal nerves divide in the sacral canal, and anterior and posterior rami emerge through the anterior and posterior sacral foramina. In presacral regions, the posterior rami pass posteriorly, skirting the articular processes, whereas the anterior rami proceed laterally to supply the body wall and the limbs.

Relations of the Roots and Spinal Nerves

The anatomic boundaries of intervertebral foramina are discussed in Chapter 12. This section examines regional differences in these boundaries to explain clinical syndromes that result from nerve compression in the foramina.

In cervical intervertebral foramina the spinal nerves are directly related anteriorly to the intervertebral disks, but in the thoracic and lumbar regions the disks are not in contact with the nerves (see Fig. 13-1). Rather, the nerves hook around the inferior border of the pedicles and are related anteriorly to the vertebral bodies. In the lumbar vertebral canal, the posterior and anterior roots of a given nerve, enclosed in their dural sleeves, cross the disk that is located above the pedicle below which the nerve exits (see Fig. 13-1). The L-2 nerve roots, for example, cross the disk between L-1 and L-2 vertebrae before reaching the appropriate intervertebral foramen, below the pedicle of the L-2 vertebra. Herniation of disks into intervertebral foramina, therefore, will have different effects, depending on the region. Protrusion of cervical disks will directly compress the exiting nerve (see Fig. 13-6A), whereas protrusion of lumbar ones will stretch the nerve roots that cross the disk in the vertebral canal (see Figs. 13-1 and 13-6B). Because cervical nerves pass above, and lumbar nerves below, the pedicles of the corresponding vertebrae, in both regions the nerve roots affected by a protruding disk bear the number of the vertebra placed just inferior to the disk. For instance, a disk lesion between C-4 and C-5 vertebrae will affect the C-5 nerve, and a disk protrusion between L-1 and L-2 vertebrae will stretch the roots of L-2.

Space-occupying lesions within the canal, or irregularities in its walls, may be demonstrated radiographically by instilling radiopaque contrast material into the subarachnoid space. Examples of such **myelograms** are shown in Figure 13-6. A frequent cause of nerve root compression is herniation or prolapse of an intervertebral disk. The resulting clinical syndrome is described briefly because it illustrates the diagnostic importance of understanding anatomic relations among virtually all the structures that have been discussed in this and the preceding chapter.

Intervertebral Disk Syndrome

Degenerative changes in a disk predispose it to prolapse. Even without prolapse, however, disk degeneration disturbs the mechanics of the back. Because the disk becomes thinner, the vertebral arch joints tend to settle. Thereafter, they have to bear an increased amount of weight, requiring adaptive changes in the capsule and ligaments. All these changes may be associated with back pain.

When a disk prolapses, parts of the nucleus pulposus, annulus fibrosus, and the hyaline cartilage plate protrude beyond their normal confines. These tissues may herniate in any direction, and they stretch and tear other tissues barring their way. This alone generates pain, because the posterior longitudinal ligament and the annulus fibrosus are themselves innervated. The prolapse attains particular clinical significance, however, when the displacement impinges upon the spinal cord, cauda equina, or, as happens most frequently, discrete nerve roots (see Fig. 13-1). Disk prolapse may occur in the lumbar and cervical regions, and much less frequently in the thoracic spine.

Clinical Picture. The dominant symptom is pain, severely limiting movement. The pain is aggravated by coughing, sneezing, or straining, all of which increase intrathecal pressure, further irritating the affected nerves. Tingling and numbness may develop in dermatomal regions served by the affected nerve. The patient's movements are hesitant and guarded, and the affected region of the spine is splinted by reflex muscle spasm. The cervical spine is usually held in some degree of lateral flexion (which maximizes the intervertebral foramen on the convex side), whereas in the lumbar spine the normal curvature is obliterated. This flattening of the back is associated with scoliosis or some lateral bend (listing). There is visible and palpable spasm in the spinal extensions. Other signs of nerve irritation include localized tenderness over these muscles. Pressure over the vertebral spines adjacent to the damaged disk may also be painful.

Diagnostic Maneuvers. Intrathecal pressure may be increased by the Valsalva maneuver or by compression of the jugular veins for about 10 seconds. Exaggeration of symptoms by either test is indicative of increased tension in an intrathecal structure. Compression of the cervical spine by pressing down on the head exaggerates the pain, owing to nerve root compression in cervical intervertebral foramina, whereas traction applied to the head tends to relieve the cervical symptoms.

The dural sleeves anchored in the intervertebral foramina may be stretched by asking the patient to raise his or her head and shoulders from the supine position and then flex the head, pressing the chin to the chest with the help of his or her own arms or those of the examiner. This maneuver pulls the thecal sac upward in the vertebral canal (owing to the attachments of the denticulate ligaments) and exaggerates the pain caused by the taut nerve root.

For testing disk herniation in the lumbar spine, the most useful diagnostic maneuver is the **straight–leg-raising test.** Figure 13-15 illustrates the anatomic mechanism by which tension is transmitted to spinal nerves L-4, L-5, and S-1 through pulling indirectly on the sciatic nerve. While the patient is lying supine, the leg on the affected side is raised passively by the examiner, keeping the knee fully extended. The range of hip flexion will be limited by pain felt in the back, which may radiate into the leg. The smaller the angle of hip flexion achieved, the more tension there is on the affected nerve root. If the leg is lowered below the point at which pain was experienced, passive dorsiflexion of the foot will elicit the pain again, because this movement also pulls on the sciatic nerve.

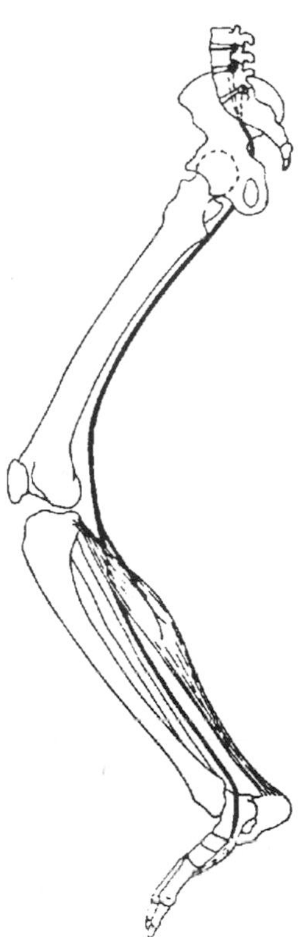

FIGURE 13-15.
The course of the sciatic nerve (*dark line*), explaining why the straight–leg-raising test increases the tension in the nerve roots of the sacral plexus. The nerve is anchored at the vertebral column and below the knee joint. It is put on tension when the hip is flexed while the knee is kept extended. The tension is further increased by dorsiflexion of the foot. (Cram TH. J Bone Joint Surg 1953; 35B: 192.)

Herniation of the upper lumbar disks may be tested by increasing the tension in the L-2 through L-4 spinal nerve roots. This can be achieved by stretching the femoral nerve, which enters the thigh over the anterior aspect of the hip. The maneuver is the mirror image of the sciatic nerve stretch. The hip is passively extended while the patient is lying prone or on his side.

A large disk prolapse in the cervical region may compress the spinal cord. Such lesions may interfere with the blood supply of the cord, or may compress some of the descending and ascending tracts, particularly in the anterior white columns. The neurologic picture may be complex; it may include weakness and incoordination in the legs, wide-based, jerky gait, and sensory disturbances.

VASCULATURE AND INNERVATION

The blood and nerve supply to the vertebral column, including structures within the vertebral canal, is furnished by the intersegmental arteries and segmental spinal nerves that develop in association with the somites (see Fig. 12-2). Although the names of these nerves and vessels may vary from region to region, and some modifications may occur in the segmental pattern laid down in the embryo, the branches of the segmental nerves and arteries that supply the spine conform to the same basic arrangement throughout the column. Many arterial branches are accompanied by corresponding veins. In addition, venous blood is collected by extensive venous plexuses that run vertically within the vertebral canal and on the surface of the vertebral column.

The clinical importance of blood vessels associated with the vertebral column is twofold: 1) arteries provide for the nutrition of neural tissues and the vertebrae; 2) veins furnish the route of access for bacteria as well as infective and neoplastic emboli to the cancellous bone of vertebrae. Relative to innervation, clinical emphasis tends to focus on pain. However, proprioceptive and motor impulses mediated by the nerves are equally important, being essential for the postural adjustments and coordinated movements that the vertebral column performs constantly and reflexly, usually without these activities ever reaching consciousness.

Arteries

Regularly spaced pairs of arteries arise from the posterior surface of the descending aorta as it lies in front of the vertebrae. Running laterally, these posterior intercostal and lumbar arteries embrace each vertebral body in the thoracic and lumbar region (see Figs. 19-10 and 25-8). On reaching the intervertebral foramen, each artery gives off a **dorsal branch** that runs with the posterior ramus of the spinal nerve. Although it is destined primarily for the muscles and skin of the back, it also gives off one or more **spinal branches** (or arteries), which enter the intervertebral foramen (Fig. 13-16A). In the cervical and sacral regions, the segmental vessels have fused into vertical arterial channels (vertebral, deep cervical, and lateral sacral arteries) which dispatch spinal branches segmentally into the vertebral canal. After entering the intervertebral foramen, spinal arteries terminate in three types of branches: one supplies the spinal cord and nerve roots (*radicular* or *neural branches*) and the other two the vertebrae, their ligaments, the dura, and epidural tissues (*postcentral* and *prelaminar branches*).

Blood Supply of Vertebrae and Associated Tissues

Minor branches of the posterior intercostal and lumbar arteries enter the anterior surface of the vertebral body (*precentral branches*), and similar twigs from the dorsal branches of these vessels penetrate the posterior surface of the laminae (*postlaminar branches*). The dorsal branches also supply the vertebral arch joints and their ligaments, and then proceed posteriorly to supply the muscles and

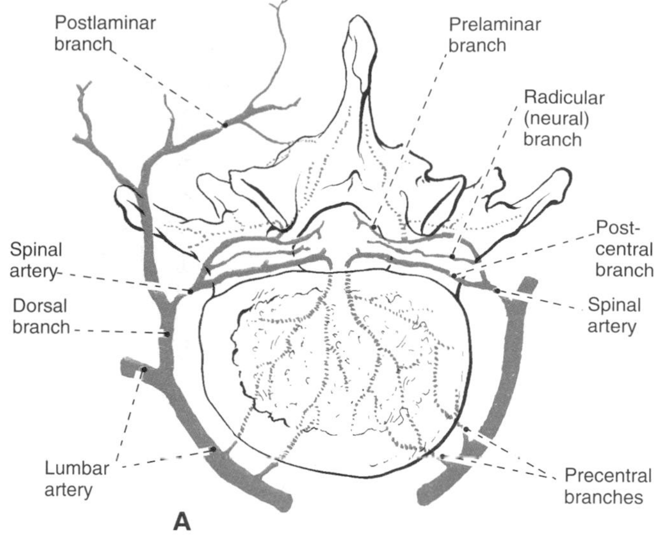

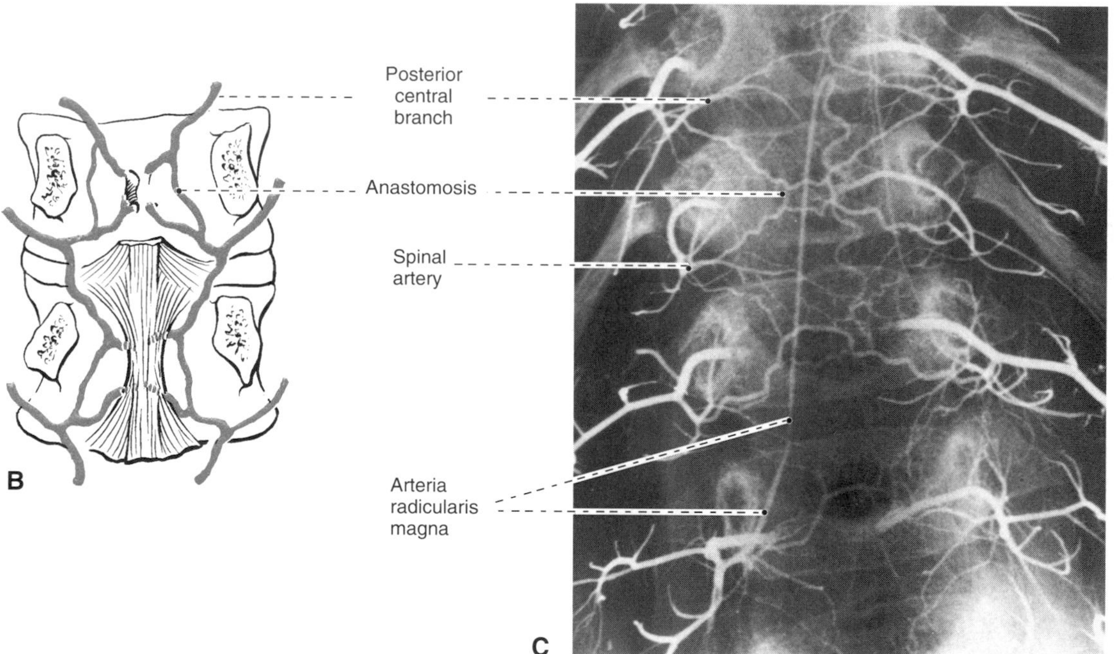

FIGURE *13-16.*
Arterial supply of the vertebrae and the contents of the vertebral canal: (A) Diagram of the branches of a segmental (in this case a lumbar) artery; (B) Anastomoses between the post-central branches of a spinal artery in the vertebral canal. The cut surfaces of the laminae are recognizable. The posterior longitudinal ligament has been removed from one vertebra. (C) Radiograph of a preparation of the lower thoracic and upper lumbar regions of the spine from the cadaver of a 6-year-old child in which the arterial system has been injected by radiopaque contrast material. Note the richness of the blood supply and the extensive anastomoses. Branches corresponding to those shown in panel A and B can be identified. Note especially the ascending *arteria radicularis magna* arising in this specimen from L-2 on the right side. (C, Parke WW, In: Rothman RH, Simeone FA., eds. The spine. Philadelphia: WB Saunders, 1975: Chap. 2.)

skin of the back. The chief nutrient arteries of all vertebrae are furnished by the **spinal arteries**, given off by the dorsal segmental branch (see Fig. 13-16A).

The *postcentral branch* of a spinal artery runs toward the back of the vertebral body (centrum) and divides into two nutrient arteries (see Fig. 13-16B). These enter the posterior surface of two neighboring vertebral bodies to supply the spongy bone and its marrow. Before doing so, however, they anastomose with one another and with arteries of the opposite side beneath the posterior longitudinal ligament. Therefore, one vertebral body is supplied by four arteries, recalling the origin of the centrum from four blocks of somatic mesenchyme (see Fig. 12-2). This anastomosis also supplies the regional dura and epidural tissues, the posterior longitudinal ligament, and the peripheral layers of the annulus fibrosus, leaving the rest of the disk avascular.

The vertebral arch, ligamenta flava, the remainder of the dura and surrounding tissues are supplied by the *prelaminar branch* of the spinal artery, which runs along the anterior surface of the lamina.

Blood Supply of the Spinal Cord

The arterial twigs that arborize in the pia mater and penetrate the spinal cord originate in three longitudinal arterial channels that descend on the surface of the cord. They are the **anterior spinal artery**, located in the anterior median fissure and a pair of **posterior spinal arteries** running along the lines of attachment of the posterior rootlets to the spinal cord (Fig. 13-17). All three begin in the posterior cranial fossa as branches of the vertebral arteries and pass down through the foramen magnum. As they descend on the surface of the cord, they receive regular infusions of blood from the radicular branches of the spinal arteries.

The anterior spinal artery supplies two-thirds of the cross-sectional area of the cord. Because no arterial anastomosis takes place in the substance of the cord, compression of a segment of the anterior spinal artery has serious consequences. The posterior spinal arteries are smaller, and each may consist of two parallel vessels that run on either side of the row of posterior rootlets.

The **radicular branches** of the spinal arteries enter the dura, proceed along the posterior and anterior roots, arborize in the pia mater and terminate by anastomosing with the anterior and posterior spinal arteries. In the lower cervical and upper thoracic regions, several of the radicular arteries may be quite large. The largest radicular artery (*arteria radicularis magna*) is unilateral and, although variable in position, is found most often at L-1 (see Fig. 13-16C). It ascends, feeding into the anterior spinal artery, and supplies the lower part of the cord. The blood supply of the lower two-thirds of the cord depends entirely on the segmental input from radicular arteries.

The Vertebral Venous Plexuses

Venous blood from the vertebrae, spinal cord, and surrounding tissues is collected by veins that correspond to the arteries. These veins empty into irregular sinuses that form cross-connected, ladderlike venous channels, both within the vertebral canal and on the external surface of the vertebral column. These are the **vertebral venous plexuses**, designated as **internal** or **external**, depending on their relation to the vertebral canal.

In the epidural space, a pair of internal plexuses run along the posterior aspect of the vertebral bodies (anterior

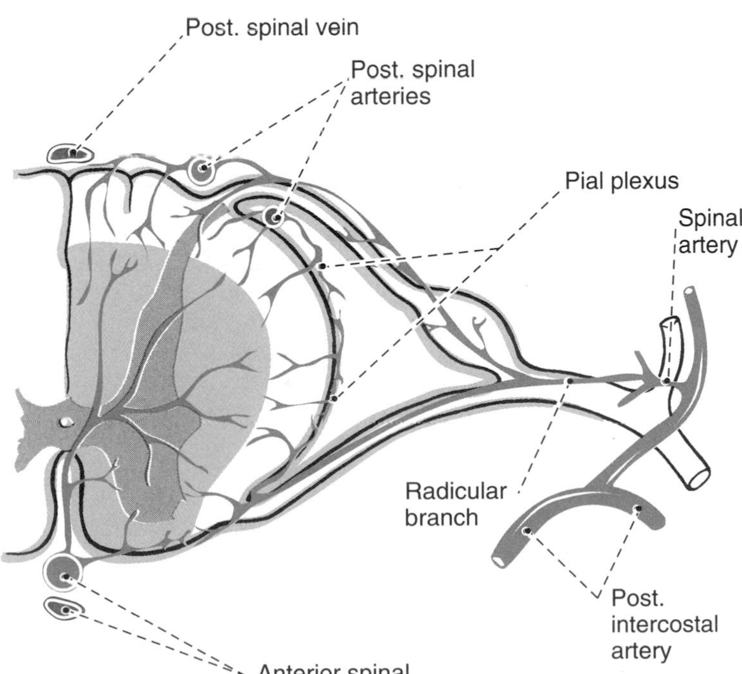

FIGURE *13-17.*
Arterial supply of the spinal cord: The size of the vessels and the thickness of the pia (*pink shading*) are exaggerated. The branches of the anterior spinal artery and those of the other arteries that supply the cord are shown in different colors to illustrate the cross-sectional area of the cord that is supplied by each of these sets of vessels. The anastomotic plexus in the pia mater is suggested.

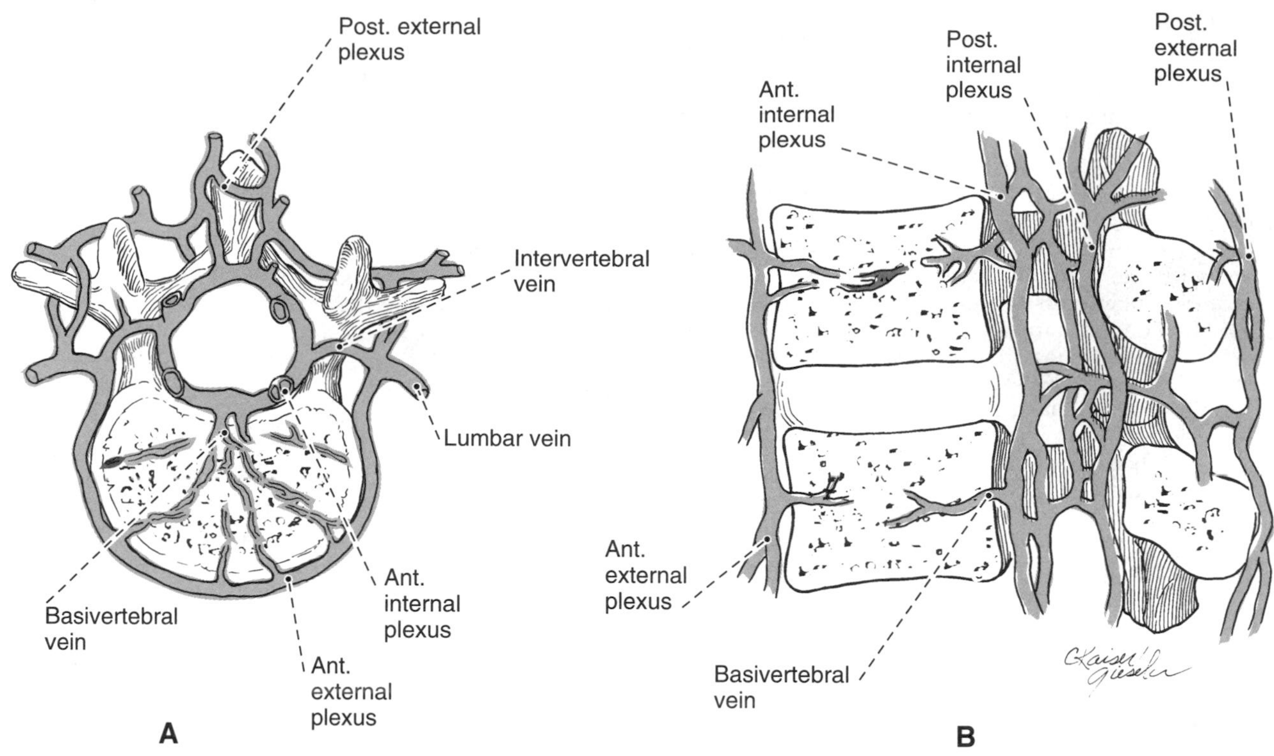

FIGURE 13-18.
The vertebral venous plexuses as seen (A) in a transverse and (B) a sagittal section.

internal plexuses), and another pair are apposed to the laminae (posterior internal plexuses; Fig. 13-18). The largest tributaries of the internal plexuses are the **basivertebral veins**, one at each vertebral level. Each vein issues from a large foramen on the posterior aspect of the vertebral body, and empties into a cross connection between the two anterior internal plexuses. The external vertebral venous plexuses are smaller than the internal ones, but otherwise similar. They connect with the internal plexuses through the intervertebral foramina. The plexuses drain into the caval and azygos systems through their connections with the intercostal and lumbar veins. They also communicate freely with the dural venous sinuses in the cranial cavity, the deep cervical and jugular veins in the neck, and veins of the pelvis.

The spacious, thin-walled irregular sinuses of the internal vertebral venous plexus can accommodate considerable volumes of blood and provide an alternative route for venous return to the caval and azygos systems in cases of venous obstruction in the body cavities or in the neck. Blood can flow freely up or down in the plexuses because these vessels lack valves. When distended, they function in the vertebral canal as a second water jacket wrapped around the one formed by the thecal sac. Fluctuations of venous pressure in the plexus are transmitted to the CSF. As discussed in relation to CSF pressure, such fluctuations are brought about by changes in intrathoracic and intra-abdominal pressure, which are freely transmitted by the connections of the valveless vertebral veins. A notable exception to the absence of valves are the small radicular veins, in which valves prevent venous congestion of the spinal cord when the internal vertebral venous plexus becomes engorged.

Because of the unimpeded, copious, to-and-fro flow of blood in the vertebral venous plexuses, septic and neoplastic emboli from pelvic, abdominal, and other organs readily sequester to venous sinusoids in the bone marrow of the vertebrae, or even proceed up into the cranial cavity. Neoplasms of the prostate, lung, breast, thyroid, and kidney metastasize to the vertebrae through these venous channels.

Innervation of the Spine

One or more **recurrent meningeal branches** are given off by each spinal nerve as soon as it is formed in the intervertebral foramen. This branch, known also as the **sinuvertebral nerve**, reenters the vertebral canal (Fig. 13-19) and carries with it sensory as well as sympathetic efferent fibers. Following the pattern of the postcentral arteries, each nerve divides into ascending and descending branches and supplies the periosteum, the posterior longitudinal ligament, and the outer laminae of the annulus fibrosus over at least two adjacent vertebrae. Nerve fibers do not penetrate the deeper layers of the annulus or the nucleus pulposus. Owing to overlapping territories of distribution, pain induced by a herniating disk is mediated by more than one sinuvertebral nerve. Sensory innervation of the cancellous bone in the vertebral bodies is suggested by the pain caused by vertebral metastases. The sinuvertebral nerves are also sensory to the meninges and

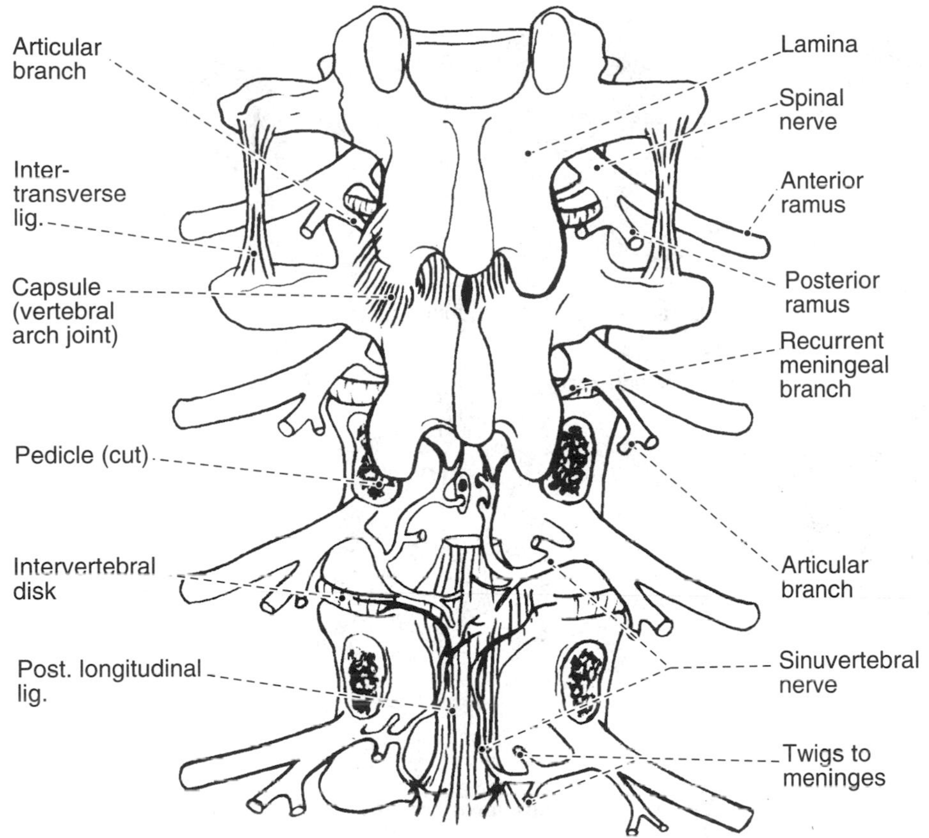

FIGURE *13-19.* **Nerve supply of the vertebral arch joints and ligaments, and some of the contents of the vertebral canal. The pedicles of the lower two vertebrae have been transected to permit a view into the vertebral canal, the contents of which have been removed.**

the walls of the vertebral venous plexuses. They furnish the vasomotor fibers that regulate blood flow in the arteries and internal vertebral venous plexuses.

As each spinal nerve's posterior ramus courses posteriorly around the articular processes, it gives off articular branches that mediate proprioceptive and pain sensations from the vertebral arch joint (see Fig. 13-19). Therefore, with a prolapsed disk, there may be three different sources of pain: 1) ruptured annulus, torn posterior longitudinal ligament and periosteum, innervated by sinuvertebral nerves of at least two segments; 2) direct compression of the spinal nerve or its roots; 3) vertebral arch joints, innervated by posterior rami, which may become painful because of their disturbed mechanics.

Developmental Defects of the Vertebral Canal

It may be deduced from developmental considerations in this chapter that the anatomy of the spinal cord, spinal nerves, and their meningeal investments within the vertebral canal results from various interrelated developmental events that are precisely regulated. Disruption of these regulatory mechanisms leads to congenital abnormalities of the vertebral canal that range in severity from those that remain asymptomatic and undiagnosed, to those that are incompatible with life (Fig. 13-20). The severe varieties of these defects involve tissues derived from both neuroectoderm and mesoderm; the less severe ones result from failure of mesodermal fusion only.

Closure of the neural tube is a critical factor for the induction of the neural arches and the development of the meninges. When the **caudal neuropore** fails to close, the central canal of the spinal cord remains splayed open, communicating with the exterior. Vertebral arch development is disrupted, and the vertebral canal and meninges do not form over the affected area. Major neurologic deficits, together with the risk of infections, reduce life expectancy. This is the most severe form of **spina bifida**. In its mildest form, *spina bifida occulta*, development is normal except for the lack of midline fusion of the two neural arches (see Fig. 13-20E). This condition usually comes to light as an incidental finding during radiologic examination. Intermediate forms of spina bifida are associated with larger vertebral arch defects. The thecal sac herniates through such defects. The spinal cord and nerve roots may remain in their normal position.

Genetic and teratogenic factors have been implicated in the etiology of spina bifida. In some European and Indian communities it has been found in over 1% of births, ten times the overall incidence in the United States, whereas African-Americans are much less frequently affected than whites. Severe forms are associated with other congenital abnormalities, such as hydrocephalus, paralysis of the limbs, and interference with bladder and bowel control.

SEGMENTAL INNERVATION

Evaluation of the anatomic and functional integrity of the spinal cord and spinal nerves relies on an understanding of the segmental innervation of the body. This section

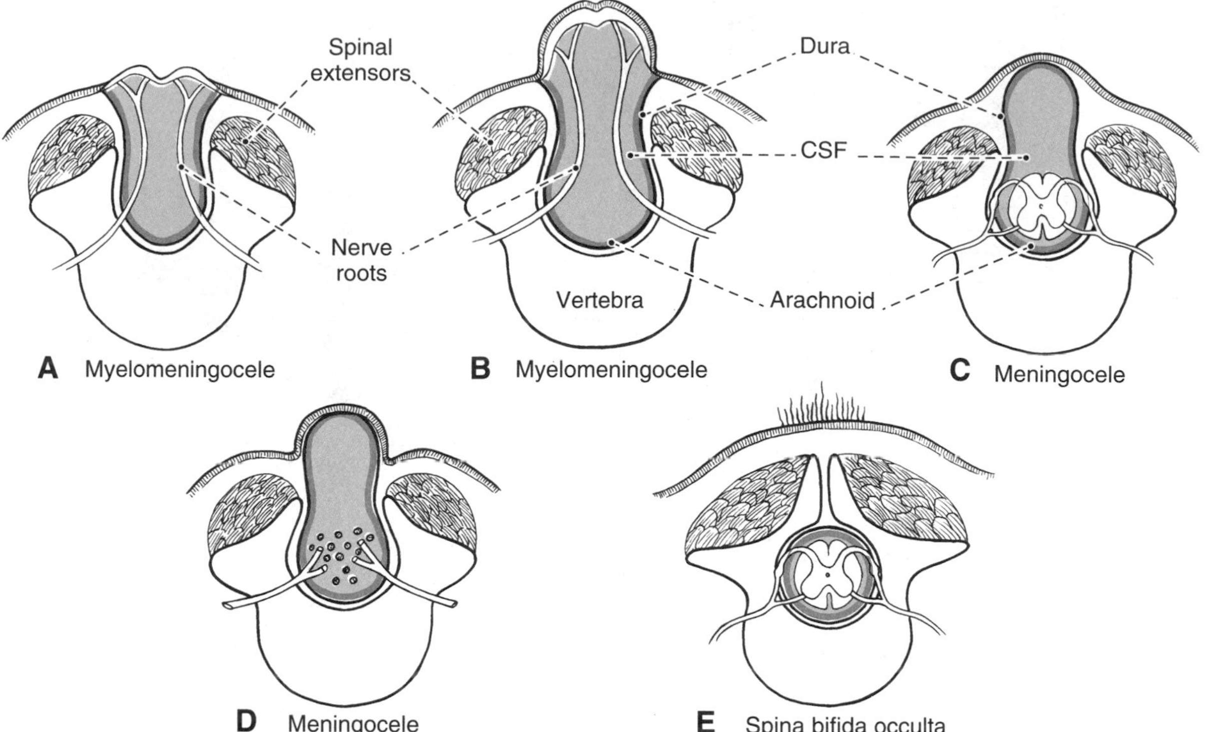

FIGURE *13-20.*
Closure defects of the vertebral canal and spinal cord, known collectively as spina bifida: (A) The spinal cord shown in *white* is completely open; until skin epithelium grows over to cover it, its surface is moistened by CSF leaking from the central canal. The CSF is also accumulating in the thecal sac subjacent to the neural tissue. (B) The dystrophic neuronal tissue (spinal cord) has been attenuated, owing to the accumulation of CSF and protrudes through the mesodermal defect as a large cyst (cele). In the instance illustrated, the cyst is completely epithelialized. (C) The defect is confined to mesodermal tissues; the spinal cord is intact. Cystic herniation of the meninges occurs through the defect and is covered by skin. (D) the same defect as in panel C, shown at the level of the cauda equina. (E) in contrast to the "overt" varieties of spina bifida (see panels A through D), in occult spina bifida there is no herniation. The inconsequential hidden mesodermal defect is often associated with tufts of hair over the cleft vertebral arch or arches.

deals with the distribution of spinal nerves to skeletal muscle and skin in the neck, the trunk, and the limbs. The cranial nerves and their territories of distribution are discussed in Chapters 7 and 32. Following a description of the body's overall segmental plan (which rationalizes much of the anatomy of the trunk and the limbs), the last section of the chapter presents the clinical evaluation of spinal nerves and associated spinal cord segments.

Development

All vertebrates are built on a basic segmental pattern. Although this segmentation is less evident in the human than in more primitive vertebrates, its existence may be readily appreciated during the period of embryonic development. Between the 21st and 31st days of gestation, the paraxial mesoderm on each side condenses into segments or **somites** (Fig. 13-21), to which reference has already been made in several contexts. Altogether, 4 pairs of somites develop in the occipital region, 8 in the cervical, 12 in the thoracic, 5 each in the lumbar and sacral regions, and as many as 10 in the coccygeal region. By the time caudal somites form, more rostral somites have differentiated. The somites give rise to **sclerotomes**, **myotomes**, and **dermatomes**. The sclerotomes are destined to become the axial skeleton (vertebrae, ribs, sternum), the myotomes skeletal muscle, and the dermatomes spread out beneath the ectoderm to form the dermis of the skin. Sets of nerve fibers that grow out of the spinal cord and the developing spinal ganglia become associated with each somite. This association defines a spinal nerve and will be retained throughout life.

Although the derivatives of a pair of somites become widely dispersed, together they define a **segment of the body**. In essence, there are segmental bone, muscle, and skin in each body segment, together with a pair each of nerves, arteries, and veins. The "segmental" blood vessels actually develop between, rather than within, segments (see Fig. 12-2), and as a rule, supply adjacent segments. Such an overlap also

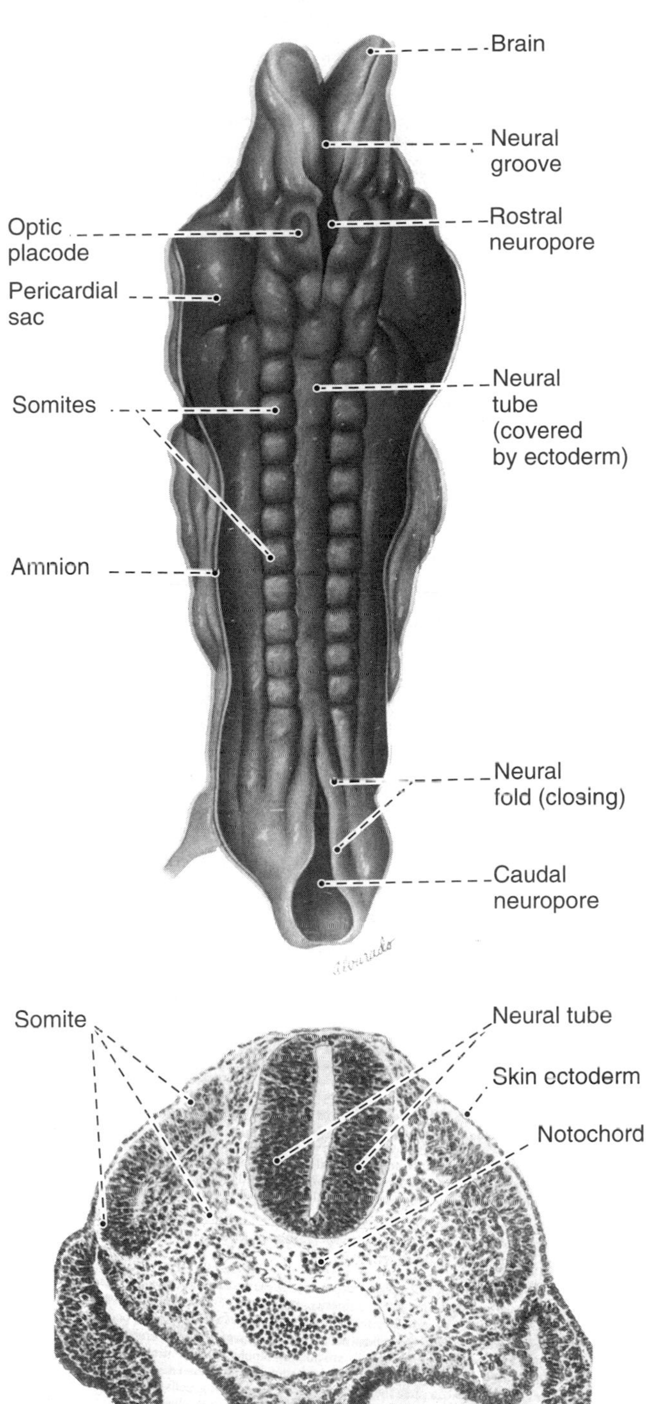

FIGURE *13-21.*
Differentiation of the segmental paraxial mesoderm: (A) Dorsal view of an embryo in which ten somites are identified; (B) transverse section of an embryo similar to that in panel A. The cells of the somite in this segment have separated into the dermomyotome and sclerotome. (A, Gasserr RF. Atlas of human embryos. Hagerstown: Harper & Rowe, 1975; B FitzGerald MJT. Human embryology. Hagerstown: Harper & Rowe, 1978. Both embryos are from the Carnegie collection.)

comes about in cutaneous innervation. The orderly segmental arrangement is clearly retained in the trunk, but is obscure in the limbs. Nevertheless, the innervation of the limbs is also segmental. Moreover, the innervation of viscera with fibers furnished by the spinal cord and spinal ganglia likewise conforms to a segmental pattern (see, for instance, Fig. 24-51).

An appreciation of the segmental distribution of nerves to muscle, skin, bone, and even viscera is not only helpful for grasping the basic anatomic structure, but is of considerable clinical importance:

1. It forms the basis of the functional interrelation between the central nervous system and the musculoskeletal system.
2. Lesions of the spinal cord or its nerve roots often manifest themselves by affecting the musculoskeletal system in a segmental fashion.
3. Pain referred from viscera may affect the cutaneous and neuromuscular segments that are innervated from the same cord segments as the viscera.

The Anatomy of a Spinal Nerve

The formation of spinal nerves from anterior and posterior roots is discussed in a preceding section. The spinal nerve emerges from the intervertebral foramen and divides almost immediately, yielding an anterior and a posterior ramus (Fig. 13-22). Before it divides, the nerve gives off one or two small meningeal branches that reenter the vertebral canal (see Figs. 13-19 and 13-22). Strictly speaking, the spinal nerve itself is a very short structure. The term, however, carries a broader connotation: as commonly used, it includes all the branches of the spinal nerve and both of its rami throughout their lengths.

Each **posterior** (dorsal) **ramus** supplies a vertebral arch joint, a segment of the extensor musculature of the spine (erector spinae), and a strip of skin on the back. In all regions, posterior rami retain a segmental arrangement. None of the posterior rami contribute nerves to the limbs.

The **anterior** (ventral) **rami** are larger; they supply the more extensive parts of the neck and the trunk located anterior to the vertebrae, and also both pairs of limbs. The structures and tissues innervated by anterior rami in these regions include the skin, muscles, bones, and joints, as well as the parietal layer of the serous sacs in the body cavity (pleura, peritoneum, and pericardium).

Anterior rami of thoracic spinal nerves retain a truly segmental arrangement, similar to that of the posterior rami, but in the cervical, lumbar, and sacral regions anterior rami form plexuses. The **cervical plexus** (C-1 through C-4) supplies all muscles of the neck, with the exception of cervical extensors, as well as the skin of the neck anterolaterally and on the posterolateral aspect of the head. Anterior rami of C-5 to T-1 are distributed to the upper limb through the **brachial plexus**, and those of L-2 through S-3 proceed through the **lumbosacral plexus** to the lower

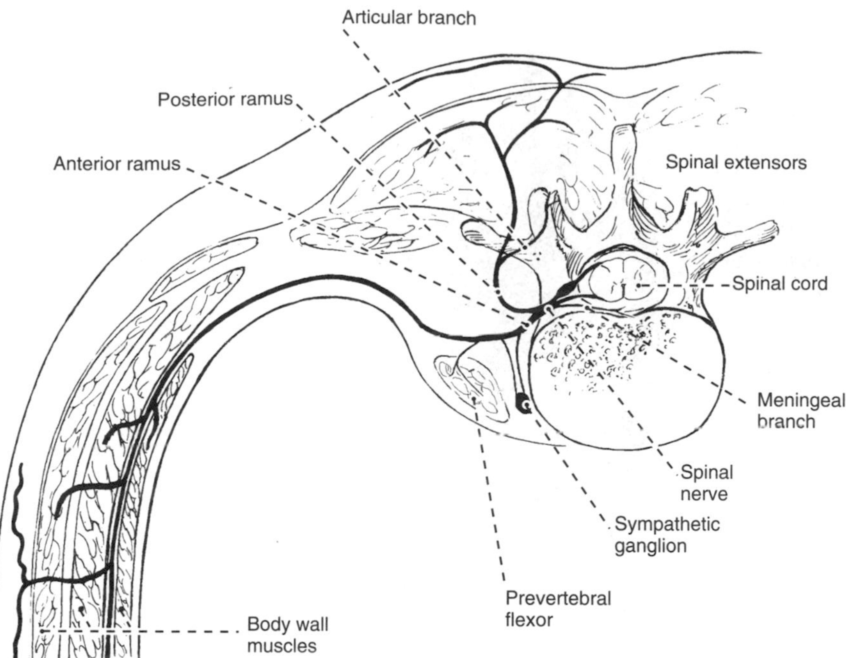

FIGURE 13-22.
Origin, division, course, and branches of a typical spinal nerve (*black line*).

limb (see Fig. 14-6). Anterior rami supplying the limbs do not innervate structures in the trunk. All the layers of the body wall are supplied by anterior rami of T-2 to L-1, including the skin down to the groin (see Fig. 13-25).

Composition of Spinal Nerves

Spinal nerves are composed preponderantly of somatic efferent and somatic afferent nerve fibers. When spinal nerves are spoken of in general terms, they are often referred to as "somatic" nerves, implying that they are made up of these two nerve fiber types exclusively. That is not true however, and in many considerations, both anatomic and clinical, it is important to realize that all spinal nerves convey visceral efferent fibers as well. Moreover, some spinal nerves are also associated with afferent fibers from viscera.

Somatic efferents are the axons of neurons in the anterior gray column contributed to the spinal nerve by its anterior root. They innervate skeletal muscle. Two types should be distinguished: *alpha efferents,* or large skeletomotor fibers, which innervate the bulk of a muscle, and *gamma efferents*, or fusimotor fibers of small diameter, which innervate the specialized intrafusal muscle fibers that regulate tension in muscle spindles (Fig. 13-10B).

Somatic afferents convey to the spinal cord, from the skin and deep structures, impulses concerned with pain, temperature, touch, pressure, vibration, and position sense. Their cell bodies are in the spinal ganglia. Passing in the posterior root, their central processes enter the spinal cord, and their peripheral processes join the spinal nerve (see Fig. 7-4).

Visceral efferent nerve fibers provide motor innervation to smooth muscle, cardiac muscle, and glands. They are of two types: *sympathetic visceral efferents,* the axons of neurons in the lateral column of spinal cord segments T-1 through L-2, and *parasympathetic efferents,* the axons of lateral column neurons in cord segments S-2 to S-4 (see Figs. 7-12 and 7-13). Both types, of visceral efferents leave the cord with somatic efferents in the anterior roots of the respective spinal nerves. There are no visceral efferents in the anterior roots of other nerves.

Parasympathetic visceral efferents enter the anterior rami of S-2 to S-4 spinal nerves, and soon branch off to supply abdominal and pelvic viscera and perineal structures (see Figs. 7-13 and 27-14). They do not distribute along branches of spinal nerves. This is quite unlike *sympathetic visceral efferents* that, despite their restricted exit from the cord in T-1 to L-2 anterior roots, pass along the anterior and posterior rami of all spinal nerves throughout the body. Such a wide distribution of sympathetic efferents is afforded through the association of all spinal nerves with the **sympathetic trunk**, or chain, composed of vertically interconnected sympathetic ganglia (see Figs. 7-11 and 22-16).

The preganglionic **sympathetic visceral efferents** enter T-1 to L-2 spinal nerves, proceed along the anterior ramus of each nerve and exit through a small branch (*white ramus communicans*) that links the anterior ramus to the sympathetic ganglion of corresponding number (T1–L2) (see Figs. 7-11 and 7-14). From upper members of these ganglia sympathetic efferents ascend to all the ganglia as far as the skull, and from lower members of the group, sympathetic efferents descend along the sympathetic trunk to all other ganglia as far as the coccyx. Sympathetic efferents leave all these ganglia for two major destinations: to innervate viscera (see Fig. 7-11) and to innervate smooth muscle and glands that are associated with somatic structures (see Fig. 7-14). A medial branch of each ganglion proceeds to viscera, and another small branch (*gray ramus communicans*) links a ganglion to each anterior ramus in the cervical, thoracic, lumbar, and sacral regions.

The sympathetic efferents that enter the anterior ramus through the gray ramus communicans are a new generation of fibers. They are the axons of autonomic ganglion cells on which the preganglionic axons of lateral column neurons terminate within the sympathetic ganglion. Some of these sympathetic efferents distribute along the anterior ramus and all its branches, others pass along the posterior ramus and its branches, having retraced their course to the point at which the spinal nerve divides. In this manner, the sympathetic ganglia provide a population of visceral efferent nerve fibers for every spinal nerve. They intermingle with somatic efferent and afferent nerve fibers, which make up the bulk of the nerve. The visceral efferents innervate sweat glands and smooth muscle associated with hair follicles (*arrectores pilorum*) and in the walls of blood vessels. Lack of sweating and vasodilatation, therefore, are useful confirmatory signs of damage to a spinal nerve or one of its branches.

Visceral afferents convey impulses from viscera and have a limited association with spinal nerves. From the viscera they enter sympathetic ganglia through their medial branches, pass along the sympathetic chain, and join the anterior rami of T-1 through L-2 spinal nerves by way of the white rami communicantes. They reach the spinal ganglia where their cell bodies are located among the ganglion cells of somatic afferents. This mingling of somatic and visceral afferents in a single posterior root and spinal cord segment provides the anatomic basis for *referred pain*. Pain that originates in a viscus (e.g., heart or uterus) is perceived as being in those somatic structures that are innervated by the same cord segments as the affected viscus.

Owing to the complexity of visceral nerve fiber distribution, any description of the components of a typical spinal nerve tends to exaggerate their presence. In both clinical and anatomic contexts, spinal nerves should be thought of primarily as somatic nerves.

Myotomes, Dermatomes, and Sclerotomes

The mass of skeletal muscle innervated by the anterior and posterior rami of a single pair of spinal nerves, or a spinal cord segment, is often spoken of as a **myotome**. Such a myotome includes portions of several muscles, and many muscles contain portions of more than one myotome. Although not a distinct physical or anatomic entity, the myotome thus defined is a useful concept in clinical anatomy. In embryology, by contrast, the term *myotome* does indeed signify a distinct physical entity, namely a specific cluster of cells making up a portion of the somite. It is this group of cells that, over the course of development, gives rise to the *myotome* of clinical anatomy.

In a similar vein, a **dermatome** in the fully developed body is defined as the area of skin innervated by one spinal cord segment (and in the embryo, a specific set of cells in the somite that gives rise to the dermis of this strip of skin). The cell bodies of the sensory nerve fibers supplying a dermatome are located in a pair of spinal ganglia.

It has been proposed that **sclerotomes** also exist in the fully developed body, in the sense that areas of bone and periosteum can be defined that are innervated by individual spinal nerves. A sclerotome defined in such a manner is not identical with the embryonic sclerotome. The bones of the limbs are not derived from embryonic sclerotomes, yet their periostea are segmentally innervated.

Segmental Innervation of Muscles

The segmental arrangement of myotomes in the trunk is clearly evident from the distribution of spinal nerves T-1 to L-1. Their posterior rami supply the thoracic and lumbar portions of the spinal extensors segmentally and their anterior rami innervate the intercostal muscles, abdominal flank muscles, and the rectus abdominis in a strictly segmental fashion.

The musculature of the limbs is also innervated segmentally. Although the segmental pattern is not immediately obvious, it can be defined by the groups of muscles that act as prime movers of major joints in the limbs.

Columns of motor neurons concerned with the supply of individual muscles in the limbs have been identified experimentally, as well as by correlating paralysis of individual muscles with the patchy distribution of motor neuron death in cases of poliomyelitis. Such cell columns in the anterior horns are constant. Depending on the muscle group, they may span two to four segments of the cord, but the greatest concentration of neurons for a particular muscle group is contained in just one or two of these segments. Thus, from a functional perspective, some segments in the motor neuron column for a given muscle are more important than others. The cell columns that innervate muscles sharing the same action at a particular joint are found in the same segments of the spinal cord. The elbow flexors, for example, are innervated from C-5 and C-6 cord segments. Therefore, a muscle group in which each muscle operates as a prime mover at a particular joint may be viewed as a segmentally innervated functional unit.

The innervation of prime movers for different joints of the upper and lower limbs is shown in Table 13-1. From an overview of these data, a few general features emerge that are helpful in understanding the basic arrangement:

1. Muscles with a common primary action on a joint share at least two adjacent segments of the spinal cord (e.g., shoulder abductors or elbow flexors).
2. Even when four or five cord segments are involved, major responsibility for the movement rests with only one or two of them, as would be expected from the distribution of motor neurons described on the foregoing.
3. The segments of the cord that supply the antagonists of a muscle group either overlap, or run in numerical sequence with the cord segments for that group. For instance, elbow flexors are sup-

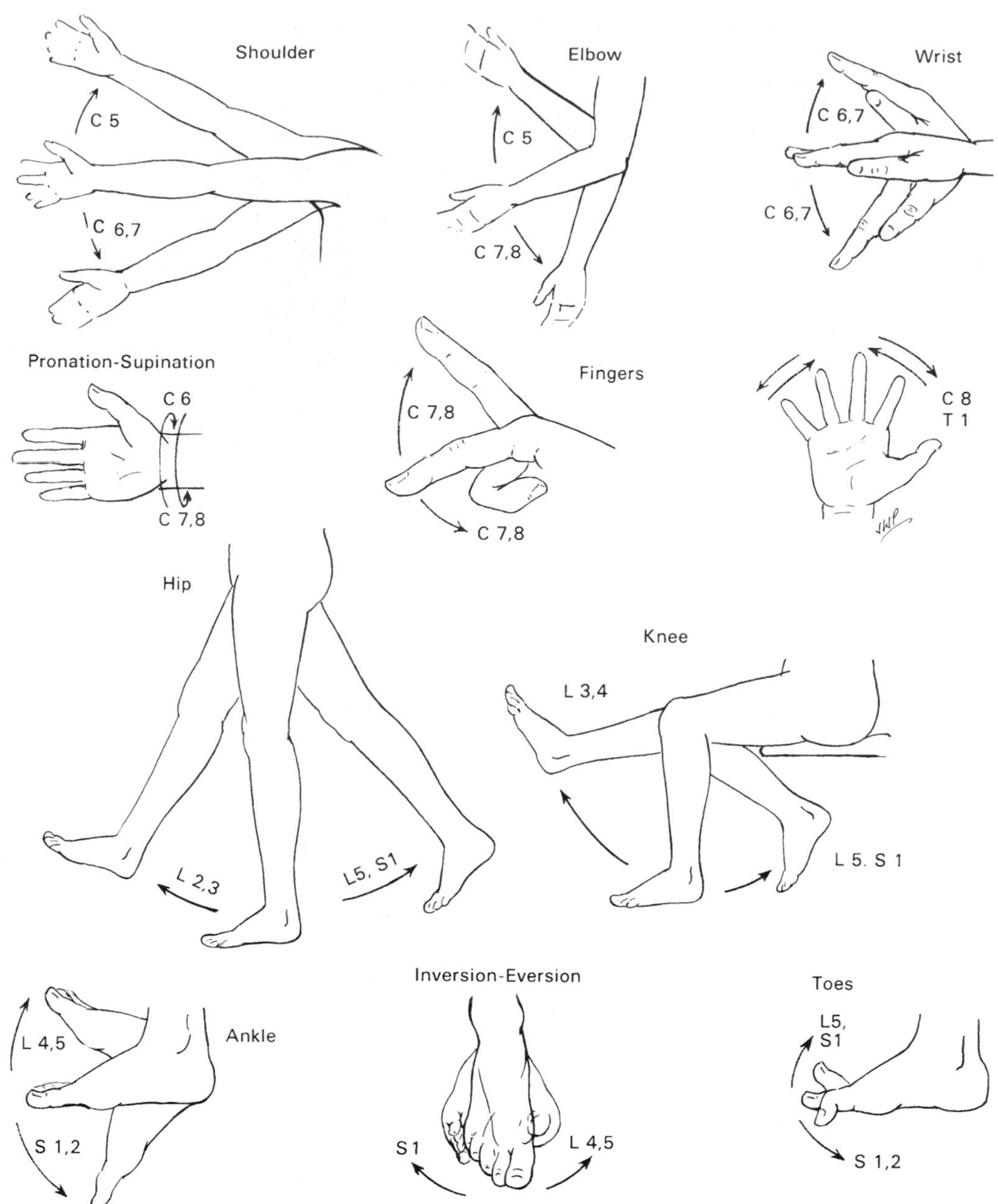

FIGURE 13-23.
Segmental innervation of the muscle groups producing movement in the limbs: Only segments principally responsible for the innervation of a movement are shown. These are the segments of greatest clinical usefulness. For a more complete account refer to Table 13-1. (Based on Last RJ. Anatomy. London: Churchill, 1972.)

plied by C-5 and C-6, whereas the chief supply of the extensors is from C-7 and C-8.

4. In general, the segments that innervate the muscles of a joint that is more distal in the limb lie en bloc more inferiorly in the cord.

The segments concerned with the chief supply of the muscles of a particular joint might be thought of as a *joint center* in the spinal cord. The joint center for the elbow, for example, resides in C-5, C-6, C-7, and C-8 segments, with C-5, C-7 and C-8 assuming the major responsibility. Figure 13-23 illustrates some of the important movements of the upper and lower limbs and the joint centers involved in producing those movements. In many clinical settings, it is important to know two things: which cord segments control a particular muscle group (e.g., L-2 and L-3 exert the predominant control over the hip flexors), and the converse: namely, which movements are controlled by a particular cord segment (e.g., L-3 is involved not only in hip flexion but also in adduction at the hip, as well as ex-

TABLE 13-1 Segmental Innervation of Limb Musculature*

Upper Limb *Joints/Prime Movers*	*C5*	*C6*	*C7*	*C8*	*T1*
Shoulder					
Abductors	X	x			
Extensors	X	X	X	x	
Lateral rotators	X	x			
Adductors		X	X	x	
Flexors	x	X	X	x	
Medial rotators	x	X	X	x	
Elbow					
Flexors	X	x			
Extensors		x	X	X	
Forearm					
Supinators	x	X			
Pronators		x	X	X	x
Wrist					
Flexors		X	X	x	x
Extensors		X	X	x	
Fingers					
Flexors		X	X	x	
Extensors		X	X	x	
Intrinsic hand muscles				x	X

(Cord Segments: C5–T1)

Lower Limb *Joints/Prime Movers*	*L2*	*L3*	*L4*	*L5*	*S1*	*S2*	*S3*
Hip							
Flexors	X	X	x				
Adductors	X	X	x				
Medial rotators	X	X	x	x	x	x	
Extensors			x	X	X	x	
Abductors			x	X	X	x	
Lateral rotators				X	X	x	
Knee							
Extensors	x	X	X				
Flexors			x	X	X	x	x
Ankle							
Extensors (dorsiflexors)			X	X	x		
Flexors (plantarflexors)				x	X	X	
Pretalar–subtalar joint							
Invertors			X	X	x		
Evertors				X	X	x	
Toes							
Extensors				X	X	x	
Flexors					X	X	x
Intrinsic foot muscles						X	x

(Cord Segments: L2–S3)

* The cord segments principally concerned with various movements are indicated by boldface capital Xs. Movements are so grouped as to make the existence of *joint centers* more readily appreciable.

tension at the knee). Such knowledge is useful, for instance, when testing the strength of particular muscle groups, or eliciting deep tendon reflexes (see following section), because it allows the examiner to gauge which spinal segments are being activated during such tests.

Deep Tendon Reflexes

Subjecting a muscle to a sudden stretch, by tapping its tendon, elicits a reflex contraction in the muscle. Such "tendon jerks" test the integrity of the anatomic components of the stretch reflex. These components are the muscle spindles that sense the stretch, the somatic afferents that transmit this information along the spinal nerve, and the specific segment of the spinal cord that innervates the muscle. In this segment, the afferent impulses elicited by the stretch are relayed by interneurons to alpha motoneurons in the anterior horn. These, in turn, discharge impulses along the spinal nerve back to the muscle, causing it to contract.

The most useful tendon reflexes are the biceps, triceps, and brachioradialis tendon jerks in the upper limb and the knee and ankle jerks in the lower limb. The biceps jerk tests spinal cord segment C-5, the biceps being a flexor of the elbow. The triceps is an elbow extensor; the triceps jerk, therefore, gives information about segments C-7 and C-8. The brachioradialis jerk involves chiefly the C-6 segment. In eliciting a knee jerk, the tendon of the extensor muscle (quadriceps) is tapped, testing segments L-3 and L-4. The ankle jerk, on the other hand, tests S-1 and S-2, because the muscles subjected to momentary stretch are the plantar flexors of the ankle.

Segmental Innervation of the Skin

In the trunk, the dermatomes, similar to the myotomes, are arranged in regular bands from T-2 to L-1 (Figs. 13-24 and 13-25). T-2 is at the sternal angle, T-10 at the level of the umbilicus, and L-1 in the region of the groin. There is considerable overlap between neighboring dermatomes of the trunk. Thus, if a single spinal nerve is blocked, the effect on the dermatome served by that nerve is undetectable clinically. Such is not true in the limbs. Limb dermatomes cover larger areas of skin and, although there is overlap between neighboring dermatomes, compression, anesthetic block, or division of a single spinal nerve that feeds into one of the limb plexuses does produce hypesthesia, or even anesthesia, over part of the appropriate dermatome.

Each of the two dermatomal maps currently in use represents the synthesis of a large number of isolated clinical observations. The map of Foerster (see Figs. 13-24 and 13-25C and D) is based largely on patients in whom specific posterior roots have been surgically divided for the treatment of pain. Keegan and Garrett's map (see Fig. 13-25A and B) is constructed largely from cases of nerve compression by herniating intervertebral disks in the cervical and lumbosacral regions, verified in most instances by surgery.

In Foerster's map, the dermatomes represented in the limbs are missing from the anterior surface of the trunk and have only limited representation on the back (see Fig. 13-25C and D). According to Keegan and Garrett, however, C-5 and T-1 are represented not only in the upper limb, but also on the anterior surface of the trunk; furthermore, their map shows a full complement of der-

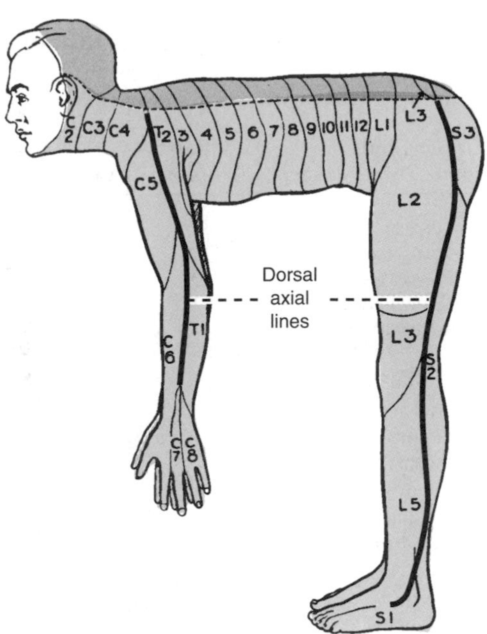

FIGURE 13-24.
Segmental innervation of the skin; dermatomal map according to Foerster: The body is shown in the quadruped position to emphasize the regular distribution of dermatomes. The dorsal axial lines are indicated; the ventral axial lines cannot be seen in this position. Nevertheless, it can be appreciated that the skin covering the preaxial border of the limbs between ventral and dorsal axial lines is innervated by the more proximal segments of the limb plexus, whereas the skin covering the postaxial border is innervated by the distal segments. For the upper limbs, skin has been borrowed from the trunk dermatomes proximally and distally (C-4 and T-2). The approximate area of skin supplied by anterior rami of spinal nerves is shaded *pink*, that supplied by posterior rami is *blue*, and the skin supplied by the trigeminal cranial nerve is *white*. (Modified from Haymaker W, Woodhall B. Peripheral nerve injuries. 2nd ed. Philadelphia: WB Saunders, 1953.)

matomes posteriorly (see Fig. 13-25A and B). Although Keegan and Garrett's map has gained wide clinical acceptance, the data on which Foerster's map is based are both anatomically and methodologically more solid, and they have been confirmed by subsequent reports.

The developmental explanation put forward by Keegan and Garrett postulates that sensory branches of limb nerves grow down the paddle-shaped limb bud along its dorsal surface and wind themselves around both its cranial and caudal borders to the ventral surface. They meet along a line down the middle of the ventral surface called the **axial line** (Fig. 13-26A). This mode of development results in contiguous dermatomes on either side of the axial line being supplied from discontinuous spinal cord segments (C-6 dermatome abuts T-1 in the forearm, for example) and overlap across the axial line is minimal. In Foerster's map there is not only a ventral axial line but a dorsal one as well (see Figs. 13-24 and 13-25C and D). He postulated that the central dermatome of each limb bud (C-7 for the upper limb and S-1 for the lower limb) becomes drawn out to cover the most distal segment of the limb, leaving behind discontinuous dermatomes in contact with one another across dorsal and ventral axial lines (see Fig. 13-26B). Whichever explanation is correct, the existence of ventral axial lines is universally accepted. Ventral axial lines are clinically useful because testing cutaneous sensation across these lines is virtually free of the complications imposed elsewhere by dermatomal overlap.

Superficial Reflexes

Stimulation of the skin by stroking or scratching in certain dermatomal areas provokes reflex muscle contraction. These so-called superficial reflexes depend on the integrity of the appropriate sensory and motor peripheral nerves and spinal cord segments. The most useful superficial reflexes are the abdominal, cremasteric, plantar, and anal reflexes.

The **abdominal reflex** is elicited by scratching the skin some distance away from the umbilicus in any one quadrant of the anterior abdominal wall. This causes contraction of the underlying abdominal muscles. In the upper quadrants of the abdomen, this reflex tests segments T-7 to T-9, and in the lower quadrants segments T-10 to T-12.

FIGURE 13-25.
Dermatomal maps according to Keegan and Garrett (A and B) based on areas of hyposensitivity to pin scratch in cases of herniated intervertebral disks; and according to Foerster (C and D), based on a method of "remaining sensitivity" (i.e., severing several posterior roots above and below the posterior root of a single spinal nerve and determining the boundaries of unaltered sensitivity). Apart from the presence or absence of dorsal axial lines, there are other notable differences between the two maps; for example, in the representation of C-3, C-4, and C-5 dermatomes in the neck and the shoulder regions, both anteriorly and posteriorly, the extent of C-6 and C-7 dermatomes in the upper limb, and assignment of the great toe to L-4 or L-5 dermatomes. The approximate area of skin supplied by anterior rami of spinal nerves is shaded *pink*, that supplied by posterior rami is *blue*, and the skin supplied by the trigeminal cranial nerve is *white*.

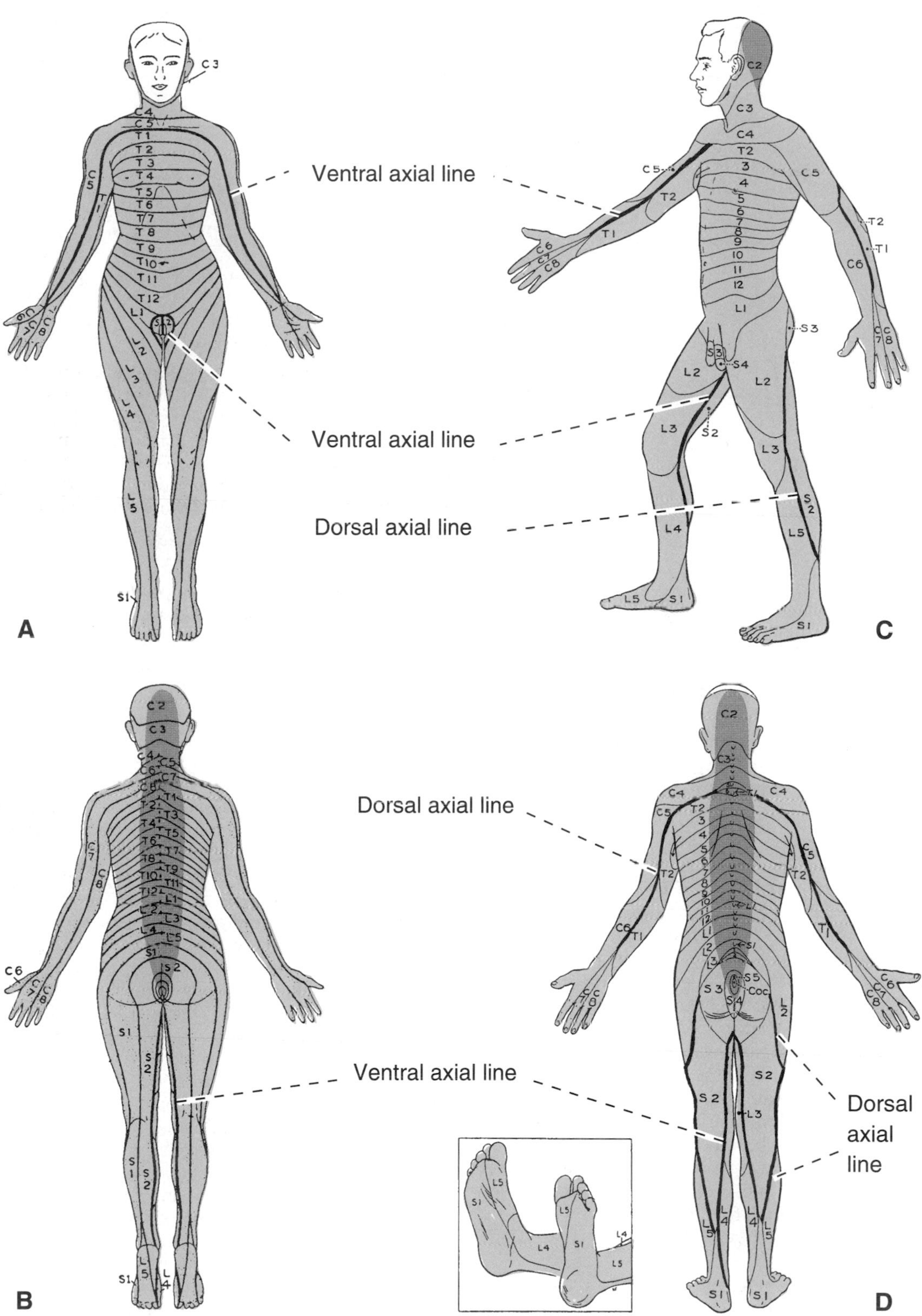
Ventral axial line
Ventral axial line
Ventral axial line
Ventral axial line
Dorsal axial line
Dorsal axial line
Ventral axial line
Ventral axial line
Dorsal axial line
A
B
C
D

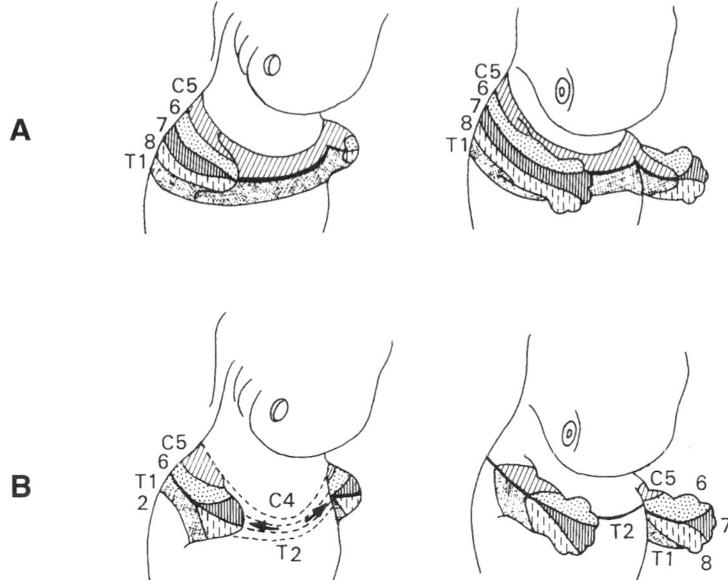

FIGURE 13-26.
Developmental explanation of the dermatomes in the upper limb: (A) According to Keegan and Garrett; (B) according to Foerster. Each is shown at two successive stages of development. (A, Bowden REM., Abdullah S, Gooding MR. In: Lord Brain, Wilkinson, M, eds. Cervical spondylosis. Philadelphia: WB Saunders, 1967.)

The **cremasteric reflex** tests L-1 and L-2 segments and is elicited in males by stroking the medial side of the thigh. This provokes reflex contraction of the cremaster muscle causing prompt and visible elevation of the testis.

The **plantar reflex** is elicited by scratching the sole along its lateral aspect from heel to toes (dermatomes L-5 and S-1), which provokes plantar flexion of the toes. The **anal reflex** is elicited by scratching the skin in the perianal region (dermatome S-3). A visible contraction of the external anal sphincter causes puckering of the anus. Segments S-2, S-3, and S-4 are involved.

Living Anatomy and Physical Examination

The demonstration of the living anatomy of the vertebral column, described in the previous chapter, and of the spinal nerves, discussed in the foregoing, constitute much of the physical examination of the spine and the neurologic screening examination. An understanding of the anatomy of the vertebral column, spinal cord, and spinal nerves will be greatly enhanced and retained if dissection of the cadaver is combined with living anatomy exercises that demonstrate functional anatomy. Similarly, the physical examination should be based on a conscious evaluation of anatomic structures, rather than on a perfunctory set of maneuvers. The diagnosis of normality through the demonstration of normal, functional anatomy should be as important an objective of the physical examination as the discovery of lesions.

In testing the movements of the vertebral column, the cutaneous sensations in dermatomes—such as pain (pinprick), temperature, touch—and the strength of muscle groups supplied by the joint centers of the spinal cord, together with the induction of deep tendon and superficial reflexes, provides a review of virtually all anatomic components of the spine and spinal nerves, as well as of the gray and white matter of the cord in discrete segments. Furthermore, because interference with descending and ascending tracts will alter muscle tone and strength, cutaneous sensations, and the character of deep tendon and superficial reflexes, the presence of lesions in the vertebral canal, spinal cord, and even the brain, may be inferred by evaluating cord segments located distal to these lesions.

RECOMMENDED READINGS

Barson AJ. The vertebral level of termination of the spinal cord during normal and abnormal development. J Anat 1970; 106: 489.

Batson OV. The function of the vertebral veins and their role in the spread of metastases. Ann Surg 1940; 112: 138.

Bonica JJ. Principles and practice of obstetric analgesia and anesthesia, vol 1. Philadelphia: FA Davis, 1967.

Bowden REM, Abdullah S, Gooding MR. Anatomy of the cervical spine, membranes, spinal cord, nerve roots and brachial plexus. In: Brain WR, Wilkinson M, eds. Cervical spondylosis. Philadelphia: WB Saunders, 1967.

Bronner-Fraser M. Origins and developmental potential of the neural crest. Exp Cell Res 1995; 218: 405.

Carlson BM. Human embryology and developmental biology. St. Louis: Mosby-Year Book, 1994.

Eckenhoff JE. The physiologic significance of the vertebral venous plexus. Surg Gynecol Obstet 1970; 131: 72.

Elliot HC. Cross-sectional diameters and areas of the human spinal cord. Anat Rec 1945; 93: 287.

Foerster O. The dermatomes in man. Brain 1933; 56: 1.

Gillilan LA. Blood vessels, meninges, cerebrospinal fluid: blood supply to the central nervous system. In: Crosby EC, Humphrey T, Lauer EW, eds. Correlative anatomy of the nervous system. New York: Macmillan, 1962: 550.

Haines DE. On the question of a subdural space. Anat Rec 1991; 230: 3.

Haley JC, Perry JG. Protrusions of intervertebral discs: study of their distribution, characteristics and effects on the nervous system. Am J Surg 1950; 80: 394.

Haymaker W, Woodhall B. Peripheral nerve injuries: principles of diagnosis. 2nd ed. Philadelphia: WB Saunders, 1953.

Hollinshead WH. Anatomy for surgeons: vol 3, the back and limbs. 3rd ed. Philadelphia: Harper & Row, 1982.

Hoppenfeld S. Orthopaedic neurology: a diagnostic guide to neurologic levels. Philadelphia: JB Lippincott, 1977.

Keegan JJ, Garrett FD. The segmental distribution of the cutaneous nerves in the limbs of man. Anat Rec 1948; 102: 409.

Last RJ. Innervation of the limbs. J Bone Joint Surg 1949; 31B: 452.

Müller F, O'Rahilly R. Occipitocervical segmentation in staged human embryos. J Anat 1994; 185: 251.

Pedersen HE, Blunck CFJ, Gardner E. The anatomy of lumbosacral posterior rami and meningeal branches of spinal nerves (sinuvertebral nerves) with an experimental study of their functions. J Bone Joint Surg 1956; 38A: 377.

Plaisant O, Cosnard G, Gillot C, Schill H, Lassau JP. MRI of the epidural space after gelatin/gadolinium venous injection. Surg Radiol Anat 1994; 16: 71.

Thron AK. Vascular anatomy of the spinal cord. New York: Springer-Verlag, 1988.

Wilson DA, Prince JR. MR imaging determination of the location of the normal conus medullaris throughout childhood. Am J Roentgenol 1989; 152: 1029.

Zhang T, Harstad L, Parisi JE, Murray MJ. The size of the anterior spinal artery in relation to the arteria medullaris magna anterior in humans. Clin Anat 1995; 8: 347.

PART IV

LIMBS

Hollinshead's Textbook of Anatomy, by Cornelius Rosse and Penelope Gaddum-Rosse.
Lippincott-Raven Publishers, Philadelphia, © 1997.

CHAPTER 14

Basic Structural Plan of the Limbs

The upper and lower limbs are distinguished by some striking morphologic and functional differences, yet both pairs of limbs are built on essentially the same basic plan. An understanding of this plan simplifies the learning of limb anatomy and provides the key for an appreciation of the anatomic adaptations that subserve the functions unique to each limb. The upper limb of *Homo sapiens* has evolved to explore as large a space as possible in which the hand can be positioned as a sensory and effector organ capable of performing innumerable complex, manipulative tasks. In comparison, freedom of movement is restricted in the lower limbs. Their robust construction ideally serves the support of the erect trunk, while giving resilience and power to the bipedal pattern of locomotion. When the normal anatomy of the limbs becomes deranged, treatment must aim to restore these respective functions.

This chapter introduces the anatomy of the limbs, emphasizing similarities, rather than differences. There is correspondence between the upper and lower limbs in their parts and segments, skeletal frame, and joints, as well as the disposition of muscle groups and the distribution of nerves and vessels. The explanation for these similarities is to be found largely in the phylogeny of tetrapods and in the morphogenetic and developmental events that transform a fin-shaped limb bud into a pentadactyl limb. The purpose of this chapter will be well served by integrating developmental considerations with a discussion of the anatomic design of the human limb.

SEGMENTS AND REGIONS OF THE LIMBS

The tetrapod limb, including that of the human primate, consists of two main parts: the **limb girdle** (*cingulum*) and the **free limb** (*pars libera*). The pectoral and pelvic girdles are incorporated into the trunk and link the free upper and lower limbs, respectively, to the axial skeleton. In the human, the pectoral girdle accounts for the squareness of the shoulders and camouflages the relatively narrow upper part of the cone-shaped rib cage. The pelvic girdle embraces the lower part of the abdominopelvic cavity and its skeleton supports the trunk in both the standing and the sitting position.

The free limbs are appendages of the trunk.* Each free limb is divided into three segments: 1) an **upper** or **proximal segment** (*stylopodium*), which corresponds to the arm and the thigh; 2) an **intermediate segment** (*zygopodium*), corresponding to the forearm and the leg; and 3) a **terminal segment** (*autopodium*), equivalent to the hand and the foot. The terminal segment itself consists of three subsegments: next to the intermediate segment is the carpus (wrist) or tarsus (ankle), followed by the midportion or *metapodium* of the terminal segment (metacarpus or metatarsus), from which project five digits.

The girdles and segments are organized around characteristic sets of skeletal elements that are homologous in the upper and lower limbs. Collectively, they constitute the **appendicular skeleton**. Adjoining parts and segments of the limbs are linked to one another by characteristic joints that also show correspondence in the upper and lower limbs. The parts of the limbs that contain some of these joints are spoken of as *regions* of the limbs (e.g., shoulder, hip, elbow, knee, wrist, and ankle). It will become evident from the next four chapters that several other regions are also described (e.g., axilla and calf). These need not be introduced here, however, as they have little bearing on the understanding of the basic plan of the limbs.

DEVELOPMENT

The Limb Bud

As soon as the trilaminar embryonic disk completes its folding, two pairs of limb buds begin to protrude from the ventrolateral parts of the newly established cylindrical body (Fig. 14-1A). Each limb bud is fin- or paddle-shaped. Its ventral and dorsal surfaces are separated by a distinct **preaxial** (cranial) and **postaxial** (caudal) **border** (see Fig. 14-1B). The borders meet in a ridge of thickened ectoderm that covers the apex of the bud (see Fig. 14-1; inset).

The elongation and development of the limb bud is governed by the interaction of this **apical ectodermal ridge** with mesenchyme contained in the limb bud. As a result, the segments of the limb become distinct within a few days of the appearance of the limb bud itself. In the terminal segment, the hand or foot plate forms (see Fig. 14-1C), and by the end of the eighth week, the digits become separated from one another by cell death in the web spaces.

The **mesenchyme** in the bud is an extension of lateral plate mesoderm, which elsewhere forms the body wall. In the limbs this mesenchyme gives rise to the bones, joints, cartilages, ligaments, tendons, and all types of fascias, as well as blood and lymph vessels. Cells or their processes invade this mesenchyme from four different sources: 1) **myogenic cells** from the somites fuse and aggregate into the muscles of the girdles and the free limbs; 2) **dermatomal cells** of the somites spread out beneath the limb ectoderm to form the dermis; 3) **axonal processes** of spinal cord and spinal ganglion neurons become organized into nerves characteristic of the limbs; and 4) **neural crest cells** differentiate into Schwann cells in the nerves and into melanocytes in the epidermis. Experiments have

* The NA term for a limb is *membrum* (Latin for *member*); the term *appendage*, and the more widely used term *extremity*, are contrived and obsolescent. The term *limb* is apt, precise, and free of ambiguity.

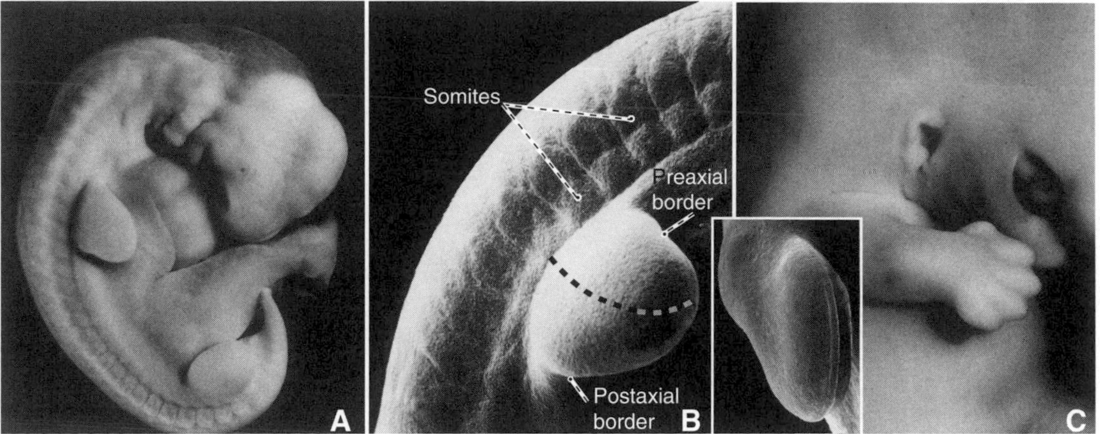

FIGURE *14-1.*
Development of the limbs: (A) The upper and lower limb buds have appeared in an embryo of 4 weeks; (B) The limb axis (*interrupted line*) and preaxial and postaxial borders are defined in the upper limb bud (inset the apical ectodermal ridge). (C) At 7 weeks the limb is cylindrical and the hand plate with its digital rays has been defined. (A and C, the Carnegie Collection, Human Developmental Anatomy Center, National Museum of Science & Medicine, Armed Forces Institute of Pathology; B, modified from Larsen WJ Human embryology. Churchill Livingstone, New York; 1993. Inset, Kelley RO. Early development of the vertebrate limb: an introduction to morphogenetic tissue interactions using scanning electron microscopy. Scanning Microsc 1985; 11: 827.)

shown that it is the limb bud mesenchyme that contains the information necessary for organizing primitive immigrant cells into the distinctive patterns that define the anatomy of limb muscles and nerves.

The Appendicular Skeleton

Condensations of limb bud mesenchyme form the skeletal primordia of the limb girdle and the segments of the free limb. All but one are soon replaced by hyaline cartilage, in which primary ossification centers appear. (The exception is the clavicle, which ossifies without chondrification.) Ossification begins during the 6th to 12th weeks of gestation in the bones of all segments except the carpus and tarsus, where it is delayed until after birth.

The skeleton of each **limb girdle** appears as three separate primordia, which become joined to one another to establish the bones and specialized joints of the girdle. One bone is placed dorsally and two ventrally (Fig. 14-2). The dorsal bone is the **scapula** in the pectoral girdle, and the **ilium** in the pelvic girdle. The ventral bones are the **clavicle** and **coracoid** (pectoral girdle), and the **pubis** and **ischium** (pelvic girdle).

In the free limb, the **upper segment** is built around a single long bone, represented by the **humerus** or **femur**, which defines the axis of the limb (Fig. 14-3A). There are two bones in the **intermediate segment** of each limb: the **preaxial bones** are the **radius** and **tibia**, and the **postaxial bones**, the **ulna** and **fibula.** In the **terminal segment**, primordia are established for sets of small bones in the carpal and tarsal subsegments. In the fully developed limb, these bones are arranged in two rows, proximal and distal, and are the homologues of the primitive pentadactylar limb. The **midportion** (*metapodium*) and **digits** of the terminal segment are made up of five rays of longitudinally linked bones. A **metacarpal bone** is lined up with the **phalanges** of a digit in the hand, and a **metatarsal bone** with the phalanges of a digit in the foot.

The digits are numbered from the preaxial border of the limb, the first being the thumb (*pollex*) or the big toe (*hallux*). There are two phalanges in the thumb and big toe, and three in each of the fingers and remaining toes. Although much shorter than the bones of the upper and intermediate segments, the phalanges, metacarpals, and metatarsals are typical long bones, whereas the bones of the carpus and tarsus are typical short bones (see Chap. 5).

Comparison of this developmental description of the appendicular skeleton with the anatomic arrangement of the bones in the fully developed limbs will indicate that the preaxial and postaxial elements retain their respective positions in the upper limb, but become reoriented relative to one another in the lower limb.

Orientation of the Limbs

Both pairs of limb buds grow ventrolaterally, more or less at right angles to the trunk (see Fig. 14-1 A and B). The **axis** of each limb runs through the bone of its upper segment and the second or third ray of bones in the terminal segment (see Fig. 14-3A). Although the limbs become cylindrical (see Fig. 14-1C), their preaxial and postaxial borders remain useful landmarks for understanding their subsequent rotation, innervation, and pattern of vascular supply. The **preaxial border** is indicated by the thumb and big toe, and the **postaxial border** by the little finger

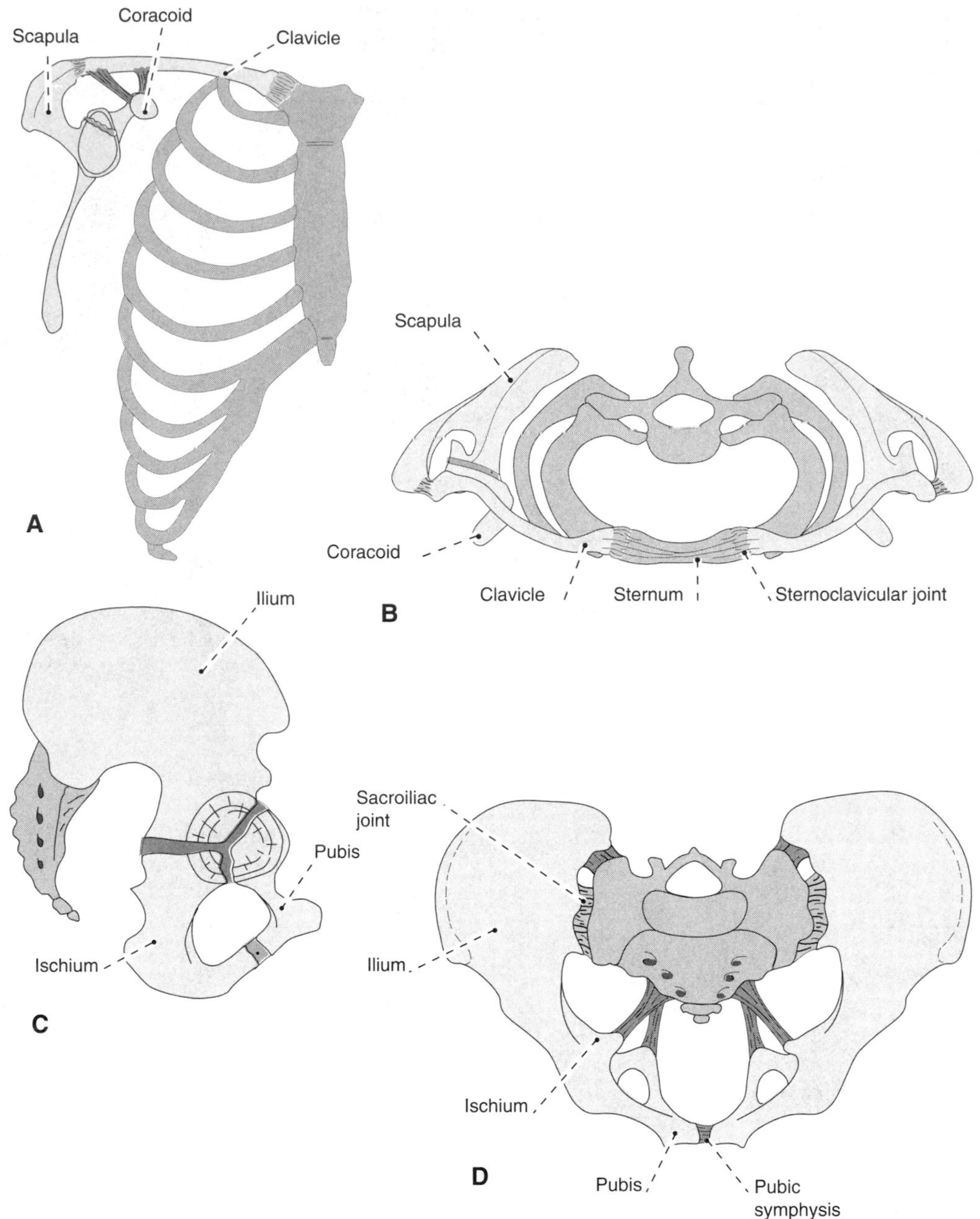

FIGURE 14-2.
Schematic representation of the bones, joints, and ligaments of (A and B) the pectoral girdle and (C and D) the pelvic girdle. The girdle skeleton is *white*, the axial skeleton is *shaded grey*, the cartilage *blue*, and synovial joints *pink*.

and little toe. The ventral and dorsal surfaces of the developing limbs, separated by these borders, will become the flexor and extensor surfaces, respectively.

Initially both the thumb and the big toe point cranially, the palmar and plantar surfaces of the hand and foot face medially, and the radius and tibia are positioned on the cranial side of the limb axis (see Fig. 14-3). In the adult, the upper limb can readily adopt this posture, but not the lower limb. Extension and adduction places the upper limb in the anatomic position: the limb axis parallels the axis of the trunk, the preaxial border is lateral and the postaxial border medial. Similarly, the preaxial bone of the intermediate segment (radius) lies lateral and the postaxial bone (ulna) medial. The flexor surface, including the palm of the hand, faces anteriorly and the extensor surface posteriorly (Fig. 14-4A).

The lower limb also becomes extended and adducted so that its axis is parallel with that of the trunk, but in addition, it rotates medially almost 180° (see Fig. 14-4A). This rotation places the big toe and the preaxial bone of the intermediate segment (tibia) medially, and the postaxial bone (fibula) and little toe laterally. The flexor surface, including the sole of the foot, faces posteriorly and the extensor surface anteriorly. Moreover, in the standing pos-

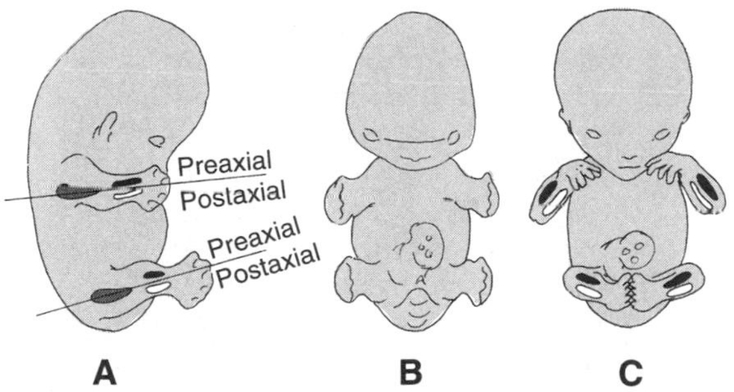

FIGURE 14-3.
(A) Development of the bones in the free limbs in relation to the limb axis: The bone primordium of the proximal segment is *stippled*, the preaxial bone of the intermediate segment *black*, and the postaxial bone *white*. (C and C) Successive stages of limb development from a ventral view before the limbs undergo rotation; the position of the preaxial and postaxial bones in the upper and lower limbs is still symmetric.

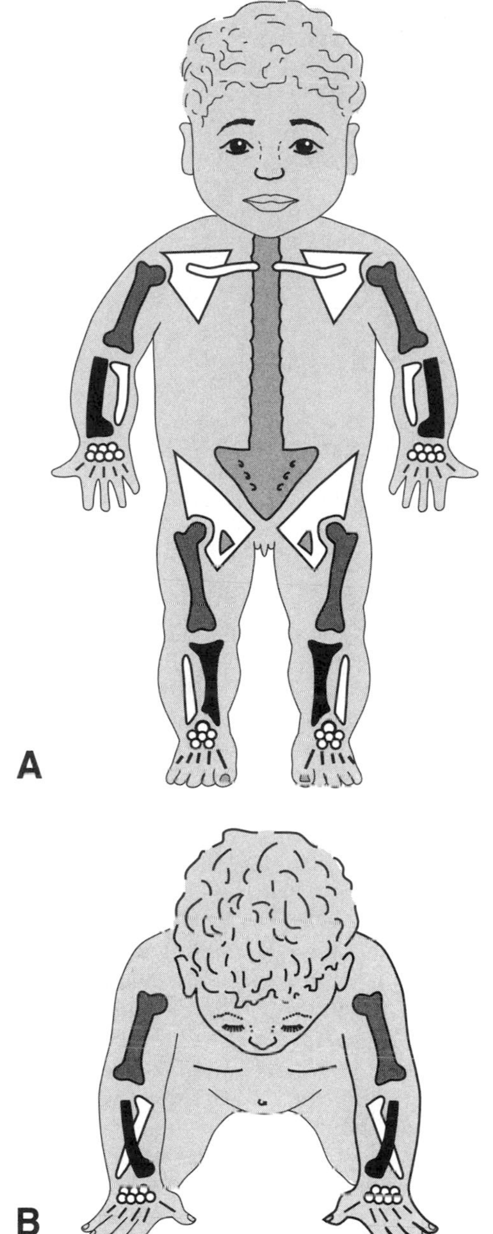

FIGURE 14-4.
Schematic representation of the orientation of the limbs after they have completed their developmental rotation, with bones of the appendicular skeleton indicated by *shading patterns* shown in the previous figure. Skeletal primordia of the terminal segment are also indicated, except for the phalanges. (A) extension and medial rotation of the lower limb has placed the preaxial border and preaxial bone medially, whereas in the upper limb the preaxial border is lateral. (B) placing the preaxial border medially in the upper limb requires crossing of the two bones of the intermediate segment (pronation).

ture, the axis of the foot assumes a right angle with the axis of the rest of the limb, placing the sole in contact with the ground (see Fig. 14-4A).

This reorientation adapts the lower limb for bipedal standing and weight bearing. The upper limb can assume a similar position, but to place the palm of the hand on the ground (creating a right angle between the axes of the forearm and hand), the radius has to cross over the ulna, placing the distal end of the preaxial bone medially (see Fig. 14-4B). The developmental rotation of the lower limb achieves this position without crossing the tibia over the fibula.

JOINTS AND FUNCTIONAL ADAPTATIONS

In contrast with the axial skeleton, in which many bones are connected by cartilaginous joints (symphyses between vertebrae, for example, and between pieces of the sternum), the appendicular skeleton is held together predominantly by synovial joints. Exceptions are the pubic symphysis, which joins the right and left pelvic girdles to one another at the front, and the fibrous joint that holds together the distal ends of the tibia and fibula at the ankle. Although there are many similarities between corresponding joints in the upper and the lower limb, there are also some differences that underlie remarkable adaptations for enhancing the mobility of the upper limb and providing stability in the lower limb. The similarities are most evident in the joints of the free limbs; the differences, on the other hand, are more evident in the joints of the girdles, as well as in the articulations of the girdles themselves with the axial skeleton.

Joints of the Girdles

In the pectoral girdle, the scapula and coracoid fuse with one another, but the clavicle remains a separate bone. A small joint between the scapula and the clavicle (acromioclavicular joint), and several ligaments that attach the scapula and coracoid to the clavicle, permit a great deal of mobility within the girdle. In addition, the girdle, as a whole, is free to move in relation to the axial skeleton (see Fig. 14-2A and B). This is made possible by the joint that links the clavicle to the manubrium sterni, the **sternoclavicular joint,** which allows a free range of movement for the clavicle. Indirectly, the mobility of the clavicle greatly enhances the mobility of the scapula, enabling it to slide freely on the rib cage. Unlike the pelvic girdle, the pectoral girdle has no direct connection with the vertebral column, nor with the pectoral girdle of the opposite side (except for the functionally unimportant interclavicular ligament). The length and the free mobility of the clavicle are the chief factors responsible for extending the operational sphere of the upper limb above the head.

By contrast, there is no movement between the bones of the pelvic girdle, and the girdle as a whole is securely linked to the axial skeleton by the massive **sacroiliac joints**, which themselves permit very little movement (see Fig. 14-2D). Up to the age of 15 to 16 years, the ilium, ischium, and pubis are united by hyaline cartilage, which ossifies thereafter, resulting in the robust coxal (hip) bone. The integrity of the bony ring formed by the sacrum and the coxal bones is assured by the **symphysis** between the pubes and is reinforced by strong ligaments that bind the coxal bones to the sacrum (see Fig. 14-2D). The bony pelvis formed in this manner surrounds the inferior part of the abdominopelvic cavity and supports the trunk on the lower limbs. It also absorbs, as well as transmits, propulsive forces between the lower limbs and the trunk.

Joints of the Free Limbs

A ball-and-socket joint links the bone of the upper segment of each free limb to the skeleton of the respective girdle (see Fig. 14-4A). Such a joint assures that the free limb, as a whole, can be flexed, extended, abducted, adducted, circumducted, and rotated. Owing to the specific anatomy of the **glenohumeral** and **hip joints**, however, the range of all these movements is far greater for the upper limb than for the lower limb. On the other hand, the strength and stability of the hip far exceed those of the joints that make up the shoulder.

There is a hinge joint between the upper and intermediate segments of each limb. Although there are differences in their specific anatomy, both the **elbow** and the **knee** function as hinges. The elbow joint involves the distal end of the humerus and both the preaxial and the postaxial bones of the forearm, whereas at the knee, in the human, the postaxial bone (fibula) has receded from the articulation (see Fig. 14-4A). As well as functioning as a hinge, the elbow joint participates in the movements of supination and pronation (see later discussion), movements that have no equivalents in the leg.

Preaxial and postaxial bones articulate with each other at both their proximal and distal ends. Reflecting the functional differences between the forearm and leg, the **radioulnar** and **tibiofibular joints** are quite distinct anatomically. The position of the tibia and fibula relative to one another is fixed, whereas the radius and ulna can move in relation to each other, rotating the hand through 180°. The proximal and distal radioulnar joints function as a pivot and produce *pronation* and *supination* of the hand. When the radius and ulna are parallel, the palm of the hand faces forward and the hand is supinated. Pronation positions the preaxial digit, the thumb, medially, and is achieved by crossing the radius over the ulna (see Fig. 14-4B).

Developmental rotation of the lower limb places the preaxial digit, the hallux, in a medial position. Owing to the fixed position of the tibia and fibula, this position cannot be reversed as it can in the upper limb. The movements of *inversion* and *eversion,* which turn the sole of the foot medially and laterally, respectively, are much more limited than, and do not correspond with, supination and pronation; they result from movements between the tarsal bones, rather than between the tibia and fibula.

Secure union between the tibia and fibula is critical for the stability of the **ankle joint**. The distal tibiofibular joint is a syndesmosis. It ties together the distal ends of the tibia and fibula, preventing their separation as they transmit the weight of the body to the talus at the ankle joint. The ankle is a hinge joint in which one tarsal bone articulates with both the tibia and fibula (see Fig. 14-4A). The corresponding joint in the upper limb is the **wrist** or **radiocarpal joint**. Here, three carpal bones articulate with the preaxial bone only, forming a condyloid joint that permits abduction, adduction, and circumduction, as well as flexion and extension.

Carpal and tarsal bones have several facets for articulating with their neighbors. The gliding motions of the **intercarpal joints** extend the range of movement at the wrist and give hand movements some of their suppleness. The largest of the **intertarsal joints** are specialized for inversion and eversion, movements necessary for adjusting the foot to uneven or sloping ground.

The **joints of the metacarpals** correspond closely to those of the **metatarsals**. Similarly, the **interphalangeal joints** of the fingers and toes are alike anatomically. The thumb is the most specialized digit. By virtue of the saddle-shaped articulation with the carpus, its metacarpal bone has greater freedom for movement than any other bone in the hand or foot. The ability to oppose the thumb to the fingers is critical for hand function, and has no equivalent in the foot.

MUSCULATURE

The anatomic and functional grouping of muscles and the distribution of nerves are similar in the upper and lower limbs. The pattern is established early in development.

The migration and proliferation of myogenic precursors derived from the somites keeps pace with the elongating limb bud. As soon as the cartilaginous primordia of the bones are formed, myogenic cells aggregate around them to form premuscle masses or blastemas. The central skeletal axis and preaxial and postaxial borders of the limb foretell a division of these blastemas into two compartments: a ventrally placed **flexor compartment** and a dorsally placed **extensor compartment** (Fig. 14-5). Under the influence of limb bud mesenchyme, ventral and dorsal premuscle masses become subdivided into the primordia of muscle groups and individual muscles, attain-

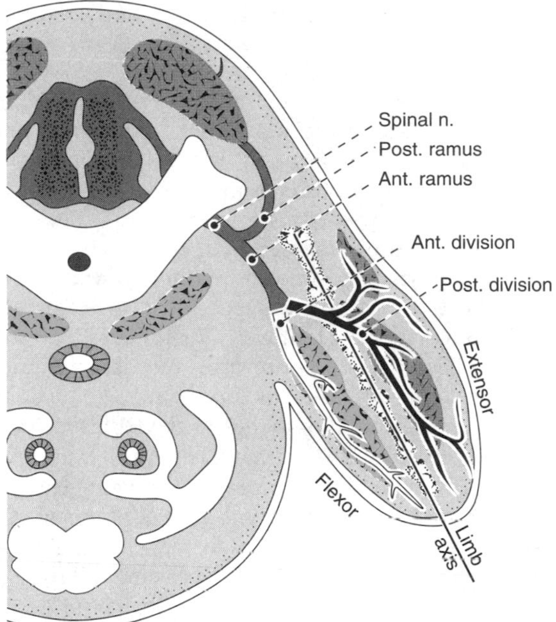

FIGURE 14-5.
Innervation of the limb bud shown in a schematic representation of a transverse section. To illustrate the basic innervation plan and compartmentalization of the limb bud, flexor and extensor compartments are demarcated by the limb bud axis, defined by the bone primordia. The anterior ramus of the spinal nerve bifurcates into an anterior division (*white*) and a posterior division (*black*). The flexor muscle mass is *pink*, the extensor muscle mass *purple*. Flexor and extensor surfaces of the limb bud, innervated by the respective divisions, are also indicated.

ing their definitive anatomy by the eighth week. Within the connective tissue framework, myoblasts proliferate, differentiate and fuse into multinucleate muscle fibers. This process is completed well before birth, and thereafter, the growth of muscles is achieved by increasing the dimensions of a fixed number of muscle fibers.

The development of muscle groups in different segments of the limb is correlated with the type of joint the muscles or their tendons will cross. If the joint permits movements other than flexion and extension, the ventral premuscle mass gives rise not only to flexors but also to muscles that can adduct and medially rotate a particular limb segment. Likewise, abductors and lateral rotators arise from the dorsal premuscle mass, along with the extensors. Some of the muscles formed in the limb bud migrate proximally and gain attachment to the axial skeleton. They produce limb movements relative to the trunk and include such muscles as the pectoralis major, latissimus dorsi, and gluteus maximus.

In the upper and lower limb, there are equivalent groups of muscles that produce flexion, extension, abduction, adduction, and rotation at corresponding joints. Comparing such groups calls for naming a lot of individual muscles, which is premature in this chapter. The same objective can be attained by explaining the innervation of corresponding muscle groups.

INNERVATION

Innervation of the Limb Bud

Mesenchyme at the root of the limb bud contains the information for guiding the axons of anterior gray column motorneurons and spinal ganglion cells into the limb bud. Invasion by the nerves formed from these axons parallels the advance of myogenic cells. By the seventh week the definitive nerves and plexuses are formed.

Only **anterior** (ventral) **rami of spinal nerves** enter the limbs, because the limb buds emerge from that part of the body wall which is served by the anterior, and not the posterior, rami (Fig. 14-5). The upper limb bud is invaded by the anterior rami of C-5 to T-1 spinal nerves and the lower one by those of L-2 to S-3 spinal nerves. At the root of the limb bud each anterior ramus splits into an **anterior** and **posterior division** (see Fig. 14-5). Nerve fibers within the anterior division are destined to innervate muscles in the flexor compartment and areas of dermis on the flexor surface of the limb. Those of the posterior division will innervate corresponding tissues of the extensor compartment. Before reaching these compartments, however, the nerve fibers for a particular limb pass through a **nerve plexus**, a network of nerves that forms at the root of the limb. The plexus permits some selective comingling of nerve fibers from several anterior rami, and their subsequent repackaging into specific, named nerves that grow distally into the limb.

Limb Plexuses and Segmental Innervation

Rearrangements of nerve fibers derived from the anterior rami destined for the limbs constitute two nerve plexuses. The **brachial plexus,** made up of C-5 to T-1 anterior rami, supplies the upper limb, and the **lumbosacral plexus,** made up of L-2 to S-3 anterior rami, supplies the lower limb (Fig. 14-6). As each plexus permits some intermingling of nerve fibers, a given anterior ramus may contribute nerve fibers to several named nerves. The innervation of both muscles and the dermis is established according to a strictly specified somatotopic pattern, the mechanism for which is not understood.

Muscular branches given off by the nerves of the limbs convey both motor and sensory fibers and enter the muscles they supply at anatomically specific sites (neurovascular hila) before the primordia of these muscles have fully formed or differentiated. Notwithstanding the mixing of axons in the nerves from several spinal cord segments, muscular branches of the nerves distribute axons to prime movers for distinct joints in a segmental pattern (see Chap. 13, Table 13-1; and Fig. 13-23). Moreover, whether an axon from a segment innervates a flexor or an extensor muscle, or a muscle in a proximal or distal segment of the limb, is also determined by the location of its cell body within the anterior gray column (see Fig. 13-10B).

The same is true of nerves destined for the skin. Cutaneous nerves reach the hand, for instance, before the

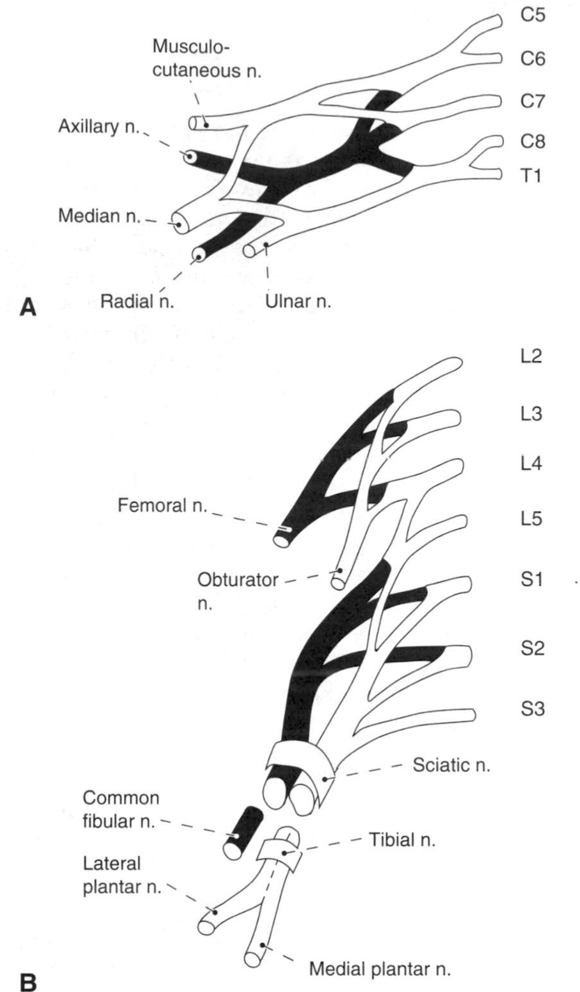

FIGURE *14-6.*
Schemes to illustrate the general plan of (A) the brachial plexus and (B) the lumbosacral plexus and the major nerves that issue from them. In each plexus, anterior rami of the contributing spinal nerves may split and recombine, but each ramus gives rise to an anterior division (*white*) and a posterior division (*black*). In each plexus two major nerves are formed by the posterior divisions, and three major nerves by the anterior divisions. The interruption in some branches of the lumbosacral plexus indicates that splitting off from a main, intermediary nerve trunk occurs some distance from the plexus.

webs between the digits regress. A given cutaneous nerve may carry axons from several spinal ganglia, but they are distributed to the dermis in a segmental manner. Such a pattern of innervation establishes the dermatomal map of the limbs (see Figs. 13-24 and 13-25).

Major Branches of the Plexuses

In each limb two major nerves are formed by the posterior divisions of its plexus. These nerves supply extensor, abductor, and lateral rotator muscles in the limb, and innervate the skin on its extensor surface. Similarly, three major nerves are formed by the anterior divisions of each plexus, and these nerves supply flexors, adductors, and medial rotators, as well as the skin on the flexor surface of the limb.

The major nerves derived from posterior divisions in the brachial plexus are the **axillary** and **radial nerves** (Figs. 14-6A and 14-7). The anterior divisions of the plexus are rearranged to form three major nerves: the **musculocutaneous**, **median**, and **ulnar nerves** (see Figs. 14-6A and 14-7). In the lumbosacral plexus the two major nerves formed from posterior divisions are the **femoral** and **common fibular** (*peroneal*) **nerves** (see Figs. 14-6B and 14-8). The three major nerves that carry the nerve fibers of the anterior divisions are the **obturator**, **medial plantar**, and **lateral plantar** nerves (see Figs. 14-6B and 14-8). The latter two nerves are terminal branches of the **tibial nerve**, and in the foot correspond to the median and ulnar nerves of the hand. This striking similarity between the major branches of the brachial and lumbosacral plexuses seems, at first glance, to be confounded by the binding together of the common fibular and tibial nerves into a large nerve trunk, known as the **sciatic nerve** (see Fig. 14-6B). From a functional point of view, however, the sciatic nerve is not a separate entity.

Comparison of the distribution of the major branches of the limb plexuses must take into consideration the developmental rotation of the lower limb. The flexor compartment, placed anteriorly in the upper limb, has rotated to the back in the lower limb; this brings the extensor compartment to the front.

The musculature of the limb girdles is supplied by minor branches of the plexuses. This nerve supply will be retained, even in those muscles that gain attachment to the vertebral column and move their sites of origin some distance from the girdle skeleton.

BLOOD SUPPLY

The main arteries and veins of the upper and lower limb are similar, although their precise development is more complex in the lower limb.

A plexus of capillaries develops in the mesenchyme of each limb bud. It is fed by branches of the aorta at the root of the limb bud. As the limb bud grows, the dynamics of flow define an **axial artery** along the limb. Vascular sprouting from the axial artery generates branches, several of which accompany the nerves of the limb. Although segments of the axial artery persist in both upper and lower limbs, the chief flow of blood proceeds through some of these branches, leading to regression of other segments of the axial artery. The resulting arterial pattern is described in the next section.

Blood drains through veins situated along the preaxial and postaxial borders of the limb bud. The **preaxial** and **postaxial veins** persist as the chief superficial veins of the fully developed limb, and serve as landmarks for its preaxial and postaxial borders. Deep veins also develop; they run along with the arteries.

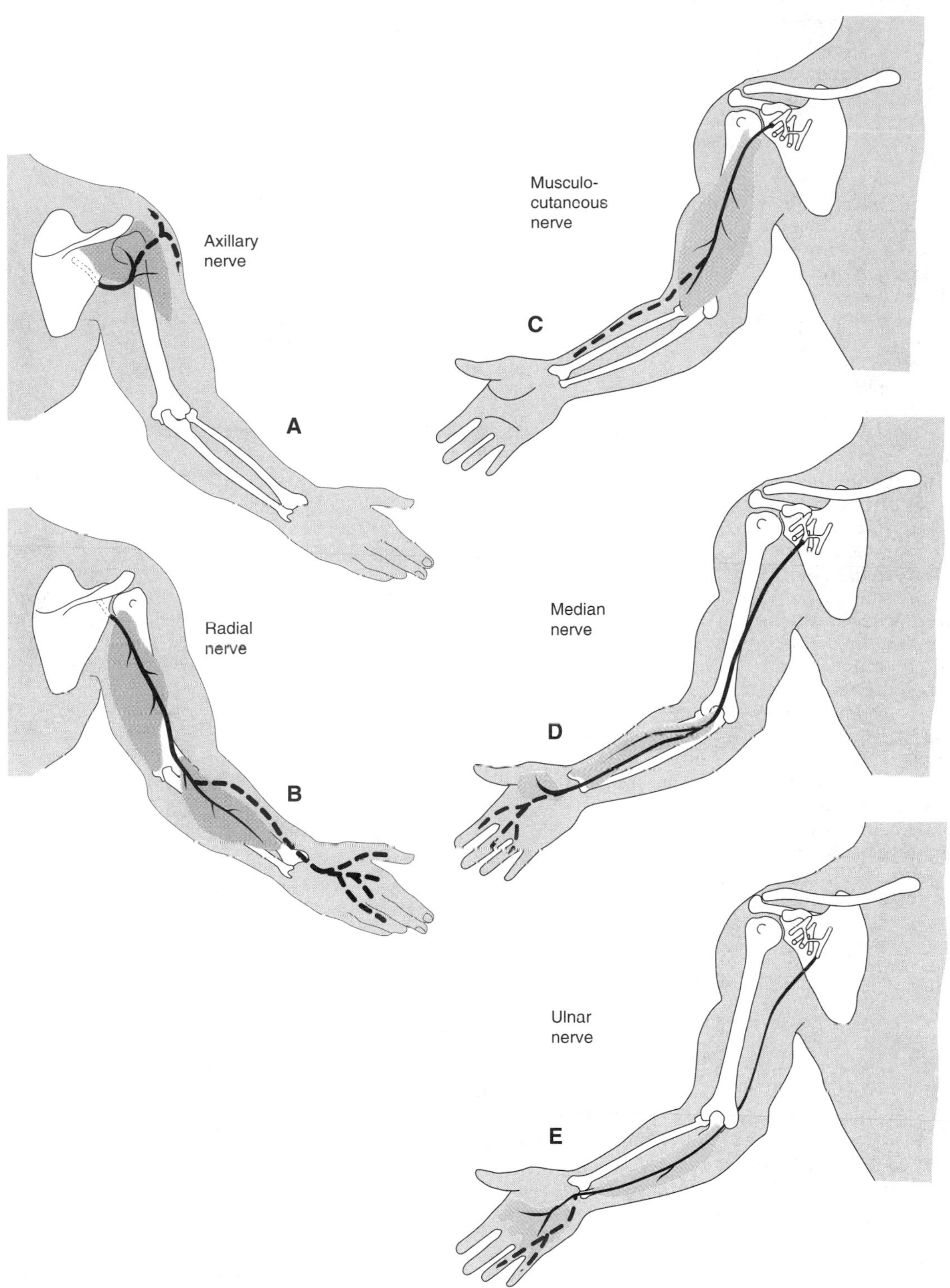

FIGURE *14-7.*
Distribution of the main nerves of the upper limb: The muscle mass innervated is *colored*; cutaneous branches are shown with *interrupted lines*. (A and B) the terminal branches of the brachial plexus formed by its *posterior* divisions (C, D, and E) those formed by its *anterior* divisions. (A) The axillary nerve supplies a powerful abductor of the shoulder (deltoid) derived from the extensor compartment, and the overlying skin. (B) The radial nerve supplies all the muscles in the extensor compartment of the arm and forearm, as well as much of the overlying skin. (C) The musculocutaneous nerve supplies the flexors of the elbow and an area of the skin on the preaxial border of the forearm. (D) The median nerve supplies the flexors of the wrist and the digits situated mainly in the preaxial two-thirds of the flexor compartment, and it is the chief sensory nerve of the palmar surface of the hand. (E) the ulnar nerve supplies the remaining flexors in the postaxial portion of the forearm, most of the small muscles in the hand, and the skin on the postaxial digits.

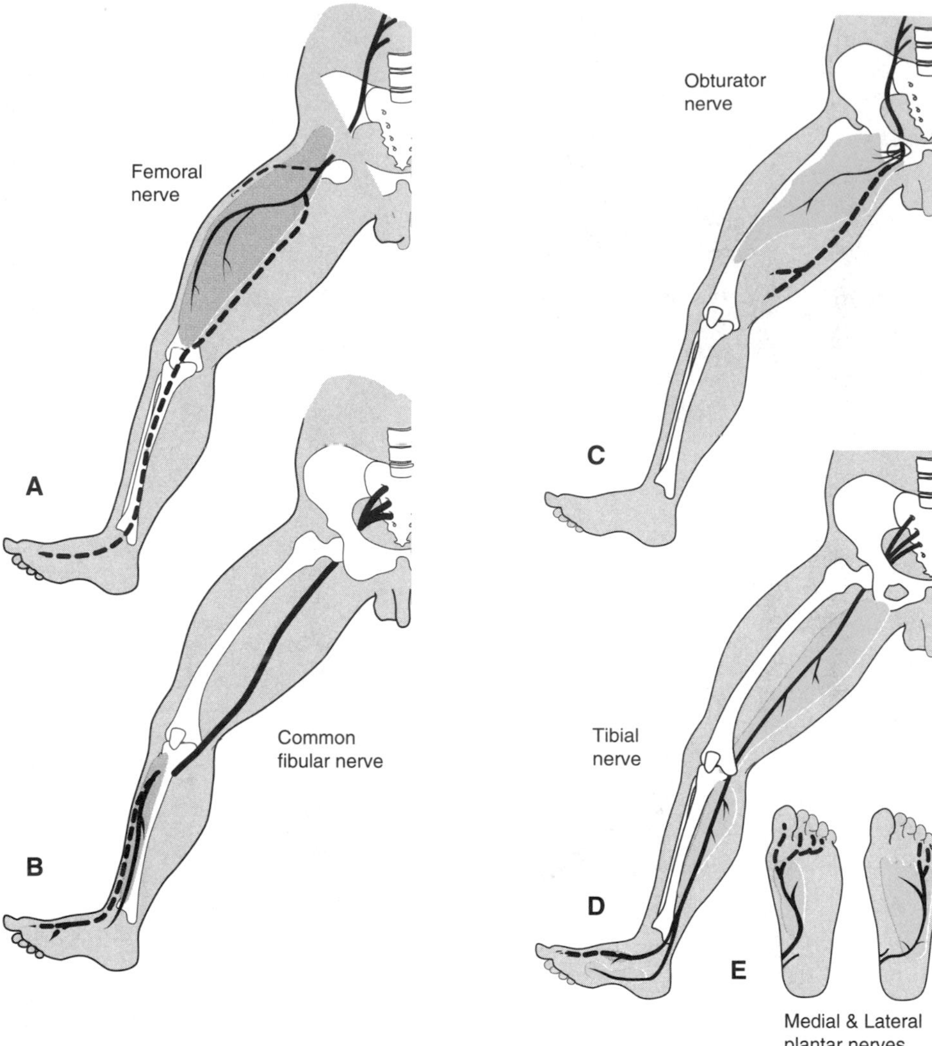

FIGURE *14-8.*
Distribution of the main nerves of the lower limb: The muscle mass innervated is *colored*; cutaneous branches are shown with *interrupted lines*. (A and B) The terminal branches of the lumbosacral plexus formed by its *posterior* divisions; (C, D, and E) those formed by its *anterior* divisions. (A) The femoral nerve supplies the extensor muscles of the knee (quadriceps) and a large area of skin; (B) the common fibular (*peroneal*) nerve is distributed to extensors of the ankle and toes and to the overlying skin; (C) the obturator nerve supplies the adductors of the thigh, which are derived from the flexor compartment, and the overlying skin; (D) the other two nerves are represented by the tibial nerve as far down as the ankle; the tibial nerve supplies the flexor muscles of the knee, ankle, and the toes in preaxial and postaxial halves of the flexor compartment. In the foot, its two components separate: the muscular and cutaneous branches of (E) the medial plantar and lateral plantar nerves resemble those of the median and ulnar nerves re-

Arteries

There is a single major arterial trunk along the proximal segment of each limb and two arteries in the intermediate segment. As these arteries enter the terminal segment, they link up with each other through a superficial and a deep anastomotic arcade or arch. The arterial arches give rise, in turn, to arteries that supply the digits (Fig. 14-9). The presence of the arches ensures that adequate arterial blood will reach the hand or foot, even if one of the proximal arteries is occluded. Anastomoses also exist around the major joints. A deep branch is given off in the proximal segment, and another in the intermediate segment, for the supply of the more deeply seated muscles and the bones. At the root of each limb, branches of the main artery establish an anastomosis with arteries of the trunk, thereby securing a potential alternative arterial route to the limb should the main artery become occluded.

The artery of the proximal segment in the upper limb is the **brachial artery** and that in the lower limb the **femoral artery**. The brachial artery is the continuation of the **axillary artery**, which itself is a continuation of the subclavian artery. The femoral artery is the continuation of the **external iliac artery**. Below the elbow, the brachial artery divides into the **radial** and **ulnar arteries**. Behind the knee the femoral artery assumes a different name (popliteal artery) and divides below the joint into the **anterior** and **posterior tibial arteries**. In the hand, the arterial arcades are the **superficial** and **deep palmar arches**, and in the foot, the **superficial** and **deep plantar arches**. Sets of **metacarpal** or **metatarsal arteries** arise from these arcades and terminate in the **digital arteries** of the hand and foot.

Of these named arteries, only the brachial artery corresponds to the original axial artery of the limb; all others have developed from branches of the axial artery. There are additional branches that have assumed functional importance. Deep structures of the proximal limb segment, for example, are supplied by the **profunda brachii** and **profunda femoris arteries**, given off by the brachial and femoral arteries, respectively. The deep branch in the forearm is the **interosseous artery** which divides into anterior and posterior branches for the supply of flexor and extensor musculature; the deep branch in the leg is the

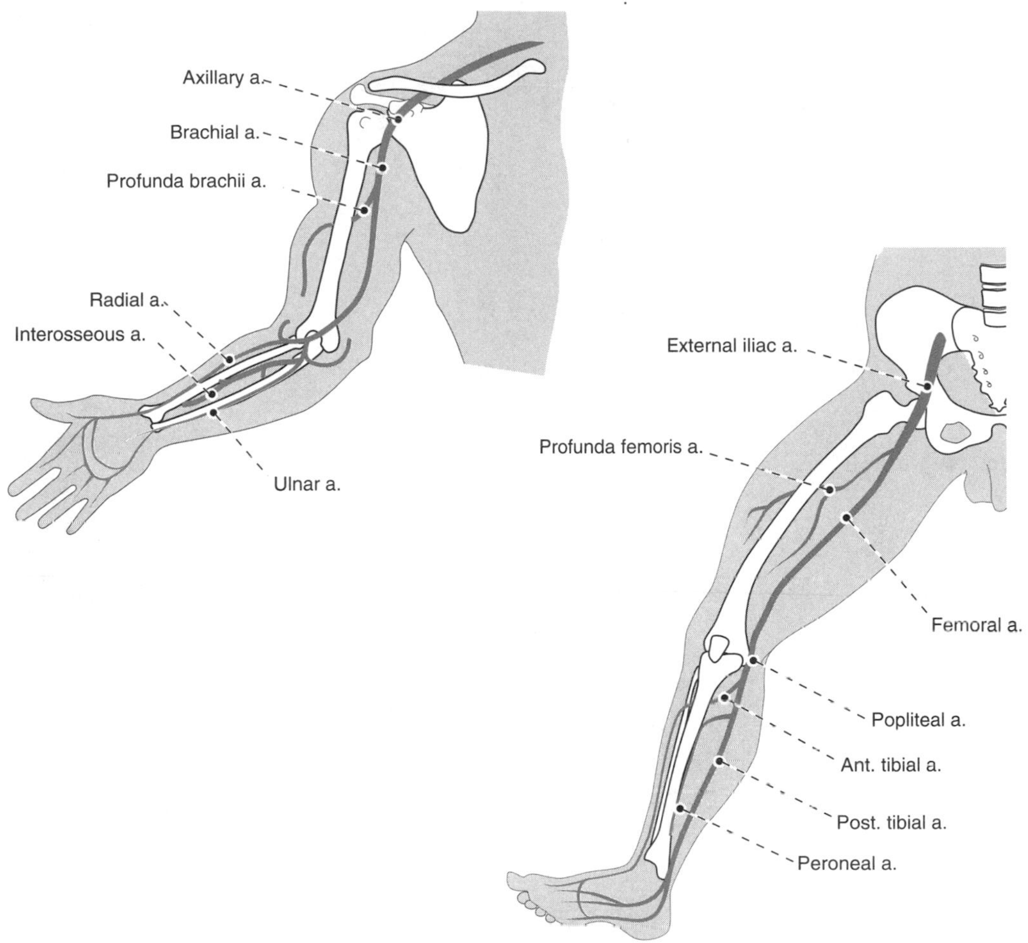

FIGURE *14-9.*
The basic plan of arterial supply in the upper and lower limbs (red lines).

peroneal artery. The interosseous and peroneal arteries correspond to portions of the axial artery that persist in the intermediate segment of each limb.

Veins

Pressure from the palm of the hand and sole of the foot diverts most of the venous blood to the dorsal aspects of the terminal segments, where the veins are visible through the skin. Blood is drained from each of these dorsal venous plexuses by superficial veins that run along the pre- and postaxial borders of the limb (Fig. 14-10).

The preaxial vein in the arm is the **cephalic vein** and in the leg the **long saphenous vein**; the postaxial veins are the **basilic vein** in the arm and the **short saphenous vein** in the leg. There are also **deep veins** that accompany the arteries in each limb. A deep vein may be single, but is frequently paired, the two members of the pair flanking the artery and being known as the **venae comitantes** of that artery (*comitans* is derived from the Latin *comes,* a companion). The two venae comitantes of the brachial artery merge to form the **axillary vein**, which receives the two superficial veins of the upper limb. The venae comitantes of the anterior and posterior tibial arteries form the **popliteal vein**, which becomes the **femoral vein** as it ascends with the femoral artery. The short saphenous vein empties into the popliteal vein, and the long saphenous vein into the femoral vein.

The veins of both the upper and the lower limb are interrupted by venous valves that prevent the retrograde flow favored by gravity. Centripetal flow in the veins is due to contractions of the limb musculature.

LYMPHATICS

Lymph drains from rich capillary plexuses of the hands and feet into lymphatic vessels that run predominantly alongside the superficial veins. A lymph node interrupts the flow at the elbow (trochlear node) and behind the knee (popliteal node). Lymph from deep structures is conveyed proximally in lymphatics that run alongside the arteries. All the lymph from the upper limb passes through groups of lymph nodes situated in the axilla. Lymph from the lower limbs is filtered by inguinal lymph nodes situated in the groin. Both the axilla and groin contain additional groups of lymph nodes that drain lymph from re-

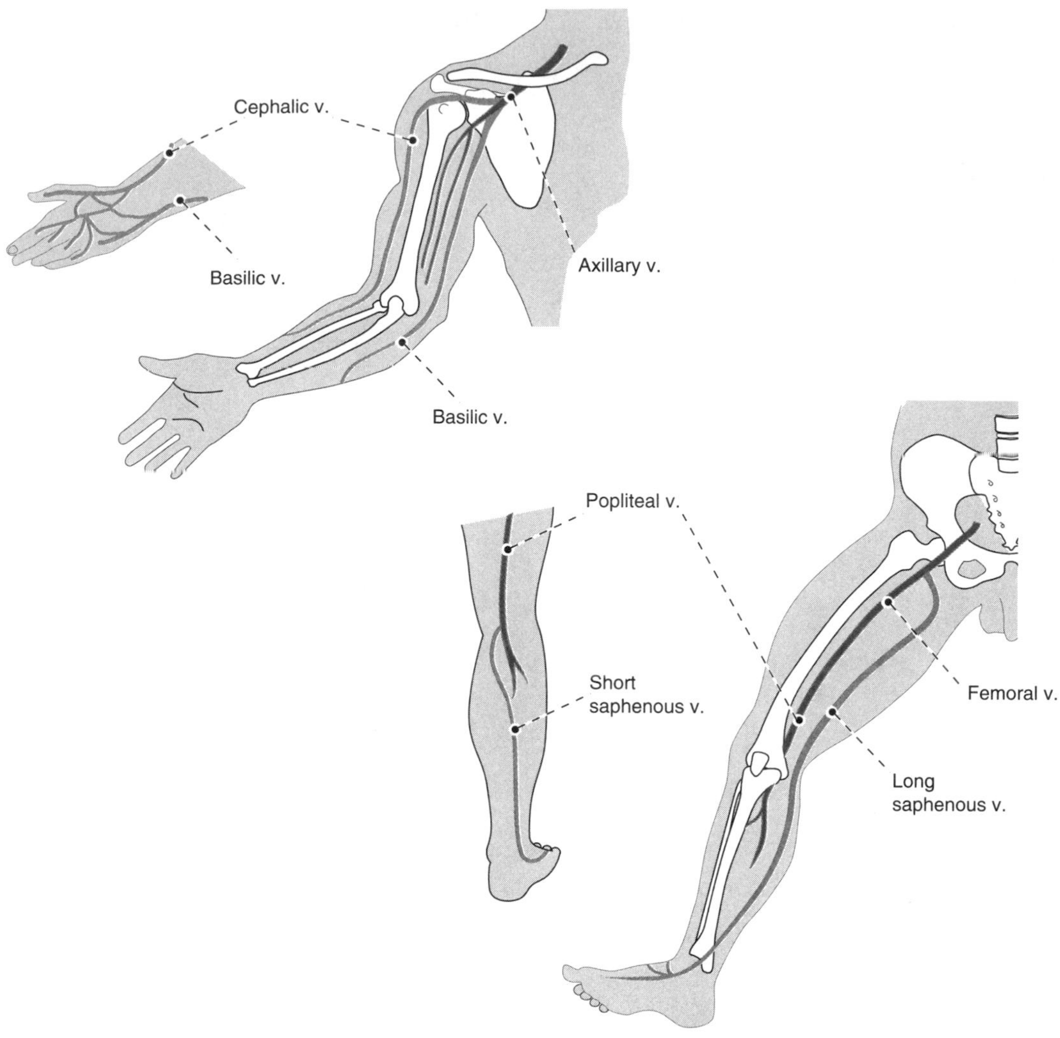

FIGURE *14-10.*
The basic pattern of venous drainage of the upper and lower limbs (blue): The dorsum of the hand shows the venous plexus and the commencement of the preaxial and postaxial veins, the continuation of which is shown on an anterior view of the forearm and arm. The dorsum of the foot is not illustrated. The preaxial and deep veins of the lower limb are shown in a medial view of the limb, and the postaxial vein in a posterior view of the leg.

gions of the trunk. Inflammation of the nodes gives rise to pain and tenderness and usually signifies infection in their drainage territory, which must, therefore, be scrutinized for evidence of infection. Painless enlargement of lymph nodes suggests neoplastic involvement caused either by metastatic spread from the drainage territory of the nodes or by primary neoplastic disease of the lymph nodes themselves.

RECOMMENDED READINGS

Bergsma D, Leuz W, eds. Morphogenesis and malformations of the limb. National Foundation-March of Dimes, Birth Defects: original article series, vol 13, no 1. New York: Alan R. Liss, 1977.

Carlson BM. Human embryology and developmental biology. St. Louis: Mosby-Year Book, 1994.

Chevallier A, Kieny M, Mauger A. Limb-somite relationship: origin of the limb musculature. J Embryol Exp Morphol 1977; 41: 245.

Duboule D. How to make a limb? Science 1994; 266: 575.

Gauffre S, Lasjaunias P, Zerah M. Sciatic artery: a case, review of literature and attempt of systemization. Surg Radiol Anat 1994; 16: 105.

Gray DJ, Gardiner G, O'Rahilly R. The prenatal development of the skeleton and joints of the human hand. Am J Anat 1957; 101: 19.

Keen JA. A study of the arterial variation in the limbs with special reference to symmetry of vascular pattern. Am J Anat 1961; 108: 245.

Lewis OJ. Evolutionary theories and comparative anatomy. In: Functional morphology of the evolving hand and foot. New York: Oxford University Press, 1989.

O'Rahilly R. Morphological patterns in limb deficiencies and duplication. Am J Anat 1951; 89: 135.
O'Rahilly R, Gardner E. The timing and sequence of events in the development of the limbs in the human embryo. Anat Embryol 1975; 148: 1.
O'Rahilly R, Müller F. Human embryology and teratology. New York: Wiley-Liss, 1992.
Rosse C. Basic structural plan and functional adaptation in the limbs. In: Rosse C, Clawson DK. The musculoskeletal system in health and disease. Hagerstown: Harper & Row, 1980.
Senior HD. The development of the arteries of the human lower extremity. Am J Anat 1919; 25: 55.
Swinyard CA, ed. Limb development and deformity: problems in evaluation and rehabilitation. Springfield: Charles C. Thomas, 1969.

Hollinshead's Textbook of Anatomy, by Cornelius Rosse and Penelope Gaddum-Rosse.
Lippincott-Raven Publishers, Philadelphia, © 1997.

CHAPTER 15

Pectoral Region, Axilla, and Shoulder

The pectoral region, axilla, and shoulder are those regions of the body that link the free upper limb to the trunk. The soft tissues of these regions are supported mainly by the bones of the pectoral girdle, the clavicle and the scapula (see Fig. 14-2), and by the upper end of the humerus. The chief aim of this chapter is to provide the anatomic information necessary for evaluating, both functionally and clinically, the movements of the pectoral girdle and the contribution of pectoral girdle mobility to the movements of the upper limb as a whole. These movements depend on three joints: the sternoclavicular joint, which allows movement between the pectoral girdle and the axial skeleton; the acromioclavicular joint, which unites the clavicle and the scapula; and the glenohumeral joint, which permits movement of the free limb relative to the pectoral girdle.

The muscles responsible for moving these joints can be classified into two major groups: those that move the shoulder girdle in relation to the axial skeleton; and those that move the free limb relative to the girdle skeleton. Muscles in the first group originate from the vertebrae, the sternum, or the ribs, and insert into the clavicle or scapula. Their actions displace the shoulder as a region or body part: the shoulder can be elevated or depressed, as well as thrust forward (protracted) or braced back (retracted). Each of these movements takes place at the sternoclavicular joint (see Fig. 14-2). Muscles in the second group originate from either the axial skeleton or the pectoral girdle (clavicle or scapula) and insert into the humerus. They act at the glenohumeral joint to cause movements of the free limb relative to the girdle. As this joint is of the ball-and-socket variety, several types of movement are possible, and the muscle groups that act on the joint are correspondingly diverse. They comprise flexors, extensors, abductors, adductors, and lateral and medial rotators.

Muscles in all these functional groups and the joints they serve receive nerve supply from the brachial plexus located in the axilla. The skin that covers these muscles, however, is innervated from a different source: namely, the segmental nerves of the trunk. The explanation for this seeming discrepancy lies in developmental events: the skin that is supplied by the brachial plexus is gradually drawn out during development to clothe the free limb, leaving the muscles of the pectoral region and shoulder to be covered by skin that, from a developmental standpoint, belongs to the trunk.

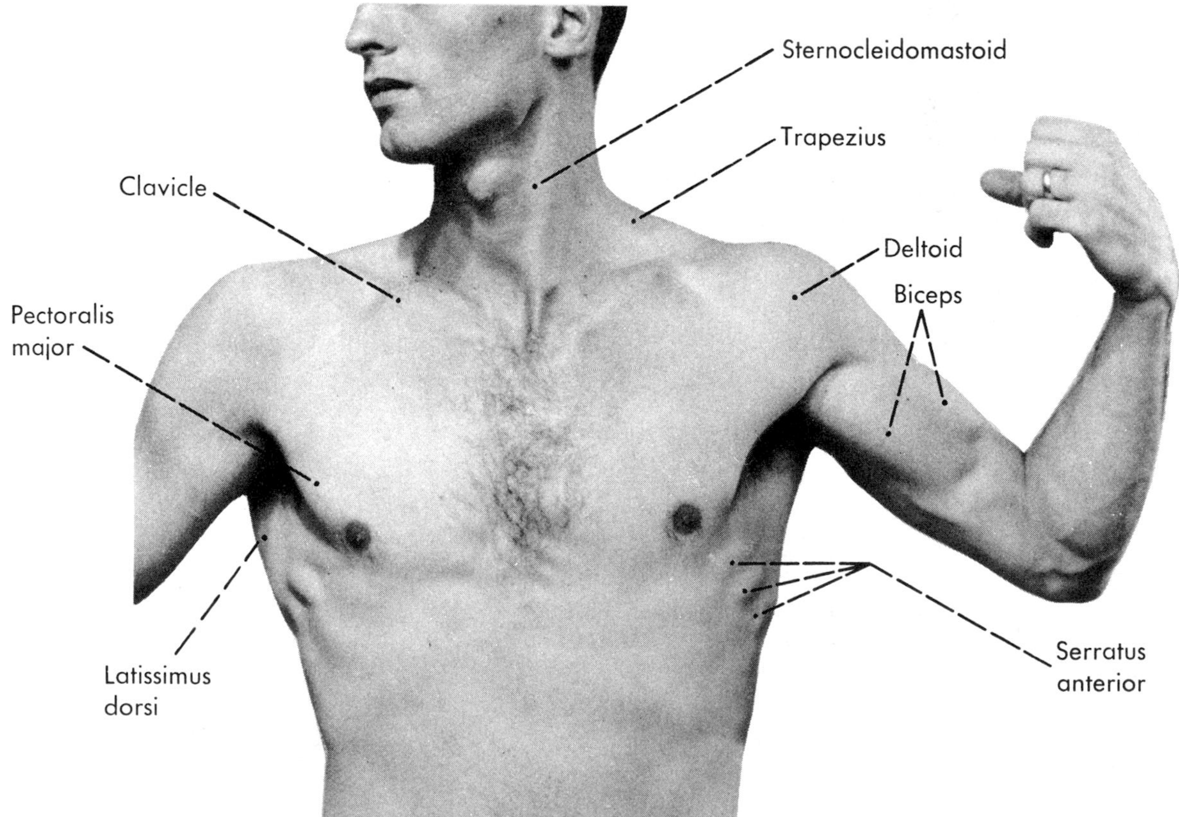

FIGURE *15-1.*
Anterior view of the thorax, shoulder, and upper limb, with several of the associated muscles contracted to make them more prominent.

The chapter begins with a general orientation to the regions, including their landmarks, cutaneous innervation and blood supply, and skeletal elements. Later sections describe the topography of individual regions. In each case the structures of importance are presented in an order that corresponds roughly to that in which they would be encountered during dissection of a cadaver. Included in these descriptions are the brachial plexus and the breast; understanding of the brachial plexus has implications not only for the pectoral and shoulder regions, but also for the free limb as a whole, and the breast in the female has particular clinical relevance. The final section of the chapter comprises a discussion of the joints and their movements, and the functional evaluation of the shoulder region.

GENERAL ORIENTATION

In addition to defining the parts and regions encompassed by the chapter as a whole, this section describes the surface landmarks, the general disposition of the major muscles, and the pattern of cutaneous innervation and blood supply over the entire area. It concludes with a description of the bones (clavicle, scapula, and humerus) and their associated ligaments.

Parts and Regions

The pectoral, shoulder, and axillary regions include the anterior, posterior, and lateral sides of the upper part of the trunk over a broad area surrounding the root of the upper limb (Figs. 15-1 and 15-2). On the anterior surface of the thorax, on each side of the sternum, is the **pectoral region** (*pectus,* Latin for chest, breast, or thorax), filled out by the pectoralis major muscle. The breast overlies the pectoralis major. In the male it is essentially limited to a small pigmented area of skin, but in the postpubertal female the breast makes up a subregion of its own, called the **mammary region**. Superiorly, the pectoral region is demarcated from the neck by the prominent clavicle. The slight hollow below the clavicle is the **infraclavicular fossa** or region, corresponding to the *supraclavicular fossa* in the neck. Inferolaterally, the pectoral region leads into the axilla or armpit over the rather fleshy border of the pectoralis major, which forms the **anterior axillary fold**.

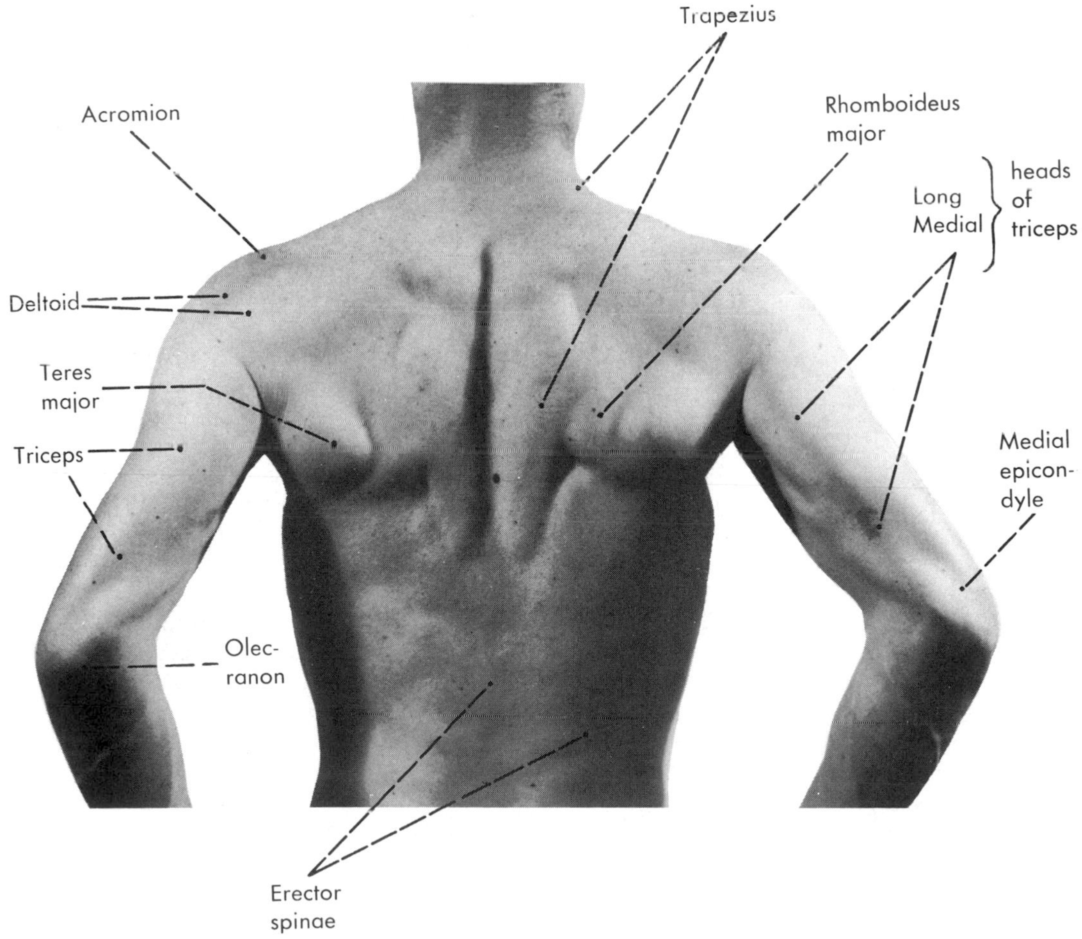

FIGURE 15-2.
Posterior view of the thorax, shoulder, and arm.

On the lateral aspect of the trunk, the armpit or **axilla** is the hollow between the rib cage and the postaxial border of the arm. The **shoulder region** is a convex area at the root of the limb, marking the junction of the limb's preaxial border with the neck. (For the definitions of "preaxial" and "postaxial" as applied to the borders of the limbs, see Chapter 14 and Figs. 14-1 and 14-3). There are several meanings to the term *shoulder*, however, and the lateral rounded part of the shoulder is perhaps better designated as the **deltoid region**, named after the muscle that occupies it. The bony prominence of the shoulder, above the deltoid region, is sometimes called the **acromial region**, named after the prominent process of the scapula.

On the posterior surface, the scapula and its associated muscles define the **scapular region**. This region is demarcated from the axilla posterolaterally by the **posterior axillary fold**, the fleshy substance of which is formed by the latissimus dorsi muscle (see Fig. 15-1). The muscles that move the bones of the pectoral girdle and the free limb span the length of the back, from skull to sacrum (see Fig. 15-23); they extend into the nuchal and occipital regions above, and the lumbar region or flank below.

Some of these anatomic regions may be subdivided by lines, defined in reference to landmarks. The **midclavicular line** runs vertically downward from the midpoint of the clavicle and divides the pectoral region into medial and lateral halves. The anterior and posterior axillary folds may be used as starting points for vertical lines projecting downward, the anterior and posterior axillary lines; midway between them is the **midaxillary line**. All are useful for locating normal anatomic structures as well as lesions and other physical signs.

Landmarks

In addition to the bony and muscular surface features just described, several bony points serve as important landmarks. Moreover, some additional muscles provide useful reference points during both dissection and the physical examination.

Bony Landmarks. The palpable bony points of the clavicle, scapula, and proximal end of the humerus are included in the general description of the bones in the concluding part of this section; those of the vertebral column relevant to the examination of the back and scapular regions are discussed in Chapter 12. The only remaining bones to be noted are the sternum and the ribs. The **sternum** or breast bone, consisting of the manubrium, body, and xiphoid process (see Fig. 19-3), lies subcutaneously in the anterior midline and is palpable throughout its length. Above the upper margin of the **manubrium** is the **jugular notch**. The junction of the manubrium with the **body** of the sternum forms a palpable ridge, the **sternal angle.** The third piece of the sternum, the **xiphoid process** (*xiphoid;* Latin for sword-shaped) is linked to the body at the **xiphisternal joint** (see Fig. 19-3), the level of which marks the lower extent of the pectoral region. The **ribs** can be felt as they approach the sternum on each side. The most relevant landmarks are the second rib, which joins the sternum at the level of the sternal angle, and the sixth rib; its union with the sternum is on level with the xiphisternal joint. The ribs are also palpable and often visible in the axilla.

Muscles. The contour of the neck is formed by the trapezius muscle (see Fig. 15-1), which may be pinched by grasping the "web" of the neck between finger and thumb. The pectoralis major, most visible in a muscular male, can be similarly identified in the anterior axillary fold, and the latissimus dorsi in the posterior axillary fold (see Fig. 15-1). Concealed by the pectoralis major are the pectoralis minor and the rather inconsequential subclavius (see Fig. 15-15). These last three are the muscles of the *pectoral region.*

The prominent deltoid (see Fig. 15-1) conceals a number of the muscles of the *scapular region* (see Fig. 15-28). Deep to the trapezius, three muscles attach to the medial border of the scapula: the levator scapulae and the rhomboid major and minor (see Figs. 15-2 and 15-23). The teres major and minor are located in the posterior axillary fold, along with the latissimus dorsi (see Figs. 15-2 and 15-23). The medial wall of the *axillary region* is formed by the serratus anterior (see Figs. 15-1 and 15-25). The muscles of the upper limb that extend into the *nuchal* and *lumbar regions* are the trapezius and latissimus dorsi, respectively (see Fig. 15-23). Muscles that descend into the *arm* from the shoulder region are the coracobrachialis, two heads of the biceps, and the long head of the triceps. These muscles are demonstrable in the arm (see Chap. 16).

Cutaneous Nerves and Vessels

Nerves

The area of skin that covers the pectoral, axillary, shoulder, and scapular regions extends to the midline in both the front and the back. Its anterior limit runs from the jugular notch to the xiphisternal joint, and its posterior limit from the external occipital protuberance on the skull to the sacrum. The inferior limit is the sixth rib anteriorly and, beyond the midaxillary line, the iliac crest. Cutaneous branches derived from both anterior and posterior rami of a large number of spinal nerves furnish the sensory innervation of the skin over this extensive area. They all run in superficial fascia (*tela subcutanea*) to reach the dermis. Because their distribution is segmental, they provide one of the means for segmental evaluation of progressive disorders of the spinal cord. Knowledge of their distribution is necessary for drawing correct inferences from the evaluation of cutaneous sensation.

Branches of Anterior Rami. The anterior rami of spinal nerves are the source of most of the cutaneous innervation of this area (Fig. 15-3). Of particular relevance are the supraclavicular nerves, the upper lateral cutaneous nerve of the arm, and cutaneous branches of the intercostal nerves, all of which are derived ultimately from anterior rami of cervical and thoracic nerves.

The **supraclavicular nerves** (branches of C-3 and C-4

anterior rami) are given off by the cervical plexus (see Fig. 30-16). They descend over the clavicle, supplying the skin over it, and continue over the upper two intercostal spaces in the pectoral region (see Fig. 15-3). Their territory of supply extends laterally over the acromion and upper part of the deltoid muscle. Farther laterally, the adjoining area of skin over the deltoid is supplied by the **upper lateral cutaneous nerve of the arm**, a branch of the axillary nerve, itself a branch of the brachial plexus. This cutaneous nerve contains C-5 fibers which, together with C-4 fibers carried by the supraclavicular nerves, account for the distribution of the C-4 and C-5 dermatomes over the shoulder region (see Figs. 13-24 and 13-25). This region is a common site for referred pain from the shoulder joint and from some internal organs which, though located some distance away, share sensory innervation from these segments. The diaphragm, together with the pleura and peritoneum that cover its surfaces, is an important example of such an organ.

Below the level of the sternal angle, the skin in the pectoral and axillary regions is supplied by branches of **intercostal nerves**, themselves the anterior rami of thoracic spinal nerves. Foerster's dermatomal maps show an abrupt transition at about this level: the C-4 dermatome adjoins the T-2 dermatome, the intervening dermatomes (C-5 to T-1) being absent from the anterior surface of the trunk and found instead in the free limb (see Chap. 13 and Fig. 13-24). Cutaneous innervation below this level, therefore, begins with the T-2 spinal segment and continues through the T-7 segment. T-2 to T-7 sensory fibers are distributed to the skin by two sets of branches from these intercostal nerves: lateral cutaneous branches, which emerge along the side of the trunk through the serratus anterior muscle; and anterior cutaneous branches, which pierce the pectoralis major near the sternum and represent the terminations of these intercostal nerves (see Fig. 13-22). The **lateral cutaneous branches**, or **nerves**, divide again into posterior and anterior branches; the posterior ones extend over the posterior axillary fold into the back, whereas the anterior ones run forward to the midclavicular line (see Fig. 15-3). The **anterior cutaneous branches**, or **nerves,** also divide: their lateral branches reach the midclavicular line, at which their territory of supply overlaps that of the lateral cutaneous nerves, and their medial branches reach the midline. One exception to this pattern concerns the second intercostal nerve: its lateral cutaneous branch, known as the *intercostobrachial nerve* (see Fig. 15-21), does not divide again and is distributed to the skin of the axilla and the arm. In the female the subbranches of both the anterior and lateral cutaneous nerves supply the breast and are sometimes referred to as the *medial and lateral mammary nerves*, respectively.

Branches of Posterior Rami. The posterior rami of spinal nerves, like the anterior ones, terminate in cutaneous branches. Typically, a posterior ramus turns toward the back and enters the extensor musculature of the spine, where it divides into a medial and a lateral branch, both of which supply the spinal extensors (see Fig. 13-22). One of these branches then goes on to supply the skin by piercing (without innervating) the superficial muscles that overlie the spinal extensors. In the cervical and upper thoracic regions it is the medial branch that takes this course, whereas lower down it is the lateral branch. In ei-

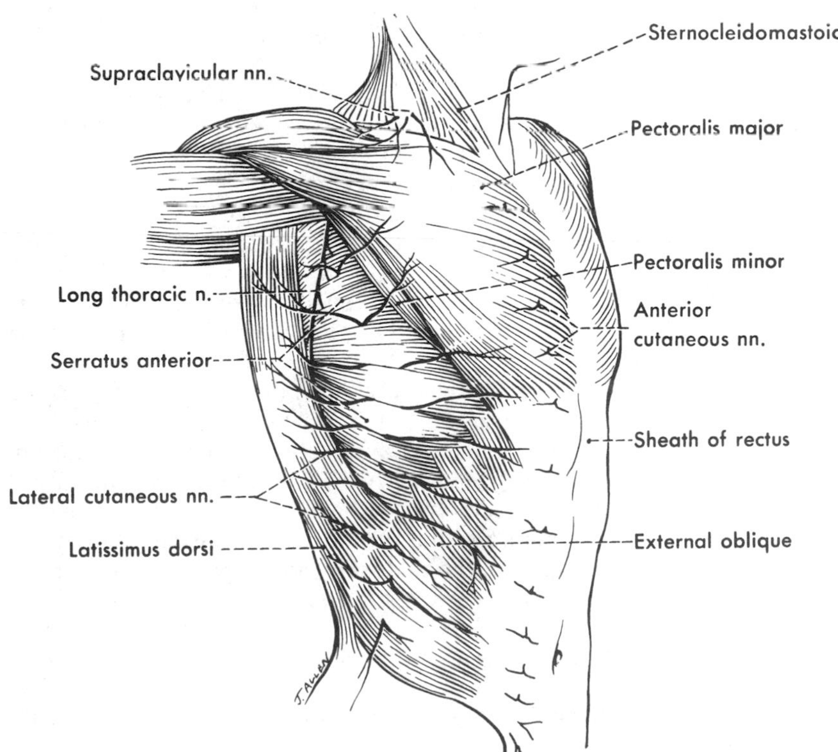

FIGURE *15-3.*
Cutaneous branches of anterior rami of spinal nerves that supply the pectoral, axillary, and shoulder regions.

ther event, on reaching the superficial fascia, the nerve divides once more into a small medial and a larger lateral subbranch. It is the latter subbranches that are responsible for innervating the skin segmentally on the back of the neck, over the scapula, and below the scapula as far down as the iliac crest. In the latter two regions they overlap the territory supplied by the lateral cutaneous branch of intercostal nerves.

Testing the posterior rami can assist in localizing a lesion to a particular spinal nerve or its anterior ramus. For instance, compression of T-1 spinal nerve in the intervertebral foramen, or of T-1 anterior ramus as it arches over the first rib, would result in paresthesia (abnormal sensation) in T-1 dermatome of the forearm and wasting of muscles in the hand (see Figs. 13-23 through 13-25). Normal sensation in the posterior part of T-1 dermatome, coupled with normal electromyographic activity in the segment of the spinal extensors innervated by T-1, would indicate that the spinal nerve is intact and the lesion must be peripheral to it.

Unfortunately, from the viewpoint of testing, not all posterior rami reach the skin of the back. The cutaneous branch of the first cervical nerve, for example, is lacking. The cutaneous branch of C-2 posterior ramus forms the **greater occipital nerve** (see Fig. 12-30), and that of C-3 the **third occipital nerve**; both ascend to supply skin on the back of the skull. Furthermore, whereas the cutaneous branches of C-4, C-5, and C-8 posterior rami do serve the skin in the back of the neck, those of C-6 and C-7 do not reach the skin at all. The cutaneous branches of the thoracic posterior rami innervate the rest of the skin; those of T-3 in the region of the scapular spine, and those of T11-12 just above the iliac crest. The upper lumbar and upper sacral posterior rami supply the skin of the buttocks (see Fig. 18-7). The lower lumbar ones do not have a cutaneous distribution and the lower sacral and coccygeal posterior rami pass to skin over the lower end of the sacrum and the coccyx.

Vessels

Arteries and veins that supply the skin correspond largely to the cutaneous nerves and run with them in the superficial fascia. Anteriorly, the *internal thoracic artery* (see Fig. 19-11) has *perforating branches* that pierce the pectoralis major along with the anterior cutaneous branches of the intercostal nerves. Similar vessels accompany the anterior branches of the lateral cutaneous nerves. As a rule, however, these vessels are rather small. Larger branches are given off from the *lateral thoracic artery* that descends from the axillary artery close to the lateral border of the pectoralis major (see Fig. 15-17B) and sends its branches forward to anastomose with those of the anterior perforating arteries. Veins follow a similar course.

The superficial arteries of the back are segmental, like the nerves, and are derived from three sources. First are the *dorsal branches* of *intercostal* and *lumbar arteries* that accompany posterior rami (see Fig. 13-16) and supply the vertebral column and the musculature of the back; they reach the skin along with the nerves. Second, in the cervical region, branches to the back are given off by the longitudinally running *vertebral* and *deep cervical arteries*. Lastly, the *lateral cutaneous branches* of the *intercostal arteries* send their posterior subbranches over the posterior axillary fold, in the company of the corresponding nerves, and supply the lateral part of the scapular region and the flank. Veins accompany the three groups of arteries.

Lymphatics pervade the superficial fascia of the pectoral region, passing toward the axilla and the sternum. Most important are those that drain the female breast; they are described later with that organ. Lymphatics of the back, from as far down as the iliac crest, drain to the posterior group of axillary lymph nodes.

Bones and Associated Ligaments

Although the humerus belongs to the free limb, rather than the limb girdle, it is included in this chapter, along with the clavicle and scapula, because learning the anatomy of its proximal end is indispensable for understanding several topics in this chapter.

Clavicle

The collar bone, or clavicle, is the anterior bone of the pectoral girdle and lies subcutaneously at the junction of the neck with the thorax (see Figs. 15-1 and 14-2). Along most of its length it is readily palpable. The **body** or shaft, more or less cylindrical, expands at its medial or **sternal end** (Fig. 15-4), terminating in a sternal articular facet. The lateral or **acromial end** is flattened, and on its tip presents the small acromial articular facet. Both sternal and acromial facets are covered by fibrocartilage. Much of the smooth *superior surface* of the bone is bare, muscles attaching mainly along its anterior and posterior rounded borders. On the *inferior surface* of the sternal end there is a roughened impression for the attachment of the *costoclavicular ligament*; the acromial end, likewise, bears a **conoid tubercle** and a **trapezoid line** for the attachment of ligaments of corresponding names.

In its medial two-thirds, the clavicle is convex anteriorly as it arches over the brachial plexus and axillary vessels; the lateral third is concave anteriorly. Fractures caused by indirect violence (sustained, for instance, during a fall on an outstretched hand) usually occur along the middle third.

The vulnerability of this region is due to not only the change in curvature, but to the absence of ligaments. Both the medial and lateral thirds of the bone, by contrast, are anchored by ligaments: two **coracoclavicular (conoid** and **trapezoid) ligaments** fix the lateral third, and the medial third is bound to the first rib and costal cartilage by the two laminae of the **costoclavicular ligament** (see Fig. 15-32). Both pairs of ligaments slant posteriorly as they approach the clavicle. Thus, when the clavicle is elevated, putting the ligaments on a stretch, it automatically rotates posteriorly. The movement is easily appreciated by placing the hand on the clavicle during abduction of the arm.

Ossification. The clavicle is an unusual bone in several

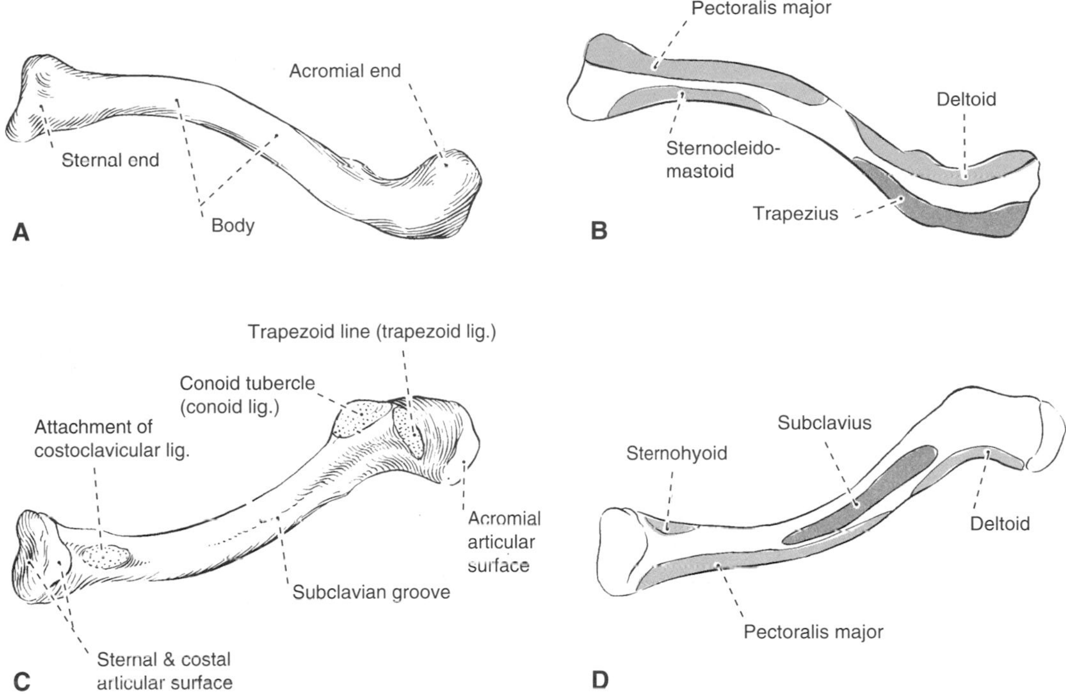

FIGURE 15-4.
(A and B) Superior and (C and D) inferior surfaces of the clavicle. Muscle origins are shown in *red*, insertions in *blue*.

respects. Two primary ossification centers appear and fuse in the mesenchymous primordium of the bone, preceding ossification and even chondrification in other parts of the skeleton. Although the bone develops largely by intramembranous ossification, both ends become cartilaginous. An epiphysis appears at the sternal end between the 18th and 20th years of life and is the last of all epiphyses in the body to unite with the shaft of its bone, at about the age of 25 years. A small epiphysis also appears at the acromial end in the 20th year and soon unites with the shaft.

The clavicle is present only in those vertebrates that use the forelimb predominantly for prehension, rather than for locomotion. It is believed to be, at least in part, a dermal bone, derived from the exoskeleton. Only a part of it (probably represented by one of its ossification centers) is likely to correspond to the pubis in the pelvic girdle (see Fig. 14-2). Failure of the two centers to unite results in *clavicular dysostosis*, which may be a component of more generalized defects in membranous bone formation (*cleidocranial dysostosis*), and may include partial or complete absence of the clavicle.

Scapula

The scapula, or shoulder blade, is the posterior component of the pectoral girdle skeleton (see Fig. 14-2). It is a flat, triangular bone that lies with its anterior surface against the thoracic cage. Although it is largely buried in muscles, its movements can readily be observed from the back. The scapula has costal and posterior surfaces; medial, lateral, and superior borders; and superior, inferior, and lateral angles (Fig. 15-5)

The **costal surface** is slightly concave, most of it occupied by the *subscapular fossa*, which gives attachment to the subscapularis muscle. The **posterior surface** is divided by the prominent scapular spine into a *supraspinous fossa* and an *infraspinous fossa*, each filled by a muscle of corresponding name. The **spine** begins as a small triangular area, the *base of the spine*, at the medial border of the scapula and continues laterally and upward, terminating in the freely projecting **acromion** (Greek: *acro* meaning extremity or tip; *omos* meaning shoulder), which forms the tip of the shoulder. The sharp forward turn of the acromion is marked posterolaterally by the *acromial angle*. The medial border of the acromion presents a small facet for articulation with the clavicle. Beneath the acromion, the supraspinous and infraspinous fossae communicate with each other around the thickened lateral edge of the scapular spine.

The **medial border** more or less parallels the spines of the vertebrae; it is often called the *vertebral border*. Several muscles attach to its anterior and posterior aspects (see Fig. 15-5). It meets the **lateral border** at the **inferior angle**. The lateral border is buried in muscles. The **superior border**, the shortest of the three, is quite sharp, but inaccessible to palpation. It meets the medial border at the **superior angle** and terminates laterally by forming the *scapular notch* (*incisura*) at the base of the coracoid process. The notch is roofed over and converted into a foramen by the *superior transverse scapular ligament* (sometimes ossified),

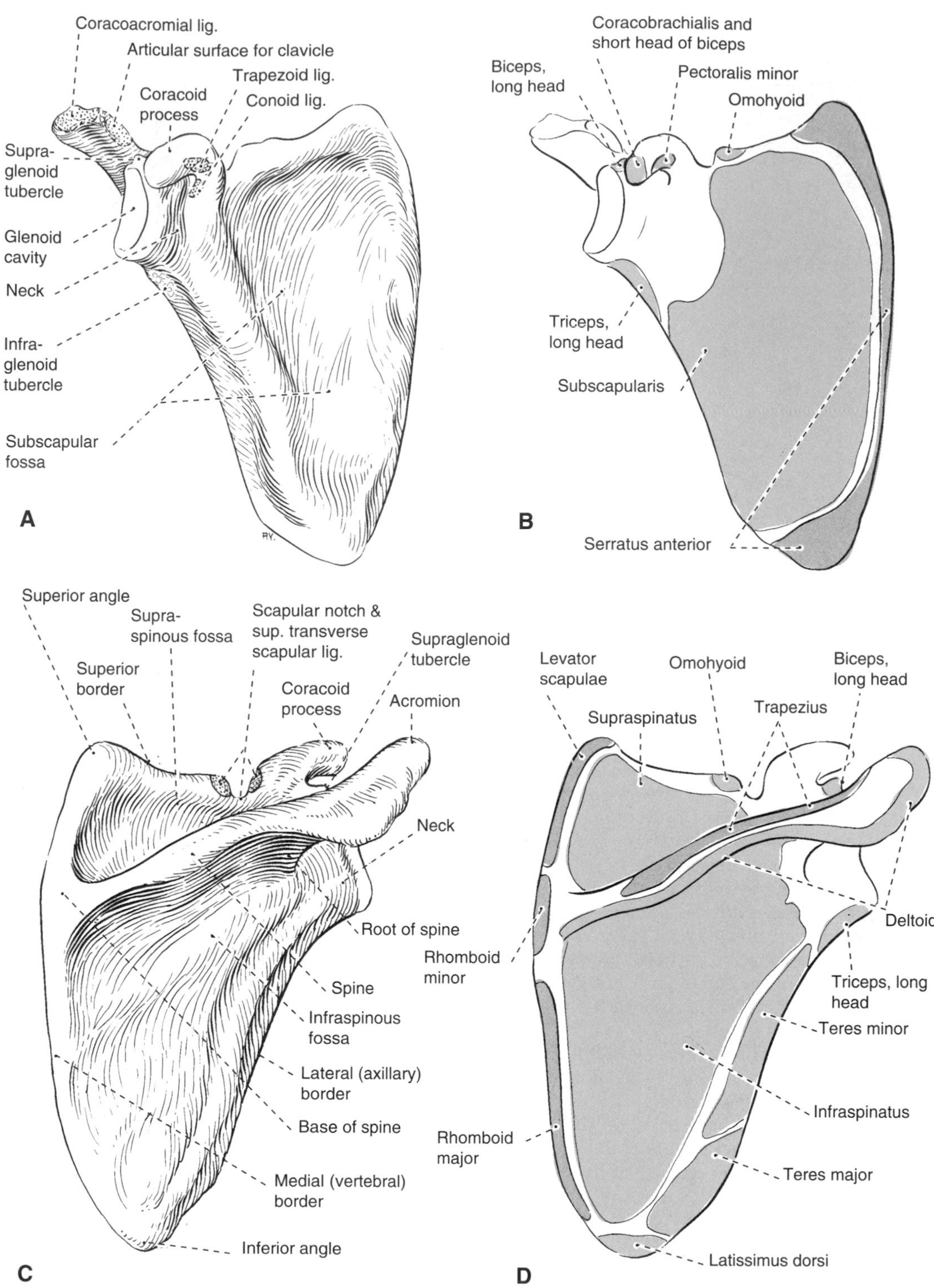

FIGURE *15-5.*
(A and B) Costal and (C and D) posterior surfaces of the scapula: Muscle origins are shown in *red*, insertions in *blue*.

through which passes the suprascapular nerve (see Fig. 15-31).

The **coracoid process** (Greek: *korakoeides;* crowlike) projects upward from the neck of the scapula, then turns anterolaterally like a beak. It arches over the major neurovascular structures of the axilla and receives the attachment of muscles and substantial ligaments. Among the latter are the coracoclavicular ligaments mentioned earlier, and the large *coracoacromial ligament* which, linking the coracoid and acromial processes of the scapula, completes an arch above the glenohumeral joint (see Fig. 15-32).

The **lateral angle** of the scapula, located where the base of the coracoid process joins the lateral border, is quite bulky. Its surface forms a large, shallow concavity, the **glenoid cavity**, for articulation with the humerus. Just above and below the rim of the cavity, the *supraglenoid* and *infraglenoid tubercles* give origin to the long heads of the biceps and triceps, respectively. Medial to the rim of the glenoid cavity, the bone narrows slightly to form the **neck** (*collum*) of the scapula. A deep notch is formed where the neck meets the root of the spine: it accommodates the suprascapular nerve and artery, and is closed over by the *inferior transverse scapular ligament*.

In contrast with the clavicle, the scapula has no direct attachment to the axial skeleton, for it is attached to the ribs and the vertebral column by muscles only. Its connection to the axial skeleton is indirect through the clavicle.

Palpation. Of its three borders and three angles, only the medial border and the inferior angle are readily palpable. Anteriorly, the acromion can be felt as it meets the clavicle at the acromioclavicular joint, which is medial to the tip of the acromion (Fig. 15-6B). On the lateral aspect of the tip of the shoulder, the acromion is subcutaneous and readily palpable between the attachments of the trapezius and the deltoid (see Figs. 15-5 and 15-6). The subcutaneous bone continues posteriorly along the crest of the spine of the scapula, all the way to the medial border. The base of the scapular spine is opposite the spinous process of T-3, and the inferior angle of the scapula is on level with T-7.

The tip of the coracoid is palpable 2.5 cm below the clavicle. It can be felt as a definite, blunt tubercle directly below the most concave point on the clavicle, a position more lateral than one might expect intuitively. It is quite sensitive to pressure. During abduction of the arm, the coracoid process can be felt moving away from the palpating finger. During the same movement, maximum excursion is shown by the inferior angle of the scapula which slides forward, around the chest wall. Fractures of the scapula are best assessed clinically by compressing the bone between the coracoid process and inferior angle. Pain with or without crepitus (grinding of bone fragments on one another) is a confirming sign.

Blood Supply. The scapula receives its blood supply from vessels that run in close contact with both its surfaces: primarily, these are the *subscapular artery* with its *circumflex scapular branch*, and the *suprascapular artery* (see Figs. 15-18 and 15-31).

Ossification. The scapula is preformed in cartilage and ossifies from a number of centers, one or two for nearly each named part of the bone. Most epiphyses appear between infancy and puberty. The largest are those for the coracoid (a true coracoid and a subcoracoid, which includes the upper part of the glenoid cavity), the acromion, the glenoid proper, and the inferior angle. The various epiphyses fuse between 15 and 20 years of age.

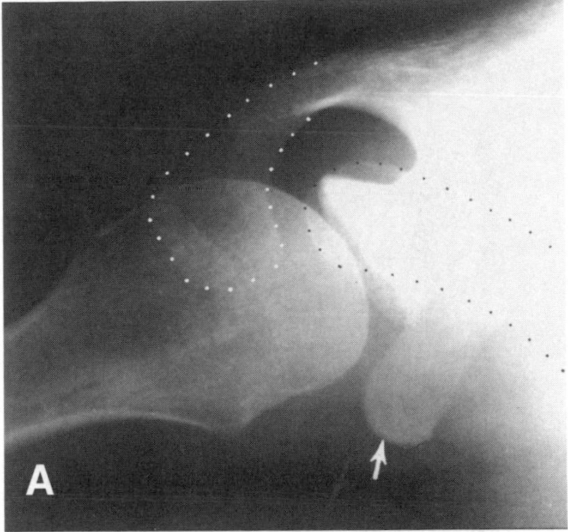

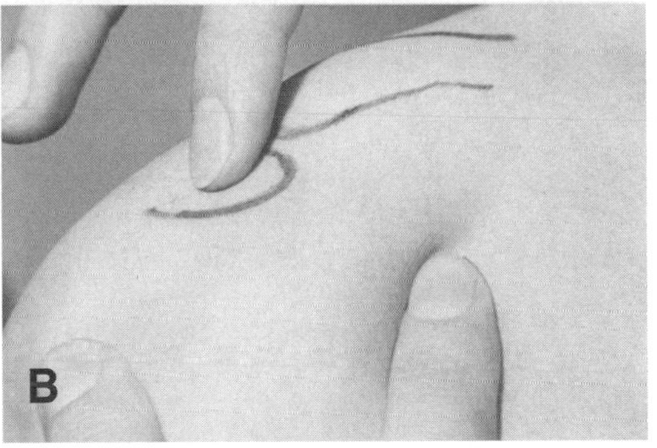

FIGURE *15-6.*
Bony points of the shoulder region: (A) a transaxillary radiograph of the shoulder region. The x-ray film is placed above the acromion and the x-rays travel through the axilla. The acromion (*white dots*) overhangs the humeral head and is separated from the lateral end of the clavicle (*black dots*) by a radiolucent gap, which is occupied chiefly by articular cartilage and an articular disk in the acromioclavicular joint. The clavicle is superimposed over the glenoid cavity, which is separated from the humeral head by radiolucent articular cartilage. The coracoid projects forward, its tip (*arrow*) being level with the lesser tubercle of the humerus. The coracoacromial ligament (invisible) bridges the gap between the coracoid and acromion. (B) the relation of the acromion, lesser tubercle, and coracoid process. The index finger of one hand is on the tip of the acromion, that of the other hand on the coracoid, and the middle finger of the same hand is on the lesser tubercle. The three bony points outline a regular triangle. This relation is disturbed when the humerus is dislocated. (A, courtesy of Dr. Rosalind H. Troupin.)

Humerus

The humerus forms the skeleton of the arm, or proximal segment of the upper limb. It is a typical long bone, with expanded upper and lower ends connected by a shaft, or body (Fig. 15-7). The proximal end of the humerus articulates with the scapula at the shoulder joint, and its distal end with the radius and ulna at the elbow joint.

The expanded **upper end** presents three promi-

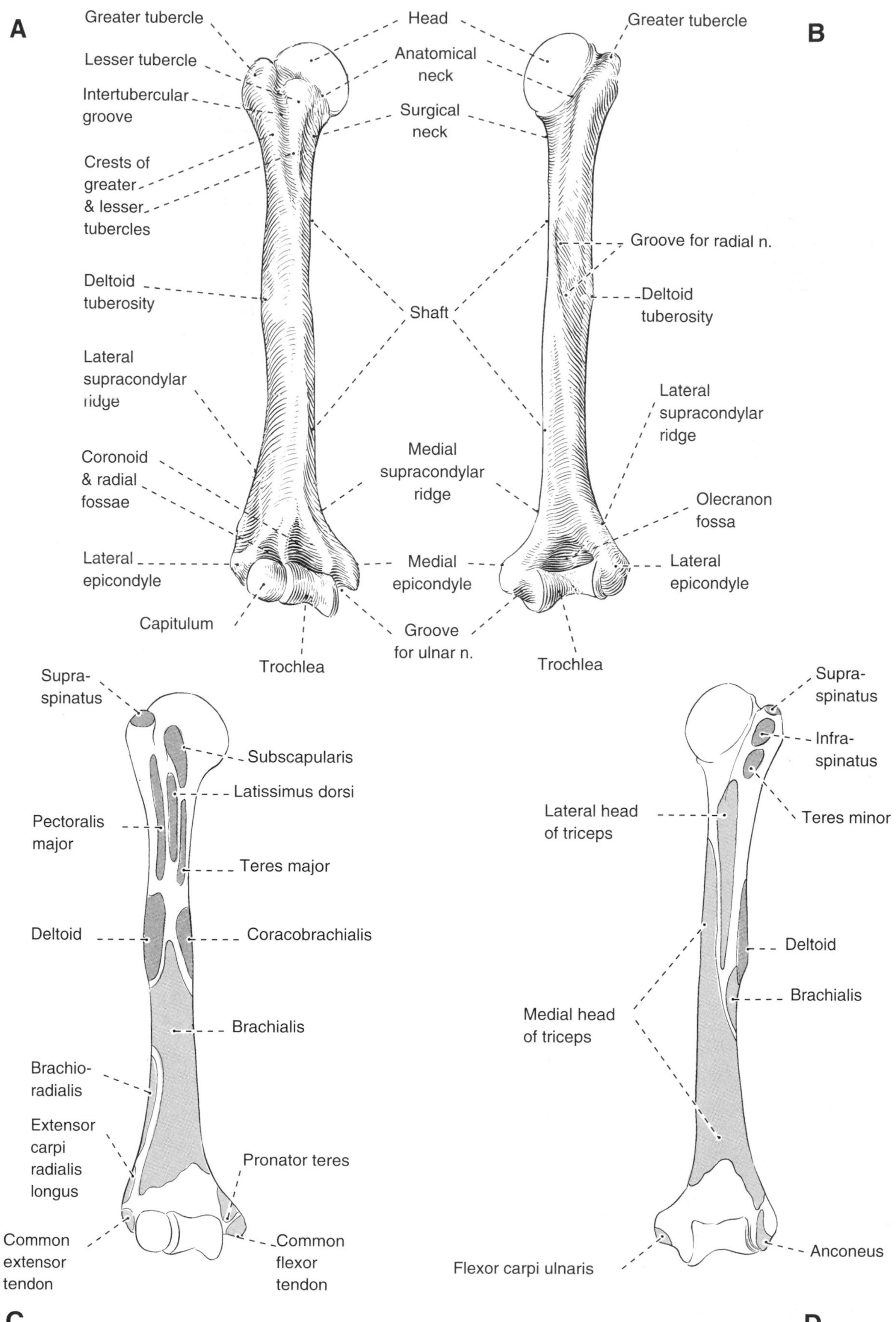

FIGURE 15-7.
(A and C) Anterior and (B and D) posterior views of the humerus: Muscle origins are shown in *red*, insertions in *blue*.

nences, the head and two tubercles. The **head** is covered by a smooth, rounded, articular surface. It joins the rest of the bone by the indistinct **anatomic neck** (*collum anatomicum*). Below the head, the **lesser tubercle** is a roughened projection on the front of the humerus, toward its medial side; a ridge of bone extending downward from it forms the *crest of the lesser tubercle.* A much larger, roughened projection just below the lateral side of the head is the **greater tubercle**; the *crest of the greater tubercle* extends downward from it. Tubercles and crests serve for the attachment of muscles. The groove between the two tubercles is the **intertubercular groove** (sulcus), often called the *bicipital groove* because it houses the tendon of the long head of the biceps muscle. The **surgical neck** (*collum chirurgicum*), so called because it is a common site of fracture, is the indefinite area below the tubercles where the bone narrows to continue as the body, or shaft.

The **body** of the humerus is roughly cylindrical but, nonetheless, does present three *borders* and three *surfaces.* The **lateral** and **medial borders**, indistinct above, become prominent edges below and form the respective *supracondylar ridges*. Each ridge ends in an **epicondyle.** On the posterior and inferior surface of the medial epicondyle is a smooth groove, the *sulcus of the ulnar nerve*. The **anterior border** begins above with the crest of the greater tubercle and becomes indistinct below, to reappear at the lower end as the ridge that separates two depressions, the *coronoid* and *radial fossae.* The smooth surfaces between these borders provide areas for muscle attachments (see Fig. 15-7). About midshaft, the anterolateral surface of the humerus presents the roughened **deltoid tuberosity**. The posterior surface is crossed spirally from its medial to lateral side by the shallow *radial groove,* which marks the course of the radial nerve.

At the expanded **lower end** of the humerus, between the epicondyles, is the **condyle** (Latin, meaning *knuckle*), bearing articular surfaces and concavities. Its convex lateral prominence, the **capitulum**, is covered by an articular surface anteriorly and inferiorly; the articular surface on the pulleylike medial prominence, the **trochlea**, is similar, but extends posteriorly as well. On the anterior surface of the condyle are two fossae, the *coronoid* and *radial fossae,* above the trochlea and capitulum, respectively. These fossae receive the coronoid process of the ulna and the head of the radius, respectively, when the elbow is flexed. On the posterior surface of the condyle, the deep *olecranon fossa* accommodates the olecranon process of the ulna when the elbow is extended.

Palpation. Palpable portions of the proximal end include the head, the greater and lesser tubercles, and the intertubercular groove. The head is accessible only in the axilla with the arm abducted. The greater tubercle is felt through the deltoid just below the acromion; 2.5 cm anterior to it is the intertubercular groove that separates the greater from the lesser tubercle (see Fig. 15-6).

Dislocations and Fractures. The location of the humeral head can be inferred from the relative positions of the lesser tubercle, the coracoid, and the tip of the acromion. With the humeral head in its normal

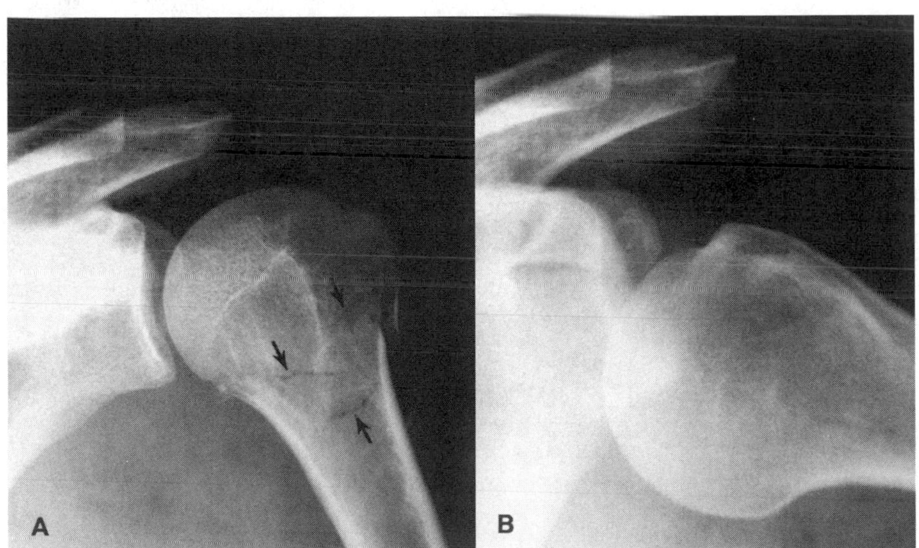

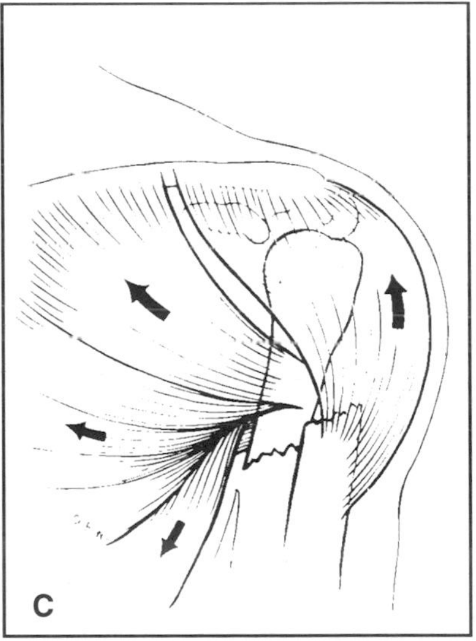

FIGURE *15-8.*
Injuries of the upper end of the humerus. (A) Fracture of the surgical neck of the humerus. The points at which the fracture line interrupts the cortex on the medial and lateral aspects of the neck are clearly seen. The fracture has been caught in two profiles between these two points because of its obliquity and is visible as an irregular streak of radiolucency (*arrows*). Note that the normal relation is retained between the humeral head, glenoid cavity, and acromion. (B) Dislocation of the humerus. Only physical examination or a transaxillary projection (*see* Fig. 15-6A) can resolve whether the dislocation is anterior or posterior. Note that the relation of the glenoid cavity and the humerus is distorted and the latter is widely separated from the acromion. (C) fracture of surgical neck of the humerus. Shortening and displacement of the fractured bone results from the pull of muscles on the bone fragments. (A and B, courtesy of Dr. Rosalind H. Troupin; C, Bickel WH. In: Morris GM, (ed). The cyclopedia of medicine, surgery, specialties. Vol 5. Philadelphia: FA Davis, 1956; 843.)

position, these three points mark the angles of a regular triangle (see Fig. 15-6). The humerus may dislocate anteriorly or posteriorly; either one results in obvious deformity. The normal relation of the three bony points will become distorted (Fig. 15-8), and the humeral head will be palpable in the abnormal position. By contrast, the relative positions of the three bony points will not be altered if the surgical neck of the humerus is fractured (see Fig. 15-8). Continuity of the proximal end of the bone with its distal end can be tested by feeling for movement at the proximal end when the humerus is rotated passively at the elbow. If the humeral neck fracture is impacted, this test will not detect the fracture. With unimpacted fractures, the broken fragments usually show some overriding and other displacements as a result of muscular pull.

Blood Supply. Several vessels contribute to the blood supply of the humerus. The upper end is supplied from numerous twigs given off by the *anterior* and *posterior circumflex humeral arteries* that encircle the surgical neck (see Fig. 15-18). The midportion of the shaft is supplied by a nutrient artery. If derived from the brachial artery, the nutrient artery enters the shaft anteromedially; if derived from the profunda brachii artery, its approach is posterior. However, both anterior and posterior nutrient arteries may be present. The lower end is supplied by twigs from the vessels forming the anastomosis about the elbow (see Fig. 16-14).

Ossification. Ossification of the humeral shaft begins in about the eighth or ninth week of embryonic life and is completed before birth. One to three epiphyseal centers appear at the upper end. There is a constant one for the head, usually present by the time of birth; the tubercles either develop from this center or from independent centers that subsequently fuse with that for the head. The upper end fuses with the shaft at about the age of 17 to 18 years in females and 18 to 21 in males. The lower end of the humerus is typically ossified from four centers, one each for the trochlea, the capitulum, and the two epicondyles. At about 14 years of age in females, 18 in males, they all fuse with each other and the shaft.

PECTORAL REGION

The pectoral region is anterior to the upper six ribs and extends from the sternum to the anterior axillary fold, and from the clavicle to the inferolateral border of the pectoralis major. Its contents are the breast, the pectoralis major, two smaller muscles (pectoralis minor and subclavius), fascias associated with the breast and the muscles, nerves, and blood and lymph vessels.

The Breast

The breast nor *mamma,* is a modified apocrine sweat gland specialized for milk production. It is the anatomic structure by virtue of which *Homo sapiens* is classified among the mammals. In both the male and female of our species the gland has grown too large to be contained in the skin, and has invaded, as do all cutaneous glands, the underlying *tela subcutanea*. The growth and accumulation of superficial fascia in association with the glandular components of the breast is a secondary sex characteristic peculiar to the female of the human species. In the latter, both the glandular and connective tissue components of the breast are subject to hormonal regulation, which results not only in physiologic but in anatomic changes. If the appropriate humoral regulatory factors are supplied, the male breast will also enlarge and can be induced to produce milk. The anatomy of the female breast assumes special importance because its distortion provides the clues for diagnosing neoplastic disease, to which this organ is particularly prone. Neoplasia can, however, occur in the male breast as well.

Developmental Considerations

During the fourth and fifth weeks of development, bilateral mammary ridges develop on the ventral surface of the embryo, extending from the root of the upper limb bud to that of the lower one and to the future perineum. They are formed by an ingrowth of thickened ectoderm into the subjacent mesenchyme. By the eighth week, these thickenings are normally restricted to ectodermal buds localized in the right and left pectoral regions where the breasts will form. In other species, and sometimes in the human as well, breast tissue also develops from ectodermal buds remaining at other locations along the "milk line." Such remnants give rise to accessory breasts in both women and men.

Branching of the epidermal buds establishes the main duct system of the gland (the lactiferous ducts) well before birth. Rudimentary depressed nipples surrounded by largely unpigmented areolae are present at birth. Only at puberty does the female breast begin the growth that distinguishes it from the male breast. This enlargement involves both glandular and connective tissue elements. Raised estrogen and progesterone levels during pregnancy cause further growth of the duct system, the development of alveoli, and an increased deposition of fat. Milk secretion begins postpartum under the influence of prolactin. Both glandular and connective tissues involute after the cessation of breast feeding.

The Male Breast

Breast tissue in the male remains rudimentary throughout life. The organ consists of the **areola**, a circular pigmented area; a papilla, the **nipple**, projects from its center (see Fig. 15-1). Usually it is impossible to discern any glandular tissue with the naked eye. The existence of such tissue subjacent to the areola is indicated, however, by its tendency to become indurated and tender in adolescent males. It may also hypertrophy, along with an increase in the surrounding adipose tissue, leading to the development of femalelike breasts, a condition known as *gynecomastia*.

In many cases the cause of gynecomastia remains unknown, and the condition may be limited to one breast. Gynecomastia may present as a complication of hormonal or other drug therapy.

The male breast has no function. It serves as a landmark on the chest. It is located in the fourth intercostal space, lateral to the midclavicular line.

The Female Breast

External Anatomy. After puberty, the breast forms a rounded eminence, the shape and size of which show considerable individual variation. The **base** of the breast, its area of attachment to the thorax, is, however, fairly constant. It extends from the second to the sixth rib in the midclavicular line (Figs. 15-9 and 15-10), and from the midline of the sternum almost to the midaxillary line. Superolaterally the breast extends over the border of the pectoralis major into the axilla; this *lateral process* is called the **axillary tail**. Most of the base overlies the pectoralis major, but inferolaterally it also covers parts of the serratus anterior and external oblique muscles. Inferiorly, the breast is demarcated rather sharply from the chest wall by a distinct **inframammary fold**, but elsewhere its contours blend smoothly with neighboring tissues. The contours of the two breasts may not be entirely symmetric, but the appearance of new asymmetries should suggest pathologic alterations in internal structure. With advancing age, and as a consequence of the hypertrophy and involution associated with pregnancies, the breasts tend to become pendulous.

The **areola**, larger than in the male, is located on the summit of the breast. In dark-skinned races it is heavily pigmented from childhood; in whites its initial pink color changes to brown during the second month of a woman's first pregnancy and does not revert to its original color again. The **nipple** (*papilla mammaria*) projecting from the center of the areola is usually cylindrical or conical. It may, however, be flat or inverted, as it often is during infancy and childhood. Inverted nipples may present difficulties in breast feeding. Recent inversion of a nipple is a sign of pathology within the breast (see following discussion). The skin of the nipple is puckered and in the crevices on its summit open some 15 to 20 lactiferous ducts. Although their orifices are too small to see with the naked eye, they may be identified by expressing some accumulated sebaceous secretion (or milk, in lactating individuals) from their openings. This maneuver aids in the identification of the ducts for ductography (Fig. 15-11).

The nipple contains an elaborate subcutaneous net-

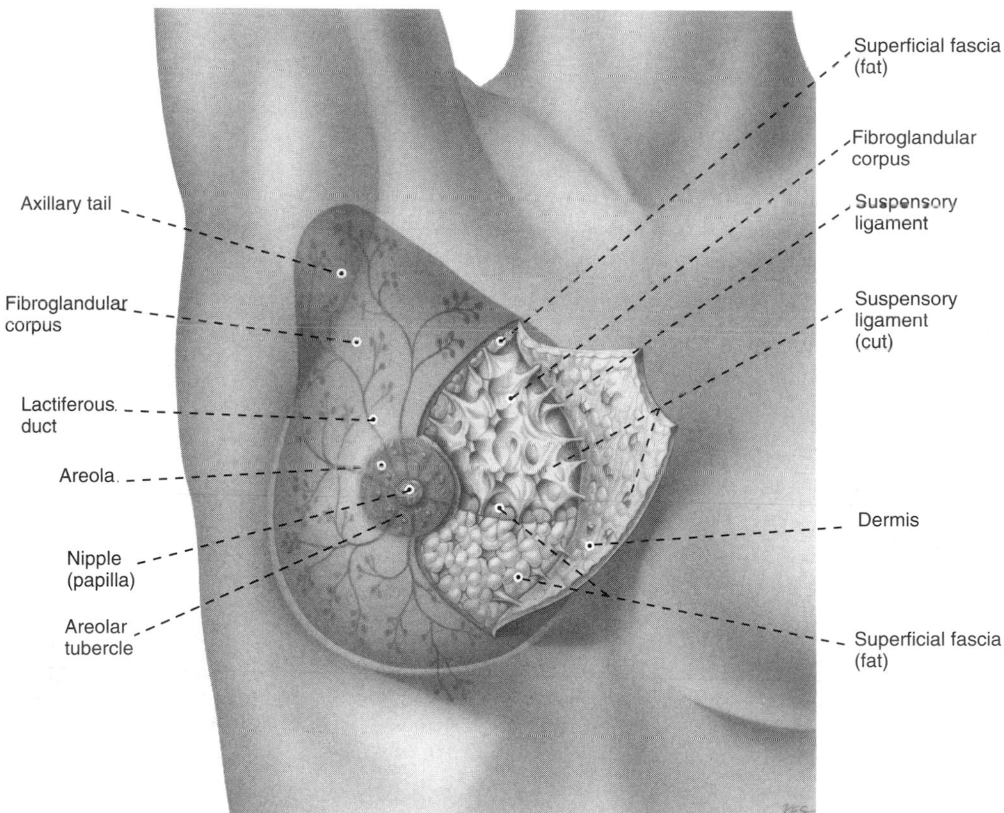

FIGURE *15-9.*
Anterior view of the female breast: The extent of the fibroglandular corpus mammae is visible through the skin. Medially the skin is reflected to show the organization of the fatty superficial fascia and suspensory ligaments. The branching of lactiferous ducts is indicated. (Note the extent of branches beyond the anatomic confines of the breast inferiorly and into neighboring "lobes"). The size of the glandular alveoli in which the ducts terminate is exaggerated; the alveoli are lacking in the nonlactating breast.

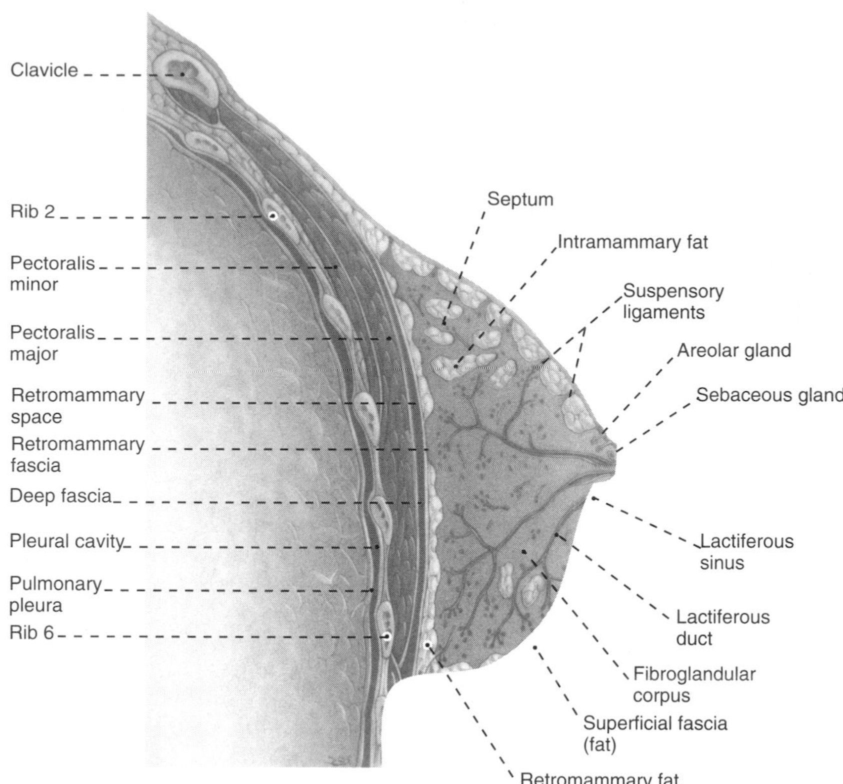

FIGURE *15-10.*
Sagittal section of the female breast (*see* explanation with Fig. 15-9).

work of smooth muscle cells and elastic fibers that encircle the terminal portions of the lactiferous ducts and attach to the skin. In the relaxed state, the network is spread flat, but its contraction transforms it into a cone-shaped cuff which is responsible for the erection of the nipple. The nipple becomes erect in response to the stimulus of suckling and also during sexual arousal. The musculoelastic cuff may also exert some sphincter action on the lactiferous ducts.

The areola contains a number of subcutaneous

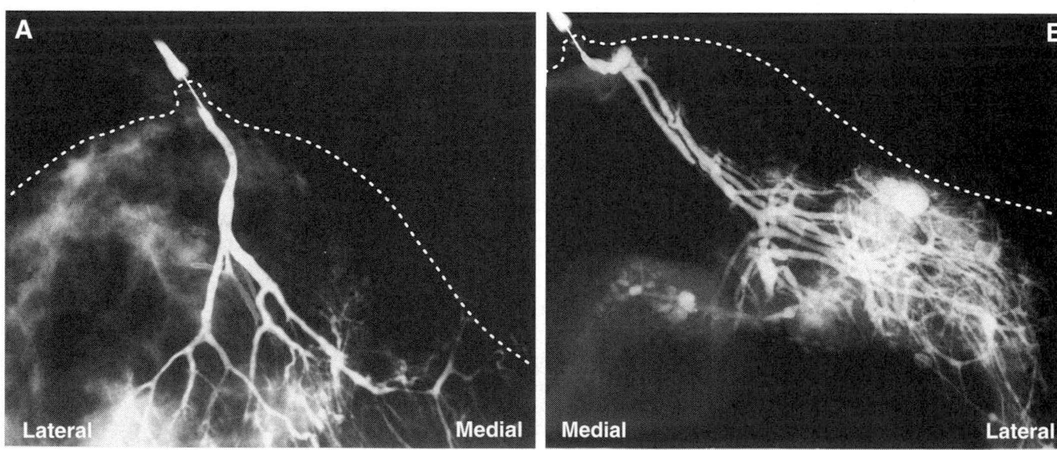

FIGURE *15-11.*
Ductograms in the breasts of two different women who show normal variation in the branching pattern. Contrast medium was injected into a lactiferous duct through the cannula under sufficient pressure to fill the terminal ducts of a lobe. The breast was compressed in a superoinferior direction and a radiograph obtained. To facilitate orientation, the outline of the breast has been superimposed on the radiograph. (A) A rather simple duct system in the breast of a postmenopausal woman. (B) A particularly well-developed duct system in the breast of a 38-year-old woman. The lactiferous duct divides under the areola and branches extensively. The cysts, filled with contrast medium, are normal findings. Although the lobe is mainly in the lateral part of the breast, some ducts (and associated cysts) extend medially beyond the quadrant occupied by most of the "lobe." Note the absence of lactiferous sinuses. (Courtesy of Dr. Mariann J. Drucker.)

glands. Some of these form small nodular elevations on the surface, known as **areolar tubercles** (of Montgomery) that enlarge during pregnancy. Their small ducts resemble lactiferous ducts; although some milk secretion may occur in these **areolar glands** during lactation, their main function is to protect the nipple during suckling by the secretions of the sebaceous glands that empty into their ducts. Sebaceous glands also open on the summit of the nipple, either directly or through the lactiferous ducts (see Figs. 15-9 and 15-10). Both sets of sebaceous glands, as well as the lactiferous ducts, are subject to infection and abscess formation.

In clinical contexts, it is customary to divide the breast into **quadrants** by lines that intersect the nipple and areola at right angles. The axillary tail is an extension of the upper outer quadrant. The remaining quadrants are also named according to their position: upper inner, lower inner, and lower outer quadrants.

Internal Structure. Although the breast begins its development as an ectodermal organ, epithelium accounts for only a small part of its substance once maturity is reached. The fully formed breast consists of glandular tissue (of epithelial origin) embedded in fibrous connective tissue, which is surrounded by fat and is connected to the dermis. To ascertain normality of the breast, and to diagnose and treat its abnormalities, it is important to understand the anatomy of both its glandular and connective tissue components, and especially the interrelation of these two components.

Beneath the skin and superficial fascia, the body of the female breast consists of a firm *fibroglandular mass* (see Figs. 15-9 and 15-10). There is considerable variation in the extent, consistency, and composition of this mass, not only during the life span of a woman but also between women of the same age, and even between the two breasts of an individual. The following account is based on the structure most typical for young, nulliparous (Latin: *nullus*, none; *parere*, to bring forth, produce [pertaining to offspring])women, as a point of reference for the variations. Only clinical experience can provide sufficient familiarity with the variations. Such familiarity is needed for distinguishing normal structure from pathologic lesions both by the physical examination and by radiologic investigations.

The fibroglandular mass of the breast consists of irregular, dense connective tissue, preponderantly composed of collagen fibers, in which the lactiferous ducts branch repeatedly. It is this fibroglandular mass that forms the **body of the breast**, or *corpus mammae* (see Figs. 15-9 and 15-10).

Glandular Tissue. The glandular tissue of the breast is usually described as consisting of some 15 to 20 **lobes**, each lobe connected to a single lactiferous duct. Although this concept has some physiologic value (see later), it is not helpful anatomically: in neither surgical nor anatomic dissections is it possible to define any lobes. Rather than being a distinct pyramidal-shaped structure, as usually described, a lobe of the breast is anatomically diffuse. It is, however, a functional unit of glandular tissue from which milk drains to the nipple through a single lactiferous duct; therefore, each lobe opens to the exterior independently of the others. Individual lobes vary in size, and usually less than half enlarge to become functional during lactation.

Because dissection of the tough corpus mammae is difficult, the extent of the glandular tissue is best demonstrated on 1- to 5-mm to thick sections of the whole breast, after the epithelium of the duct system has been stained and the fibrous tissue rendered transparent. Such preparations, however, do not give information about the lobular organization of glandular tissue. Injection of a lactiferous duct with contrast medium can reveal the extent of its branching on a radiograph, known as a ductogram (see Fig. 15-11). Each lactiferous duct is said to dilate as it passes deep to the areola to form a **lactiferous sinus** in which milk can accumulate. Such dilations, however, are not seen on ductograms. Beyond the areola, lactiferous ducts branch repeatedly, tapering to form smaller and smaller ducts. The finest of these, the terminal ductules, appear to end blindly. Some authorities describe small, solid masses of cells on the tips of the terminal ductules. These structures enlarge and acquire lumina during pregnancy, eventually differentiating into secretory alveoli. In the nonpregnant state, however, they are only "potential alveoli." Indeed, the term *alveolus* should perhaps be avoided in this context.

A cluster of terminal ductules, together with the duct that drains them, constitutes a **mammary lobule**. The terminal duct and its ductules are embedded in relatively loose connective tissue that, during pregnancy, allows proliferation and growth of ductules and alveoli, and an increase in vasculature. In histologic sections, many lobular units appear to be surrounded by dense fibrous connective tissue; a few are in adipose tissue. Some may even extend into superficial fascia outside the breast. Cyst formation in some of the lobular units is a normal finding in the breasts of most women. The lobules involute with advancing age, but can regrow in response to medications used in the treatment of some systemic diseases.

Most malignant neoplasms of the breast are carcinomas, resulting from neoplastic change in the epithelium of lactiferous ducts or their larger, extralobular branches (ductal carcinomas); some arise from epithelium within the lobules (lobular carcinomas). In this context, it is relevant that glandular tissue extends beyond the gross outline of the breast. Regardless of the presence of a demonstrable axillary tail, there is nearly always an extension of breast tissue into the axilla, and even into the posterior axillary fold. Similarly, tissue from one breast may reach or cross the anterior midline or extend downward and medially beyond the inframammary fold. Neoplastic change can occur in such extensions of breast tissue (Fig. 15-12), as well as in ectopic or supernumerary breasts.

Lactation. Following the differentiation and growth of alveoli during pregnancy, secretion of *colostrum*, a milklike fluid, begins a few days before delivery and is replaced by secretion of milk a few days after delivery. The alveolar cells become distended by the proteins and fat they synthesize. Fat droplets surrounded by cell membrane are discharged into the alveolar lumen

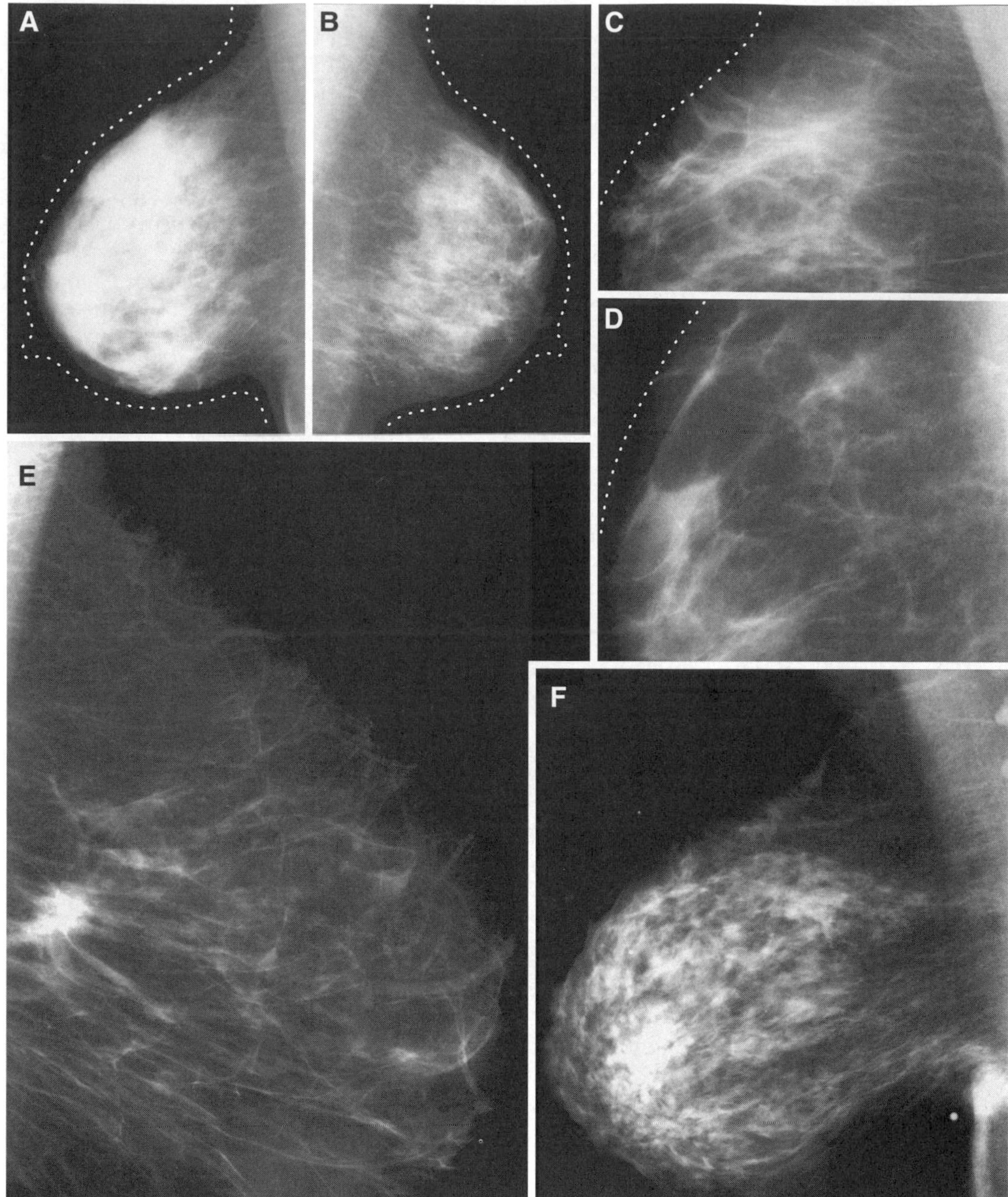

FIGURE 15-12.
Radiologic anatomy of the breast: mammograms. In each case, the breast was compressed in a mediolateral direction and a radiograph obtained. The contrast between radiolucent fat and radiopaque fibroglandular tissue produces a pattern that varies from breast to breast. All the patterns illustrated are normal except in panel E. (A and B) Right and left breasts of the same individual; note the asymmetries in the size and shape and the pattern of radiopacities and radiolucencies. (C) Extensions of the fibroglandular mass to the dermis (*dotted line*) in the upper portion of the breast produce the suspensory ligaments. (D) Radiolucent fat lobules in the fibroglandular mass demarcate pseudosepta. (E) The "spiculated mass" in the breast of this 65-year-old patient is a ductal carcinoma. Note the virtual absence of fibroglandular tissue, and the distortion of the remaining "septa" by the neoplasm. (F) Normal breast of a 52-year-old woman, with a substantial amount of fat between the fibroglandular mass and the pectoralis major. Note the round radiopacity in the inframammary fold, beyond the anatomic confines of the breast. The lesion was detected as a lump by physical examination, and a small radiopaque marker was affixed to the skin over the palpable lump. (Courtesy of Dr. Mariann J. Drucker.)

(apocrine secretion), whereas protein products are released by exocytosis (merocrine secretion). Milk secretion is a continuous process. The secreted milk accumulates, distending the gland and its duct system, until suckling activates the *let-down reflex*. This reflex is mediated by nerves and hormones. Nerves of the nipple and areola relay the stimulus through the spinal cord to the hypothalamus, leading to the secretion of oxytocin by the pituitary gland which, in turn, causes the contraction of myoepithelial cells that surround the alveoli and ducts. Milk may flow from both breasts, not just the one that is being suckled.

Connective Tissue Framework. The connective tissue framework of the breast extends from the dermis to the deep fascia of the pectoralis major, and is made up of the fatty superficial fascia and the dense fibrous tissue of the corpus mammae. A radiograph of the breast, called a mammogram, provides information about the internal structure of the breast because of contrasts between the radiolucencies generated by fat, and the radiopacities produced by the dense fibrous tissue containing the duct system and most of the lobular units (see Fig. 15-12).

The **superficial fascia** in which the body of the breast is embedded is fatty beneath the skin, except under the areola and nipple, and merges with the surrounding tela subcutanea. Posteriorly, at the base of the breast, it forms a limiting membrane called the **retromammary fascia** (see Fig. 15-10). This membrane is analogous with the membranous layer of superficial fascia over the abdominal wall (see Fig. 23-2), and resembles the deep fascia of the pectoralis major. However, it is separated from pectoralis fascia by the **retromammary space**, which contains a small amount of loose areolar tissue. The fibroglandular mass of the breast rests on the retromammary fascia; a variable amount of fat intervenes between the two (see Fig. 15-10).

The retromammary fascia may be demonstrated by peeling away the whole body of the breast from the pectoralis major. Incising the fibrous sheet on the posterior aspect of the breast will demonstrate its membranelike character. The extent of the retromammary space may also be explored. The presence of a space between the two adjacent layers of fascia accounts for the mobility of the breast on the pectoralis major, an important sign in the physical examination of the breast.

Anteriorly, the **fibrous tissue of the body of the breast** sends extensions through the superficial fascia to attach to the dermis, thereby subdividing the superficial fascia into lobules of fat. These fibrous extensions form peaklike projections, resembling the roofs of tents; their apices are anchored to the dermis (see Figs. 15-9 and 15-12). Best developed over the upper quadrants, they are known as the **suspensory ligaments** of the breast. They are associated with the name of Astley Cooper (whose description, however, includes most of the fibrous framework of the breast, not just the so-called suspensory ligaments). Although they are equivalent to retinacula cutis of the superficial fascia, the suspensory ligaments may contain glandular tissue, and cancer may extend into them.

The spaces demarcated in the superficial fascia by the suspensory ligaments are filled by **lobules of fat**. In a dissection, the fat lobules may be scooped out of the fibrous tissue spaces as the skin is being reflected, thus displaying the irregular surface of the fibroglandular corpus (see Fig. 15-9). The irregularity is due to variations in size of both the ligaments and the fat lobules, which partly account for the uneven or lumpy texture of the breast on palpation. Another factor contributing to lumpy texture is the accumulation of fat lobules within the fibroglandular mass itself (see Figs. 15-9 and 15-12). Such islands of fat are present within the mass of a young woman's breast; they increase in size and number as the fibroglandular corpus becomes progressively replaced by adipose tissue with the advancement of age. The fibrous tissue that remains between the fat lobules creates the appearance of **septa**, which seem to connect the dermis to the retromammary fascia. Such septa, however, cannot be defined in the body of the breast unless there is fat accumulation.

Nerve and Blood Supply. The nerve supply of the breast is provided by the anterior and lateral cutaneous branches of the upper six intercostal nerves, described in a preceding section (see Fig. 15-3). The arteries and veins of the breast accompany these nerves in the superficial fascia. Enlarged lateral branches of the *anterior perforating arteries* (from the internal thoracic) run to the breast as *medial mammary arteries*. They are from any combination of the first four perforating arteries. The *lateral mammary arteries* are usually derived from the *lateral thoracic artery* (see Fig. 15-17B). Typically, a single branch of this vessel rebranches as it approaches the breast from the axilla over the lateral border of the pectoralis major muscle. *Lateral cutaneous branches of the posterior intercostal arteries* that emerge in the axilla with the corresponding branches of the intercostal nerves also run forward and contribute to the supply of the breast. All these arteries enlarge during lactation. The superficial veins of the breast form a variable anastomotic pattern and drain along the arterial paths. The chief venous drainage is toward the axilla.

Lymphatic Drainage. The lymphatic drainage of the breast has particular clinical relevance because the primary route for the spread of breast carcinoma is through lymphatic vessels. Drainage begins in deep lymphatic plexuses around the lobes and ducts. The efferent lymph vessels draining these plexuses pass through the body of the breast to the axillary and parasternal lymph nodes. A superficial plexus beneath the areola drains only the terminal portions of the lactiferous ducts and the subcutaneous tissues. There is but little communication between the deep and subareolar plexuses. Although some efferent vessels pierce the pectoralis major to reach the axilla, the principal drainage is along longer and larger vessels that run laterally and medially in the subcutaneous tissues.

More than 75% of the total drainage from the breast passes to groups of lymph nodes located in the axilla, and this includes lymph from all quadrants. The medial quadrants of the breast also drain to the **parasternal** (sternal, internal mammary) **nodes** situated along the internal thoracic vessels on the internal surface of the anterior thoracic wall. The lymphatics pierce the pectoralis major and enter the thorax alongside the anterior cutaneous nerves (see Fig. 15-3) and medial mammary arteries. Similarly, of the lymphatics that pass laterally, a few enter the intercostal spaces alongside the lateral cutaneous nerves and follow the intercostal vessels forward to the parasternal nodes, or posteriorly to the intercostal nodes adjacent to the vertebrae. Most of the efferent lymphatics, however, drain to lymph nodes in the axilla.

The **axillary lymph nodes** are disposed in several groups (described in the section on the axilla). The largest lymphatics of the breast end in the *pectoral group*, which lies between the pectoralis major and minor in the anterior wall of the axilla (Fig. 15-13). Those that perforate the pectoralis major pass to the apex of the axilla and terminate in the *apical group*. Some lymph from the breast may even reach the *subscapular group* in the posterior wall of the axilla. The wide distribution of nodes that receive lymph from the breast indicates the extent of the dissection that must be performed to surgically eradicate metastases of a breast carcinoma.

Surgeons divide axillary lymph nodes that drain the breast into three levels. Level I nodes, numbering a dozen, lie lateral to the pectoralis minor (brachial, subscapular, and pectoral nodes); Level II nodes, about half as many, lie deep to the pectoralis minor (central nodes); level III nodes constitute the two to three apical nodes that lie between the medial border of the pectoralis minor and the first rib. Usually lymph passes from level I to levels II and Ill in a sequential manner. Therefore, few patients have lymph node metastases at levels II and III without involvement at level I. Lymph can, however, enter level II or III nodes from the breast through interpectoral nodes without passing through level I. This explains the approximately 5% of cases with breast cancer in whom metastases exist at level II or III without involvement at level I (*skip metastases*).

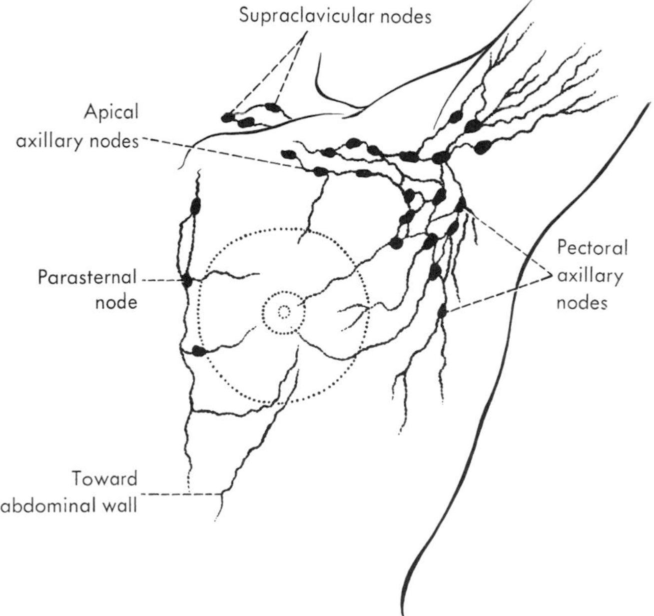

FIGURE *15-13.*
Schema of lymph drainage of the breast.

Although **subcutaneous lymphatics** drain relatively little lymph from the breast, their importance lies in the anastomoses they make with other lymphatics, opening up potential routes for the more distant spread of cancer from the breast. Starting from the subareolar plexus, they spread across the midline to anastomose with lymphatics of the other side; upward across the clavicle; and downward over the costal margin into the abdominal wall. These anastomoses explain how a breast carcinoma may metastasize to the opposite axilla or to lymph nodes in the groin. Such a wide spread of cancer cells is enhanced if major lymph vessels are blocked by the cancer: lymph finds alternative routes around the blockage.

Physical Examination of the Breast

As in other parts of the body, the physical examination of the breast is a demonstration of its anatomy in a living subject. Self-examination relies on the evaluation of the same anatomic components and concepts as examination by a physician. Women should be familiar with the appearance and feel (texture) of their breasts, take note of any changes, and seek medical advice.

The contours of the breasts are best examined (either in front of a mirror, or by a physician standing in front of the subject) with both arms raised above the head, or bending forward and letting the breasts hang down. Pull on the lactiferous ducts by a neoplasm may change the angle of the nipple or may retract it. Pull on the suspensory ligaments, or other retinacula cutis, may flatten the rounded contour. Blockage of lymphatics results in accumulation of tissue fluid (edema) causing puffiness of the skin. Anchoring of the dermis by the suspensory and retinacular ligaments causes pitting of the edematous skin, resembling orange peel.

The breast should be palpated systematically in concentric circles, or quadrant by quadrant, not overlooking the axillary tail. Breast tissue should be rolled gently but firmly, using the pads of the fingers, against the rib cage. The fibrous framework of the breast imparts to it an inherent lumpiness. Changes in this texture, and the appearance of lumps not previously present, are indications for investigation. Lumps are usually discernible in the normal breast if a part of it is rolled between the thumb and the fingers. The breasts may be tender, particularly during certain phases of the menstrual cycle. Although malignant neoplasms themselves are usually not tender, they may coexist with other causes of breast tenderness. The fibrous framework of the breast is subject to a variety of pathologic changes that include benign neoplasms of fibrous tissue presenting as single or multiple lumps.

The retromammary space and fascia, and the fibrous framework of the breast itself, allow the breast, as a whole, to be moved freely on the chest wall, particularly when the pectoralis major is contracted and provides a firm base for it. When the retromammary fascia becomes tethered to the deep fascia of the pectoralis major by cancer cells invading the space by direct spread, or from blocked lymphatics that pass through it, the mobility of the breast is lost. This can be detected by moving the whole breast on the contracted pectoralis major, or by the change in the contour and movement of the breast on the chest wall when the arms are raised or when the subject bends forward.

The axillae and supraclavicular fossae should be meticulously palpated for enlarged lymph nodes. Normal lymph nodes may be palpable in some individuals. Knowing the location of the groups of axillary lymph nodes (see also axilla section), the tissues of the axilla should be rolled against the ribs and the humerus, and also against the anterior and posterior axillary folds. The arm should be supported at the elbow so that the muscles in these folds can be relaxed. The rationale for examining both axillae, as well as the neck and the groins, is provided by the anatomy of the lymphatic drainage.

Muscles and Associated Structures

Deep to the breast or, in the male, to the superficial fascia, the pectoralis major covers all the remaining structures in the pectoral region. These include the pectoralis minor and the subclavius muscles, the clavipectoral fascia stretching between them, and the branches of the brachial plexus and axillary artery that pass through or around the pectoral muscles, emerging from the axilla to supply them.

Pectoralis Major

The pectoralis major is a muscle of the pectoral girdle; it attaches the humerus to the clavicle and the axial skeleton and produces movement at the shoulder joint. The large fan-shaped muscle covers the front of the rib cage from the clavicle to the sixth or seventh rib. From this wide area of origin, its fibers converge and twist upon themselves in the anterior axillary fold before inserting into the humerus as a ribbonlike tendon (Fig. 15-14).

The pectoralis major will spring into prominence when the hands are pressed together in the position of prayer, some distance in front of the body. It has three parts: the *clavicular part* arises from the medial third of the clavicle, the *sternal part* from the manubrium and body of the sternum, and the *costal part* from the cartilages of the first six or seven ribs (see Fig. 15-14). The latter two parts are often referred to collectively as the *sternocostal* part. As they converge toward their insertion, the clavicular fibers blend with the upper sternal ones, to form an *anterior lamina* to the tendon. The lower portion of the muscle forms the *posterior lamina*; its fibers run laterally and upward, twisting as they pass behind the anterior lamina so that the fibers of lowest origin insert highest on the humerus. The *bilaminar tendon* passes behind the anterior border of the deltoid muscle, crosses the intertubercular groove, and inserts on its lateral lip, the crest of the greater tubercle (see Fig. 15-7).

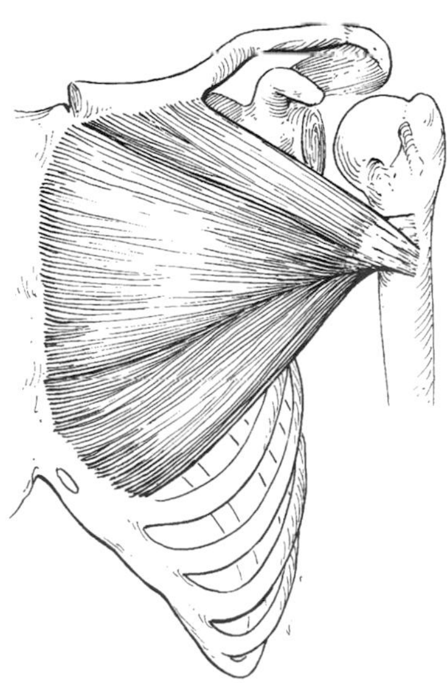

FIGURE ***15-14.***
The pectoralis major.

The muscle is a powerful adductor and flexor of the arm. The sternal part of the muscle is most active in adduction. The clavicular part, on the other hand, is the prime mover in flexion. The lower portion of the sternocostal part (attached only to the ribs) extends the flexed humerus. These fibers also depress the shoulder, acting via the humerus. Because the muscle inserts anterior to the long axis of the humerus, it medially rotates it.

The pectoralis major is supplied segmentally by C-5 to T-1 through two branches of the brachial plexus (lateral and medial pectoral nerves). The central portion, concerned chiefly with adduction, receives C-7 and C-8.

Pectoralis Minor

Lying deep to the pectoralis major, the pectoralis minor attaches the scapula to the axial skeleton. It arises from three consecutive ribs, between the second and the sixth, and tapers toward its insertion on the medial side of the coracoid process (Fig. 15-15). By acting via the scapula, the muscle depresses the shoulder and assists in its protraction; it also functions in rotation of the scapula. The muscle cannot be demonstrated in a living subject, neither can its action be tested independently. It is supplied by the same branches of the brachial plexus as the pectoralis major (lateral and medial pectoral nerves; C-6, C-7, and C-8).

Subclavius

The subclavius is a small, rounded muscle, hidden by the clavicle, that arises by a tendon from the first rib and inserts on the lower surface of the clavicle (see Fig. 15-15). It can depress and rotate the clavicle, but is probably more important in shunting the clavicle toward the manubrium in violent movements of the arm (throwing or hitting out). A small branch of the brachial plexus, named after the muscle, innervates it (C-5 and C-6).

Variations. Occasionally a part of the pectoralis major, or even the entire muscle, may be absent. Most common is absence of the sternocostal part. The pectoralis minor is sometimes absent. Truly anomalous muscles are sometimes found in the pectoral region. The **sternalis** is a small muscle lying superficial to the sternum (see Chap. 23). So-called **axillary arch muscles** represent remains of a *panniculus carnosus*, similar to the platysma (see Fig. 30-11). They usually form an arch across the axilla between the pectoralis major and the latissimus dorsi, and can be an extension of either muscle.

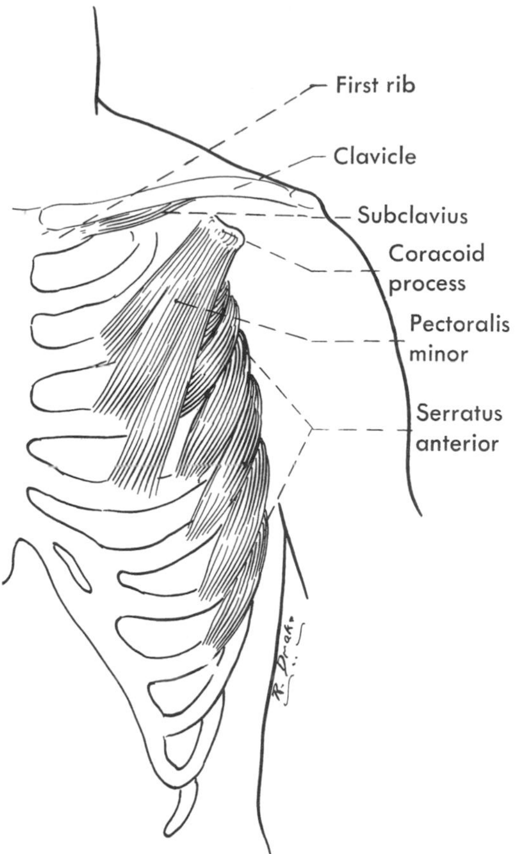

FIGURE *15-15.*
The pectoralis minor and subclavius muscles: The anterior part of the serratus anterior is also shown.

Fascias

Each of the muscles discussed in the foregoing is invested in its own fascia. In addition, a separate layer of fascia, similar in nature to deep fascia, is associated with the pectoralis minor and subclavius, namely the **clavipectoral fascia** (Fig. 15-16). Together with the muscles, it helps complete the anterior wall of the axilla and, through its attachment to the axillary fascia (see following), helps maintain the concavity of the armpit.

When anterior and posterior layers of the deep fascia of the pectoralis minor meet at the upper border of the muscle, they fuse and continue upward as the clavipectoral fascia, to split again around the subclavius, before attaching to the clavicle (see Fig. 15-16). Lateral to the subclavius muscle, the fascia attaches to the coracoid process and the first rib, and is particularly strong; this part is sometimes called the *costocoracoid ligament.* Beyond the inferolateral edge of the pectoralis minor, its deep fascial laminae likewise extend downward and become continuous with the axillary fascia (see section on the axilla). This sheet (strictly speaking, no longer a part of the clavipectoral fascia), functions as a suspensory ligament for the floor of the axilla.

Nerves and Vessels

Branches of the brachial plexus and the axillary artery, together with tributaries of the axillary vein, as well as lymphatics and lymph nodes (described with the breast) are topographically related to the pectoral muscles and their fascias. They include the *lateral and medial pectoral nerves* (the nerve to the subclavius has its course entirely in the neck), and the *thoracoacromial and lateral thoracic arteries and veins* that supply the pectoral muscles. These structures originate in the axilla and are dealt with in the next section.

AXILLA

The axilla is a pyramidal space through which pass the major vessels and nerves that run between the upper limb and the neck and trunk. The apex of the pyramid points into the neck, behind the clavicle, and its base is formed by the skin of the armpit and the attached fascia, the axillary fascia.

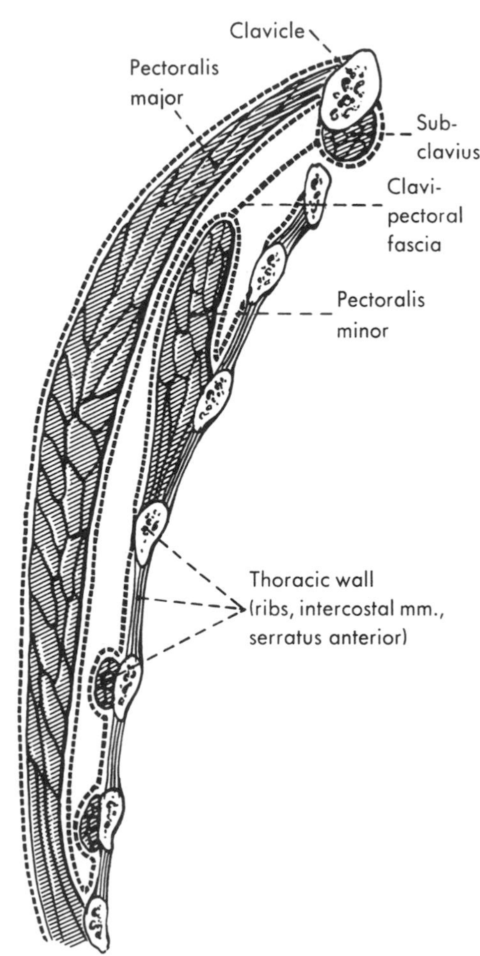

FIGURE *15-16.*
Diagram of the clavipectoral and related fascias (*broken lines*).

Boundaries

As discussed in the previous section, the anterior wall of the axilla is formed by the pectoral muscles, the clavipectoral fascia, and the clavicle. Its medial wall is made up of the serratus anterior, which covers the thoracic cage (Fig. 15-17). Much of its posterior wall is composed of the subscapularis muscle on the costal surface of the scapula and, more laterally, the muscles of the posterior axillary fold (teres major and latissimus dorsi). Because its anterior and posterior walls converge laterally, the lateral wall is narrow. It is the portion of the humerus between the insertions of the anterior and posterior axillary fold muscles, essentially the intertubercular groove. The curved base, or floor, of the axilla consists of the axillary fascia, a fairly thick sheet that extends between the deep fascial layers of the axillary fold muscles, the thoracic wall, and the arm. The apex opens into the root of the neck between the subclavius muscle and clavicle, and the first rib.

Contents

The contents of the axilla are the axillary artery and vein, lymph nodes, and the brachial plexus with its branches. The axillary artery, the brachial plexus, and the main branches of the plexus are closely grouped together in the axilla and are enclosed in the **axillary sheath**, a sleeve of rather tough fascia. It is an extension of the prevertebral fascia of the neck (see Fig. 30-3) and gradually fades out as its contents proceed into the arm. The sheath, the axillary vein (which is outside it), the groups of lymph nodes, and the minor branches of the main vessels and nerves that leave the axilla through its walls, all are embedded in a rather large amount of loosely lobulated fat that is partially subdivided by fibrous strands and septa. This tough and abundant fatty tissue make anatomic and surgical dissection in the axilla quite challenging.

Examination of the axilla should include palpation of the axillary artery and the axillary lymph nodes. The artery is best felt by compressing it against the humerus. Palpation of the lymph nodes is described in the section on the breast.

Owing to the presence of the fat and its rather poor compartmentalization by fibrous tissue, an **axillary abscess** may grow to considerable size before it builds up sufficient tension to cause pain. Pus may track to the neck, or into the arm (if it enters the axillary sheath), or between the pectoral muscles (if it breeches the clavipectoral fascia). The axillary sheath, on the other hand, forms a complete investment around its contents. Local anesthetics may be injected into it to block all motor and sensory nerves to the entire limb (*axillary block*).

Blood Vessels and Lymph Nodes

Axillary Artery

The axillary artery is the continuation of the subclavian artery and itself becomes the brachial artery (Fig. 15-18). The first change in name occurs as the continuous arterial trunk crosses the first rib, and the second as it leaves the axilla at the lower border of the teres major muscle. Branches of the axillary artery supply the muscles and joints of the shoulder and pectoral regions. They establish a free anastomosis around the scapula between branches of the subclavian and brachial arteries (**circumscapular anastomosis**) so that occlusion of the axillary artery itself does not interfere seriously with the blood supply of the upper limb.

Course and Relations. The axillary artery is the central structure of the axilla. Its passage behind the pectoralis minor provides a convenient basis for dividing it into three parts: a first part above the muscle, a second part behind it, and a third part below the muscle. All three parts are related to other muscles in the walls of the axilla as well as to the brachial plexus (see Fig. 15-17B). In fact, the cords of the brachial plexus (described in the next section) are named *posterior*, *lateral*, and *medial cords* because of the relation they bear to the second part of the artery.

The *first part* of the artery lies on the upper digitations of the serratus anterior muscle, the medial cord of the plexus being interposed between the artery and the muscle; here, the lateral and posterior cords are above the artery (see Fig. 15-17B). The *second part* lies on the subscapularis muscle, and the cords surround the artery in the manner indicated by their names. The *third part* has behind it the teres major muscle as well as the subscapularis; it is surrounded by the major nerves of the limb as they issue from the plexus. The artery is paralleled by the axillary vein, which lies anterior to it. The medial cord and its branches lie between the artery and the vein.

Branches. The axillary artery is usually described as giving off six branches: one from the first part, two from the second, and three from the third.

The *first part* gives off the **superior thoracic artery**, a small vessel that runs medially to be distributed over the first two intercostal spaces; it also supplies the pectoralis major and the sternoclavicular joint. The two branches of the *second part* are the short thoracoacromial and long lateral thoracic arteries, both mentioned in connection with the blood supply of the pectoral region. The three branches of the *third part* of the axillary artery are the subscapular artery and two circumflex humeral arteries (see Fig. 15-18).

The **thoracoacromial artery** originates close to the upper border of the pectoralis minor, runs forward to pierce the clavipectoral fascia, and divides into clavicular, pectoral, acromial, and deltoid branches (see Figs. 15-17B and 15-18).

The small clavicular branch runs toward the sternoclavicular joint, supplying it and a part of the thoracic wall. The pectoral branch is the largest branch and runs downward with the lateral pectoral nerve on the deep surface of the pectoralis major. The deltoid branch runs between the clavicular head of the pectoralis major and the deltoid muscle to supply both. The small acromial branch, often arising from the deltoid branch, emerges between the pectoralis major and the deltoid and enters into an anastomotic network

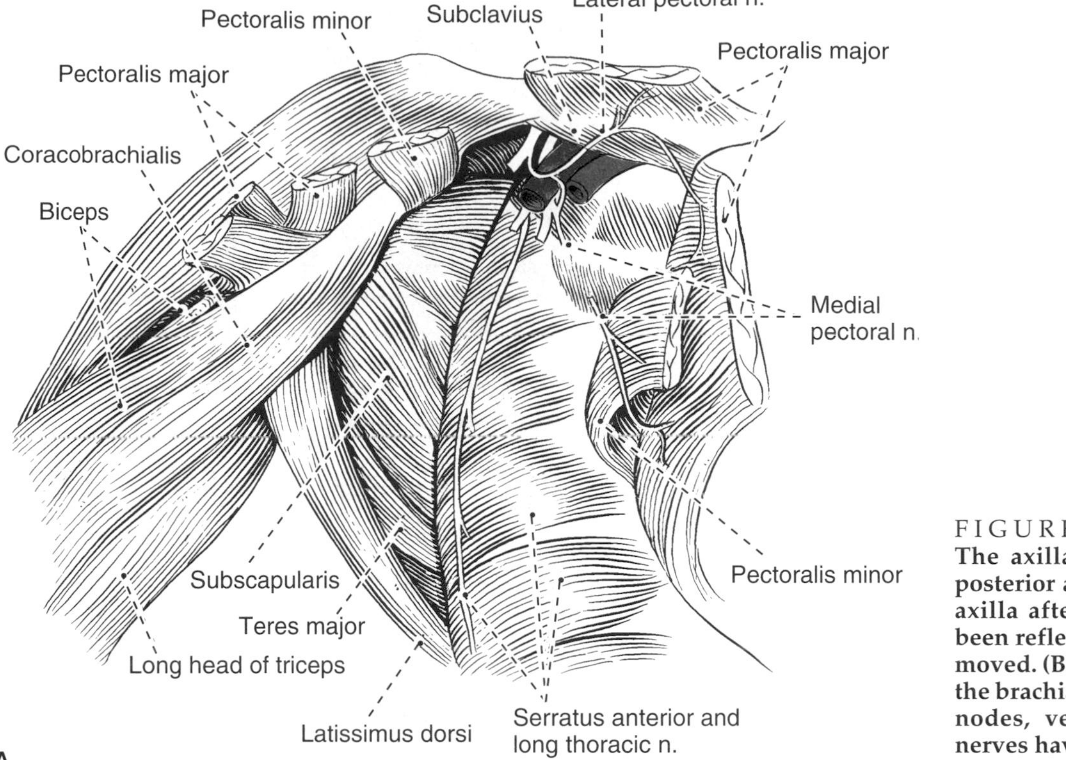

FIGURE *15-17.* **The axilla and its contents: (A) posterior and medial walls of the axilla after its anterior wall has been reflected and its contents removed. (B) The axillary artery and the brachial plexus in situ. Lymph nodes, veins, and the pectoral nerves have been removed.**

over the acromion, called the *acromial rete* (*rete;* Latin for net). The rete also receives branches from the suprascapular and posterior circumflex humeral arteries, to be discussed later. All branches supply the structures along their path.

The **lateral thoracic artery** typically arises close to the lower border of the pectoralis minor and runs downward for a variable distance on the serratus anterior (see Fig. 15-17B). The artery was formerly called the external mammary artery because, through its *lateral mammary branches*, it is a chief source of blood for the breast. In addition, it gives branches to the pectoral and serratus muscles, and the contents of the axilla.

The **subscapular artery** is usually the largest branch of the axillary artery. It passes backward to descend on the subscapularis (see Fig. 15-17B) and soon divides into two trunks: the **circumflex scapular artery** that passes around the lateral border of the scapula to supply muscles in the infraspinous fossa (see Fig. 15-31); and the **thoracodorsal artery** that continues downward along the muscles of the posterior axillary fold and is distributed to them. The artery is joined in its course by the thoracodorsal nerve, a branch of the brachial plexus (see Fig. 15-17B). These two branches of the subscapular artery sometimes arise separately from the axillary artery.

The **anterior** and **posterior circumflex humeral arteries**, the last branches of the axillary artery, may arise independently or by a common stem. The anterior circumflex humeral passes around the front of the surgical neck of the humerus. The larger posterior circumflex humeral skirts the surgical neck around its posterior aspect, where it is joined by the axillary nerve (see Figs. 15-29 and 15-31). Both artery and nerve run under the deltoid muscle, supply it, and send twigs to the upper end of the humerus and the shoulder joint. Anterior and posterior circumflex humeral arteries anastomose around the humerus.

Variations and Anomalies. As the foregoing account implies, there are variations in the branches of the axillary artery. Branches may arise together, or their subbranches may be given off directly by the main artery. Thus, instead of 6, the branches may total anywhere from 5 to 11. A rare but striking **anomaly** arises when, instead of continuing as a single brachial artery, the axillary artery divides in the axilla into two branches. On entering the arm, one of the branches usually runs more superficially and may represent the radial or ulnar arteries; the deeper branch usually corresponds to the brachial artery proper.

Axillary Vein

The axillary vein (Fig. 15-19) is a segment of the chief venous channel that collects blood from all parts and regions of the upper limb. It is the direct upward continuation of the basilic vein, the postaxial vein of the upper limb (see Fig. 14-10). The basilic vein enters the axilla along the brachial artery and becomes known as the axillary vein as it crosses the lower border of the teres major. After proceeding through the axilla along the axillary artery, the axillary vein becomes the subclavian vein as it crosses the first rib. The axillary vein lies below, and ante-

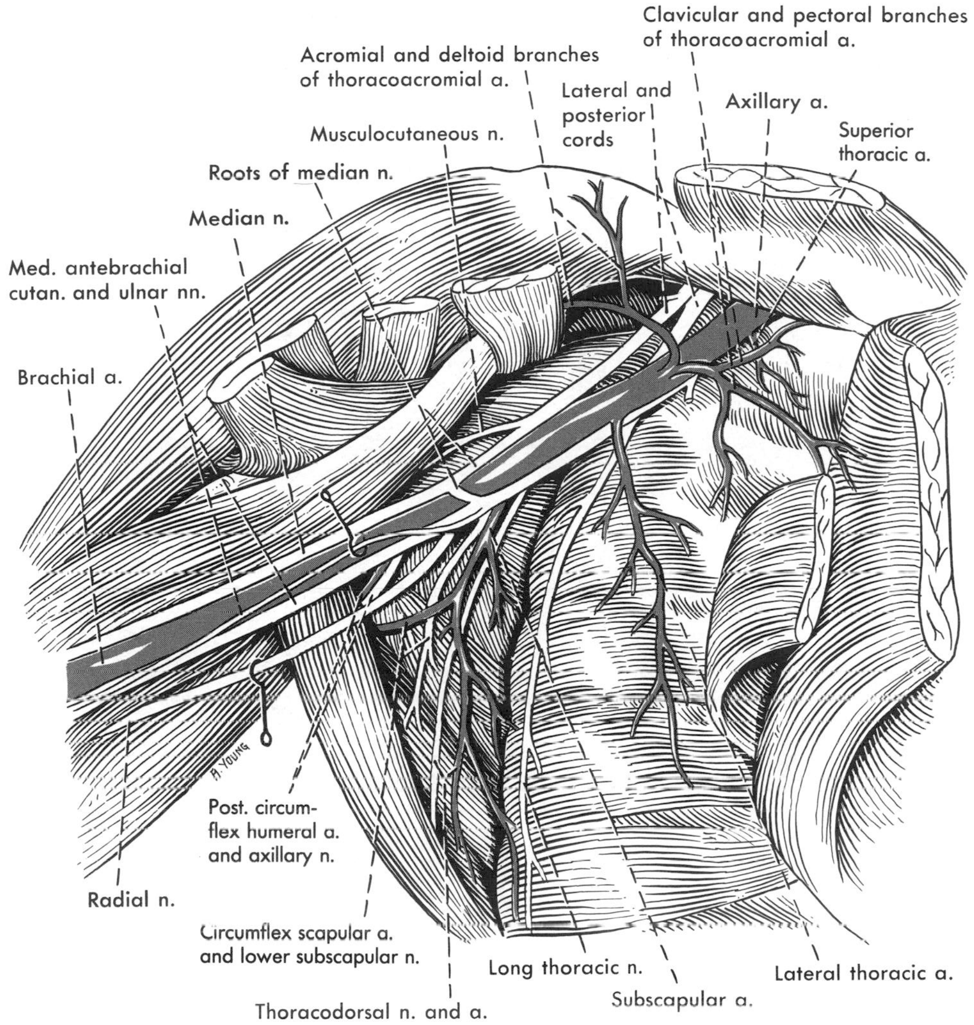

B

rior to, the axillary artery. Between the two vessels lie the medial cord of the brachial plexus and the ulnar and medial cutaneous nerves of the arm. The vein is outside the axillary sheath, and the central group of axillary lymph nodes is located on its surface.

Tributaries of the axillary vein include two brachial veins, the cephalic vein, and veins that correspond largely to the branches of the axillary artery. There is no thoracoacromial vein, however; the veins that correspond to the branches of the thoracoacromial artery join the cephalic vein or terminate in the upper part of the axillary vein as independent tributaries.

The **cephalic vein**, the preaxial vein of the upper limb (see Fig. 14-10), runs in the superficial fascia between the pectoralis major and the deltoid and then turns deeply between them to join the axillary vein. It receives veins from these muscles. The **lateral thoracic vein** communicates with the superficial epigastric vein of the abdominal wall and provides one of the potential alternative routes for venous return to the heart from the lower part of the body when the inferior vena cava is blocked (see Chap. 21).

Axillary Lymph Nodes

Lymph nodes of the axilla receive and filter the lymph from the upper limb and from the anterior and posterior aspects of the trunk as far distal as the umbilicus and iliac crest. As described earlier, lymph from the breasts drains predominantly to the axillary nodes.

The nodes are embedded in the fatty connective tissue of the axilla and are related to its blood vessels (see Fig. 15-19). They may number fewer than a dozen or up to about three dozen. Their dissection and removal may be required in the surgical treatment of breast cancer. The larger ones are usually fairly obvious during dissection of a cadaver, but many smaller nodes are removed with the surrounding fat in the process of cleaning the vessels and nerves of the axilla.

The nodes form a rather straggling chain from the base of the axilla to its apex. Despite their numerous interconnections, the nodes are usually subdivided into groups relative to both the territories they drain and their location; such divisions aid their identification during a

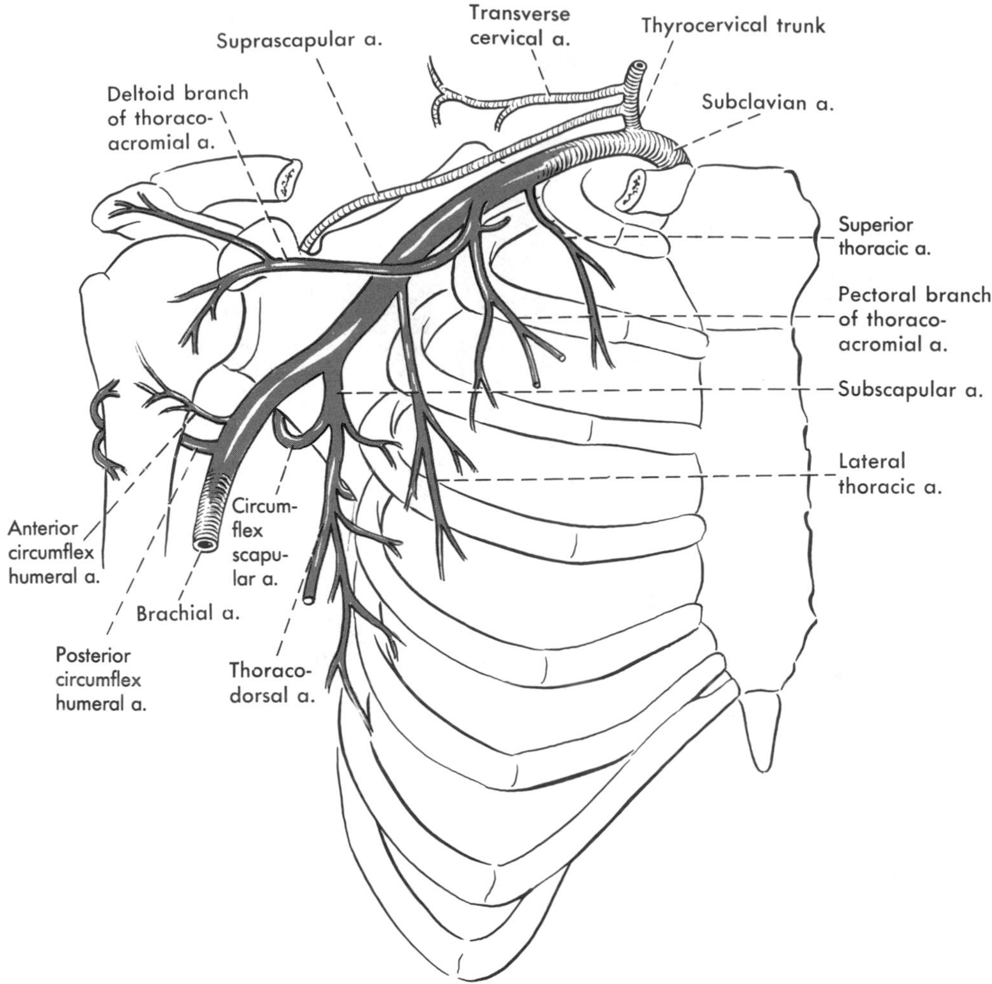

FIGURE *15-18.*
Diagram of the axillary artery and its branches.

dissection. Afferent lymphatics from the periphery are received predominantly by three groups of nodes: those from the arm by the **brachial** (*lateral*) **group**; those from scapular region and the back by the **subscapular** (*posterior*) **group**; and those from the anterior abdominal and thoracic wall, between the clavicle and the umbilicus, by the **pectoral** (*anterior*) **group**. These three peripheral groups drain into the **central group** of nodes which, in turn, transmits lymph to the **apical group**. The latter give rise to the *subclavian lymphatic trunk.* On the left side, this trunk commonly joins the thoracic duct; on the right side, it joins the right lymphatic duct, or the jugular duct from the neck, or it may enter the subclavian vein independently (see Chap. 30).

There are exceptions to this orderly pattern of drainage, the most important involving the lymphatics of the breast. As described earlier, these drain primarily to the pectoral nodes, but some also enter other groups directly. Furthermore, when the primary nodes of drainage become blocked by cancer cells, alternative routes of flow open up and carry metastases to nodes outside the usual territory of drainage.

The **brachial nodes** are the most lateral and lie on the lower part of the axillary vein (see Fig. 15-19). With the exception of lymphatics that run along the cephalic vein (see later discussion), all the lymphatics that ascend through the arm terminate in them. The **subscapular nodes** are grouped around the subscapular vessels and the subscapularis muscle. The **pectoral nodes** are situated along the lateral border of the pectoralis minor around the lateral thoracic vessels. Outlying members of this group, the *interpectoral nodes,* are between the two pectoral muscles. The **central nodes** lie on the axillary vein, somewhat behind the pectoralis minor. The **apical nodes** are associated with the upper part of the axillary vein in the apex of the axilla. They receive lymph that has passed through all the other axillary nodes. In addition, some lymphatics from the breast drain directly to the apical nodes, as do the lymphatics that course along the cephalic vein from the preaxial border of the free limb. The latter may be interrupted by the *infraclavicular subgroup* of nodes, located along the vein in the groove between the deltoid and pectoralis major in the infraclavicular fossa. Some of the lymphatics from the apical group, instead of joining the subclavian lymphatic trunk, drain into the *supraclavicular* or *deep cervical lymph nodes* in the root

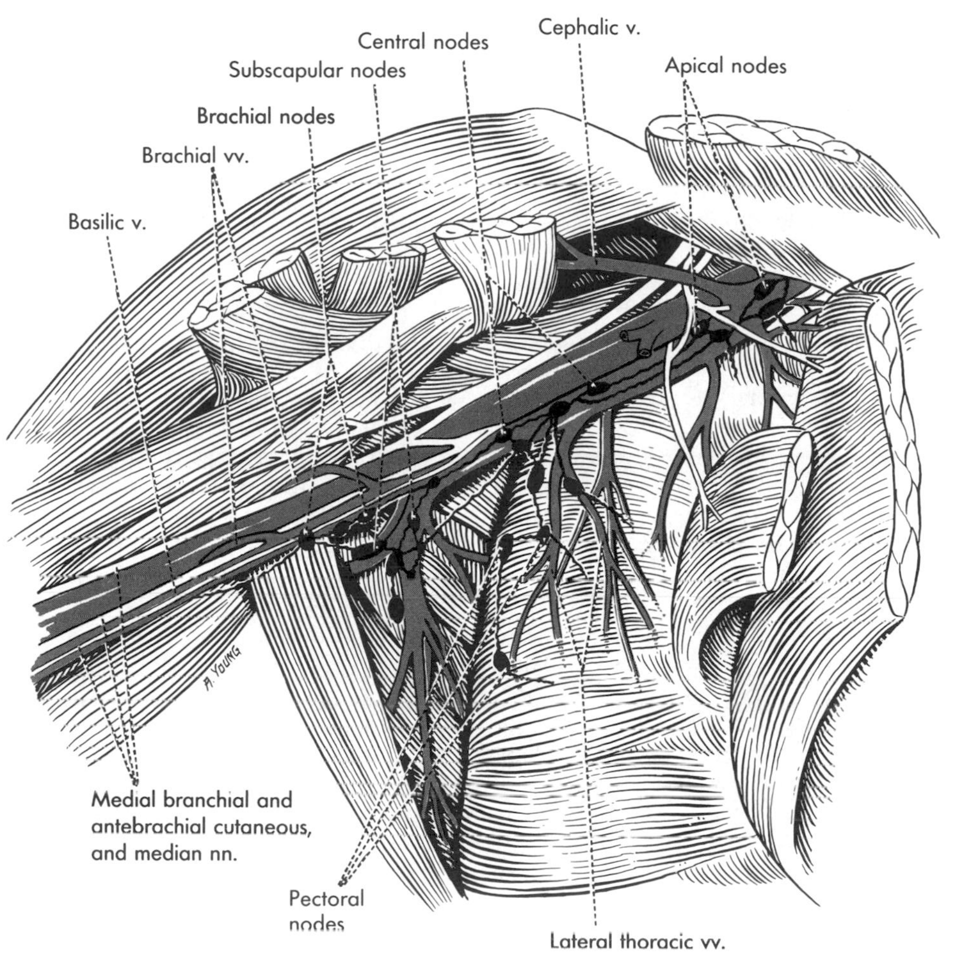

FIGURE *15-19.*
Veins and lymph nodes of the axilla.

of the neck. Therefore, metastases from the drainage territory of the axillary lymph nodes may spread to some of the lower deep cervical nodes as well.

The Brachial Plexus

The brachial plexus is an ordered network of large nerves through which the sensory and motor nerve supply is distributed to all structures that constitute the upper limb. It is formed by the anterior rami of C-5 to T-1 spinal nerves and conforms to the general plan of a limb plexus already discussed in Chapters 13 and 14 (see Fig. 14-6). Understanding of the plexus is essential for comprehension of normal and disordered neuromuscular and sensory functions in the upper limb.

Contributing Nerve Fiber Types

The brachial plexus is composed preponderantly of somatic nerve fibers, both efferent and afferent, but nerves from the sympathetic component of the autonomic nervous system also join the plexus and are distributed to the limb with its branches (see Chap. 13).

Somatic efferent fibers destined for skeletal muscle of the upper limb arise in anterior horn cells of cord segments C-5 to T-1. Groups of these motor neurons constitute the lateral portions of the anterior gray columns in these segments (see Fig. 13-10). They serve all the motor units in upper limb musculature.

Somatic afferent fibers that convey exteroceptive (pain, temperature, pressure, touch, and vibration) and proprioceptive (joint and position sense, and muscle spindle) impulses from the limb have their cell bodies in spinal ganglia C-5 to T-1.

Presynaptic **sympathetic nerve fibers** for the upper limb originate in lateral gray column neurons of upper thoracic segments (T-2 to T-1), pass along the sympathetic chain, and relay in the inferior cervical and upper thoracic sympathetic ganglia. Postsynaptic fibers reach the brachial plexus by gray rami communicantes associated mainly with C-8 and T-1 spinal nerves. The sympathetic fibers are distributed with the branches of the brachial plexus to smooth muscle of blood vessels and hair follicles, and to sweat glands.

Removal of the lower cervical and upper thoracic sympathetic chain (sympathectomy) has been performed surgically to induce vasodilation, particularly in the hand, in cases of constrictive peripheral vascular disease (e.g., Raynaud's disease) or for the elimination of excessive sweating of the hands. This procedure simultaneously deprives the head and neck of their sympathetic input.

Formation and Component Parts

The plan and composition of the plexus are shown in Figure 15-20, and some of its anatomic relations in Figure 15-21. The anterior rami of C-5 to T-1 spinal nerves are known as the **roots** of the plexus. They unite to form three **trunks**: C-5 and C-6 form the **upper trunk**, C-7 continues alone as the **middle trunk**, and C-8 and T-1 unite into the **lower trunk**. The regrouping of nerve fibers destined for the flexor and extensor compartments of the limb begins at this level (see Figs. 14-5 and 14-6). Each trunk splits into an **anterior** and a **posterior division**, the former carrying fibers for the flexor compartment and, the latter, fibers for the extensor compartment. The divisions unite to form the cords of the plexus. All three posterior divisions merge to form the **posterior cord**; in it are gathered all C-5 to T-1 nerve fibers for the extensor compartment. The posterior cord lies behind the axillary artery. Owing to the presence of this artery, there is no corresponding **anterior cord**: rather, the anterior divisions form two cords, one on either side of the artery, the **lateral** and **medial cords**, respectively. The lateral cord gathers the anterior divisions of the upper and middle trunks (C-5, C-6, and C-7), and the medial cord is the continuation of the anterior division of the lower trunk (C-8 and T-1). Lateral and medial cords together supply the flexor compartment of the limb.

Thus, the trunks mix the fibers together from selected roots, the divisions sort out the fibers destined for the flexor and extensor compartments, and the cords maintain this sorting. They also provide for the regrouping of fibers from different spinal cord segments for distribution along the major branches of the plexus.

The spinal cord segments that contribute to the plexus are surprisingly constant, as is the organizational plan of the plexus. Rarely, there may be a substantial input from C-4, in which case the plexus is said to be *prefixed*. When T-2 contributes significantly, the plexus is *postfixed*. Both instances result in appropriate shifts in the apportionment of different segments to the cords and main branches. Although connective tissue that defines the usual anatomic subdivisions of the plexus may not separate them according to the plan described, the normal subdivisions are usually demonstrable by splitting connective tissue planes in the plexus. Sometimes a true **anterior cord** occurs, without the usual splitting into lateral and medial cords.

Relations

The roots, trunks, and divisions of the brachial plexus are located above the clavicle in the neck. Their relations are important and are described in Chapter 30. Only the cords are truly within the axilla (see Fig. 15-21). In the neck, the plexus may be palpated posterior to the sternocleidomastoid muscle and feels like a bunch of tense cords. The cords of the plexus, however, are not discernible in the axilla.

The roots of the plexus emerge between the anterior and middle scalene muscles (see Figs. 30-20 and 30-21). The prevertebral fascia continues laterally with the roots of the plexus and encloses the entire plexus, together with the axillary artery, in a fascial sleeve, the *axillary sheath*. During movements of the arm the fascial sleeve facilitates sliding of the brachial plexus in the axilla. It will also confine local anesthetic injected around the plexus.

The relations of the plexus, and some of its branches, to the axillary artery are shown in Figure 15-17B (see also Fig. 30-21). The posterior cord, visible above the first part of the artery, becomes hidden lower down. Conversely, the medial cord, formed behind the first part of the artery, emerges along its medial border lower down; here, it lies between the artery and the axillary vein. The lateral cord approaches the artery from above and continues parallel with it. The artery is crossed anteriorly by a large nerve that joins the distal ends of the lateral and medial cords; it is the medial root of the median nerve.

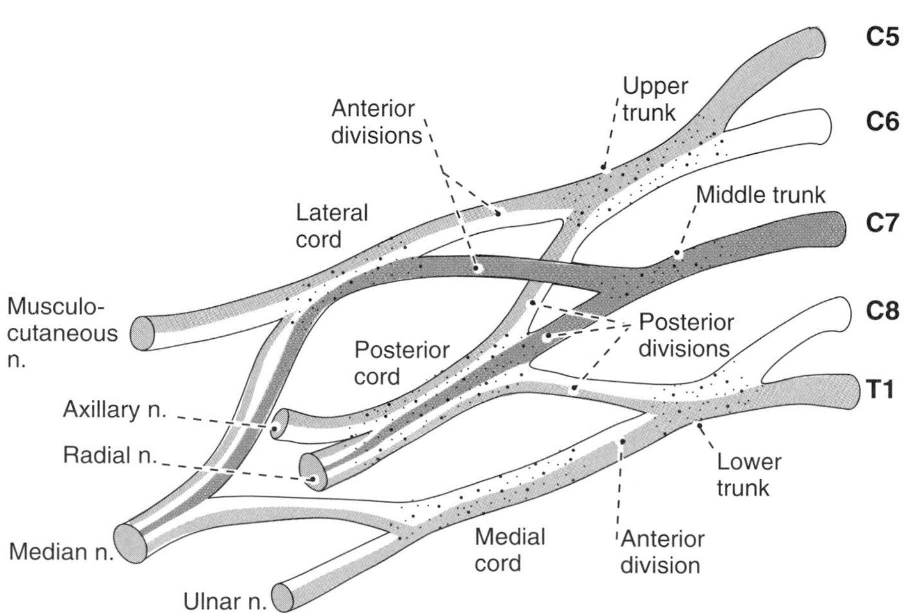

FIGURE 15-20.
The basic plan of the brachial plexus and its major terminal branches: The roots of the plexus are identified by *different colors* to illustrate the manner in which the components of each root are distributed through the plexus and emerge in its major branches. The trunks of the plexus are *stippled*.

Branches

The main nerves of the upper limb are terminal branches of the cords (see Chap. 14; Fig. 14-7). In addition, several small branches are given off to supply the pectoral girdle musculature and skin along the medial aspect of the limb (Fig. 15-22). Some of these minor branches arise from the roots and trunks in the neck (supraclavicular branches of the plexus) and others from the cords below the clavicle (infraclavicular branches). There are no branches from the divisions.

Main Terminal Branches. Each cord contributes to the formation of two major branches (see Figs. 15-20 and 15-21). The *posterior cord* terminates in the **axillary** and **radial nerves**, the *lateral cord* in the **musculocutaneous**

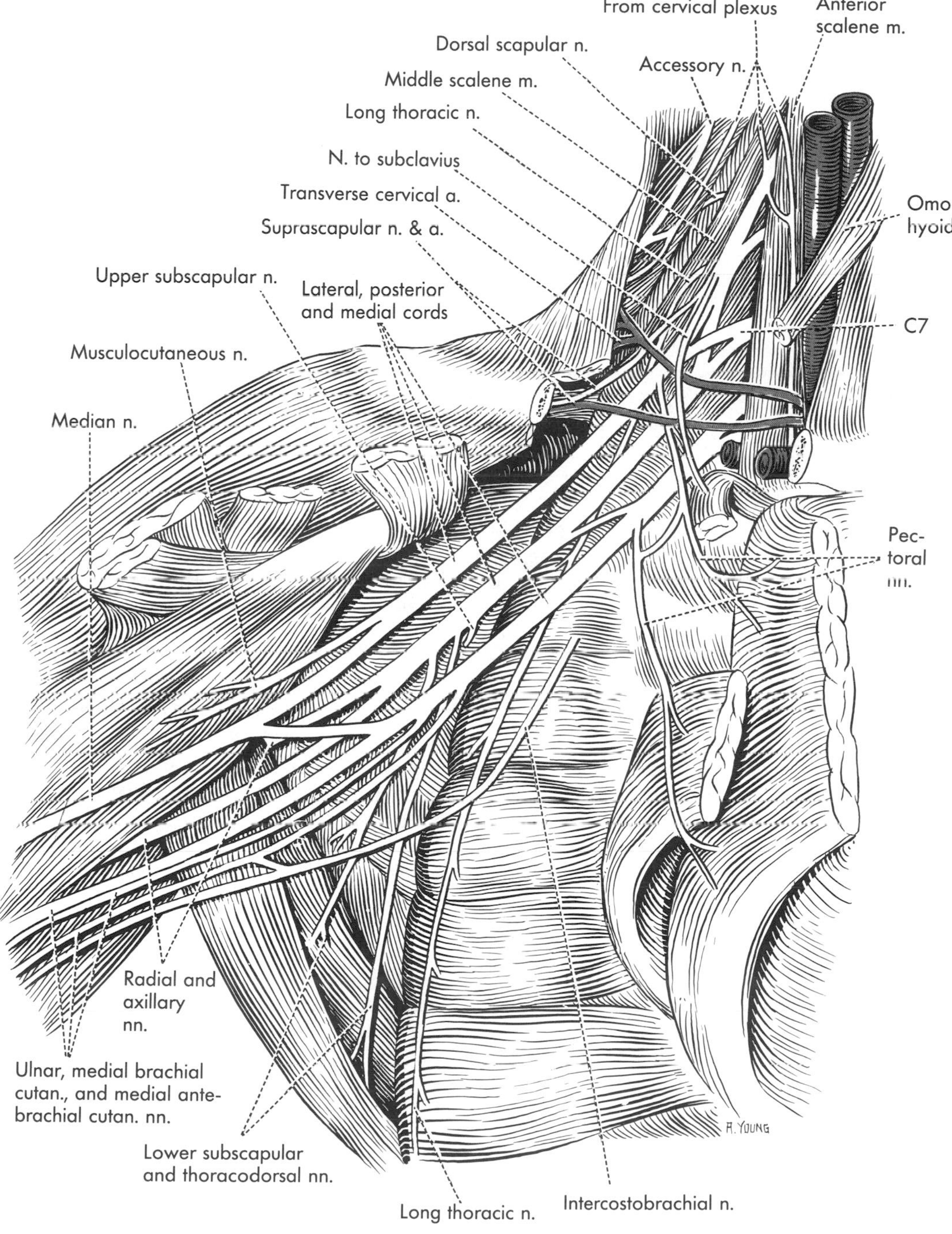

FIGURE *15-21.*
The brachial plexus and its branches in a dissection of the axilla and neck: In this specimen, the lateral pectoral nerve arises higher than usual, above the clavicle instead of from the lateral cord in the axilla.

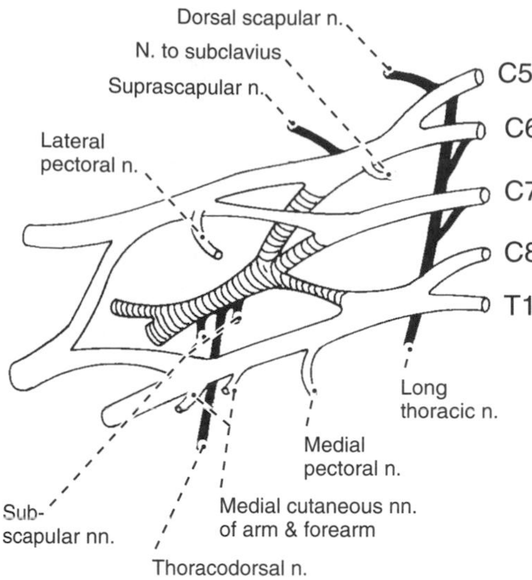

FIGURE *15-22.*
Smaller branches of the brachial plexus from roots, trunks, and cords: The posterior divisions and the posterior cord are *shaded.*

nerve and the **lateral root** of the median nerve; the *medial cord* gives off the **medial root of the median nerve** and the **ulnar nerve**. Thus nerve fibers derived from the posterior divisions are distributed along two major nerves (axillary and radial), and fibers from the anterior divisions are carried in three major nerves (musculocutaneous, median, and ulnar). Even before describing their mode of origin, it is useful to attach from the outset a broad functional designation to each of these nerves.

The **radial nerve** (C-5 to T-1) supplies the extensor musculature of the elbow, wrist, and digits. It is sensory to the skin on the extensor surface of the arm, forearm, and hand. The *radial nerve is the nerve of extension.*

The **axillary nerve** (C-5 and C-6) *supplies the chief abductor of the shoulder,* the deltoid, and the skin overlying it. It is also sensory to the shoulder joint.

The **musculocutaneous nerve** (C-5 and C-6) *is the chief nerve of elbow flexion.* It also supplies skin on the preaxial border of the forearm.

The **median nerve** (C-6, C-7, C-8, and T-1) *is the chief nerve of sensation in the hand* because it supplies the pulp of the digits commonly used for feeling. It is also the *chief nerve for pronation* and for *flexion of the wrist and of the digits.* It supplies the bulk of the muscles in the flexor compartment of the forearm and, in the hand, most of the muscles of the thumb.

The **ulnar nerve** (C-8, T-1, and C-7) *is the chief nerve of the intrinsic muscles of the hand.* It also supplies some forearm muscles in the flexor compartment and skin over the postaxial half of the hand. (The nerve receives a contribution from the anterior division of C-7, sometimes as a delicate slip in the plexus, at other times lower down, as a communicating branch from the median nerve).

Testing the functional integrity of these nerves is discussed with the appropriate regions in this chapter and the next one.

Origin, Course, and Relations. Figures 15-17B and 15-21 illustrate the origin and topographic relations of branches of the plexus. From the *posterior cord* the **radial nerve** proceeds distally behind the axillary artery (see also Fig. 30-21); it may give off one or more small branches before it leaves the axilla. The **axillary nerve** turns posterolaterally from the posterior cord to disappear with the posterior circumflex humeral vessels between the subscapularis and teres major muscles. The **musculocutaneous nerve** diverges laterally from the *lateral cord* and leaves the axilla by passing through the coracobrachialis, a muscle on the medial side of the arm. The **lateral root of the median nerve** (see Fig. 15-17B) crosses to the front of the axillary artery from the lateral cord, as does the **medial root** from the *medial cord.* Their union forms the **median nerve** in front of, or lateral to, the axillary artery. The two roots of the median nerve vary in length, but often form the middle *V* of the letter *M*, the vertical limbs being the musculocutaneous and ulnar nerves (see Fig. 15-21). The **ulnar nerve** leaves the axilla as the continuation of the medial cord between the axillary artery and vein. C-7 fibers usually pass from the lateral cord to the ulnar nerve either along the roots of the median nerve, or as an independent fascicle ("lateral root" of the ulnar) in the axilla or in the arm.

Small Branches of the Plexus. Knowing the site of origin and distribution of the minor branches of the brachial plexus (see Figs. 15-21 and 15-22) is of value in localizing injuries of the plexus. Testing these nerves is discussed with the functional evaluation of the muscles they supply. Above the clavicle, two small nerves arise from the roots and two from the upper trunk; below the clavicle, the lateral cord gives off one small nerve, and the medial and posterior cords each give off three.

From the C-5 root, the **dorsal scapular nerve** proceeds posteriorly to the rhomboids and levator scapulae; C-5, C-6 and C-7 roots give origin to the **long thoracic nerve**, which descends behind the roots, continuing in the axilla on the surface of the serratus anterior and distributing its fibers in a segmental fashion to the muscle.

Two branches arise from the upper trunk. The **suprascapular nerve** (C-5 and C-6) supplies the supraspinatus and infraspinatus muscles and is sensory to the shoulder and acromioclavicular joints. Its course is described in a later section. The **nerve to the subclavius**, the second small branch, crosses in front of the upper part of the plexus to reach its muscle.

The small branch of the lateral cord is the lateral pectoral nerve; the three minor branches of the medial cord are the medial pectoral nerve and two cutaneous nerves, one for the arm and the other for the forearm.

The **lateral pectoral nerve** (C-5, C-6, C-7), given off by the *lateral cord,* is connected to the **medial pectoral nerve** (C-8 and T-1) by a communicating loop close to the origin of that nerve from the *medial cord* (see Fig. 15-21). Both pectoral nerves supply both pectoral muscles, and both terminate in the pectoralis major without any cutaneous distribution. They are named according to their cords of origin, not their positions in the pectoral region.

The **lateral pectoral nerve** pierces the clavipectoral fascia close to the medial border of the pectoralis minor and then descends on the posterior surface of the pectoralis major as it branches and distributes segmental fibers to that muscle. The **medial pectoral nerve** leaves the axilla along the lateral border of the pectoralis minor, passes through or around that muscle, and ends in the pectoralis major (see Fig. 15-21).

The remaining two branches of the medial cord, the **medial brachial cutaneous nerve** and the **medial antebrachial cutaneous nerve**, head distally in the company of the ulnar nerve. As their names imply, they innervate the skin on the medial side of the arm and forearm, respectively. The **intercostobrachial nerve**, not a branch of the plexus, but the lateral cutaneous branch of the second intercostal nerve, anastomoses with the medial brachial cutaneous nerve and contributes T-2 fibers for the supply of the skin on the medial side of the arm (see Fig. 15-21).

The three minor branches of the *posterior cord* are the two subscapular nerves and the thoracodorsal nerve between them. The **thoracodorsal nerve** (C-6, C-7, and C-8) descends on the posterior wall of the axilla and supplies the latissimus dorsi (see Fig. 15-21). The **upper** and **lower subscapular nerves** (C-5 and C-6) supply the subscapularis. In addition the lower subscapular nerve, the longer of the two, supplies the teres major. (The teres minor is supplied by the axillary nerve.) Their course is described later in the chapter.

Compression and Injuries

Compression Syndromes. The brachial plexus is subject to compression in three general areas: 1) between the scalene muscles, over the first thoracic rib, by a cervical rib or its fibrous vestige; 2) behind a deformed clavicle; and 3) underneath the coracoid process and pectoralis minor.

Arterial compression is usually part of the syndrome in all three instances. When the subclavian or axillary artery is compressed, the pulse at the wrist is weaker, or may disappear on the affected side. The vein may also be compressed by the coracoid or the clavicle, resulting in swelling and edema of the hand and arm. Pain and paresthesia (tingling or numbness) occur over the area of distribution of the affected nerves, as do muscle weakness and atrophy.

Most commonly the T-1 root is compressed, either by a rib or by increased tone in the scalene muscles (**scalene syndrome** or **thoracic outlet syndrome**). The symptoms and signs are exaggerated by extension of the arm and retraction of the shoulder. Irritation of the sympathetic fibers in the affected roots may result in vasoconstriction, leading to painful ischemic changes in the hand (Raynaud's disease). The condition may culminate in gangrene. Hyperextension of the arm at 45° abduction will reproduce the syndrome of clavicular or coracoid compression of the neurovascular structures. The radial pulse may be obliterated by this maneuver in many normal individuals who have no symptoms or signs.

Injuries. In addition to compression, the brachial plexus may be injured by penetrating wounds or by traction on the upper limb. Penetrating injuries are localized and may occur anywhere in the plexus; traction injuries usually affect the roots of the plexus. The latter are more common and more serious.

Traction force may be applied to the plexus in two ways: 1) by increasing the angle between the neck and the shoulder, and 2) through the abducted arm. When the body is forcefully thrown and lands with the shoulder against the ground, neck and shoulder will be forced apart and the upper roots of the plexus (C-5 and C-6) will become avulsed. The same type of injury may result from pulling on the fetal head during delivery. On the other hand, when the arm is wrenched or when it catches the weight of the body falling from a height, the lower roots (C-8 and T-1) will suffer damage. The C-5 or C-6 lesions will leave the patient with a greatly disabled shoulder, but a reasonably functional hand, whereas damage to C-8 or T-1 will produce the opposite result.

The prognosis is influenced by the actual site of the tear. This may be located fairly precisely with knowledge of the anatomic distribution of the sensory and motor components of the affected roots, and of the branches of the brachial plexus. With the aid of Chapters 13 and 14 and this chapter, it should be possible to construct the clinical picture that results from interruption of individual roots, trunks, or cords of the plexus. This diagnostic exercise has to be performed in the reverse in clinical practice in which the lesion has to be identified from the clinical picture.

SHOULDER

The shoulder is a large and poorly defined region. In the most inclusive sense, the term encompasses the square prominence of the shoulder made up of the acromial and deltoid regions, the glenohumeral (shoulder) joint along with the acromioclavicular joint, and the scapular region in the back, including the muscles that attach the scapula to the vertebral column from the skull to the sacrum. The contents of this large region include the scapula, the lateral end of the clavicle, and the proximal end of the humerus (all discussed in the introductory section of the chapter); joints, which are discussed in the last section; and the muscles, nerves, and blood vessels that are associated with these bones and joints. As in the pectoral region, the nerve and blood supply of the skin and superficial tissues is different from that of the deep structures. These tissues are discussed in the general orientation section of this chapter, as are the surface features and landmarks of this region (see Figs. 15-1, 15-2, and 15-6). The **superficial fascia** presents no notable feature. It is rather adherent to the deep fascia and, over the acromion, contains a *subcutaneous bursa,* which facilitates sliding of the skin over this bony prominence. Some features of the deep fascia are discussed with the relevant muscles.

Muscles and Associated Structures

The muscles of the shoulder region, like those of the pectoral region, fall into two functional groups in accordance with the classification given in the introductory section to this chapter. The topographic arrangement of these muscles, however, is more complex than that of the pectoral muscles (Fig. 15-23). They are all associated with the scapula and are important for the mobility of the upper limb as a whole. To evaluate limitations of movement, or to localize lesions to parts of the brachial plexus and its branches, it is often necessary to assess the function of individual muscles. Twelve in number, they are grouped according to their function and topographic arrangement.

The muscles that move the pectoral girdle and humerus in relation to the axial skeleton are aptly designated the extrinsic muscles of the shoulder; those that move the humerus in relation to the scapula are the intrinsic muscles. The **extrinsic muscles** are disposed in a superficial and a deep subgroup. The *superficial* extrinsic muscles, consisting of the trapezius and latissimus dorsi, cover not only the extensor musculature of the spine (see Fig. 12-32), but also the deep extrinsic muscles and most of the intrinsic shoulder muscles as well. The *deep subgroup* includes the levator scapulae and two rhomboid muscles, each of which attaches the scapula to the vertebral column, and the serratus anterior, which attaches the scapula to the rib cage (see Fig. 15-25). The **intrinsic muscles** include the deltoid, three muscles that fill the fossae on the surfaces of the scapula (subscapularis, supraspinatus, and infraspinatus), and two that attach to its lateral border (teres major and minor) (see Fig. 15-23). With one exception (the trapezius), all of these muscles receive innervation from the brachial plexus.

Superficial Extrinsic Muscles

Trapezius. The trapezius attaches the clavicle and scapula to the vertebral column. It is the most superficial muscle in the hack and plays an important role in elevation and retraction of the shoulder as well as in rotation of the scapula. Each muscle is shaped like a large triangle with its base along the midline and its apex pointing toward the tip of the shoulder (see Fig. 15-23). Taken together, the two muscles present a trapezoid shape on the back, which accounts for their name.

The **origin** of the trapezius is from the skull along the medial part of the *superior nuchal line* and the *external occipital protuberance;* in the neck, it is attached to the *ligamentum nuchae;* over the thorax, it originates from all the *thoracic vertebral spinous processes* and their connecting supraspinous ligaments. Occasionally, the muscle fails to reach the skull. The uppermost fibers

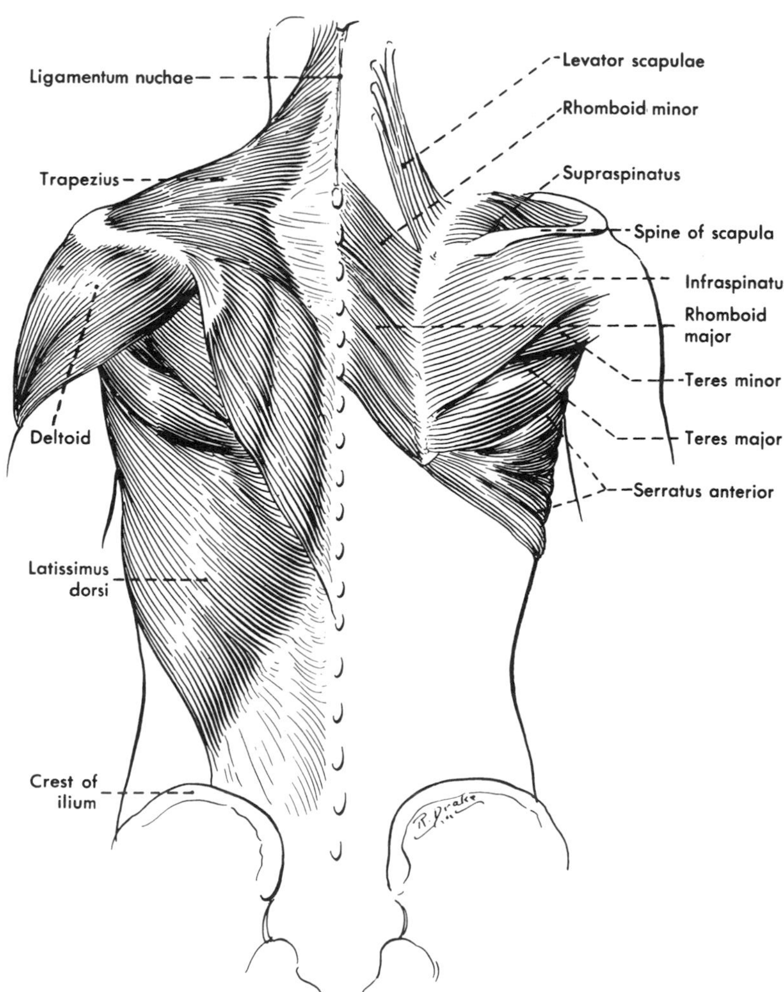

FIGURE *15-23.*
Posterior view of the muscles of the shoulder; the trapezius, latissimus dorsi, and deltoid have been removed from the *right side*.

run downward and forward to **insert** on the lateral third of the *clavicle* (see Fig. 15-4); the fibers arising from the lower cervical and upper thoracic region, usually the thickest part of the muscle, maintain a downward slope and insert on the *acromion* (see Fig. 15-5); the fibers arising from most of the thoracic region pass laterally and upward to insert along the length of the *spine of the scapula*.

The upper fibers that slope downward work together with the levator scapulae and rhomboids to elevate the pectoral girdle; those that are directed upward depress the girdle; the central horizontal fibers retract the shoulder. Acting together, the upper and lower parts of the muscle rotate the scapula (see under section: Movements at the Shoulder Joint). The muscle is readily demonstrated by observing its contraction in the lateral contour of the neck when the shoulders are elevated. Its power can be tested by pressing down on the shoulder while the subject is attempting to elevate it; or better, by palpating its contraction while opposing abduction of the arm. When the muscles of the two sides contract, lack of symmetry of the upper fibers along the contour of the neck is the best indication of weakness or paralysis.

The trapezius is innervated by the *spinal accessory nerve* (which originates in upper cervical cord segments, and leaves the cord independently between the posterior and anterior roots), and by sensory (proprioceptive) branches of the anterior rami of C-2, C-3, and C-4 spinal nerves. Unlike the other shoulder muscles, it receives no fibers from the brachial plexus, a curious finding that has not been explained.

Latissimus Dorsi. The latissimus dorsi attaches the humerus to the axial skeleton (Fig. 15-24). It has migrated farther from the upper limb bud than any other upper limb muscle. The muscle is superficial to the spinal extensors and covers the lower half of the back (see Fig. 12-32). From a very extensive origin, the thin muscular sheet converges toward the posterior axillary fold where it twists around the teres major in a manner analogous to the twist of the pectoralis major upon itself. Together with the teres major, the latissimus dorsi inserts into the humerus (see Fig 15-7). It is supplied by the *thoracodorsal nerve* (C-6, C-7, and C-8), a branch of the posterior cord.

The **origin** of the latissimus dorsi is from the *spinous processes* of the lower six thoracic, all the lumbar, and the upper sacral vertebrae; from the posterior part of the *iliac crest;* and from the lower *three* or *four ribs* by muscular slips that interdigitate here with slips of origin of the external oblique muscle of the abdomen. Close to its insertion, the muscle's twist causes the distal end of its anterior surface to be turned posteriorly. The muscle fibers end in a flattened tendon, separated from that of the teres major by a bursa (subtendinous bursa of the latissimus). It **inserts** into the *crest of the lesser tubercle* and the floor of the intertubercular groove of the humerus.

The latissimus dorsi participates in adduction and extension of the arm. Because it inserts on the front of the humerus, anterior to its axis, it also medially rotates the arm. It participates in a combination of these movements as in a swimming stroke. By exerting force on the humerus, it can depress the shoulder, or prevent its up-

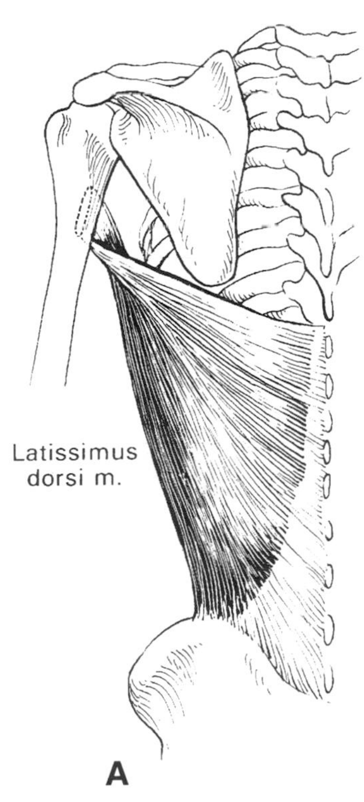

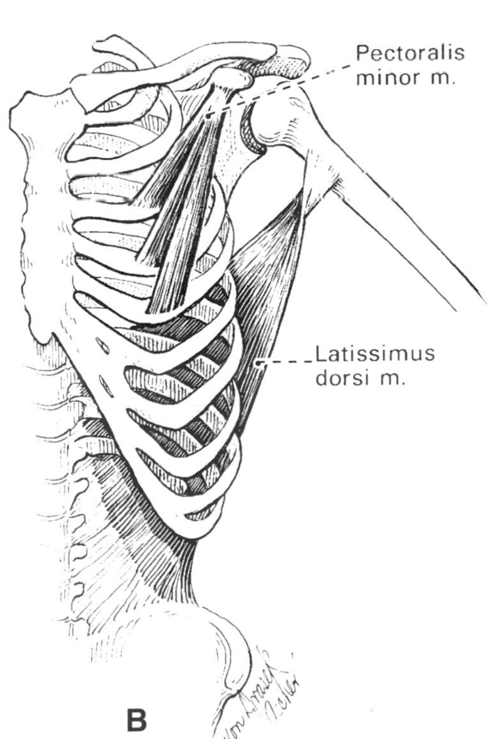

FIGURE *15-24.*
The latissimus dorsi muscle seen (A) from the back and (B) from the front.

ward displacement, which would tend to occur when an individual hangs by the arms or uses a crutch, for example.

Deep Extrinsic Muscles

The levator scapulae, the two rhomboids, and the serratus anterior all attach to the medial border of the scapula and are responsible for moving this bone while retaining it in apposition with the rib cage.

Levator Scapulae and Rhomboids. These three muscles (see Fig. 15-23) elevate and retract the shoulder. The **levator scapulae** arises from the transverse processes of the first three or four cervical vertebrae; the **rhomboid major and minor** arise from the spinous processes of C-7 to T-5 vertebrae and the supraspinous ligaments associated with them. The levator is a distinct muscle, but the two thomboids may be difficult to separate from one another. The three muscles insert in continuity into the medial border of the scapula (see Fig. 15-5): the levator from the superior angle to the base of the scapular spine, and the rhomboids from here to the inferior angle. The levator, being the highest, has the greatest advantage for scapular elevation; the rhomboids are mainly active in retracting the shoulder. All of them are innervated by the *dorsal scapular nerve* (C-5), although the levator also receives fibers directly from cervical anterior rami above the brachial plexus.

Because the upper fibers of the trapezius also elevate the shoulder, it is difficult to assess the levator scapulae independently. The rhomboids, and the dorsal scapular nerve, however, may be tested by having the subject place the forearm horizontally across the back and having the examiner resist the subject's attempt to push the hand posteriorly. To retain the medial border of the scapula close to the spine, the rhomboids contract and spring into prominence.

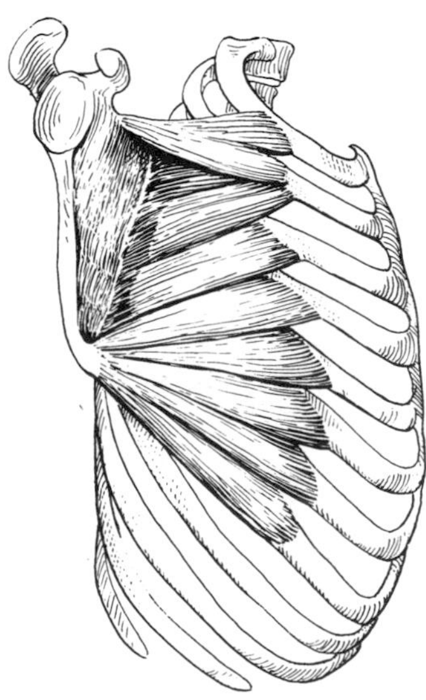

FIGURE *15-25.*
The serratus anterior muscle.

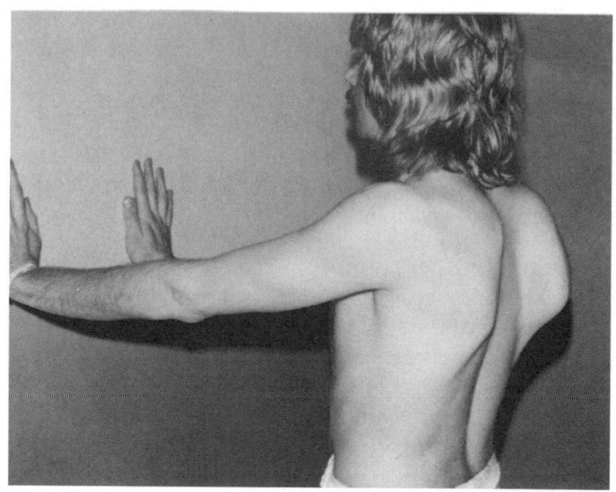

FIGURE *15-26.*
Winging of the scapula caused by paralysis of the serratus anterior. The patient is pushing against the wall. (Courtesy of Dr. David M. Chaplin.)

Serratus Anterior. The serratus anterior attaches the scapula to the axial skeleton. Even at rest, it is chiefly responsible for retaining the scapula in apposition with the chest wall. It is a complex, fan-shaped muscle consisting of eight fleshy digitations (Fig. 15-25). They arise from the anterolateral aspects of the upper eight to ten ribs and converge on the anterior lip of the medial border of the scapula (see Fig. 15-5). The muscle hugs the rib cage, forming the medial wall of the axilla (see Fig. 15-17), before it inserts into the scapula. In muscular subjects, its serrations are readily seen in the axilla (see Fig. 15-1). The origins of its lower slips interdigitate with those of the external oblique muscle of the abdomen (see Fig 15-3).

The muscle's insertion into the scapula is not evenly arranged: the upper four digitations attach along most of the medial border, whereas the lower (and, therefore, the larger) four digitations insert into a relatively small area on the anterior surface of the inferior angle (see Fig. 15-25). By exerting force at this point, they are important in scapular rotation. The upper half of the muscle is responsible mainly for protraction of the shoulder.

The muscle is supplied segmentally (C-5, C-6, and C-7) by the *long thoracic nerve,* a branch of the brachial plexus arising from its roots. The muscle and the nerve are best tested by demonstrating the muscle's ability to keep the scapula in apposition with the chest wall; when weak or paralyzed, *winging of the scapula* will occur when the subject pushes against an immovable object in front of him or her (Fig. 15-26). The less force used, the more sensitive the test. It is chiefly the serratus anterior that prevents the scapula from being pushed away from the trunk during push-ups, when the body weight is supported on the arms.

Intrinsic Shoulder Muscles

The intrinsic muscles of the shoulder attach the humerus to the pectoral girdle. Largest and most superficial among them is the deltoid, which provides the power for abducting the arm. The subscapularis, supraspinatus, infraspinatus, and the two teres muscles stabilize and retain the head of the humerus in the shallow glenoid cavity. Forming a musculotendinous cuff around the shoulder joint, these short muscles, largely hidden by the trapezius and deltoid, are critical for the normal functioning of this joint (see Fig. 15-28).

A relatively dense layer of **deep fascia** covers the subscapularis muscle on the anterior surface of scapula and similar layers invest the supraspinatus and infraspinatus muscles in the respective fossae of the scapula. Fibrous septa extend from the fascia to the underlying bone, separating these muscles from their neighbors. In a similar manner, septa extend from the deep fascia of the deltoid into its fleshy substance. All these septa provide additional surfaces for the attachment of muscle fibers, thereby increasing the bulk of each muscle.

Deltoid. The large size of the deltoid and the prominent acromion, from which the deltoid largely arises, are features characteristic of the shoulder in the human. Although it is the largest abductor of the shoulder, the deltoid has to rely on synergy with other intrinsic shoulder muscles to exert its force (as explained later).

The triangular, bulky mass of the deltoid is composed of three parts. (Fig. 15-27). Anterior and posterior parts of the muscle, which arise from the clavicle and scapular spine, respectively (see Figs. 15-4 and 15-5), are composed of parallel fibers and are more suited for flexing and extending the arm than abducting it. The central portion of the muscle takes origin by shorter fibers from the acromion, and these fibers insert into *tendinous septa* within the muscle from which, in turn, new fibers originate. This multipennate arrangement lends power to the muscle, and it is this central portion that is most active in abduction. All three parts of the muscle insert into the *deltoid tuberosity* half way down the shaft of the humerus (see Fig. 15-7). Thus the general direction of all the fibers is vertical.

Although activity is evident in the muscle from the beginning of abduction, it can only exert abductive power if the humeral head is stabilized by the other intrinsic muscles. If it is not, the deltoid simply elevates the humerus in the pendant position without causing any abduction. Once the arm has been raised above the head, the deltoid largely relaxes.

The deltoid is innervated by the *axillary nerve,* (C-5 and C-6). Integrity of the nerve (which is prone to injury; see later) and the power of the deltoid is best tested by opposing abduction at about 45°. When the deltoid is weak and wasted as a result of nerve injury, or of disuse because of a painful shoulder, the point of the shoulder becomes prominent.

Supraspinatus. The supraspinatus is active throughout abduction. The muscle has been called the *workhorse of abduction*. It fills the supraspinous fossa, where its hard muscle belly may be palpated through the trapezius during abduction (Fig. 15-28, and also see 15-23). The muscle takes its origin from the fossa (see Fig. 15-5) and from the fascia that covers the muscle, and inserts on the greater tubercle of the humerus (see Fig. 15-7). Before doing so, its tendon fuses with the capsule of the shoulder joint. It is separated from the overlying acromion, the coracoacromial ligament, and the deltoid muscle by the subacromial and subdeltoid bursae (see Fig. 15-28 and 15-33).

The muscle is ideally placed for initiating abduction by spurt action, and its contraction is necessary for the deltoid to obtain a purchase (see Fig. 15-33). The supraspinatus is innervated chiefly by C-5 through the *suprascapular nerve*, given off by the upper trunk of the brachial plexus.

Infraspinatus and Teres Minor. Because they are placed on the posterior aspect of the shoulder joint (see Fig. 15-28), these two muscles produce lateral rotation of the humerus. The method for assessing their power is de-

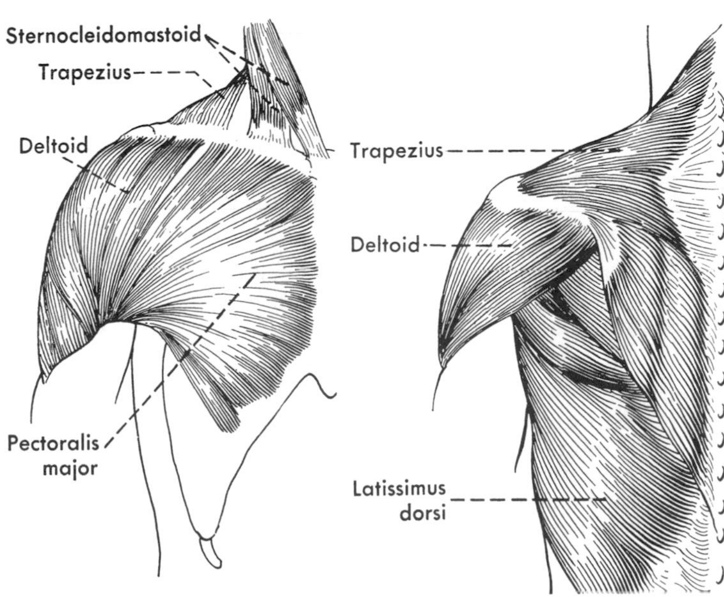

FIGURE 15-27.
The deltoid muscle seen in an *anterior view* of the right shoulder and a *posterior view* of the left.

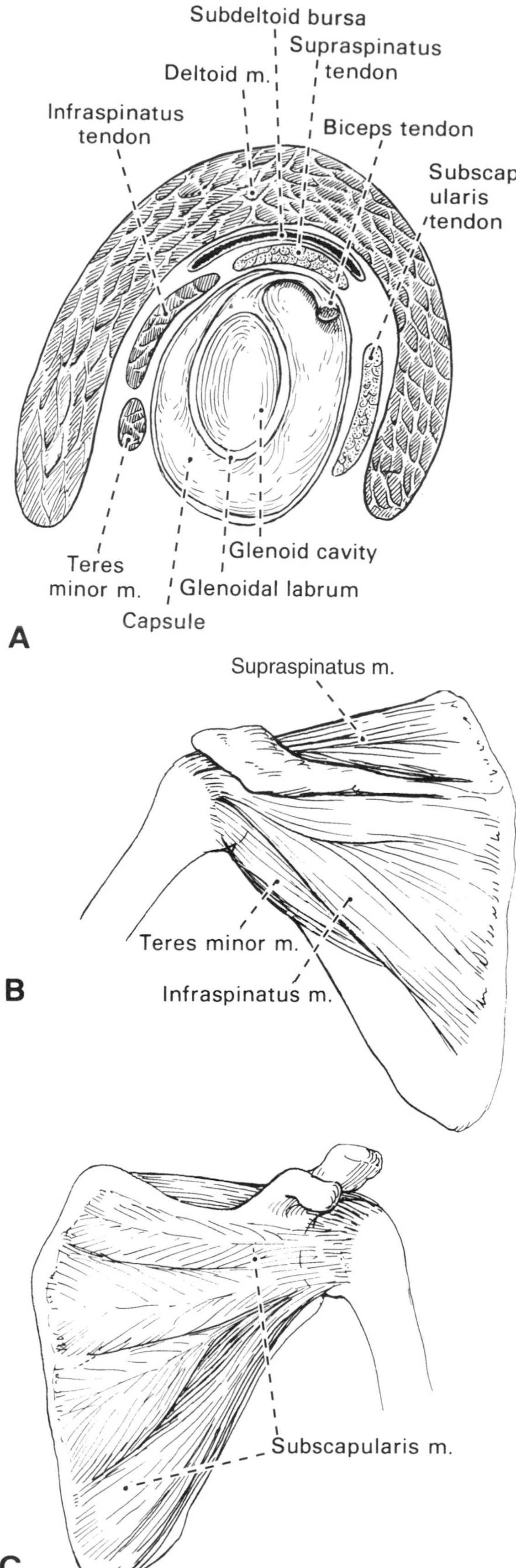

scribed with the evaluation of the movements of the shoulder joint (see Fig. 15-37). Owing to the upward slope of their fibers, both muscles contribute an important downward vector to counterbalance the upward pull exerted on the humerus by the powerful deltoid, thereby assuring that the humeral head is optimally positioned in the glenoid cavity during abduction.

The infraspinatus arises from the infraspinous fossa and the teres minor from an adjoining area on the lateral border of the scapula (see Fig. 15-5). The two muscles are separated by a fascial septum, to which both attach, and they insert into the greater tubercle of the humerus, posterior to the supraspinatus (see Fig. 15-7). The infraspinatus is innervated by the *suprascapular nerve* and the teres minor by the *axillary nerve* (Fig. 15-29).

Teres Major. The teres major, located in the posterior axillary fold, is an adductor and extensor of the shoulder (see Figs. 15-23 and 15-29). The muscle arises from the lateral border of the scapula below the teres minor (see Fig. 15-5) and inserts with the latissimus dorsi into the crest of the lesser tubercle of the humerus (see Fig. 15-7). Because it passes to the anterior surface of the humerus, it also medially rotates that bone. The muscle is innervated from the posterior cord of the brachial plexus by the *lower subscapular nerve* (C-5, C-6, and C-7). The visible and palpable contraction of the muscle can be distinguished in the axilla and in the back when adduction of the elevated arm is resisted by the examiner. Curiously, the teres major seems to function in adduction only when resistance to the movement is offered.

Relations. The teres major is related to several muscles, and some of these relations are useful landmarks for locating the nerves and vessels. The lower border of the teres major is considered the boundary line between the axilla and the arm. The anterior surface of the muscle is crossed by the nerves and vessels continuing from the axilla into the arm (see Figs. 15-17B and 15-21).

As the teres major approaches the humerus, it passes in front of the long head of the triceps (see Fig. 15-29). Two small gaps are delineated above the teres major, one on either side of the long head of the triceps. The more medial is the triangular space, bounded by the teres major, the teres minor, and the long head of the triceps. The more lateral is the quadrangular space, bordered above and below by the teres muscles and, on its sides, by the humerus and the long head of the triceps. The axillary nerve and posterior circumflex humeral artery pass through the quadrangular space, and the circumflex scapular artery through the triangular space.

The teres major is separated from the teres minor, the infraspinatus, and the subscapularis by *intermuscular septa.* As noted earlier, the latissimus

FIGURE *15-28.*
Intrinsic muscles of the shoulder that contribute to the formation of the tendinous cuff, sheltered by the deltoid: (A) Lateral view of the socket of the glenohumeral joint after the humerus, with its muscles; has been removed; (B) Posterior and (C) anterior aspects of the intrinsic muscles of the shoulder.

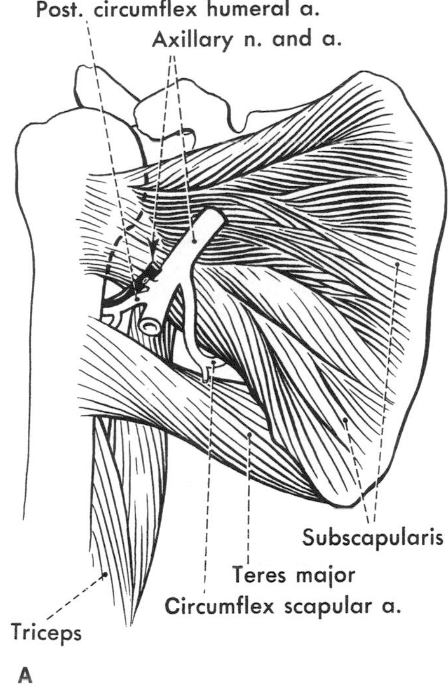

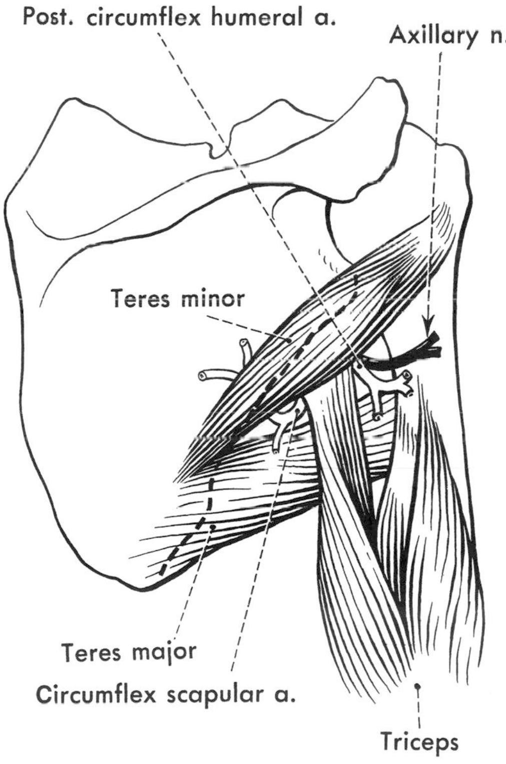

FIGURE *15-29.*
The subscapularis and teres major and minor muscles, with the triangular and quadrangular spaces bordered by them: (A) Anterior view; (B) posterior view. The axillary nerve and the posterior circumflex humeral artery traverse the quadrangular space, whereas the circumflex scapular artery passes through the triangular space.

dorsi approaches the teres major from behind and below, twists around it, giving a rounded contour to the posterior axillary fold, and inserts anterior to it. A bursa intervenes between the two muscles close to their insertion.

Subscapularis. The muscle arises from the costal surface of the scapula (see Fig. 15-5), its broad tendon passing across the front of the shoulder joint to insert into the lesser tubercle of the humerus and its crest (see Fig. 15-7). The *subscapularis bursa* intervenes between the muscle and the neck of the scapula (see Fig. 15-32). The subscapularis muscle completes the musculotendinous cuff around the shoulder joint anteriorly (see Figs. 15-28 and 15-29). Being the anterior counterpart of the infraspinatus and teres minor, it medially rotates the humerus as well as holds the head of the humerus against the glenoid cavity. The fibers of its lower half exert a downward pull on the humerus, assisting the infraspinatus in counterbalancing the upward pull of the deltoid. The subscapularis is supplied by both *upper and lower subscapular nerves* as they branch off from the posterior cord, and by the *subscapular artery.*

Tendinous Cuff. The supraspinatus, infraspinatus, teres minor, and subscapularis all converge on the greater and lesser tubercles of the humerus. Before reaching them, their tendons fuse with the underlying capsule of the shoulder joint and with each other, forming in effect a cuff around the superior aspect of the joint (see Fig. 15-28). The integrity of this structure, known as the **rotator cuff,** is essential for abduction and plays an important stabilizing role in all movements of the humerus. The muscles operating at the shoulder through the cuff dynamically stabilize and steer the head of the humerus. They balance the forces to which the shoulder joint is subjected by its powerful prime movers, in particular the deltoid and the pectoralis major.

Although the term *rotator cuff* is widely used, not all the muscles contributing to it are actually rotators of the humerus. Notably the supraspinatus, most frequently involved in rotator cuff lesions, is purely an abductor. *Tendinous cuff* is a preferable term. Functionally speaking, the tendon of the long head of the biceps, which passes through the shoulder joint between the greater and lesser tubercles of the humerus (see Figs. 15-32 and 15-33), can be considered part of the tendinous cuff. It assists the cuff muscles in stabilizing the humeral head.

The tendinous cuff is subject to degenerative changes, calcification, and rupture. Tears and defects have been found in more than 25% of cadaver specimens. The microscopic anatomy and microvasculature of the cuff have been studied extensively to explain the etiology of "rotator cuff tendon failure." Repetitive traumatization of the cuff owing to its impingement on the acromion and coracoacromial ligament during abduction is believed to be a predisposing factor. The site of rupture may be at the attachment to bone or along the tendon. Extension of the humerus rotates the greater tubercle forward, freeing it from the shelter of the acromion. This allows palpation of the site of insertion of the supraspinatus. Tenderness is suggestive of damage to the tendinous cuff.

Nerves and Vessels

Because they are related to the muscles, all the deep nerves and vessels of the shoulder have been encountered in the preceding section. A summary may, however, serve a useful purpose.

Nerves

The nerves of the shoulder region include the spinal accessory nerve to the trapezius, the dorsal scapular nerve to the rhomboids, C-3 and C-4 additional branches to the trapezius and levator scapulae, the long thoracic nerve to the serratus anterior, the suprascapular nerve to the supraspinatus and infraspinatus, the axillary nerve to the deltoid and teres minor, the thoracodorsal nerve to the latissimus dorsi, and the upper and lower subscapular nerves to the subscapularis, the latter also supplying the teres major.

The **spinal accessory nerve** is an atypical nerve. Its rootlets emerge from the lateral surface of C-1 to C-5 spinal cord segments and unite as they ascend in the subarachnoid space, entering the skull through the foramen magnum. For a short distance the spinal accessory nerve becomes attached to the cranial accessory nerve (the 11th cranial nerve, so named because it is accessory to the vagus nerve). However, as soon as they leave the skull together through the jugular foramen, the two nerves part company, and the spinal accessory nerve descends in the neck behind the sternocleidomastoid. It supplies that muscle as well as the trapezius. Its course is described with the trapezius (see Figs. 30-8 and 30-9). Branches from the third and fourth cervical anterior rami join the accessory nerve; they contain only proprioceptive fibers for the trapezius.

The **dorsal scapular nerve**, derived from C-5 root of the brachial plexus (see Fig. 15-22), runs downward and backward through the scalene muscles and the levator scapulae, to which it gives a branch, and then descends parallel to the medial border of the scapula on the deep surface of the rhomboids to end in them (Fig. 15-30). **Nerves to the levator scapulae** also arise from the third and fourth cervical anterior rami and enter the anterior surface of the levator scapulae close to its origin.

The **long thoracic nerve**, derived from C-5, C-6, and C-7 roots of the brachial plexus (see Fig. 15-22), runs down in the neck on the middle scalene muscle to reach the first digitation of the serratus anterior (see Fig. 15-21). As described earlier, it descends on this muscle in the axilla.

The **suprascapular nerve** (C-5 and C-6), a branch of the upper trunk of the brachial plexus (see Fig. 15-22), runs laterally under cover of the trapezius and clavicle to reach the suprascapular notch (see Fig. 15-21). It passes through the foramen created by the notch and the superior transverse scapular ligament to enter the supraspinous fossa, where it gives branches to the supraspinatus. It then passes beneath the inferior transverse scapular ligament, skirting the root of the scapular spine to enter the infraspinous fossa and end in the in-

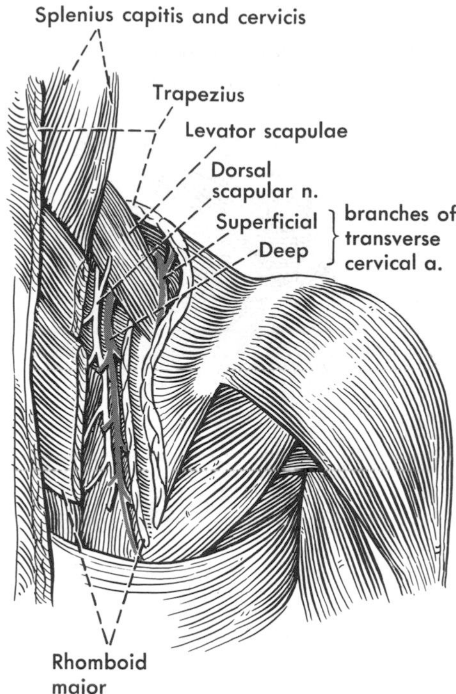

FIGURE *15-30.*
The dorsal scapular nerve and branches of the transverse cervical artery.

fraspinatus muscle (Fig. 15-31). Through most of its course, the nerve is accompanied by the suprascapular artery.

The **axillary nerve** (C-5 and C-6) arises as a terminal branch of the posterior cord (see Figs. 15-20 and 15-21) behind the axillary artery. It leaves the axilla with the posterior circumflex humeral artery (see Fig. 15-17B) by passing along the inferior aspect of the shoulder joint capsule and then through the quadrangular space (see Fig. 15-29). Here it gives a branch to the teres minor and then, running deep to the deltoid, skirts around the posterior aspect of the surgical neck of the humerus. It gives off the *upper lateral brachial cutaneous nerve* to skin overlying the deltoid before it continues forward around the surgical neck of the humerus where it breaks up into branches for the deltoid. The axillary nerve is susceptible to injury in shoulder dislocation, in humeral neck fracture, and when injections are delivered into the deltoid.

The **thoracodorsal nerve** (C-6, C-7, and C-8) leaves the posterior cord of the brachial plexus (see Fig. 15-22) behind the axillary artery, descends on the subscapularis muscle, crosses the teres major and ends in the latissimus dorsi (see Figs. 15-17B and 15-21). The **upper and lower subscapular nerves** arise from the posterior cord on either side of the thoracodorsal nerve (see Fig. 15-22). Both subscapular nerves receive fibers from C-5 and C-6. The upper subscapular nerve passes directly into the subscapularis muscle, but the lower subscapular nerve descends on the subscapularis parallel to the thoracodorsal nerve, giving branches to that muscle and ending in the teres major (see Fig. 15-21).

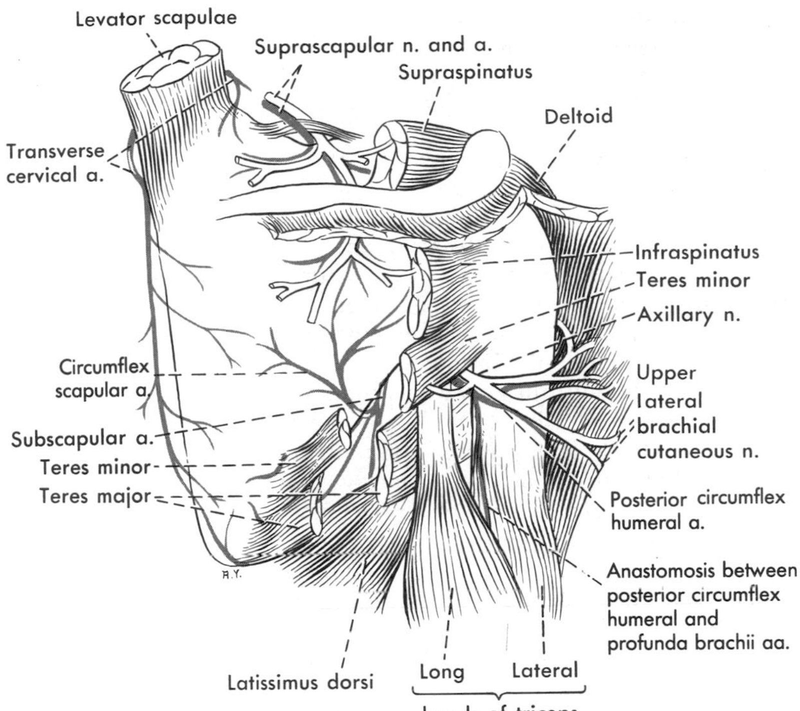

FIGURE *15-31.*
Nerves and vessels of the posterior aspect of the shoulder.

Blood Vessels

The branches and tributaries of the axillary vessels that supply the shoulder are described in earlier sections of this chapter; others arise from and terminate in the subclavian vessels in the root of the neck. Because the arteries are usually accompanied by corresponding veins, the following account deals only with arteries. The arteries to be summarized include two branches derived from the subclavian artery: the transverse cervical and suprascapular arteries, which accompany the dorsal scapular and suprascapular nerves, respectively; and several primary and secondary branches of the axillary artery: subscapular and circumflex scapular arteries, the thoracodorsal artery, and the posterior circumflex humeral artery, as well as the lateral thoracic and thoracoacromial arteries.

In addition to providing the blood supply for the structures in the shoulder region, these arteries form an anastomotic system that establishes a potential alternative route for blood flow between the first part of the subclavian artery in the neck and the third part of the axillary artery just before it enters the arm. This system is known as the **circumscapular anastomosis** and allows blood to reach the arm should the intervening arterial trunk become blocked.

Course of the Arteries. The **transverse cervical** (*transverse colli*) and **suprascapular arteries** originate in the root of the neck from the *thyrocervical trunk,* a branch of the subclavian artery (see Figs. 15-18 and 30-23). Running parallel with each other in front of the brachial plexus, they cross the lower part of the neck (see Fig. 15-21) and turn posteriorly. The transverse cervical artery heads toward the levator scapulae and rhomboids to join the dorsal scapular nerve. The suprascapular artery joins the suprascapular nerve and heads toward the scapular notch.

As the transverse cervical artery reaches the levator scapulae, it divides into a *superficial branch* that runs on the deep surface of the trapezius and a *deep branch* that descends on the deep surface of the rhomboids with the dorsal scapular nerve (see Fig.15-30). The two branches of the transverse cervical artery may arise separately from the thyrocervical trunk. As it crosses the scapular notch, the *suprascapular artery* runs above the superior transverse scapular ligament, which separates it from the nerve (see Fig. 15-31). They then rejoin one another and ramify in the supraspinous and infraspinous fossae, the contents of which they supply.

The **subscapular artery** arises from the third part of the axillary artery and soon divides into two branches, the thoracodorsal and circumflex scapular (see Figs. 15-17B and 15-18). The **thoracodorsal artery** continues downward on the subscapularis muscle, supplying it and the teres major. The **circumflex scapular artery** turns posteriorly through the triangular space around the lateral border of the subscapularis muscle and the scapula (see Fig. 15-29). It passes upward in the infraspinous fossa, supplies the muscle and the scapula, and anastomoses with other vessels.

The **posterior circumflex humeral artery** arises from the third part of the axillary artery (see Fig. 15-17B) and passes posteriorly through the quadrangular space with the axillary nerve (see Figs. 15-29 and 15-31). It runs around the surgical neck of the humerus, giving off branches into the deltoid muscle, and ends by anastomosing with the much smaller *anterior circumflex humeral artery.*

Two branches from the second part of the axillary artery also contribute to the supply of the structures around the shoulder. These are the deltoid branch of the **thoracoacromial artery**, which helps to supply the deltoid muscle, and the **lateral thoracic artery**, which supplies the serratus anterior (see Fig. 15-18).

Anastomoses. Most vessels of the pectoral and shoulder regions can participate in collateral circulation, but the anastomoses are particularly well developed on the posterior surface of the scapula (see Fig. 15-31). Branches of the transverse cervical and suprascapular arteries anastomose with those of the circumflex scapular artery. The smaller **acromial anastomosis** (*acromial rete;* discussed earlier) links branches of the suprascapular artery with those of the thoracoacromial and circumflex humeral vessels. The latter also anastomose with branches of the brachial artery (profunda brachii).

Should the third part of the subclavian artery become compressed as it crosses the first rib (thoracic outlet syndrome; see foregoing), or the axillary artery be ligated or blocked in its first or second part, blood can flow from the transverse cervical and suprascapular vessels retrogradely along the circumflex scapular and subscapular arteries. From these it can be distributed to the other vessels, either through the axillary artery or through direct connections between the branches of neighboring vessels themselves.

Moreover, because the branches of several arteries in this region (transverse cervical, lateral thoracic, and thoracodorsal) also anastomose with perforating branches of the intercostal arteries, blood can reach the pectoral and scapular regions from the aorta through these channels as well. More importantly, when there is an obstruction in the aorta (see Chap. 22; Fig. 22-10), blood may circumvent the obstruction by flowing from the arch of the aorta through the subclavian vessels, the circumscapular anastomosis, the perforating branches of the intercostal arteries, and back to the aorta. Thus, parts of the body distal to the obstruction may still be perfused. The enlarged perforating vessels may, over time, erode the bone, causing notching of the ribs (evident on radiographs).

Lymphatics

The deep lymphatic vessels of the shoulder follow the blood vessels. Most drain into axillary lymph nodes. Some, however, drain along the transverse cervical and suprascapular vessels into deep cervical lymph nodes that lie under cover of the trapezius and in the posterior triangle of the neck.

JOINTS AND MOVEMENTS

The chapter on the Basic Structural Plan of the Limbs (see Chap 14), as well as the general orientation section of this chapter, introduced the sternoclavicular, acromioclavicular, and glenohumeral joints and the types of movements permitted by each. This section describes the anatomy of these joints as the foundation for analyzing their movements and evaluating their functional integrity.

Movements between the scapula and clavicle take place at the **acromioclavicular joint**. The clavicle, in turn, articulates with the manubrium at the **sternoclavicular joint**. In addition, several muscles link the scapula and clavicle to the axial skeleton. By definition, this linkage can be considered a joint and is designated the *scapulothoracic joint*. In all movements of the shoulder, the scapulothoracic, sternoclavicular, and acromioclavicular joints work together with the **glenohumeral joint** in a synchronized rhythm (Fig. 15-32). The glenohumeral joint is known colloquially as the *shoulder joint*. However, the term *shoulder* is also used to designate the region that encompasses the glenohumeral, acromioclavicular, and scapulothoracic joints (see section entitled Parts and Re-

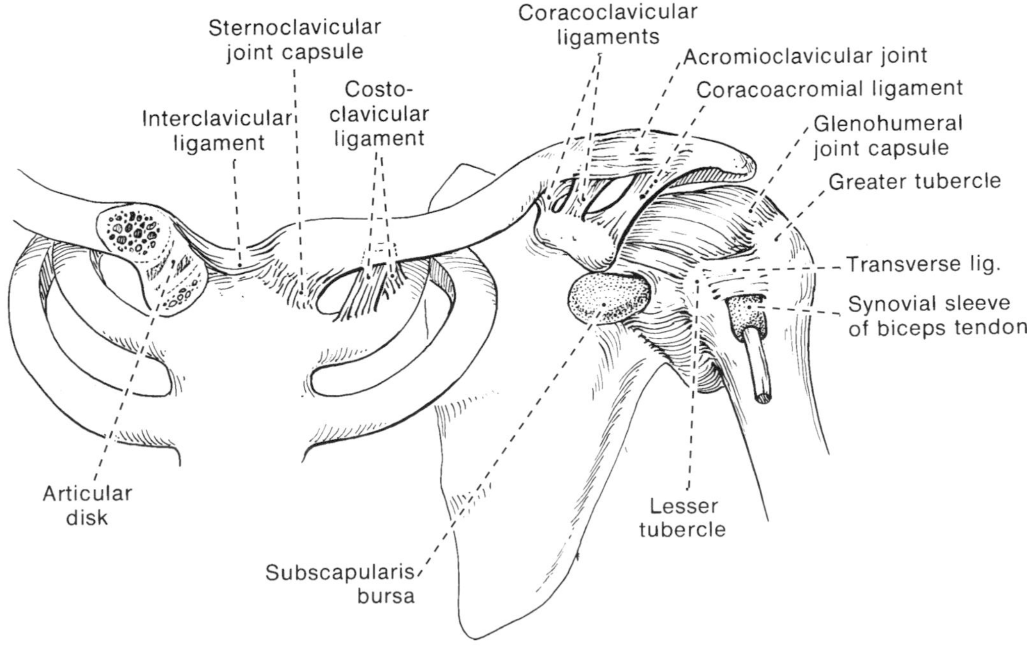

FIGURE *15-32.*
The sternoclavicular, acromioclavicular, and glenohumeral joints, with associated ligaments seen from the *front*.

gions). Therefore, when speaking of movements of the shoulder, or when clinically evaluating them, it is important to be clear about the context in which the term is being used.

Sternoclavicular Joint

This synovial joint is formed by the articulation of the sternal end of the clavicle with the clavicular notch of the manubrium sterni (see Fig. 15-32). The joint allows the shoulder to be moved up and down, forward and backward, or in a combination of these movements.

Although the articular surfaces of the two bones are reciprocally saddle-shaped, they are quite flat and disparate in size. In fact, they do not actually come in contact with one another, being separated by an *articular disk.* The comparatively large sternal end of the clavicle rocks and rotates on the smaller fulcrum provided by the manubrium and the adjoining first costal cartilage, the medial end of which is frequently included in the joint. The joint is readily located in the living subject by the prominent medial end of the clavicle, which projects above the manubrium, and on each side forms the lateral boundaries of the jugular notch.

The *articular disk* divides the joint into two entirely separate synovial cavities. It is attached above to the clavicle, and below to the cartilage of the first rib at its articulation with the sternum. These attachments tend to resist medial displacement of the clavicle. Around its periphery the disk is also attached to the joint capsule. In addition to stabilizing the clavicle, the disk acts as a hinge upon which the clavicle can move. The lower part of the articular surface of the clavicle swings laterally and away from the disk as the shoulder is elevated, and back toward the disk as the shoulder is depressed. This is the freest movement of the clavicle, but protraction (thrusting the shoulder forward) and retraction (bracing the shoulder back) also take place at this joint. Rotation of the clavicle about its long axis accompanies elevation of the shoulder and abduction of the arm. This movement is typically not permitted in a saddle joint, but is made possible here by the presence of the articular disk.

The **fibrous capsule** of the sternoclavicular joint is the key structure in supporting the weight of the entire upper limb. It is strengthened by **anterior** and **posterior sternoclavicular ligaments**, of which the posterior is the thicker. The two clavicles are also joined to one another across the upper surface of the sternum by an **interclavicular ligament** which, together with the sternoclavicular ligaments, tends to prevent lateral and upward displacements of the clavicle. The joint is further reinforced by the **costoclavicular ligament** that is attached to the first rib and its cartilage and to the inferior surface of the clavicle (see Fig. 15-32). As explained earlier (see section entitled Clavicle), the two laminae of this ligament limit elevation and rotation of the clavicle. The orientation of their fibers, sloping upward and backward, is responsible for backward rotation of the clavicle during elevation of the shoulder and abduction of the arm.

Acromioclavicular Joint

The acromion meets the lateral tip of the clavicle at this small synovial joint (see Fig. 15-32). It is located medial to the tip of the acromion and is not readily discerned by palpation. The small, flat articular facets provide for a certain amount of play between the scapula and the clavicle. The articular capsule, known as the **acromioclavicular ligament**, is rather thin and somewhat lax to permit this movement. An *articular disk* subdivides the joint cavity; the division is usually partial, but occasionally, is complete.

The chief bracing that holds the clavicle and scapula together is not the acromioclavicular joint itself, but rather, the **coracoclavicular ligament**. This structure reinforces the acromioclavicular joint and may be consided a fibrous joint in its own right, connecting the clavicle and the coracoid process of the scapula. It consists of two parts, the trapezoid and conoid ligaments, each named for its distinctive shape. The quadrangular **trapezoid ligament** is attached to the coracoid process for about an inch of its length and runs upward and laterally to attach to the trapezoid line on the inferior surface of the clavicle (see Figs. 15-4 and 15-32). The cone-shaped **conoid ligament** lies partly behind the trapezoid ligament, and its fibers pass upward and backward. The apex of the cone is attached to the bend or knuckle of the coracoid process, and its base to the conoid tubercle on the undersurface of the clavicle (see Figs. 15-4 and 15-32). These two ligaments resist separation of the clavicle and scapula, and assure that the movement of the two bones is coordinated during movements of the shoulder.

Dislocations

The clavicle may become dislocated or subluxed at either end as a result of forces transmitted to it from the free limb. Dislocation at the sternoclavicular joint causes particular concern when the clavicle is displaced posteriorly because it may compress the trachea. Such displacement may result from both direct and indirect violence to the joint. Distracting forces applied to the upper limb commonly injure the acromioclavicular joint, resulting in its dislocation, known as *acromioclavicular separation.* The weight of the arm then pulls the scapula down, leaving the lateral end of the clavicle abnormally prominent. When the distracting force is large, the capsule of the joint (acromioclavicular ligament) is usually torn, as may be the conoid and trapezoid ligaments as well.

Blood Supply and Innervation

The **sternoclavicular** and **acromioclavicular joints** receive their blood supply from twigs of vessels that run close to them. The *clavicular branch of the thoracoacromial artery,* the *internal thoracic artery,* and the *suprascapular artery* furnish such articular branches to the sternoclavicular joint. The acromioclavicular joint is supplied from a network of small vessels (*acromial rete*) lying superficially over the acromion, formed by several arteries of the shoulder. The innervation of the joints is provided by articular branches of the nerves that supply the muscles that move the joints, or by nerves running close to them. The sternoclavicular joint receives twigs from the nerve to the *subclavius muscle* and the *medial supraclavicular nerve*. The acromioclavicular joint is innervated by the *suprascapular, axillary*, and *pectoral nerves*.

Movements of the Pectoral Girdle

The movements of the pectoral girdle comprise elevation, depression, protraction, retraction, and rotation. Typically, these movements are invoked to enhance the functional range obtained at the glenohumeral joint. It is instructive, however, as well as clinically important, to analyze these movements independently of glenohumeral motion.

In the normal limb, the scapula and clavicle always move together; the limits of scapular mobility are actually imposed by the clavicle. The sternal end of the clavicle moves in a direction opposite that of its lateral end, similar to two ends of a lever moving around a fulcrum, which is provided by the taut costoclavicular ligament. This relation no longer exists if 1) the clavicle is fractured, 2) the coracoclavicular or costoclavicular ligaments are torn, or 3) the acromioclavicular joint is dislocated.

Elevation. The scapula and clavicle become elevated in full arm abduction. However, the movement can be performed independently during shrugging of the shoulders. The muscles concerned are the levator scapulae, the rhomboid major and minor, and the upper portion of the trapezius (see Fig. 15-23). The strength of the elevators of the shoulder can be assessed by opposing the subject's attempts to shrug the shoulder.

Depression. Gravity and the weight of the arm depress the scapula and clavicle. Only during climbing, or walking on crutches, is active depression of the pectoral girdle required. In the back, the lower fibers of the trapezius and the latissimus dorsi (by its attachment to the humerus) are the muscles concerned (see Figs. 15-23 and 15-24). Anteriorly, the pectoralis minor and the lower portion of the pectoralis major (through the humerus) assist in the movement (see Figs. 15-14, 15-15, and 15-24).

Protraction. The shoulder is thrust forward by the serratus anterior and pectoralis minor (see Figs. 15-15 and 15-25). The movement commonly accompanies shoulder flexion as in reaching forward, throwing, or stabbing. Sliding of the scapula around the rib cage is governed by the serratus anterior. The lateral end of the clavicle moves passively with the scapula.

Retraction. The rhomboids and the horizontal fibers of the trapezius brace the shoulders back (Fig. 15-23).

Rotation. Scapular and clavicular rotation form such an integral part of arm abduction that the movement is described in that context.

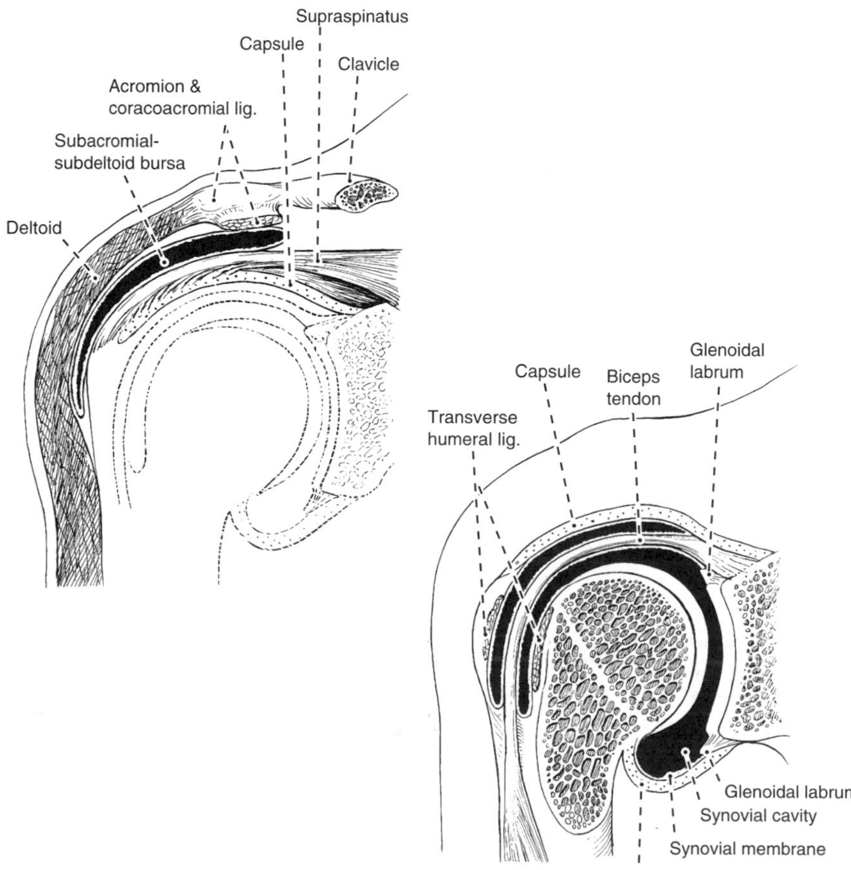

FIGURE 15-33.
Schematic diagram of a coronal section of the shoulder region to show anatomic relations: (A) The position of the deltoid and supraspinatus in relation to the subacromial bursa and the shoulder joint capsule; (B) relations of the glenoidal cavity, labrum, capsule, and biceps tendon.

Glenohumeral Joint

The shoulder is a **polyaxial synovial joint** of the **ball-and-socket** variety, linking the head of the humerus to the glenoid cavity of the scapula.

Articular Surfaces. The roughly hemispheric articular surface on the humeral head, limited by the anatomic neck of the humerus, is approximately four times larger in surface area than the shallow, ovoid socket formed by the glenoid cavity. The latter is slightly enlarged and deepened by a rim of fibrocartilage, the **glenoidal labrum** (Fig. 15-33 and see 15-28). Hyaline articular cartilage covers the bony surfaces. Because neither the ball nor the socket represents a segment of a perfect sphere, only limited areas of the mating surfaces are in contact in any position, permitting the humeral head to slide or spin or both, freely on the glenoid surface. Maximum congruity is obtained between ball and socket in abduction and lateral rotation, which tightens the ligaments of the joint and transforms the humerus and scapula into a single rigid unit. The joint is then said to be in a close-packed position.

Fibrous Capsule and Ligaments. The thin fibrous capsule forms a loose sleeve and puts no restraints on joint movement except in the close-packed position. The capsule is attached just peripheral to the glenoidal labrum. On the humerus, it follows the articular margin around the anatomic neck except inferiorly, where it extends to the surgical neck, thus enclosing the epiphyseal line of the humeral head within the joint cavity (see Fig. 15-33).

The joint capsule hangs loosely below the joint, but is strengthened above and posteriorly by thickened capsular bands and by both extracapsular and intracapsular structures. The **coracohumeral ligament** is a thickening in the capsule between the base of the coracoid process and the greater tubercle. It helps support the weight of the pendant arm; however, with the arm abducted, the ligament is lax and the strength of the joint depends entirely on the muscles of the tendinous cuff. Two to three less well-developed bands (**glenohumeral ligaments**) reinforce the capsule posteriorly. The **tendinous cuff** strengthens the capsule superiorly by fusing with it (see Figs. 15-28 and 15-33). The **coracoacromial arch** made up by the coracoid process, **coracoacromial ligament** and the acromion, overhangs the capsule and tendinous cuff, and forms a large secondary socket for the head of the humerus (see Figs. 15-28 and 15-33). Movement beneath the arch is aided by the presence of the **subacromial and subdeltoid bursae**, which often fuse with each other.

Within the joint, the **tendon of the long head of the biceps** is attached to the upper lip of the glenoid fossa and labrum; it passes over the humeral head and, on leaving the joint, descends in the intertubercular groove (see Figs. 15-28 and 15-33). The fibers of the capsule bridging the groove form the **transverse ligament**, mainly responsible for retaining the tendon in place (see Fig. 15-32). The tendon is a chief stabilizer of the joint. Lateral rotation of the humerus makes the intertubercular groove better accessible for palpation, permitting examination of the tendon, which is subject to degeneration, even a tear, and also dislocation from its groove when the transverse ligament is ruptured.

Synovial Membrane. The capsule is lined by synovial membrane. Within the synovial cavity, a sleeve of synovial membrane invests the tendon of the long head of the biceps (see Figs. 15-32 and 15-33). The synovial membrane of the joint is continuous with that of the subscapularis bursa, which always communicates with the joint (see Fig. 15-32); there is no communication with the subacromial–subdeltoid bursa.

Nerve and Blood Supply. The capsule is supplied by sensory nerves and the synovial membrane predominantly by sympathetic vasomotor nerves. Both types are derived from articular branches of the nerves that supply the prime movers of the joint. Most important are the *axillary* and *suprascapular nerves*, but some contribution is also made by the lateral pectoral nerve and sometimes by independent twigs from the posterior cord or the radial nerve. The **blood supply** to the shoulder joint is from the *suprascapular, subscapular,* and the two *humeral circumflex arteries.*

Relations. In addition to the tendinous cuff, the coracoacromial arch and subacromial–subdeltoid bursa, described in the foregoing, the shoulder joint is covered more superficially by the deltoid muscle. Under cover of the deltoid, the coracobrachialis muscle and the short head of the biceps (see Fig. 16-11A), arising together from the coracoid process, are related to the joint anteromedially. The long head of the triceps, arising from the infraglenoid tubercle, is related posteromedially (see Fig. 15-29). The axillary nerve runs posteriorly along the inferior aspect of the shoulder joint capsule as it passes through the quadrangular space. It may be injured here by the dislocated humerus.

Movements at the Shoulder Joint

Practically all movements in which the humerus swings or slides on the glenoid fossa are accompanied by scapulothoracic and sternoclavicular movements. Scapular and clavicular movements become more pronounced as the humeral swing increases and may continue after the close-packed position has been obtained at the shoulder joint. For an understanding of shoulder mechanisms, and also in clinical evaluation of this region, glenohumeral movements are more profitably analyzed by considering the joints in succession, rather than simultaneously. The shoulder joint may be abducted and adducted, flexed and extended, and laterally and medially rotated. An uninterrupted succession of these movements produces circumduction.

Although the scapula is placed obliquely, for most purposes it is adequate to consider abduction and adduction as raising and lowering the arm at the side of the trunk in the coronal plane, and considering flexion and

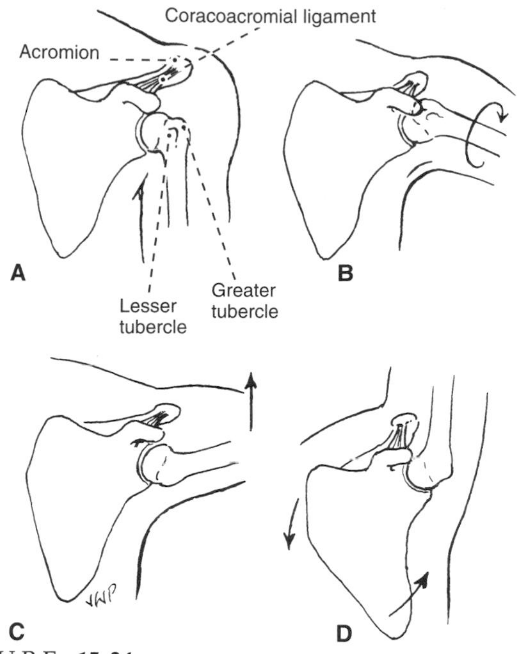

FIGURE *15-34.*
Abduction of the shoulder: starting from the (A) neutral position, (B and C) conjunct rotation of the humerus laterally, places a large area of articular surface above the glenoid cavity, extending the range of glenohumeral abduction from 90° to 120°. (D) An additional 60° of movement is attained by scapular rotation. (Based on McMinn RMH. Last's anatomy. 8th ed. London: Churchill Livingstone, 1990.)

extension as moving the arm forward and backward in a sagittal, rather than an oblique plane.

Abduction. The total range of abduction is 180°. At its maximum the medial surface of the arm can touch the ear. The harmony between glenohumeral and scapulothoracic movement is particularly well illustrated during abduction of the arm. For every 15° of movement, 10° occur at the glenohumeral joint and 5° at the scapulothoracic joint. Clinically, abduction is the most useful movement to test. A significant anatomic defect of the shoulder may be ruled out if the arm can be abducted through 180° without pain and under perfect control.

When abduction is analyzed on the skeleton, it is easy to appreciate that moving the humerus from a pendant position to one in which the humeral and glenoid articular surfaces come edge to edge superiorly, will result in 90° of abduction (Fig. 15-34). This range can be increased to 120° by rotating the humerus laterally, so that the large area of the humeral head now facing downward comes to lie superiorly. The remaining 60° of abduction are accounted for by scapular and clavicular movement.

At 120° of abduction, the close-packed position of the glenohumeral joint is secured. During further abduction, therefore, the humerus and the scapula will be moved as one unit. The abduction force is provided by rotator muscles of the scapula that increase the angle between the superior border of the scapula and the clavicle. This angulation generates tension in the coracoclavicular ligaments; therefore, the clavicle will be elevated and rotated mainly by forces acting on the scapula.

It was emphasized at the outset that movement occurs simultaneously at all joints almost from the start of abduction. However, it is possible to restrain scapular and clavicular movements by grasping the scapula firmly by its inferior angle. Glenohumeral movement can then be assessed independently.

The **rotation element** of humeral abduction needs clarification. The humerus *rotates laterally* during abduction. In most individuals (though not in all), voluntary medial rotation of the humerus restricts glenohumeral abduction. Contrary to common opinion, the cause of lateral rotation is not impingement of the greater tubercle on the acromion. In all instances, the tubercle slides under the acromion (Fig. 15-35), its passage facilitated by the subacromial–subdeltoid bursa. The rotatory element in abduction is an inevitable outcome of the geometric properties of the articulating surfaces. In the loose-packed position of the joint, the point of contact between humerus and glenoid fossa slides along a succession of arcs on an ovoid surface. The rotation will occur *passively* (consequential movement or **conjunct rotation**) as a result of the abduction force without the assistance of lateral rotators.

> The point in question is demonstrated by an interesting exercise (see Fig. 5-14). Standing up, press the palm of the hand against the thigh and, henceforth, keep the hand in this orientation. Now flex the arm to the horizontal and then swing it out laterally (i.e., extend it). When the hand is returned to the thigh, the palm of the hand faces forward. Repeating the same cycle all over, starting from this position, will place the back of the hand against the thigh. The humerus has clearly rotated laterally as a consequence of flexion, extension, and adduction without any *active* rotation. It can be made to rotate medially in a similar manner by performing the exercise in the reverse sequence.

Force of Abduction. The prime movers of glenohumeral abduction are the supraspinatus and the deltoid (see Fig. 15-33). The deltoid provides the power of abduction, whereas the supraspinatus is particularly important in initiating abduction and stabilizing the humeral head in its shallow socket. The supraspinatus is assisted in the latter task by the other intrinsic muscles of the shoulder (see Fig. 15-28). Both the supraspinatus and deltoid exert an upward force on the humeral head, which has to be counterbalanced if the humerus is to remain stabilized on the glenoid fossa. The weight of the arm provides such a counterforce; furthermore, the contractions of the subscapularis, infraspinatus, and teres minor, owing to the obliquity of their fibers, exert a force on the humeral head that has a downward component (see Fig. 15-28). Normal shoulder abduction depends on the operation of these **force couples**. One vector is provided by the prime movers of abduction and the other by the weight of the arm plus the remaining muscles of the tendinous cuff.

Consideration of the force couples explains why tears or paralysis in the musculotendinous cuff (not only in the

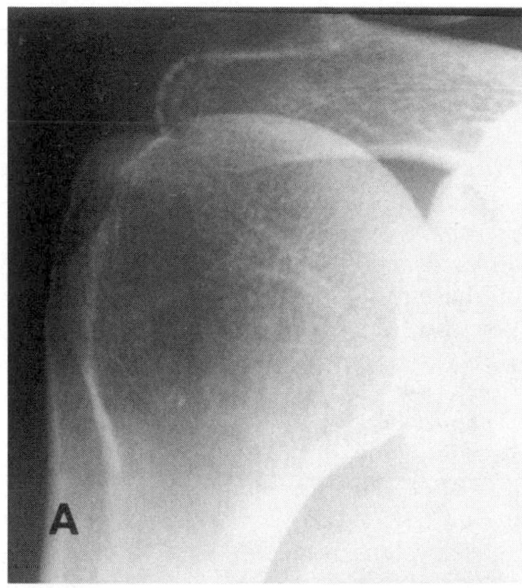

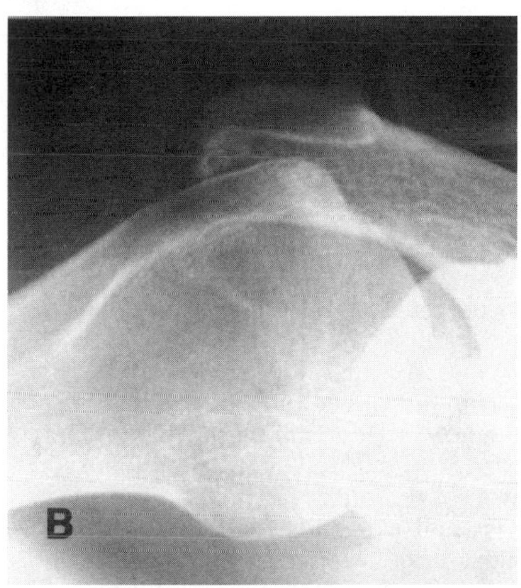

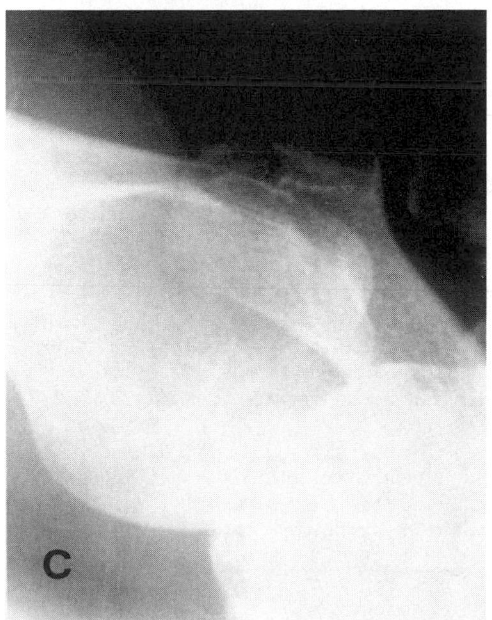

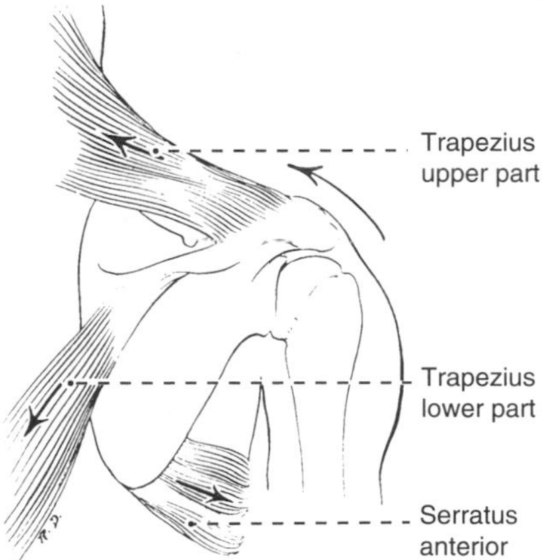

FIGURE *15-36.*
The muscles that rotate the scapula upward during abduction of the arm.

supraspinatus) seriously impair shoulder abduction. In cases of acute tears the limiting factor is pain; once the acute lesion heals, however, the disability is the result of imbalance in the force couples.

> In typical cases of supraspinatus tendon tear or paralysis, abduction cannot be initiated actively, but will proceed normally through deltoid action if the limb is moved passively into 20° to 30° abduction. The subject may achieve this much abduction by automatically leaning toward the affected side and letting the arm hang. Some patients with rotator cuff lesions may be able to abduct the arm and support it above the head without difficulty. However, such individuals will be unable to support the arm at 90° of abduction because one member of the force couple is missing.

Scapular rotation, the final element of arm abduction, is also achieved through force couples, in this case forces that pull tangentially on prominences of the scapula to bring about its rotation (Fig. 15-36). The upper part of the trapezius and the lower half of the serratus anterior turn the scapula like a wing-nut, the wings being the acromion and the inferior angle of the scapula. The portion of the trapezius that attaches to the base of the scapular spine also aids this action.

FIGURE *15-35.*
Sequential radiographs taken during abduction of the humerus to show that the greater tubercle slides under the acromion and that impingement of the tubercle on the acromion, plays no part in bringing about lateral rotation of the humerus. (A) Neutral position; (B) at approximately 90° abduction, the greater tubercle has passed well beyond the lateral margin of the acromion; (C) at about 120°, the acromion shelters a large part of the proximal end of the humerus. Scapular rotation has already taken place. (Courtesy of Dr. Rosalind H. Troupin.)

Adduction. The powerful axillary fold muscles adduct the arm. Anteriorly, the pectoralis major, and posteriorly, the latissimus dorsi and teres major, are the prime movers. A functionally insignificant muscle, the coracobrachialis, which originates from the coracoid and inserts into the humeral shaft (see Figs. 15-7 and 15-17), is also an adductor and represents the only counterpart in the upper limb of the massive adductor musculature of the lower limb.

Adduction is limited by contact between the arm and the rib cage, but the movement may be continued in front of the chest. Protraction of the pectoral girdle contributes significantly to the latter phase of the movement. Powerful adductor movements are required in climbing. The adductor muscles may also be called into action as accessory muscles of respiration when a breathless individual leans on the arms. The points of insertion being now stabilized, these attachments function as points of origin, and the chest wall will be lifted by contraction of the adductor musculature.

Flexion–Extension. In full flexion the arm assumes the same position as at the limit of abduction: the arm contacts the ear. Starting from the neutral position, extension is limited to about 45°. The flexors are the clavicular portion of the pectoralis major and clavicular fibers of the deltoid. The extensors are the latissimus dorsi, teres major, and posterior fibers of the deltoid. The power for extending the flexed arm is provided chiefly by the latissimus dorsi and the sternocostal fibers of the pectoralis major.

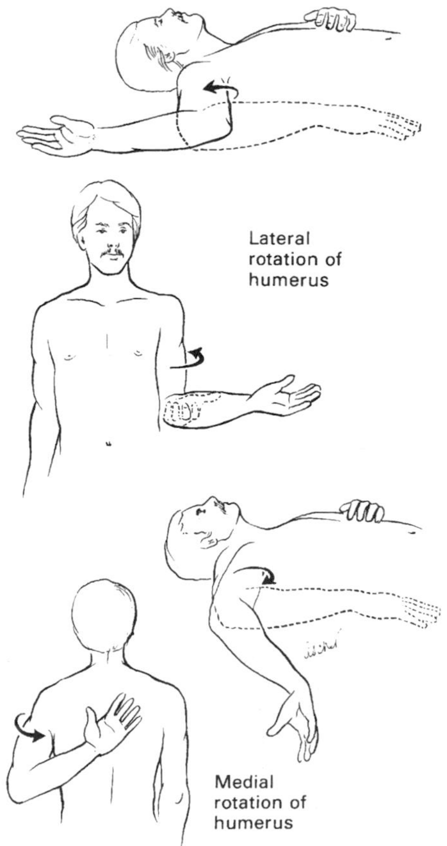

FIGURE *15-37.*
Methods of testing lateral and medial rotation (*arrows*) of the humerus in the erect and supine subject.

Rotation. Lateral rotation may be tested by swinging the forearm laterally when it is flexed in the horizontal position. A simple way of assessing medial rotation is to ask the patient to place his or her hand between his two scapulae. These movements may also be checked in the supine position (Fig. 15-37). Lateral rotation is brought about by muscles from which attachment to the humerus is posterior to the vertical axis of the humerus: these are the infraspinatus, teres minor, and posterior fibers of the deltoid (see Figs. 15-27 and 15-28B). Medial rotation, on the other hand, requires muscles that attach anteriorly to the vertical axis. Prime movers here are the subscapularis, pectoralis major, latissimus dorsi, teres major, and clavicular fibers of the deltoid.

Factors of Stability

Bony contours of the shoulder joint, unlike those of the hip joint, do not contribute anything to stability. Of the capsular ligaments, only the coracohumeral ligament plays a significant role in supporting the weight of the arm. Stability is effected mainly by muscle action. The chief muscular stabilizers are the tendinous cuff muscles. The coracoacromial arch, the tendinous cuff, and the biceps tendon reinforce the joint on its upper aspect. They have no counterparts inferiorly; hence, dislocation usually occurs in this direction. In most cases, the head of the dislocated humerus rests in the axilla just below the coracoid (anterior or subcoracoid dislocation; see Fig. 15-8), where it may be palpated. Compression of the brachial plexus, the axillary artery, and particularly the axillary nerve, must be looked for in these cases. The muscles that run in relation to the inferior aspect of the joint (long head of triceps, short head of biceps, and coracobrachialis) play no active role in stabilizing the joint.

RECOMMENDED READINGS

Basmajian JV, Bazant FJ. Factors preventing downward dislocation of the adducted shoulder joint: an electromyographic and morphological study. J Bone Joint Surg 1959; 41A: 1182.

Basmajian JV, DeLuca CJ. Upper limb. In: Muscles alive: their functions revealed by electromyography. 5th ed. Baltimore: Williams & Wilkins, 1985.

Bateman JE, Fornasier VL. The shoulder and neck. 2nd ed. Philadelphia: Saunders, 1978.

Bennet JD, Vallet AD. US and MR imaging of the axilla. Radiology 1989: 173.

Bundred NJ, Morgan DAL, Dixon JM. Management of regional nodes in breast cancer. BMJ 1994; 309: 1222.

Collins JD, Shaver ML, Disher AC, Miller TQ. Compromising abnormalities of the brachial plexus as displayed by magnetic resonance imaging. Clin Anat 1995; 8: 1.

Egan RL. Breast imaging: diagnosis and morphology of breast disease. Philadelphia: WB Saunders, 1988.

Egan RL. Mammography. 2nd ed. Springfield, IL: Charles C Thomas, 1972.

Gagey N, Quillard J, Gagey O, Meduri G, Bittoun J, Lassau JP. Tendon of the normal supraspinatus muscle: correlations between MR imaging and histology. Surg Radiol Anat 1995; 17: 329.

Gagey N, Gagey O, Bastian G, Lassau JP. The fibrous frame of the supraspinatus muscle. Surg Radiol Anat 1990; 12: 291.

Gagey N, Ravaud E, Lassau JP. Anatomy of the acromial arch: correlation of anatomy and magnetic resonance imaging. Surg Radiol Anat 1993; 15: 63.

Gardner E. The innervation of the shoulder joint. Anat Rec 1948; 102: 1.

Gowan ID, Jobe FW, Tibone JE, Perry J, Moyaes DR. A comparative electromyographic analysis of the shoulder during pitching: professional versus amateur pitchers. Am J Sports Med 1987; 15: 586.

Halsell JT, Smith JR, Bentlage CR, et al. Lymphatic drainage of the breast demonstrated by vital dye staining and radiography. Ann Surg 1965; 162: 221.

Haymaker W, Woodhall B. Peripheral nerve injuries: principles of diagnosis. 2nd ed. Philadelphia: WB Saunders, 1953.

Hollinshead WH. Anatomy for surgeons: vol 3, the back and limbs. 3rd ed. Philadelphia: Harper & Row, 1982.

Hoppenfeld S. Orthopaedic neurology: a diagnostic guide to neurologic levels. Philadelphia: JB Lippincott, 1977.

Hoppenfeld S. Physical examination of the spine and extremities. New York: Appleton-Century-Crofts, 1976.

Huelke DF. A study of the transverse cervical and dorsal scapular arteries. Anat Rec 1958; 132: 233.

Huelke DF. Variation in the origins of the branches of the axillary artery. Anat Rec 1959; 135: 33.

Kelkar R, Newton PM, Armengol J, et al. Three-dimensional kinematics of the glenohumeral joint during abduction in the scapular plane. Trans Orthop Res Soc 1993; 39: 136.

Kerr AT. The brachial plexus of nerves in man: the variations in its formation and branches. Am J Anat 1918; 23: 285.

Liou JTS, Wilson AJ, Totty WG, Brown JJ. The normal shoulder: common variations that simulate pathologic conditions at MR imaging. Radiology 1993; 186: 435.

MacConaill MA, Basmajian JV. Pectoral girdle, arm and forearm. In: Muscles and movements: a basis for human kinesiology. Baltimore: Williams & Wilkins, 1969.

Makhoul RG, Machleder HI. Developmental anomalies of the thoracic outlet syndrome: an analysis of 200 consecutive cases. J Vasc Surg 1992; 16: 534.

Miller RA. Observations upon the arrangement of the axillary artery and brachial plexus. Am J Anat 1939; 64: 143.

Moriggl B, Steinlechner M. Ultrasono-anatomy for evaluation of the local lymphatic groups of the mamma. Surg Radiol Anat 1994; 16: 77.

Moseley HF, Goldie I. The arterial pattern of the rotator cuff of the shoulder. J Bone Joint Surg Br 1963; 45B: 780.

Murakami G, Shimada K, Sato I, Kunieda H, Suzuki S, Hoshi H. Typology of the subclavian and axillary lymphatics. Clin Anat 1994; 7: 204.

Poppen NK, Walker PS. Normal and abnormal motion of the shoulder. J Bone Joint Surg 1976; 58A: 195.

Ranney D. Thoracic outlet: an anatomical redefinition that makes clinical sense. Clin Anat 1996; 9: 50.

Rockwood CA Jr, Matsen FA, III eds. The shoulder. Philadelphia: WB Saunders, 1990.

Seeger LL, Ruszowski JT, Bassett LW, Kay SP, Kathmann RD, Ellman H. MR imaging of the normal shoulder: anatomic correlation. Am J Roentgenol 1987; 148: 83.

Stanwood JE, Kraft GH. Diagnosis and management of brachial plexus injuries. Arch Phys Med Rehabil 1971; 52: 52.

Turkel SJ, Panio MW, Marshall JL, Girgis FG. Stabilizing mechanisms preventing anterior dislocation of the glenohumeral joint. J Bone Joint Surg 1981; 63A: 1208.

Vendrelle-Torne E, Setoain-Quinguer J, Domenech-Torne FM. Study of normal mammary lymphatic drainage using radioactive isotopes. J Nucl Med 1973; 13: 801.

Vorherr H. The breast: morphology, physiology, and lactation. New York: Academic Press, 1974.

Warner JJP, McMahon PJ. The role of the long head of the biceps brachii in superior stability of the glenohumeral joint. J Bone Joint Surg Am 1995; 77A: 366.

Hollinshead's Textbook of Anatomy, by Cornelius Rosse and Penelope Gaddum-Rosse.
Lippincott-Raven Publishers, Philadelphia, © 1997.

CHAPTER 16

The Free Upper Limb: Arm, Forearm, and Hand

continued

The arm, forearm, and hand are the segments of the free upper limb. The free upper limb is an extension of the pectoral and shoulder regions: there is both anatomic and functional continuity between the pectoral girdle and the free limb, as there is between the regions and segments of the free limb itself. The shoulder, elbow, and wrist joints that link the pectoral girdle and the segments of the free limb to one another are crossed from one region to the next not only by muscles and tendons that move these joints, but also by nerves and vessels.

The functional integrity of the hand, the ultimate effector and sensory organ of the upper limb, depends as much on structures that constitute or traverse the more proximal regions as it does on structures within the hand itself. Indeed, several major nerves and vessels that originate in the neck and axilla are best evaluated by testing hand function; the same is true for muscle groups of the arm and forearm. In many instances, however, elucidating the causes of functional loss requires an understanding of spatial relations within the discrete regions.

Chapter 14 deals with the basic anatomic plan of the limbs and provides an introduction to the segments, bones, joints, muscle groups, innervation, and vasculature of the free upper limb. That general overview is helpful for understanding the more detailed considerations of the upper limb in this chapter. The chapter begins with a general orientation, including a description of the skeleton of the entire free limb, an overview of major muscle groups and fascial compartments, and a summary of cutaneous nerves and vessels. It proceeds to the more detailed regional anatomy of the arm, forearm, and hand. Those sections are followed by a description of the joints of the free limb, and the chapter concludes with a discussion of the movements of the hand.

GENERAL ORIENTATION

Parts and Regions

Except for its terminal segment, the free upper limbs' shape is more or less cylindrical. Nevertheless, it is both possible and customary to define **anterior** and **posterior surfaces**, as well as **lateral** and **medial borders**, on each of its segments when the limb is in the anatomic position. These surfaces and borders are established early in development and are indeed more obvious at the limb bud stage (see Fig. 14-1). The **arm** (*brachium,* in Latin), built around the humerus, is the proximal segment of the free limb; proximally it includes the deltoid region along its lateral border (described in Chap. 15) and on its medial side, it leads into the axilla. The **forearm** (*antebrachium*), built around the radius and ulna, is the intermediate segment; it is joined to the arm at the elbow (*cubitus,* in Latin) and at the wrist (*carpus*) to the **hand** (*manus*), the terminal segment of the limb. The anterior surface of the hand is the **palm**, and its posterior surface the **dorsum**, or back, of the hand.

Colloquially, the **elbow** refers to the posterior aspect of the region constituted by the bony prominences of the humerus and ulna (see Fig. 16-3). Anteriorly, the elbow region presents the **cubital fossa**; less of a depression on the surface, it is actually an intermuscular space filled by vessels and nerves passing between the arm and forearm. Unlike the elbow, the **wrist** has its own skeletal frame made up of the eight carpal bones, the **carpus**. The **metacarpus**, built around five metacarpal bones, supports the palm and dorsum of the hand. Five **digits** project from the metacarpus: the first is the **thumb** (*pollex*), the second the **index**, the third the **middle finger** (*digitus medius*), the fourth the **ring finger** (*digitus anularis*), and the fifth the **little finger** (*digitus minimus*). Each finger consists of a proximal, middle, and distal **phalanx** (Latin: a line of soldiers); the thumb comprises only a distal and proximal phalanx. Each phalanx has a bone in it, also called a phalanx.

The palm of the hand is bordered by two fleshy eminences: the **thenar eminence** at the base of the thumb and the **hypothenar eminence** at the base of the little finger.

The lateral and medial borders of the forearm and hand are usually referred to as their **radial** and **ulnar borders**, respectively. The radial border corresponds to the preaxial border, and the ulnar to the postaxial border, of the developing limb (see Figs. 14-1 and 14-3). Both the English and the Latin names of the segments, regions, and subregions are adapted freely as adjectives and other descriptive terms, and are used commonly in both anatomic and clinical contexts. Familiarity with all of them is a requirement for effective communication.

Skeletal Anatomy

The bones and joints of the hand, forearm, and arm are frequently injured. However, x-rays films of the site of injury may be negative, particularly when there is no displacement of the fragments and before bone repair produces a radiolucent zone at the fracture site. The diagnosis, therefore, must often be made on physical signs, and both students and clinicians need to be familiar with the anatomy of the bones, not only on the skeleton, but also in the living limb and on radiographs.

Humerus

Because an understanding of the shoulder requires knowledge of the humerus, it is described in Chapter 15 (see Fig. 15-7). The anatomy of its lower end is further examined with the elbow joint (see under Joints). Only those parts accessible to palpation in the arm need be described here.

Palpation. The cylindrical shaft of the humerus is palpable through the muscles of the arm from the surgical neck of the bone to the elbow. The shaft is most accessible medially, between the flexor and extensor muscles. The palpable features of the proximal end are described in Chapter 15. The lower end of the humerus flares out, and its sharp edges project laterally and medially as the **supracondylar ridges** (Fig. 16-1). Both are palpable. They terminate in bony prominences, the **medial** and **lateral epicondyles**. The **condyle**, or articular portion of the lower end, is between the epicondyles and is out of reach (see Chap. 15; Fig 15-7).

Radius and Ulna

The radius is the preaxial bone of the forearm and the ulna its postaxial bone (see Figs. 14-3 and 14-4). Each is a long bone, the more or less cylindrical shaft, or body, of which terminates in an expanded and a narrow end (Fig. 16-2).

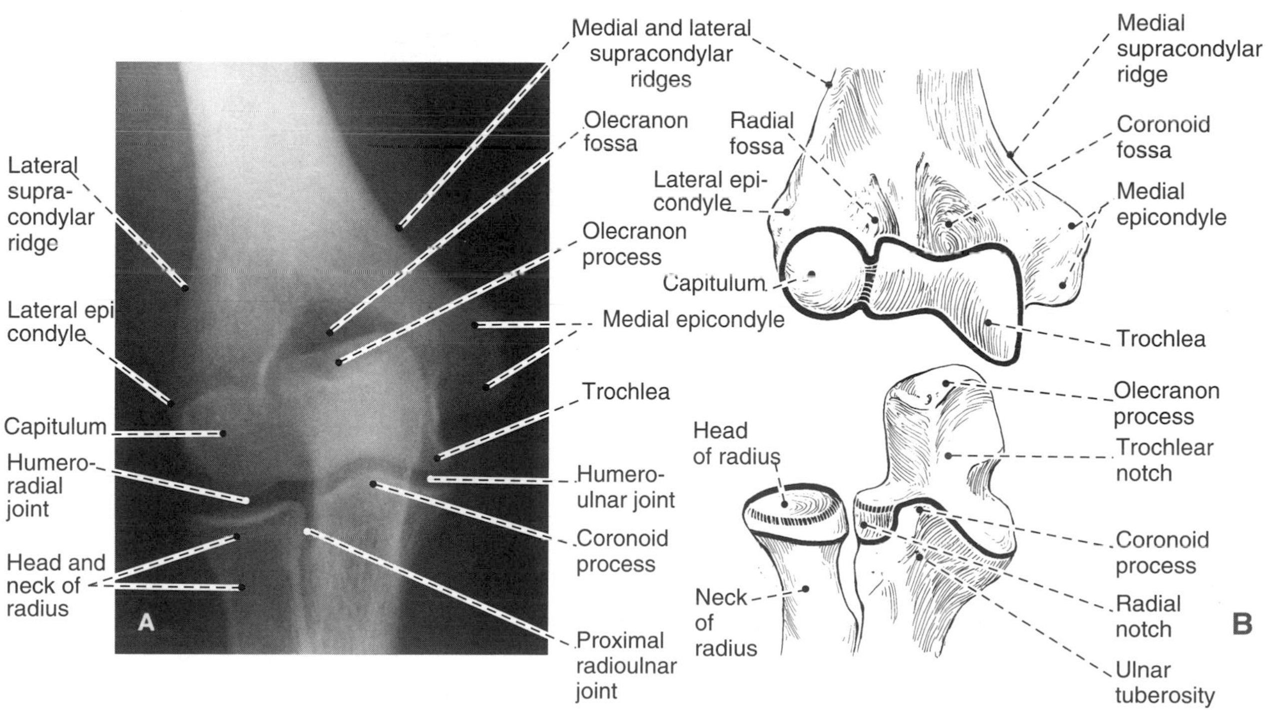

FIGURE *16-1.*
(A) A radiograph of the right elbow region compared with (B) a schematic drawing of the bones. On the drawing, the articular facets are accentuated by *heavy lines*. (A, courtesy of Dr. Rosalind H. Troupin.)

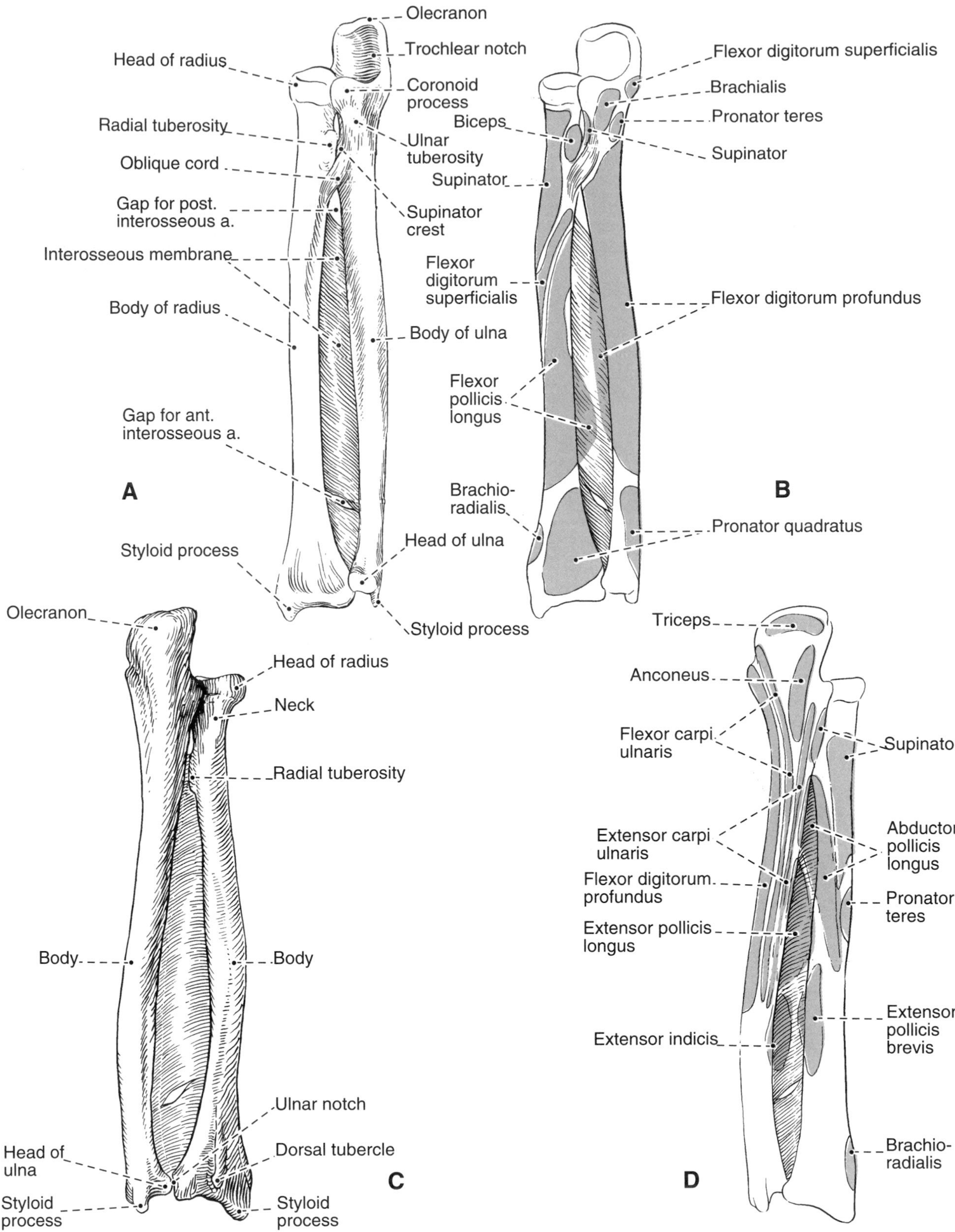

FIGURE *16-2.*
The bones of the forearm seen from (A and C) the front and from (B and D) the back. Areas of muscle origin are *red*, insertions are *blue*.

The narrow end of each bone is its *head*. The head of the radius is at the elbow, whereas the head of the ulna is at the wrist. The expanded end of the radius articulates with the carpal bones at the wrist (radiocarpal) joint, whereas that of the ulna articulates with the humerus at the elbow.

The two bones move together when the elbow is flexed and extended; both articulate with the condyle of the humerus. They also articulate with one another at each end: the proximal and distal **radioulnar joints** permit the movement of the radius and ulna in relation to one another, resulting in pronation and supination of the forearm and hand. The head of the radius is received by the *radial notch* of the ulna (see Fig. 16-1), whereas the head of the ulna is accommodated by the *ulnar notch* of the radius (see Fig. 16-6A). In the resting position of the limb, and also during the performance of most common tasks, the radius is crossed over the ulna, and the forearm and hand are pronated. The supinated position places the bones parallel to one another and is the *anatomic position,* but not the natural position, of the limb.

The **antebrachial interosseous membrane** stretches between the shafts of the two bones and provides additional area for muscle attachment. Although the radius and ulna receive the insertions of a few muscles, a great many more muscles take their origins from the bones, as well as from the interosseous membrane (Fig. 16-2).

Radius. The disklike **head** of the radius is covered with articular cartilage (see Figs. 16-1 and 16-2). Its flat, slightly concave upper surface articulates with the capitulum of the humerus. Around its circumference it articulates with the radial notch of the ulna and with the *annular ligament,* a tough band that forms a sling around the head of the radius and holds it in position against the ulna's radial notch (see Figs. 16-61 and 16-63). The narrowed portion of the radius immediately below the head is the **neck**. The *radial tuberosity* is a raised projection, facing toward the ulna, at the junction of the neck and the body; the tendon of the biceps brachii inserts into it.

The expanded **distal end** of the radius presents a slightly concave *carpal articular surface* through which the radius participates in the wrist joint (see Fig. 16-6). The articular surface extends onto the ulnar side of the bone as the *ulnar notch,* which helps form the distal radioulnar joint. On the lateral side, the bluntly pointed **styloid process** projects downward beyond the carnal articular surface. The posterior surface presents a small, sharp projection, the *dorsal tubercle,* which functions as a pulley for the tendon of the long extensor of the thumb (see Figs. 16-2 and Fig. 16-20).

Between the radial tuberosity and the distal end, the **body** (diaphysis) of the radius has ill-defined anterior, posterior, and lateral **surfaces**, demarcated by anterior, posterior, and interosseous **borders**. The lateral surface is slightly convex and presents a rough area at about its midpoint, the *pronator tuberosity,* for the insertion of the pronator teres muscle (see Fig. 16-2). The interosseous membrane attaches along the interosseous border and closes the space between the radius and ulna.

Ulna. The expanded **proximal end** of the ulna terminates in two stout projections, the **olecranon** posteriorly and the **coronoid process** anteriorly. Between them, the deep *trochlear notch* grasps the trochlea of the humerus (see Fig. 16-1). The articular surface extends from the trochlear notch into the *radial notch* on the lateral side of the ulna and accommodates the head of the radius. Anteriorly, at the base of the coronoid process, the insertion of the brachialis muscle is marked by the *ulnar tuberosity.* The **body** (diaphysis) of the ulna, similar to that of the radius, has anterior, posterior, and interosseous **borders**, the first two being rather indistinct and the last, more sharply defined. They separate the anterior, posterior, and medial **surfaces** of the bone. At the narrow distal end, the **styloid process** projects beyond the head of the ulna toward the carpal bones (see Figs. 16-2 and 16-5).

Palpation. Parts of both the radius and the ulna are subcutaneous and palpable. Their bony projections serve as useful landmarks for ascertaining anatomic relations around the elbow and wrist, where injuries are common.

The **olecranon** forms the bony projection of the elbow. It is subcutaneous; only the *olecranon bursa* separates it from the skin. The bursa normally contains only enough fluid to lubricate the movement of the skin over the bone. In the extended elbow, the tip of the olecranon is more or less level with the two epicondyles of the humerus (see Fig. 16-1), but when the elbow is flexed, these three bony points outline an equilateral triangle (Fig. 16-3). The triangle remains unaltered in supracondylar fractures of the humerus, but is distorted by dislocation of the elbow. The resulting deformity should not be confused with a

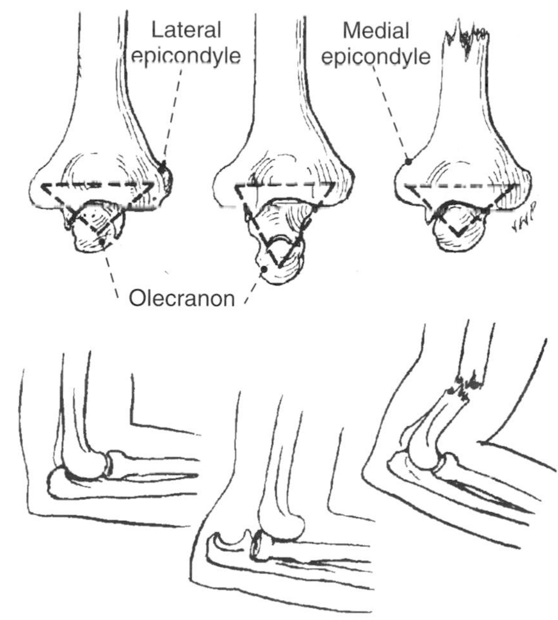

FIGURE *16-3.*
Relation of the olecranon and medial and lateral epicondyles to one another in the normal joint, in posterior dislocation of the elbow, and in supracondylar fracture of the humerus.

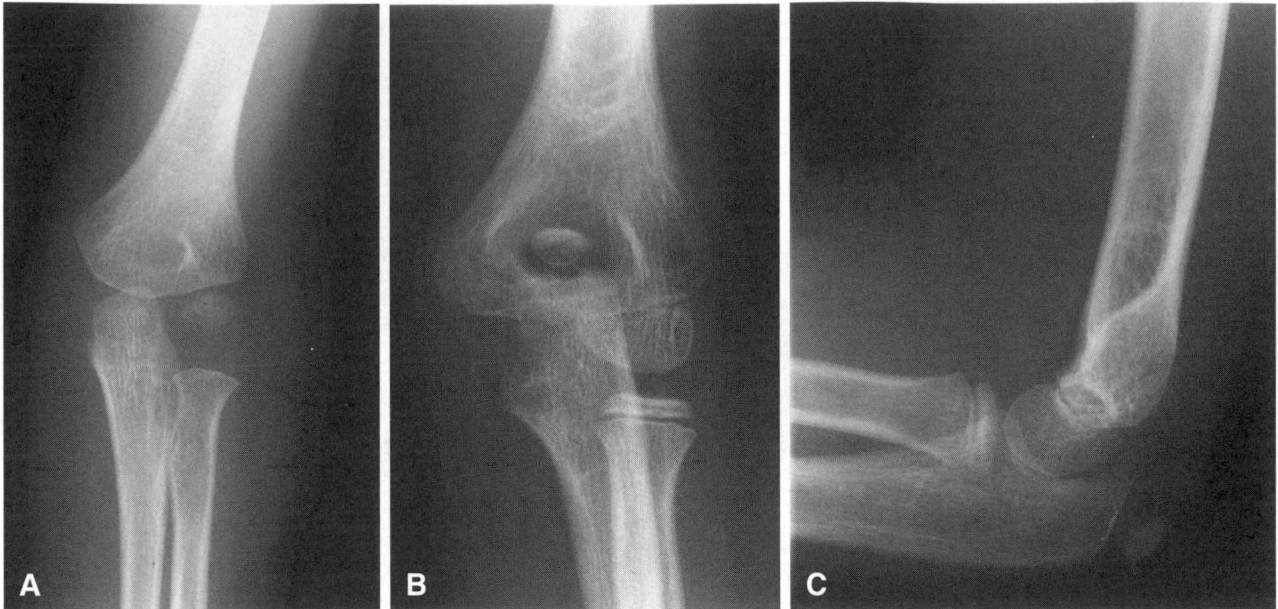

FIGURE 16-4.
Radiographs of ossification around the elbow. (A) At 4 1/2 years of age, note center for capitulum; (B and C) an 8 years of age, note centers for head of radius and olecranon. (Courtesy of Dr. Eric L Effmann.)

swelling over the olecranon itself caused by distension of the olecranon bursa (student's elbow). The other bony projection on the ulna's proximal end, the **coronoid process**, is buried in muscles in the depth of the cubital fossa and is inaccessible to palpation.

The **head of the radius** is just distal to the lateral epicondyle. When the index finger is placed on the epicondyle, the middle finger can feel the head rotating during pronation and supination. The rotating head is also visible. If it is pulled out of the sling formed by the annular ligament, as may happen when a child is jerked by the arm, its absence can be verified by palpation.

The palpable bone along the back of the forearm is the ulna, which is subcutaneous from the olecranon to the styloid process. The shaft of the radius is covered in muscles.

In the pronated forearm the **head of the ulna** is visible as a smooth prominence on the back of the wrist in line with the little finger. In the supinated hand it is no longer visible, but may be grasped between finger and thumb if the tendons around the wrist are relaxed. The **ulnar styloid process** is more readily felt in the supinated forearm, just above the most distal skin crease of the wrist. The **styloid process of the radius** is blunter than that of the ulna and its tip is at a slightly lower level (see Figs. 16-5 and 16-6). On the dorsal aspect of the wrist, the radius feels superficial, but it is actually only its styloid process and **dorsal tubercle** that are truly subcutaneous. The tubercle is in line with the index finger. The anterior surface of the radius is inaccessible at the wrist owing to the presence of the flexor tendons.

Ossification. The appearance and fusion of ossification centers around the elbow are used for estimation of bone age in children (Fig. 16-4). The radius and the ulna are each ossified from three centers, one for the diaphysis and one at each end for the epiphyses. The diaphyseal centers for both bones appear during the eighth or ninth week of embryonic life, but the epiphyseal centers appear from 1 to 9 years after birth and join the diaphyses between the 14th and 21st years.

Very rarely, the radius or the ulna fails to form, or the distal part of one or both bones may be lacking.

Carpus

The carpus is the proximal region of the hand built around a set of eight irregular bones. The carpal bones are arranged in two rows of four each (Fig. 16-5). In the *proximal row*, beginning on the radial side, the **scaphoid,** the **lunate**, and the **triquetral** bones articulate proximally with the radius and the articular disk of the ulna to form the **radiocarpal** or **wrist joint.** The **pisiform,** the fourth bone in the proximal row, lies on the anterior surface of the triquetrum and articulates only with that bone. The *distal row*, starting on the radial side, is made up of the **trapezium**, **trapezoid**, **capitate**, and **hamate** bones. They articulate with the proximal row at the **midcarpal joint** and with the metacarpal bones at the **carpometacarpal joints**. Members of each row articulate with their neighbors at the **intercarpal joints.** Constituted of these numerous bones and joints, the carpus is a pliable region, and its movements amplify those that occur at the radiocarpal joint.

In the proximal row, the following features of individual bones are noteworthy. The **scaphoid** (Greek: *skaphe*, skiff plus *eidos*, form; i.e., boat-shaped) is the largest carpal bone (Fig. 16-6). Shaped more like a dumbbell than a boat, it has expanded ends and a narrow waist. It is covered by articular cartilage on all surfaces except over its waist. It is only here that blood vessels have access to it. During a fall on the outstretched hand, this is the area where the bone fractures (see Fig. 16-6B),

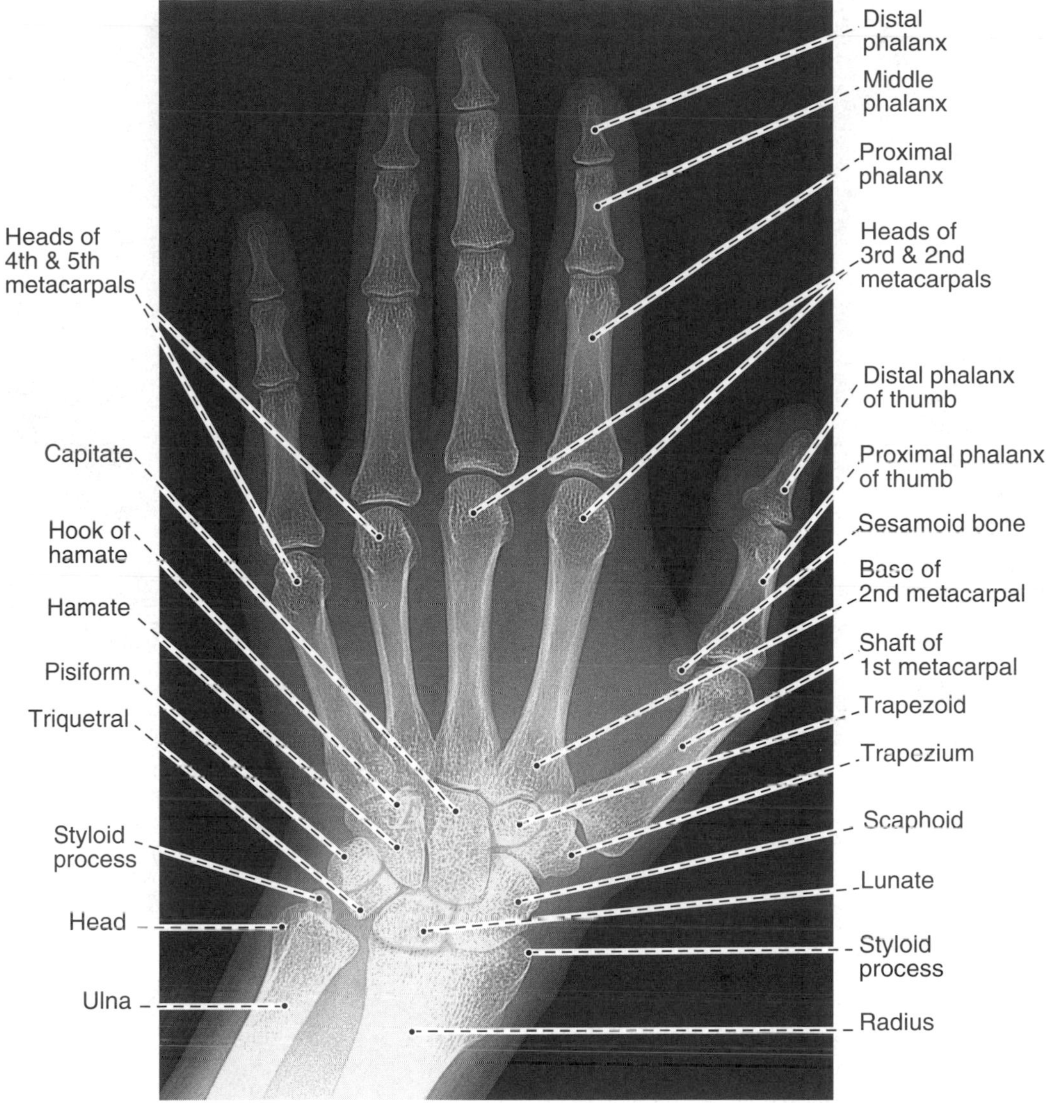

FIGURE *16-5.*
Bones of the wrist and hand seen on radiograph from the palmar aspect. (Courtesy of Dr. Thurman Gillespy III.)

and this is the reason for the ischemic necrosis that often follows. The convex surface of the half-moon–shaped **lunate** faces into the wrist joint and it is perched with its concavity on the "head" of the capitate (see Fig. 16-6A). A fall on the outstretched hand may cause the lunate to slip from this position: it usually dislocates in a palmar direction into the carpal canal (see following). The pyramidal or "three-cornered" **triquetrum** bears a small facet for the articular disk that separates it from the ulna, and a cup-shaped facet on its palmar surface for the **pisiform bone**. So named because of its resemblance to a pea, the pisiform has long been considered a sesamoid bone, but some studies suggest that it is a bona fide member of the carpus.

Distinguishing features of the bones in the distal row include the bulky "head" of the **capitate**, a *tubercle* on the palmar surface of the **trapezium**, the saddle-shaped articular surface on the trapezium for the first metacarpal, and the *hook* (hamulus) of the **hamate**, which projects into the palm just below the pisiform (see Fig. 16-6B).

Carpal Arch. Held together by their ligaments, the carpal bones form an arch: the dorsal aspect of the carpus is convex, whereas its palmar aspect is deeply concave. The concavity constitutes the carpal sulcus, or groove (*sulcus carpi*; Fig. 16-7). The sulcus is deepened by bony prominences on either side: on the radial side, the tubercles of the scaphoid and trapezium, and on the ulnar side, the pisiform and the hook of the hamate. A strong ligament, the **flexor retinaculum**, attaches to these four bony prominences and converts the carpal sulcus into the **carpal canal** (or carpal tunnel), the contents of which are described in a later section (see under The Wrist). The existence of the carpal arch has important consequences for hand function (see under Movements of the Hand).

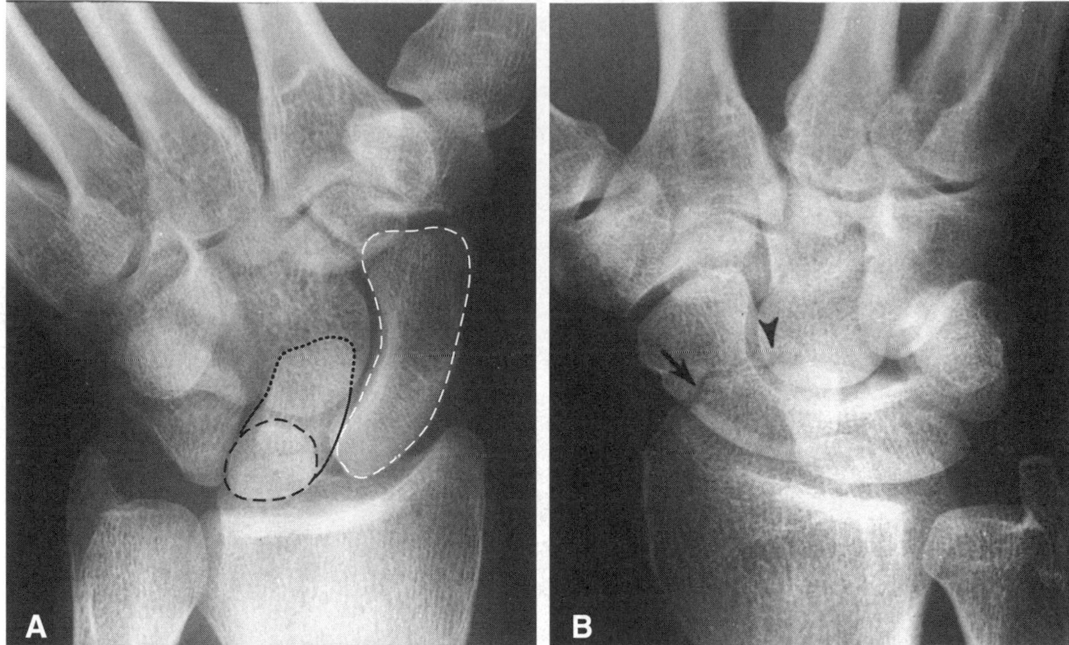

FIGURE *16-6.*
Radiographs of (A) a left and of (B) a right wrist taken in abduction to give a complete view of the scaphoid. In panel A, which is normal, the surfaces of the scaphoid that are covered by articular cartilage are indicated by white lines. The profile of the lunate facing toward the dorsum of the wrist is identified by a *black interrupted* line and the *black dots* outline the rest of the bone perched on top of the capitate. Panel B was taken 14 days after the patient fell on his outstretched hand and sprained his wrist. A fracture of the scaphoid is identified at the waist of the bone by an *arrow*, and its extension into the surface that articulates with the capitate is marked by an *arrowhead*. (Courtesy of Dr. Rosalind H. Troupin.)

Palpation. The position of the carpal bones is more proximal than commonly appreciated. The level of the radiocarpal joint is about 2 cm above (or proximal to) the distal skin crease of the wrist (see Fig. 16-32), and the plane of the carpometacarpal joints is level with the proximal border of the outstretched thumb.

Most of the carpal bones, although palpable, cannot be separately identified. On the **dorsum of the hand**, the scaphoid and the lunate can, however, be precisely palpated. They are the bones most frequently affected in traumatic injuries and by ischemic necrosis. The *scaphoid* is palpable just distal to the styloid process of the radius in a depression called the *anatomic snuff box* (see Fig. 16-33). This depression is demarcated by tendons that spring into prominence when the thumb is extended. Tenderness in the snuff box is suggestive of a scaphoid fracture. The *lunate* is easily felt during flexion and extension of the wrist with the middle finger when the index finger is placed on the dorsal tubercle of the radius.

In the **palm of the hand** only those bony prominences of the carpus are palpable to which the flexor retinaculum attaches. The blunt *tubercle of the scaphoid* can be felt at the distal skin crease on the radial side of the midline of the wrist, when the wrist is extended. Distal to it, the *tubercle of the trapezium* can be discerned through the thenar eminence. On the ulnar side, the *pisiform bone* is easily palpated in the "heel" of the hand and the *hook of the hamate*

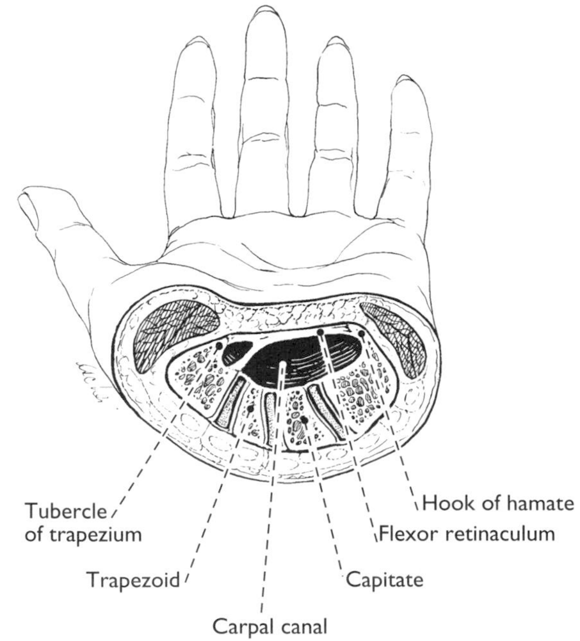

FIGURE *16-7.*
A schematic representation of a section cut across the distal row of carpal bones to show their anterior concavity. The flexor retinaculum converts this carpal sulcus into the carpal canal (carpal tunnel).

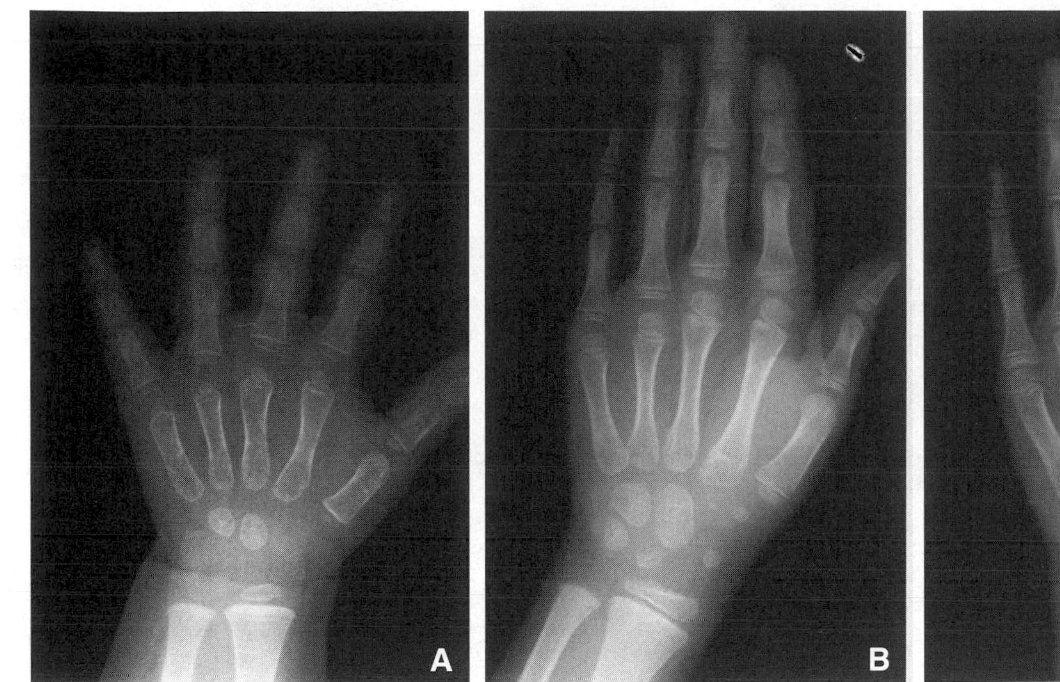
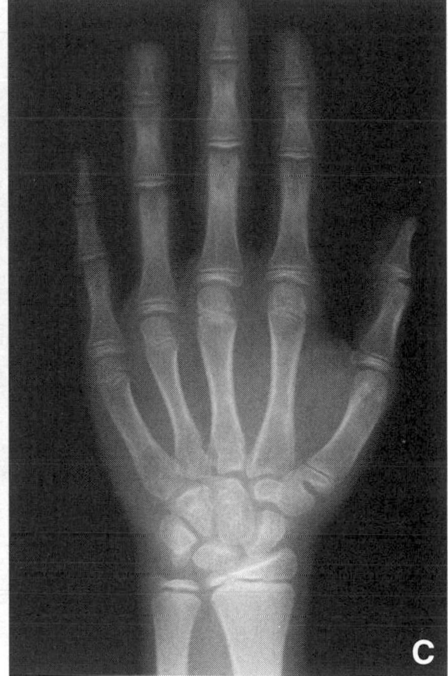

FIGURE 16-8.
Radiographs of ossification centers at the wrist: (A) 2 years of age; (B) 5 1/2 years; (C) 9 1/2 years. (Courtesy of Dr. Eric L. Effmann.)

offers resistance a short distance lower, in the hypothenar eminence. Pressure exerted between these four bony points compresses the contents of the carpal tunnel, and can induce or exaggerate the symptoms of carpal tunnel syndrome (see under The Wrist).

Ossification. Each carpal bone ossifies typically from a single center. Some of these bones begin to ossify soon after birth, but others are delayed until the early teenage years. The appearance and fusion of these ossification centers is used to determine the bone age of children radiologically (Fig. 16-8). Confusion with supernumerary carpal bones can readily occur.

Variations. More than 20 different types of supernumerary carpal bones have been described, but most wrists have none. Some of these accessory bones are believed to be sesamoid bones, some to be true accessory carpals (arising from accessory cartilages unconnected with tendons), and some to represent failure of fusion of two centers of ossification arising abnormally within a normal cartilaginous carpal element. Congenital fusion of two or more carpal bones, although rare, most often involves the lunate and triquetral bones. This does not interfere with movement of the wrist and is usually detected as an incidental finding on radiographs.

Metacarpals and Phalanges

The intermediate subsegment of the skeleton of the hand is represented by the metacarpals and the distal subsegment by the phalanges (see Fig. 16-5). The metacarpals form the skeleton of the palm, and the phalanges of the digits. All are miniature long bones. Each has a *body* or shaft, the proximal expanded end of which is the *base* and the distal end, the *head*. The bases of the metacarpals contact each other, but their heads are spread apart. The bases articulate with the distal row of carpal bones at the **carpometacarpal joints** as well as with each other at the **intermetacarpal joints**. The **metacarpophalangeal joints** link the metacarpal heads to the bases of the proximal phalanges, and the **interphalangeal joints** provide for movement between the phalanges of individual digits.

The five **metacarpals** resemble one another closely. They are identified by Roman numerals, starting from the radial side. Metacarpal I is that of the thumb, and metacarpal V, that of the little finger. The shaft of each is gently curved, presenting a concavity toward the palm. Each bone is triangular in cross section, providing two palmar surfaces for the attachment of muscles and a bare subcutaneous surface on the back of the hand. The articular surfaces on the bases of metacarpals II to V are rather flat, permitting slight gliding movements between the articulating bones. The metacarpal bone of the thumb is separated from the other four and, together with its carpal bone (trapezium), it has rotated into a plane that is at right angles to that of the others (see Fig. 16-34). Its base presents a saddle-shaped articular surface for a corresponding facet on the trapezium. These anatomic features account for the enhanced mobility of the thumb.

The head of metacarpal I is also specialized: it presents a pulley-shaped articular surface that permits only flexion and extension. The articular surfaces on the heads of the other metacarpals, by contrast, are condyloid, extend onto their palmar surfaces, and permit abduction, adduction and passive rotation of the fingers, in addition to flexion and extension.

The two **phalanges** of the thumb are named *proximal* and *distal;* the three of each finger are named *proximal, middle*, and *distal*. The expanded *base* of each phalanx presents a shallow, concave articular facet, and the heads of the proximal and middle phalanges have pulley-shaped facets for articulation with the bases of the more distal phalanges. The interphalangeal joints are hinge joints, allowing only flexion and extension. The roughened head of each distal phalanx bears a raised *tuberosity* on its palmar aspect that supports the connective tissue of the pulp of the digits (see Fig. 16-55).

Two small **sesamoid bones**, one on the ulnar side and another on the radial, typically lie on the palmar surface of the metacarpophalangeal joint of the thumb (see Fig. 16-5). Occasionally, there are one or more sesamoids at other metacarpophalangeal or interphalangeal joints.

Ossification. Each metacarpal or phalanx ossifies from two centers. The one for the body appears early, approximately in the ninth week of fetal life; the single epiphyseal center usually appears after the first year of postnatal life. The single epiphysis is typically in the head of each metacarpal and at the base of each phalanx (see Fig. 16-8). The exception is the metacarpal of the thumb: its epiphysis is at the base. The sesamoid bones usually begin to ossify at or after the age of 18 years.

Transverse Metacarpal Arch. When the wrist and fingers are extended, the palm of the hand is flat and the heads of the metacarpal bones lie in one plane. Flexion of the wrist causes cupping of the palm and the metacarpal heads come to lie in an arc. This reflects the presence of the *carpal arch* (see Fig. 16-7) with which the metacarpals articulate.

In the extended position, the fingers are of different lengths and are spread apart. Flexion of the fingers brings them together, and their tips contact the palm along a straight line. The knuckles, which represent the metacarpal heads, form an arc in this position. The curvature of the arc becomes exaggerated as the power of the grip is increased. The arc described by the metacarpal heads in the clenched or cupped hand is the *transverse metacarpal arch.* The relative mobility of the fourth and fifth metacarpal bones is largely responsible for changes in the arch.

The transverse metacarpal arch permits the tips of the fingers to meet and work together in any position of flexion. It provides an important mechanism for the effectiveness of both the power grip and the precision grip (see under Movements of the Hand).

Clinically it is important to note that, owing to the metacarpal arch, each finger when flexed individually contacts the ball of the thumb and points toward the tuberosity of the scaphoid. Fractures of the metacarpals should be immobilized using this relation as a guide; otherwise, the fracture will unite with the distal fragment rotated and the resulting finger deformity will interfere seriously with hand function. Furthermore, in the treatment of hand injuries, the position chosen for immobilization must maintain the metacarpal arch. Scar formation and fibrosis in the flat position will prevent reformation of the arch and will compromise hand function.

Skeletal Injuries

The bones of the upper limb may break owing to direct or indirect violence. The upper limb is not constructed for weight bearing. A fall on the outstretched hand may sprain ligaments of the wrist, elbow, and shoulder, but it may also fracture or dislocate some of the bones through which the major component of the force is transmitted. The more common sites of injury are along the line through which force is transmitted from the hand to the axial skeleton. These sites, and the injuries sustained, some of which have been mentioned already, include fracture of the scaphoid (see Fig. 16-6), dislocation of the lunate, fracture of the distal end of the radius (Colles' fracture), intra-articular fracture of the radial head, dislocation of the elbow, and supracondylar fracture of the humerus (see Fig. 16-3). The same force may dislocate the shoulder (see Fig. 15-8B) or break the clavicle. Several of these injuries are prone to serious complications because of the involvement of nerves, blood vessels, and muscles. Knowledge of topographic relations within the segments of the limb is a requirement for diagnosing and minimizing such injuries.

Muscle Groups and Fascial Compartments

A large number of muscles are responsible for executing movements in the upper limb. In the free limb, they can be categorized according to their prime mover actions exerted at particular joints and also according to the compartments they occupy. The compartments are defined by bony and fascial boundaries. This section is an introductory overview of the functional grouping and topographic compartmentalization of the muscles, from the shoulder to the hand. More detailed descriptions of individual muscles will be found in the various sections devoted to the individual regions of the limb.

Muscle Groups

Conforming to the developmental compartmentalization of the limb (see Fig. 14-5), flexor muscles for joints between the limb segments occupy the anterior compartment of the segment proximal to the joint, and extensor muscles occupy the posterior compartment. The boundary between these major compartments is represented by the skeleton of the segment, which develops along the limb's axis (see Chap. 14). Many muscles originate and insert on these bones, but the areas available for muscle attachment are further increased by fascial septa, such as the interosseous membrane. The septa also help to demarcate the compartments from one another.

In accordance with this general plan, the large muscles that flex the elbow arise from the humerus and intermuscular septa (attached to the supracondylar ridges of the humerus) and occupy the anterior compartment of the arm, whereas the elbow extensors are located in the posterior compartment. There are two **elbow flexors**, the *brachialis* and *biceps*, and one **extensor**, the *triceps*, a composite muscle made up of three parts or heads. The flexor compartment also contains a small adductor of the arm, the *coracobrachialis*, and the extensor compartment contains a small muscle, the *anconeus*, insignificant in both function and size. Muscles in the flexor compartment are innervated by the musculocutaneous nerve, those in the extensor compartment by the radial nerve (see Fig. 14-7).

In the forearm, the two compartments are separated by two bones, rather than one, with the interosseous membrane stretching between them. The **flexors of the carpus**, located in the anterior compartment, bear names that reflect their attachment to either the radial or the ulnar side of the wrist: *flexor carpi radialis* and *flexor carpi ulnaris*. Likewise, the **extensors of the carpus,** *extensor carpi radialis* and *extensor carpi ulnaris*, lie in the posterior compartment and attach to the radial and ulnar sides of the wrist, respectively. Although the carpus can also be abducted and adducted, there are no specific muscles for these movements. Abduction and adduction at the wrist are performed by the combined action of carpal flexors and extensors on the radial or ulnar side of the limb, respectively.

The forearm also accommodates the bellies of those muscles that provide power to the hand; their tendons cross the carpus and metacarpus and insert on the digits. These so-called **extrinsic muscles of the hand** include the flexors and extensors of the digits (*flexor digitorum* and *extensor digitorum*) located in the anterior and posterior compartments, respectively. Specializations (best explained in a later section) exist in both sets. Because of its independence of the other digits, the thumb is served by a separate set of flexors and extensors (*flexor pollicis* and *extensor pollicis*) located in the appropriate compartments of the forearm. The extrinsic muscles of the thumb also include an abductor (*abductor pollicis longus*) that originates in the posterior compartment. The third group of muscles accommodated in the forearm move the radius and ulna in relation to one another: **pronators** are in the anterior compartment and a **supinator** in the posterior compartment.

Muscles in the posterior compartment of the forearm, similar to those of the arm, are supplied by the radial nerve. The innervation of the anterior compartment is shared by the median and ulnar nerves (see Fig. 14-7).

In summary, three functional groups of muscles are contained in the forearm: 1) flexors and extensors of the wrist; 2) extrinsic muscles of the hand that chiefly flex and extend the digits (including the thumb); and 3) muscles of pronation and supination. Not included in these categories is a rather large muscle located on the radial side of the forearm, the brachioradialis. It is between the two compartments, having been displaced from the extensor compartment during development. Owing to its site of origin, however, it is supplied by the radial nerve, even though it assists in elbow flexion.

The *intrinsic muscles of the hand* allow precision of hand movement. The bellies of these muscles are confined to the palm, but their tendons proceed to the digits. They consist of three major groups: 1) the **interosseous muscles** that fill the spaces between the shafts of the metacarpals; 2) muscles serving the thumb, which make up the **thenar eminence**; and 3) those serving the little finger, located in the **hypothenar eminence**. These muscle groups are demarcated from one another by fascial septa. The interosseous muscles are named according to the numbers of the interosseous spaces they occupy, and the thenar and hypothenar muscles according to the movements they produce. There is a flexor and an abductor for the thumb and for the little finger. The thumb also has an adductor and an "opponens" responsible for opposition of the thumb. As some thumb movements can be produced by both extrinsic and intrinsic muscles, distinction is made by designating the respective muscles as long or short. For instance, the extrinsic flexor is the flexor pollicis *longus*, whereas the flexor contained in the thenar eminence is the flexor pollicis *brevis*. A set of slender muscles associated with the tendons of the digital flexors is separate from the three main groups. These are the **lumbrical** muscles.

The innervation of the intrinsic muscles of the hand is shared unequally between the median and ulnar nerves (see Fig. 14-7). Generally speaking, those in the thenar eminence are supplied by the median nerve and the remainder by the ulnar nerve.

Fascias

The **superficial fascia** of the arm and forearm, composed of loose areolar tissue, contains a variable amount of fat. Cutaneous nerves and vessels run in it (see later discussion). Over the olecranon, the fascia forms the *olecranon bursa*. On the dorsum of the hand, the fascia is thin and loose, allowing the skin to be moved easily. In the palm, it shows specializations, which are described later (see under The Hand).

The **deep fascia** of the upper limb is a dense connective tissue membrane. Similar to a long glove, it ensheathes the structures of the limb subjacent to the superficial fascia, from the fingers to the axilla. By its attachments to bones, the deep fascia helps form the compartments of the limb. Because of its inelastic nature, it limits swelling and distension in some of these compartments. Indeed, it may need to be incised if pressure threatens to endanger the blood supply and viability of the contents of a compartment. Such may be the case, for instance, in the anterior compartment of the forearm.

The membranous nature of the deep fascia is most evident in the arm and forearm where it is known, respectively, as the **brachial** and **antebrachial fascia**. At the elbow, the brachial fascia blends with the epicondyles of the humerus. More proximally it sends bilateral membranous extensions inward to attach to the supracondylar ridges; these are the **lateral** and **medial intermuscular septa** (see Figs. 16-10, 16-11, and 16-15). Together with the humerus, they divide the arm into anterior (flexor) and posterior

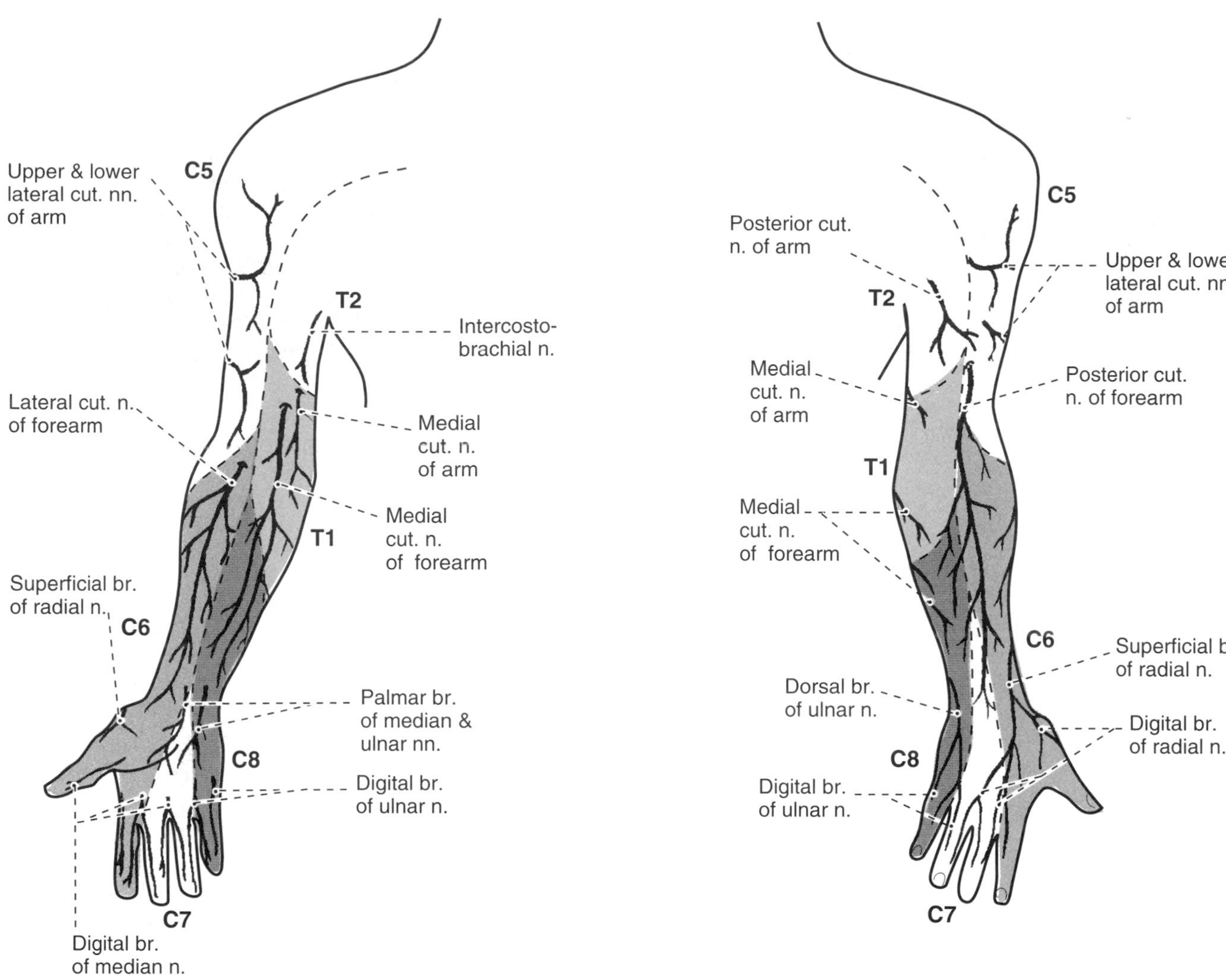

FIGURE *16-9.*
Cutaneous nerves of the free limb: The dermatomal areas are shown to provide an indication of the approximate spinal cord segments to which specific cutaneous nerves relay sensory information.

(extensor) compartments. The antebrachial fascia serves a similar purpose in the forearm. Laterally, it extends inward to reach the radius, whereas on the ulnar side, it is fused to the entire subcutaneous length of the ulna. The interosseous membrane, together with the bones themselves, completes the separation into anterior and posterior compartments. Additional inward extensions of the fascia form septa between individual muscles. In the lower anterior part of the forearm, the antebrachial fascia splits into two layers. The deeper layer subdivides the muscles of the anterior compartment into superficial and deep subgroups.

Around the wrist, the deep fascia forms retaining bands for the tendons, known as *flexor* and *extensor retinacula* (*retinaculum;* Latin for rope or retaining band) (see Figs. 16-31 and 16-32). In the palm of the hand, it invests and defines the thenar and hypothenar eminences; between them, it blends with the *palmar aponeurosis,* a triangular, sheetlike tendon. It also blends with the superficial fascia in the digits. These specializations of the deep fascia around the wrist and in the hand are examined further in subsequent sections.

Cutaneous Nerves and Vessels

Most of the nerves and vessels that supply the skin are given off by their parent trunks as they proceed through the segments of the limb. In the course of a dissection, however, they are often destroyed by the time the parent trunk is displayed. Therefore, a summary of the cutaneous nerves and vessels of the whole limb seems desirable at this point.

Nerves

The segmental innervation of the skin from the anterior rami of spinal nerves C-5 to T-1 is described in Chapter 13 (see Figs. 13-24 and 13-25). These segmental somatic afferent fibers are distributed to the skin of the arm and forearm by several *brachial* and *antebrachial cutaneous nerves*, named according to their positions in the limb (Fig. 16-9). They pierce the deep fascia and arborize in the superficial fascia. The hand, in which cutaneous sensibility is particularly important, is supplied by cutaneous branches of the median, ulnar, and radial nerves (see Fig. 16-45).

The **medial cutaneous nerve of the arm** (*medial brachial cutaneous nerve*) and the **medial cutaneous nerve of the forearm** (*medial antebrachial cutaneous nerve*) are branches of the medial cord of the brachial plexus (see Figs. 15-20 and 15-21). Both convey T-1 and C-8 fibers, distributed sequentially in a proximal to distal direction, to the medial aspect of the limb almost as far as the wrist, where the ulnar nerve takes over. Their supply territory extends approximately as far as the anterior (ventral) axial line. (For a description of the axial lines, see Chap. 13 and Figs. 13-24 and 13-25.) The remainder of the skin on the arm and forearm is served by lateral and posterior cutaneous nerves named after each segment. In the arm, the lateral surface is supplied by the **upper lateral** and **lower lateral cutaneous nerves of the arm** (see Fig. 16-9), the former a branch of the axillary nerve and the latter of the radial nerve. Both convey predominantly C-5 fibers to the deltoid region and the lateral side of the arm as far down as the elbow. The small **posterior cutaneous nerve of the arm** is also a branch of the radial nerve. Below the elbow, the **lateral cutaneous nerve of the forearm** is a terminal branch of the musculocutaneous nerve (see Figs. 14-7 and 16-12), and it brings preponderantly C-6 fibers to the radial side of the forearm as far as the wrist, where the radial nerve takes over. The **posterior cutaneous nerve of the forearm**, much larger than its counterpart in the arm, is a branch of the radial nerve and delivers preponderantly C-6 and C-8 fibers to either side of the posterior (dorsal) axial line, as well as some C-7 fibers to the back of the wrist.

The innervation of skin of the hand is shared by digital, palmar, and distal dorsal branches of the median, ulnar, and radial nerves (see Fig. 16-45). The C-6 fibers are delivered to the radial side of the hand by the median and radial nerves, C-7 fibers to the palm by the palmar branches of the median and ulnar nerves, and to the dorsum by the radial nerve. The dorsal and digital branches of the ulnar nerve bring C-8 and some C-7 fibers to the ulnar side of the hand and to the ulnar two or three fingers.

Vessels

Arteries that run in the superficial fascia and supply the skin are branches of the main arterial trunks in the respective limb segments (see Fig. 14-9). They are described for the hand in a later section. In regions other than the hand, cutaneous arteries are relevant to the transplantation of large skin flaps, when major injuries of the limb have to be repaired, but for the purposes of this chapter they may be ignored.

Superficial veins, on the other hand, are large vessels; many are visible through the skin. They are usually the first choice for venipuncture, either to obtain blood samples for laboratory analysis or to administer drugs and fluids intravenously. For these purposes they must be located with care, especially when obscured by fatty superficial fascia, not only to puncture them, but to avoid concomitant injury to neighboring vessels and nerves.

The veins begin in the hand. Those in the palm form a delicate network that drains the fingers as well as the tissues of the palm. From this plexus blood drains through veins passing largely between the metacarpal heads into a larger, subcutaneous **dorsal venous network**. The network is visible on the back of the hand and presents many different patterns. It gives rise to two large veins, the basilic vein and cephalic vein (see Fig. 14-10). Both proceed through the superficial fascia of the forearm and arm into the axilla, and collect venous blood from all superficial structures of the free limb. The **basilic vein** starts on the ulnar side, winds its way to the front of the forearm before it reaches the elbow, and then continues along the medial side of the arm. It pierces the brachial fascia and completes its ascent to the axilla in the anterior compartment of the arm. It is the main tributary of the axillary vein (see Fig. 15-19). The **cephalic vein** begins on the radial side of the dorsal venous plexus, winds its way to the front of the forearm above the wrist, and ascends on the lateral side of the elbow and arm. It reaches the axillary vein by passing along the sulcus between the deltoid and pectoralis major and piercing the clavipectoral fascia. The basilic and cephalic veins are interconnected over the cubital fossa by the **median cubital vein** (see Fig. 16-26).

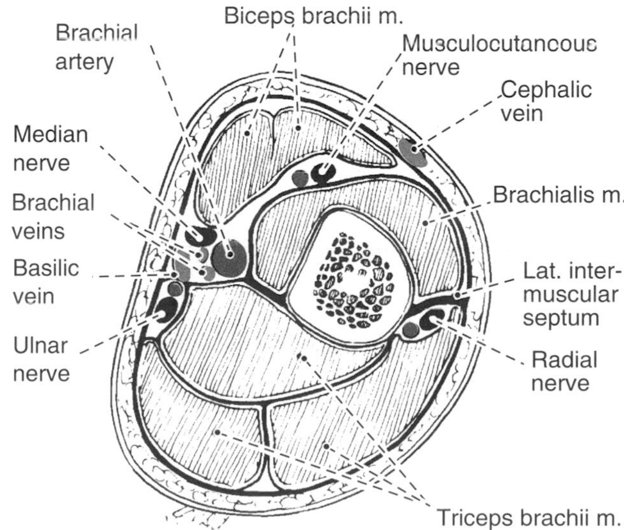

FIGURE *16-10.*
A transverse section across the lower third of the arm.

Lymphatic vessels form a rich subcutaneous plexus, particularly in the hand. Several of them ascend in the superficial fascia of the forearm and arm; on the way they are joined by numerous lymphatic afferents. Those draining the radial side of the hand are uninterrupted until they reach the lateral group of lymph nodes in the axilla. Lymphatics draining the ulnar side of the hand and forearm, however, terminate in one or two small lymph nodes at the elbow. These are the **supratrochlear nodes**, lying along the basilic vein. When enlarged or inflamed, they are palpable just above the medial epicondyle.

THE ARM

The general anatomic plan of the arm is simple (Fig. 16-10). The anterior and posterior compartments, separated from one another by the humerus and the medial and lateral intermuscular septa, are occupied by the large flexor and extensor muscles, respectively. Between these muscles, the brachial artery approaches the elbow in the anterior compartment on the medial side of the arm, and it is accompanied by the median and ulnar nerves. Concerned with the innervation of the forearm and hand, neither nerve gives off any branches in the arm. Emerging from the axilla, the musculocutaneous and radial nerves make their way through the flexor and extensor compartments, respectively. They distribute their branches in a lateral direction as they pass toward the elbow.

Anterior Compartment

Muscles

Of the three muscles that occupy the anterior compartment of the arm (Fig. 16-11), the coracobrachialis assists adduction at the shoulder, whereas the brachialis and biceps are powerful flexors of the elbow. The biceps also provides the chief force for supinating the forearm. All three muscles are supplied by the musculocutaneous nerve (C-5 and C-6), from the lateral cord.

Coracobrachialis. From its origin at the coracoid process and insertion half way down into the medial border of the humerus (see Figs. 15-5, 15-7, and 16-11), the coracobrachialis can produce adduction and some flexion at the glenohumeral joint. Its contracted belly can be observed in the lateral wall of the axilla when adduction of the arm is opposed. This maneuver is useful to confirm the integrity of the musculocutaneous nerve before it enters the arm. Because its action is more powerfully executed by muscles in the axillary folds, the significance of the coracobrachialis is mainly as a landmark. The muscle may vary in size, and sometimes it inserts close to the elbow.

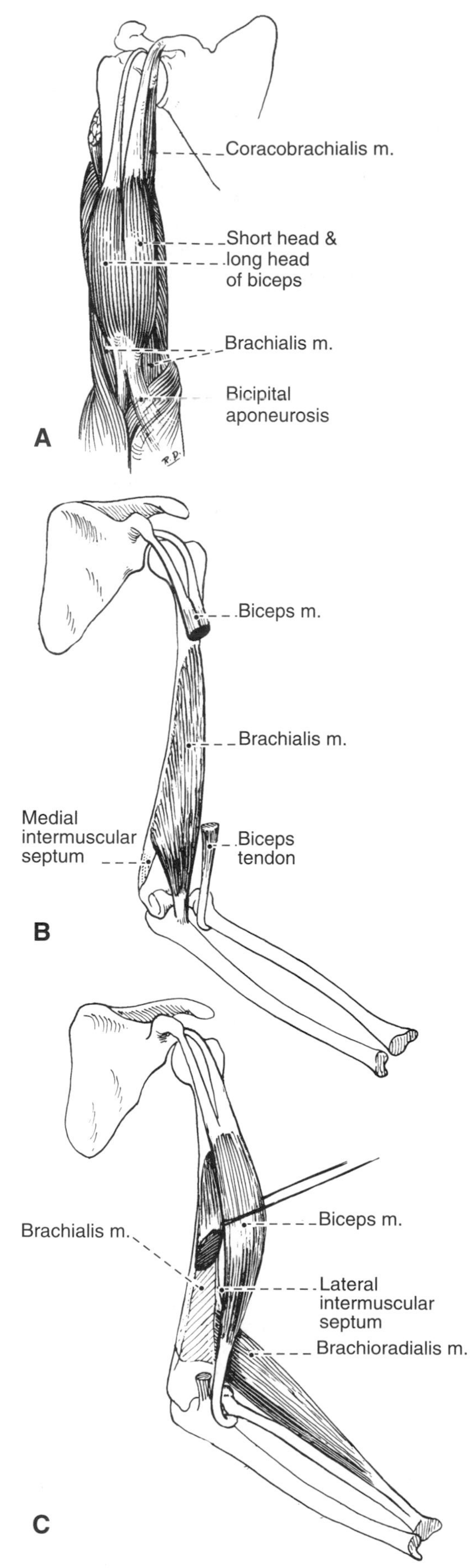

FIGURE *16-11.*
Flexor muscles of the elbow from (A) an anterior view; (B) with the bulk of the biceps resected; and (C) with the bulk of the brachialis resected.

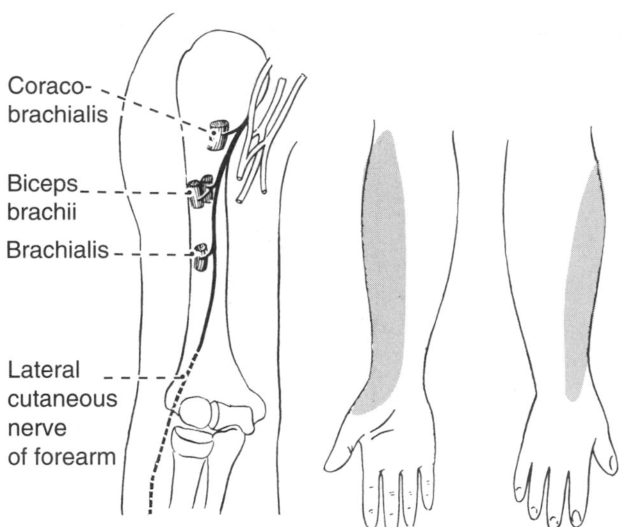

FIGURE **16-12.**
Distribution of the musculocutaneous nerve to muscles and skin (*shaded* areas).

Brachialis. As obscured by the superficial bulk of the biceps, the brachialis is often insufficiently appreciated (see Fig. 16-11B). It is the most important flexor of the elbow. It participates in this act whether the movement is performed slowly or rapidly, whether the forearm is pronated or supinated, and whether a load is being lifted, or it is only the force of gravity that has to be overcome. It has been aptly named the workhorse of elbow flexion.

The brachialis arises from the anterior surface of the lower half of the humeral shaft (see Fig. 15-7) and from the two intermuscular septa (see Fig. 16-11B and C). Its fibers converge on a short tendon, deep in the cubital fossa, which inserts into the coronoid process of the ulna (see Fig. 16-2). The muscle is ideally placed for fast or spurt action, but gives power to elbow flexion under all circumstances. By its isometric contraction it maintains the flexed position, especially when resistance or weight is applied to the forearm. When the flexed forearm is extended by the force of gravity, it is the brachialis that controls elbow extension by gradual relaxation while the triceps is quiescent. The hardened belly of the brachialis may be palpated on either side of the biceps and its tendon when flexion is opposed.

The chief segmental nerve supply from C-5 and C-6 reaches the muscle by the **musculocutaneous nerve**. Paradoxically, the radial nerve also gives a minor branch (C-7) to the brachialis, an anomaly that is probably explained by the derivation of the lateral portion of the muscle from the extensor premuscle mass. This branch of the radial nerve may actually proceed through the muscle, without innervating it, to supply the elbow joint.

Biceps Brachii. The chief function of the biceps is to supinate the pronated forearm. This will be apparent from its mode of insertion. However, the biceps is also a powerful prime mover when the supine or semiprone forearm is flexed. The muscle remains largely quiescent during flexion if full pronation is maintained. It functions chiefly as a reserve muscle of elbow flexion, being called into action when power is required.

The name of the muscle is derived from its two heads of origin, a short head and a long head. Both heads begin as tendons at their scapular attachments, under cover of the deltoid, and give rise to separate muscular bellies that then fuse with one another in front of the brachialis (see Fig. 16-11A). The fused belly terminates in a rounded, stout tendon above the elbow. It crosses the joint and inserts into the tuberosity of the radius (see Fig 16-2).

The **short head** of the biceps is fused with the coracobrachialis as the latter arises from the tip of the coracoid process (see Figs. 15-5 and 16-11). The **long head** is attached by a long tendon to the supraglenoid tubercle of the scapula (see Fig. 15-5). This tendinous long head passes through the glenohumeral joint and is invested by a sleeve of synovial membrane as it traverses the intertubercular groove (see Fig. 15-32).

Emerging beneath the transverse ligament of the joint capsule, the tendon carries with it a diverticulum of the synovial sheath (see Fig. 15-32). The transverse ligament helps retain the long head tendon in the groove. The **biceps tendon** of insertion passes deeply into the cubital fossa and is attached to the posterior lip of the radial tuberosity. In the supinated position, the tuberosity faces toward the ulna, but in pronation it is rotated posteriorly, and the tendon is wrapped around the radial neck, with a bursa intervening between tendon and bone (*bicipitoradial bursa*). Contraction of the biceps, therefore, first reverses rotation of the radius (i.e., supinates) before causing elbow flexion.

A fibrous band, the **bicipital aponeurosis**, arises from the medial border of the bicipital tendon and the lower, medial part of the muscle; it crosses over the forearm muscles that originate from the medial epicondyle (see Fig. 16-11A). The aponeurosis fuses with the deep fascia of the forearm, thereby gaining attachment to the ulna. Through this second insertion, the biceps exerts only its flexor action.

In addition to providing power to supination and elbow flexion, the biceps also contributes to glenohumeral flexion by its short head and to glenohumeral abduction by its long head. However, these actions acquire significance only when the chief prime movers for these actions are paralyzed.

Like the brachialis, the biceps is innervated by C-5 and C-6 through the **musculocutaneous nerve**, which sends a separate branch into each belly. A tap on the biceps tendon (palpable in the cubital fossa) elicits the *biceps reflex*. This reflex tests spinal cord segments C-5 and C-6, but chiefly C-5, as well as both afferent and efferent limbs of the reflex arc that involve the musculocutaneous nerve and the brachial plexus.

Nerves

The musculocutaneous, median, ulnar, and radial nerves, four major branches of the brachial plexus that continue into the free limb (see Fig. 14-6A), all pass through the anterior compartment of the arm. It seems that the boundary between the flexor (anterior) and extensor (posterior) compartments of the embryonic limb (see Fig. 14-5) shifts during development. A consequence of the resulting displacement is that the **radial nerve**, derived from the posterior divisions of the plexus, winds its way from the posterior to the anterior compartment of the arm, and the **ulnar nerve**, although derived from the anterior divisions of the plexus, passes from the anterior into the posterior compartment. Both remaining nerves, derived from the anterior divisions, stay in the anterior compartment. However, only one of them, the **musculocutaneous nerve,** is concerned with supplying the muscles of the anterior compartment of the arm (Fig. 16-12); the median nerve, together with the ulnar nerve, is destined for the forearm and hand, and accompanies the brachial artery through the arm without innervating any structures in it (Fig. 16-13). Therefore, the only nerve important to the function of anterior compartment muscles in the arm is the musculocutaneous nerve. Nonetheless, the course of the other three nerves through the anterior compartment needs to be appreciated.

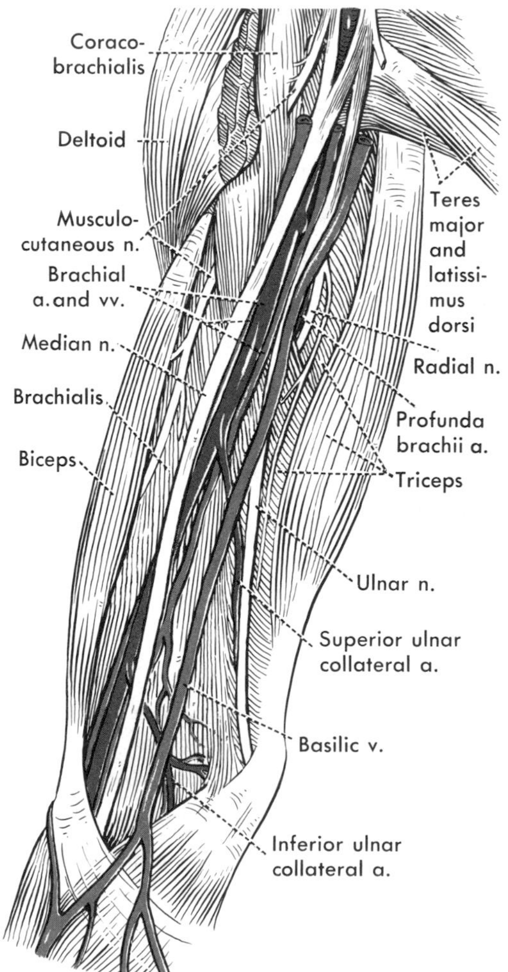

FIGURE *16-13.*
Anatomic relations in the arm, showing the chief nerves and vessels.

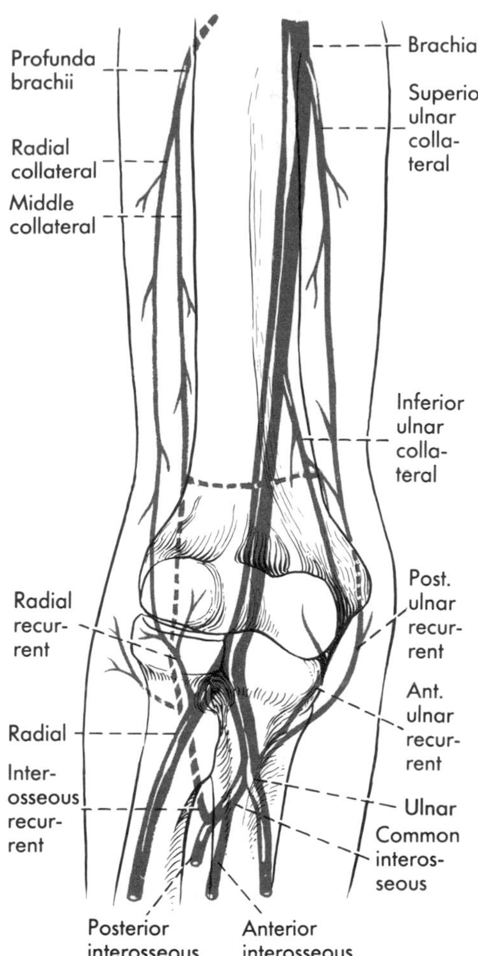

FIGURE *16-14.*
Diagram of the lower part of the brachial artery and the circumarticular anastomoses around the elbow joint.

Musculocutaneous Nerve. In functional terms, the musculocutaneous nerve is best thought of as the nerve of elbow flexion. It also provides the power for supination and, through its terminal branch, supplies an extensive area of skin on the preaxial border of the forearm (see Fig. 16-12).

The nerve is given off by the lateral cord of the brachial plexus and carries C-5 and C-6 fibers to the free limb. In the axilla, the nerve diverges laterally and gives off one or more branches to the coracobrachialis before it penetrates the muscle. Emerging on the lateral side of the coracobrachialis, the nerve gives off branches to the biceps and brachialis muscles as it descends between them (see Fig. 16-13). After having spent all its muscular fibers, it then continues downward to emerge lateral to the tendon of the biceps as the **lateral cutaneous nerve of the forearm** (see Fig. 16-9).

In addition to supplying muscles and skin, the musculocutaneous nerve also sends branches to the elbow joint and the humerus. They convey somatic afferent and visceral efferent fibers. Sometimes the nerve is connected to the median nerve by a communicating branch in the arm. Such a branch may represent fibers that failed to join the median nerve in the axilla through its lateral root. Likewise, but less frequently, fibers may pass from the median nerve to the musculocutaneous nerve.

Course of the Median, Ulnar, and Radial Nerves. The **median nerve** commences on the anterolateral aspect of the axillary artery and descends with that vessel into the arm. It continues its course parallel to the brachial artery on the medial side of the arm (see Fig. 16-13). It gradually crosses the brachial artery anteriorly to lie medial to the artery at the elbow. Although it does not supply any structures in the arm, it gives off some branches before it crosses the elbow. These include a branch to the pronator teres (a muscle of the forearm), and an articular branch to the elbow joint. Through much of their course in the arm, the median nerve and brachial artery lie on the surface of the brachialis muscle and are sheltered by the biceps (see Fig. 16-10).

The **ulnar nerve** leaves the axilla lying posteromedial to the axillary artery (see Fig. 15-17B). In the arm, the nerve lies parallel to the median nerve, with the brachial artery and brachial veins between them (see Fig. 16-13). At about the middle of the arm, the ulnar nerve inclines posteriorly, piercing the medial intermuscular septum to continue its course in the posterior compartment on the medial aspect of the triceps. Passing behind the medial epicondyle, the nerve enters the forearm. Here the nerve is subcutaneous, can be rolled and compressed against the bone, and accounts for the colloquial name of the epicondyle: "funny bone."

The **radial nerve** descends through the posterior compartment of the arm, but enters the anterior compartment by perforating the lateral intermuscular septum just above the elbow. It is described in the next section (see under Posterior Compartment).

Vessels

Arterial blood is distributed to all segments of the free limb by the **brachial artery** and its branches. Venous blood is drained from superficial structures by the **cephalic** and **basilic veins**, discussed in the previous section, and from deep structures by the **brachial veins**.

The **brachial artery** begins at the lower border of the teres major muscle as the direct continuation of the axillary artery. It terminates in the cubital fossa by dividing into the radial and ulnar arteries. The artery runs down on the medial side of the arm, lying first on the coracobrachialis and then, for most of its course, on the brachialis (see Fig. 16-13). Its pulsations can be palpated along the medial border of the biceps when the artery is compressed against the humerus.

Sphygmomanometer readings of arterial blood pressure are usually obtained by placing a stethoscope over the brachial artery as it enters the cubital fossa on the surface of the brachialis, along the medial side of the biceps tendon (see Figs. 16-25 and 16-26). The artery is deep to the bicipital aponeurosis. Verification of the pulsations of the artery in this position is also important before venipuncture is attempted in or close to the cubital fossa. The neurovascular relations are further described in the appropriate section (see under Cubital Fossa).

In its descent through the arm, the brachial artery is closely associated with veins and nerves (see Fig. 16-13). Two brachial veins are apposed to the artery, and in the upper part of the arm, the basilic vein, having pierced the brachial fascia, runs medial to it (see Fig. 16-10). The median nerve, anterior to the artery at its commencement, runs along its lateral side in the upper part of the arm. It then crosses in front of the artery to enter the cubital fossa along its medial side. Proximally, the ulnar nerve is posterior to the artery, but it turns backward from it at about the middle of the arm.

In addition to unnamed **branches** that supply muscles, fascia, and skin, there are three named branches of the brachial artery: the **profunda brachii artery**, and the **superior** and **inferior ulnar collateral arteries** (Fig. 16-14). They all contribute to an anastomosis around the elbow joint, as well as supplying soft tissues and bones.

The **profunda brachii** (deep brachial), given off near the commencement of the brachial artery, leaves the anterior compartment as it passes posteriorly in company with the radial nerve. Its course is described with the structures of the posterior compartment. The **superior ulnar collateral artery** arises at about the middle of the arm and passes posteriorly along with the ulnar nerve. The **inferior ulnar collateral artery** arises only a little above the elbow. These last two arteries anastomose with **posterior** and **anterior recurrent branches** of the ulnar artery, establishing an alternative path for blood flow around the elbow joint. A **nutrient artery**, given off by the brachial artery, usually enters the humerus close to the insertion of the coracobrachialis.

The paired **brachial veins** arise by the union of the radial and ulnar veins and collect blood from deep tissues of both the anterior and posterior compartments of the arm (see Fig. 16-13). They ascend, one on each side of the brachial artery, and are linked to one another by anastomotic interconnections (not shown in Fig. 16-13). They terminate in the axillary vein, which is formed by the union of the two brachial veins with the basilic vein. Sometimes there is only one brachial vein.

Anomalous Brachial Vessels. In approximately 30% of individuals, there are two arteries that proceed down the arm in one or both limbs. This anomaly may arise in two ways. Most commonly, the brachial artery gives off its radial or ulnar branch at a higher level than usual, well above the cubital fossa. Thus, only one of the two vessels in the arm is truly the brachial artery. Less frequently, there is a true doubling of the brachial artery, the axillary artery having given rise to two vessels, rather than one. The two brachial arteries usually unite in the cubital fossa before dividing into radial and ulnar arteries. Occasionally they do not: one divides in the usual way and the other continues, without division, as the common interosseous artery of the forearm (the embryonic axial artery; see Chap. 14).

The identity of the vessels is determined by their relation to the median nerve and their fate in the forearm. The normal artery, representing the axial artery of the limb, takes the usual course of the normal brachial artery and is crossed superficially by the median nerve. The anomalous artery lies in a more superficial position and is named either a *superficial brachial artery*, or a *superficial radial* or *superficial ulnar artery*, depending on the branching pattern and course it pursues in the forearm.

Posterior Compartment

Muscles

The large muscle mass in the back of the arm is the **triceps brachii**, which covers the posterior aspect of the humerus below the deltoid. Associated with the triceps at the elbow are two small muscles, the **articularis cubiti** and the **anconeus**.

Triceps Brachii. As its name implies, the triceps has three heads of origin: the medial head, the lateral head, and the long head (Fig. 16-15). The three heads unite and function as the extensor of the elbow.

The true functional counterpart to the chief flexor of the elbow (the brachialis) is the **medial head** of the triceps. The muscle is misnamed; the head lies deep, not medial, and is the mirror image of the brachialis in the extensor compartment of the arm. It originates from the humerus and intermuscular septa below the radial groove (see Fig. 15-7D); the other two heads of the triceps are superficial to it. The **lateral head** originates from a narrow area on the humerus above the radial groove (see Fig. 15-7D) and from part of the lateral intermuscular septum. The **long head** lies medially and arises by a strong tendon from the infraglenoid tubercle of the scapula just outside the shoulder joint. It passes downward between the teres minor and teres major, separating the quadrangular space from the triangular space (see Fig. 15-29). The lateral and long heads merge half way down the arm, giving rise to a flat tendon that remains superficial to the fleshy medial head. Lower down it is joined by some of the medial head fibers. The three heads insert by a stout tendon into the upper surface of the olecranon. The tendon of insertion is separated from the capsule of the elbow joint by the **subtendinous bursa** of the triceps muscle.

The three heads participate in elbow extension in an unequal manner. The medial head is always active, the long head is quiescent during active extension, and the lateral head shows minimal activity. However, when resistance has to be overcome, the lateral and long heads are recruited. (In this manner they resemble the two heads of the biceps.) For instance, all parts of the triceps are active during push-ups or when a heavy object is being pushed with the arms. The triceps is called into action as a synergist when the semiflexed forearm is forcefully supinated (e.g., undoing a tight screw). It cancels out the flexor action of the biceps. The muscle is quiet, however, when the forearm is extended by the force of gravity. Therefore, when

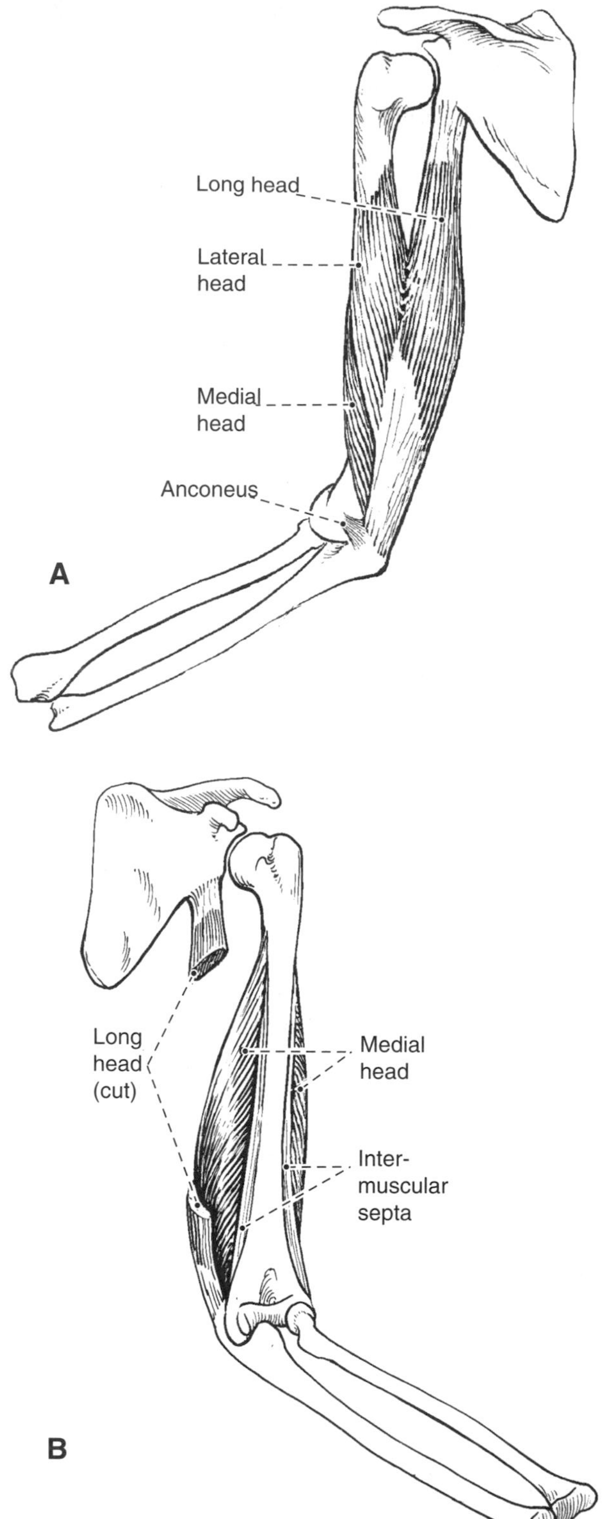

FIGURE *16-15.*
Extensor muscles of the elbow from (A) a posterior view, and (B) from an anterior view, with the brachialis and biceps removed.

testing the power of the triceps, the limb should first be abducted to 90°; the elbow is then extended, moving the forearm in a transverse, rather than a sagittal, plane.

Because the long head of the triceps crosses the shoulder joint, it can assist slightly in adduction and extension the arm.

The triceps is supplied by several branches of the **radial nerve** (C-6, C-7, and C-8). The course of the nerve and its pattern of branching in the posterior compartment are described in the following section. The *triceps reflex* can be elicited by tapping the tendon of the triceps (best done with the limb abducted to 90°); it tests cord segments C-7 and C-8, which are the predominant segments for extension in the joint center of the elbow (see Table 13-1 and Fig. 13-23). The peripheral afferent and efferent pathways of the reflex involve the radial nerve and respective parts of the brachial plexus.

Articularis Cubiti and Anconeus. These two small muscles are considered parts of the triceps. The **articularis cubiti** is made up of some deep fibers of the medial head of the triceps. It inserts into the capsule of the elbow joint, preventing it from being caught by the olecranon. The **anconeus** is a small, flat, triangular muscle arising from the lateral epicondyle of the humerus and inserting on the lateral side of the olecranon and an adjacent part of the body of the ulna (see Figs. 16-15 and 16-27). Its upper border blends with the medial head of the triceps. Both muscles are supplied by the radial nerve.

Nerves and Vessels

The radial nerve and the profunda brachii artery pass through the posterior compartment of the arm. The ulnar nerve, which winds its way into the distal part of the compartment, is discussed in the foregoing.

Radial Nerve. In functional terms, the radial nerve is the extensor nerve of the elbow, wrist, and digits: it innervates muscles in the posterior compartment of the arm and forearm and supplies skin over the posterior surface of the arm, forearm, and hand (Fig. 16-16). As the direct continuation of the posterior cord of the brachial plexus, the radial nerve carries fibers from C-5 through T-1 cord segments into the free limb (see Fig. 15-21). In its course through the axilla and the posterior compartment of the arm, it gives off both muscular and cutaneous branches. After entering the anterior compartment of the arm, however, its muscular and cutaneous fibers part company when the nerve divides at the elbow into a deep and a superficial branch. The deep branch carries with it all the fibers that innervate muscles in the posterior compartment of the forearm (see Fig. 16-16), and the superficial branch conveys fibers to the skin on the back of the hand.

Course. The radial nerve enters the arm behind the brachial artery. Below the lower border of the teres major, the nerve turns posterolaterally with the profunda brachii artery, entering the posterior compartment of the arm between the long head of the triceps and the humerus (Fig. 16-17). It continues its downward and lateral course in the middle third of the arm, passing between the deep and superficial heads of the triceps. The nerve lies on the most proximal fibers of the medial head of the triceps as they arise from the radial groove, which keep it away from contact with the bone (see Fig. 16-17). Nevertheless, it is much closer to the bone than the musculocutaneous nerve and, hence, more vulnerable in humeral fractures. It may be rolled against the humerus in this position. When it reaches the lateral edge of the humerus, it pierces the lateral intermuscular septum and continues inferiorly in the

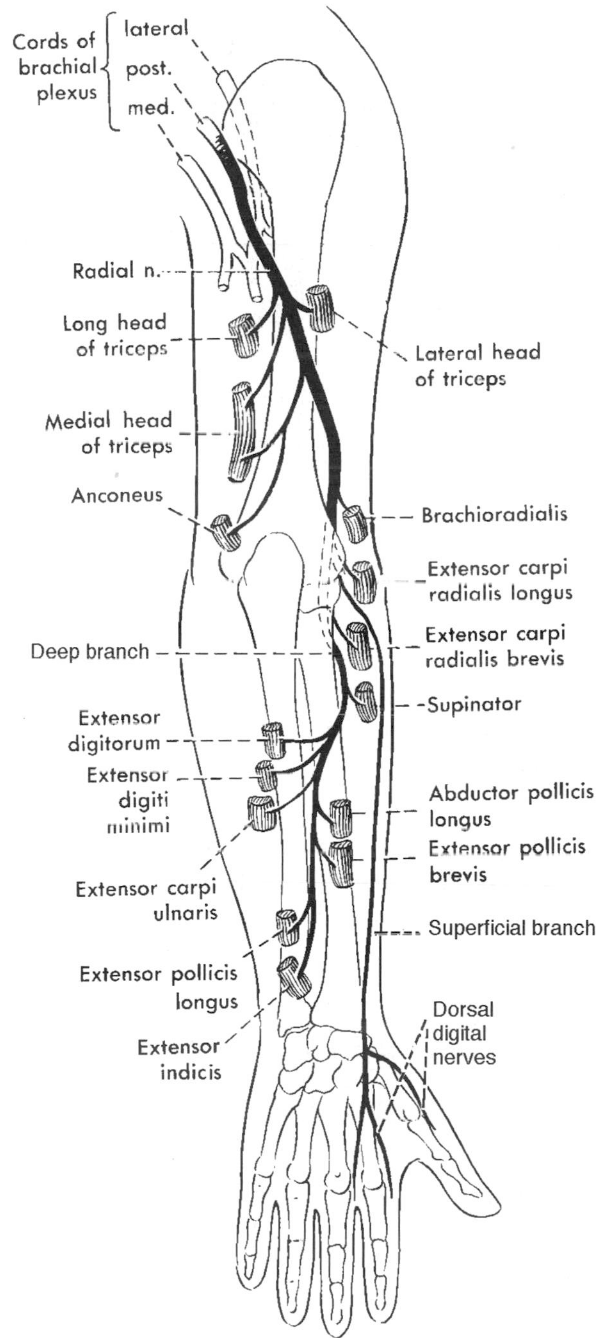

FIGURE *16-16.*
Distribution of the radial nerve.

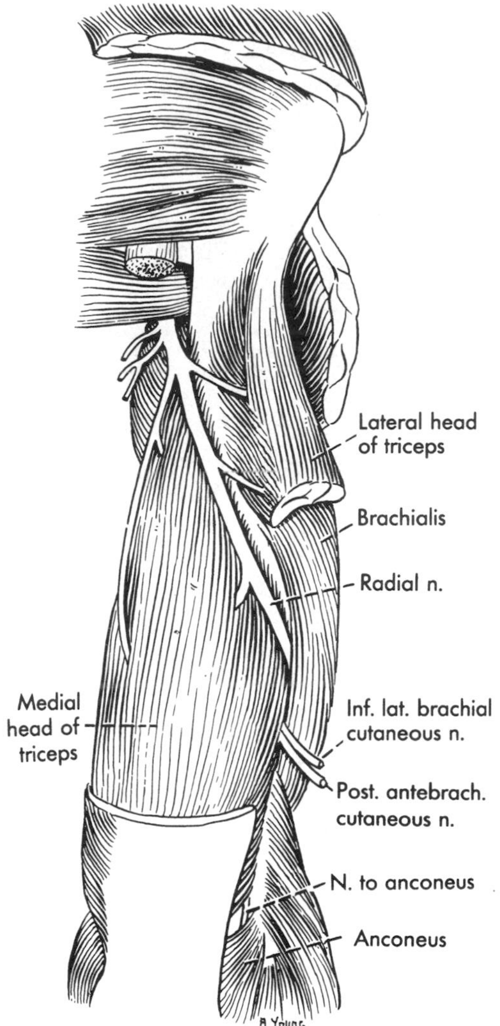

FIGURE *16-17.*
The course of the radial nerve through the posterior compartment of the arm.

anterior compartment, lying between the brachialis and brachioradialis. Here the nerve divides in front of the lateral epicondyle; its superficial branch continues down in the anterior compartment of the forearm, whereas its deep branch turns posteriorly (see Fig. 16-26).

Branches. The levels at which the branches of the radial nerve arise is of clinical importance in cases of radial nerve injury (see Figs. 16-16 and 16-17). The medial head receives two branches: one given off in the axilla, which descends with the ulnar nerve (ulnar collateral nerve); the other originates in the radial groove. One of these also supplies the brachialis and the elbow joint, the other the anconeus. The branches to the long head also originate at a high level, before the nerve enters the radial groove, whereas the lateral head receives its branch in the radial groove. Before the nerve divides, in the anterior compartment, it gives branches to the forearm muscles that originate from the lateral supracondylar ridge of the humerus (brachioradialis and extensor carpi radialis longus; see Fig. 16-16). Three cutaneous branches are given off high in the axilla and upper part of the arm: the *posterior cutaneous nerve of the arm*, the *lower lateral cutaneous nerve of the arm*, and the *posterior cutaneous nerve of the forearm* (see Fig. 16-9).

Injuries. The radial nerve is subject to injury in the arm owing to its compression or to fractures of the humerus. Compression results in transient paralysis; it may be caused in the axilla, for instance, by the use of a crutch, or in the radial groove by the arm of a chair while the subject is asleep. When the fragments are displaced, fracture of either the surgical neck or the shaft of the humerus may damage the radial nerve. Because of considerable overlap in cutaneous innervation, testing skin sensibility is likely to give equivocal results. Even in cases of relatively high injury, elbow extension may be obtained, if pain permits assessment of the movement. Gravity acting as an extensor must, however, be ruled out, and the movement should be tested in an abducted position of the arm. If the nerve is injured, wrist extensors will be paralyzed, resulting in the characteristic posture of "wristdrop."

Profunda Brachii Artery and Its Anastomoses. The profunda brachii artery (see Fig. 16-14), a branch of the brachial artery, is the chief source of arterial blood for the arm musculature. It accompanies the radial nerve throughout its course in the arm and is parallelled by one or two corresponding veins. In addition to supplying muscles, it supplies a nutrient artery to the humerus and contributes to the anastomoses around both the shoulder and elbow joints. The artery ends by dividing above the elbow into two branches: the **radial collateral artery**, which anastomoses in front of the elbow with a branch of the radial artery (*radial recurrent artery*), and the **middle collateral artery,** which anastomoses behind the elbow with a branch of the interosseous artery (*interosseous recurrent artery*; see Fig. 16-14). An ascending *deltoid branch* of the profunda brachii anastomoses with the posterior circumflex humeral artery, a branch of the axillary artery.

The profunda brachii artery provides a potential alternative route of blood flow from the axillary artery to the arteries below the elbow. The brachial artery may be compressed, temporarily or permanently, without endangering the blood supply of the forearm and hand. This happens, for instance, when, wearing a thick garment, the elbow is maximally flexed. Owing to compression of the brachial artery in the cubital fossa, the radial and ulnar pulses disappear, yet enough blood reaches the hand to maintain sufficient capillary perfusion and maintain the normal pink color of the skin. The anastomoses between the ulnar collateral branches of the brachial artery and the recurrent branches of the ulnar artery (see Fig. 16-14) serve the same function on the medial side of the elbow. Permanent occlusion of the brachial artery results in the enlargement of all these anastomoses.

THE FOREARM

The forearm, like the arm, is divided into an anterior and a posterior compartment. Its anatomy is much more com-

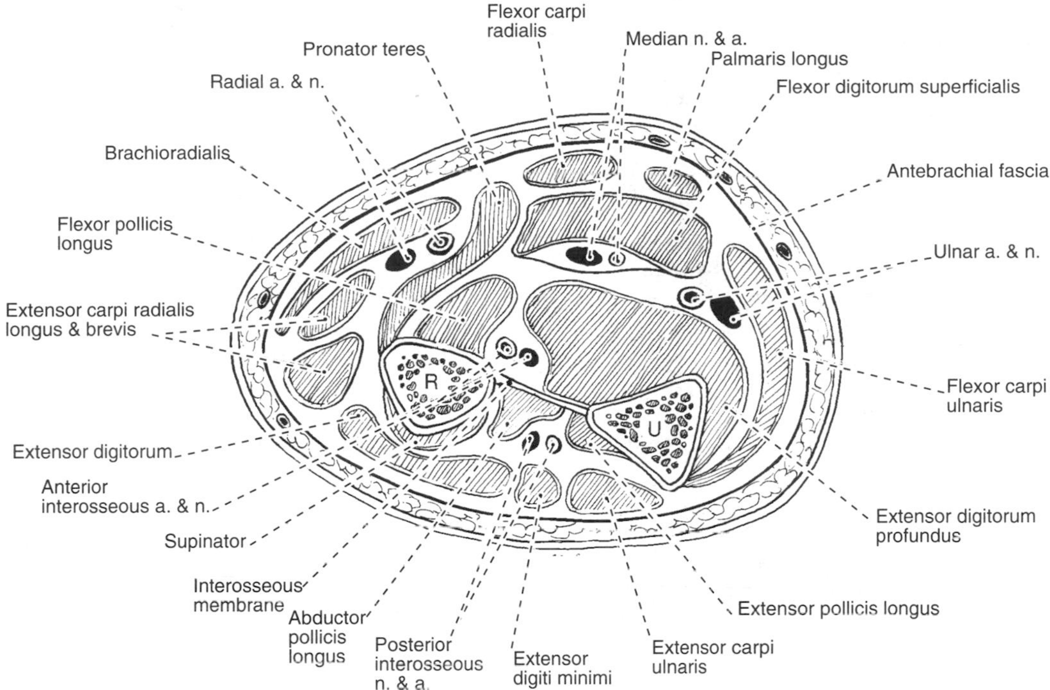

FIGURE 16-18.
Transverse section at the junction of the middle and upper thirds of the forearm drawn to show the layering of muscles and the relations of nerves and arteries to the muscles. *R*, radius; *U*, ulna.

plex, however, because it contains the prime movers for not one but several joints. These muscles are packed into layers in each compartment (Fig. 16-18). The radial, median, and ulnar nerves, after entering the forearm, pass down to the hand beneath the superficial muscles of the anterior compartment. They dispense most of their branches to the superficial muscles in the region of the elbow; a deep branch of the median nerve (*anterior interosseous nerve*) supplies the deep muscles anteriorly, whereas the deep branch of the radial and its *posterior interosseous branch* supply the remaining muscles in the back of the forearm. Each deep nerve is accompanied by an artery of corresponding name (*anterior and posterior interosseous arteries*), both derived from the ulnar artery. Similar to the main nerves, the radial and ulnar arteries descend to the wrist in the anterior compartment.

During dissection or surgery, the display of muscles, nerves, and arteries in the forearm must take into account the layering of the muscles, and the descriptions that follow take such a topographic approach. However, understanding the nearly 20 individual muscles contained in the forearm will be facilitated by first considering their functional grouping relative to their prime mover action at the radioulnar, wrist, and interphalangeal joints. The added advantage of such a consideration is that it forms the basis for assessing movements and muscle power during the physical examination of the forearm and hand.

Functional Grouping of Muscles

Pronation and supination, the two movements possible at the radioulnar joints, are performed by two pairs of muscles: the *pronator teres* and *pronator quadratus* forming one pair (Fig. 16-19A and B), and the *biceps* and *supinator* the other. Both pronators are in the anterior compartment (the pronator teres in the superficial, and the pronator quadratus in the deep muscle layer); the supinator is located deep posteriorly (Fig. 16-20), and the biceps is in the arm.

The chief **prime movers of the wrist** are named according to their actions at the wrist joint and the positions of their tendons, which cross the wrist along either its radial or its ulnar aspect. They are the *flexor carpi radialis* and *flexor carpi ulnaris* anteriorly, and the *extensor carpi radialis* (*longus* and *brevis*) and *extensor carpi ulnaris* posteriorly (see Fig. 16-19). A functionally inconsequential flexor, the slender *palmaris longus*, lies between the radial and ulnar flexors. All these muscles are superficial.

Movements of the digits result from the coordinated action of the extrinsic and intrinsic muscles of the hand. The **extrinsic prime movers of the fingers** are located between the ulnar and radial prime movers of the wrist in both the anterior and posterior forearm compartments. There are two flexor muscles for the fingers, one superficial (*flexor digitorum superficialis*), the other deep (*flexor digitorum profundus*) (see Fig. 16-20A and B). The superficial extensor of the fingers is the *extensor digitorum*, which sends a tendon to the dorsum of each of the four fingers. The little and index fingers each receive an additional extensor tendon from the *extensor digiti minimi* and *extensor indicis* muscles, respectively. These two muscles represent remaining parts of a second or deep extensor that is present in the foot (extensor digitorum brevis) and in the upper limb of some primates and other vertebrates.

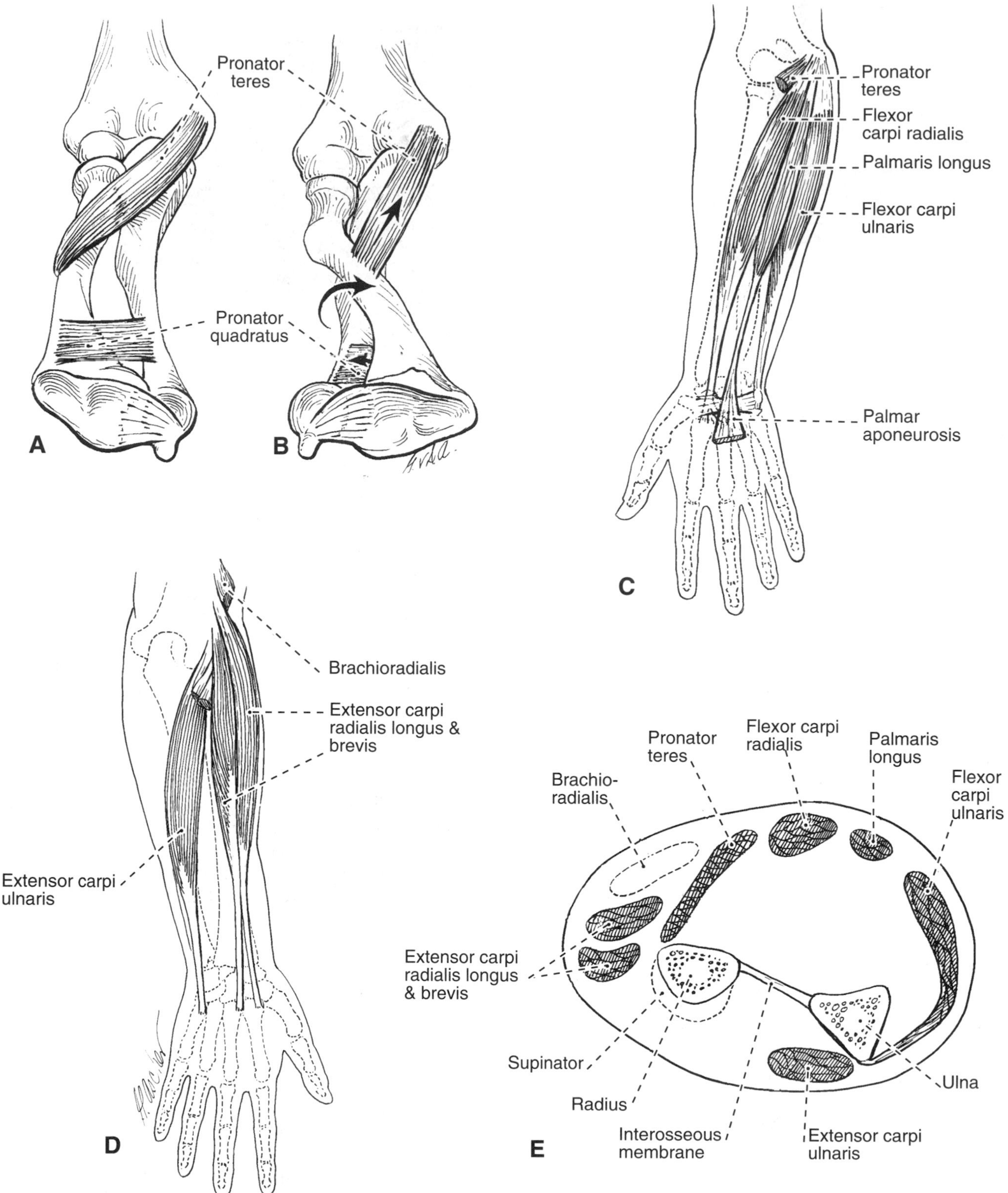

FIGURE *16-19.*
Functional grouping of muscles in the forearm: (A and B) pronators; (C and D) prime movers of the wrist; (E) transverse section identifying the muscles in the superficial layer of the flexor and extensor compartments.

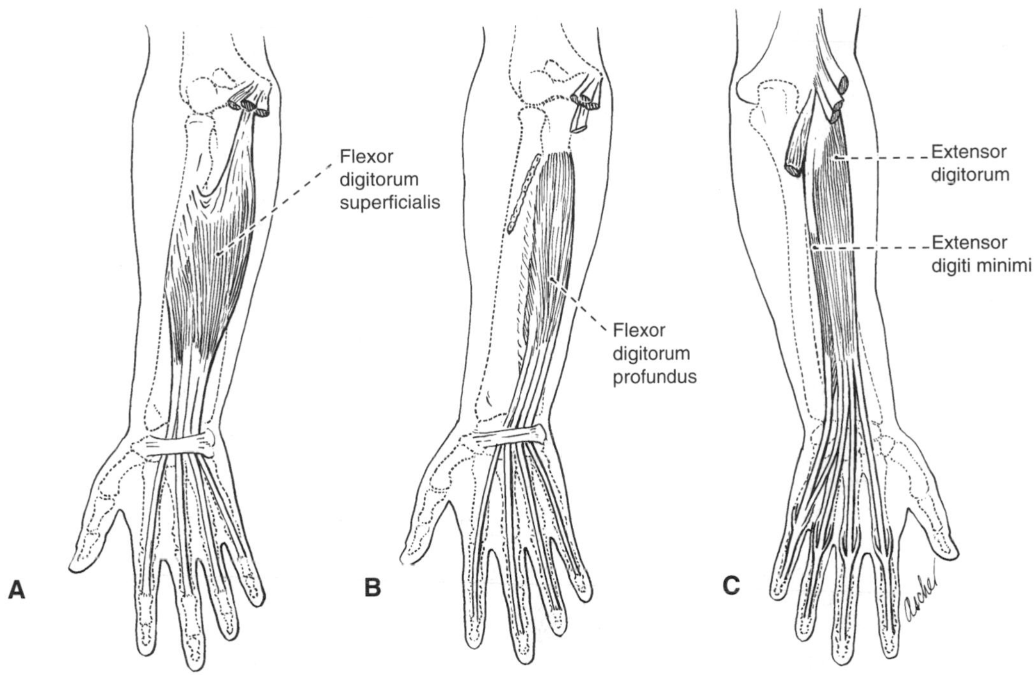

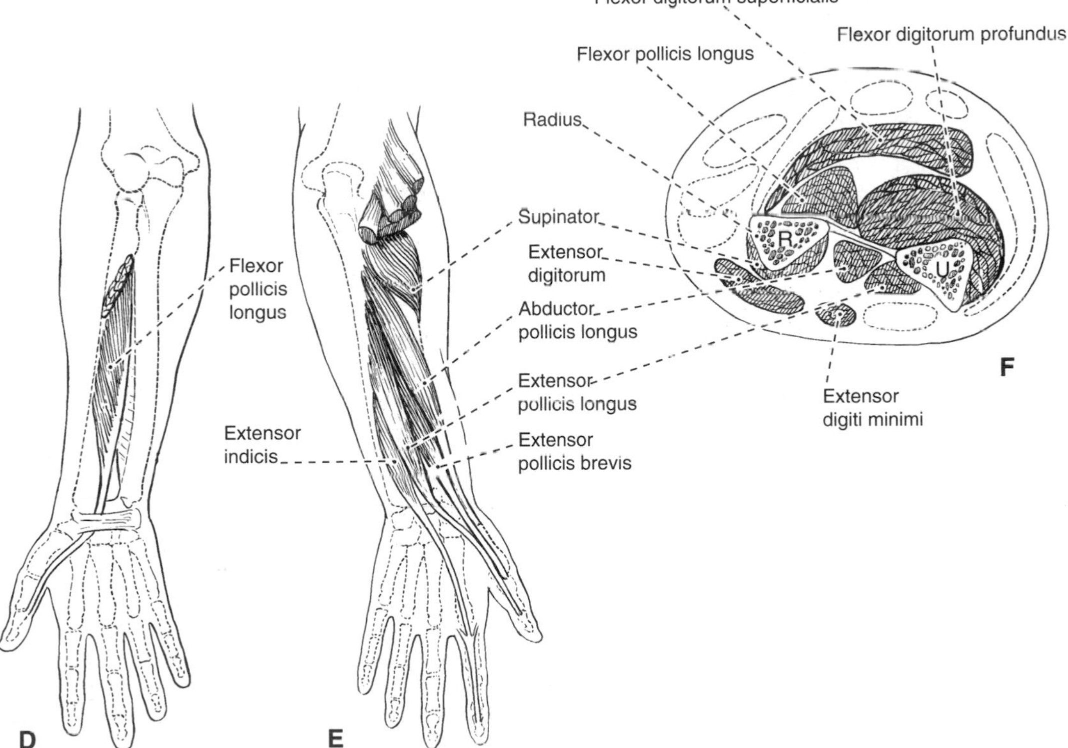

FIGURE *16-20.*
Functional grouping of muscles in the forearm: prime movers of the digits. (A through **C).** Extrinsic muscles of the
fingers, (D and E) of the thumb and index finger, and (F) a transverse section showing the position of the muscles in the intermediate and deep layers of the flexor and extensor compartments. The supinator is shown in panels E and F.

Extrinsic prime movers of the thumb include one flexor, the *flexor pollicis longus* (the flexor pollicis brevis is an intrinsic muscle of the hand), two extrinsic extensors (*extensor pollicis longus* and *brevis*), and an extrinsic abductor as well (*abductor pollicis longus*). They are all in the deep layer.

Anterior Compartment

Superficial Muscles

All superficial muscles attach superiorly to the medial epicondyle of the humerus by a mass of dense connective tissue, often called the *common flexor tendon*. Many of their fibers arise, in addition, from the overlying antebrachial fascia and the fascial septa that separate the muscles. Because their attachment by way of the common flexor tendon is proximal to the elbow joint, these muscles can assist in elbow flexion, in addition to their principal action. The five muscles in this group are readily located by placing the "heel" of one hand on the opposite medial epicondyle: the thumb corresponds to the *pronator teres*, the index finger to the *flexor carpi radialis*, the middle finger to the *palmaris longus*, the ring finger to the *flexor digitorum superficialis* (which is beneath the latter two muscles), and the little finger to the *flexor carpi ulnaris*.

Pronator Teres. The muscle arises by two unequal heads, the larger *humeral head* from the upper part of the medial epicondyle, and the smaller *ulnar head* from the coronoid process of the ulna (see Figs. 15-7 and 16-2). The two heads pass downward and laterally, forming the medial boundary of the cubital fossa. Before they unite, the median nerve passes between them (see Fig. 16-26) and supplies both (C-6 and C-7). The muscle inserts deep to the brachioradialis on the point of greatest convexity of the radial shaft (see Fig. 16-2).

The attachments of the pronator teres offer certain mechanical advantages (see Fig. 16-19 A and B) which explain why the muscle is well suited for quick and powerful pronation (spurt action). The pull of the muscle generates a significant force vector along the shaft of the radius, which ensures good contact between the capitulum and the radial head (shunt action) when pronation is performed rapidly. The pronator teres is readily demonstrated by opposing pronation. Injury to the median nerve above the elbow results in a complete loss of active pronation.

Flexor Carpi Radialis. The radial flexor of the wrist arises from the medial epicondyle by the common flexor tendon (see Fig. 15-7). Its substantial belly terminates in a tendon half way down the forearm (see Fig 16-19). At the wrist, the tendon passes beneath the flexor retinaculum in a compartment of its own, formed by the splitting of the retinaculum just before it attaches to the trapezium (see Fig. 16-30). The tendon inserts on the base of the second metacarpal, sometimes sending a slip to the third metacarpal as well. The muscle receives a branch from the median nerve near the elbow (C-7 and C-8). Its action is demonstrated by opposing wrist flexion and feeling its tendon on the radial side of the wrist (see under The Wrist). Acting together with the radial extensors, it produces abduction at the wrist.

Palmaris Longus. In many species, the palmaris longus operates the claws. In the human, it is vestigial and can act only at the wrist joint. Its short muscular belly arises in common with the other superficial muscles from the medial epicondyle and is soon succeeded by a long slender tendon that crosses the wrist superficial to the flexor retinaculum (see Fig. 16-19). The tendon ends by fanning out and blending with the palmar aponeurosis. The power it contributes to wrist flexion is inconsequential in comparison with that of the other wrist flexors. Its tendon at the wrist serves as a useful landmark both for locating and testing the median nerve (see Fig. 16-43), which supplies the muscle. The muscle, or its tendon, may be absent unilaterally or bilaterally. Conversely, its tendon, or the entire muscle, may be duplicated.

Flexor Carpi Ulnaris. The ulnar flexor of the wrist arises by *two heads*, one from the medial epicondyle by way of the common flexor tendon, the other from the ulna through an aponeurosis that is attached to the upper three-fifths of the ulna's posterior border (see Figs. 16-2D and 16-19). The two heads join just below the medial epicondyle and the ulnar nerve, having passed behind the epicondyle, runs between them and continues toward the wrist lying deep to the muscle. The tendon, which replaces the belly of the muscle some distance above the wrist, inserts on the pisiform bone. The pisiform is in turn stabilized on the hamate bone by the *pisohamate* and *pisometacarpal ligaments*, which may be considered the continuation of the tendon. The muscle is innervated by the ulnar nerve (C-7 and C-8) close to the elbow. Its contraction may be demonstrated by opposing wrist flexion, which throws its tendon into prominence on the ulnar margin of the wrist. By acting together with the ulnar extensor, the flexor carpi ulnaris contributes to adduction at the wrist.

Flexor Digitorum Superficialis. As its name implies, this muscle is considered a member of the superficial muscle group. It is, however, located deep to the four superficial muscles discussed earlier, and actually forms an *intermediate muscle layer* in the forearm (see Figs. 16-18 and 16-20). It arises by two heads and inserts by four tendons on the middle phalanx of each of the four fingers. Although it is primarily the flexor of the proximal interphalangeal joints, it contributes to flexion of all the joints it crosses, including the elbow, the wrist, and the metacarpophalangeal joints.

The large *humeroulnar head* of the muscle arises from the medial epicondyle by way of the common flexor tendon and from the medial border of the coronoid process of the ulna. Its *radial head* arises from the upper part of the anterior border of the radius (see Fig. 16-2). The two heads are united high in the forearm by a dense membrane, behind which the *median nerve* and *ulnar artery* run downward (see Fig. 16-22). In the lower part of the forearm, the muscle gives rise to its four tendons; those that proceed to the middle and ring fingers are placed in front of those that pass to the index and little fingers. Retaining this arrangement, the tendons enter the hand through the carpal canal and fan out in the palm to reach their respective fingers. In both the canal and the palm, they are superficial to the tendons of the flexor digitorum profundus. A large bursa, the *common synovial tendon sheath,* is wrapped around both sets of tendons to facilitate their sliding in the canal (see Figs. 16-30 and 16-32). Similar sheaths invest the tendons in the fingers as well (digital sheaths). The arrangement of the tendon sheaths, as well as that of the tendons, is described in later sections (see under The Wrist and The Hand).

The flexor digitorum superficialis is innervated by the median nerve through branches that enter its deep surface and supply it with fibers derived from C-7, C-8 and, to some extent, T-1.

Deep Muscles

The flexor digitorum profundus, the flexor pollicis longus (see Fig. 16-20), and the pronator quadratus (see Fig. 16-19) make up the deep layer of muscles in the anterior compartment. They lie deep to the flexor digitorum superficialis and flexor carpi ulnaris, and cover the anterior surface of the forearm bones and the interosseous membrane. The pronator quadratus is confined to the forearm, whereas the other two muscles send their tendons through the carpal canal into the hand to insert on the distal phalanges of the digits. The median nerve innervates most of this muscle mass, leaving to the ulnar nerve only the ulnar half of the flexor digitorum profundus.

Flexor Digitorum Profundus. The deep flexor of the fingers has an extensive origin from much of the anterior and medial surfaces of the ulna and from the adjacent interosseous membrane (see Fig. 16-2). The muscle divides into two parts some distance above the wrist: the smaller radial part gives rise to a tendon to the index finger, and the larger ulnar part continues into three tendons for the remaining fingers (see Fig. 16-20). The level of this division may vary from above the wrist to the palm of the hand.

Located deep to the tendons of the flexor digitorum superficialis, the profundus tendons pursue a similar course through the carpal canal, the palm of the hand, and the fingers, except that they insert on the distal phalanx, rather than the middle one.

The ulnar portion of the flexor digitorum profundus is supplied by the *ulnar nerve* and the radial portion by the *anterior interosseous branch of the median nerve.* Both bring C-8 and T-1 fibers to the muscle; C-7 fibers are contributed by the latter. The muscle flexes primarily the distal interphalangeal joints of the fingers. In so doing, however, it also produces an equal amount of flexion at the proximal interphalangeal joints. It is a less effective flexor at the metacarpophalangeal joints and can contribute to wrist flexion only when the fingers are kept extended.

Flexor Pollicis Longus. The long flexor of the thumb arises from the anterior surface of the radius and from the adjacent interosseous membrane (see Fig. 16-2). The unipennate muscle belly gives rise to a tendon that passes through the carpal canal (see Fig. 16-20) on the radial side of the digital flexor tendons. The tendon inserts on the base of the distal phalanx of the thumb. It is surrounded by its own synovial tendon sheath, which extends from above the wrist almost to the point of insertion (see Figs. 16-30 and 16-32).

The C-7, C-8, and T-1 fibers are distributed to the flexor pollicis longus by the *anterior interosseous branch of the median nerve.* Although the primary action of the muscle is to flex the distal phalanx of the thumb, its continued action will flex the proximal phalanx as well.

Pronator Quadratus. The pronator quadratus, lying posterior to the flexor pollicis longus and the flexor digitorum profundus, is the deepest muscle in the forearm. Its parallel fibers form a broad band that runs over the anterior surfaces of the radius and ulna, reaching about a hand's breadth above the wrist (see Fig. 16-19). Its ulnar attachment is the more stable one (see Fig. 16-2), representing its origin; its radial attachment moves along an arc as the muscle contracts. The fibers are at their greatest length when the hand is supinated and the radius and ulna are, therefore, uncrossed (see Fig. 16-19). The anterior interosseous nerve supplies the muscle (C-8). The pronator quadratus is always active in pronation, the pronator teres being recruited during swift or powerful pronation. For this reason, and because it is deeply sealed, its contraction is difficult to demonstrate by opposing pronation.

Nerves

The median and radial nerves enter the anterior compartment of the forearm through the cubital fossa, the ulnar nerve emerges from behind the medial epicondyle to regain its rightful place in the flexor aspect of the limb.

Median Nerve. In functional terms, the median nerve is the chief nerve responsible for innervating the pronators of the forearm, the flexors of the wrist and digits, and the area of skin most critical for relaying sensations from the hand (Fig. 16-21 and see Fig. 14-7). It is formed in the axilla by the union of its lateral and medial roots, and it conveys anterior division fibers from all the spinal nerves that contribute to the brachial plexus (see Fig. 15-20). After its descent in the arm, it gives off muscular branches as it passes through the cubital fossa and the forearm. It leaves the forearm by entering the carpal canal. Its further course and distribution are described in the section on the hand.

Course. The median nerve enters the forearm on the front of the brachialis muscle, medial to the brachial

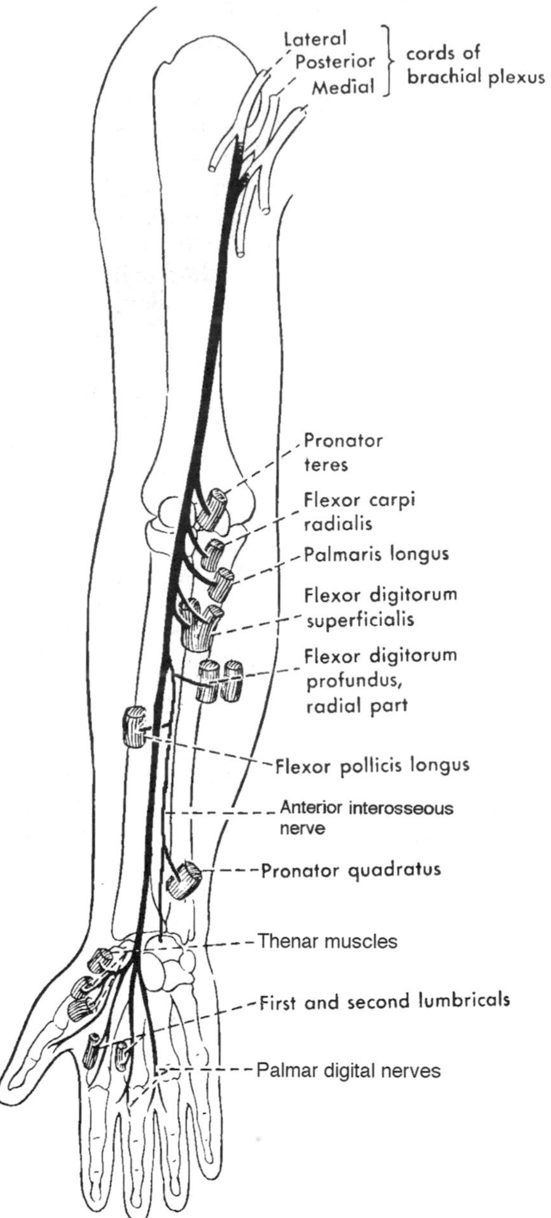

FIGURE *16-21.*
Distribution of the median nerve.

artery and deep to the bicipital aponeurosis (Fig. 16-22). It passes down the midline of the forearm, leaving it equidistant between the styloid processes of the radius and ulna as it dips behind the flexor retinaculum. On exiting the cubital fossa, the nerve passes between the two heads of the pronator teres; the ulnar head of the muscle separates it from the deeply lying ulnar artery. The nerve continues between the flexor digitorum superficialis and profundus, being held to the deep surface of the superficial flexor by connective tissue (see Fig. 16-18). Here, the *median artery*, a small branch of the anterior interosseous artery, accompanies the median nerve. A little above the wrist, the median nerve becomes superficial between the tendons of the flexor digitorum superficialis and flexor carpi radialis. The prominent tendon of the palmaris longus, when present, is a good guide to the nerve (see Fig. 16-43).

Branches. The median nerve gives an *articular branch to the elbow joint* as it crosses that joint. Its remaining branches in the forearm are muscular. Except for the flexor carpi ulnaris (supplied by the ulnar nerve), each of the superficial muscles receives one or two branches as the median nerve passes through, or shortly after it leaves, the cubital fossa. The largest branch of the median nerve is the **anterior interosseous nerve** (Fig. 16-23). It supplies all the deep muscles in the anterior compartment: the flexor pollicis longus, the radial half (or more) of the flexor digitorum profundus, and the pronator quadratus. The nerve runs down in the groove between the flexor digitorum profundus and the flexor pollicis longus with the anterior interosseous artery, dips behind the pronator quadratus, and then proceeds on the interosseous membrane to supply the wrist. A short distance above the flexor retinaculum, the median nerve gives off a small **palmar branch**, which is distributed to skin in the central part of the palm.

Ulnar Nerve. In functional terms the ulnar nerve is the chief motor nerve of the intrinsic muscles of the hand. In addition, it supplies the ulnar flexor of the wrist and the part of the flexor digitorum profundus that serves the ulnar one or two fingers (Fig 16-24). It is also sensory to the skin on the ulnar side or the hand (see Figs. 14-7 and 16-45). The nerve commences as the continuation of the medial cord of the brachial plexus, and conveys C-8 and T-1 fibers to the forearm and hand. The C-7 fibers join it in the axilla from the lateral root of the median nerve or through the ulnar collateral branch of the median nerve in the arm. These fibers are distributed to mainly the flexor carpi ulnaris. In the forearm, the nerve runs under cover of this muscle, from the medial epicondyle to the flexor retinaculum. The nerve crosses the reticulum superficially to enter the hand. Its further course and distribution are described in the section on the hand.

Course. After entering the flexor compartment between the two heads of the flexor carpi ulnaris, the ulnar nerve descends toward the wrist between that muscle and the flexor digitorum profundus (see Fig. 16-23). It emerges with the ulnar artery from behind the flexor ulnaris just above the wrist, and crosses the anterior surface of the flexor retinaculum close to the pisiform bone (see Fig. 16-22). In the lower two thirds of the forearm, the ulnar artery runs along the lateral side of the nerve.

Branches. The ulnar nerve supplies an *articular branch to the elbow joint* and muscular branches to the *flexor carpi ulnaris* and the ulnar side of the *flexor digitorum profundus* (see Figs. 16-23 and 16-24). Two cutaneous branches are given off about a hand's breadth above the wrist: the **dorsal branch** winds around the ulna to supply the back of the hand; a small **palmar branch** runs down on the ulnar artery to supply skin over the hypothenar eminence.

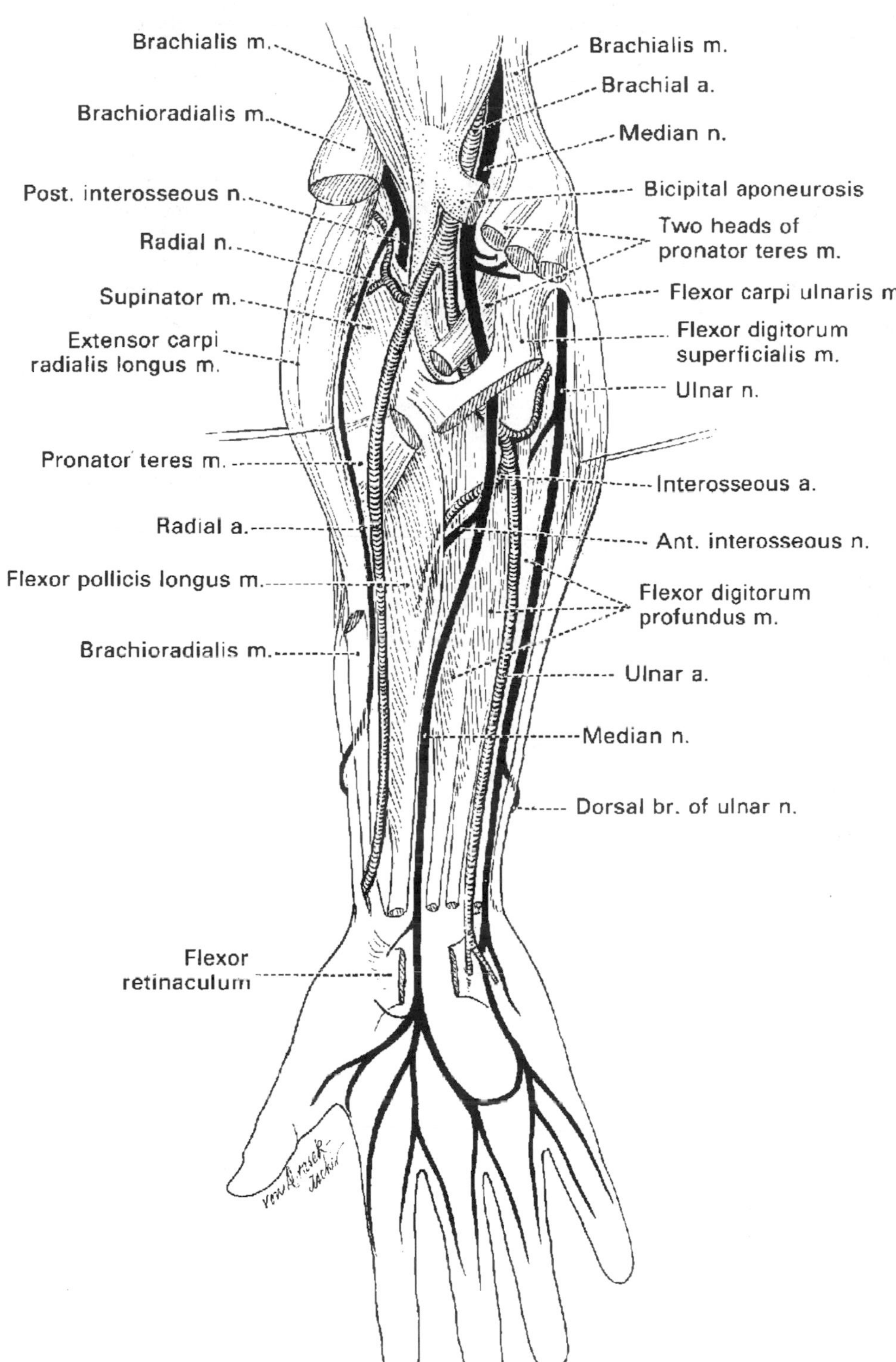

FIGURE *16-22.* **Anatomic relations in the forearm, showing the chief nerves and vessels in the anterior compartment.**

Radial Nerve. Only the superficial branch of the radial nerve, which is entirely cutaneous, passes down the anterior compartment of the forearm (see Fig. 16-22); the deep, muscular branch is in the posterior compartment. In the proximal two-thirds of the forearm, the superficial radial nerve is deep to the brachioradialis and crosses over the supinator, the pronator teres, and the flexor pollicis longus. The radial artery runs along its medial side. A hand's breadth above the wrist, the nerve turns laterally, winds around the radius, passing deep to the tendon of the brachioradialis, and descends to supply the back of the hand. It has no branches in the anterior compartment of the forearm.

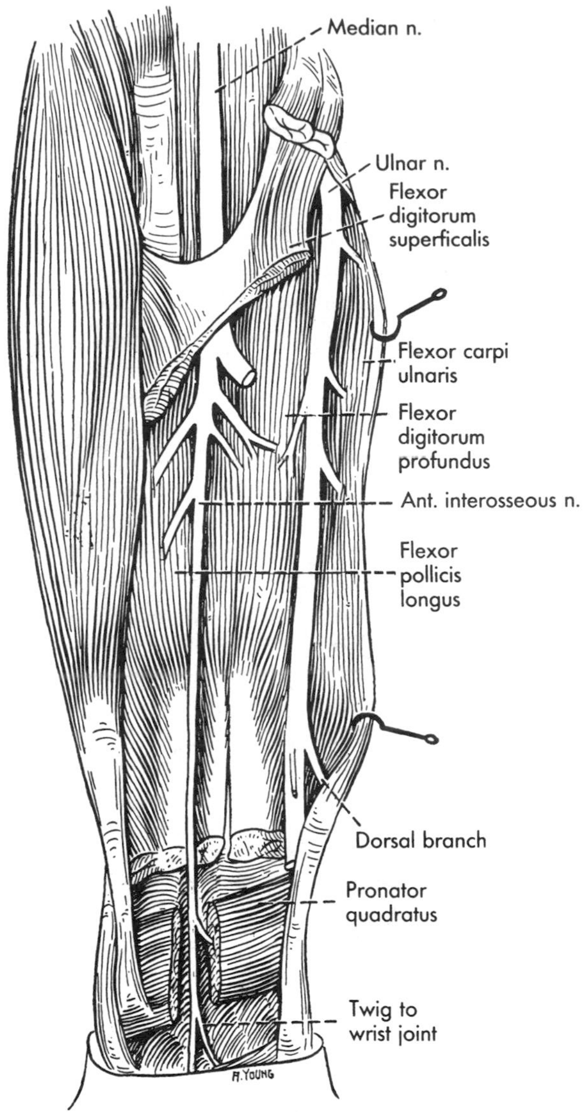

FIGURE *16-23.*
Anatomic relations in the forearm: the anterior interosseous branch of the median nerve, the ulnar nerve, and the deep muscles in the anterior compartment.

Vessels

After the brachial artery divides in the cubital fossa, its two terminal branches, the **radial** and **ulnar arteries**, diverge toward each side of the forearm and descend toward the styloid processes of the radius and ulna (Fig. 16-25). On entering the hand, the arteries terminate by anastomosing with each other through the palmar arches (see Fig. 14-9). Each artery is accompanied by one or two veins of corresponding name and, through much of its course, is paralleled by the nerve of corresponding name (see Fig. 16-22). The vessels run through the anterior compartment of the forearm between the deep and superficial muscle layers (see Fig. 16-18).

Radial Artery. The radial artery is the smaller, lateral terminal branch of the brachial artery. At its commencement it lies level with the radial tuberosity, deep in the cubital fossa, medial to the biceps tendon, on the anterior surface of the brachialis muscle (see Fig. 16-22). While heading laterally to descend under cover of the brachioradialis, it crosses over the biceps tendon, and then over all the muscles that attach to the anterior and lateral surfaces of the radius: the supinator, the radial head of the flexor digitorum superficialis, the pronator teres, the flexor pollicis longus, and above the wrist, the pronator quadratus. In the middle third of the arm, the radial artery is joined along its lateral side by the superficial branch of the radial nerve. In the lower third of the forearm, the artery appears

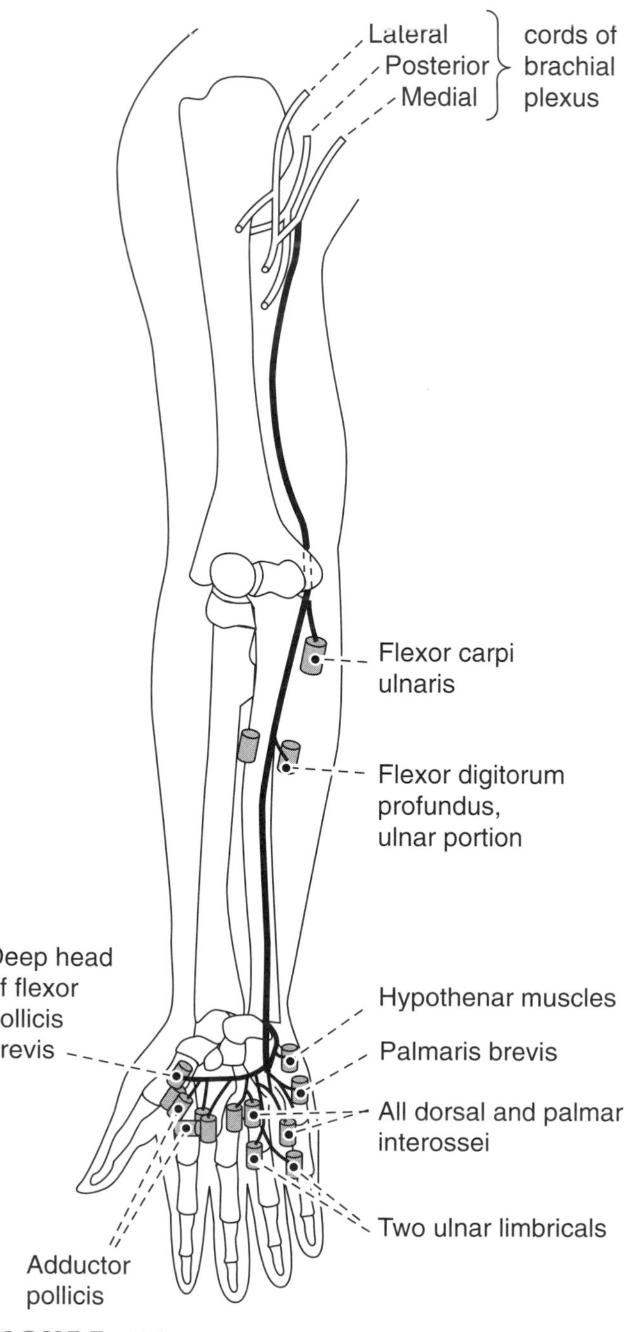

FIGURE *16-24.*
Distribution of the ulnar nerve.

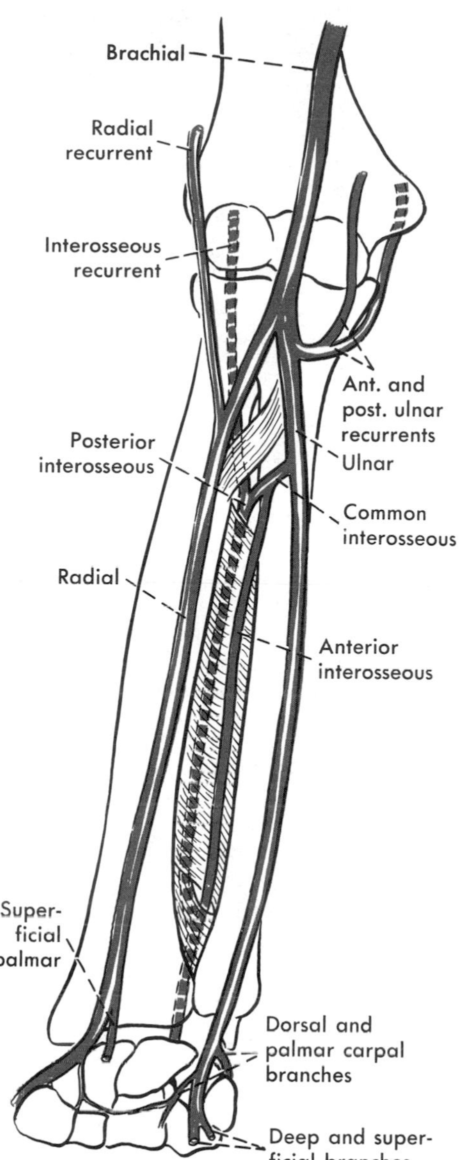

FIGURE *16-25.*
Diagram of the chief arteries of the forearm and the branches around the elbow and wrist.

between the tendons of the brachioradialis and the flexor carpi radialis; only fascia and skin cover it. Here, the artery may be compressed against the radius (and the pronator quadratus, which covers the bone) and its course verified for some distance by feeling its pulsations. After reaching the radial styloid process, the artery turns posteriorly, passing deep to the tendons of the extensor pollicis brevis and abductor pollicis longus. Its pulsations may be felt against the scaphoid as it crosses the anatomic snuff box (see Fig. 16-33), and enters the hand between the first two metacarpal bones. Its further course and branches are described later in the section on the hand.

Branches. Throughout its course the radial artery gives off unnamed branches to muscles, joints, and superficial tissues of the forearm. A little below its origin, it gives off the **radial recurrent artery** that runs upward, following the course of the radial nerve, to anastomose with the radial collateral branch of the profunda brachii artery (see Figs. 16-14 and 16-25). At the wrist, just before the radial artery turns posteriorly, it gives off two small branches: the **superficial palmar branch** enters the thenar eminence, and the **palmar carpal branch**, passing behind the flexor tendons, helps supply the bones and joints of the wrist.

Ulnar Artery. The ulnar artery is the larger, medial terminal branch of the brachial artery. It inclines medially as it leaves the cubital fossa, passing from the anterior surface of the brachialis to that of the flexor digitorum profundus. It descends on this muscle to the wrist, sheltered by the flexor carpi ulnaris (see Fig. 16-25).

In the cubital fossa, the artery is lateral to the median nerve; after exiting the fossa, it crosses behind the nerve, but is separated from it by the ulnar head of the pronator teres. The artery passes deep to the membranous arch between the two heads of the flexor digitorum superficialis and is joined on its lateral side by the ulnar nerve, which accompanies it to the wrist. The ulnar artery emerges from under cover of the flexor carpi ulnaris in the vicinity of the wrist, where it is palpable against the ulna on the radial side of the flexor carpi ulnaris tendon. At the wrist the artery passes superficial to the flexor retinaculum along the lateral side of the pisiform bone and, entering the hand, continues as the *superficial palmar arch.*

Branches. Like the radial artery, the ulnar artery distributes numerous unnamed branches in the forearm. Its first named branch at the elbow is the **ulnar recurrent artery**, which soon divides into anterior and posterior branches. These branches ascend, skirting the medial epicondyle, to anastomose with branches of the brachial artery (see Figs. 16-14 and 16-25). The anterior branch anastomoses with the inferior ulnar collateral artery, and the posterior branch with the superior ulnar collateral artery, completing the *circumtrochlear anastomosis* around the medial side of the elbow.

The largest branch, the **common interosseous artery**, arises on the lateral side of the ulnar artery as it passes behind the flexor digitorum superficialis (see Figs. 16-22 and 16-25). After crossing deep to the median nerve, this short, stout vessel divides into the anterior and posterior interosseous arteries. The **posterior interosseous artery** immediately passes posteriorly between the flexor digitorum profundus and the flexor pollicis longus to traverse the gap at the upper end of the interosseous membrane (see Fig. 16-25). Its course in the posterior compartment is described in the next section. The **anterior interosseous artery** descends on the interosseous membrane between the flexor digitorum profundus and the flexor pollicis longus. It serves as the chief source of blood for the deep muscles. The artery ends by passing behind the pronator quadratus and dividing into anterior and posterior branches. The small anterior branch continues to the front of the wrist, and the posterior one passes through a hole in the lower part of the interosseous membrane to the back of the wrist. Both contribute to an anastomosis around the carpal bones, called the *carpal rete* (*rete;* Latin for net).

A small branch, the **median artery**, is given off by the anterior interosseous artery. It accompanies and supplies the median nerve. Occasionally, the median artery is large and continues with the median nerve into the hand, where it joins the superficial palmar arch. At an early stage of development, the interosseous and median arteries serve as the axial artery of the intermediate segment of the limb.

Two small branches are given off by the ulnar artery before it crosses the flexor retinaculum: the **palmar carpal branch** runs behind the flexor tendons to reach the floor of the carpal canal; the **dorsal carpal branch** runs around the ulnar side of the wrist to join the anastomosis on the dorsal aspect of the carpus.

Veins. The radial artery is accompanied by two **radial veins,** and the ulnar artery by two **ulnar veins**. These veins have tributaries corresponding to the branches of the arteries, and drain the deep tissues of the forearm. Radial and ulnar veins unite in the cubital fossa to form the brachial veins (see Fig. 14-10).

Cubital Fossa

The cubital fossa is an intermuscular space in the proximal part of the anterior compartment of the forearm. It is important anatomically and clinically because, with the exception of the ulnar nerve, it contains all the major nerves and vessels that supply the forearm and hand. The apex of the triangular fossa points inferiorly, and its base is formed by a line connecting the two epicondyles of the humerus (Fig. 16-26). As the biceps and brachialis pass to their insertions in front of the elbow, they lead into the cubital fossa from the arm. The greater part of the floor of the fossa is formed by the brachialis and supinator muscles; the roof is the antebrachial fascia, medially reinforced by the bicipital aponeurosis. The brachioradialis forms the lateral boundary and the pronator teres the medial boundary.

The biceps tendon is a useful guide to the contents of the cubital fossa (see Fig. 16-26). The **brachial artery** enters the fossa along the medial side of the tendon, and divides into the **ulnar** and **radial arteries** deep in the fossa. The **median nerve** accompanies the brachial artery into the fossa, lying just medial to it, and lower down crosses the ulnar artery superficially, close to the origin of that vessel. Just above this point, several motor branches are given off by the nerve to muscles that arise from the medial epicondyle. Just distal to this point, the **anterior interosseous nerve** branches off. Both the brachial artery and the median nerve are held down in the cubital fossa by the bicipital aponeurosis that crosses superficial to

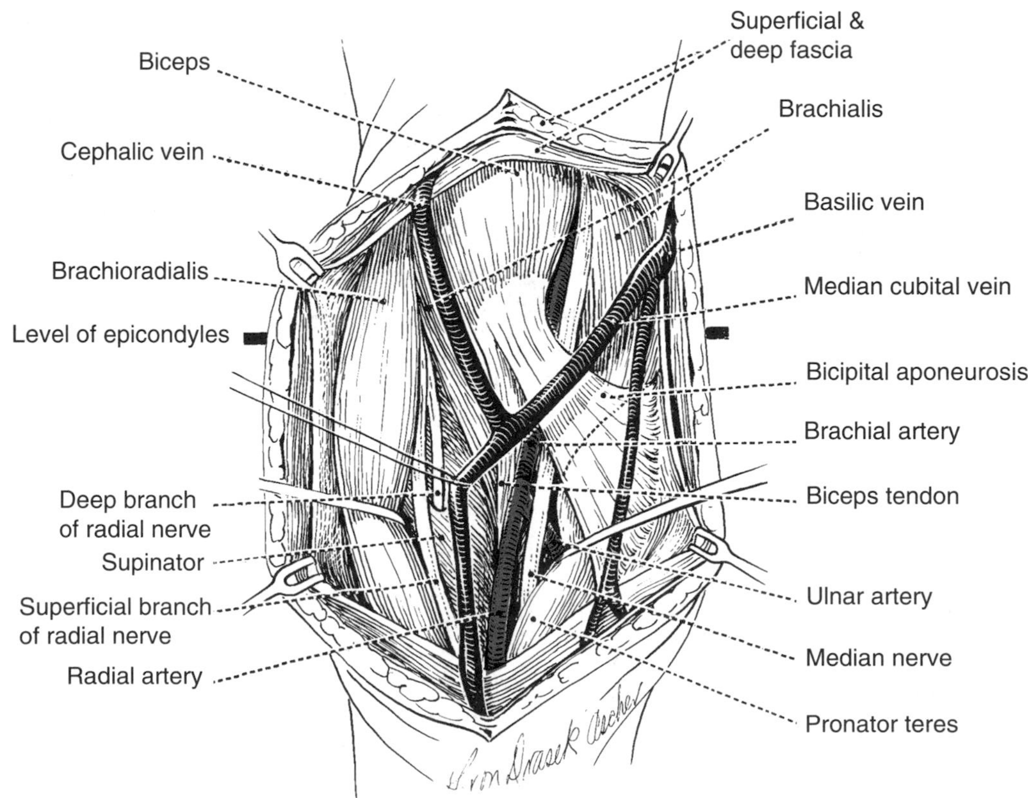

FIGURE *16-26.*
The contents of the cubital fossa exposed by pulling the brachioradialis and pronator teres to the side. The level of the epicondyles, shown in the intact arm by a skin crease, is indicated by a *black bar*.

them and to the pronator teres. The **radial nerve** divides into superficial and deep terminal branches in the lateral corner of the fossa, being sheltered by the brachioradialis. The superficial branch descends in the lateral boundary of the fossa underneath that muscle, but the deep branch turns posteriorly and exits from the fossa. Embedded in the superficial fascia overlying the cubital fossa, the **cephalic vein** passes upward on the lateral side and the **basilic vein** on the medial side. The two veins are interconnected by the **median cubital vein**.

During venipuncture and other manipulations around the elbow, it is useful to bear in mind the relation of nerves and vessels to one another across a line that joins the two epicondyles (see Fig. 16-26). The line is marked by a skin crease. Proceeding from the lateral to the medial epicondyle, the order of structures is as follows: 1) superficial to the brachioradialis over the lateral epicondyle is the cephalic vein, and deep to the muscle is the radial nerve; 2) in the center is the biceps tendon; 3) medial to the tendon is the brachial artery, with the median nerve on its medial side; 4) the bicipital aponeurosis separates the artery and nerve from the median cubital vein; and 5) the basilic vein is superficial to the pronator teres over the medial epicondyle.

Posterior Compartment

Superficial Muscles

The superficial muscles posteriorly include the brachioradialis, the extensor carpi radialis longus and brevis, the extensor digitorum and extensor digiti minimi, and the extensor carpi ulnaris (Fig. 16-27). Except for the brachioradialis, which is a flexor of the elbow, these muscles extend the wrist or the fingers (see Fig. 16-19 and 16-20). The muscles originate from the lateral epicondyle of the humerus and the lateral supracondylar ridge above it. Those that arise from the lateral epicondyle fuse with each other and with the antebrachial fascia and its intermuscular septa to form a *common extensor tendon* attached to the epicondyle. All muscles terminate in tendons, which are held in place on the posterior aspect of the wrist by the *extensor retinaculum.* The retinaculum is a band of fibrous tissue responsible for preventing the tendons from bow stringing when the muscles contract. Synovial sheaths invest the tendons as they pass through compartments created by attachments of the retinaculum to the radius and ulna (see Fig. 16-31).

The muscles that attach to the supracondylar ridge (brachioradialis and extensor carpi radialis longus) are innervated by the **radial nerve** before it divides into its superficial and deep branches; the muscles attached to the epicondyle are supplied by the deep branch of the nerve. The spinal cord segment distributed to the brachioradialis is chiefly C-6, those to the carpal extensors are C-6 and C-7, and those to the digital extensors C-7 and C-8.

Brachioradialis. Although classified among the posterior muscles, the brachioradialis spans the preaxial border of the forearm. It originates from the proximal part of the lateral supracondylar ridge and from the lateral intermuscular septum of the arm; it inserts into the lower end of the radius just proximal to the styloid process (see Fig. 16-11). Above the styloid process, the flat tendon of the brachioradialis, and those of the carpal extensors, are crossed superficially by the thumb muscles (see Fig. 16-27). By virtue of its attachments, the brachioradialis functions as a flexor of the elbow, but its action is different from that of the biceps and brachialis. It is a typical example of a shunt muscle, whereas the biceps and brachialis flex the elbow by spurt action.

The pull of the brachioradialis on the radius is greater *along* the shaft of the radius than *across* it (the reverse of the dominant direction of pull exerted by the biceps or by the brachialis). In any position of the elbow, it tends to pull the radius toward the humerus. On the other hand, once a certain degree of flexion is attained, the biceps and brachialis tend to pull the radius and ulna away from the humerus. Owing to the spurt action of these muscles, any point on the forearm will move on a curved path, and a centripetal force directed toward

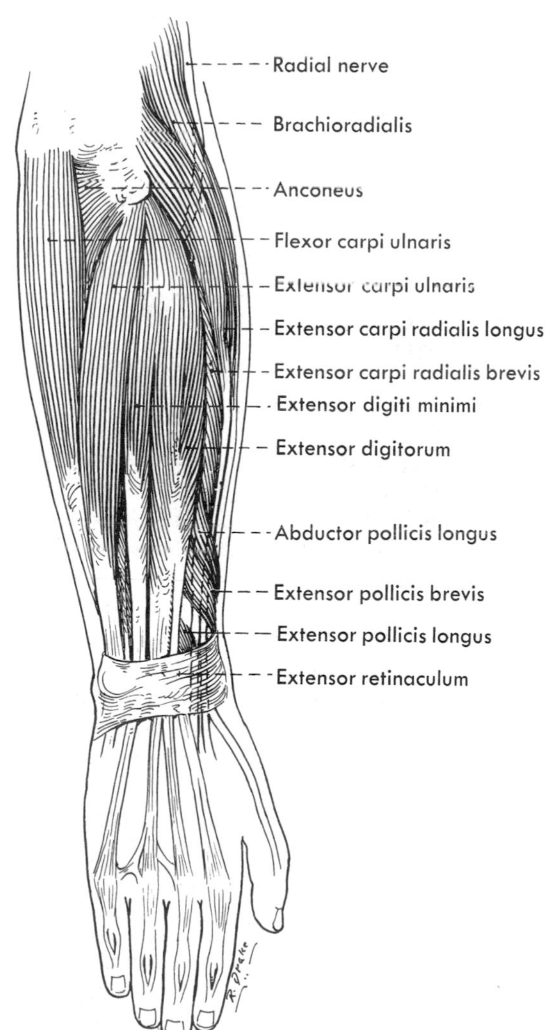

FIGURE *16-27.*
The extensor muscles in the back of the forearm.

the axis of movement is required if the point is not to fly off at a tangent to the curved path. This centripetal force at the elbow is provided by the brachioradialis which is called into action when the movement is rapid, be it flexion or extension. During slow movement at the elbow, the brachioradialis is quiescent.

The brachioradialis is active when weight is lifted while the forearm is in the semiprone position. When elbow flexion is restrained in this position by an examiner, the muscle is thrown into prominence. Contrary to previous teaching, the brachioradialis is inactive during pronation and supination.

The brachioradialis receives a branch from the **radial nerve** (C-5, C-6, and C-7) just above the elbow before the nerve divides. The muscle is used clinically for eliciting a tendon reflex, which tests the same cord segments as the biceps tendon reflex, but chiefly C-6. The reflex, however, assesses different pathways through the brachial plexus and peripheral nerves from those tested by the biceps reflex.

Extensor Carpi Radialis Longus and Brevis. The long extensor of the carpus arises from the lateral supracondylar ridge just distal to the brachioradialis (see Fig. 15-7). It passes across the lateral aspect of the elbow joint and tapers to a flat tendon. The tendon shares a synovial sheath beneath the extensor retinaculum with the extensor carpi radialis brevis (see Fig. 16-31) and then inserts on the base of the second metacarpal. The extensor carpi radialis brevis arises from the lateral epicondyle by the *common extensor tendon,* lying at first largely deep to the long extensor and then on its ulnar side. Its tendon inserts on the base of the third metacarpal. In addition to extending the wrist, the two radial extensors are also prime movers in wrist abduction, a movement in which they act together with the flexor carpi radialis.

Extensor Digitorum and Extensor Digiti Minimi. The extensor digitorum arises from the lateral epicondyle of the humerus by the common extensor tendon and forms a centrally placed superficial mass on the posterior surface of the forearm (see Fig. 16-27). On its ulnar side, it gives rise to the extensor digiti minimi muscle, which has its own separate tendon of insertion. The extensor digitorum itself usually terminates in four tendons (occasionally, only three) which pass through a large compartment of the extensor retinaculum and then diverge toward the fingers over the dorsum of the hand. They join the extensor expansion of the fingers and produce extension at the metacarpophalangeal and interphalangeal joints (see under The Hand). They are active also in wrist extension when the fingers are extended.

Extensor Carpi Ulnaris. The extensor carpi ulnaris arises by two heads, one from the lateral epicondyle through the common extensor tendon (see Fig. 16-27), the other from the posterior border of the ulna (see Fig. 16-2). Its tendon passes through a special compartment of the extensor retinaculum and inserts into the medial side of the base of the fifth metacarpal. In addition to extending the wrist, acting with the ulnar flexor of the carpus, it also produces wrist adduction.

Deep Muscles

The deep extensor muscles are the supinator, three muscles to the thumb (a long and a short extensor and a long abductor), and the extensor indicis (Fig. 16-28 and see 16-20). The supinator is completely covered by overlying muscles. The extensor indicis and the muscles of the thumb arise deeply, but emerge in the lower part of the forearm from under the cover of the extensor digitorum (see Fig. 16-27) and send their tendons, encased in synovial sheaths, through the compartments of the extensor retinaculum to their respective insertions. These muscles are innervated by the deep branch of the radial nerve, which conveys predominantly C-6 fibers to the supinator and C-7 and C-8 fibers to the other muscles.

Supinator. Deeply placed in the extensor compartment of the forearm, the supinator wraps itself around the

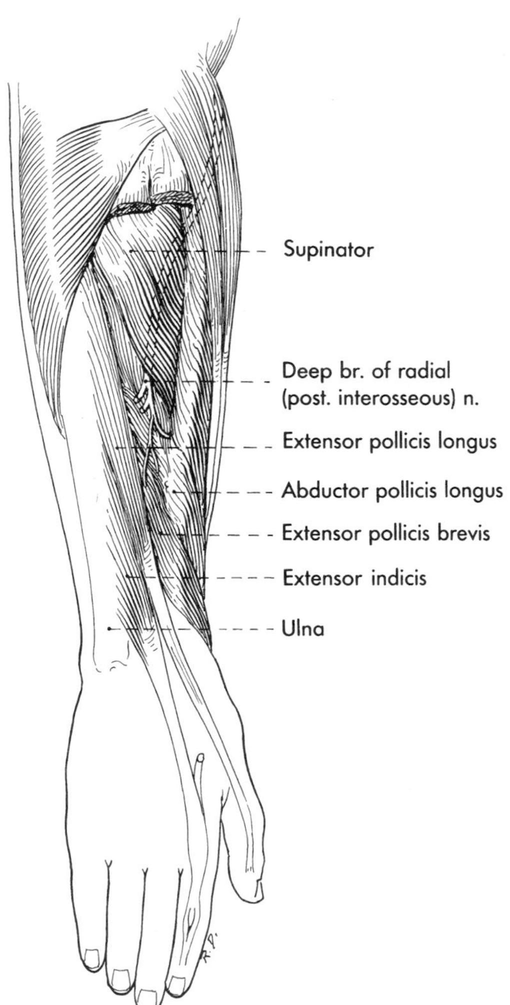

FIGURE *16-28.*
Deep muscles of the extensor group in the forearm.

upper third of the radius (see Fig. 16-28). The muscle originates from the posterior aspect of the lateral epicondyle, the radial collateral ligament of the elbow joint, and the lateral surface of the ulna below the radial notch (see Fig. 16-2). The ulnar fibers encircle the neck of the radius and are deep to those that originate on the epicondyle. The muscle inserts into the radius over a wide area between the neck and the point of insertion of the pronator teres (see Fig. 16-2). The fibers are at maximum length when the forearm is pronated, and their contraction restores the radius into a position parallel with the ulna. The deep branch of the radial nerve and posterior interosseous vessels pass between the deep and superficial parts of the muscle. The nerve supplies the supinator before it enters it.

Abductor Pollicis Longus. The long abductor of the thumb arises from the posterior surfaces of the ulna and radius and from the intervening interosseous membrane (see Fig. 16-2). Its tendon inserts on the radial (anteriorly directed) surface of the base of the first metacarpal. To reach this point, after the muscle has emerged from under cover of the extensor digitorum, it spirals distally around the radius (see Figs. 16-2 and 16-28), crossing over the radial extensors of the carpus. Its tendon (often double or triple) and that of the closely associated extensor pollicis brevis usually share the same tendon sheath deep to the extensor retinaculum (see Fig. 16-31). When the thumb is abducted, the prominent tendon of the muscle forms the lateral boundary of the anatomic snuff box (see Fig. 16-33).

The muscle abducts, extends, and laterally rotates the first metacarpal to draw the thumb away from the position of opposition. It can also contribute to abduction of the wrist.

Extensor Pollicis Brevis. The short extensor of the thumb accompanies the abductor pollicis longus (see Fig. 16-27). It arises from the posterior surface of the radius and from the adjacent interosseous membrane below the origin of the long abductor (see Fig. 16-2). Its tendon inserts on the base of the proximal phalanx of the thumb, often sending a slip to the long extensor tendon as well. It is an extensor of the proximal phalanx of the thumb.

Extensor Pollicis Longus. The long extensor of the thumb arises from the posterior surface of the ulna and the adjacent interosseous membrane (see Fig. 16-2); its tendon inserts on the distal phalanx of the thumb (see Fig. 16-28). The muscle runs obliquely from the ulna toward the thumb and, shortly after it emerges from beneath the extensor digitorum, it is replaced above the wrist by its tendon. The tendon skirts around the dorsal tubercle of the radius, which functions as a pulley. The tendon crosses the tendons of the radial extensors of the carpus, along with the other thumb muscles (see Fig. 16-31). Beneath the extensor retinaculum, its tendon sheath typically communicates with that of the carpal extensors. The muscle extends the distal phalanx of the thumb and all the other joints that its tendon crosses. Because of its obliquity, it can contribute to adduction of the thumb.

At the base of the thumb, the tendon of the extensor pollicis longus forms the ulnar border of the anatomic snuff box (see Fig. 16-33). Along the dorsal aspect of the first metacarpal and proximal phalanx, the tendon frequently receives a slip from the extensor pollicis brevis and abductor pollicis brevis, and also from the adductor pollicis. When inflammatory joint disease (e.g., rheumatoid arthritis) involves the tendon sheaths, the extensor pollicis longus tendon is susceptible to rupture.

Extensor Indicis. The extensor of the index finger is the most inferior muscle to arise from the posterior surface of the ulna (see Figs. 16-2 and 16-28). It crosses the wrist in the tendon sheath of the extensor digitorum. On the back of the hand, its tendon joins the tendon of the extensor digitorum that passes to the index finger. The two tendons blend into the dorsal digital expansion (see Fig. 16-58), through which they extend all the joints of the index finger.

Nerves and Vessels

The radial nerve itself does not enter the posterior compartment of the forearm, although it supplies the brachioradialis and the extensor carpi radialis longus as it descends in front of the elbow (see Fig. 16-16). It is the **deep branch of the radial nerve** that enters the posterior compartment of the forearm to supply the remaining superficial and deep muscles. The **posterior interosseous vessels** accompany the deep branch of the radial nerve and its continuation to the wrist, the posterior interosseous nerve (Fig. 16-29). The arterial supply to the posterior aspect of the forearm is provided by the posterior interosseous artery. A terminal branch of the anterior interosseous artery also enters the posterior compartment (see Fig. 16-25). Both vessels are accompanied by corresponding veins.

Deep Branch of the Radial Nerve. Originating at the bifurcation of the radial nerve in the lateral part of the cubital fossa, the deep branch of the radial nerve enters the upper border of the supinator muscle on the anterior aspect of the forearm. After curving through the muscle between its superficial and deep laminae, the nerve emerges from its inferior border in the posterior compartment of the forearm (see Fig. 16-29). Its terminal branch, the **posterior interosseous nerve**, reaches the wrist and ends by supplying the wrist and the intercarpal joints. Most of its branches, however, are muscular; none are distributed to skin.

Branches. Before entering the supinator, the nerve gives a branch to the extensor carpi radialis brevis. It supplies several branches to the supinator as it passes through it. After emerging from that muscle, it breaks up into a number of branches to supply most of the remaining muscles (see Fig. 16-29). The descending long branch, the posterior interosseous nerve, passes superficial to the long abductor and short extensor of the thumb, but dips beneath the extensor pollicis longus and extensor indicis muscles to reach the wrist joint. In its course, it supplies some of the deep muscles as well.

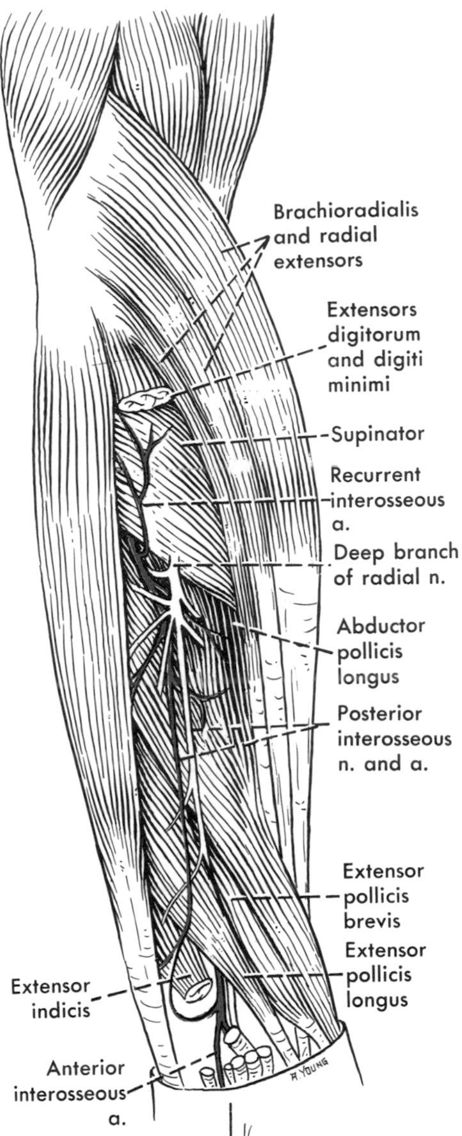

FIGURE *16-29.*
Anatomic relations in the posterior compartment of the forearm: the deep branch of the radial nerve and the posterior interosseous artery.

Lesions. Different patterns of paralysis result from lesions of the radial nerve and its deep branch. Damage to the radial nerve after it has pierced the lateral intermuscular septum of the arm may paralyze all the extensor muscles of the forearm, producing a *wristdrop* (inability to extend the hand against the force of gravity) as well as inability to extend the metacarpophalangeal joints of the digits. Lesions of the deep branch may have varying effects. When the lesion is complete, extension at the metacarpophalangeal joints of the digits is abolished, whereas the radial extensors can still extend the wrist. The deep branch may be damaged by fracture of the radius. Surgical repair of the nerve is difficult because of the numerous branches into which it breaks up at the lower border of the supinator muscle.

Posterior Interosseous Artery. A branch of the common interosseous artery (itself a branch of the ulnar artery), the posterior interosseous artery reaches the posterior aspect of the forearm by passing over the upper border of the interosseous membrane (see Fig. 16-25). It then runs downward on the membrane deep to the supinator muscle. On emerging at the lower border of the muscle, it gives off the **interosseous recurrent artery**, which passes upward, on or through the supinator, and deep to the anconeus, to anastomose behind the lateral epicondyle with the middle collateral branch of the profunda brachii (see Figs. 16-25 and 16-29). Other branches are given off directly to the extensor muscles, and the remaining part of the artery descends across the thumb muscles, where it terminates by anastomosing with the posterior branch of the anterior interosseous artery. This anastomosis contributes to the dorsal *carpal rete.*

THE WRIST

The wrist is the region that transmits from the forearm to the hand the tendons of the extrinsic muscles, as well as the major nerves and vessels of the hand. These soft tissues are grouped around the distal ends of the radius and ulna, the radiocarpal joint, and the carpal bones, the latter forming the proximal subsegment of the skeleton of the hand (see Chap. 14). Anatomic relations around the wrist have clinical significance as landmarks for the physical examination and also because direct and indirect trauma commonly damage structures around the wrist. These relations are best examined in the context of the retinacula that retain the relative positions of the long tendons as they pass the wrist invested in their synovial sheaths.

Retinacula

The flexor and extensor retinacula represent reinforcements in the deep fascia that invests the upper limb. The flexor retinaculum is distal to the radiocarpal joint and is attached only to carpal bones. The extensor retinaculum, on the other hand, crosses the wrist joint and the distal radioulnar joint. Its bony attachments are to the radius and to the carpal bones on the ulnar edge of the hand.

The **flexor retinaculum** is the heavy thickening of the antebrachial fascia at the front of the wrist that converts the carpal sulcus into the carpal canal, known conventionally as the *carpal tunnel* (see Fig. 16-7). Located deep in the palm of the hand between the thenar and hypothenar eminences, it is less than 4 cm^2 in size and 2 to 3 mm thick. The retinaculum is attached on the radial side to the tubercles of the scaphoid and the trapezium, and on the ulnar side to the pisiform and the hook of the hamate (Fig. 16-30, and see Fig. 16-32). Superiorly, the retinaculum blends with the deep layer of the antebrachial fascia and inferiorly with the fascia that invests the thenar and hypothenar muscles, both of which take origin from the retinaculum. At a rough approximation, the superior limit of

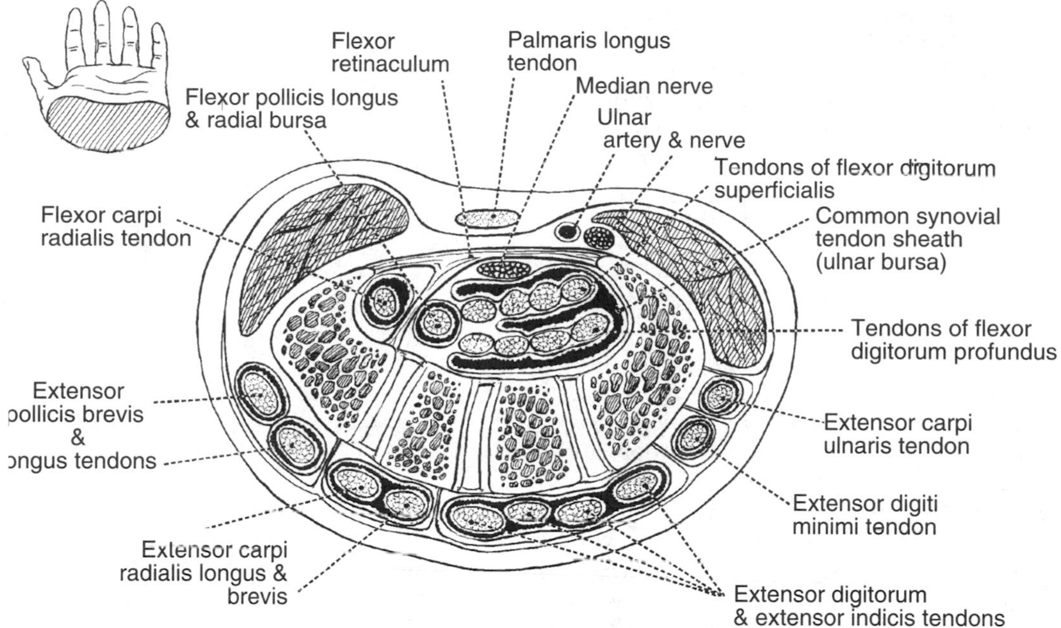

FIGURE *16-30.*
Transverse section of the wrist across the carpal canal: Synovial membrane is indicated as a ruffled white line. Synovial fluid within synovial sheaths is shown in *black*; for purposes of clarity, its quantity is exaggerated. The inset shows the level of the section.

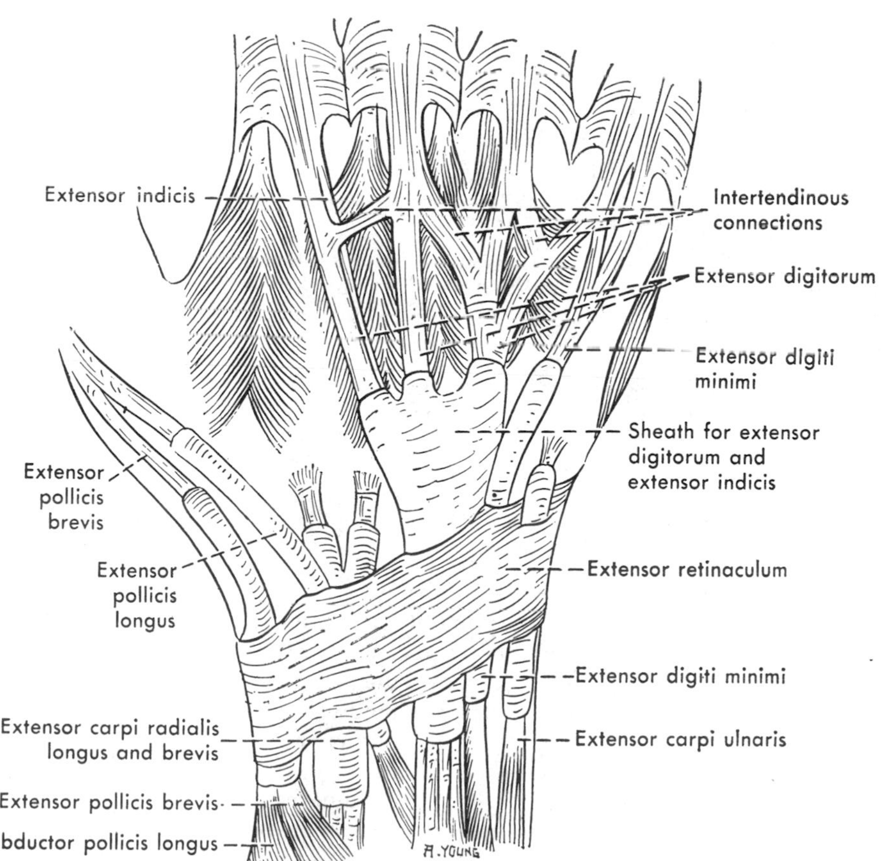

FIGURE *16-31.*
The extensor retinaculum, with the tendons and their synovial sheaths on the dorsum of the wrist.

the retinaculum is on level with the distal skin crease at the wrist, and its inferior limit with the distal margin of the abducted thumb. The tendons retained by the retinaculum in the carpal tunnel are those of the flexor digitorum superficialis and profundus and flexor pollicis longus (see Fig. 16-30). The flexor carpi radialis longus tendon occupies a separate compartment in the groove of the trapezium. The median nerve passes through the tunnel on the palmar surface of the flexor digitorum superficialis tendons, and is immediately deep to the retinaculum. The ulnar artery and nerve, by contrast, are superficial to the retinaculum (see Fig. 16-30).

The **extensor retinaculum** is a ribbonlike band, thinner, broader, and longer than its flexor counterpart (Fig. 16-31). Its attachments are such it does not restrict movements of the radius during pronation and supination, nor does it become slack. From its attachment to the anterior border of the radius above the styloid process, the retinaculum slopes downward to blend with the deep fascia and periosteum over the pisiform and triquetral bones. Fibrous septa bind it down to bony prominences on the dorsal aspect of the radius, preventing side-to-side displacement of the extensor tendons. These bony attachments convert the space beneath the retinaculum into compartments through which pass the tendons of the muscles from the posterior compartment of the forearm. The dorsal branches of the radial and ulnar nerves are superficial to the retinaculum.

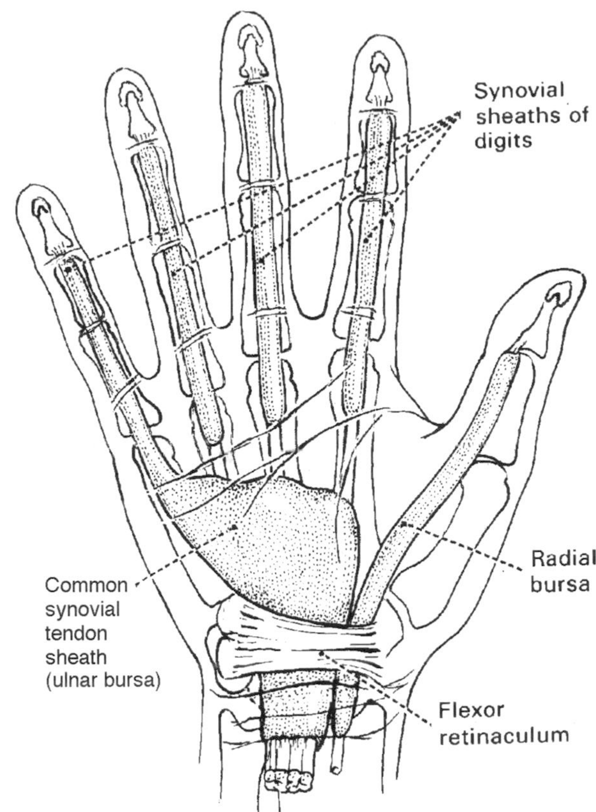

FIGURE *16-32.*
Synovial sheaths of the flexor tendons in the carpal canal and the hand: Note the proximal extent of the radial and ulnar bursae in relation to skin creases of the wrist, the upper limit of the retinaculum, and the joint line of the wrist joint. Note also the relation of the digital synovial sheaths to skin creases of the palm and to the joints.

Synovial Sheaths

All tendons that pass beneath the flexor and extensor retinacula are invested in bursae formed by synovial membrane (see Fig. 4-2). These so-called synovial sheaths contain sufficient synovial fluid to lubricate the adjacent surfaces of the membrane. Wrapped around the tendons, the bursae facilitate the movement of the tendons beneath the retinacula. The general arrangement of synovial sheaths in the wrist region is illustrated in Figure 16-30. The anatomic location of these sheaths has clinical importance.

> Inflammation caused by irritation or infection (tenosynovitis) will distend the sheaths. The pressure must be relieved surgically or the tendons will die owing to ischemia. Because of the slow turnover of collagen, tendon rupture may not occur for several weeks, but the median nerve will suffer damage in the carpal canal in a very short time.

All eight tendons of the flexor digitorum superficialis and profundus share a **common synovial tendon sheath** (often called the *ulnar bursa*) in the carpal canal, as do the four tendons of the extensor digitorum on the back of the wrist (see Figs. 16-30, through 16-32). The tendons of the flexor carpi radialis and flexor pollicis longus are enveloped by individual synovial sheaths. However, communications may exist between the sheaths underneath the retinacula. None of the synovial sheaths extends into the fingers on the dorsal aspect. In the palm, however, the common synovial tendon sheath extends into the little finger, and the independent sheath of the flexor pollicis longus (often called the *radial bursa*) covers the tendon to the terminal phalanx of the thumb (see Fig. 16-32). The flexor tendons in the remaining three digits are also invested in synovial sheaths. Only rarely does one of these sheaths retain continuity with the ulnar bursa. Such a possibility, however, has to be kept in mind in connection with penetrating wounds of any finger, not just the little finger and thumb. Both palmar and dorsal tendon sheaths end blindly proximal and distal to the retinacula, except as described on the palmar side for the thumb and little finger.

> Distension of the common flexor sheath may present as a tender swelling in the palm of the hand or proximal to the skin crease of the wrist. Painful irritation of the synovial sheath is common at the point where the tendons of the extensor pollicis brevis and abductor pollicis longus cross over those of the extensor carpi radialis longus and brevis (see Fig. 16-31).

Location of Tendons, Nerves and Arteries

Tendons

In locating the tendons around the wrist, on either the anterior or the posterior aspect, it is best to proceed from the styloid process of the radius to that of the ulna. On the anterior aspect, the tendons of the flexor carpi radialis, palmaris longus, and flexor carpi ulnaris are the important landmarks. On the dorsum, the boundaries of the anatomic snuff box are helpful in physical examination.

Placing the index finger on the subject's radial styloid process anteriorly, the examiner may palpate with the middle finger the stout tendon of the flexor carpi radialis while the subject flexes the wrist. In the center of the wrist, the slender tendon of the palmaris longus springs into prominence when the wrist is flexed with the fingers extended and the hand cupped, or when abduction of the thumb is opposed (see Fig. 16-43). The tendon of the flexor carpi radialis, attached to the pisiform, becomes prominent when abduction of the little finger is opposed (see Fig. 16-44). Anteriorly, the only tendons that do not pass through the carpal canal are those of the palmaris longus and the flexor carpi ulnaris.

The **anatomic snuff box** is a triangular fossa that appears on the dorsum of the wrist when the thumb is extended and abducted. The radial boundary of the fossa is formed by the tendons of the extensor pollicis brevis and abductor pollicis longus, and the ulnar boundary by the extensor pollicis longus tendon (Fig. 16-33). The latter leads proximally to the dorsal tubercle of the radius. On the radial side of the tubercle, the tendons of the long and short extensors of the carpus become palpable when the wrist is extended; on the ulnar side are the tendons of the extensor digitorum.

Nerves and Arteries

Pulsations of the **radial artery** can be felt against the radius between the radial styloid process and the tendon of the flexor carpi radialis. After it has turned dorsally, the artery is also palpable in the floor of the anatomic snuff

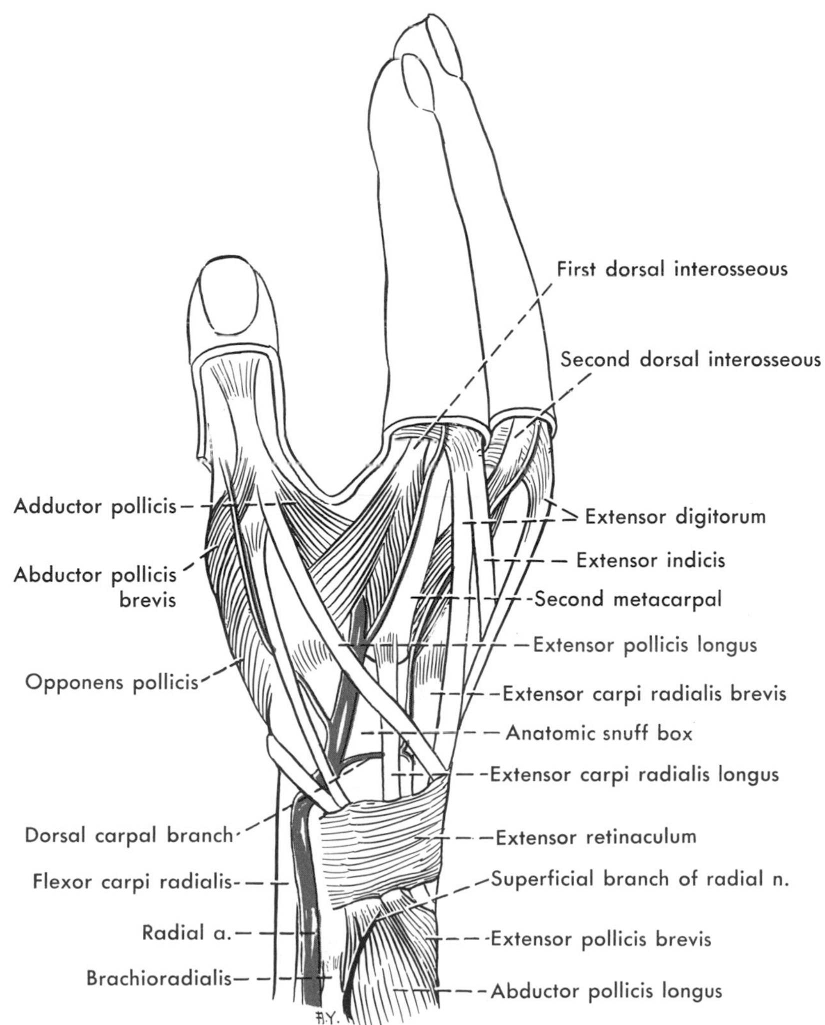

FIGURE *16-33.*
Anatomic relations on the radial side of the wrist.

box and between the bases of the first and second metacarpals. The **median nerve** lies immediately deep to the tendon of the palmaris longus, just before the nerve enters the carpal tunnel at the distal skin crease of the wrist. If the palmaris longus is absent, the nerve can be located on the medial side of the flexor carpi radialis. It is superficial to the tendon of the flexor pollicis longus. The palmar cutaneous branch of the radial artery enters the palm parallel to the median nerve, but remains superficial to the retinaculum. In lacerations, this small vessel may bleed profusely.

The **ulnar nerve** is located adjacent to the lateral side of the tendon of the flexor carpi ulnaris. Here it may be rolled against the head of the ulna. The **ulnar artery** is lateral to the nerve. Both structures remain superficial to the retinaculum.

THE HAND

Anatomically, the hand of *Homo sapiens* is a relatively primitive structure. It is less specialized than the foot, or indeed the hand of several other primates. Yet the attainments of our civilization in science, technology, and art must be largely attributed to the infinite variety of purposeful actions that the human hand is capable of performing. The versatility of the manipulative and prehensile functions of the hand is a reflection, not of functional adaptations within the hand itself but rather, of the complexity of humans' cerebral cortex. The movements comprise flexion, extension, abduction, and adduction of all the digits and, in addition, opposition of the thumb. While testing the individual movements of the digits is a requisite in clinical evaluation of the hand, the overall assessment of hand function must recognize the manner in which these movements are combined in using the hand for power grip and precision grip.

The hand is a sensory organ as well as a manipulative tool. In the manipulation of the environment, the hand relies on sensation for gathering information and for execution of tasks that require precision grip. Precision and power are integrated by the interplay of the extrinsic and intrinsic muscle groups as they operate the adaptable skeletal framework of the hand.

General Anatomic Plan

The **metacarpal bones**, the **phalanges**, and the joints connecting them form the anatomic foundation of the hand. Dorsal to this foundation, the only major structures are the extensor tendons and the dorsal digital expansions of the fingers; everything else is contained in the palm of the hand in clearly ordered layers (Fig. 16-34). Deepest are the **interosseous muscles**, associated with the metacarpal bones. Only potential fascial spaces (the midpalmar and

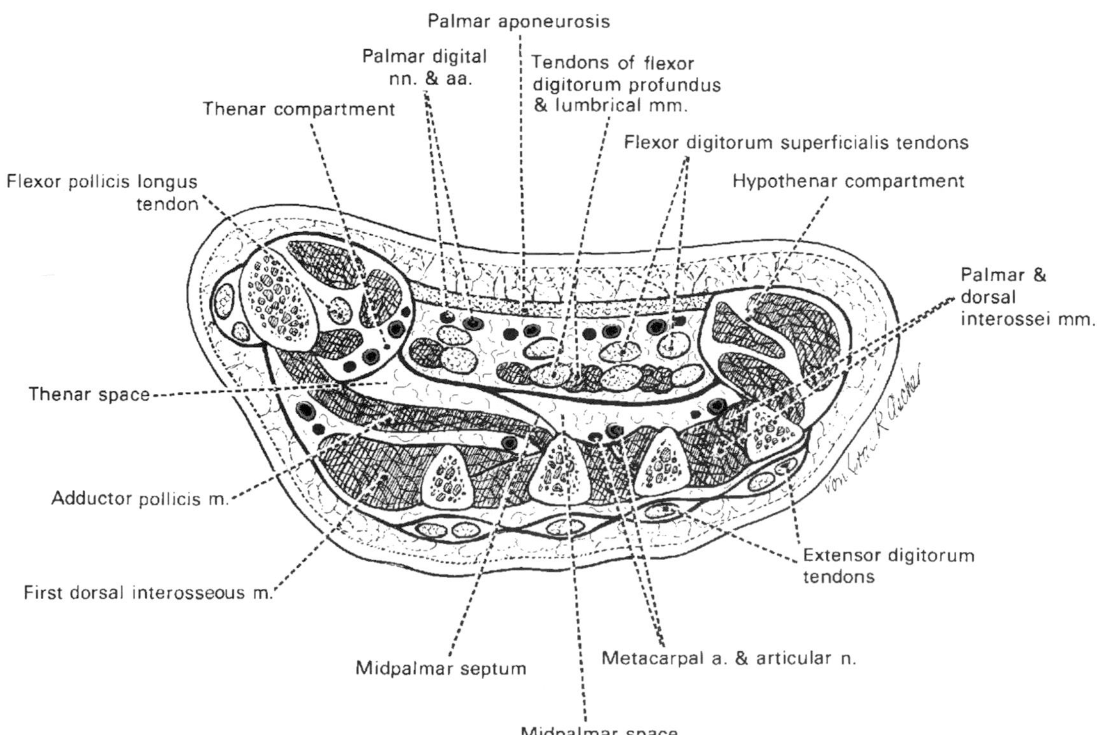

FIGURE *16-34.*
A section of the hand across the metacarpal bones to show the anatomic relation of various layers and the fascial spaces in the palm. The extent of the spaces is exaggerated.

thenar spaces) intervene between this layer and the next, which contains the **long flexor tendons** with the associated lumbrical muscles. Most superficial is the palmar aponeurosis. The vessels and nerves run in two planes. The **deep branch of the ulnar nerve** and the **deep palmar arch** (one of the two arterial arcades in the hand) lie between the interossei and the flexor tendons; branches of the **median nerve** and of the **superficial branch of the ulnar nerve,** as well as the **superficial palmar arch**, are between the flexor tendons and the palmar aponeurosis. Branches of each arterial arch (metacarpal arteries and palmar digital arteries, respectively) proceed toward the digits accompanied by branches of the ulnar and median nerves (see Fig. 16-34).

On each side of the palm are the muscles of the **thenar** and **hypothenar eminences** with the nerves and vessels of the thumb and little finger. The fingers contain the flexor tendons in their osseofascial tunnels (see Figs. 16-36 and 16-37) and the digital nerves and vessels.

The following sections present groups of structures in the approximate order in which they would be encountered during dissection of the hand. The superficial and deep fascia of the hand have been introduced in the General Orientation section, and mention has also been made of the cutaneous branches of arteries and nerves (see Chap. 14 and Fig. 16-9). All these structures receive further consideration in the sections dealing with the palm and the dorsum of the hand.

The Palm

Fascia

The **superficial fascia** over the palmar aspect of the hand forms lobulated pads of fat subdivided by fibrous septa. Cutaneous nerves, blood vessels, and superficial lymphatics run in the superficial fascia. Over the hypothenar eminence, the fascia also contains the **palmaris brevis muscle** (Fig. 16-35). Dense connective tissue septa in the superficial fascia tether the skin to the deep fascia. They are particularly well developed along permanent *flexion lines* or palmar creases and in the pulps of the fingers (see Fig. 16-55). The septa prevent sliding of the skin when an object is grasped.

The septa also localize edema, hematomas, or pus. As pressure builds up in the spaces between the septa, considerable pain is generated. The septa have to be divided by a horizontal cut when such abscesses are drained to open up discrete spaces in the superficial fascia.

The **deep fascia** shows a number of specializations (see Figs. 16-34 and 16-35). The **flexor retinaculum**, located in the hand, is described in the foregoing with the wrist. In the center of the palm, the deep fascia blends with the tendon of the palmaris longus, forming the **palmar aponeurosis**. On either side of the aponeurosis, the muscles of the thumb and little finger are covered by the much thinner **thenar** and **hypothenar fascias**, respectively. These fascias and their extensions are examined further in relation to the fascial spaces of the palm. In the digits, the deep fascia blends with the fibrous tissue of the superficial fascia and the fibrous digital sheaths.

Palmar Aponeurosis. The palmar aponeurosis, located in the central part of the palm, is a triangular, tendinous sheet formed by the fusion of the deep fascia with tendon fibers of the palmaris longus (see Fig. 16-35). The aponeurosis is present even if the palmaris longus itself is lacking. At its apex it is continuous with the palmaris longus tendon, and at its base it breaks up into a pair of slips for each finger. Some fibers of the slips insert into the fibrous sheaths of the flexor tendons; others pass dorsally around the sheaths to attach to the metacarpals and to the deep transverse metacarpal ligaments (Fig. 16-36), forming a gateway for the tendons as they enter their fibrous sheaths in the fingers. In the connective tissue between the slips, the palmar digital nerves and vessels emerge from beneath the aponeurosis and enter the fingers.

Most fibers of the aponeurosis run longitudinally. They are bound together by transverse fasciculi, which merge along the margins of the aponeurosis with the thenar and hypothenar fascias. The most distal transverse fibers form a continuous band, which becomes conspicu-

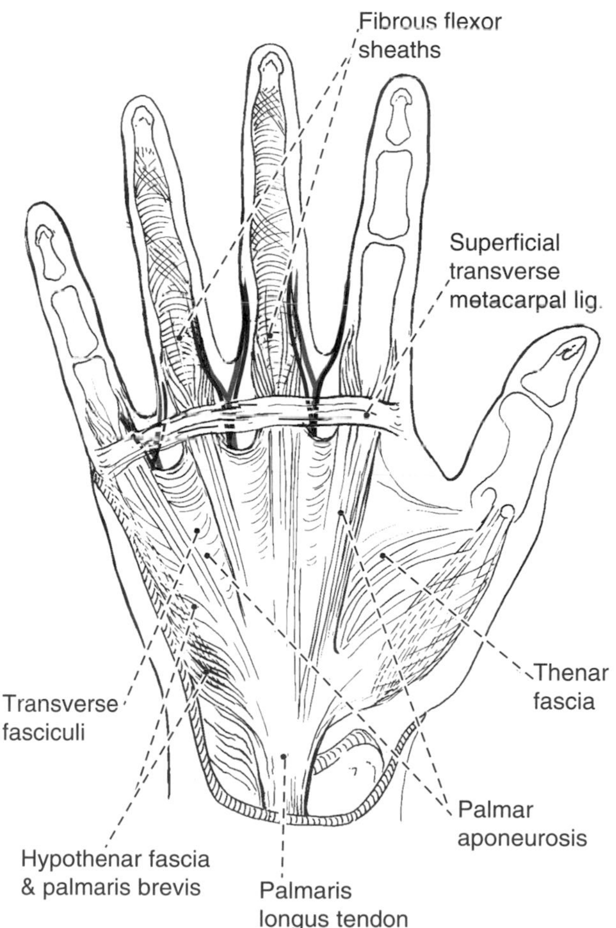

FIGURE *16-35.*
The palmar aponeurosis.

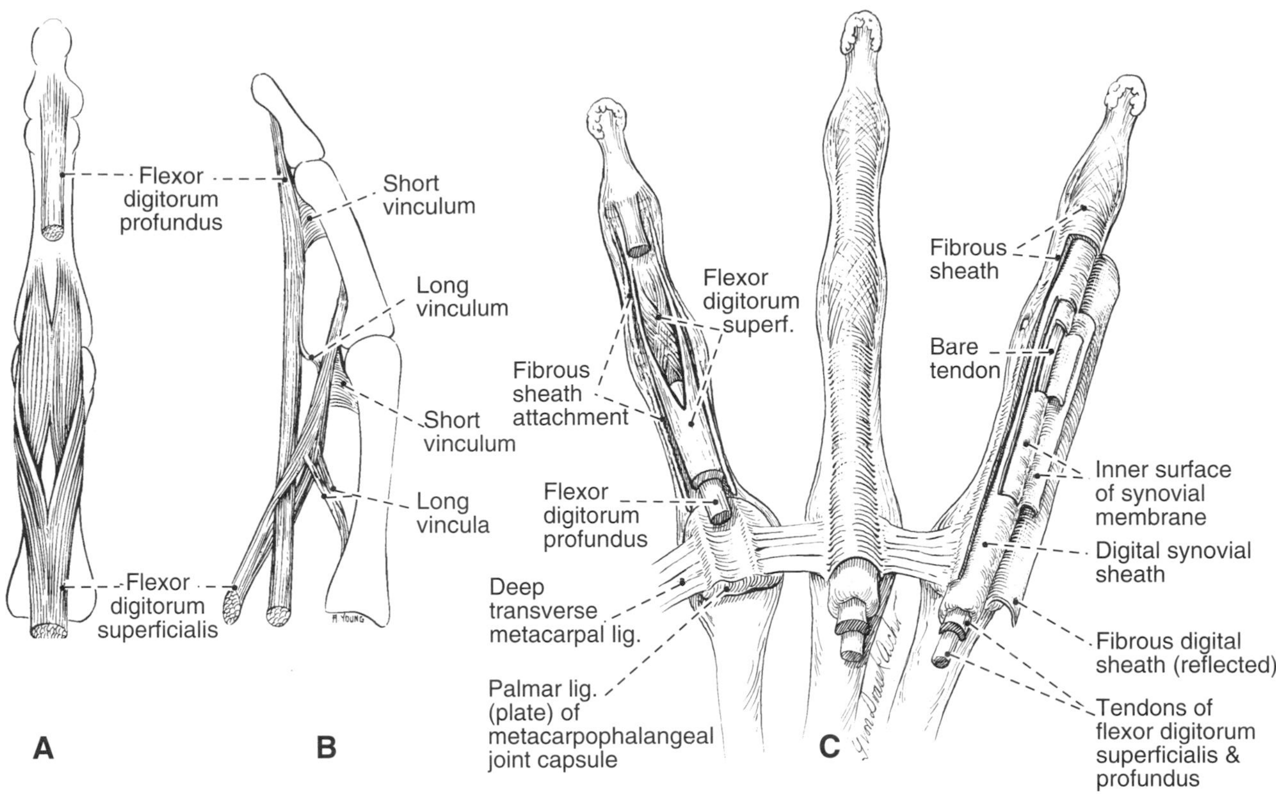

FIGURE *16-36.*
The arrangement of (A and B) the flexor tendons and (C) digital synovial sheaths and fibrous digital sheaths in the fingers.

ous across the finger webs once the skin is reflected. This structure is the **superficial transverse metacarpal ligament** (see Fig. 16-35). It differs from the deep ligament of the same name (see Fig. 16-36) in that it is uninterrupted and lies both more superficially and more distally, reaching almost to the free edge of the finger webs.

When a metacarpophalangeal joint dislocates, the metacarpal head may become caught in the space between the superficial and deep transverse metacarpal ligaments. Reduction will not be possible until the metacarpal head has been eased out of the clasp of the two ligaments.

The palmar aponeurosis may undergo fibrosis and contracture, producing dense fascial bands that look like tendons. Because of the attachment of the aponeurosis to the fibrous digital sheaths, the contracture leads to flexion deformity of the fingers. This condition is called **Dupuytren's contracture** and is common in middle-aged or older men. It usually affects the ring and little fingers but may affect any part of the palm. The joints and tendons are normal, but the fibrous digital sheaths may be affected by the same process. The etiology of the condition is unknown.

Flexor Tendons and Digital Sheaths

After the tendons of the flexor digitorum superficialis and profundus emerge from the carpal canal, they proceed in pairs toward the metacarpophalangeal joints. Here, each pair of tendons (one from the superficial flexor and one from the deep) enters another osseofibrous tunnel formed by a fibrous digital sheath. Between these two tunnels in the palm of the hand, the tendons are covered by the palmar aponeurosis. Within each fibrous digital sheath, the tendon of the flexor digitorum superficialis inserts into the middle phalanx and that of the profundus into the distal phalanx (see Fig. 16-36).

Flexor Tendons. The synovial sheaths covering the tendons of the flexor digitorum superficialis and profundus and flexor pollicis longus in the hand are described in the section on the wrist (see Fig. 16-32). In the palm of the hand, the lumbrical muscles arise from the bare regions of the flexor digitorum profundus tendons.

As the tendons reach the thickened anterior capsule of the metacarpophalangeal joints (the so-called *palmar plates*), they enter *the fibrous digital sheaths* (see Fig. 16-36). The tendons of the flexor digitorum superficialis are superficial (anterior) to those of the profundus. Over the proximal phalanges they becomes deeply grooved and each then splits into two parts to allow the profundus to pass through. The two parts of the superficialis tendon spiral posteriorly on each side of the profundus tendon and come together dorsal to it. After crossing the proximal interphalangeal joint, the two halves of the superficialis tendon interchange a few fibers and insert on the

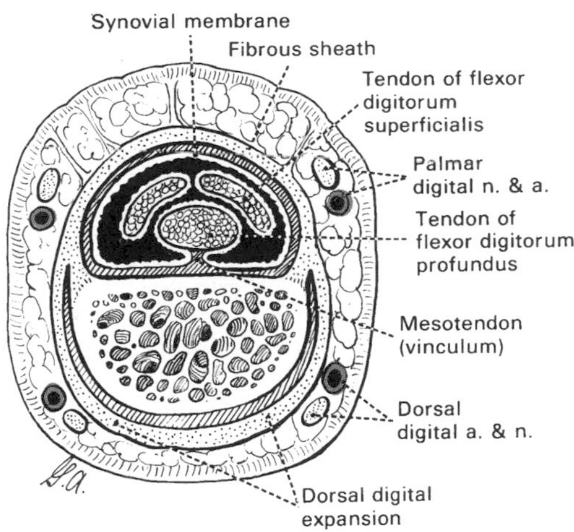

FIGURE *16-37.*
A transverse section across the proximal phalanx of a finger to show the arrangement of flexor tendons and their synovial sheaths within the fibrous flexor sheaths.

middle phalanx. The tendon of the profundus continues across the distal interphalangeal joint to its insertion on the distal phalanx. In the thumb, only one tendon occupies the osseofibrous tunnel, that of the flexor pollicis longus.

Before they reach their sites of insertion, the tendons of both digital flexors give off a few delicate tendon fibers that attach directly to the phalanx. These slender bands function as *mesotendons* and are called vincula (*vinculum;* Latin, meaning *band*). There is a **short vinculum** and a **long vinculum** for each tendon. The vincula provide routes for blood vessels to reach the tendons from the periosteum.

Testing of the Flexor Tendons. It is evident from the attachment of the tendons that the distal phalanx can only be flexed by the flexor digitorum profundus. The integrity of the muscle and tendon can be tested by holding all the joints of a given finger in extension, releasing the distal interphalangeal joint, and then asking the subject to flex the tip of the finger.

Both the superficial and the deep flexor tendons produce flexion at the proximal interphalangeal and metacarpophalangeal joints. The flexor digitorum superficialis can, however, be tested in the middle, ring, and little fingers independently of the profundus by the following maneuver. Holding all fingers in extension at all joints immobilizes the flexor digitorum profundus. If the finger to be tested is freed, and the subject is asked to flex it, flexion will occur at the proximal interphalangeal and metacarpophalangeal joints owing to contraction of the flexor digitorum superficialis. Under these conditions, the profundus cannot flex the finger at either the distal or the proximal interphalangeal joint because its individual tendons cannot be operated separately by its muscle belly. This is demonstrated in the normal hand by the inability to flex the distal interphalangeal joint of a finger when the other fingers are immobilized in extension.

Testing the profundus tendon in the index and middle finger demonstrates the integrity of the anterior interosseous branch of the median nerve (C-8 and T-1); testing the tendon in the little and ring fingers provides the same information for the ulnar nerve (C-8 and T-1) in the forearm. The flexor digitorum superficialis is innervated by the median nerve in the forearm (C-7 and C-8). The flexor pollicis longus (anterior interosseous nerve, C-8 and T-1) inserts into the distal phalanx of the thumb and is tested in the same way as the flexor digitorum profundus. When a finger remains in extension in the resting hand, it is an indication that a flexor tendon of that finger is interrupted.

Digital Sheaths. Dense fibrous tissue covers the flexor tendons from the metacarpal heads to the bases of the distal phalanges and forms the **fibrous digital sheaths** (*vaginae tendinum digitorum manus*). In each digit, the sheet of fibrous tissue attaches along either side of the row of phalanges and also to the palmar plates of the metacarpophalangeal and interphalangeal joints. It thus creates a roof over the pair of tendons (see Fig. 16-36). Transverse (annular) fibers located over the phalanges act as retinacula (often called "pulleys") for the moving tendons, and thinner, cruciate fibers over the joints ensure that the sheaths do not interfere with flexion. The synovial membranes that line the fibrous sheaths form the **digital synovial sheaths** (*vaginae synoviales digitorum manus*); (see Figs. 16-32 and 16-36). Each synovial sheath reflects from the inner aspect of its fibrous sheath onto the phalanx and then onto the tendons (Fig. 16-37), allowing the vincula to reach the tendons. Filled with synovial fluid, the synovial sheaths protrude at the proximal ends of the fibrous sheaths, which open into fascial spaces of the palm (see later discussion).

> **Trigger Finger.** Swelling or nodule formation in one of the flexor tendons or its synovial sheath, or a narrowing of the fibrous digital sheath, may produce a *trigger finger* (Fig. 16-38). During flexion, the swelling may be pulled out of the osseofascial tunnel of the finger into the palm of the hand. Its reentry into the tunnel during extension will be retarded, but when the resistance is overcome by extension force, the finger will snap into extension (sometimes audibly). This is painful and commonly occurs in traumatic or degenerative conditions.

Intrinsic Muscles of the Hand

The intrinsic muscles of the hand may be divided into four groups: 1) the lumbrical muscles; 2) the muscles of the thumb (thenar muscles); 3) the muscles of the little finger (hypothenar muscles); and 4) the interosseous muscles. The lumbricals are associated with the tendons of the flexor digitorum profundus; the thenar and hypothenar muscles produce fleshy eminences on the radial and ulnar side of the palm, respectively; the interosseous muscles are the deepest structures in the palm, filling the spaces between the metacarpal bones. Although hand function, in terms of movements, is described in a later section, the

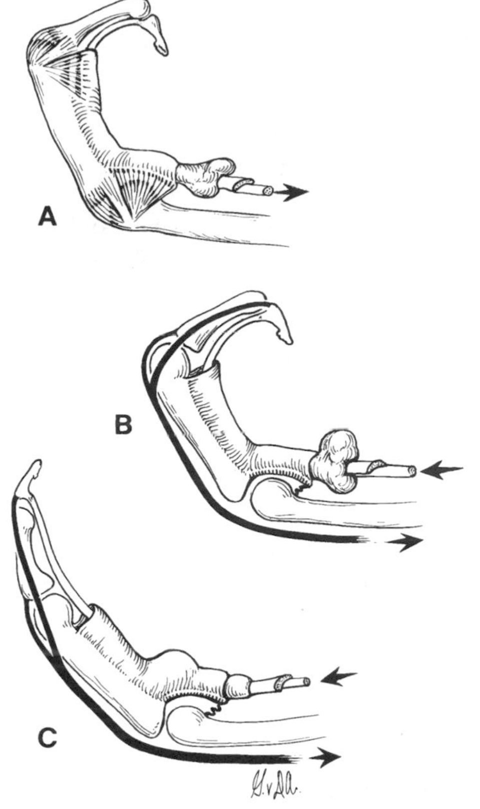

FIGURE *16-38.*
Trigger finger: (A) flexion displaces a swelling in the synovial sheath of the flexor tendon from the digital fibrous sheath into the palm; (B) extension is limited by the resistance the swelling encounters in reentering the narrow osseofibrous tunnel. (C) when this resistance is overcome by extensor force, the finger snaps into extension.

movements of the digits need to be defined to comprehend the action of intrinsic hand muscles. This is particularly true for the thumb.

Movements of the Digits. It is intuitively obvious that *flexion* of the fingers closes the hand and their *extension* opens it. *Abduction* of the fingers spreads them apart, that is, moves them away from the axis of the hand, the axis being represented by the third metacarpal and the anatomic position of the middle finger; *adduction* returns the fingers toward this axis. The palmar and dorsal surfaces of the **thumb** are oriented at right angles to the corresponding surfaces of the fingers (Fig. 16-39). Therefore, *flexion of the thumb* bends it across the palm toward the ulnar side; *extension* reverses this movement and carries the thumb away from the index finger in the plane of the palm. *Abduction* moves the thumb away from the index in a plane perpendicular to that of the palm; *adduction* returns it to the neutral position. The movement of *opposition,* characteristic of the human thumb, is a combination of flexion, medial rotation, and adduction that brings the palmar surface of the thumb in contact with the palmar surfaces of the fingers. The reverse movement, carrying the thumb away from opposition, is known as *reposition.* The joints that allow these movements are considered in a subsequent section.

Lumbricals. The lumbricals are four slender muscles that arise from the tendons of the flexor digitorum profundus in the palm of the hand (see Fig. 16-34; see also Figs. 16-47 and 16-52). Their tendons pass along the palmar surface of the deep transverse metacarpal ligaments, on the radial sides of the fingers, and join the dorsal digital expansion (see Figs. 16-58 and 16-59). Thus, they can flex the metacarpophalangeal joints indirectly, but they are more important in extension of the interphalangeal joints. Because they link flexor and extensor tendons, their action is complex.

The lumbricals of the index and middle fingers arise from the radial side of their respective tendons, whereas those of the ring and little fingers attach to two neighboring tendons of the profundus. They extend the interphalangeal joints through their insertion into the dorsal digital expansion (see Fig. 16-58). Because of the

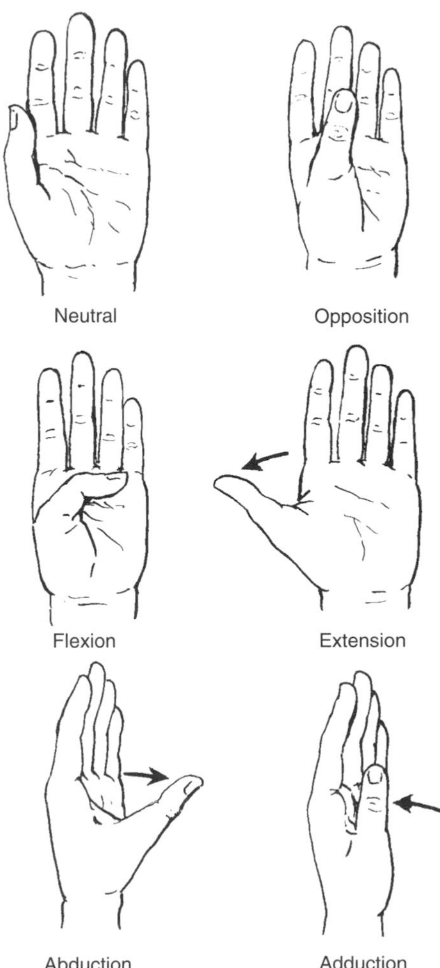

FIGURE *16-39.*
Movements of the thumb.

manner in which they pass the proximal interphalangeal joint, they prevent its hyperextension by the extensor digitorum. As a rule, the radial two lumbricals are innervated by the median nerve and the other two by the deep branch of the ulnar nerve.

Thenar Muscles. Movements of the thumb are controlled not only by extrinsic muscles (two extensors, a flexor, and an abductor), but also by four short intrinsic muscles in the hand. In the thenar eminence the **abductor pollicis brevis** and **flexor pollicis brevis** are superficial (Fig. 16-40A); deep to them is the **opponens pollicis** (see Fig. 16-40B). A fourth muscle, the **adductor pollicis**, is the largest. Because it is more deeply placed than the others, it does not contribute to the eminence but is nonetheless considered a thenar muscle. The principal actions of these muscles are implied by their names. However, they can and do contribute actively to other thumb movements. In terms of innervation, the usual rule is that a branch of the median nerve supplies those thumb muscles that form the thenar eminence, whereas the deep branch of the ulnar nerve supplies the adductor and the deep head of the flexor brevis (which adjoins the adductor).

Abductor Pollicis Brevis. The short abductor is located on the radial border of the thenar eminence. Most of its fibers originate from the flexor retinaculum and the trapezium (see Fig. 16-40A), but some of the superficial ones arise from the palmar aponeurosis and the thenar fascia (see Fig. 16-43). Its short tendon inserts into the radial side of the base of the proximal phalanx of the thumb. It may send a superficial lamina around the radial border of the thumb to attach to the tendon of the extensor pollicis longus.

Flexor Pollicis Brevis. The short flexor is located medial to the abductor brevis (see Fig. 16-40A) and has two heads. The larger *superficial head* arises from the flexor retinaculum and the trapezium and the *deep head* from the floor of the carpal canal. Here the deep head is closely associated with the adductor pollicis and is considered by some as a component of that muscle. The two heads are

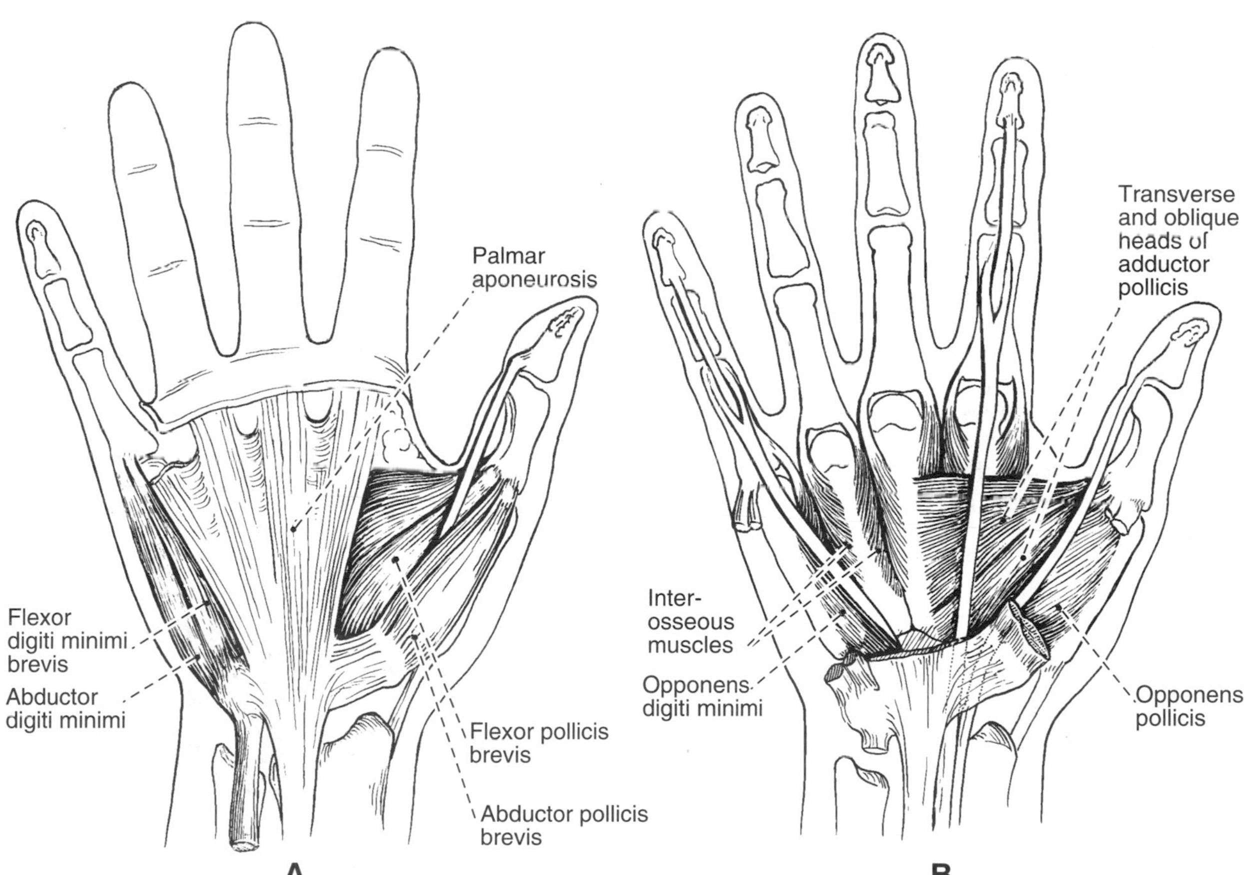

FIGURE *16-40.*
The thenar and hypothenar muscles: (A) The superficial fascia of the palm and the thenar and hypothenar fascias have been removed; (B) the dissection has been carried further by removing the palmar aponeurosis as well as the flexor tendons of the middle and ring fingers. In addition, the two superficial muscles in both thenar and hypothenar eminences have been resected.

separated by the tendon of the flexor pollicis longus. After they have joined, the muscle inserts on the radial side of the flexor surface of the base of the proximal phalanx. The tendon of insertion contains the radial sesamoid of the metacarpophalangeal joint (see Fig. 16-5).

Opponens Pollicis. Largely covered by the two muscles just described, the opponens pollicis arises, like them, from the flexor retinaculum and inserts along the radial side of the body of the first metacarpal (see Fig. 16-40B). It pulls and rotates the metacarpal in an ulnar direction across the palm, opposing the pulp of the thumb against the fingers.

Adductor Pollicis. The adductor of the thumb is a fan-shaped muscle that extends across the center of the palm deep to the flexor tendons (see Fig. 16-40B). Its proximal fibers constitute the *oblique head* and arise from the floor of the carpal canal and the bases of the first three metacarpals. The distal fibers originate along the palmar surface of the shaft of the third metacarpal and represent the *transverse head*. Both heads converge on the sesamoid bone on the ulnar side of the metacarpophalangeal joint and insert into the base of the proximal phalanx.

Thus, of the four thenar muscles, only the opponens inserts on the metacarpal shaft; the remaining three insert through sesamoid bones into the base of the proximal phalanx. However, directly or indirectly, all these muscles can move the carpometacarpal joint, the most important joint of the thumb (see under Joints).

Innervation. The innervation pattern of thenar muscles is important in the diagnosis of nerve injuries. As a rule, the adductor is supplied by the ulnar nerve and the other three by the median nerve; however, there are exceptions. Most constant is the innervation of the adductor by the deep branch of the ulnar nerve (97%), and the abductor pollicis brevis by the median nerve (95%). The deep head of the flexor brevis is usually supplied by the ulnar nerve and the superficial part by the median. The opponens is innervated in 80% of cases by both the median and the ulnar nerve, and only in the remaining 20% is it supplied entirely by the median nerve. Rarely, the opponens is supplied completely by the ulnar nerve. The segmental supply to thumb muscles (as to all intrinsic hand muscles), is overwhelmingly from T-1, with some input from C-8.

Hypothenar Muscles. The hypothenar eminence, like the thenar eminence, consists of three muscles. These are the **abductor digiti minimi**, **flexor digiti minimi brevis**, and **opponens digiti minimi**. Their arrangement and mode of insertion mirror those of the thenar muscles (see Fig. 16-40). Their actions are implied by their names. There is no named adductor for the fifth digit; its adduction is obtained by one of the interossei. The functionally inconsequential **palmaris brevis** forms a thin muscle sheet located in the superficial fascia over the hypothenar eminence (see Fig. 16-35). It has no counterpart on the thenar side but, similar to some of the superficial fibers of the abductor pollicis brevis on the thenar side, it helps tether the skin. The palmaris brevis is the only muscle supplied by the superficial division of the ulnar nerve; all the others are innervated by the deep branch of the ulnar nerve (C-8 and T-1).

The **abductor digiti minimi** arises from the pisiform bone, the adjacent tendon of the flexor carpi ulnaris, and also from the hypothenar fascia. It joins the flexor digiti minimi to insert into the medial side of the base of the proximal phalanx of the little finger (see Fig. 16-40A). It frequently sends a slip of insertion around the ulnar border of the finger to attach to the extensor tendon. The **flexor digiti minimi brevis** arises from the flexor retinaculum and the hamulus of the hamate bone. It fuses with the abductor and inserts with it. It flexes the metacarpophalangeal joint. The **opponens digiti minimi** is largely covered by the abductor and the flexor. It arises from the flexor retinaculum and from the hook of the hamate. Similar to the opponens of the thumb, it inserts on the palmar surface of the body of the fifth metacarpal, and its action is restricted to the carpometacarpal joint of the little finger. It rotates the fifth metacarpal, thereby enhancing the cupping of the hand and increasing the power of grip. The *deep branches of the ulnar nerve* and *artery* enter the hypothenar muscles between the abductor digiti minimi and the flexor; they supply both muscles, as well as the deeper-lying opponens.

Interosseous Muscles. The interosseous muscles are so named because they fill the spaces between the metacarpal bones (see Fig. 16-34). They consist of two sets: the palmar and dorsal interossei. Both groups are located in the palm of the hand, where they form the deepest muscle layer (Fig. 16-41).

The dorsal interossei are larger, and are visible on the back of the hand as well as in the palm. Each dorsal interosseous originates by two heads from adjacent sides of

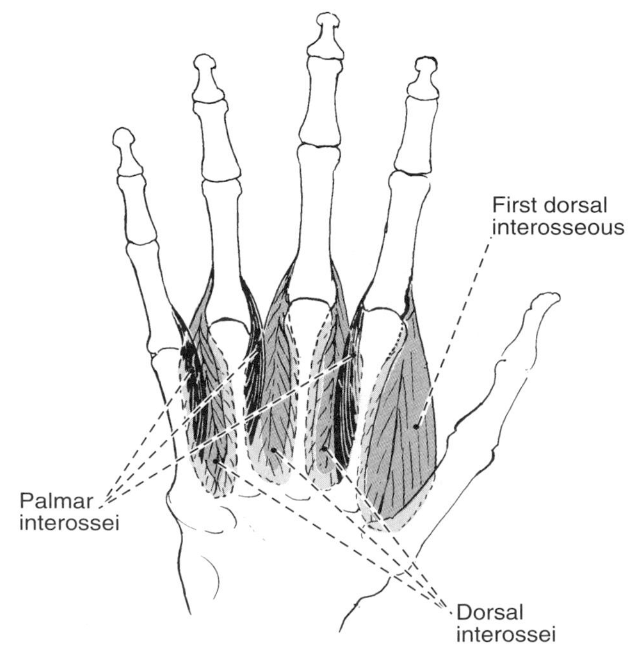

FIGURE *16-41.*
Palmar and dorsal interosseous muscles.

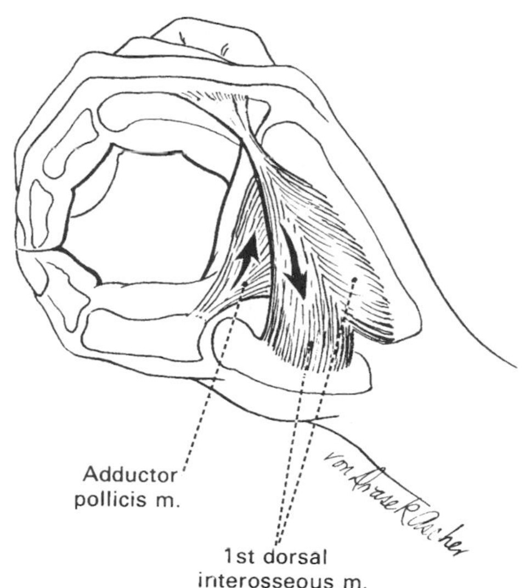

FIGURE *16-42.*
The first dorsal interosseous and adductor pollicis contracting (*arrows*) during precision grip.

two metacarpal bones and inserts into the proximal phalanx and dorsal digital expansion. The tendons leave the palm by passing dorsal to the deep transverse metacarpal ligaments, but their line of pull is such that they flex the metacarpophalangeal joints (see Figs. 16-58 and 16-59). There are four dorsal interossei. The first is the largest; it fills the space between the metacarpal bone of the thumb and that of index finger, and inserts into the radial side of the index finger (Fig. 16-42). The muscles of the next two spaces insert on either side of the middle finger; the one in the last space inserts into the ulnar side of the ring finger (see Fig. 16-41). This pattern of insertion can be reasoned from one of the actions exerted by the dorsal interossei at the metacarpophalangeal joint: they *abduct* or spread all fingers away from the imaginary axis of the hand represented by the middle finger. No dorsal interossei are associated with the thumb or the little finger as these possess their own abductors.

There are only three **palmar interossei** (see Fig. 16-41). Each originates from a single metacarpal bone anterior to the attachment of the dorsal interosseous. The tendon leaves the palm by passing dorsal to the deep transverse metacarpal ligament and inserts into the dorsal digital expansion (see Fig. 16-58 and 16-59). Acting together with the dorsal interossei, they flex the metacarpophalangeal joints. The palmar interossei *adduct* the fingers at the metacarpophalangeal joint, moving them toward the imaginary axis of the middle finger. The palmar interosseous of the index passes the metacarpophalangeal joint on its ulnar side and those of the ring and little finger on the radial side of the respective joint (see Fig. 16-41). The middle finger has none, as the dorsal interossei can deviate it from the axis in either direction. The arrangement of the two sets of interossei is such that one tendon joins the dorsal digital expansion on each side in each finger (see Fig. 16-41) except in the fifth, where there is no interosseous on the ulnar side.

Action. The interossei are responsible for three distinct types of finger movements: 1) flexion of the metacarpophalangeal joint; 2) abduction–adduction of the metacarpophalangeal joint; and 3) by virtue of their insertion into the dorsal digital expansion, extension of the proximal and distal interphalangeal joints.

Innervation. As a rule, all interossei are innervated by the deep branch of the ulnar nerve (C-8 and T-1). The first dorsal interosseous, however, is sometimes innervated (wholly or in part) by the median nerve. This muscle becomes hard and prominent when the index is abducted against resistance or when it is pinched hard against the thumb (see Fig. 16-42).

Variations. A certain amount of fusion may occur among either the thenar or the hypothenar muscles. This is particularly true of the adductor and short flexor of the thumb. The flexor digiti minimi brevis may be either absent or so fused with the abductor or the opponens that it is unrecognizable. Sometimes a vestigial palmar interosseous muscle is associated with the thumb, but it may be considered a component of the adductor pollicis.

Testing of the Intrinsic Muscles. Functional evaluation of the intrinsic hand muscles is useful clinically. Information is gained not only about the muscles but also about the nerves and spinal segments that supply them.

The **thenar muscles** are best evaluated with the hand resting palm up on a table. The subject is asked to touch with the thumb an object, such as a pen, held by the examiner in positions requiring, in turn, abduction, extension, and flexion. (These movements are illustrated in Fig. 16-39.) *Abduction* is produced by both the abductor pollicis longus and brevis. Verifying the contraction of the latter is important because, of all hand muscles, the **abductor pollicis brevis** is the most informative in the evaluation of the median nerve. Because its superficial fibers arise from the palmar aponeurosis and the thenar fascia, contraction of the muscle will pull on these structures; the palmaris longus contracts reflexly to hold the aponeurosis in position, and its tendon springs into prominence (Fig. 16-43). If the distal phalanx is kept extended, the **flexor pollicis brevis** flexes the carpometacarpal joint. The belly of the **adductor pollicis** can be palpated as it hardens during precision grip (see Fig. 16-42).

Opposition of the thumb to the index and little fingers should be tested. For assessing the power of this movement, the subject firmly opposes the thumb against the tip of the index finger, the two digits describing a circle (see Fig. 16-42). The examiner interlocks his index and thumb in a similar position with those of the subject and attempts to force them through between the subject's index and thumb. The test assesses the power of precision grip, and requires the integrity of a complex set of muscles, prominent among which is the first dorsal interosseous. Furthermore, nervous pathways for proprioception and muscle coordination must also be intact.

To test the **adductor pollicis**, the subject holds a card firmly between the side of the thumb and index

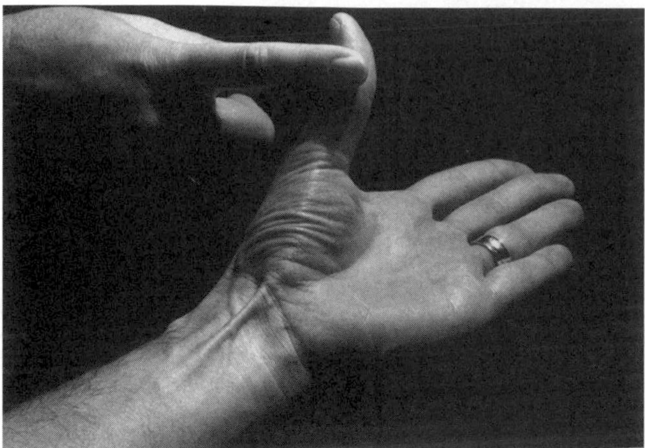

FIGURE *16-43.*
Contraction of the abductor pollicis brevis plicates the skin of the thenar eminence and reflexly invokes the contraction of the palmaris longus, throwing its tendon into prominence. The latter muscle contracts to stabilize the palmar aponeurosis from which the short abductor arises. The test, as demonstrated, verifies the integrity of the median nerve, both in the proximal forearm and at the wrist. Abduction of the thumb is opposed by the examiner.

finger. If the adductor is intact, the thumb is stabilized with its interphalangeal joint in extension as the subject resists the examiner's attempt to pull the card away. If the muscle is weak or paralyzed, the subject will flex the interphalangeal joint and try to retain the card by flexion power.

Of the hypothenar muscles, testing of the **abductor digiti minimi** is particularly useful because it provides information about the ulnar nerve in both the hand and the forearm. When the muscle contracts, the pisiform, from which the muscle arises, has to be stabilized on the triquetral bone. Therefore, as soon as abduction of the little finger is initiated, the tendon of the flexor carpi ulnaris reflexly springs into prominence in a manner analogous to that of the palmaris longus during testing of the abductor pollicis brevis (Fig. 16-44).

The adductor action of the **dorsal interossei** is best evaluated by the examiner attempting to pull a card away that is firmly held between the sides of two of the subject's extended fingers. The contraction of the first dorsal interosseous is readily verified during precision grip (see Fig. 16-42). **Palmar interossei** are tested by the subject spreading (abducting) the extended fingers and resisting the examiner's attempt to push them together. Normally, considerable resistance is encountered. Both maneuvers evaluate the deep branch of the ulnar nerve. As noted in the foregoing, however, the first dorsal interosseous is sometimes supplied by the median nerve.

Nerves

A brief summary of the overall pattern of innervation of the hand may be helpful as an introduction to the more detailed descriptions of individual nerves and their distribution patterns.

The **median nerve** is the chief nerve of sensation in the hand because it supplies the palmar surfaces of the digits most commonly employed for feeling and for precision grip. In addition, it is motor to the thenar eminence musculature. The **ulnar nerve** is the chief motor nerve of the intrinsic muscles of the hand, and it is sensory to only the ulnar one and a half fingers. The **radial nerve** supplies no muscles in the hand and its sensory distribution is confined to the dorsum. Division of either the median or ulnar nerves seriously impairs hand function, whereas interruption of the superficial branch of the radial nerve above the wrist is barely perceptible. In the diagnosis of nerve injuries, motor, sensory, and sympathetic components of the nerves must be taken into account. Innervation by the three nerves is also shared by the joints of the hand.

The motor distribution of the median nerve is essentially confined to the thenar muscles, all other muscles being supplied by the ulnar nerve. The ulnar nerve frequently encroaches on the motor territory of the median nerve, but the reverse hardly ever occurs. There is considerable overlap in the cutaneous distribution of the three nerves on both the palmar and the dorsal aspect of the hand, owing to communicating branches as well as to some variation in the true anatomic distribution pattern. Therefore, the typical sensory distribution of the three nerves, shown in Figure 16-45, contrasts with the skin areas, the supply of which is always derived from only one nerve (Fig. 16-46). Clearly, the latter areas are the most valuable in discriminatory testing.

Cutaneous sensitivity to light touch is tested with the back of the examiner's fingers; pinprick is used for pain perception. Two-point discrimination is tested by asking the subject whether he or she feels one or two points of a bent paper clip touching the skin, as the

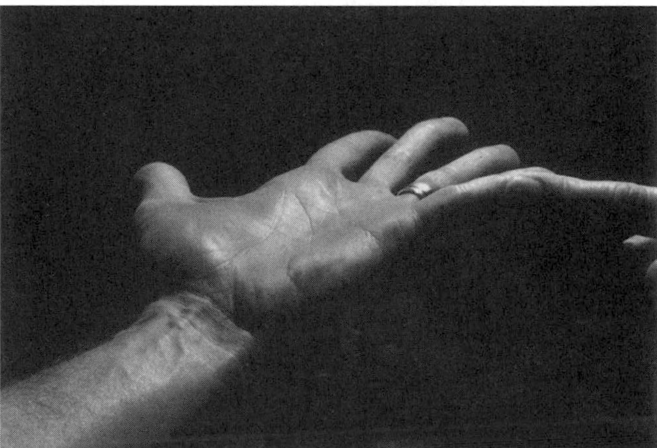

FIGURE *16-44.*
Abduction of the little finger is opposed. Contraction of the abductor digiti minimi plicates the skin of the hypothenar eminence and reflexly invokes the contraction of the flexor carpi ulnaris to stabilize the pisiform bone from which the abductor muscle originates. The test, as demonstrated, verifies the integrity of the ulnar nerve in the proximal forearm and at the wrist.

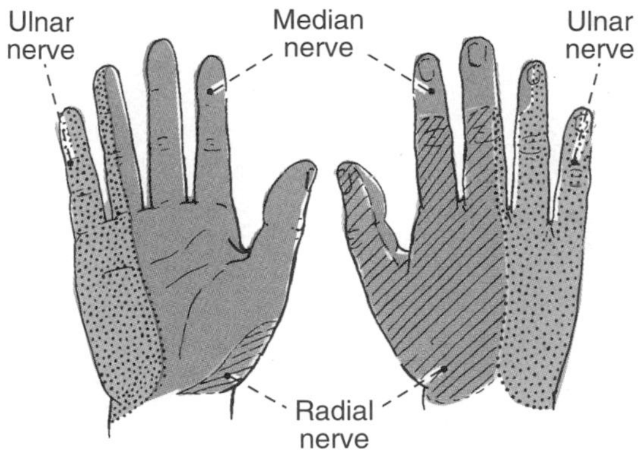

FIGURE *16-45.*
The typical sensory distribution of the median, ulnar, and radial nerves in the hand. The considerable overlap between these areas is not indicated.

examiner varies the distance between the points. Normally, points 2 to 6 mm apart can be resolved on the flexor surface, but the distance is much greater on the dorsum. It is important to remember that ischemia seriously impairs cutaneous sensitivity.

To test higher integrated sensory function, the subject should feel and identify such common objects as coins, keys, or a pen, keeping the eyes closed. In cases of cerebral damage, the patient may be unsuccessful, even though touch and pain sensation may be unimpaired. Integrated motor and sensory function is further assessed by asking the patient to pick up a pen and sign his or her name.

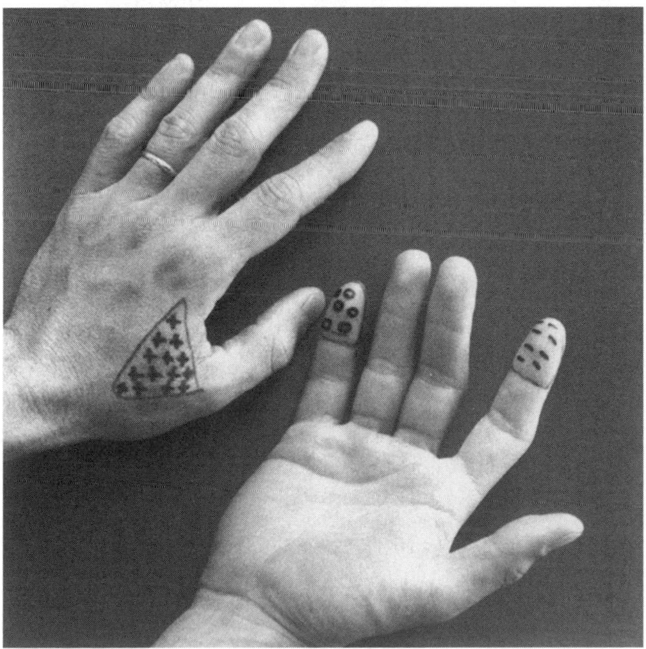

FIGURE *16-46.*
The clinically most reliable cutaneous areas for testing the radial (*purple*), ulnar (*blue*), and median nerves (*red*) in the hand. In these areas there is the least likelihood of overlapping innervation from the neighboring nerves. (Courtesy of Dr. Frederick A. Matsen III.)

Median Nerve. The median nerve enters the hand on the radial side of the palmaris longus tendon (or, if that muscle is lacking, on the radial side of the flexor digitorum superficialis tendons) by passing deep to the flexor retinaculum (Fig. 16-47). In the carpal canal, the nerve lies between the flexor retinaculum and the tendons of the flexor digitorum superficialis, the latter wrapped in the common synovial sheath. As soon as the nerve emerges at the distal border of the retinaculum it breaks up into branches. A *muscular branch* (sometimes called recurrent branch) goes to the thenar eminence; the remaining branches terminate in *palmar digital nerves* for the thumb, and the index, middle, and ring fingers. A *communicating branch* usually links the nerve to the ulnar nerve.

At their origin, the branches are embedded in loose connective tissue on the deep surface of the palmar aponeurosis. Those for the fingers continue in this layer and are accompanied by the common palmar digital arteries, branches of the superficial palmar arch (Fig. 16-48; see also Fig. 16-52). The muscular and digital branches to the thumb turn laterally and enter the fascial envelope which encloses the thenar eminence.

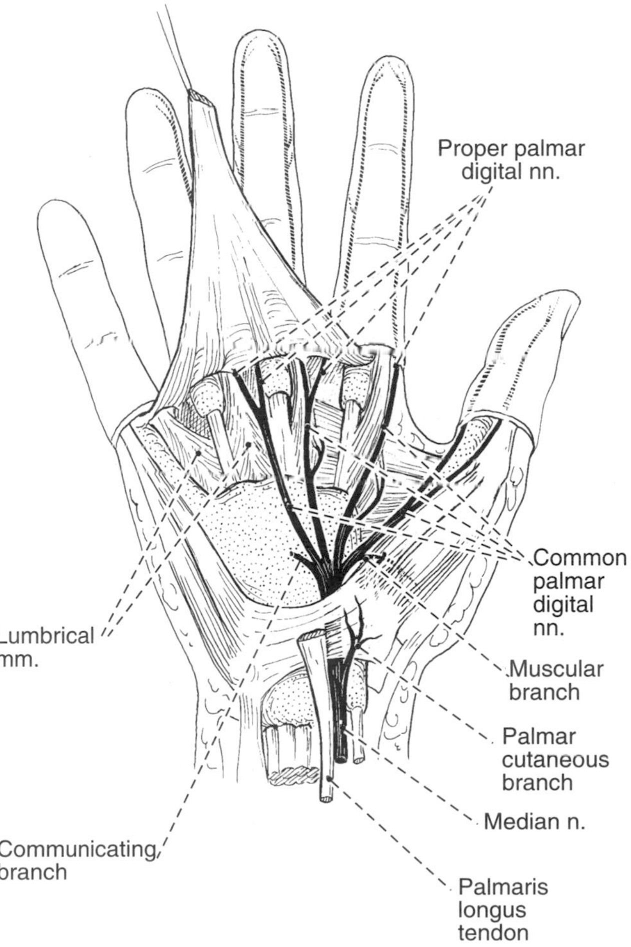

FIGURE *16-47.*
The median nerve in the hand: The palmar aponeurosis has been reflected.

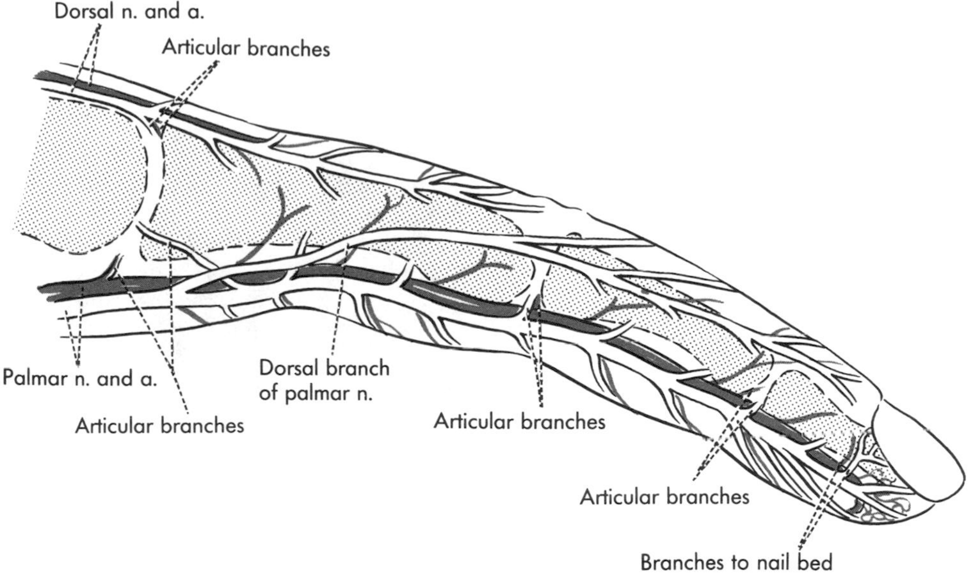

FIGURE *16-48.* **Digital nerves and vessels on one side of a finger.**

Branches. Before the median nerve enters the carpal canal, it sends a **palmar cutaneous branch** over the anterior surface of the retinaculum. The branch remains in the superficial fascia and is distributed to skin over the thenar eminence and the center of the palm (see Fig. 16-47).

The **muscular branch** turns anteriorly and curves around the flexor retinaculum. It is the first or most lateral branch of the median nerve in the palm. It crosses the surface of the flexor pollicis brevis before penetrating it (see Fig. 16-47). The superficial portion of that muscle, as well as the abductor pollicis brevis and opponens, are supplied by the nerve. The muscle most consistently supplied by the median nerve is the abductor pollicis brevis.

The common branching pattern of the **palmar digital nerves** is shown in Figures 16-47 and 16-52. Two *proper palmar digital nerves* pass to the thumb. They may originate by a common stem or independently, as does the next proper palmar digital nerve that proceeds to the radial side of the index. Two *common digital nerves* pass toward the finger webs between the index, middle, and ring fingers. In the webs each divides into two *proper palmar digital nerves,* one for each adjacent side of these digits.

The proper palmar digital nerves have a similar course and distribution in the thumb and all fingers. They proceed with the palmar digital arteries along the sides of the fibrous digital sheaths and terminate in the nailbed and pulp of the digits (see Figs. 16-48 and 16-52). Their branches are distributed to the skin on the palmar surface of the thumb, index, and middle fingers and on the radial half of the ring finger. A larger dorsal cutaneous branch of each nerve supplies the dorsal aspect of the distal and middle phalanges. In addition to their cutaneous afferents, the palmar digital nerves supply the digital arteries with sympathetic vasomotor fibers, and the sweat glands with sudomotor fibers.

While in the palm, the nerve to the radial side of the index finger gives a branch to the first lumbrical muscle. The common digital nerve to the index and middle fingers likewise gives a branch to the second lumbrical. The proper palmar digital nerves also supply the joints they pass.

The **communicating branch** between the median and ulnar nerves accounts for some of the anomalous muscular and cutaneous distributions of these nerves that have been reported in different surveys. Such exchange of fibers can occur in both the forearm and hand. A loop connecting the two nerves (Fig. 16-49) is present in more than 75% of hands.

Compression and Injuries. The median nerve is prone to compression in the carpal canal. The **carpal tunnel syndrome** provides an instructive demonstration of the distribution of the median nerve. Only by knowing its anatomy is it possible to distinguish this condition from other syndromes that cause paresthesias and muscle atrophy in the hand.

The condition is more common in women and often there is no identifiable cause. The syndrome may be precipitated by arthritis of the wrist or intercarpal joints (e.g., rheumatoid arthritis), dislocation of the lunate, distension or swelling of the synovial sheaths (tenosynovitis or rheumatoid arthritis), a tumor (ganglion), or by diseases in which there is generalized swelling (myxedema or toxemia of pregnancy) or overgrowth of bone (acromegaly). Initially, irritation of the nerve causes tingling in the sensory distribution area of the nerve, and twitching of the thenar muscles may be experienced. These symptoms can be reproduced by pressure over the flexor retinaculum. With nerve paralysis the thenar muscles atrophy and there is anesthesia in the sensory distribution area of the median nerve. Movements of the fingers are unaffected, and even those of the thumb are not

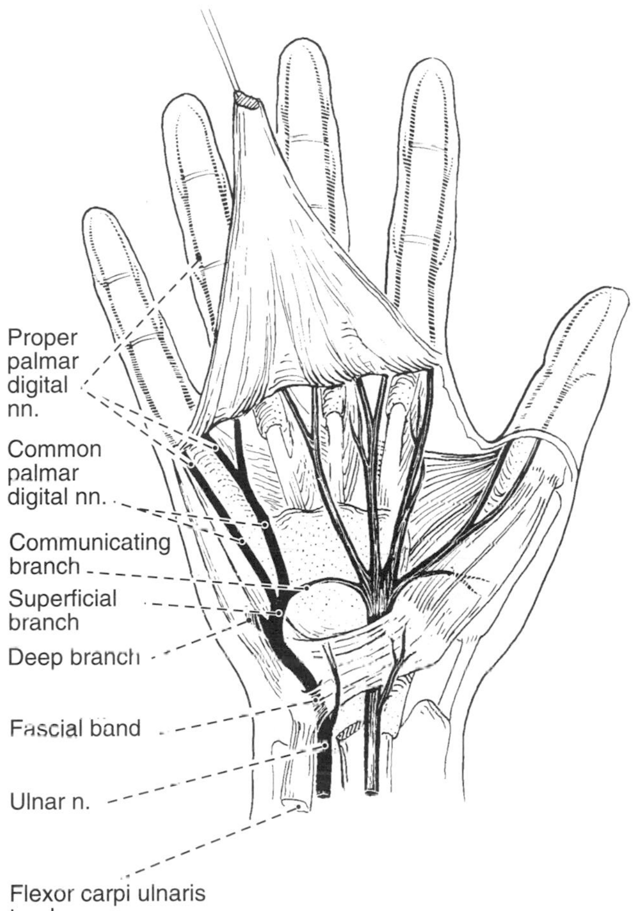

FIGURE 16-49.
The ulnar nerve (*solid black*) at the wrist and its superficial branches in the hand: The palmar aponeurosis has been reflected.

seriously impaired. Flexion is accomplished by the flexor pollicis longus (anterior interosseous nerve) and by the deep head of the flexor pollicis brevis (ulnar nerve). Although the action of the opponens pollicis is lost, opposition is obtained by the pull of the flexor muscles, and abduction is provided by the abductor pollicis longus (deep branch of radial nerve). Fine, coordinated movements of the hand may suffer because of the loss of proprioception.

Symptoms and signs of the compression syndrome are relieved by division of the flexor retinaculum at the wrist. In long-standing cases, nerve regeneration may not take place.

When the **median nerve is cut** at the wrist, the clinical picture is identical with that of complete compression in the carpal canal. In both conditions there will be, in addition, vasodilation and lack of sweating in the cutaneous distribution area. The best muscle to test in this case is the abductor pollicis brevis (see Fig. 16-43). Even though the thumb possesses another abductor, the test, if properly performed, provides unambiguous information about the status of the abductor pollicis brevis.

If the nerve is cut in the forearm above the level of innervation of the long flexor muscles, the resulting hand disability and deformity will be much more severe. In addition to the sensory and motor loss described for the carpal tunnel syndrome, flexion will be impossible in the thumb, index, and middle fingers except at the metacarpophalangeal joints. The latter can be flexed by the interossei. The ulnar half of the flexor digitorum profundus will be unimpaired and flexion of the ring and little fingers will not be seriously affected by paralysis of the flexor digitorum superficialis. The position of the hand has been likened to that assumed in the act of dispensing blessing; therefore, the deformity is known as the *benediction attitude.*

Ulnar Nerve. The ulnar nerve enters the hand on the lateral side of the pisiform bone with the ulnar artery. Although both structures are in front of the flexor retinaculum, they are partially covered by a fascial band (see Fig. 16-49). This tissue, sometimes identified as the *palmar carpal ligament* or the *superficial lamina of the flexor retinaculum,* is merely a reinforcement in the deep fascia that in-

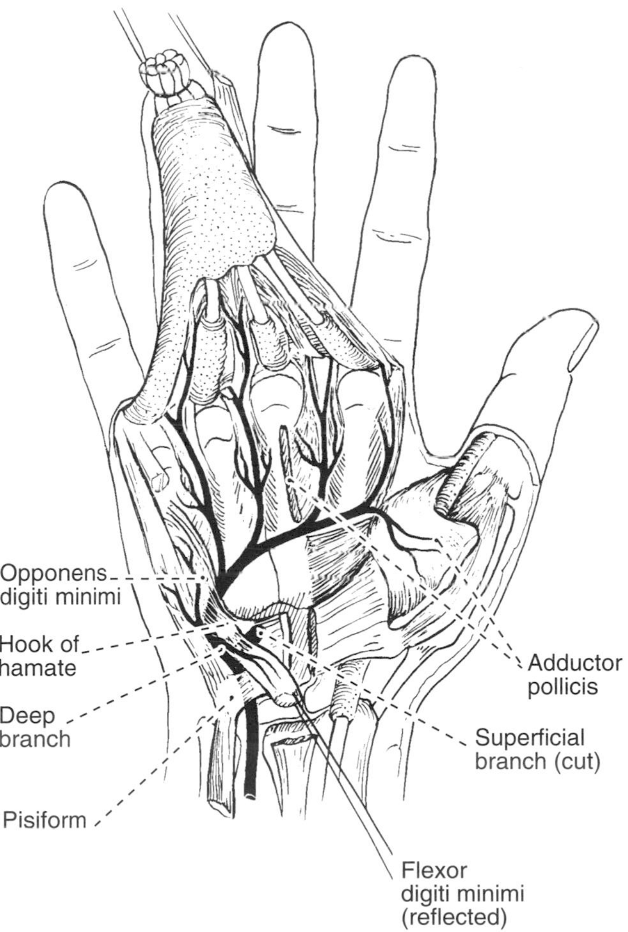

FIGURE 16-50.
The ulnar nerve at the wrist and its deep branch in the hand: After reflecting the palmar aponeurosis, the flexor retinaculum was divided and all flexor tendons were pulled distally. In addition, the muscle bellies of the flexor digiti minimi and abductor pollicis (transverse head) have been divided and elevated to reveal the nerve deep to them.

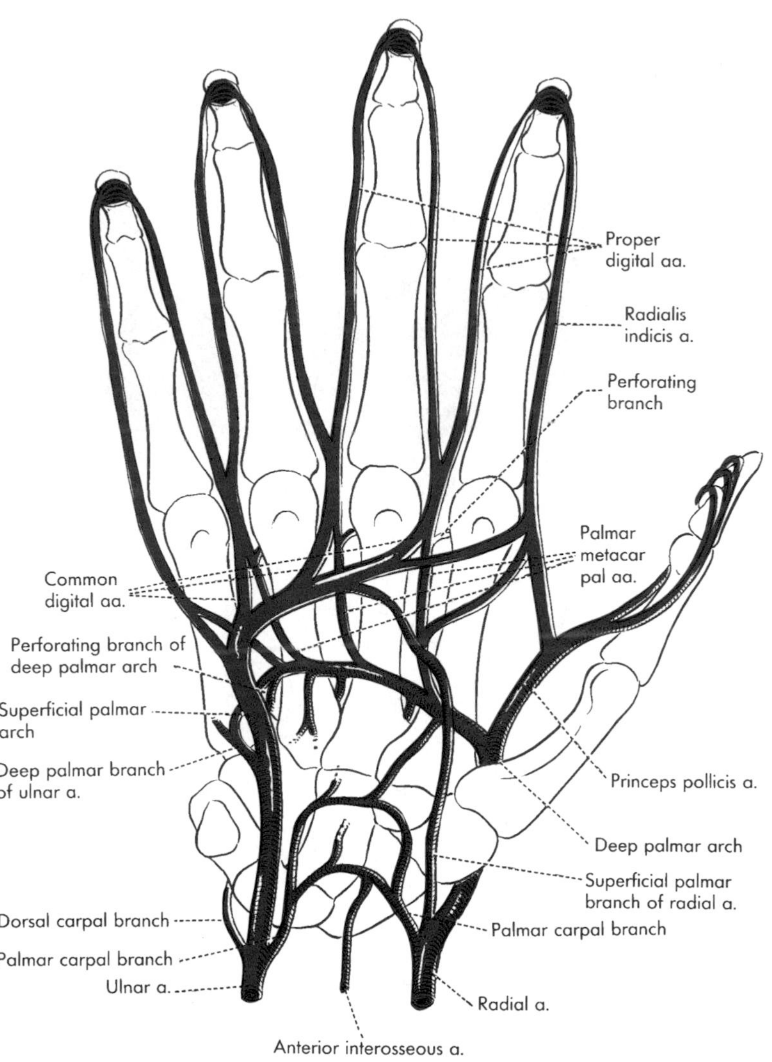

FIGURE *16-51.*
The arterial supply of the hand: superficial and deep palmar arches.

vests the forearm and hand. A triangular space deep to this ligament is bounded, in addition, by the pisiform and the flexor retinaculum proper. The space is known as the *canal of Guyon*. The nerve may suffer compression underneath the ligament.

At the level of the pisiform the ulnar nerve splits into a *superficial* and a *deep branch* (see Figs. 16-49 and 16-50). The superficial division contains motor fibers for the palmaris brevis, but is otherwise cutaneous. The deep branch supplies all the hypothenar muscles, all the interossei, the ulnar two lumbricals, and the adductor pollicis. In addition, it usually innervates the deep head of the flexor pollicis brevis and, more rarely, the opponens pollicis. It supplies no skin. A communicating branch links the superficial division to a corresponding branch of the median nerve.

Branches. Before the ulnar nerve enters the hand, it gives off a small **palmar cutaneous branch**, which passes over the flexor retinaculum and shares the supply of the skin in the palm with a similar branch of the median nerve (see Fig. 16-49).

The **superficial division** or branch (see Fig. 16-49) passes over the hypothenar eminence, where it divides into palmar digital nerves. A *proper palmar digital nerve* proceeds along the hypothenar muscles to the ulnar side of the little finger, and a *common palmar digital nerve* passes deep to the palmar aponeurosis to the web between the ring and little fingers. Here it divides into proper palmar digital nerves, one for each of the adjacent sides of these fingers. The course, distribution, and fiber composition of these nerves corresponds with those derived from the median nerve (see Fig. 16-48). All these branches run with common and proper palmar digital arteries, branches of the superficial palmar arch (see Fig. 16-52).

The **deep division** or branch of the ulnar nerve heads toward the depth of the palm with the deep branch of the artery. They pass between the abductor digiti minimi and flexor digiti minimi brevis. At the root of the hook of the hamate, a fibrous arch (from which these muscles arise) normally protects the nerve, but occasionally may compress it (see Fig. 16-50). The nerve dispenses its branches to the hypothenar muscles and then runs across the sur-

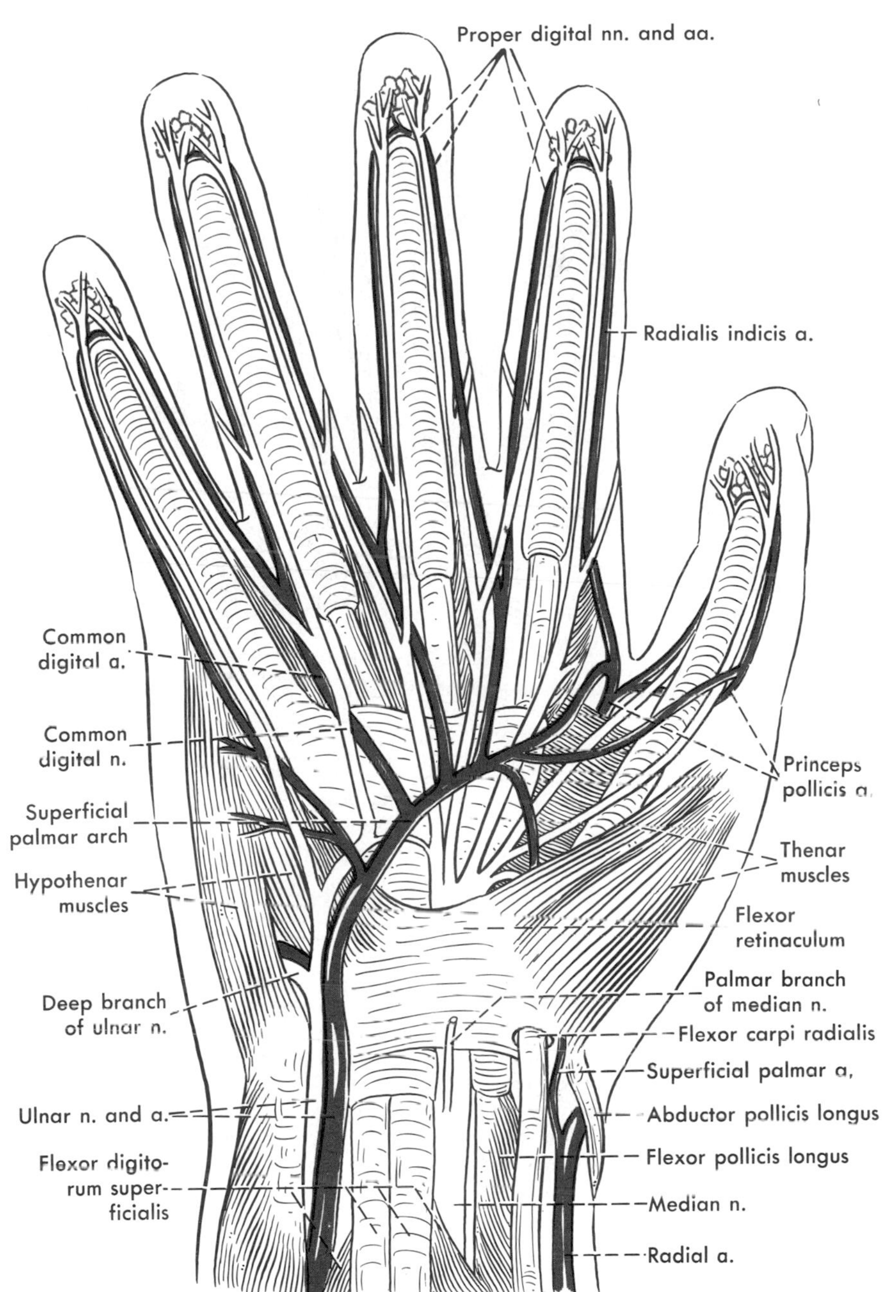

FIGURE *16-52.*
Anatomic relations in the palm of the hand: superficial branches of the median and ulnar nerves and the superficial palmar arch.

face of the interossei, lying deep to the flexor tendons. Its course follows the deep palmar arch and is close to the bases of the metacarpals (see Fig. 16-53). In its course across the palm, it distributes its branches to the palmar and dorsal interossei and the ulnar two lumbricals, and then ends in the adductor pollicis. Here the nerve may communicate with the muscular branch of the median nerve. Its long articular branches pass to the metacarpophalangeal joints and shorter ones to the joints of the carpus (see Fig. 16-53).

Compression and Injuries

The most serious effects of compression or injury of the ulnar nerve are on the intrinsic musculature of the hand. These lesions lead to muscle imbalance at the metacarpophalangeal and interphalangeal joints and consequent deformities of the hand, the severity of which depends in part upon the level of the lesion. In contrast with the clinical picture associated with median nerve injury described earlier, compression or even section of the ulnar nerve near the elbow has less

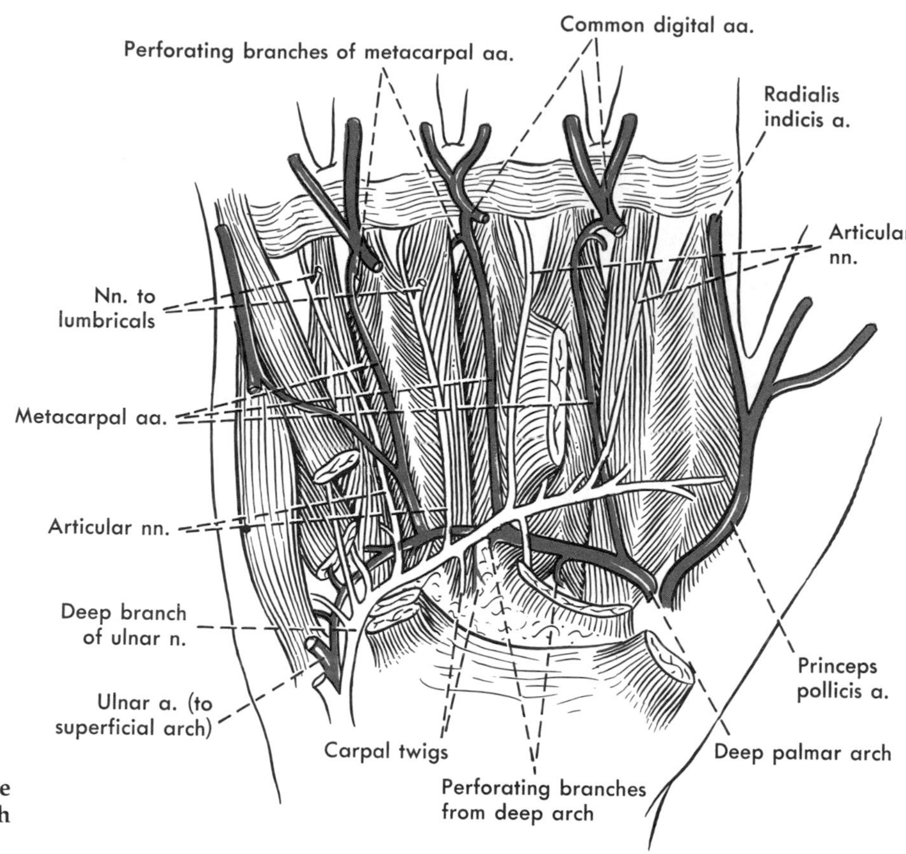

FIGURE *16-53.*
Anatomic relations in the hand: the deep palmar arch and the deep branch of the ulnar nerve.

severe consequences than lesions of the nerve near the wrist. The explanation lies in the degree of muscle imbalance at joints in the hand, and whether or not the flexor digitorum profundus has been affected.

When the ulnar nerve is damaged in the region of the wrist, the ulnar half of the flexor digitorum profundus remains unaffected (as it receives its innervation as the nerve courses through the forearm), but the hypothenar muscles, interossei, ulnar two lumbricals, and the adductor pollicis are paralyzed. Owing to the loss of the interossei, the metacarpophalangeal joints become hyperextended caused by overpull by the extensor digitorum. Inaction of the interossei also leads to flexion of the interphalangeal joints, chiefly caused by overpull by the flexor digitorum profundus. Interphalangeal flexion is less pronounced in the index and middle fingers because their intact lumbricals provide some balance. Muscle imbalance at the thumb leads to abduction of this digit. The transverse metacarpal arch becomes flat. The characteristic, composite deformity is known as the *ulnar claw hand.* Sensation is lost in the distribution area of the nerve distal to the lesion, and the corresponding area of the skin is dry and vasodilated. The ulnar nerve may be injured directly at the wrist or it may be compressed by the fascial band that binds it down to the pisiform, or by the other band that arches over its deep division at the hook of the hamate.

The ulnar nerve is also in a vulnerable position behind the medial epicondyle. Owing to deformity or previous trauma in the elbow region, or to unknown causes, the nerve may become loose and habitually dislocate from its groove. This traumatizes it, leading to neuritis and sometimes paralysis. The arrangement of fasciculi within the nerve is such that those supplying the hand may be affected before those that supply the flexor carpi ulnaris and the flexor digitorum profundus. When the nerve supply of the latter muscle is lost, the muscle imbalance observed in the ulnar two fingers will improve and the degree of clawing will be reduced.

Vessels

Blood is delivered to the hand by the **radial** and **ulnar arteries**. Two anastomotic arcades connect these two vessels in the palm of the hand: the **superficial** and **deep palmar arches** (Fig. 16-51). They ensure that occlusion of one artery does not impair blood supply to the hand, a function that can be demonstrated by a simple test. Powerful clenching of the fist squeezes blood out of the cutaneous capillary bed; while doing so, either the radial or the ulnar artery should be compressed above the wrist. When the hand is opened, the blanched skin becomes pink owing to filling of the peripheral vascular bed from the unoccluded vessel. However, if both arteries are compressed simultaneously, the hand will remain blanched when opened. The patency of one or the other vessel can thus be readily assessed.

Conforming to the branching pattern of the palmar digital nerves, **common palmar digital arteries** pass from

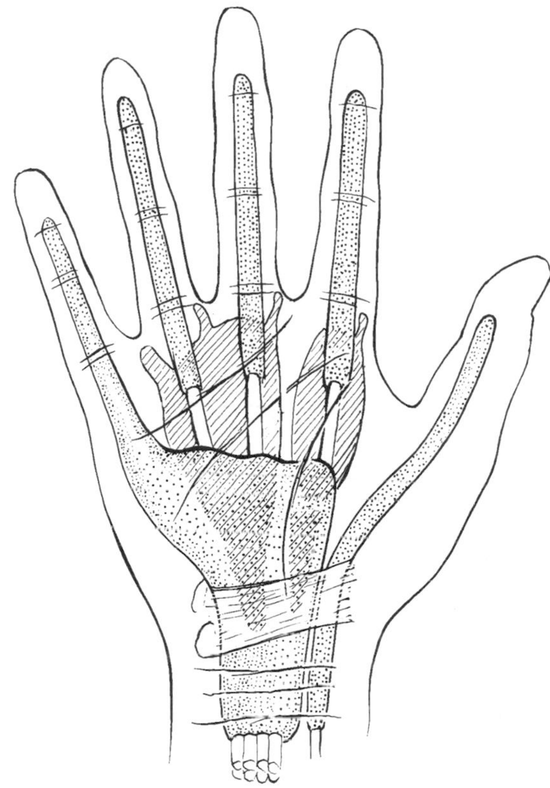

FIGURE *16-54.*
The thenar and midpalmar spaces in relation to the synovial sheaths of the flexor tendons: The fascial spaces are *shaded by lines*; the synovial bursae are *stippled*.

the superficial palmar arch to the finger webs and divide into **proper palmar digital arteries** (Fig. 16-52). **Palmar metacarpal arteries**, arising from the deep palmar arch, anastomose with the digital vessels (Fig. 16-53). Only smaller branches reach the dorsum of the hand from these vessels. The large venous channels, on the other hand, are on the dorsum, and the veins that accompany the main arteries in the palm are relatively small.

The multiple anastomoses between all vessels of the hand explain why bleeding is so profuse from lacerations in any part of the hand. Bleeding usually cannot be controlled by compression or ligation of one major vessel alone. The brachial artery may have to be compressed.

Superficial and Deep Palmar Arches. Although two arteries contribute to each palmar arch, the superficial arch is formed mainly by the ulnar artery and the deep arch by the radial artery. The superficial arch and its branches are embedded in a layer of loose connective tissue and fat between the palmar aponeurosis and the flexor tendons. The deep arch and its branches are located between the flexor tendons and the interossei. The arches are described in the following as continuations of the arteries that primarily form them.

Ulnar Artery. Just before it crosses the flexor retinaculum, the ulnar artery gives off a small *palmar carpal branch* that runs behind the flexor tendons to reach the floor of the carpel canal and a *dorsal carpal branch* that runs around the ulnar side of the wrist to join the dorsal carpal rete (see Fig. 16-51). After crossing the retinaculum, the ulnar artery divides into a *superficial* and a *deep branch* just distal to the pisiform bone. The **superficial palmar arch** is the continuation of the superficial division of the ulnar artery (see Figs. 16-51 and 16-52). The arch is completed by anastomosis with several branches of the radial artery. It is level with the distal border of the extended thumb and is deep to the palmar aponeurosis. Its branches are the **common palmar digital arteries** that divide into **proper palmar digital arteries** at the finger webs. The pulsations of the latter may be palpated along the sides of the fingers against the phalanges (see Fig. 16-48). They are the chief source of blood to the fingers. In the palm and fingers, branches of the superficial arch are accompanied by the digital nerves (see Fig. 16-52).

Radial Artery. Before the radial artery turns dorsally at the radial styloid process, it sends two branches into the palm: the *palmar carpal branch*, which anastomoses with the corresponding branch of the ulnar artery, and the *su-*

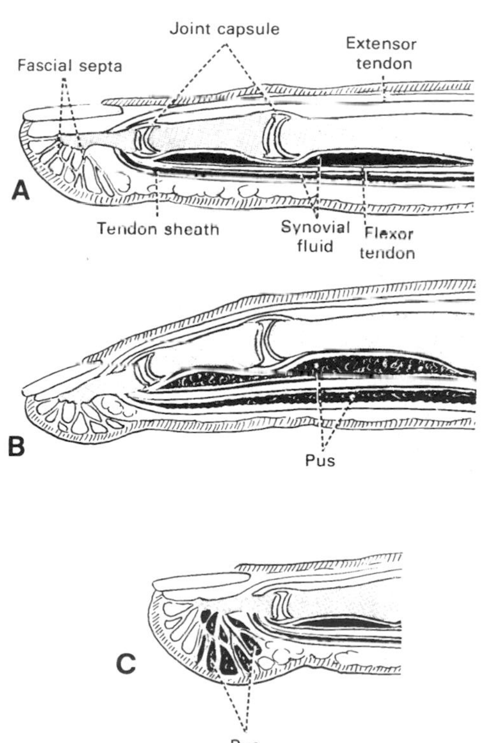

FIGURE *16-55.*
Fascial spaces of a finger commonly involved in local infections: (A) normal anatomy; (B) tenosynovitis; (C) felon. Synovial membrane is indicated as a ruffled white line. Synovial fluid and exudate or pus within the synovial sheath and fascial spaces is shown in *black*.

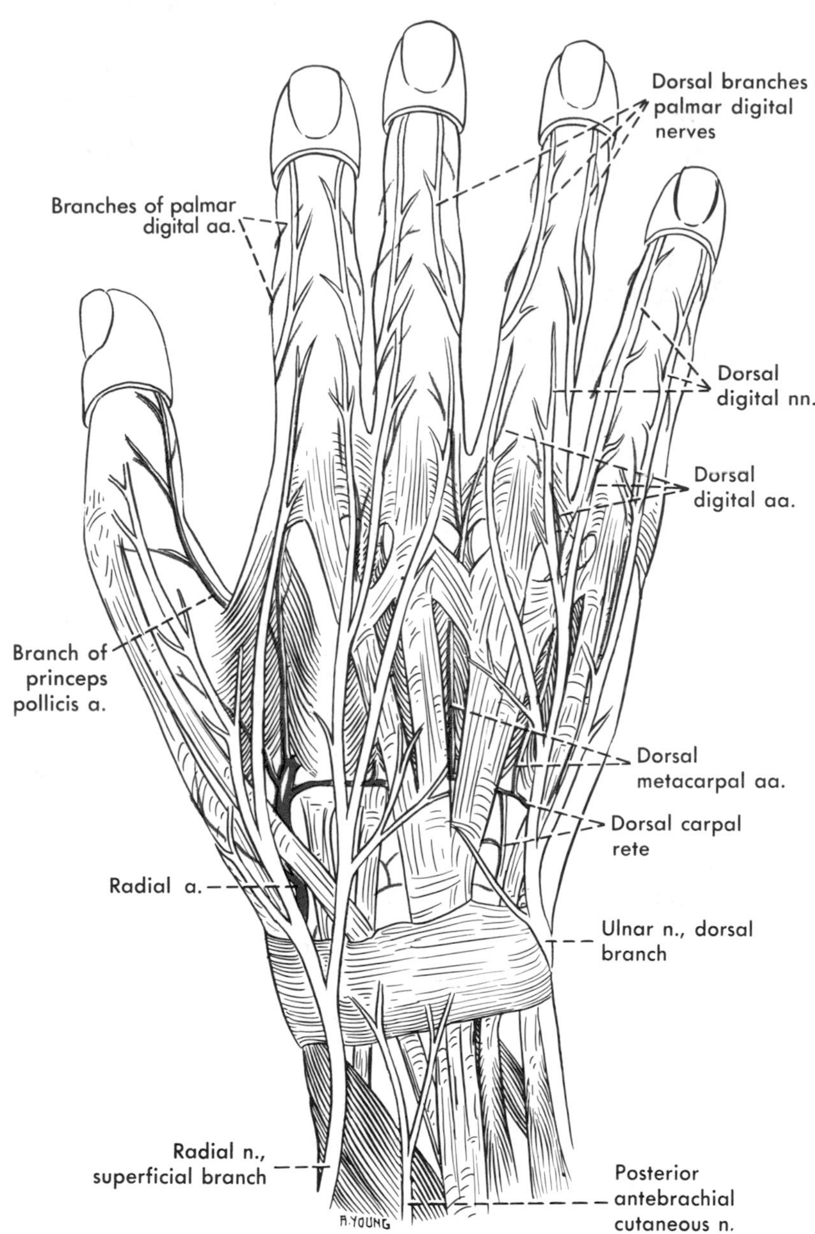

FIGURE *16-56.*
Anatomic relations on the dorsum of the hand.

perficial palmar branch (see Fig. 16-51). This branch passes through the thumb muscles and, on emerging from them, is one of the vessels that completes the superficial palmar arch (see Figs. 16-51 and 16-52). After it has passed around to the dorsum of the carpus, the radial artery enters the hand between the first and second metacarpal bones, through the interval between the two heads of the first dorsal interosseous (see Fig. 16-33). It continues across the anterior surface of the interossei as the **deep palmar arch** and anastomoses with the deep branch of the ulnar artery (see Figs. 16-51 and 16-53). The arch is on level with the hook of the hamate and is deep to the flexor tendons. The **palmar metacarpal arteries** arise from its convexity and anastomose in the finger webs with the common palmar digital arteries. They also send *perforating branches* to the dorsum of the hand, where they anastomose with the dorsal metacarpal arteries (see Fig. 16-57). The digital artery of the thumb (*princeps pollicis*) and of the radial side of the index finger (*radialis indicis*) originate separately from the deep palmar arch. These vessels, or the common stem they may share, frequently contribute to the superficial palmar arch (see Figs. 16-51 and 16-52).

Fascial Spaces and Septa of the Palm and Digits

Between the palmar aponeurosis and the deep fascia that covers the interossei, the palm is filled by loose connective tissue containing some fat. In it are embedded the long flexor tendons, the lumbricals, nerves, and blood vessels (see Fig. 16-34). Sliding of these structures on one another during movements of the hand is facilitated by the connective tissue. Compartments are delineated by more or less well-defined connective tissue condensations or septa that connect the deep surface of the palmar aponeurosis to the deep fascia of the interosseous muscles. Effusions or

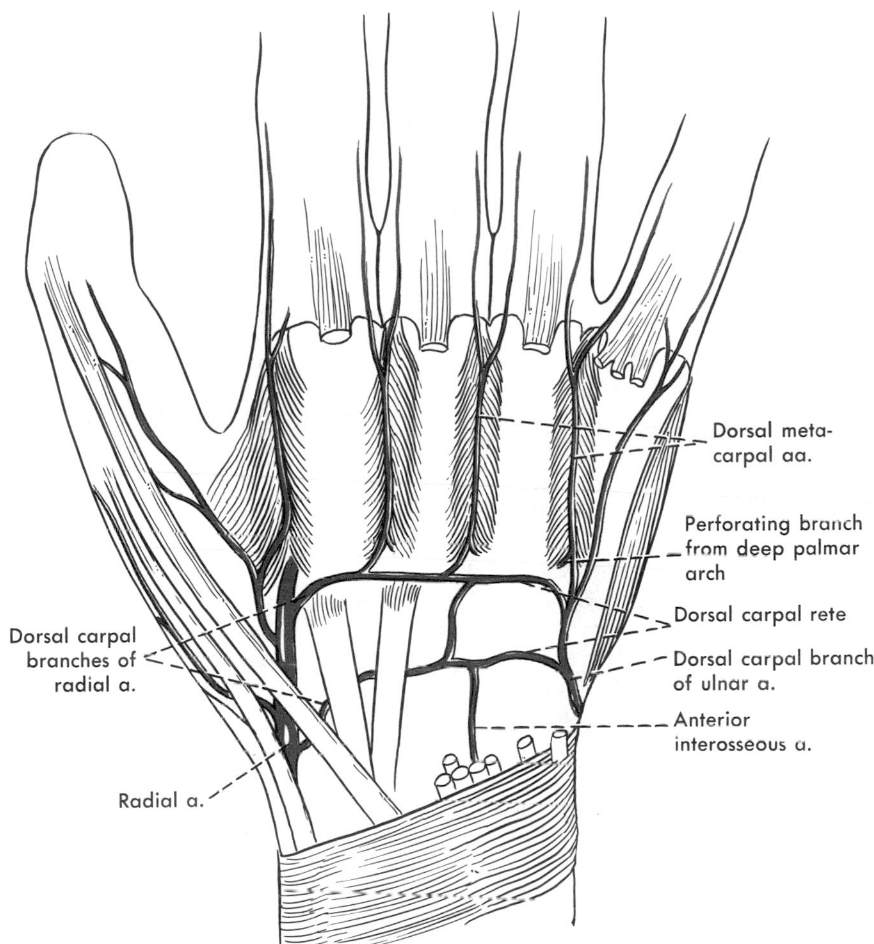

FIGURE 16-57.
Arteries of the dorsum of the hand.

pus can open up potential spaces in this loose tissue and better define the spaces and the septa. Clinically, these spaces have become less important since antibiotics became available; out of 1000 cases of hand injuries, for instance, in only 6 were the fascial palmar spaces involved.

Several such spaces have been described in the palm of the hand. The best-defined and largest are the thenar space and the midpalmar space (see Figs. 16-34 and 16-54). The **thenar space** is between the anterior surface of the adductor pollicis and the flexor tendons of the index finger. The **midpalmar space** is between the interossei and the deep surface of the tendons of the middle and ring fingers. They are closed in the normal hand, are not lined by synovial membrane, and no structures run through them. The connective tissue lamina that separates the two palmar spaces forms the so-called *midpalmar* or *oblique septum* (see Fig. 16-34). The proximal ends of the digital synovial sheaths of the ring and middle fingers protrude into the midpalmar space, and that of the index into the thenar space (see Fig. 16-54). When these sheaths become infected, pus may burst into the palmar spaces from the related sheaths.

Lying deep to the flexor digitorum profundus, the thenar and midpalmar spaces extend proximally into the carpal canal, where their connective tissue walls come together and blend above the retinaculum with connective tissue in the forearm. Short extensions continue from the spaces into the finger webs. These extensions probably act as bursae between the lumbrical muscles and the deep transverse metacarpal ligaments.

Alternative concepts of the fascial spaces have been proposed. One such proposal holds that all the loose connective tissue of the central compartment occupies a single fascial space in which the long tendons and lumbricals are embedded; only distally is the compartment divided by septa that extend around the flexor tendons and the lumbrical muscles.

Fascial Spaces of the Digits

In penetrating injuries of the digits, the synovial sheaths and tendon spaces in their superficial fascia are susceptible to infection and suppuration. Most often involved are the pulps of the digits and tissues under the nail or the nail fold (Fig. 16-55). Much of the relevant anatomy has already been discussed (see Figs. 16-36 and 16-37). When a digital synovial sheath is distended by exudate or pus (**tenosynovitis**), the entire finger is swollen, but tenderness is chiefly confined to the palmar aspect along the digital tendon sheath (see Fig. 16-55B). In draining the sheath, the incision must avoid the fibrous sheath on the flexor surface, because scarring will lead to contracture. The incision should be made on the side of the finger, dorsal to the palmar digital nerves and vessels (see Fig. 16-37). An abscess in the finger pulp is localized by the septa of superficial fascia and is known as a **felon** (see Fig.16-55C). Its drainage must avoid infection of the synovial sheath. A transverse incision is made through the side of the finger, severing the fibrous septa that localize the abscess, and avoiding scar formation over the finger's sensory surface.

Dorsum of the Hand

In comparison with its palmar aspect, the dorsum of the hand is bony and hard. The skin slides freely over the thin, deep fascia and can be pinched up between finger and thumb. It can also be lifted up by edema, hematoma, or pus. The dorsal digital nerves and vessels and the superficial lymphatics run in the scanty superficial fascia. Beneath the deep fascia are the tendons of the extrinsic extensor muscles of the digits. They terminate in a complex aponeurosis known as the *dorsal digital expansion*.

Nerves

The nerves to the dorsum of the hand are derived from the superficial radial nerve and the dorsal branch of the ulnar nerve (Fig. 16-56; and see Fig. 16-45). Above the wrist, the **superficial branch of the radial nerve** emerges from under cover of the brachioradialis muscle and divides into *dorsal digital nerves*. These supply the radial side of the dorsum of the hand and proceed to the thumb and the index and middle fingers. The dorsal digital nerves to the thumb supply skin as far as the nail bed; those to the other digits go little beyond the proximal interphalangeal joints. The **dorsal branch of the ulnar nerve** also originates above the wrist, winds its way around to the dorsum of the hand and breaks up into dorsal digital nerves that supply the ulnar one and a half or two and a half fingers (see Figs. 16-45 and 16-56). Their distribution over their respective fingers corresponds to that of the radial branches. There is a good deal of variation in the apportionment of the fingers between these radial and ulnar digital nerves.

Vessels

The arteries on the dorsum of the hand are derived from the radial artery and from the dorsal carpal rete (Fig. 16-57 and also see 16-56). In its course through the anatomic snuff box, and before it passes between the two heads of the first dorsal interosseous (see Fig. 16-33), the **radial artery** gives off *dorsal digital arteries* to the thumb and the radial side of the index (see Fig. 16-57). It also gives *dorsal carpal branches* to the **dorsal carpal rete**, a rather simple anastomotic network that receives additional input from the *dorsal carpal branch* of the **ulnar artery** and the terminal posterior branch of the *anterior interosseous artery*. Slender **dorsal metacarpal arteries** are given off by the rete. They divide close to the heads of the metacarpals into small **dorsal digital arteries** that enter the digits, but are soon replaced by branches of the proper palmar digital vessels (see Fig. 16-48). Close to their points of division, the dorsal metacarpal arteries receive *perforating branches* from the palmar metacarpal arteries (see Fig. 16-53); these may be the chief source of blood for the dorsal digital vessels.

Venous blood is collected from dorsal digital veins into a superficial venous plexus on the dorsum of the hand (see Fig. 14-10). The plexus also drains blood from the palm of the hand through *intercapitular veins*, so named because they pass between the heads of the metacarpals. The cephalic and basilic veins drain the dorsal venous plexus to the axillary vein (see section on cutaneous nerves and vessels).

Lymphatics ascend along the cephalic and basilic veins, draining rich lymphatic plexuses on both the dorsum and palm of the hand. They are described in the section on cutaneous nerves and vessels.

Extensor Tendons and the Dorsal Digital Expansion

After the extensor tendons of the digits emerge from underneath the extensor retinaculum, they fan out across the back of the hand toward the digits (see Fig. 16-31). **Intertendinous connections** join the four tendons of the *extensor digitorum* to one another just proximal to the metacarpophalangeal joints. This explains why independent extension of the middle and ring fingers is difficult and unnatural. The index and little fingers, by contrast, enjoy much greater independence in extension because they are served by additional extensors, the *extensor indicis* and *extensor digiti minimi*, the tendons of which are not bound to those of the extensor digitorum. The thumb has its own extensors, the *extensor pollicis longus* and *brevis*. Thus extension of the middle or ring finger is served by a single muscle (extensor digitorum) whereas that of each of the other fingers or the thumb is served by two.

The cutting of any one of the extensor digitorum tendons proximal to the intertendinous connections results in little or no loss in finger extension, but if the tendon of the middle or ring finger is cut distal to the connections, extension of the relevant metacarpophalangeal joint will no longer be possible.

The insertion of the extensor tendons of the thumb is relatively simple: the extensor pollicis brevis attaches to the base of the proximal phalanx and the long extensor to the distal phalanx. (Sometimes the extensor brevis continues to the distal phalanx and is capable of extending it even when the tendon of the extensor pollicis longus is cut.) Aponeurotic expansions from the tendons of the abductor pollicis brevis and adductor pollicis contribute some transverse fibers to the long extensor tendon. The extensor tendons of the fingers insert on the middle and distal phalanges through a more complex arrangement that forms the dorsal digital expansion.

Dorsal Digital Expansion. The dorsal digital expansion is a triangular aponeurosis through which the extensor digitorum, the interossei, and the lumbricals exert their coordinated actions at the metacarpophalangeal and interphalangeal joints. In clinical contexts it is often called the **extensor hood** or **extensor aponeurosis**. It is located over the metacarpophalangeal joints and the proximal and middle phalanges and is formed by aponeurotic expansions of the extensor digitorum tendons, the tendons of the interossei, and lumbricals, and some intrinsic bands of connective tissue.

The ribbonlike **tendon of the extensor digitorum** trifurcates over the proximal phalanx (Fig. 16-58). The **central slip** inserts into the base of the middle phalanx and the two **lateral bands** pass on either side of the proximal interphalangeal joint, fuse with each other beyond it, and insert into the base of the distal phalanx. The trifurcate tendon is held centered over the midline of the finger by transverse fibers in the expansion (transverse retinacular ligaments).

On each side, the **tendon of an interosseous muscle** commingles with the lateral band of the extensor digitorum and becomes an integral part of it (see Figs. 16-58 and 16-59). The fusion occurs over the middle phalanx. Proximal to this point, the interosseous tendon fans out into an aponeurosis, some fibers of which fuse with the central slip of the extensor digitorum, whereas others arch over it and blend with the interosseous aponeurosis from the other side of the finger. On the radial side, the tendon of a lumbrical joins the expansion in the region of the proximal interphalangeal joint, just distal to the interosseous tendon.

This arrangement allows each trifurcate extensor digitorum tendon to transmit forces generated by two interossei and a lumbrical as well as its own muscle belly. These forces extend the proximal and distal interphalangeal joints. Extension of the metacarpophalangeal joint is also mediated by the dorsal digital expansion. The extensor digitorum tendon sends a fibrous slip from its deep surface into the capsule of the metacarpophalangeal joint and, from there, to an insertion on the base of the proximal phalanx (see Fig. 16-59). This slip, however, plays little or no role in metacarpophalangeal extension because it remains lax during all phases of the movement. Only in hyperextension, when the tendon is pulled even further proximally, does the fibrous slip become taut. A series of fibers, derived from the dorsal digital expansion, encircle the metacarpophalangeal joint and the proximal phalanx and fuse on the palmar aspect of the finger with the deep transverse metacarpal ligament and the fibrous digital sheaths (see Fig. 16-59). It is these fibers, rather than the fibrous slip, that transmit the pull of the extensor digitorum to the proximal phalanx and bring about extension of the metacarpophalangeal joint.

Several other components have been described in the dorsal digital expansion (e.g., retinacular ligaments, oblique cord) the functional importance of which remains controversial except when they limit movement owing to their scarring or contracture. The normal function and the disorders of the extensor mechanism in the fingers can be explained by understanding the interplay of the major components described in the foregoing.

Integration of Finger Movements by the Dorsal Digital Expansion. The metacarpophalangeal joint may be flexed or extended whatever the position of the interphalangeal joints. On the other hand, movement at the proximal and distal interphalangeal joints is always synchro-

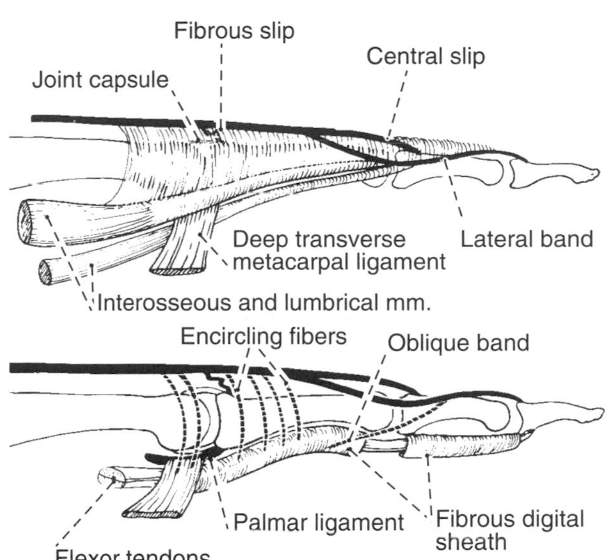

FIGURE *16-59.*
The dorsal digital expansion seen from the side and some of its components illustrated schematically.

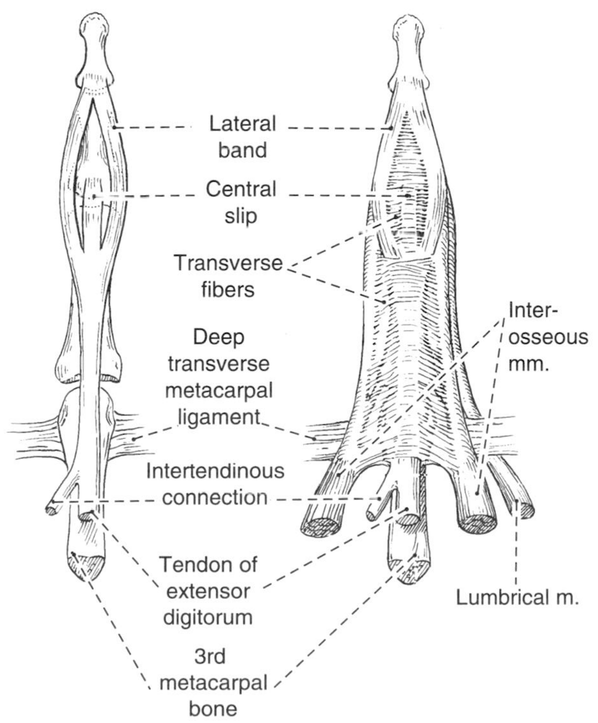

FIGURE *16-58.*
Components of the dorsal digital expansion seen from the dorsal aspect.

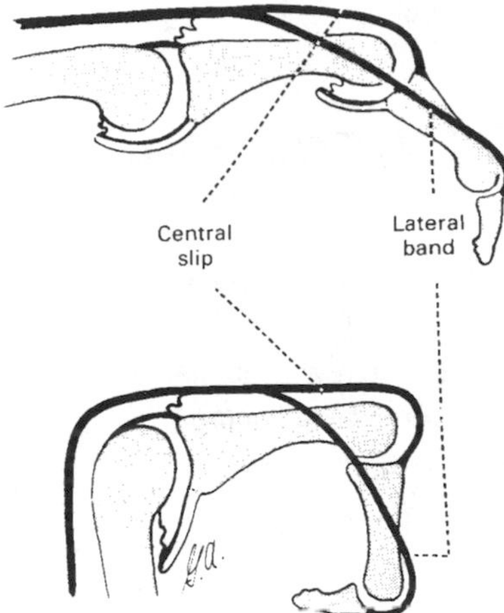

FIGURE *16-60.*
Integration of movements at the interphalangeal joints by components of the dorsal digital expansion. For explanation see text. (Adapted from Harris C, Rutledge GL Jr. J Bone Joint Surg 1972; 54-A: 713.)

nized. The middle phalanx cannot be extended without extending the distal phalanx as well, and the same is true in reverse. This is because the muscles that exert force through the central slip of the expansion also exert force along the lateral bands. The mechanism requires that the lengths of these tendons be precisely balanced.

During flexion of the interphalangeal joints, the two lateral bands of the dorsal digital expansion bowstring in a palmar direction because flexion shifts their point of distal attachment in this direction (Fig. 16-60). The bands slide onto the wider palmar aspect of the head of the proximal phalanx which prevents their slackening. When the proximal interphalangeal joint is flexed completely, the distal phalanx cannot be extended because the central slip of the expansion has been put under tension passively and, therefore, fixes the entire extensor hood. In the reverse of the movement, the middle phalanx comes into extension first as the central slip of the expansion extends the proximal interphalangeal joint. Then the lateral bands approximate each other on the dorsum of the finger as the pull is transmitted along them. The lumbricals may play a role in integrating flexor and extensor mechanisms as they are attached to both flexor and extensor tendons. Some fibrous bands in the digital expansion (oblique and retinacular ligaments), which run between the lateral bands and the fibrous flexor sheaths (see Fig. 16-59), may have a similar function.

Finger Deformities Caused by Disrupted Extensor Mechanisms. Some common finger injuries emphasize the functional importance of the dorsal digital expansion and its components.

When the extensor tendon is avulsed from the distal phalanx, with or without a chip of bone, or when the lateral bands are ruptured or cut, a flexion deformity results at the distal interphalangeal joint (*baseball or mallet finger*). The torn ligament or the fracture may heal if the finger is immobilized with the distal interphalangeal joint in extension. The deformity will not be completely corrected, however, if the healed ligament is longer than the normal structure.

If the central slip of the digital expansion is ruptured, minimal deformity results as long as the transverse fibers of the expansion remain intact. If they are also torn, a characteristic deformity is produced at the proximal interphalangeal joint called (somewhat paradoxically) the *boutonniere* deformity by English-speaking medical practitioners and *button hole* by the French. In this case, all extensor force is transmitted to the distal phalanx by the intact lateral bands, producing hyperextension of the distal interphalangeal joint. The proximal interphalangeal joint buckles into flexion and protrudes through the breech in the extensor hood. The two lateral bands now run on the palmar aspect of the proximal interphalangeal joint and exaggerate flexion. Correction of the deformity must aim at reattachment of the central slip without interfering with the lateral bands.

Hyperextension of the proximal interphalangeal joint with associated flexion of the distal interphalangeal joint is known as the *swan neck* deformity. Some young subjects can produce it voluntarily. Hyperextension at the proximal interphalangeal joint allows the lateral bands to bowstring on the dorsal aspect of the middle phalanx, giving them sufficient slackness to permit the flexor digitorum profundus to flex the distal interphalangeal joint. When due to trauma or disease, the cause is evulsion or rupture of the palmar plate of the proximal interphalangeal joint. The deformity is commonly seen in rheumatoid arthritis.

The dorsal digital expansion and the extensor tendons are often severely involved in inflammatory changes associated with rheumatoid arthritis. In this case, the extensor tendons usually slip in an ulnar direction from their central position at the metacarpophalangeal joints. Flexion of the fingers displaces the tendons further. Extension at these joints becomes impossible unless the tendon snaps back into a more central position.

JOINTS

The general arrangement of the joints of the free upper limb is described in Chapter 14. The glenohumeral joint, discussed in Chapter 15, links the free limb to the pectoral girdle. This section deals with the elbow joint and the wrist joint, the radioulnar joints (which are integrated with the elbow and wrist), the joints of the carpus (intercarpal, carpometacarpal, and intermetacarpal joints), and the joints of the digits (metacarpophalangeal and interphalangeal joints).

Elbow Joint

The elbow joint (*articulatio cubiti*) is a compound synovial joint in which the radius and ulna articulate with the humerus (Fig. 16-61 and see 16-1). The joint cavity is continuous with that of the proximal radioulnar joint, and the

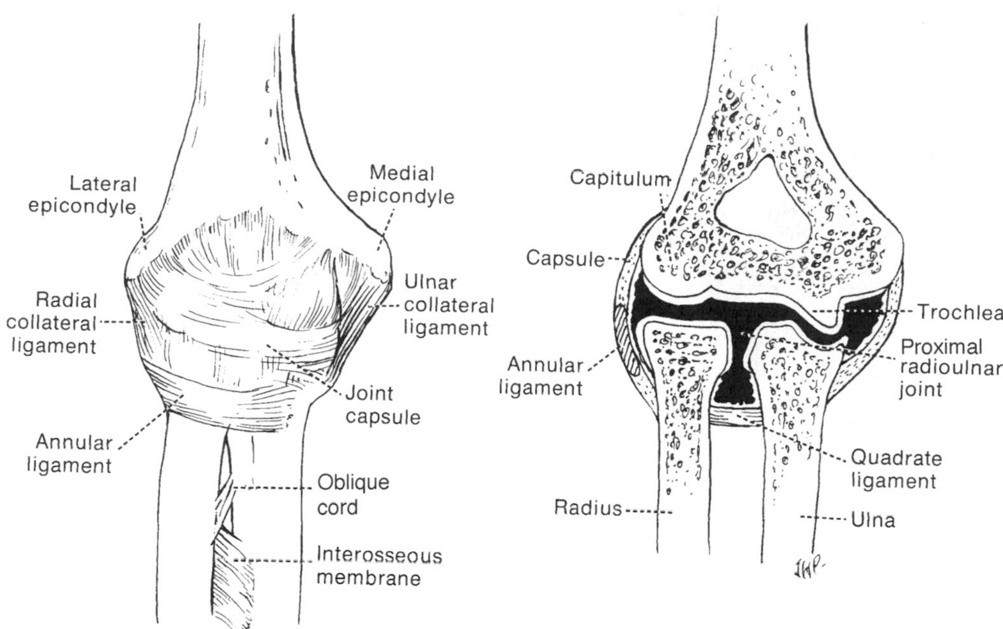

FIGURE *16-61.*
The elbow joint: On the left, the joint capsule is shown with its associated ligaments. The coronal section of the joint on the right shows the relation of the proximal radioulnar joint to the elbow. Articular cartilage is shown as an *even white line*; synovial membrane as a *ruffled white line*; synovial fluid is *black*.

two joints are enclosed by a single capsule. Though anatomically integrated, the two joints function independently. The elbow is a uniaxial joint that acts as a hinge, permitting flexion and extension of the forearm.

Articular Surfaces

The proximal articular surface consists of the **capitulum** and the **trochlea of the humerus**. The distal articular surface is represented by the **head of the radius** and the **trochlear notch of the ulna**. Whereas the proximal surface is covered by uninterrupted articular cartilage, the continuity of the distal articular surface is broken by the proximal radioulnar joint (see Figs. 16-1 and 16-61). The integrity of the latter is clearly essential for elbow flexion and extension, and ligaments normally hold the radial head in close apposition to the ulna's radial notch.

The elbow joint essentially has two parts: *laterally*, the humeral capitulum articulates with the radial head (*humeroradial joint*), whereas *medially*, the trochlea of the humerus articulates with the ulna's trochlear notch (*humeroulnar joint*). For purposes of description, the four bony structures are sometimes referred to as the *lateral* and *medial condyles* of the elbow joint.* Only if a joint is subluxed and abnormal movements take place does a lateral condyle come into contact with the medial condyle on the opposite side of the elbow joint. In normal movements, the two lateral condylar surfaces remain in contact with one another and the same is true for the two medial condylar surfaces.

The slightly concave superior surface of the radial head slides on the spheroidal capitulum during elbow flexion, and spins on it during pronation and supination. Both the trochlea and the trochlear notch are divided into unequal medial and lateral facets (see Fig. 16-1B). The trochlea is shaped like a pulley; its medial portion projects further inferiorly than the lateral portion. The trochlear notch occupies the upper surface of the coronoid process and the anterior surface of the olecranon process. A smooth ridge on the trochlear notch corresponds to the groove on the trochlea. The coronoid articular surface is level with the plateau of the radial head, but the articular surface on the olecranon reaches upward behind the trochlea. The latter is essentially grasped by the two ulnar processes (Fig. 16-62 and see 16-1).

Maximum congruity between the trochlea and trochlear notch is obtained when the elbow is fully extended. This is the close-packed position of the joint in which its stabilizing ligaments become taut. In all positions between full extension and full flexion, some abduction and adduction can be elicited passively in the joint because the articular surfaces on the two medial condyles are not congruent. This incongruity also permits some movement of the ulna during active pronation and supination.

The articular surfaces of the two lateral condyles

* Relative to the structures that make up the elbow joint the term *condyle* should, strictly speaking, refer only to the expanded lower end of the humerus, itself comprising the capitulum and trochlea as well as other structures (see Chap. 15). The terms *lateral* and *medial condyle* are sometimes used in a rather loose, general sense to refer to the four structures that participate in flexion and extension, not only at the elbow joint but also at the knee joint (see Chap. 18).

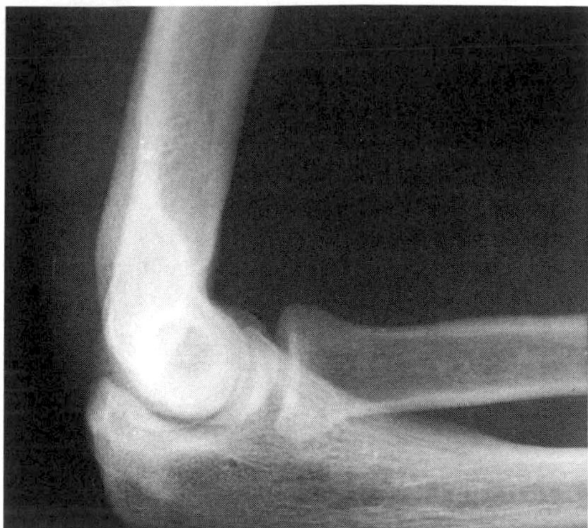

FIGURE *16-62.*
Lateral radiograph of the elbow joint.

(capitulum and radial head) lie more or less at right angles to the long axes of the bones on which they lie (the humerus and radius, respectively); however, the same is not true for the medial condyles. The larger, more medial part of the articular surface on each medial condyle is slanted relative to the long axis of its bone. As a result, when the elbow is fully extended, with the hand in the supinated (anatomic) position, the forearm diverges laterally. The medial border of the hand does not touch the side of the thigh. The long axis of the forearm makes an angle of 150° to 160° with that of the humerus; this is the **carrying angle**. When the forearm is pronated, it falls into line with the arm and the carrying angle disappears. The same is true when the elbow is flexed, because flexion brings the less-angulated lateral facets of the trochlea and trochlear notch into contact. This movement places the supinated hand over the shoulder or in front of the face. If fractures of the humeral shaft are allowed to unite with the distal fragment rotated, this relation is distorted and difficulty may be experienced in performing such essential movements as placing food in the mouth.

Capsule and Ligaments

The capsule of the elbow joint is thin anteriorly and posteriorly, but the *radial* and *ulnar collateral ligaments* reinforce the joint on its sides (Fig. 16-63 and see 16-61). Anteriorly, the capsule's attachment to the humerus encloses the coronoid and radial fossae; posteriorly the attachment is to the upper margin of the olecranon fossa (see Figs. 15-7 and 16-61). Both epicondyles are outside the capsule. The epiphyseal line of the distal epiphysis is intra-articular, but that of the medial epicondyle is outside the capsule. Inferiorly, the capsule attaches to the articular margins on the coronoid and olecranon processes but, over the radius, it blends with the ligaments that retain the radius and ulna in apposition at the proximal radioulnar joint. These ligaments are the **annular** and **quadrate ligaments** (see Figs. 16-61 and 16-63). The annular ligament is a strong, nearly complete fibrous circle that attaches to the margins of the ulna's radial notch and encircles the head of the radius. The quadrate ligament connects the lower edge of the radial notch to the neck of the radius. It forms the inferior part of the joint capsule and bridges the gap between the two bones. The **ulnar collateral ligament** is a triangular fibrous band that spans the space between medial epicondyle, the subcutaneous edge of the olecranon, and the coronoid process. The **radial collateral ligament** fans out from the lateral epicondyle and blends with the annular ligament.

The integrity of the collateral ligaments is tested in the following manner. The examiner grasps the subject's wrist with one hand and then, while stabilizing the humerus with the other hand, applies force to the wrist in a lateral or medial direction. With the subject's elbow extended, no side-to-side movement is possible if the ligaments are intact.

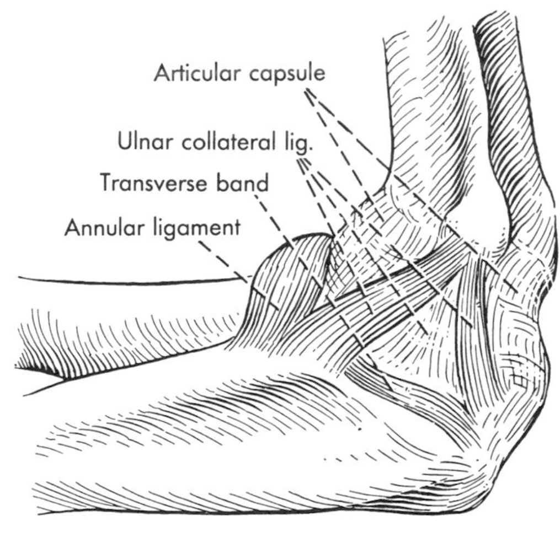

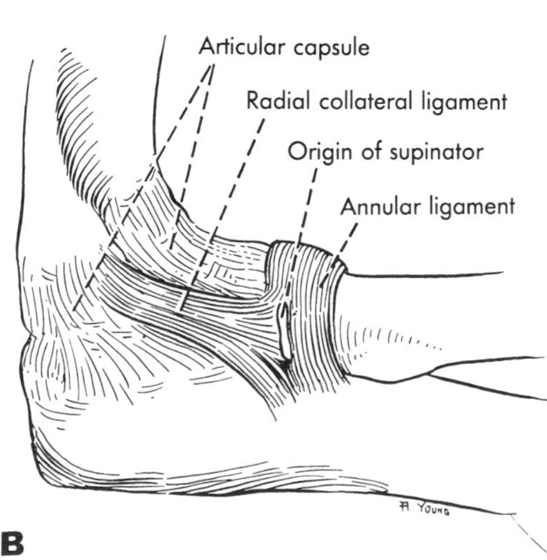

FIGURE *16-63.*
Ligaments of the elbow joint: (A) medial view; (B) lateral view.

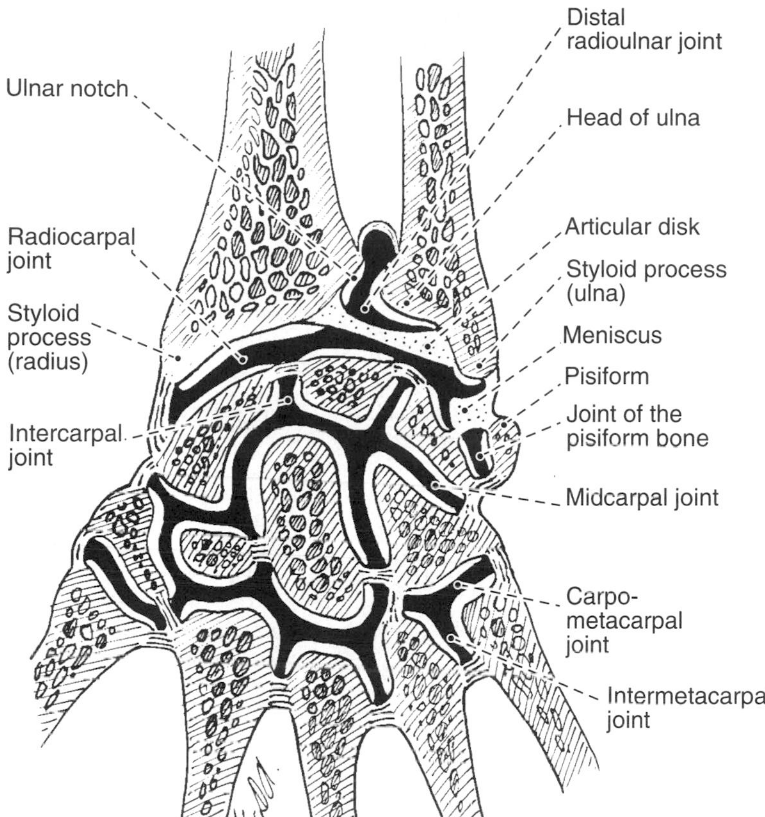

FIGURE 16-64.
The joints of the wrist and carpus. (Adapted from Lewis OJ, Hamshere RJ, Bucknill TM. J Anat 1970; 106: 539.)

Synovial Membrane

The capsule is lined by synovial membrane that is attached to the articular margins. It encloses a synovial cavity common to the humeroulnar, humeroradial, and proximal radioulnar joints. The membrane doubles back on itself at the lines of capsular attachment and is draped over the *fat pads* that occupy the coronoid, radial, and olecranon fossae. The fat pads are compressed by the radius and ulna and function to spread the synovial fluid when they are allowed to expand. They also retain the synovial membrane in contact with the articular cartilage of the condyles where they are free from contact with the apposing articular surface.

Movements

In full extension the arm and forearm make an angle of 180°. Full flexion is limited by contact between the arm and forearm. Flexion is carried out primarily by the brachialis and biceps muscles and by the brachioradialis (see Fig. 16-11). Their contributions to the movement are described in the respective sections. Extension is brought about by the triceps and anconeus (see Fig. 16-15). Other muscles of the forearm that originate from the humerus and cross the joint (see Fig. 16-19) can also produce movement at the elbow, but they become important in flexion and extension only when the chief prime movers are paralyzed. In both flexion and extension, gravity plays an important part and must be taken into account when the muscles are being tested.

Nerve and Blood Supply. All four nerves that pass the elbow joint send twigs to it; the musculocutaneous and the median supply it anteriorly, the radial and ulnar posteriorly. The elbow joint receives twigs from the vessels that form the collateral circulation about the elbow (see Fig. 16-25A).

Injuries. Most **dislocations** at the elbow are posterior (see Fig. 16-3); the ulna cannot be anteriorly dislocated without a concomitant fracture. The ulnar nerve is frequently injured by such dislocation. In **fractures of the humerus** close to the elbow, the brachial vessels are susceptible to injury. The resulting pressure of blood in the cubital fossa and spasm of collateral vessels may obliterate most of the circulation to the muscles of the forearm.

Radioulnar Joints

Both proximal and distal ends of the radius and ulna articulate with one another by uniaxial synovial joints of the pivot variety; these are the proximal and distal radioulnar joints, respectively (see Figs. 16-61 and see 16-64). In addition, the two bones are joined to one another by the *interosseous membrane* (see Fig. 16-2), which may be considered a fibrous joint (syndesmosis) between the two bones. At all three articulations, the radius is the moving bone.

The movements of supination and pronation take place around a vertical axis that runs through the proximal and distal radioulnar joints.

The vascular supply and innervation of the proximal radioulnar joint correspond to those of the elbow; the distal joint is supplied by the same nerves and vessels as the wrist joint; the anterior and posterior interosseous nerves and vessels supply the interosseous membrane.

Proximal Radioulnar Joint

The disk-shaped radial head is covered by articular cartilage, not only on its upper surface, but around its entire circumference, where the radius articulates with the radial notch of the ulna and the inner aspect of the annular ligament (see Figs. 16-1 and 16-61). Superiorly, the joint communicates with the elbow joint and, inferiorly, it is closed by the *quadrate ligament*. The chief structure responsible for the integrity of the joint is the **annular ligament**. Its strong fibers make up about four-fifths of a circle; the last fifth is represented by the radial notch. The inferior fibers of the ligament embrace the neck of the radius and form a narrower circle than those that surround its head. Laterally the ligament is held in place by the *radial collateral ligament* (see Fig. 16-63). When stabilized by the capitulum superiorly, the radial head and neck spin in the funnel-shaped articular collar made up of the annular ligament and the radial notch. This arrangement prevents distal displacement of the head of the radius. In children, however, before the radial head is fully developed, it may be pulled out of its osseoligamentous collar without tearing the ligament.

Distal Radioulnar Joint

In this pivot joint, three quarters of the circumference of the ulnar head is covered by articular cartilage, upon which slides the articular facet of the radius, which is limited to the concave ulnar notch. The chief structure responsible for the integrity of the distal radioulnar joint is a triangular **articular disk**. Composed of fibrocartilage, it retains the two bones in apposition and, at the same time, permits the radius to move (see Fig. 16-19). The apex of the disk is attached to the root of the ulnar styloid process and the base to the radius along the inferior edge of the ulnar notch (see Figs. 16-19 and 16-64). Twisting at its apex, the disk moves with the radius while its upper surface slides on the inferior aspect of the ulnar head, which is covered by articular cartilage. Inferiorly, the disk faces into the wrist (radiocarpal) joint. The disk normally separates the synovial cavities of the radiocarpal and distal radioulnar joints. Occasionally, it may be perforated. The *synovial membrane* extends upward between the radius and ulna beyond their articular margins and forms the *sacciform recess*. Although their synovial cavities are usually separate, the distal radiocarpal joint and the wrist joint are enclosed by the same capsule, formed largely by the *palmar* and *dorsal radiocarpal ligaments* (Fig. 16-65).

Interosseous Membrane

In addition to providing areas for the attachment of the deep muscles of the forearm (see Fig. 16-2), the interosseous membrane transmits to the ulna some of the forces absorbed at the wrist by the radius. Most fibers of the membrane slope downward from the radius to the ulna, and apparently become taut when the radius is subjected to an upward thrust, as it would be when, to break a fall, body weight is supported by an outstretched hand. The membrane is relatively lax during the movements of supination and pronation. It is most tense when the hand is in the midprone position.

The interosseous membrane stops short of the neck of the radius, permitting passage of the posterior interosseous vessels to the posterior compartment of the forearm. The gap is crossed by the **oblique cord** (see Fig. 16-2), which joins the neck of the radius to the ulnar tuberosity. Inferiorly, the interosseous membrane blends with the capsule of the distal radioulnar joint. Proximal to this, an aperture in the membrane transmits the terminal branches of the anterior interosseous artery to the back of the wrist (see Fig. 16-25).

Movements

The movements of supination and pronation, defined in Chapter 14, are unique to the forearm. The essence of the movement in either direction is rotation of the radius. Whereas the head and neck of the radius spin around a fixed axis, the distal end of the bone describes an arc of about 180° around the head of the ulna, carrying the hand with it. When the radius and ulna are crossed, the back of the hand looks forward, or upward if the elbow is flexed. This is the position of **pronation**. In **supination**, the two bones are parallel and the palm now looks forward or, with elbow flexion, upward. The muscle groups responsible for active pronation and supination are discussed under Functional Grouping of Muscles in the Forearm, as well as with the individual muscles (see Figs. 16-19 and 16-20).

Proximally the axis of pronation and supination passes through the center of the head of the radius; the distal end of the axis is not fixed. The hand can be supinated and pronated with the ulna lying on the table. The finger tips will move along arcs, the largest of which is described by the thumb, whereas the little finger has practically no excursion. Objects grasped by the index finger and thumb can thus be manipulated in a large volume of space with great precision. When the forearm is free, supination and pronation carries the thumb and little finger along arcs of similar radius. In this instance, the palm of the hand and the middle finger move the least. Thus a twisting force can be exerted on an object such as a doorknob or a screwdriver.

Slight movements of the head of the ulna are synchronized with excursions made by the distal end

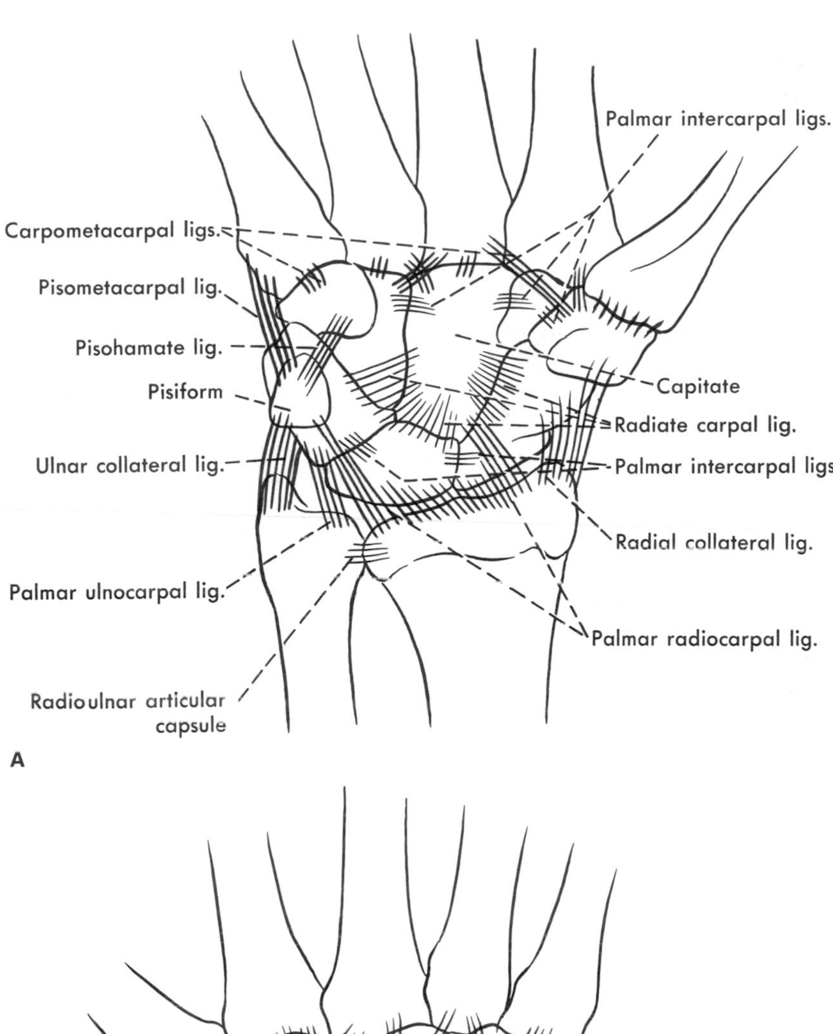

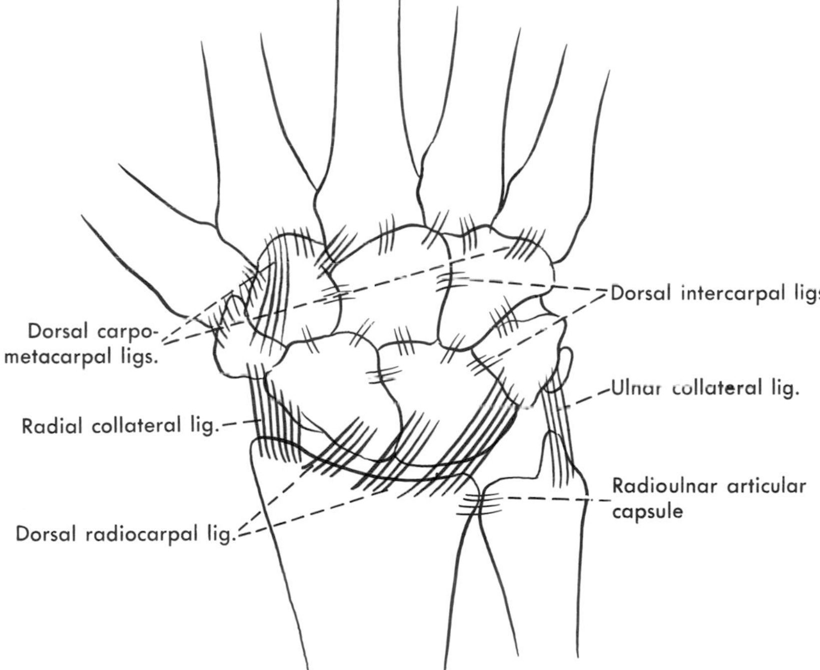

FIGURE *16-65.*
Diagrams of the capsular ligaments attaching to the bones of the wrist and carpus: (A) palmar view; (B) dorsal view. Intercarpal ligaments are *black*, others are *red*.

of the radius. The movements are an exaggeration of the slight play permitted by the incongruity between the medial condyles in the elbow joint.

The **range** of pronation and supination should be measured from the midprone position. This should be done with the elbow flexed. The normal range is 90° in either direction, whether performed actively or passively. When the forearm is extended, the range of supination and pronation is considerably augmented by rotation of the humerus. In this position, the latter movement can mask, or compensate for, a reduced range of supination or pronation.

Joints of the Wrist and Carpus

The types of movements possible at the wrist are determined by the **radiocarpal** or **wrist joint**. The range of motion, however, is a summation of movement obtained at the radiocarpal, **midcarpal**, **intercarpal**, **carpometacarpal**, and **intermetacarpal joints**. It will be evident from the anatomy of the radiocarpal joint that the wrist may be flexed, extended, abducted, and adducted. True rotation is not possible. The combination of all movements produces circumduction. Functional rotation of the hand is amply provided for by the radioulnar joints (pronation and supination).

The **range of movement** at the wrist can be tested by placing the hands together in the position of prayer (extension) and then reversing the position by putting the backs of the hands together (flexion). The range of wrist abduction (radial deviation) and adduction (ulnar deviation) may be measured by placing the supine hand on a piece of paper and drawing a line along the little finger in full abduction and adduction while keeping the forearm fixed. Wrist abduction is much more limited than adduction. There is considerable variation in the range of all movements from individual to individual. The progress of a disease or healing process can, however, be monitored in any patient by making such measurements from time to time.

The landmarks for testing the radiocarpal and carpometacarpal joints are described under Skeletal Anatomy.

Radiocarpal Joint

The wrist, or radiocarpal joint is a biaxial synovial joint of the ellipsoid variety. The proximal, concave articular surface is shallow and consists of the distal surface of the radius and the triangular articular disk. The scaphoid, lunate, and triquetral bones are held together by *intercarpal interosseous ligaments* and present a continuous, convex, distal articular surface (see Fig. 16-64; see also Figs. 16-5 and 16-6). Because the transverse diameter of each articulating surface is much longer than its anteroposterior diameter, rotation of the carpus as a whole is not possible in the shallow socket.

Although the head of the ulna is excluded from the radiocarpal joint by the articular disk, the ulnar styloid process, covered by articular cartilage on its tip and along its lateral side, completes the socket medially. The ulnar styloid articulates with a **meniscus** which is distinct from the articular disk and usually separates the small joint of the pisiform bone (pisotriquetral joint) from the wrist joint (see Fig. 16-64). Ossification may occur in the meniscus.

The stability of the joint depends on its capsular ligaments (see Fig. 16-65) and the tendons that surround the wrist. The *radial* and *ulnar carpal collateral ligaments* of the capsule are not well developed. More important are the *palmar radiocarpal* and *radioulnar ligaments;* they are positioned to absorb hyperextensive forces at the wrist that are sustained, for instance, during a fall on the outstretched hand. Corresponding ligaments on the dorsum complete the fibrous capsule. The capsule also encloses the distal radioulnar joint.

The synovial cavity of the wrist joint does not communicate with the more distal joints of the carpus. The meniscus or the articular disk may, however, be perforated, allowing communication between the wrist joint and the joint of the pisiform bone or the distal radioulnar joint, respectively.

Intercarpal, Carpometacarpal, and Intermetacarpal Joints

The carpus and metacarpus are a deformable unit, the plasticity of which is essential for normal hand function. This plasticity results from the presence of about a dozen joints between the carpal bones (intercarpal joints) and the bases of the metacarpals (intermetacarpal joints) and between carpal and metacarpal bones (carpometacarpal joints). The **carpal arch**, and the **transverse metacarpal arch**, described in the section, Skeletal Anatomy, depend on the integrity and coordinated movement of these joints. The carpal arch is formed by the carpal bones and intercarpal joints; the transverse metacarpal arch, formed by the heads of the metacarpals, exists because of the shape of the articular surfaces at the intermetacarpal joints. Grasping by the hand depends on the pliability of the transverse metacarpal arch. The free range of movement that distinguishes the thumb from the other digits is determined by its carpometacarpal joint.

Intercarpal synovial joints separate the carpal bones from one another in both the distal and the proximal row (see Fig. 16-64). The joints of the proximal row communicate with the *midcarpal joint*, which is largest intercarpal joint and intervenes between the proximal and distal rows. This joint especially contributes to the range of wrist flexion. In abduction and adduction, the sinuous outline of the midcarpal joint locks the distal and proximal rows of carpal bones together and ensures that the hand moves as a whole.

The intercarpal joints of the distal row communicate with the carpometacarpal joints and intermetacarpal joints. Thus, there is a continuous synovial cavity between the carpal bones and the bases of the metacarpals. There are two exceptions: the carpometacarpal joint of the thumb and the joint of the pisiform bone (pisotriquetral joint) are separate. *Capsular ligaments* are attached to the palmar and dorsal surfaces of all bones in continuity with the capsule of the wrist joint (see Fig. 16-65). The bones are further secured by *interosseous ligaments* that run between their nonarticular deep surfaces (see Fig. 16-64).

Carpometacarpal Joint of the Thumb. The freedom of thumb movement is due to the independence of the first metacarpal bone from the others, and to the saddle-shaped articular surfaces between the trapezium and the first metacarpal.

The trapezium is set in the carpus in such a manner that the long axis of its sellar (saddle-shaped) articular surface makes an angle of nearly 90° with the palm. This determines the orientation of the first metacarpal and the neutral or resting position for describing thumb movements (see Fig. 16-39). The joint is biaxial (see Fig. 5-12), but the curvatures of the articular surface on the metacarpal are greater than those on the trapezium; therefore, the joint is very loose in all positions except in full abduction and adduction. Joint stability in these positions is essential for hand function. In precision grip the thumb metacarpal is abducted and the joint is stabilized, whereas in power grip, the joint becomes stable in the adducted position. In both positions, the thumb is opposed as well. The taut capsular ligaments on the dorsal and lateral aspects of the joint are the chief stabilizing factors in abduction and adduction. In the neutral position, the capsule is very loose and free passive movements are permitted.

When the thumb moves in an ulnar direction, the nature of the incongruous articular surfaces dictates that the metacarpal bone will rotate medially along its long axis. This results in the opposition of the pulp of the thumb against the palm or against the pulp of any of the fingers. A special muscle exists for bringing about this movement actively, the opponens pollicis. However, rotation of the metacarpal is inevitable and even if the opponens is paralyzed, the thumb will swing into opposition when the flexor muscle pulls the metacarpal in an ulnar direction (consequential movement). The carpometacarpal joint of the thumb is chiefly responsible for opposition, abduction, adduction, and circumduction of this digit. It also contributes to flexion and extension, but these movements occur mainly at the more distal joints.

Blood Supply and Innervation. The ligaments and bones of the wrist are supplied by twigs from the dorsal carpal rete and, on the palmar side, by palmar carpal branches of the radial and ulnar arteries and twigs from the anterior interosseous artery and the deep palmar arch. The nerve supply is from both anterior and posterior interosseous nerves and from the dorsal and the deep palmar branches of the ulnar nerve.

Movements at the Wrist. The muscles that move the wrist are described in the section on the forearm; Functional Grouping of Muscles (see Figs. 16-19 and 16-20). The chief **flexors** of the wrist are the *flexor carpi radialis*, the *flexor carpi ulnaris*, and the *palmaris longus*. The abductor pollicis longus, an accessory flexor at the wrist, is the only flexor that is not innervated by either the median or the ulnar nerve. The flexor digitorum superficialis and profundus muscles, and the flexor pollicis longus, are effective as wrist flexors only when the digits are kept extended. The chief **extensors** are the *extensor carpi radialis longus* and *brevis* and the *extensor carpi ulnaris*. The extensors of the digits can help extend the wrist only when the digits themselves are flexed. All the extensors are innervated by the radial nerve. The chief **abductors** are the *flexor carpi radialis* and the *extensor carpi radialis longus* and *brevis*. Electromyographic studies have assigned variable roles to the other muscles capable of producing abduction or radial deviation at the wrist. These muscles include the abductor pollicis longus, and the extensor pollicis longus and brevis. The **adductors** are the *extensor and brevis carpi ulnaris* and the *flexor carpi ulnaris*.

In addition to producing movements, prime movers of the wrist **stabilize** the joint while other muscles act on the digits. When the fingers are flexed, flexion of the wrist is prevented by contraction of the extensors carpi radialis and ulnaris. Their contraction is readily verified. Similarly, when the fingers are extended without extending the wrist, contraction of the flexors carpi radialis and ulnaris becomes palpable. The prime movers of the wrist are also called into action to increase the mechanical advantage of the finger muscles to ensure maximum power of grip. This is **synergistic action**. Its importance becomes evident when one compares the power of grip while the wrist is flexed or extended. The tendons of the extensor digitorum are not long enough to allow maximum flexion of the fingers and the wrist simultaneously. In fact, the range of wrist flexion is limited by tension in the extensor digitorum: more flexion is possible at the wrist when the fingers are extended than when they are flexed. Conversely, when complete finger flexion is required for a powerful grip, the wrist is automatically extended.

Metacarpophalangeal and Interphalangeal Joints

The metacarpophalangeal joints of the fingers permit flexion, extension, abduction, adduction, and circumduction. The laxity of the ligaments and disparity of the articular surfaces at these joints permits a considerable range of passive movement in all positions of these joints, except in full flexion. Together with the transverse metacarpal arch, these passive movements enhance the plasticity of the hand and facilitate its adaptability to the shape and size of objects being grasped. Movement at the interphalangeal joints is confined to flexion and extension. Continued flexion of the metacarpophalangeal and interphalangeal joints brings all the finger tips in contact with the distal palmar crease; a sum of approximately 90° flexion at all the joints.

Metacarpophalangeal Joints

The condyloid articular surface on the metacarpal heads extends farther on the palmar aspect than it does dorsally; it is also wider in the palm than on the knuckles (Fig. 16-66). The shallow, ovoid facet of the proximal phalanx is much smaller than the metacarpal head and, when the ligaments are lax, accessory movements are freely elicited at the joint, including rotation. The latter movement cannot be performed actively. The joint line is palpable on the knuckles, but in the palm it is about 2 cm proximal to the free edge of the finger web.

On the palmar aspect the capsule has thickened into a stiff, fibrocartilaginous plate called the **palmar ligament** or **palmar plate** (see Figs. 16-66 and also 16-36). The plate is grooved by the flexor tendons as they cross the joint, and its deep surface articulates with the metacarpal head. The palmar plate is firmly attached to the base of the phalanx and always moves with it (see Fig. 16-66). A much thinner portion of the capsule attaches the proximal edge of the palmar plate to the metacarpal. The thin portion of the capsule may become torn and, when a dislocated joint

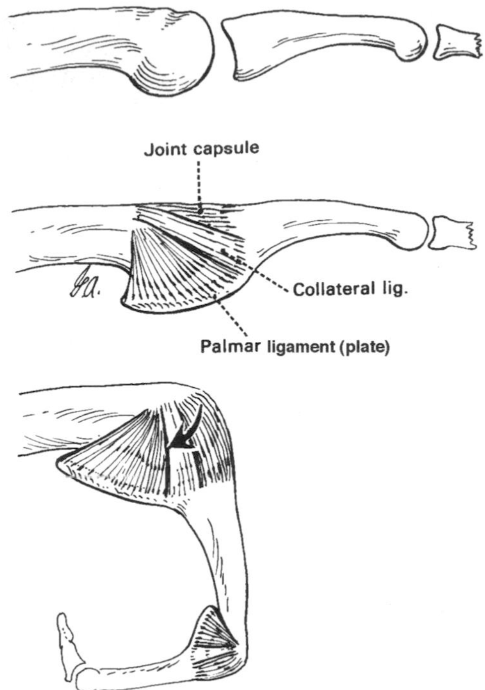

FIGURE *16-66.*
The metacarpophalangeal and interphalangeal joints: The attachment of the deep transverse metacarpal ligament to the palmar plate of the metacarpophalangeal joint is not shown.

is reduced, the palmar plate may become caught between the metacarpal head and the phalanx. Three types of ligaments attach to the palmar plate: collateral ligaments, deep transverse metacarpal ligaments, and the fibrous digital sheaths (see Figs. 16-36 and 16-66).

The oblique, cordlike portion of the **collateral ligament** is attached dorsally to the metacarpal head and distally to the base of the phalanx (see Fig. 16-66); a fan-shaped portion blends with the palmar plate. The collateral ligaments are lax in extension, permitting abduction, adduction, and passive rotation. As the phalanx is flexed, the cordlike ligament is drawn over the broader portion of the metacarpal head and becomes increasingly tight. Because of this tension, the fingers cannot be spread apart (actively or passively) in the fully flexed position (90°) and no accessory movements can be elicited. If an injured ligament is allowed to heal with the joint in extension, it will be too short to permit flexion and the fingers will become stiff in the extended position. Therefore, an injured hand should be immobilized with the metacarpophalangeal joints in approximately 90° flexion.

The **deep transverse metacarpal ligaments** are in the depth of the finger webs and run between the edges of the neighboring palmar ligaments of the four fingers (see Fig. 16-36). These connections restrict independent flexion of the middle and ring fingers, and prevent separation of the metacarpal heads. However, they permit the required mobility of these bones during changes of the transverse metacarpal arch. The deep transverse metacarpal ligament is not to be confused with the *superficial transverse metacarpal ligament* that is part of the palmar aponeurosis (see Fig. 16-35).

Two **sesamoid bones** articulate with the palmar aspect of the head of the first metacarpal (see Fig. 16-5); rarely, such bones may also be present at other metacarpals.

Interphalangeal Joints

The pulley-shaped articular surfaces of the proximal and distal interphalangeal joints function as pure hinge joints. Only flexion and extension are possible. The structure of the joints and the arrangement of the ligaments, including the palmar ligaments (plates), resemble those of the metacarpophalangeal joints (see Fig. 16-66), except that there is no equivalent of the transverse metacarpal ligaments. The palmar ligaments are important factors in preventing hyperextension of the interphalangeal joints.

Blood Supply and Innervation. The blood supply of the metacarpophalangeal and interphalangeal joints is from the metacarpal and digital arteries. Their nerve supply is from the digital nerves. The metacarpophalangeal joints of the more medial fingers often receive additional innervation from the deep branch of the ulnar nerve.

MOVEMENTS OF THE HAND

The normal attitude of the hand is the **position of rest** in which the wrist is slightly extended, the metacarpophalangeal and interphalangeal joints of all fingers are partially flexed, and the thumb rests in the neutral position against the index and middle fingers; the transverse metacarpal arch is quite pronounced, cupping the palm of the hand noticeably. The hand deviates from this position if some of the deep flexor tendons are cut, if the median or ulnar nerves are interrupted, or if the radial nerve is damaged at or above the elbow. Injury to the lower roots of the brachial plexus deprives the hand of its intrinsic muscles, leading to flattening of the metacarpal arch and to clawing (as seen in ulnar nerve lesions).

Finger deformities characteristic of the more common tendon injuries have been described in earlier sections.

Movements of the Digits

Although anatomists of antiquity had a fair knowledge of the actions of specific hand muscles, much research has been done in recent times to provide an understanding of the interplay of various muscle groups during movements of the digits.

Finger Movements

In the position of rest, all muscles are relaxed and the fingers are held partially flexed owing to what has been called the viscoelastic properties of the flexor digitorum profundus. In natural or habitual movements of the hand, the four fingers tend to move together and under these circumstances, only the prime movers contract; their antagonists remain quiescent. When only one finger is moved, most commonly the index or little finger, the others have to be immobilized; in this case there is activity in both prime movers and antagonists. Opening and closing the hand is a function of the extrinsic muscles. The intrinsic muscles modify these basic movements. They do not participate in closing the hand fully, but come into play when different movements are required at different joints. The interossei and lumbricals are responsible for producing the combined position of metacarpophalangeal flexion and interphalangeal extension. This posture is an important component of numerous activities, such as writing, drawing, cutting with a knife and fork, or holding a spoon. The interossei also produce controlled abduction and adduction of the fingers. These movements are components of such complex activities as playing musical instruments or using a keyboard. In the extended hand, uncontrolled abduction of the fingers can result from the pull of the extensor digitorum tendons as they fan out from the wrist. Likewise, uncontrolled adduction of the fingers occurs during flexion.

The sole extensor of the metacarpophalangeal joints is the extensor digitorum. This muscle is also active in interphalangeal extension, whatever the position of metacarpophalangeal joints. The interossei and lumbricals, in addition to contributing to interphalangeal extension as prime movers, render the action of the extensor digitorum at the distal interphalangeal joints more efficient because they prevent hyperextension at the proximal interphalangeal joints. These joints would tend to hyperextend owing to the attachment of the central slip of the digital expansion to the base of the middle phalanx. Hyperextension is prevented as the interossei and lumbricals pull the extensor expansion in a palmar direction on each side of the finger.

Thumb Movements

The importance of thumb movements in hand function is emphasized in several sections of this chapter. The natural movement of the thumb is opposition. The opponens pollicis controls this movement when the thumb is gently opposed to the index and middle fingers. However, when the thumb approaches the ring and little finger, the latter begin to move reflexly toward the thumb from the inception of thumb movement. Thus, thenar and hypothenar muscles contract in unison.

When firm opposition is required, not only does the opponens pollicis become active, but also the abductor and flexor pollicis brevis, as well as the adductor pollicis. Interestingly, the hypothenar muscles are recruited during firm opposition, even when this movement is performed against the radial two fingers. The thenar and hypothenar muscles acting together exaggerate the transverse metacarpal arch. These muscle groups are ideally positioned for this purpose as they diverge from their attachment to the flexor retinaculum toward the metacarpophalangeal joints of the first and fifth digits.

Movements of the Hand as a Whole

Individual digits can be tested separately, and the range of each movement can be recorded in degrees, but the movements that transform the hand into the functional unit it is cannot be measured in this way. These movements are complex biomechanical operations involving all joints at the same time. Most important of these are the movements concerned with prehension, which involve grasping an object. Although they are complex, they can be broken down into two basic acts: power grip and precision grip. The thumb and the radial two fingers are chiefly (but not exclusively) concerned with precision grip; the ulnar half of the hand contributes greatly to power grip. Because both types of grip require that the object be held securely, joint stability is an important factor in hand function.

In **power grip** the fingers form one jaw of a clamp, the other jaw being the palm. The thumb is wrapped around the dorsum of the clenched fingers and serves as a buttress. It is powerfully adducted. If precision needs to be combined with power, it is the thumb that supplies precision as it shifts its point of contact to the side of the index finger and comes to direct the object that is grasped. These movements may be observed when a rope, hammer, steering wheel, or the handle of a pitcher are held in the hand. During these movements, the wrist is stabilized in the neutral position.

Precision grip employs the pulp of the thumb, index, and middle fingers, that is, the sensory surface of the digits (see Fig. 16-42). The wrist is stabilized in extension, the position most advantageous for the action of extrinsic hand muscles. The carpometacarpal joint of the thumb becomes stable in abduction and opposition. The ulnar half of the hand may retain power grip over an object while the thumb and radial fingers manipulate it with precision. These basic movements can be combined in a constantly changing sequence of actions.

Movements of the hand as a whole become impaired by pain and by anatomic defects in the hand. To diagnose such defects it is necessary that individual movements are understood in appropriate detail. A second major cause of functional impairment of the hand is interference with its central control. In cerebral palsy and other diseases of the central nervous system, the complicated hand movements suffer the greatest loss, and during recovery they are the last to return.

RECOMMENDED READINGS

Al-Qattan MM, Robertson GA. An anatomical study of the deep transverse metacarpal ligament. J Anat 1993; 182: 443.

Atkinson WB, Elftman H. The carrying angle of the human arm as a secondary sex character. Anat Rec 1945; 91: 49.

Basmajian JV, DeLuca CJ. Muscles alive: their functions revealed by electromyography. 5th ed. Baltimore: Williams & Wilkins, 1985.

Bojsen-Möller F, Schmidt L. The palmar aponeurosis and the central spaces of the hand. J Anat 1974; 117: 55.

Brand PW. Clinical mechanics of the hand. 2nd ed. St. Louis: Mosby-Year Book, 1993.

Bugbee WD, Botte MJ. Surface anatomy of the hand: the relationships between palmar skin creases and osseous anatomy. Clin Orthop 1993; 296: 122.

Campero M, Verdugo RJ, Ochoa JL. Vasomotor innervation of the skin of the hand: a contribution to the study of human anatomy. J Anat 1993; 182: 361.

Charles CM. On the arrangement of the superficial veins of the cubital fossa in American white and American Negro males. Anat Rec 1932; 54: 9.

Coleman SS, Anson BJ. Arterial patterns in the hand. Surg Gynecol Obstet 1961; 133: 409.

Eyler DL, Markee JE. The anatomy and function of the intrinsic musculature of the fingers. J Bone Joint Surg 1954; 36A: 1.

Flynn JE. Clinical and anatomical investigations of deep fascial space infections of the hand. Am J Surg 1942; 55: 467.

Fröber R, Linss W. Anatomic bases of the forearm compartment syndrome. Surg Radiol Anat 1994; 16: 341.

Gardner E. The innervation of the elbow joint. Anat Rec 1948; 102: 161.

Gray DJ, Gardiner G, O'Rahilly R. The prenatal development of the skeleton and joints of the human hand. Am J Anat 1957; 101: 19.

Gray DJ, Gardner E. The innervation of the joints of the wrist and hand. Anat Rec 1965; 151: 261.

Greulich WW, Pyle SI. Radiographic atlas of skeletal development of the hand and wrist. 2nd ed. Stanford: Stanford University Press, 1959.

Guéro S, Guichard S, Fraitag SR. Ligamentary structure of the base of the nail. Surg Radiol Anat 1994; 16: 47.

Haymaker W, Woodhall B. Peripheral nerve injuries: principles of diagnosis. 2nd ed. Philadelphia: WB Saunders, 1953.

Hollinshead WH. Anatomy for surgeons: vol 3, the back and limbs. 3rd ed. Philadelphia: Harper & Row, 1982.

Hoppenfeld S. Orthopaedic neurology: a diagnostic guide to neurologic levels. Philadelphia: JB Lippincott, 1977.

Hoppenfeld S. Physical examination of the spine and extremities. New York: Appleton-Century-Crofts, 1976.

Ip MC, Chang KSF. A study on the radial supply of the human brachialis muscle. Anat Rec 1968; 162: 363.

Johnson MK, Cohen MJ. The hand atlas. Springfield, IL: Charles C. Thomas, 1975.

Kaplan EB. Functional and surgical anatomy of the hand. 3rd ed. Philadelphia: JB Lippincott, 1984.

Kauer JMG. The interdependence of carpal articulation chains. Acta Anat (Basel) 1974; 88: 481.

Kjaer I. Skeletal maturation of the human fetus assessed radiographically on the basis of ossification sequences in the hand and foot. Am J Phys Anthropol 1974; 40: 2577.

Kuczynski K. Carpometacarpal joint of the human thumb. J Anat 1974; 11: 119.

Landsmeer JMF. The coordination of finger-joint motions. J Bone Joint Surg 1963; 45A: 1654.

Lewis OJ, Hamshere RJ, Bucknill TM. The anatomy of the wrist joint. J Anat 1970; 106: 539.

Long C. Intrinsic-extrinsic muscle control of the fingers. J Bone Joint Surg 1968; 50A: 973.

Manchot C. The cutaneous arteries of the human body. New York: Springer-Verlag, 1983.

McCormack LJ, Cauldwell EW, Anson BJ. Brachial and antebrachial arterial patterns: a study of 750 extremities. Surg Gynecol Obstet 1953; 96: 43.

Mezzogiorno A, Passiatore C, Mezzogiorno V. Anatomic variations of the deep palmar arteries in man. Acta Anat 1994; 149: 221.

Misra BD. The arteria mediana. J Anat Soc India 1955; 4: 48.

Morrey BF, ed. The elbow and its disorders. 2nd ed. Philadelphia: WB Saunders, 1993.

Murphy F, Kirklin JW, Finlayson AI. Anomalous innervation of the intrinsic muscles of the hand. Surg Gynecol Obstet 1946; 83: 15.

Napier JR. The prehensile movements of the human hand. J Bone Joint Surg 1956; 38B: 902.

O'Rahilly R. A survey of carpal and tarsal anomalies. J Bone Joint Surg 1953; 35A: 626.

Oberlin C, Salon A, Pigeau I, Sarcy J-J, Guidici P, Treil N. Three-dimensional reconstruction of the carpus and its vasculature: an anatomic study. J Hand Surg Am 1992; 17: 767.

Ranney D, Wells R. Lumbrical muscle function as revealed by a new and physiological approach. Anat Rec 1988; 222: 110.

Ranney D. The hand as a concept: digital differences and their importance. Clin Anat 1995; 8: 281.

Schmidt H-M, Lanz U. The surgical anatomy of the hand. Stuttgart: Hippokrates, 1992.

Stopford JSB. The variations in distribution of the cutaneous nerves of the hand and digits. J Anat 1918; 53: 14.

Sunderland S. The actions of the extensor digitorum communis, interosseous and lumbrical muscles. Am J Anat 1945; 77: 189.

The puzzle of Dupuytren's contracture [editorial]. Lancet 1972; 2: 170.

Toft R, Berme N. A biomechanical analysis of the joints of the thumb. J Biomech 1980; 13: 353.

Tountas CP, Bergman RA. Anatomic variations of the upper extremity. New York: Churchill, Livingstone 1993.

Whitson RO. Relation of the radial nerve to the shaft of the humerus. J Bone Joint Surg 1954; 36A: 85.

Wright RD. A detailed study of movement of the wrist joint. J Anat 1935; 70: 137.

Hollinshead's Textbook of Anatomy, by Cornelius Rosse and Penelope Gaddum-Rosse.
Lippincott-Raven Publishers, Philadelphia, © 1997.

CHAPTER 17

Gluteal and Hip Regions

The gluteal and hip regions are those parts of the body that link the free lower limb to the trunk. Their soft tissues are supported mainly by the bones of the pelvic girdle (ilium, ischium, and pubis; see Fig. 14-2) and the upper end of the femur. The chief aim of this chapter is to provide the anatomic information necessary for evaluating, both functionally and clinically, the role of the gluteal and hip regions in stabilizing the trunk on the lower limbs, and the contributions of these regions to the movements of the lower limb as a whole. The joints at which stability and movements need to be controlled are the hip joints, which link the free limb to the pelvic girdle, and the sacroiliac joints, which unite the girdle to the axial skeleton. Because all the major nerves of the lower limb pass through the gluteal and hip regions, this chapter also deals with the general organization of the lumbosacral plexus from which these nerves issue. The anatomic relations of the plexus, however, are deferred to Chapters 25 and 27, because the plexus itself is located on the posterior walls of the abdominal and pelvic cavities.

In contrast with the upper limb, with its prehensile and sensory functions, the lower limb of *Homo sapiens* bears the entire body weight and serves the purpose of locomotion. The basic structural plan common to the upper and lower limbs (see Chap. 14) is adapted to meet these functional requirements. The adaptations are most evident in the pelvic girdle, the hip, knee, and ankle joints, and in the architecture of the foot.

In the static, erect position, the body is usually supported on both legs. The entire body weight can, however, be transferred to one leg; during locomotion, for example, such a transfer takes place from one leg to the other during the gait cycle (see Chap. 18). Whether static or moving, the body must be stabilized on one or both supporting legs, and stability is thus a crucial factor at all joints. Of particular importance are the sacroiliac joints and the

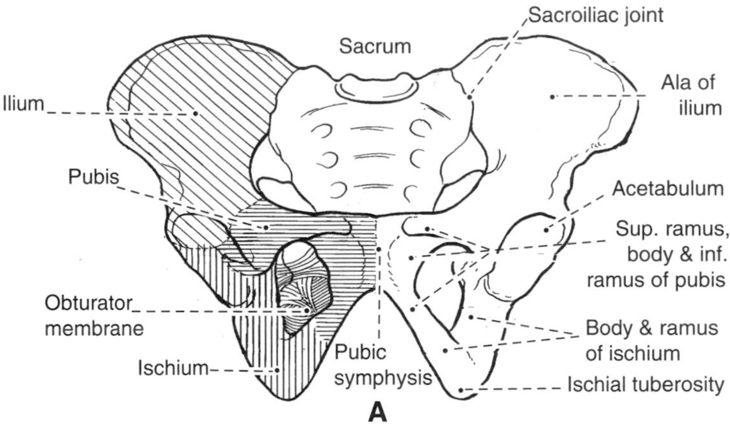

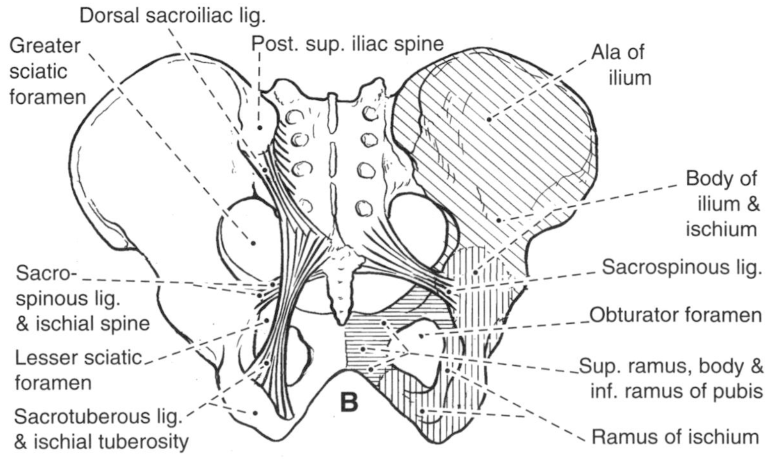

FIGURE *17-1.*
The bony pelvis, tilted slightly backwards and seen from (A) an anterior and (B) a posterior view. The three component bones of the pelvic girdle are *shaded differently*. The posterior view shows the chief bracing ligaments between the sacrum and the coxal bone.

pubic symphysis, which unite the two hip bones and the sacrum into the **bony pelvis** (Fig. 17-1). The movements of the bony pelvis consist chiefly of side-to-side and anteroposterior tilts, both of which occur at the hip joints. The pelvis transmits the body weight through the hip joints and the bones of the free limbs to the ground. In the standing position, the line of gravitational force passes through a series of links made up of the hip, knee, and ankle joints and the joints of the foot (Fig. 17-2). The direction of pelvic tilt and the tendency of the various links to buckle are determined by gravity's line of force in relation to the various joints. The hip is a ball-and-socket joint: therefore, the pelvis may tilt or rotate at the hip in any direction. Consequently, it is important to appreciate that the function of muscle groups serving the hip is not only to initiate movement, but also to stabilize the hip, controlling and preventing its tilt in those positions where its ligaments alone cannot counterbalance the gravitational force.

The chapter begins with a general orientation to the gluteal and hip regions. The soft tissue structures of importance are presented in subsequent sections in an order that roughly corresponds to that in which they would be encountered during a dissection. As a summary, the final section discusses the functional evaluation of the hip and gluteal regions.

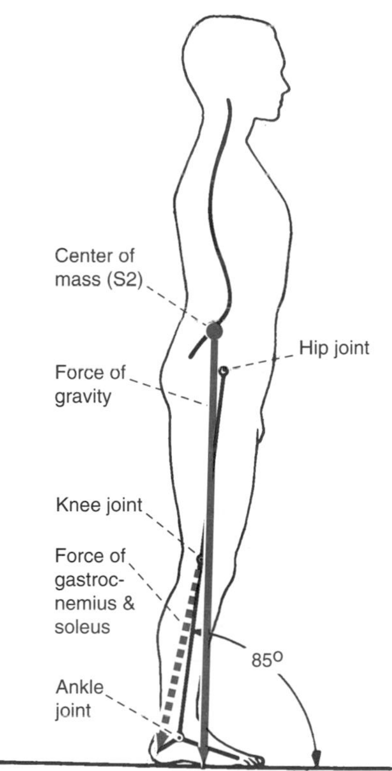

FIGURE 17-2.
The line of gravitational force shown in relation to the body's center of mass and the hip, knee, and ankle joints in the position of relaxed standing. The line passes behind the hip joint, in front of the knee joint, and in front of the ankle joint. Of all muscle groups in the lower limb, only those of the calf muscles are required to contract to maintain this posture.

GENERAL ORIENTATION

In addition to defining the parts and regions, this section describes the skeleton and surface landmarks of the gluteal and hip regions and concludes with an account of the lumbosacral plexus.

Parts and Regions

The gluteal and hip regions include the posterior and anterolateral aspects of the lower part of the trunk. Posteriorly, the bulging buttocks make up the **gluteal region** (*gloutos,* Greek for the buttock; *clunis* or *natis,* equivalent Latin terms). Gluteal, cluneal, and natal, all are used as adjectives pertaining to this region. Right and left buttocks are separated from one another by the *gluteal cleft,* known also as the *natal cleft.* A horizontal skin crease, the *gluteal sulcus* or *gluteal fold,* separates the buttock from the posterior aspect of the *femoral region* (*femur* or *regio femoralis*), known colloquially as the thigh. In Latin, *femur* means both the thigh and the femoral bone (*os femoris*). The **thigh** is the proximal segment of the free lower limb. Anterolaterally the buttock continues into the **hip region** (*regio coxalis: coxa,* Latin for hip) that comprises the hip joint and the soft tissues around it. Located mainly laterally, the hip region also extends anteriorly and merges with the lateral portion of the inguinal region. The **inguinal region** marks anteriorly the junction of the abdomen with the thigh, and forms a deep furrow when the thigh is flexed. There is no clear demarcation between the gluteal, hip, and femoral regions.

Bones and Joints of the Pelvic Girdle

The general anatomy of the pelvic girdle is described in Chapter 14 and compared with that of the pectoral girdle (see Fig. 14-2). At birth, the pelvic girdle consists of three bones, the **ilium**, **ischium**, and **pubis**, held together by a Y-shaped hyaline cartilage (see Fig. 14-2). These three entities remain individually recognizable even after puberty, when ossification of the cartilage converts the pelvic girdle into a single bone called the **hip bone** or **coxal bone** (*os coxae*). The area of fusion between ilium, ischium, and pubis presents a large cup-shaped fossa, the *acetabulum,* which faces laterally and articulates with the head of the femur (*acetabulum;* Latin for vinegar cruet). From their fused acetabular portions, the three bones diverge in different directions (Fig. 17-3 and see 17-1). The ilium is the upper, larger part of the os coxae and forms the upper part of the acetabulum. The pubis forms the anterior part of the acetabulum and the anteromedial part of the hip bone. The ischium forms a posteroinferior part of the acetabulum and the lower, posterior part of the hip bone.

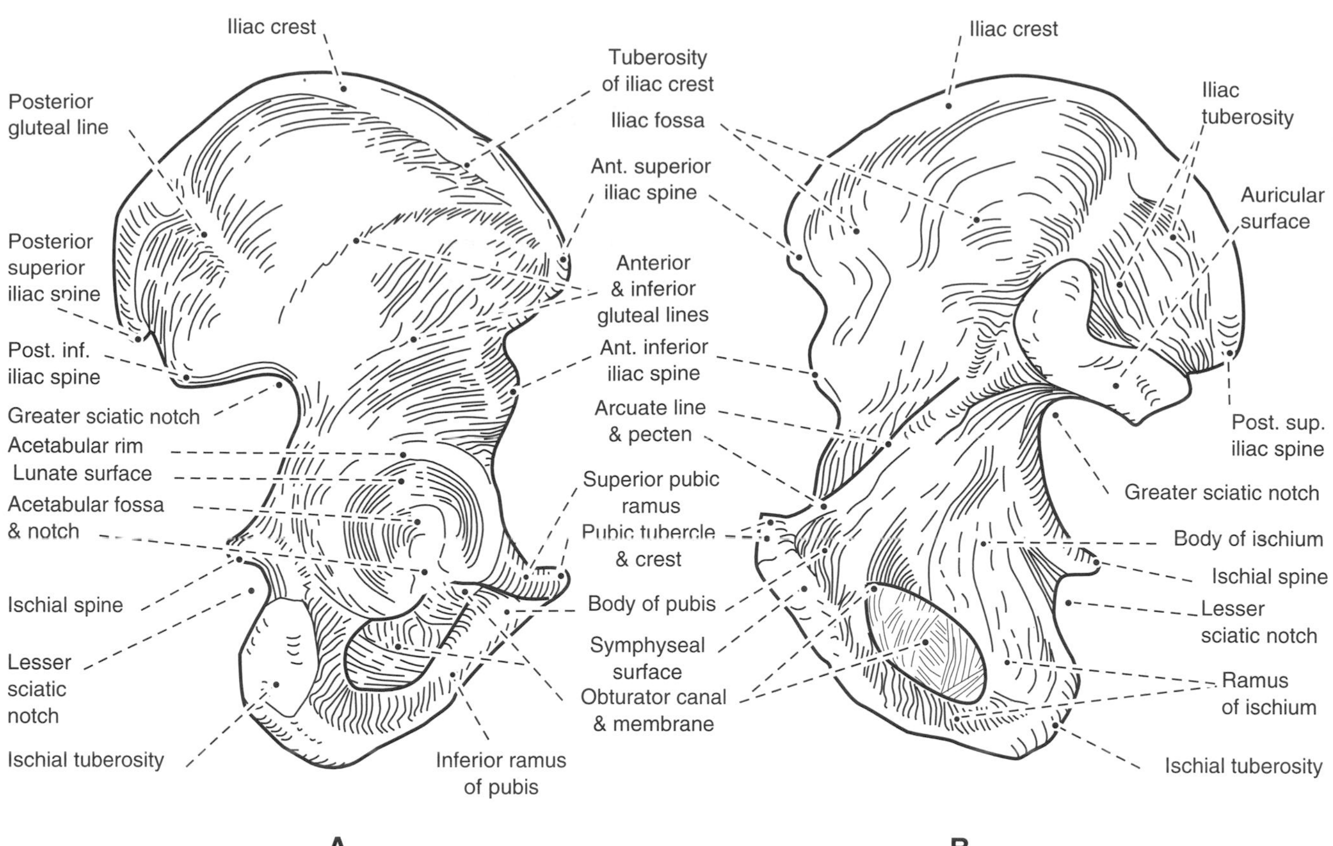

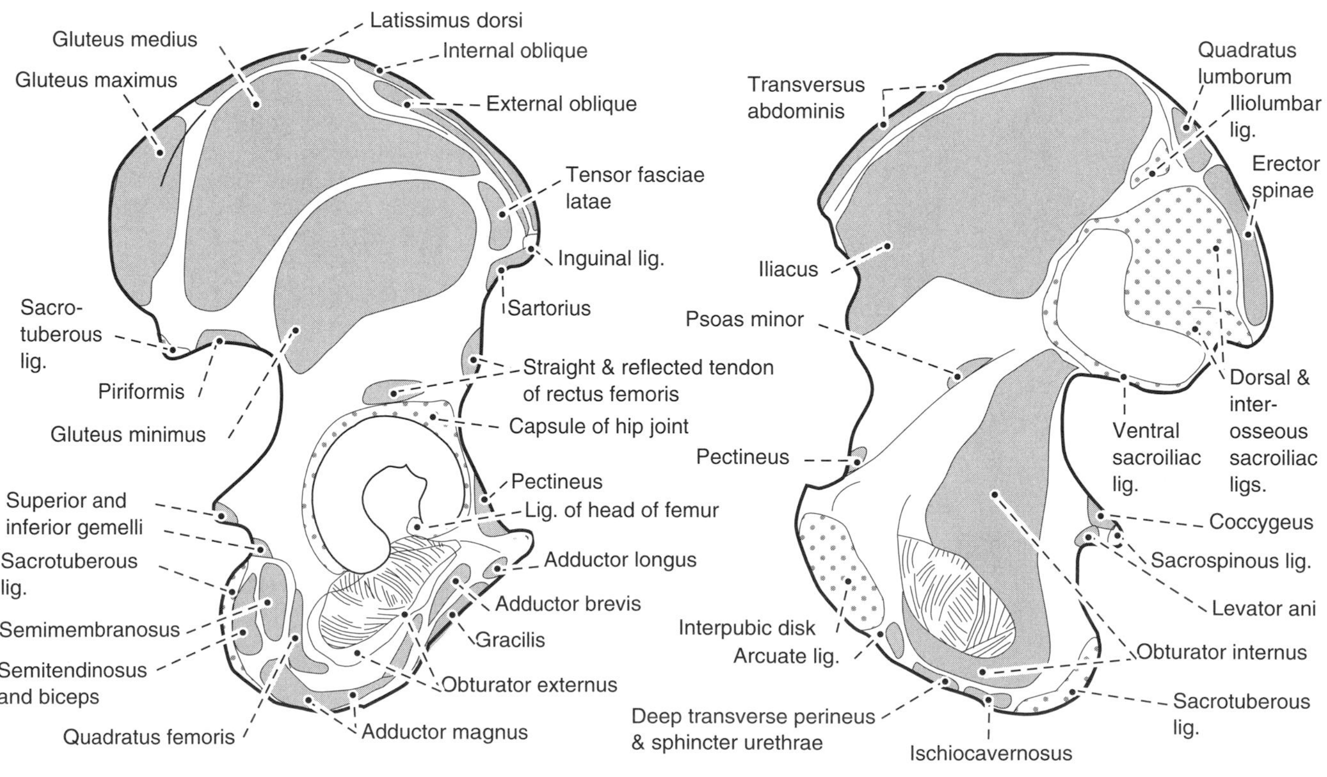

FIGURE *17-3.*
The right coxal bone with its anatomic features seen (A) in a lateral view and (B) in a medial view; muscular and ligamentous attachments to (C) the lateral surface and (D) the medial surface are also illustrated. Sites of muscle origin are *red* and insertions *blue*.

The **acetabulum** faces not only laterally but also downward and forward. Around most of its circumference is a heavy bony rim (*limbus acetabuli*). The rim is incomplete inferiorly, presenting the so-called *acetabular notch* (*incisura acetabuli*) that leads into the *acetabular fossa*. A rough area in the center of the fossa is surrounded by a smooth *lunate surface* covered by articular cartilage (see Fig. 17-3A). The articular surface is incomplete inferiorly where the notch opens into the fossa.

There is a large, somewhat oval foramen in the coxal bone, the **obturator foramen**. It lies below the acetabulum and is bounded by the pubis and ischium. Its name in Latin implies that it is closed. Indeed the **obturator membrane** does close it almost completely; a small aperture remains anterosuperiorly (the *obturator canal*) through which the obturator nerve and vessels pass as they leave the pelvis to enter the thigh.

The remaining features of the coxal bone are best described in connection with the individual bones that compose it (see Fig. 17-3A and B). Many of these features are palpable and are of special importance, because it is in reference to these bony landmarks that various degrees of pelvic tilt, deformity, and limb shortening can be determined. Because of its situation between the trunk and the free limb, the hip bone provides attachment for muscles of both. The muscular and chief ligamentous attachments are shown in Figure 17-3C and D.

The component bones and the joints of the pelvic girdle are described in the following. Further details of the complete bony pelvis, such as the anatomy of the pelvic apertures and sex differences in the skeletal pelvis, are given in Chapter 27 (The Pelvis).

Ilium

The ilium has two parts. That which contributes to the acetabulum is the **body** of the ilium; its medial surface forms the wall of the pelvic cavity. The rest of the bone projects upward from the acetabulum, like a wing, and is named accordingly the **ala** of the ilium; its medial surface flanks the abdominal cavity and forms the *iliac fossa*. The iliacus muscle, a flexor of the hip, arises from the fossa. The lateral or gluteal surface of the ala is marked by the *inferior, anterior,* and *posterior gluteal lines* which demarcate areas of origin for the abductor muscles of the hip (gluteal muscles).

The upper margin of the ala is thickened and forms the **iliac crest** (see Fig. 17-3A and B). The *inner* and *outer lips of the crest,* and the *intermediate line* between them, provide attachment for the three layers of abdominal wall muscles. The crest forms an arc, the summit of which is in the midaxillary line. Anterior to the summit, the external lip of the crest presents the **tubercle of the iliac crest**. The crest itself terminates anteriorly in the **anterior superior iliac spine**, and posteriorly in the **posterior superior iliac spine**. Below the anterior superior iliac spine, on the anterior border of the bone, is the *anterior inferior iliac spine*. In like manner, the *posterior inferior iliac spine* is located below the posterior superior iliac spine on the posterior border of the bone. This point marks the commencement of the **greater sciatic notch**, a concavity along the inferior margin of the ilium.

The portion of the ilium superior to the greater sciatic notch is thickened and presents the **sacropelvic surface,** which faces medially. On the lower part of this surface is the **auricular facet**, so called because of its fancied resemblance to an ear. Covered with articular cartilage, the facet articulates with the sacrum (sacroiliac joint). The rest of the sacropelvic surface is occupied by a rough protuberance, the **iliac tuberosity**. Attached to the tuberosity are the strong *sacroiliac ligaments*, of major importance for assuring a stable union between the pelvic girdle and the sacrum (Fig. 17-4 and see 17-1B). A smooth ridge, the **arcuate line**, begins at the anterior border of the auricular facet and extends forward and downward, separating the iliac fossa from the medial surface of the body of the ilium. It continues across the line of bony fusion onto the pubis, becoming known as the pecten of that bone (see later discussion).

Palpation. The iliac crest is palpable along its entire length. In most individuals, the anterior superior iliac spine is visible as a prominence and can be readily palpated. The posterior superior iliac spine cannot be distinguished by palpation but its position is usually marked in both genders by a dimple (dimples of Venus). The anterior and posterior inferior iliac spines are inaccessible because of the overlying muscles. The tubercle of the iliac crest is readily palpable along the lateral lip of the crest, anterior to its summit.

The palpable points of the iliac crest are useful landmarks for vertebral levels. The posterior superior iliac spines are on level with S-2 and indicate the position of the body's center of mass (see Fig. 17-2) and of the sacroiliac joints (which cannot be palpated). The summit of the iliac crest is level with L-4 spinous process, and its tubercle with L-5.

Ischium

The parts of the ischium are the body and the ramus. The **body** helps form the acetabulum and the lateral wall of the pelvic cavity. Its posterior margin borders the *greater sciatic notch.* The **ramus** extends inferiorly from the body and then curves anteriorly to form the posteroinferior boundary of the obturator foramen. The junction of the ramus and body is marked on the posterior margin of the ischium by a sharp bony spur, the **ischial spine**. The **ischial tuberosity** is a large and rough bony swelling located on the posteroinferior margin of the ramus as it turns anteriorly. The concavity of the posterior margin of the ramus between the ischial spine and tuberosity forms the **lesser sciatic notch**.

Ligaments. Two stout ligaments attach to the ischial spine and tuberosity and secure the ischium to the sacrum, thereby strengthening the union between the pelvic girdle and the sacrum; these are the **sacrospinous ligament** and the **sacrotuberous ligament** respectively (see Fig. 17-1B). Together with the sacrum itself, they con-

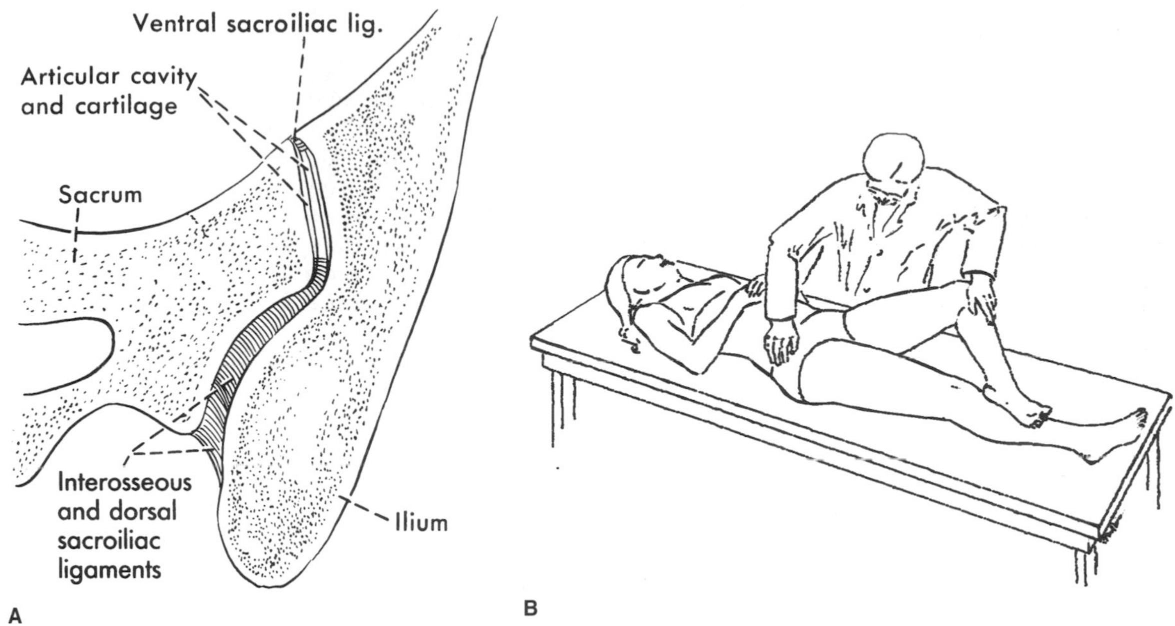

FIGURE 17-4.
The sacroiliac joint: (A) a schematic transverse section through the right sacroiliac joint; (B) testing the right sacroiliac joint. The joint is subjected to stress by pressing on the right anterior superior iliac spine and on the distal end of the left femur after the left hip has reached its limit of movement in the position shown.

vert the greater sciatic notch into the **greater sciatic foramen** and the lesser sciatic notch into the **lesser sciatic foramen** (see Fig. 17-1B). Each foramen allows muscles, nerves and vessels to leave the pelvis: those passing through the greater sciatic foramen reach the lower limb, and those traversing the lesser sciatic foramen end in the perineum.

Palpation. Only the most posteroinferior part of the ischium is palpable: the ischial tuberosity may be palpated through the substance of the buttock when the hip is flexed. In the sitting position, the body is largely supported by the tuberosities. Extending forward from the tuberosity, the ramus of the ischium is palpable in the perineum as it forms the posterolateral boundary to the urogenital region (see Fig. 28-1). The ischial spine is on level with the center of the acetabulum and can be palpated by a rectal or a vaginal examination.

Pubis

The pubis forms the anterior or most ventral component of the pelvic girdle (see Fig. 14-2). It consists of a body and two rami (see Fig. 17-1 and 17-3). The **body** is a flat, somewhat triangular piece of bone that forms the narrow anterior wall of the pelvic cavity. Its pelvic surface faces upward and posteriorly, and its perineal surface downward and anteriorly. Medially, the body presents a rough and narrow *symphyseal surface* (see Fig. 17-3B) at which it is firmly bound by the *pubic symphysis* to the pubis of the other side. The symphysis is in the median plane. The anterosuperior margin of the body is thickened and forms the **pubic crest**. The crest ends laterally as the prominent **pubic tubercle**.

The two rami of the pubis diverge from the body. The **superior ramus** passes laterally and upward to fuse with the ilium and ischium in the acetabulum. The **inferior ramus** passes downward and fuses with the ramus of the ischium below the obturator foramen, thus forming the **conjoint ramus**.

A sharp ridge, the *pecten*, runs along the superior ramus and becomes continuous with the arcuate line of the ilium, the two together forming the *linea terminalis*. A roughened area, the *iliopubic* (iliopectineal) *eminence*, marks the junction of the superior pubic ramus with the ilium. As the obturator nerve and vessels pass toward the obturator canal, they produce a small groove on the posteroinferior surface of the superior ramus (*obturator sulcus*); the groove is guarded by a small ridge (*obturator crest*).

Palpation. When a finger is run medially along the crease of the groin from the anterior superior iliac spine toward the pubic symphysis, the pubic tubercle is the first bony landmark encountered. The *inguinal ligament* connects these two bony points (see Fig. 17-22). The ligament is not palpable, but the tubercle is a useful landmark for the examination of the groin. The pubic crest and symphysis can be felt but indistinctly through the fat pad that covers them. In the male, the tubercle and crest are more easily palpated through the loose skin of the scrotum (see Chap. 26). The conjoint ramus is palpable in the perineum from the body of the pubis to the ischial tuberosity.

Ossification of the Coxal Bone

Ossification occurs from three primary centers, one each for the ilium, ischium, and pubis. In the infant or child, the three bones are still widely separated by cartilage (see Fig. 17-7A). The ramus of the ischium and the inferior ramus of the pubis unite at about the seventh or eighth year. One or more secondary centers appear in the acetabulum. The bodies of the ilium and ischium fuse here with the superior ramus of the pubis, and with the minor secondary centers, by about the age of 15 years. Secondary or epiphyseal ossification centers appear for the iliac crest and the ischial tuberosity, and sometimes for the symphyseal end of the pubis and for the anterior inferior iliac spine. These centers fuse over a considerable range of time. Ossification is essentially complete by the age of 20 to 21.

Fractures of the Coxal Bone

Fracture of the hip bone may result from a blow, but the most common cause is compression of the ringlike bony pelvis by a crushing force; such as can occur, for instance, in an automobile accident. The fracture normally occurs across a weak part of the bone and, therefore, most likely involves the wing of the ilium, the superior pubic ramus or the conjoint ramus. If the broken bones become displaced by the fracture, damage to pelvic viscera may occur.

Joints of the Pelvic Girdle

The pelvic girdle and the sacrum are united into the bony pelvis by three joints: the pubic symphysis, which unites the two hip bones to one another in the anterior midline; and the right and left sacroiliac joints, which unite the two bones to the vertebral column. All are strong, and on them depends the stability of the bony pelvis in supporting the weight of the trunk on the femoral heads. Indeed, the important movements of the pelvis occur not at these joints, but at the hip joint; the pelvis moves as a whole on the stabilized femurs.

Pubic Symphysis. The pubic symphysis is a fibrocartilaginous joint. The symphyseal surfaces of the pubic bones are covered by hyaline cartilage and are secured to one another by the *interpubic disk,* which consists of fibrocartilage. The disk may contain a small cavity. At its superior and inferior margins, the disk is reinforced by some functionally inconsequential ligaments: the *superior pubic ligament* between the two pubic crests, and the *arcuate pubic ligament* between the two inferior pubic rami. No perceptible movements are permitted by the symphysis. However, during the later stages of gestation, the interpubic disk tends to become more pliable and allows some separation of the pubes, particularly during parturition.

Sacroiliac Joint. The sacroiliac joint is a synovial joint formed between the auricular surfaces of the sacrum and ilium (see Fig. 17-4A). It is located at the level of the first three sacral vertebrae. The reciprocally shaped articular surfaces are irregular and permit only minimal gliding and rotational displacements. In a young person, such movements probably occur normally during locomotion. In the later months of pregnancy, the range of these movements becomes greater, owing to the laxity of the ligaments. Even in the mobile joint, however, the sacral and iliac articular surfaces become locked together when the weight of the body is transmitted from the sacrum to the ilia; the sacrum, in effect, becomes wedged between the ilia. At about the age of 50 years, the joint tends to become fused, with gradual obliteration of the joint cavity.

The articular capsule is thin; the *ventral sacroiliac ligament* reinforces it anteriorly (see Fig. 17-4A). The stability of the joint is chiefly assured by its strong extracapsular ligaments. The **interosseous sacroiliac ligament** occupies the posterior two-thirds of the space between the sacropelvic surface of the ilium and the lateral mass of the sacrum (see Fig. 17-4A). Its robust fibers run between the iliac tuberosity and the tuberosity of the sacrum. It blends posteriorly with the more superficially lying *dorsal sacroiliac ligament* (see Figs. 17 1B and 17-4A). Less important is the *iliolumbar ligament,* attached to the transverse process of the fifth lumbar vertebra and the anterior or pelvic surface of the ilium and sacrum. In the back, the sacroiliac joint is reinforced by two additional ligaments (see Fig. 17-1B). Attached above to the sacrum and below to the ischial tuberosity, the **sacrotuberous ligament** forms a strong brace for the joint. The smaller and more rounded **sacrospinous ligament** attaches above to the sacrum and coccyx and below to the ischial spine. All of these ligaments, but particularly the interosseous one, tend to prevent movement between sacrum and ilium.

Movements. The weight transmitted to the first sacral vertebra tends to force the sacrum downward and forward, causing its lower end to rotate upward and backward. The sacrotuberous and sacrospinous ligaments anchor the lower end and resist rotation of the sacrum between the coxal bones. This movement of the sacrum puts tension on the interosseous sacroiliac ligaments which, in turn, tend to draw the two ilia closer together. Thus the bony pelvis behaves essentially as a single bony unit. Nevertheless, slight movements are possible between the pelvic girdle and the sacrum before the sacroiliac joints become obliterated. Abnormal mobility or subluxation may be a cause of low back pain. The joint can be tested by subjecting it to a distracting force through pressure applied to the anterior superior iliac spine, using the opposite femur as a lever (see Fig. 17-4B). If pathology in the hip joint can be excluded, pain elicited in the sacral region is indicative of disease in the sacroiliac joint.

Orientation of the Bony Pelvis

Knowledge of the correct orientation of the pelvis is important not only in the physical examination, but for explaining and appreciating various movements and actions of the muscles. In the normal erect position the four superior iliac spines (right and left anterior and right and left posterior) lie in one and the same transverse (horizontal) plane (Fig. 17-5). If this requirement is met, the pelvis

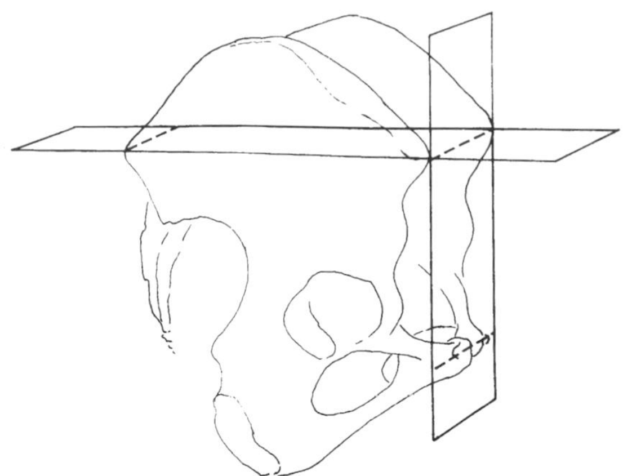

FIGURE *17-5.*
Orientation of the bony pelvis: The four superior iliac spines lie in one and the same horizontal plane. The anterosuperior iliac spines and the pubic tubercles are in the same vertical plane.

is said to be *level* or *neutral.* In a level pelvis, furthermore, the anterior superior iliac spines and the pubic tubercles lie in the same vertical plane (see Fig. 17-5).

A pelvic dip to one side is detected by inspecting the standing patient from the front and noting the deviation of the anterior superior iliac spines from their horizontal alignment. The same may be done with reference to the posterior spines. Anterior or posterior tilts are detected with reference to the alignment of the anterior and posterior superior iliac spines. Such tilts are effectively camouflaged by compensatory spinal curvatures (see Figs. 12-35 and 17-20).

Femur

Although the femur belongs to the free limb, rather than the limb girdle, it is included in this chapter, along with the bones of the pelvic girdle, because learning the anatomy of its proximal end is indispensable for understanding several topics in this chapter.

The femur forms the skeleton of the thigh, the proximal segment of the free lower limb (Fig. 17-6). It is a long bone with a body or shaft, an expanded upper end, which participates in forming the hip joint, and an expanded lower end, which articulates with the tibia and patella at the knee joint.

The **upper end** consists of a *head, neck,* and two *trochanters* (Greek for runner). The shape of the femur departs from that of most long bones in that the head and neck make an angle with the long axis of the shaft. This allows greater mobility at the hip joint, but also imposes unusual strains on the neck of the femur, because the body weight has to be transmitted through an arc. In accordance with engineering principles for bearing such an oblique thrust, the bony trabeculae in the neck are arranged in arcs that fall along the lines of calculated stress and strain (see Figs. 5-4 and 5-5).

The ball-like **head** of the femur is covered with cartilage except in a depression, the *fovea capitis,* on its medial side. The fovea serves for the attachment of the *ligament of the head.* The **femoral neck**, smaller in diameter than the head, is about 5 cm long and projects from the shaft medially, upward, and also forward. These angulations between the neck and shaft are important because they influence the relation of the line of gravitational force to the hip and knee joints. The **greater trochanter** is located where the upper margin of the neck joins the shaft (see Fig. 17-6A and B). It is a rugged, pyramidal process that projects upward. The *trochanteric fossa* is a well-defined pit, facing medially, where the trochanter joins the neck. The **lesser trochanter**, a smooth, rounded eminence, is located where the lower margin of the neck joins the shaft. It faces posteriorly and medially. Both trochanters, as well as the trochanteric fossa, serve for the attachment of several muscles (see Fig. 17-6C and D). The two trochanters are connected by bony ridges both posteriorly and anteriorly: the posterior ridge is the **intertrochanteric crest** and the less distinct anterior ridge, the **intertrochanteric line**. At the midpoint of the intertrochanteric crest is a smooth elevation, the *quadrate tubercle,* named for the muscle attached to it. Lateral to the tubercle is a larger and rougher elevation, the **gluteal tuberosity** (named after the insertion of the gluteus maximus), which may be sufficiently prominent to be termed the *third trochanter.* The anterior part of the hip joint capsule attaches to the intertrochanteric line. The continuation of this line below the lesser trochanter onto the back of the femoral shaft becomes the *pectineal line;* the pectineus muscle is attached to it.

Below the trochanters, the **body** or shaft of the femur is roughly cylindrical until it expands at the lower end to form the condyles. Most of its circumference is smooth where a large fleshy muscle attaches to it (see Fig. 17-6C). Several muscles attach by sheetlike tendons to a narrow longitudinal ridge of bone on its posterior surface (see Fig. 17-6B and D). This is the **linea aspera**, along which a medial and a lateral lip (*labium*) may be defined. The *medial lip* of the linea aspera begins above at the pectineal line; the *lateral lip* begins at the gluteal tuberosity. At the lower end of the femur, the two lips diverge as the medial and lateral *supracondylar lines;* between them is the broad and smooth *popliteal surface.*

The expanded **lower end** of the femur terminates in two rounded **condyles**, a lateral and a medial, for articulation with corresponding condyles of the tibia. The articular surfaces on the condyles blend together anteriorly to form the *patellar articular surface.* Posteriorly, the condyles are separated by a deep **intercondylar fossa**. An *intercondylar line* demarcates the fossa from the femur's popliteal surface. On the sides of the condyles are roughened **lateral** and **medial epicondyles**. The medial epicondyle is surmounted by a projection, the **adductor tubercle.** The femoral condyles are further discussed in Chapter 18 in connection with the knee. In addition to the ligaments of the knee, a number of muscles attach to the lower end of the femur (see Fig. 17-6C and D).

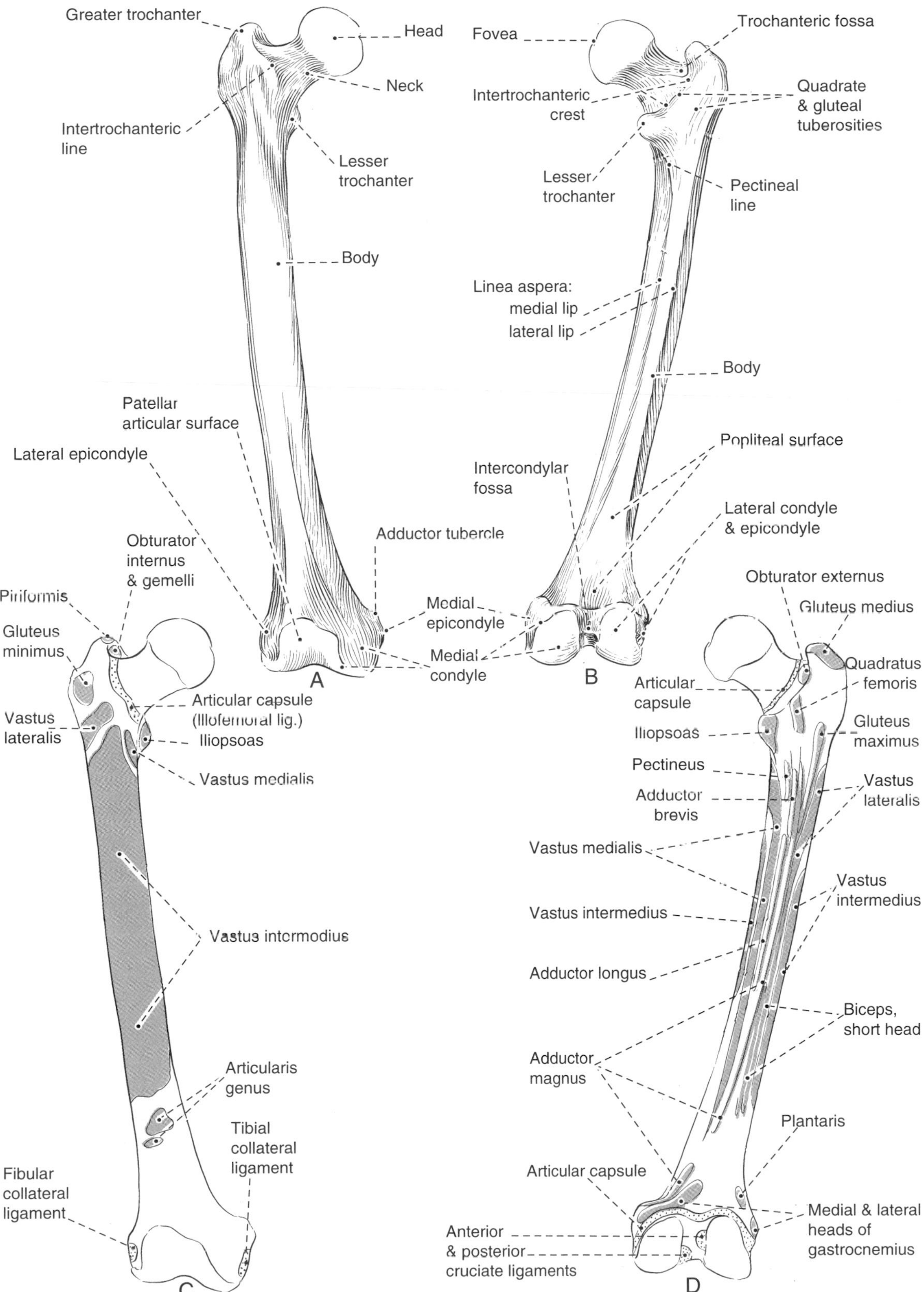

FIGURE 17-6.
The right femur, showing its anatomic features in (A) an anterior and (B) a posterior view, and the muscles that are attached to its (C) anterior and (D) posterior surfaces. Sites of origin are *red*, insertions *blue*.

Angles of the Femur. There are three angulations in the femur: the angle of inclination, the angle of torsion, and the angle of the shaft. The angle between the neck and body of the femur is the **angle of inclination**. It decreases from about 150° at birth to 126° to 128° in adulthood, reaching 120° in old age. A deformity caused by a decrease in the angle of inclination is known as *coxa vara*; it essentially shortens the leg and also limits abduction at the hip. Because of the medial displacement of the line of force acting on the hip joint in relation to the knee, the knee tends to be forced into a so-called *valgus deformity* (bowlegs). An increase in the angle of inclination (*coxa valga*) lengthens the limb and mimics contracture of the hip abductors (see Fig. 17-19). Because of the relative lateral displacement of the weight-bearing force line, the knee becomes predisposed to a *varus deformity* (knock-knees).

The forward projection of the femoral neck is described as the **angle of torsion**. This angle is measured between the axis of the neck and the transverse axis that passes through the femoral epicondyles; it is normally about 12° to 14°. An increase (*anteversion*) or decrease (*retroversion*) in the angle of torsion influences rotation of the limb at the hip and produces a gait with "toeing in" or "toeing out," respectively. In addition, anteversion displaces the body's center of mass anteriorly in relation to the knee, predisposing the latter to hyperextension. Retroversion, on the other hand, tends to produce knee flexion and recruits the knee extensors to stabilize the joint.

Finally, the shaft of the femur makes an angle of about 10° with the vertical tibia. During normal standing, the medial condyles of the two femora contact one another at the knee, but the upper ends of the femoral shafts are separated by the width of the pelvis and the lengths of the femoral necks. Rotatory movements of the weight-bearing femur take place not around the long axis of the shaft, but around the axis that connects the femoral head and the medial condyle. This distinction is important in considering muscle action at the hip.

Palpation

At the upper end of the femur, palpable bony points include the greater trochanter and the head. The trochanter is directly inferior to the tubercle of the iliac crest and its tip is on level with the anterior superior iliac spine and the ischial tuberosity (Nélaton's line). The femoral head, neck, and lesser trochanter are deeply buried in muscles; the head, however, may be palpated through the overlying muscles, halfway between the pubic symphysis and the anterior superior iliac spine. None of the shaft is directly palpable. Palpable points at the lower end are discussed with the knee.

Ossification. The body of the femur begins to ossify from a primary center, which appears in the seventh or eighth prenatal week. A secondary center appears for the distal end just before full term is reached, and another one develops in the cartilaginous head during the first postnatal year. The presence of the distal epiphysis is one reference by which the age of a viable fetus can be estimated. During years 4 to 5, an epiphysis appears for the greater trochanter (Fig. 17-7A), and after the age of 10 years, one for the lesser trochanter as well. The epiphyses of the head and the trochanters fuse with the shaft between the 16th and 18th year, and the lower end joins a year or so later.

A so-called **slipped femoral epiphysis** results when

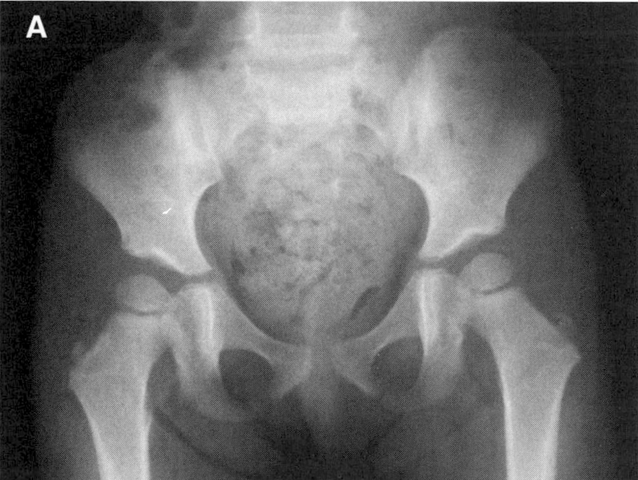

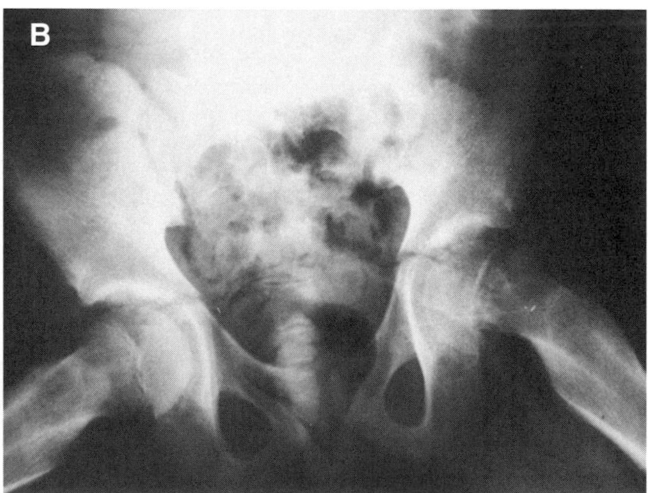

FIGURE *17-7.*
Ossification of the coxal bone and the upper end of the femur: (A) In a 5-year-old child, the ilium is separated from the pubis and ischium in the acetabulum by radiolucent hyaline cartilage; the same is true for the inferior ramus of the pubis and the ramus of the ischium. Growth plate cartilage separates the epiphysis of the head of the femur from the femoral neck; secondary ossification centers have appeared for the greater trochanters. (B) Slipped epiphysis of the left femur. The radiograph was taken in the so-called frog-leg position, with the thighs abducted and laterally rotated. Compare the normal epiphysis on the right with that of the left. Note also that bony union has not yet taken place in the acetabulum. (A, courtesy of Dr. Eric L. Effmann; B, courtesy of Dr. Rosalind H. Troupin.)

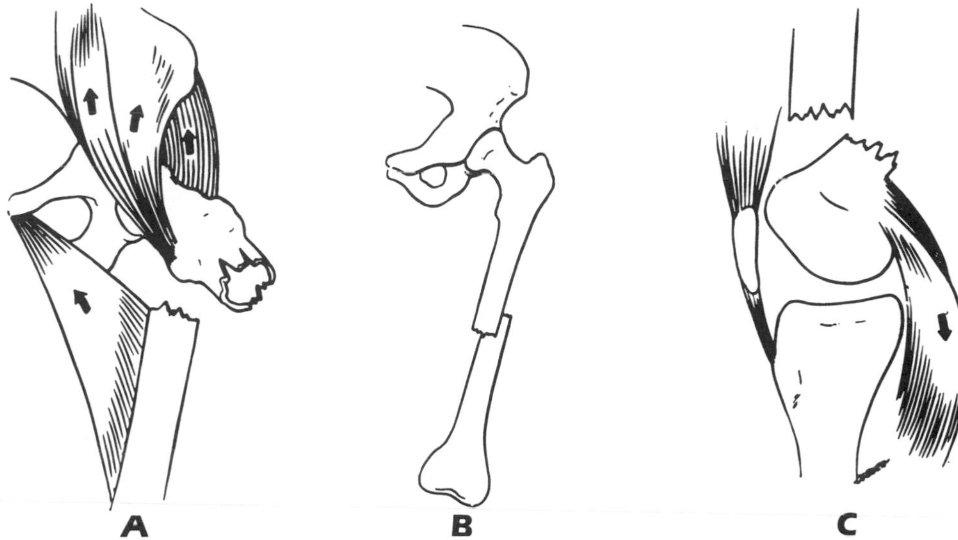

FIGURE 17-8.
Typical displacement in fractures in the upper, middle, and lower parts of the shaft of the femur. (A) The upper fragment is flexed, abducted, and laterally rotated; the lower fragment is adducted, and the limb is shortened. (B) Overriding of the fragments is shown. (C) A lateral view; the lower fragment is rotated backwards (flexed). (Ivins JC. Modern medicine annual. New York: Harcourt Brace Jovanovich, 1951; 222.)

the forces to which the head of the femur is subjected during weight bearing displace the epiphysis of the head before its bony union with the neck is established (see Fig. 17-7B). The displacement may damage the blood vessels that supply the head, and the ischemic changes may result in softening and degeneration of the epiphysis (ischemic or avascular necrosis). As a consequence of abnormal growth, there will be permanent deformity even though, with time, the deformed femoral head becomes revascularized. In many cases, ischemic necrosis of the proximal femoral epiphysis occurs without any demonstrable slip of the epiphysis. This condition is known as *osteochondrosis* or Legg-Calvé-Perthes disease.

Blood Supply. Multiple arteries enter the proximal and distal epiphyses of the femur and one or two enter its shaft. The nutrient arteries of the shaft are usually derived from branches of the *profunda femoris artery* (see Figs. 14-9 and 18-19). They enter the femur close to the linea aspera and run up and down in the marrow cavity. The arteries that supply the head and neck of the bone are particularly important, owing to their vulnerability in cases of slipped femoral epiphysis and femoral neck fracture. These vessels are related to the hip joint and are discussed with the blood supply of that joint (see Fig. 17-17).

Fractures. Fracture of the femur as a result of violence may occur at any level. Because of the pull of muscles that are attached to the fractured pieces of bone, rotation and displacement of the fragments occurs in a characteristic fashion, depending on the site of the fracture. Fractures of the femoral neck occur in the elderly because the bone, weakened by osteoporosis, cannot withstand the forces to which it is subjected. The complications of this fracture are a consequence of injury to the vessels that supply the femoral neck (see Fig. 17-17) and of the intra-articular location of the fracture (further discussed with the hip joint).

Fractures below the trochanters are accompanied by displacement of the upper fragment owing to the pull of the numerous muscles attaching here. The limb is also shortened as a result of the upward pull of muscles attaching to the femur below the fracture (Fig. 17-8A). Fractures a little above the condyles are accompanied by a posterior displacement of the lower fragment by muscles of the calf that originate from the femur (Fig. 17-8C). This displacement is particularly dangerous because the sharp edge of bone may damage the popliteal vessels as they lie close to the femur's popliteal surface.

Lumbosacral Plexus

The lower limb, like the upper limb, is innervated through a nerve plexus derived from anterior rami of spinal nerves (see Chap. 14). This is the lumbosacral plexus; the lumbar part is located in the abdomen, the sacral part in the pelvis (Fig. 17-9). The major nerves that issue from it to supply the lower limb are derived from the **anterior rami of L-2 to S-3** spinal nerves (see Figs. 14-6 and 17-9). Although L-1 and S-4 are often included in representations of the lumbosacral plexus, they usually supply only a limited area of skin in the inguinal (L-1) and perianal (S-4) regions, and have no muscular distribution in the limb. On occasion, however, one or the other may supply both muscle and skin in the limb. If such is the case for L-1, the plexus is said to be *prefixed;* if S-4 is a major contributor, the plexus is *postfixed*.

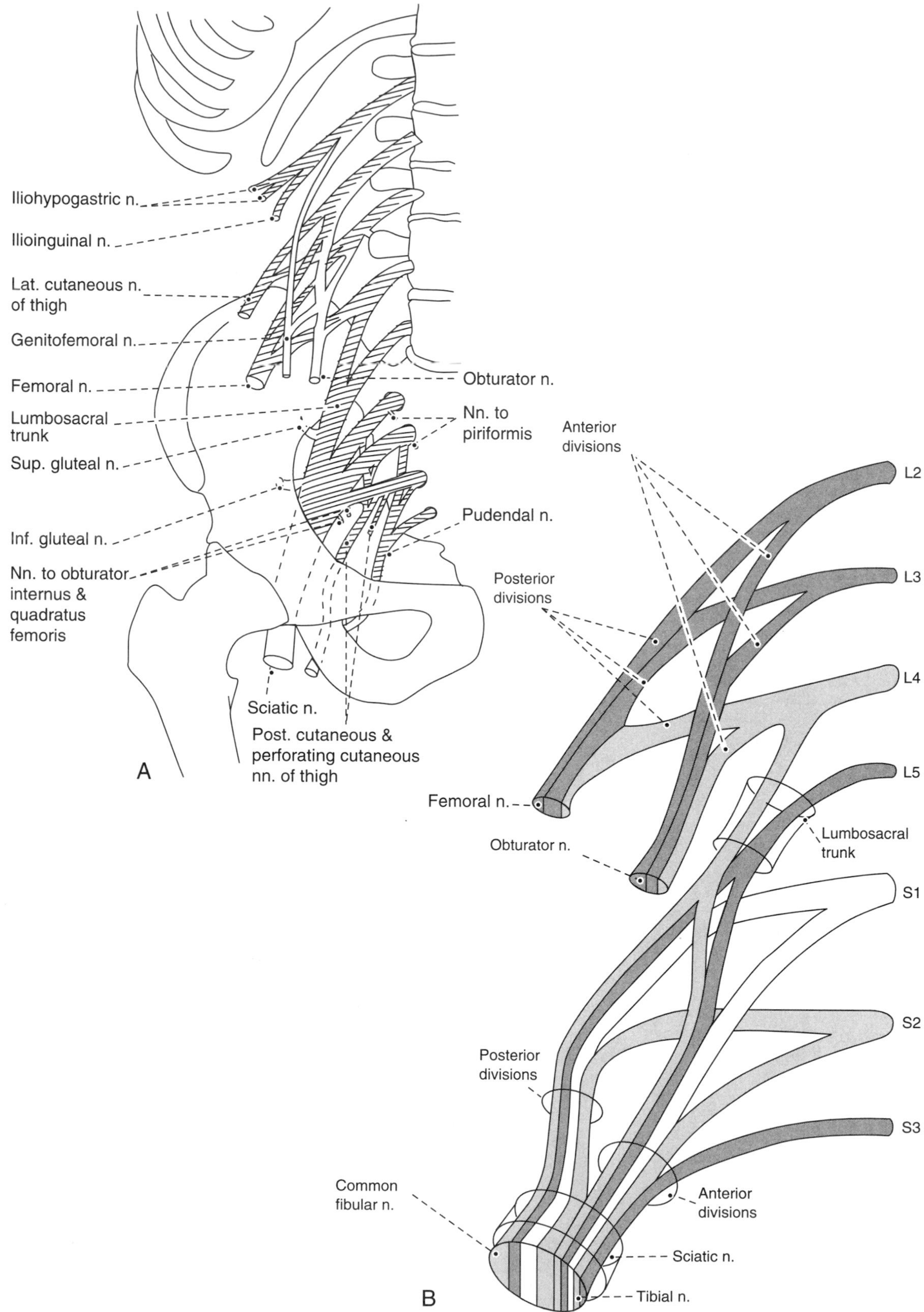

FIGURE *17-9.*
Location, formation, and branches of the lumbosacral plexus. (A) Diagrammatic representation of the lumbosacral plexus in relation to the vertebral column and the bony pelvis. All branches of the plexus are indicated. (B) The basic plan of the lumbosacral plexus and its main terminal branches. Each root of the plexus is designated by a *different color* to illustrate the manner of its distribution.

The lumbosacral plexus conforms to the basic plan of a limb plexus, discussed in Chapter 14. Each **root,** representing an anterior ramus, splits into an **anterior** and a **posterior division** for the respective supply of the flexor or extensor compartment of the limb. The divisions are then regrouped into the definitive major nerves that proceed to the lower limb. In contrast with the brachial plexus (see Chap. 15), there are no trunks or cords interposed between the divisions and the definitive nerves.

Contributing Nerve Fiber Types

The lumbosacral plexus is composed preponderantly of somatic nerve fibers. The **somatic efferents** are the axons of neurons in the lateral portions of the anterior horns of gray matter in spinal cord segments L-2 to S-3. These groups of neurons are chiefly responsible for the lumbar enlargement of the cord (see Chap. 13; Fig. 13-14). The cell bodies of **somatic afferents** concerned with exteroceptive (pain, temperature, pressure, and touch) and proprioceptive (joint position sense and muscle spindle) impulses from the lower limb are located in L-2 to S-3 spinal ganglia. **Sympathetic efferents** control vasomotor activity and sweating in the lower limb. They enter the plexus as postsynaptic fibers through gray rami communicantes contributed to each root of the plexus by lumbar and sacral sympathetic chain ganglia. The presynaptic neurons for the sympathetic outflow to the lower limb are located in the lateral column of gray matter in T-10 to L-2 segments (see Chap. 13). All presynaptic fibers that relay to the lower limb enter the sympathetic chain through white rami communicantes at or above the anterior ramus of the L-2 spinal nerve. Therefore, resection of the upper three lumbar sympathetic ganglia with the intervening sympathetic trunk deprives the lower limb of all sympathetic innervation. Severe and chronic vasospasm, one of the causes of painful ischemic changes in the foot, which can lead to gangrene (Raynaud's disease), may be eliminated by such a *lumbar sympathectomy.*

Formation

Lumbar Plexus. As soon as L-2, L-3, and L-4 roots of the lumbar plexus split off from their spinal nerves and emerge from the intervertebral foramina, they are engulfed by the psoas major muscle, because this muscle is attached to the lateral surfaces and transverse processes of the lumbar vertebrae (see Fig. 25-2). Within the psoas, the roots split into anterior and posterior divisions, which then reunite to form the branches of the plexus; the latter emerge from the muscle along either its lateral or medial border. The **femoral nerve,** formed by the posterior divisions of L-2, L-3, and L-4, descends from the plexus lateral to the psoas muscle. The anterior divisions of the same roots unite to form the other major branch of the lumbar part of the plexus, the **obturator nerve,** which leaves the psoas major medially (see Fig. 25-2).

Only a portion of the L-4 anterior ramus contributes to the lumbar plexus; the remaining smaller part, along with L-5 root, forms the **lumbosacral trunk** that descends into the pelvis and feeds into the sacral plexus (see Fig. 17-9B). The lumbosacral trunk and the obturator nerve enter the pelvis on the ala of the sacrum, medial to the psoas major.

Sacral Plexus. The anterior rami of S-1, S-2, and S-3 emerge from the anterior (pelvic) foramina of the sacrum and proceed laterally on the anterior surface of the piriformis (see Fig. 27-11). The lumbosacral trunk joins the sacral roots and fuses with S-1. The plexus lies in the posterior wall of the pelvic cavity; its relations are described in Chapter 27.

All the roots, including L-4 and L-5 contained in the lumbosacral trunk, split into anterior and posterior divisions (see Fig. 17-9B). However, the separation of these divisions is not apparent without dissection. Anterior and posterior divisions converge laterally to form a large nerve trunk, the **sciatic nerve,** which leaves the pelvis through the greater sciatic foramen. As explained in Chapter 14, the sciatic nerve is actually composed of two nerves that usually separate from one another just above the knee. Sometimes, however, they may issue independently from the plexus and leave the pelvis as separate entities. They are the common fibular and tibial nerves. The posterior divisions of L-4, L-5, S-1, and S-2 form the **common fibular** (*common peroneal*) **nerve;** the corresponding anterior divisions, plus the anterior division of S-3, form the **tibial nerve** (see Fig. 17-9B). The posterior division of S-3 is represented in minor, cutaneous branches of the plexus.

Branches

Main Terminal Branches. The lumbosacral plexus has four main terminal branches: the femoral and obturator nerves and the common fibular and tibial nerves. These nerves are introduced in general terms in Chapter 14 (see Fig. 14-8). Although the course and branching pattern of each are described with the regions of the lower limb in the next chapter, it is useful to attach functional labels to them at this juncture.

The **femoral nerve** (L-2, L-3, and L-4) is the nerve of knee extension and hip flexion (see Figs. 14-8A and 18-13). It also supplies a large area of skin on the anteromedial aspect of the thigh and the medial aspect of the leg and foot. Clinically, it is best evaluated by testing the power of knee extension and cutaneous sensitivity over the medial side of the ankle.

The **obturator nerve** (L-2, L-3, and L-4) is the nerve of the adductors of the hip and is best evaluated clinically by testing the power of adduction (see Figs. 14-8C and 18-21). Its cutaneous distribution is restricted to a small area on the medial side of the thigh.

The **common fibular nerve** (L-4, L-5, S-1, and S-2; see Figs. 14-8B and 18-31) is the chief nerve of ankle dorsiflexion (i.e., extension) and is best evaluated by testing the power of ankle dorsiflexion. Its cutaneous distribution is limited to the lateral aspect of the calf and the dorsum of the foot.

The **tibial nerve** (L-4, L-5, S-1, S-2, and S-3) is the chief nerve of flexion of the knee, ankle, and toes, as well as the nerve of the intrinsic muscles of the foot (see Figs. 14-8D and E and 18-28). In the foot it splits into the *medial* and *lateral plantar nerves,* equivalents of the median and ulnar nerves. Its clinical evaluation is complex and can be meaningful only after the regional distribution of the nerve is understood.

Minor Branches. In addition to the four major nerves, there are several small lumbar and sacral branches given off by the plexus; they supply skin and muscle in the limb and also in the perineum (see Fig. 17-9A). The names of most of these nerves are derived from the structures they innervate. The minor branches include four *cutaneous nerves,* the first of which has a minor muscular distribution as well (genitofemoral nerve, lateral cutaneous nerve of the thigh, and posterior and perforating cutaneous nerves of the thigh), four *muscular branches* (superior and inferior gluteal nerves, nerve to the obturator internus muscle, and nerve to the quadratus femoris muscle), and a mixed muscular and cutaneous branch destined for the perineum, the *pudendal nerve.* Omitted from Figure 17-9A is an occasional branch of the lumbar plexus, the *accessory obturator nerve* (which, if present, supplies the pectineus muscle). The *ilioinguinal* and *iliohypogastric nerves,* both derived from L-1, do not properly belong to the lower limb plexus, although they are customarily included among its branches. All these nerves are best dealt with after the muscles and skin they innervate have been discussed.

Injuries

Gunshot wounds are the most frequent cause of discrete lesions within the lumbosacral plexus or its branches. Dislocation of the hip, fracture of the pelvis, or pelvic neoplasms may also compromise various nerves. The functional loss associated with nerve lesions is discussed with the respective nerves.

GLUTEAL REGION

The soft tissues of the gluteal region include deep and superficial fascia with associated cutaneous nerves and vessels, muscles with their associated nerves and vessels, and

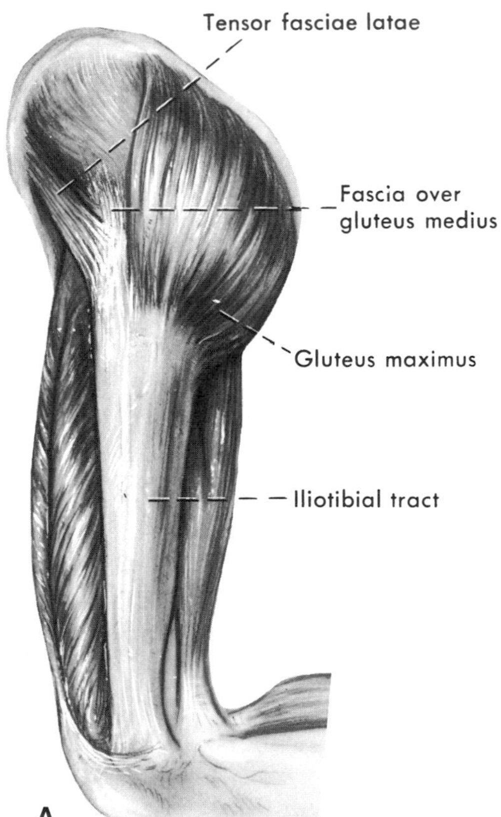

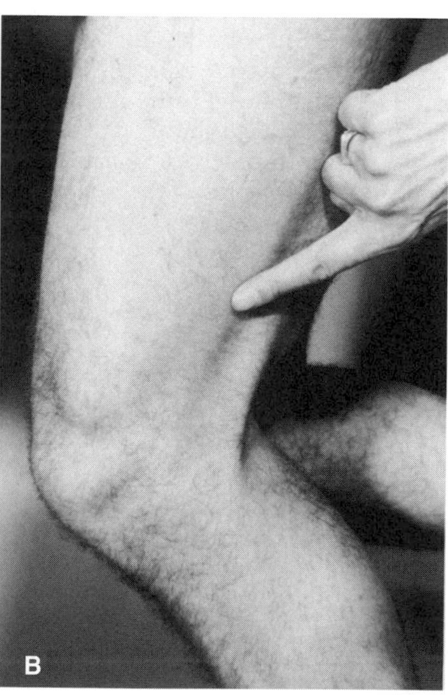

FIGURE *17-10.*
The iliotibial tract and the muscles associated with it: (A) Lateral view of the thigh and gluteal region showing the iliotibial tract, tensor fasciae latae, and gluteus maximus. (B) The iliotibial tract, seen anterior to the tendon of the biceps femoris, is an important factor in stabilizing the flexed knee when it is supporting the body weight (Note, the right leg is off the ground.)

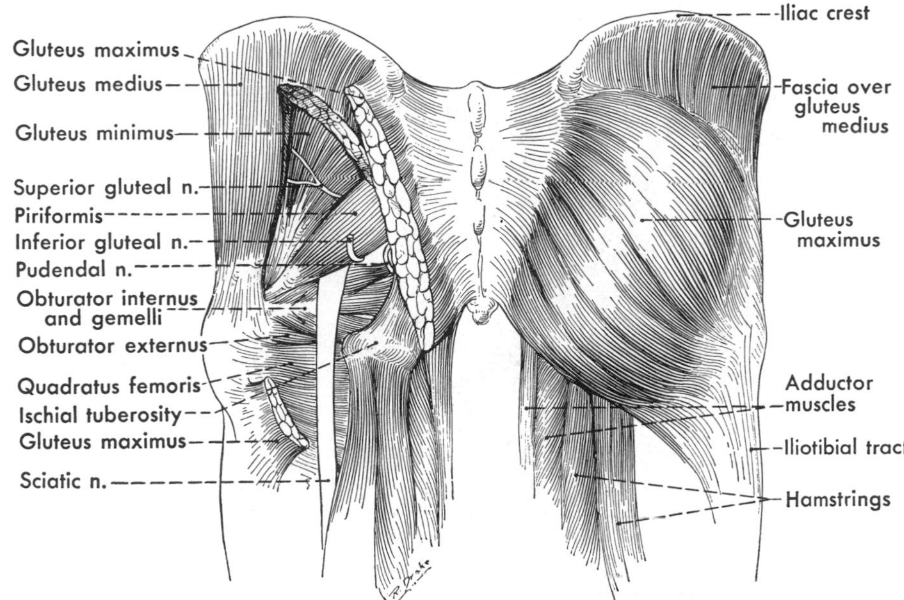

FIGURE *17-11.* **Muscles of the gluteal region seen from the back. On the *left side* the gluteus maximus has been resected and a wedge has been removed from the gluteus medius.**

the sciatic nerve that passes through the region on its way to supply the free limb.

Fascia

Superficial Fascia

The characteristic shape of the buttock is largely due to the pad of adipose tissue that occupies the gluteal region. Large lobules of fat are supported by coarse fibrous septa of the tela subcutanea. The quantity of fat decreases as the fascia continues into the neighboring regions of the back, the lateral and anterior aspects of the abdomen and the thigh. Small nerves and blood vessels reach the skin through the superficial fascia after they have pierced the deep fascia.

Deep Fascia

Like the upper limb, the lower limb is invested in a sheath of deep fascia composed of a rather substantial and inelastic connective tissue membrane. Although it forms a more or less continuous stocking, it is known by different names in different regions. It is called the **fascia lata** (*lata;* Latin for broad) over the thigh. The fascia lata extends into the hip and gluteal regions to attach to bony prominences and ligaments associated with the pelvis. These include the length of the iliac crest, the inguinal ligament, the conjoint ramus and ischial tuberosity, the sacrotuberous ligament, and the sacrum. In the gluteal region, the deep fascia splits into two laminae around the gluteus maximus, the large, superficial muscle of the buttock (Figs. 17-10 and 17-11). A strong tendinous reinforcement, the **iliotibial tract,** commences in the fascia lata in the region of the greater trochanter (see Fig. 17-10). A substantial part of the gluteus maximus, as well as another muscle known as the *tensor fasciae latae,* inserts into the tract, which then descends along the lateral aspect of the thigh and inserts on the lateral condyle of the tibia.

Cutaneous Nerves and Vessels

As in the pectoral and shoulder regions, most of the skin over the buttock is supplied by nerves of the trunk, rather than branches of the limb plexus. Two groups of cutaneous nerves enter this region: the **clunial nerves** given off by posterior rami of lumbar and sacral nerves, and cutaneous branches of the **subcostal** and **iliohypogastric nerves**, which are the anterior rami of T-12 and L-1 spinal nerves (see Figs. 17-9 and 18-7).

The *superior clunial nerves* (see Fig. 18-7) are lateral branches of the posterior rami of the upper three lumbar nerves. They cross the posterior part of the iliac crest and descend into the buttock. The **middle clunial nerves**, lateral branches of the posterior rami of the first three sacral nerves, pass laterally from the posterior sacral foramina into the buttock. The **inferior clunial nerves** curve around the lower border of the gluteus maximus and are derived from the *posterior cutaneous nerve of the thigh,* a branch of the lumbosacral plexus (see Fig. 18-7).

The small vascular twigs that are embedded in the superficial fascia are branches of the **gluteal vessels.** These enter the buttock through the greater sciatic foramen and supply all its contents. **Lymphatics** from the superficial and deep tissues of the entire region, commencing in the posterior midline within the natal cleft, drain to the lateral group of inguinal lymph nodes (see Fig 18-9).

Muscles

The gluteal region contains the chief abductor and extensor muscles of the hip joint, as well as a group of muscles that

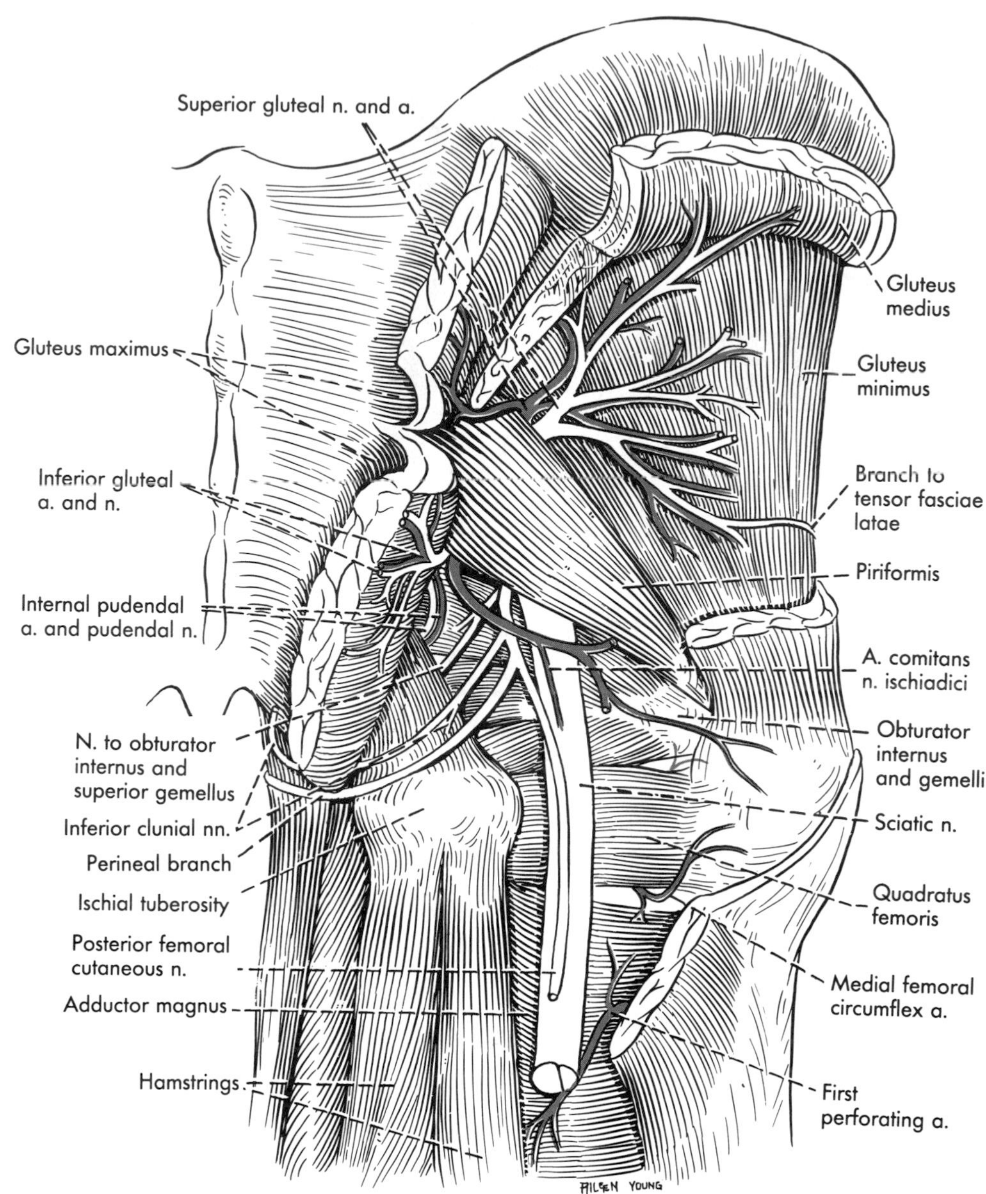

FIGURE *17-12.*
Nerves and vessels of the gluteal region in relation to the piriformis and other muscles.

contribute to rotation of the femur. Some of these muscles also participate in flexion and extension of the hip.

The most superficial muscles are the large **gluteus maximus** posteriorly and the smaller **tensor fasciae latae** anteriorly (see Fig. 17-10). The chief action of the former is hip extension, and of the latter, hip flexion. In a deeper layer beneath are the **gluteus medius** and **gluteus minimus** muscles, the main abductors of the hip (see Fig. 17-11). Five short muscles constitute the deepest layer: the **piriformis**, the **obturator internus**, and the two **gemellus** muscles associated with it, and the **quadratus femoris** (Figs. 17-11 and 17-12). They form a muscular cuff around the posterior aspect of the hip joint capsule and the neck of the femur. Their chief action is implied by the name given to this group: **short rotators** of the hip. All are innervated from the sacral plexus by minor branches which, as a rule, bear names that reflect the muscles they supply (see Fig. 17-9).

Tensor Fasciae Latae

This muscle's name acknowledges its insertion into the iliotibial tract (see Fig. 17-10). However, the function implied by its name is much less important than its action as a hip flexor, and an antagonist of the gluteus maximus (see next section). It arises from the anterior part of the iliac crest (see Fig. 17-3C) and passes downward and backward. Just below the level of the greater trochanter, its tendon helps form the iliotibial tract. The *superior gluteal nerve* (see Figs. 17-9A and 17-12) terminates in it and supplies it (L-4 and L-5).

Gluteus Maximus

The largest single muscle in the body, the gluteus maximus is the most powerful extensor of the hip. It originates over a wide area on the back of the bony pelvis (see Fig. 17-11), including the posterior end of the iliac crest and ilium (see Fig. 17-3C), the sacrum, coccyx, and the sacrotuberous ligament. Only the deep fibers of the lower half of this thick, quadrangular muscle insert into the gluteal tuberosity of the femur (see Fig. 17-6D); the remaining and far greater number insert into the iliotibial tract. The *inferior gluteal nerve* (see Figs. 17-9A and 17-12) conveys L-5, S-1, and S-2 fibers to it (see Table 13-1 and Fig 13-23).

The gluteus maximus covers most of the muscles, and all nerves and vessels, in the buttock. Of the two layers of the fascia lata that invest the muscle, the deep one is thickened and contains the inferior gluteal nerve and vessels. There are usually two **bursae** associated with the gluteus maximus over the greater trochanter: one between the trochanter and the muscle (*gluteus maximus bursa*), and the other between the muscle and the skin (*subcutaneous trochanteric bursa*). Either of these bursae may become inflamed and give rise to hip pain (see Functional Evaluation). The diagnosis is made by localizing tenderness to the region of the bursae by palpation.

Action. Despite its preeminence among hip extensors, the gluteus maximus is called into action only during rapid and powerful extension or when resistance has to be overcome. In the normal gait cycle, hip extension is achieved primarily by the *hamstring muscles* (see Figs. 17-11 and 18-17) that arise from the gluteal tuberosity. Paralysis of the gluteus maximus does not seriously compromise ambulation on level ground. Where the muscle is definitely required is for hip extension in such actions as climbing, going upstairs, or getting up from a squatting position. Furthermore, both the hamstrings and the glutei contract when the trunk is swayed forward and will continue to be active as long as the gravitational force line from the body's center of mass falls anterior to the hip. They stop contracting as soon as the trunk is restored to a vertical position above the hip. The gluteus maximus can extend the femur not only through its bony attachment but also through the iliotibial tract. Although the latter descends to the tibia and crosses the knee joint, the gluteus maximus does not move the knee because the tract is fixed along its length to the femur through the lateral intermuscular septum of the thigh (see Fig. 18-10). Acting through the iliotibial tract, the gluteus maximus, together with the tensor fasciae latae, controls anteroposterior tilting of the pelvis when the body weight is supported on one leg. These two muscles are recruited when the leg is slightly flexed at the hip and knee, thereby foregoing the stabilizing effect of the ligaments at these joints. Although the tensor fasciae latae is a flexor of the hip, it controls hip extension produced by the force of gravity, just as the gluteus maximus controls hip flexion, counterbalancing the gravitational pull.

Gluteus Medius and Minimus

These two fan-shaped muscles are the chief abductors of the hip (see Figs. 17-11 and 17-12). They originate on the lateral surface of the ilium (see Fig. 17-3C), the minimus anterior and deep to the medius, and insert by separate tendons into the greater trochanter (see Fig. 17-6C and D).

The **gluteus medius** arises from the ala of the ilium between the iliac crest, the anterior gluteal line, and the posterior gluteal line, and also from the deep fascia covering the muscle. It inserts into the large posterior part of the upper surface of the greater trochanter. The **gluteus minimus** arises from the ilium between the anterior and inferior gluteal lines and inserts in front of the gluteus medius on the upper and anterior surface of the greater trochanter.

Action. The gluteus medius and minimus are relaxed when the body weight is supported on both legs; otherwise, however, they are in constant use despite that abduction of the femur, as such, seems an unusual movement in everyday activity. During walking, the two abductors on one side alternate with those of the other side, a fact that may be confirmed if the hands are placed over the muscles just below the iliac crests. The contraction occurs on the side of the stance leg, its purpose being to prevent the pelvis from sagging on the opposite side. When standing on one leg, voluntary relaxation of the abductors results in tilting of the pelvis downward on the unsupported side, mimicking abductor weakness or paralysis. Voluntary increase in the contraction of these muscles tilts the pelvis upward, mimicking contracture of the abductor musculature. The importance of such pelvic tilts relative to ambulation is considered in Chapter 18. During clinical evaluation, the efficiency of the abductors may be tested by observing the level of the two anterior and posterior superior iliac spines (see Fig. 17-5) while the subject is standing on one leg. If the abductors are weak, the anterior and posterior superior iliac spines will sag on the opposite side. This maneuver is known as the Trendelenburg test. The test is positive when the pelvis tilts downward on the unsupported side, signifying weakness of the abductors. The power of the abductors of one side may be assessed more accurately when the subject, lying on the contralateral side, abducts the thigh against gravity and against resistance applied by the examiner.

Both abductors are supplied from L-4, L-5, and S-1 segments by the superior gluteal nerve (see Table 13-1). The tensor fasciae latae (sharing the same nerve) and the upper fibers of the gluteus maximus (supplied by the inferior gluteal nerve) can assist in abduction.

Short Rotators

Numerous muscles, including those discussed in the foregoing, have a rotatory action on the femoral shaft, but only a few function primarily as rotators. These are the short muscles situated deep to the gluteus maximus: the **piriformis, obturator internus**, the **superior and inferior gemelli**, and the **quadratus femoris** (see Figs. 17-11 and 17-12). All insert around the trochanteric fossa (see Fig. 17-6C and D) and rotate the femur laterally. They are assisted by the *obturator externus* (located in the upper part of the thigh) and the gluteus maximus. The piriformis is supplied by twigs given off by the S-1 and S-2 roots of the sacral plexus; the *nerve to the obturator internus* supplies that muscle and the superior gemellus; the *nerve to the quadratus femoris* serves the inferior gemellus as well as its own muscle (see Fig. 17-12).

The **piriformis** arises from the anterior surface of the lateral mass of the 2nd, 3rd, and 4th sacral segments. The pyramid-shaped muscle exits the pelvis through the greater sciatic foramen and inserts on the summit of the greater trochanter (see Fig. 17-6C). The sacral plexus is formed largely on the pelvic surface of the piriformis, and the branches of the plexus emerge in the gluteal region along the superior and inferior margins of the muscle (see Fig. 17-12). The sciatic nerve, or a part of it, may pass through the piriformis, splitting the muscle into two.

The **obturator internus** has an extensive area of origin from the medial surface of the obturator membrane and part of the coxal bone that surrounds it (see Fig. 17-3D). The muscle tapers posteriorly to a narrow belly and tendon, and makes a sharp turn around the lesser sciatic notch to head toward its insertion just above the trochanteric fossa. The tendon is separated from the ischium by a large bursa and is joined posteriorly by the two gemellus muscles. The **superior gemellus** arises from the ischial spine, and the **inferior gemellus** from the ischial tuberosity. They insert into the tendon of the obturator internus (see Fig. 17-12). Below the obturator internus and the gemelli is a short, quadrangular muscle, the **quadratus femoris**. It arises from the ischial tuberosity and inserts on the quadrate tubercle and adjoining parts of the intertrochanteric crest (see Fig.17-6D).

Nerves and Vessels

With the exception of the cutaneous nerves discussed earlier, the nerves of the buttock are branches of the sacral plexus. The vessels of the region are branches of the internal iliac artery (see Figs 27-8 and 27-9) or tributaries of the internal iliac vein. Both the plexus and the internal iliac vessels are located in the pelvic cavity. Nerves and vessels leave and enter the pelvis with the piriformis muscle (see Fig. 17-12). Those for which distribution is primarily confined to the buttock are the superior and inferior gluteal nerves and vessels and the two small nerves to the obturator internus and quadratus femoris. Those that pass through the buttock to another distribution are the internal pudendal vessels, the pudendal nerve, the posterior cutaneous nerve of the thigh, and the sciatic nerve.

The **superior gluteal nerve** contains fibers from the fourth and fifth lumbar and first sacral roots of the plexus. It enters the buttock with the **superior gluteal artery** above the piriformis, lying deep to the gluteus maximus and medius (see Fig. 17-12). The artery sends a superficial branch into the overlying gluteus maximus, and its deep branch passes upward and laterally, along with the nerve, in the fascial plane between the gluteus medius and minimus. They supply these muscles and the nerve continues beyond them into the tensor fasciae latae. The **inferior gluteal nerve** and **vessels** enter the buttock below the piriformis muscle (see Fig. 17-12). The nerve contains fibers from the fifth lumbar and first two sacral roots of the plexus, and the artery is a branch of the internal iliac artery. Both nerve and artery supply the gluteus maximus. The artery gives off other muscular twigs and unnamed anastomotic branches that join the **cruciate** or **crucial anastomosis** formed by a number of vessels around the upper end of the femur (see later). The **arteria comitans nervi ischiadici** is a small branch of the inferior gluteal artery. As its name implies, it accompanies the sciatic nerve (*nervus ischiadicus*), and is the remnant of the *axial artery* of the developing lower limb (see Chap. 14).

The **nerve to the obturator internus** receives fibers from the fifth lumbar and first two sacral roots of the plexus. It enters the buttock below the piriformis muscle and crosses the posterior surface of the superior gemellus, giving off a twig into it. It then reenters the pelvis on the surface of the obturator internus muscle (see Fig. 17-12) and supplies its fan-shaped belly on the lateral wall of the pelvis. The **nerve to the quadratus femoris** receives fibers from the fourth and fifth lumbar and first sacral roots of the plexus, and also emerges below the piriformis muscle. It passes downward and deep to the obturator internus and the sciatic nerve, and enters the deep surface of the inferior gemellus and quadratus femoris.

Of the nerves and vessels that pass through the buttock without supplying structures in it, the pudendal nerve and the internal pudendal vessels are the most medial and have the shortest course in the buttock. The **pudendal nerve** is a branch of the sacral plexus, and the **internal pudendal artery** a branch of the internal iliac. They serve the perineum. They leave the pelvis with the piriformis, appear in the buttock at the lower margin of the muscle and descend, crossing the posterior surface of the superior gemellus (see Fig. 17-12) and, deep to it, the spine of the ischium. To reach the perineum, the nerve and artery pass medially through the lesser sciatic foramen. The **internal pudendal vein** runs with the artery and nerve.

The **posterior cutaneous nerve of the thigh** is a branch of the sacral plexus, made up predominantly of S-2 and S-3 fibers. It enters the buttock at the lower border of the piriformis, medial to the sciatic nerve. While still under cover of the gluteus maximus, it gives off several *inferior clunial nerves* and some perineal branches. The clunial branches round the lower border of the gluteus maximus to reach skin over part of the buttock. The perineal branches pass medially and supply the medial side of the thigh and the perineum. The main posterior cutaneous nerve of the thigh runs down along the posterior midline of the thigh (see Fig. 18-7) and supplies an extensive area of skin.

The **sciatic nerve** is the largest nerve in the body. Its origin is described earlier (see under Lumbosacral Plexus and Fig. 17-9). Formed in the pelvis on the anterior surface of the piriformis, it emerges in the buttock below the piriformis (see Fig. 17-11). Here it is located half way between the ischial tuberosity and greater trochanter. Pressure may be applied on it through the gluteus maximus. As the nerve descends into the thigh under cover of the gluteus maximus, it runs across the posterior surfaces of the obturator internus, gemelli, and quadratus femoris (see Fig. 17-12). Entering the thigh, it disappears deep to (anterior to) the hamstring muscles, inferior to their origin from the ischial tuberosity. It does not supply any structures in the buttock, but its upper branches to the hamstring muscles may arise at or above the level of the ischial tuberosity.

There are variations in the course of the sciatic nerve through the gluteal region. Only in approximately 85% of cases does it pursue the course just described. In some 12% to 15% of instances, the nerve is divided by the piriformis muscle: the common fibular part comes through the muscle or above it, and only the tibial part passes below the muscle. When the two components of the sciatic nerve are thus kept apart, they may remain separate throughout their course, or they may unite below the piriformis. In rare cases (less than 1%) the entire sciatic nerve passes through the piriformis.

HIP REGION

The hip region includes the hip joint itself and the muscles, nerves, and vessels that are associated with its anterior and medial aspects. Many structures of the hip region proceed into the thigh. Describing them with the hip region, rather than with the thigh is more a matter of logistics than a true anatomic division between the hip and the thigh as distinct body regions. The attachments and actions of those muscles that move the hip can be reasoned from the examination of the skeleton. This information is presented in this section, whereas the anatomic relations of these structures (to be studied in the course of a dissection) are deferred for the next chapter.

Hip Joint

Without the stabilizing effect of surrounding muscles, the shoulder joints would dislocate if they had to sustain the weight of the body as in a handstand. The hip joints, on the other hand, are so constructed that the body weight can be supported on the femoral heads with minimal or no expenditure of muscular energy. Deeply molded articular surfaces and strong ligaments are the key factors in the stability of the hip joint.

Anatomy of the Joint

The hip is a **polyaxial synovial joint** (see Fig. 5-10) that joins the free lower limb to the pelvic girdle. The closely fitting ball-and-socket–shaped articular facets of the femoral head and acetabulum permit movement in all directions. In contrast with the shoulder joint, however, movements at the hip are limited by strong ligaments and interlocking articular surfaces.

Articular Surfaces. The head of the femur constitutes more than a hemisphere (see Figs. 17-6 and 17-13). With the exception of the **fovea**, a central, small, navel-like recess, it is completely covered by articular cartilage. By contrast, in the acetabulum, only the horseshoe-shaped **lunate articular surface** is covered by articular cartilage (see Fig. 17-3A). The central *acetabular fossa* and the *acetabular notch* below it lack cartilage. The bare bone is in contact with an intra-articular pad of fat (see Figs. 17-13 and 17-14). On both the femoral head and the acetabulum the cartilage is thickest superiorly, where the greatest weight is borne. This may be appreciated from a radiograph of the hip joint, which shows a band of radiolucency between the coxal bone and the femur. Although referred to by radiologists as the "joint space," it is filled by cartilage, which is radiolucent (see Fig. 17-13A). Only during squatting is the inferior aspect of the femoral head exposed to any weight-bearing.

The femoral head is retained in the acetabulum even after the capsule and muscle attachments around the joint have been severed. This is largely due to the **acetabular labrum**, a fibrocartilaginous lip that is attached to the bony rim of the acetabulum and increases the extent of the articular socket (see Fig. 17-14). The labrum is completed inferiorly by the **transverse ligament** of the acetabulum that bridges over the acetabular notch, a deficiency in the lower part of the bony rim. The labrum must be stretched or torn to pull the head from the acetabulum.

Capsule and Ligaments. The thick, fibrous capsule encloses a voluminous joint cavity containing the head and neck of the femur, as well as the *ligament of the head* with a fat pad surrounding it (see Fig. 17-14). Proximally, the capsule is attached to the bony rim of the acetabulum (see Fig. 17-3C), the acetabular labrum and the transverse ligament of the acetabulum. The femoral attachments are far beyond the articular margins; anteriorly, the capsule is attached between the bases of the two trochanters along the intertrochanteric line (see Fig. 17-6C); posteriorly, the attachment is to the base of the neck, thus excluding the trochanteric fossa from the joint cavity (see Fig. 17-6D). Up to the age of 18 to 19 years, the epiphyseal cartilage of the greater trochanter is partially intracapsular and that of the femoral head, completely intracapsular.

Bacteria carried by the blood may seed to the vascular region of the metaphysis in the femoral neck (Fig. 17-15A). Unless diagnosed early and treated appropriately, the focus of infection established in the growing bone (osteomyelitis) will expand, and the pus formed will burst through the cortex of the femoral neck, resulting in septic arthritis of the hip joint (see Fig. 17-15B). The destruction of intra-articular tissues such as articular cartilage will follow, with an end result of permanent disability. This outcome is a consequence of the epiphyseal plate at the proximal end of the femur being located within the hip joint cavity.

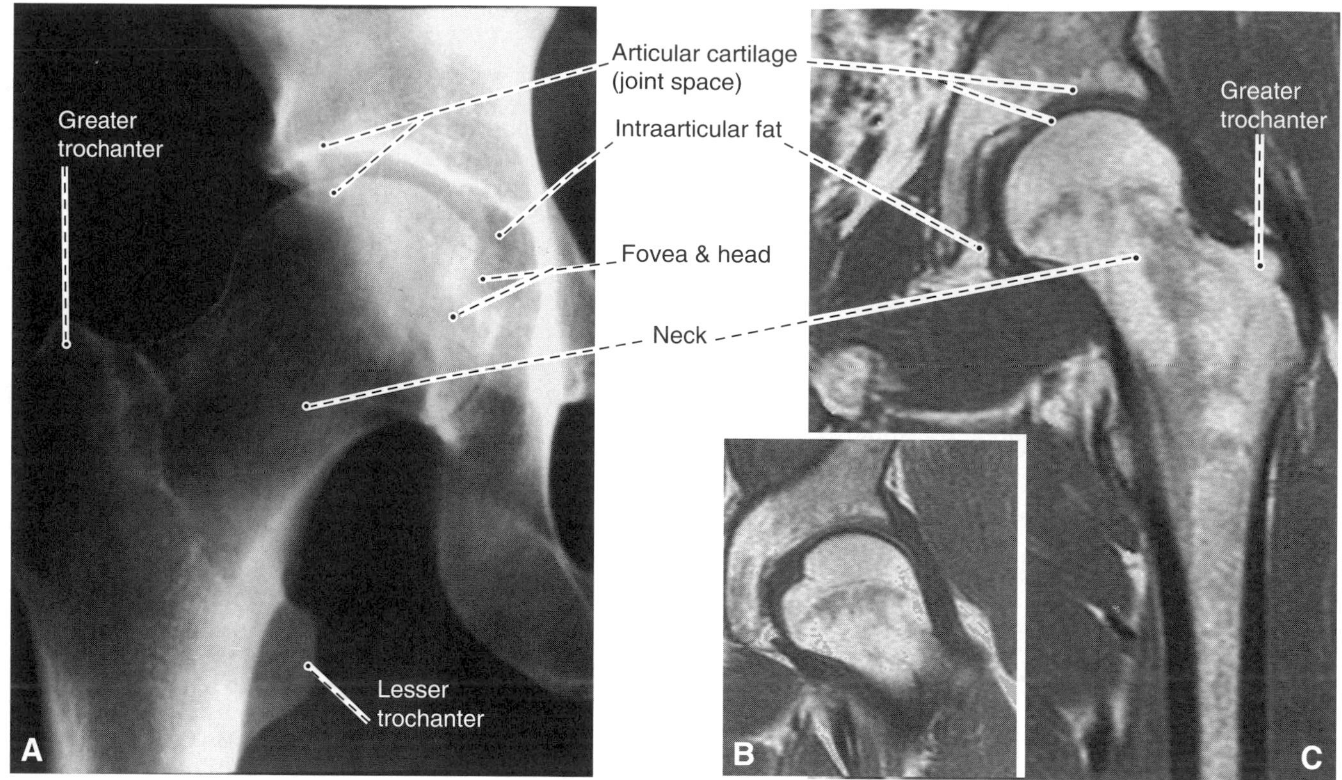

FIGURE *17-13.*
The anatomy of the hip joint revealed on (A) a radiograph and (B and C) by magnetic resonance imaging scans taken in the coronal plane. The imaging plane in panel B is anterior to that in panel C and cuts through the femoral head only. (A, courtesy of Dr. Rosalind H. Troupin; B and C, courtesy of Dr. Thurman Gillespy III.)

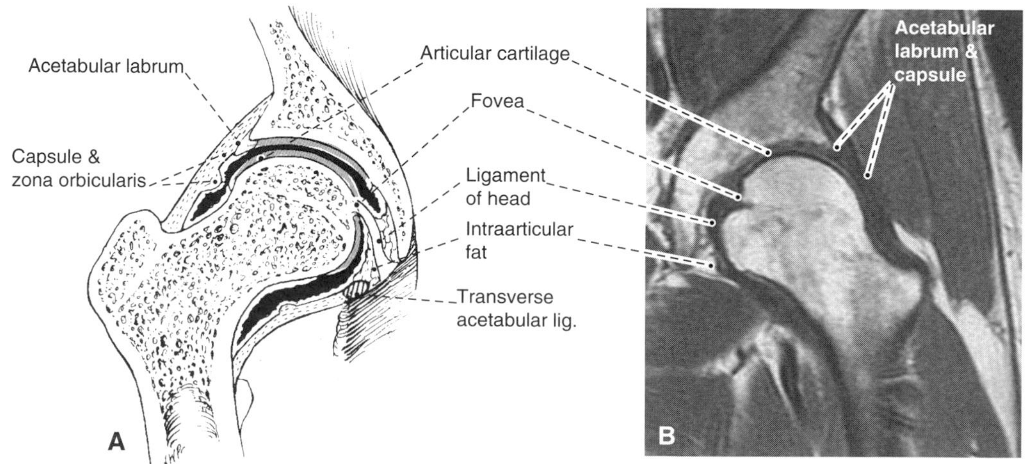

FIGURE *17-14.*
Coronal sections through the hip joint, shown (A) diagrammatically and (B) by a magnetic resonance imaging scan. In panel B, the fibrous tissue of the capsule appears dark. Adjacent to it superolaterally is the gluteus minimus, and inferiorly, the obturator externus. (B, courtesy of Dr. Thurman Gillespy III).

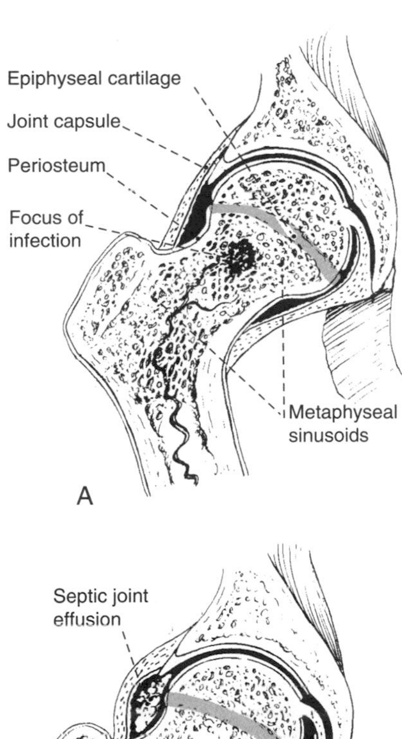

FIGURE 17-15.
Two stages of acute osteomyelitis in the upper end of the femur of a child illustrating the clinical relevance of intraarticular growth plates: (A) establishment of the infection in the metaphyseal sinusoids; (B) a stage reached in 2 to 3 weeks with extension of the pathologic process into the joint cavity. (Courtesy of Dr. D. Kay Clawson.)

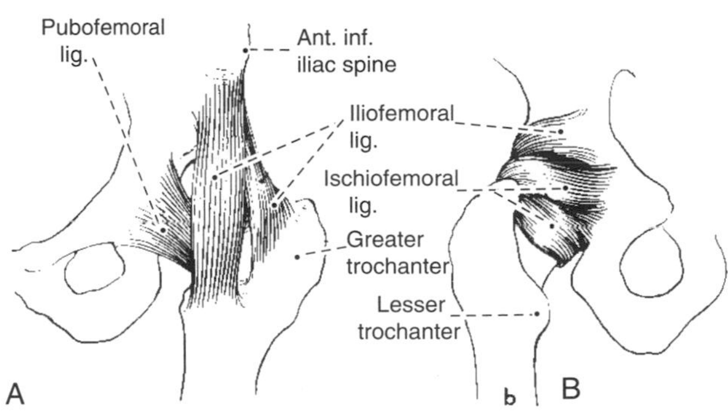

FIGURE 17-16.
Chief ligaments of the capsule or the hip joint (A) from in front and (B) from behind.

Although some of the circular fibers of the capsule form a thickened ring around the femoral neck (*zona orbicularis*), the main reinforcements run longitudinally and obliquely (Fig. 17-16). Most important of these is the **iliofemoral ligament**, the strongest ligament in the body. Shaped like an inverted Y (and referred to sometimes as the "Y ligament"), its stem attaches to the anterior inferior iliac spine and its two arms insert in continuity along the intertrochanteric line. It is the chief factor in counterbalancing the gravitational force during relaxed standing. Because the line of gravitational force falls behind the transverse axis of the hip joints (see Figs. 17-2 and 17-19A), the force tends to tilt the pelvis backward on the femoral heads. The iliofemoral ligament becomes maximally taut in extension and medial rotation, that is, in the close-packed position of the hip. Indeed, it is the chief factor limiting the ranges of these movements. The **pubofemoral** and **ischiofemoral ligaments** (see Fig. 17-16) limit abduction and lateral or medial rotation.

The **ligament of the head** is intracapsular (see Fig. 17-14). Surrounded by a sleeve of synovial membrane, it passes from the acetabular notch and transverse ligament to the fovea. It is of doubtful importance and, occasionally, may absent. Along it runs the *artery of the ligament of the head,* which enters the head at the fovea. It has been claimed that the ligament stabilizes the head of the femur in the fetus, because a long ligament tends to be associated with congenital dislocation of the hip (see later discussion).

Synovial Membrane. The capsule is lined by synovial membrane that reflects at the femoral capsular attachments and invests the femoral neck in a synovial sleeve (see Fig. 17-14A). The blood vessels that supply the femoral neck (see following section on blood supply) tend to raise folds in the membrane. The synovium is attached to the edges of the articular margins on both femur and acetabulum, and thus, excludes the intra-articular fat, the ligament of the head, and the femoral neck from direct contact with synovial fluid. The membrane may protrude anteriorly through a defect in the capsule between the iliofemoral and pubofemoral ligaments and may communicate with a bursa that lies deep to the tendon of the iliopsoas muscle.

Nerve Supply. Sensory (proprioception and pain) and vasomotor fibers reach the hip joint in the articular branches of the nerves that supply the prime movers of the joint. These include the **femoral** and **obturator nerves**, as well as smaller branches of the sacral plexus (superior gluteal nerve, nerve to quadratus femoris). The precise distribution of these nerves has been worked out, and some have been severed in attempts to relieve hip pain.

The anterior part of the joint capsule and its ligaments are supplied by one or more branches of the *femoral nerve*. They may arise directly from the nerve itself or from its muscular branches. The *obturator nerve* also innervates the anteroinferior part of the joint. The posterior aspect of the capsule is supplied by a twig

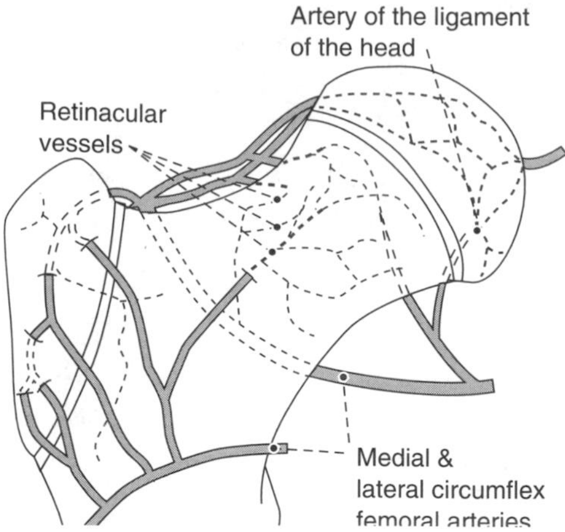

FIGURE *17-17.*
Arterial anastomosis that supplies the upper end of the femur and the hip joint.

from the *nerve to the quadratus femoris*. Sometimes, a branch of the superior gluteal nerve reaches the upper lateral part of the joint.

The significance of joint pain for hip function is considered in a later section (see Functional Evaluation).

Blood Supply. The hip, as do all other joints, receives its blood supply from a periarticular arterial anastomosis (Fig. 17-17). The anastomosis is fed by the articular branches of various arteries. Described more fully elsewhere, these vessels include the **medial** and **lateral circumflex branches of the femoral artery** and its perforating branch, and branches of the **obturator** and **gluteal arteries**, given off by the internal iliac artery. Although the vasculature of the ligaments and capsule of the hip joint is quite sparse, all intra-articular structures depend on this anastomosis for their blood supply. Of these, the most critical is bone, especially the proximal femoral epiphysis during its growth. Vessels enter the neck of the femur as well as the greater trochanter.

The periarticular anastomosis is formed around the upper end of the femur. Branches of the anastomosis pierce the capsule at its femoral attachment and surround the femoral neck as they proceed toward the head beneath the synovial membrane, supplying the underlying bone. These are the **retinacular vessels**. Before closure of the growth plate, the retinacular vessels can reach the femoral head only through the periosteum, which bridges the avascular epiphyseal cartilage between the neck and the head of the femur. After closure, anastomosis is established between epiphyseal and metaphyseal vessels within the cancellous bone, but further distally there is little or no anastomosis between the nutrient artery of the shaft and the vascular bed of the neck. The **artery of the ligament of the head**, a small inconstant branch of the obturator or medial circumflex femoral artery, contributes little to the blood supply of the head. Therefore, if the retinacular vessels in the periosteum are damaged, the epiphysis of the femoral head becomes predisposed to ischemic (avascular) necrosis. Femoral neck fracture, dislocation of the hip, and slipping of the femoral epiphysis (see Fig. 17-7) can all conceivably injure the retinacular vessels and lead to bone death.

Dislocation of the Hip

Despite the robust construction of the hip, its dislocation is common in traffic accidents. When the flexed knee hits the dashboard, the femur dislocates posteriorly. It may fracture the posterior rim of the acetabulum and compress or damage the sciatic nerve as it lies on the short rotator muscles underneath the gluteus maximus (see Fig. 17-12). Anterior dislocation could potentially harm the femoral nerve and femoral artery, which cross the joint anteriorly. However the iliopsoas, on which they lie, effectively guards them (see Figs. 17-22 and 18-14).

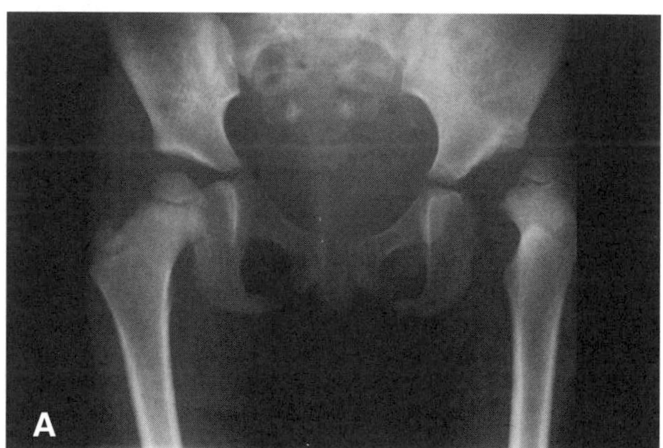

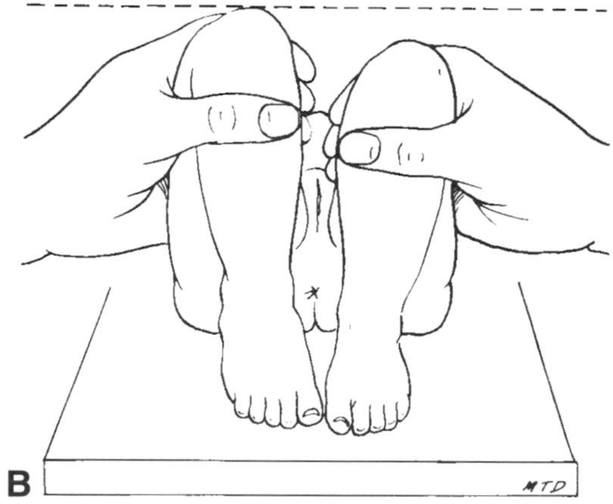

FIGURE *17-18.*
Congenital dislocation of the hip: (A) In the radiograph, the head of the left femur is dislocated. Note the wide open acetabulum and the smaller epiphysis of the femoral head on the *left* compared with that on the *right*. Note also that the inferior edge of the right femoral neck forms a smooth arch together with the inferior margin of the superior ramus of the pubis. This arch is distorted on the *left*. (B) Physical sign indicative of dislocation of the left hip: The femur appears shorter on the side of the dislocation because the femoral head has been displaced upward. (A, courtesy of Dr. Rosalind H. Troupin.)

Dislocation of the hip is one of the most common congenital anomalies, with drastic consequences for later life if not diagnosed during the first few days of life. **Congenital dislocation of the hip** entails spontaneous dislocation of the femoral head, either before or during birth (Fig. 17-18). It is five times more common in the female than in the male. Multiple factors contribute to the etiology. Dislocation of the hip should be looked for in every newborn child. The diagnosis is established by the physical signs.

The dislocated limb appears shortened. This may be apparent by an alteration in the number and symmetry of the skin creases in the thigh and by a difference in the level of the knees when both hips and knees are flexed with the infant supine (see Fig. 17-18B). Abduction of the affected hip is limited, as the femoral head impinges on the ilium. Telescoping of the femur also indicates instability and dislocation. This is elicited by grasping the knee and thigh in one hand and the pelvis in the other. If dislocation is present, the thigh will shorten and lengthen when the examiner pushes up and pulls down on the limb. *Ortolani's click sign* is the most important diagnostic test for hip subluxation or dislocation in the newborn. Usually it is impossible to elicit the sign later than 5 days after birth. The examiner grasps both thighs with the knees flexed so that his or her fingers follow along the femur to the greater trochanter, the thumbs placed on the medial side of the thighs. The palms cradle the knees and the flexed legs. The examiner fixes the pelvis of the newborn by fully abducting the opposite hip. The head of the femur on the side of the suspected dislocation is made to move out of the acetabulum as the examiner adducts the flexed hip and presses the thigh posteriorly. The reverse movement attempts to replace the head into the acetabulum by abducting the hip and pulling the thigh forward. A click is palpable or audible when the head of the femur enters or leaves the acetabulum.

Movements

Movements of the hip joint are a critical element in ambulation. Several abnormalities of gait are associated with deranged anatomy of the hip and its associated structures. Not only paralysis and injury, but even immobilization, lead to fibrosis and shortening of ligaments, tendons, and muscles, resulting in so-called *contractures.* These limit the range of motion and perturb the balance of forces that come into play at the hip during ambulation. The purpose of discussing hip movements in this section is to lay the anatomic foundation for clinical evaluation of the hip. Some clinical examples are included to illustrate how the normal anatomy of the hip region may be verified by physical examination.

Because it is a ball-and-socket joint, the hip permits flexion–extension, abduction–adduction, lateral and medial rotation, and circumduction. Flexion and extension are produced by the spin of the femoral head within the acetabulum around a mechanical axis that passes through the femoral neck. Abduction, adduction, and medial and lateral rotation are the result of swings and slides of the femoral head and neck. The femoral shaft, to which most of the muscles attach, serves as a lever for these movements. All these movements come into play during the normal gait cycle (see Chap. 18). Testing their passive ranges is discussed before considering the muscle groups capable of producing them actively. The soft tissues that may limit hip movements can be appreciated with reference to the simplified schematic diagrams of Figure 17-19.

Flexion–Extension. The range of active flexion is in excess of 100° and falls short of bringing the thigh and the abdomen in contact with each other unless the lumbar spine is also flexed. A greater range of passive hip flexion can be obtained when the examiner applies force to the flexed knee of a supine subject (see Fig. 17-20C). When the knee is extended, on the other hand, hip flexion is limited by tension in the hip extensors, chiefly the hamstrings (see Fig. 17-19A). Contracture of the hip extensors reduces the range even further.

Extension is limited to about 15°, but its apparent range can be increased spectacularly by extension of the lumbar spine, as in an arabesque performed by a ballet dancer. The passive range of hip extension, though small, is an important requirement for normal ambulation. The movement is limited by the length of the iliofemoral ligament and the hip flexors (see Fig. 17-19A). Pathologic shortening of these muscles or of the ligament (hip flexion contracture) reduces the range of extension, causing the pelvis to tilt forward, thus displacing the gravitational force line forward. Compensation for the resultant imbalance takes the form of an increased lumbar lordosis; abnormal gait ensues. A normal extension range can be verified by eliminating the lumbar lordosis with a maneuver called the Thomas test (Fig. 17-20).

Abduction–Adduction. The abduction–adduction range required for normal ambulation is quite small. The thighs are abducted when standing with the legs apart, and are adducted when the legs are crossed over each other, a position commonly assumed during sitting. The range of movement in abduction and adduction is limited by the ultimate length of the muscles, for ligamentous restraints of the joint in this plane are minimal. It may be appreciated from Figure 17-19B, F, and G that abduction is limited by the length of the adductors and vice versa. If the adductor muscle group is pathologically shortened, as in adductor contracture, not only is the range of abduction limited, but a deformity also results (see Fig. 17-19F and G).

Rotation. Medial and lateral rotation of the femoral shaft result from anteroposterior swings and slides of the femoral head in the acetabulum, which may occur in any position of flexion–extension. The range of rotation increases as flexion is increased owing to relaxation of the ligaments. The rotational range should be tested both in the flexed position of the hip, while the subject is sitting on the examination table with the legs hanging over the edge (Fig. 17-21), and also in the extended position, with the subject lying prone on the table and knees bent to 90°.

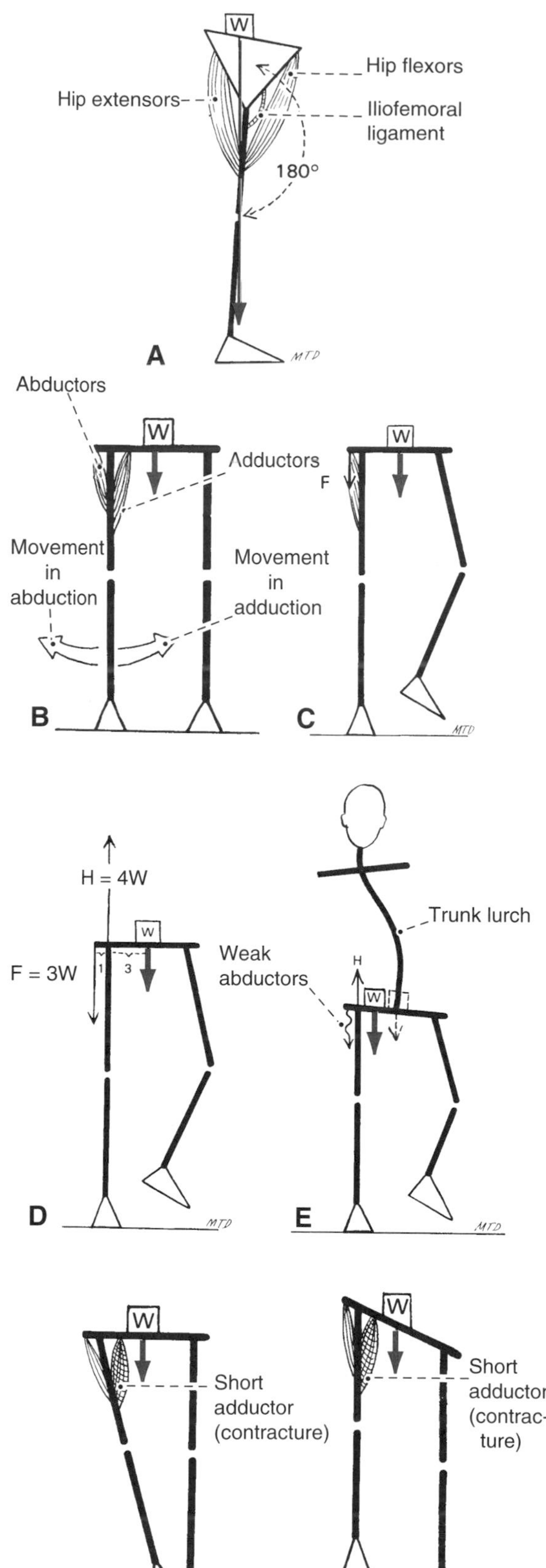

FIGURE 17-19.
Simplified schematic representations of the pelvis and the lower limbs with the major muscle groups and forces that are active at the hip: (A) Lateral view; the pelvis is represented as a triangle; *W* = the body's center of mass and gravity's line of force acting from it. (B) anterior view; the pelvis is represented here and in the subsequent figures as a *bar*. (C) Abductors of the hip on one side balance the pelvis when the opposite leg is lifted. *F* = the force exerted by abductor muscles that operates at the hip in addition to *W*. (D) The hip compression force on the side of the stance leg is nearly four times body weight. (*F* = hip abduction force; *H* = hip compression force, *W* = body weight). For instance, in a subject weighing 74.8 kg (165 lb), 299 kg (660 lb) compression force would be acting at the hip when the subject stands on one leg. (E) When the abductors are paralyzed or weak, the trunk lurches toward the weak side when that leg supports the body, shifting the center of mass over the hip, thereby reducing the force required for the abductors to balance the pelvis. (F) Contracture of the hip adductors prevents the leg from achieving the neutral (vertical) position in the abduction–adduction plane. (G) For walking, the limb must be vertical; therefore, the pelvis must be elevated, which produces a fixed tilt. An apparent shortening of the leg is the result. (Courtesy of Dr. Walter C. Stolov.)

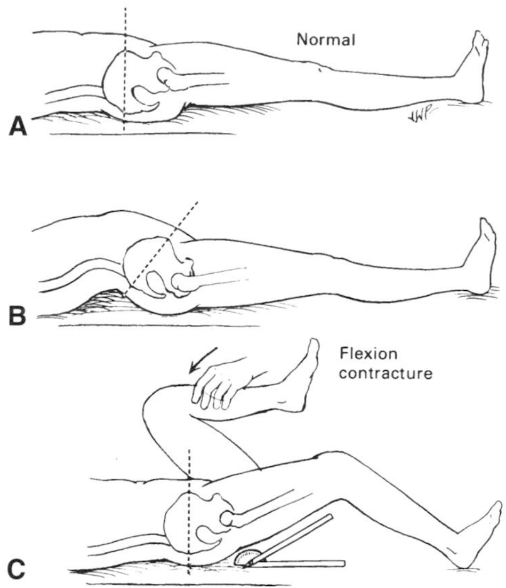

FIGURE 17-20.
The Thomas test for the detection of hip flexion contracture. The subject is lying supine on a hard surface with hips and knees extended. (A) If there is no contracture, the pelvis remains neutral with the anterior superior iliac spine lying vertically above the posterior superior iliac spine. (B) If a flexion contracture is present, to keep the legs on the table, the subject arches his or her back, compensating for the forward tilt of the pelvis. (C) To test the right hip, the left thigh is flexed passively until the anterior superior iliac spine directly overlies the posterior superior iliac spine. This places the pelvis in the neutral position and brings the lumbar spine down flat on the table. If there is a flexion contracture, the right thigh cannot remain on the table and will make an angle with it that equals the angle of the deformity. (Courtesy of Dr. D. Kay Clawson.)

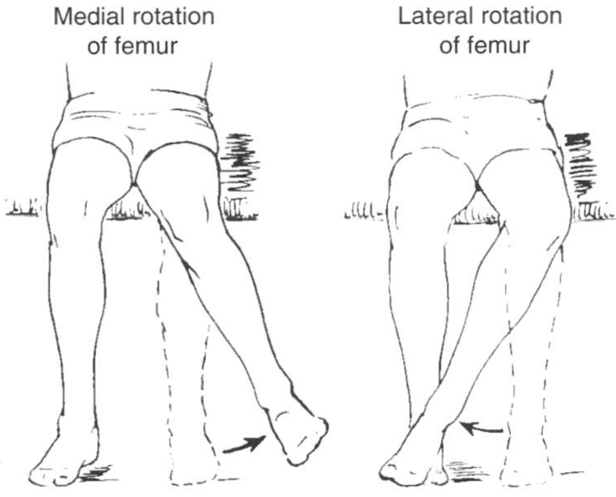

FIGURE 17-21.
Medial and lateral rotation of the femur with the subject sitting, requiring the hips to be flexed. Medial and lateral rotation should also be tested similarly with the hip extended, when the subject is lying prone with knees flexed 90° (Courtesy of Dr. D. Kay Clawson.)

Muscles

Muscles Related to the Hip

The hip joint is surrounded on all sides by muscles. Therefore, unlike the shoulder joint, it is not accessible by direct palpation: swelling and distention of the hip joint are difficult to detect clinically. Behind the joint is the gluteal region, containing the gluteal muscles and the short rotators, some of them closely apposed to the posterior aspect of the joint capsule (see Fig. 17-12). Anteriorly, the joint is covered by its flexors (Fig. 17-22). These include the psoas major and the iliacus, both arising within the abdominal cavity and reaching their femoral insertion by passing under the inguinal ligament. Their fused bellies rest on the iliofemoral ligament; a bursa is interposed between the muscles and the ligament. They are directly anterior to the femoral head. The femoral nerve enters the thigh in the sulcus between the two muscles (see Fig. 17-22) and the femoral artery and vein lie medial to the nerve (see Fig. 18-14). The more superficial muscles located anterior to the joint are the tensor fasciae latae, the sartorius, and the rectus femoris. They arise from the ilium, descend through the thigh and insert into bones around the knee.

Inferiorly, the joint capsule is skirted by the obturator externus (see Fig. 17-14B) that passes from the external surface of the obturator membrane (see Fig. 17-3C) to the trochanteric fossa (see Fig. 17-6D). The pectineus and adductor muscles occupy the medial compartment of the thigh and conceal the obturator externus from the front. Superiorly, the gluteus minimus is in contact with the joint capsule (see Fig. 17-14B).

Prime Movers of the Hip

Functionally, the most important muscle groups around the hip are its flexors and abductors. The flexors accelerate the thigh as it is swung into motion during the gait cycle and the abductors stabilize the pelvis when the body is supported on only one leg (see Fig. 17-19C). Other prime movers include extensors, adductors, and lateral and medial rotators. More often than not, several of these muscles are called into action as antagonists to the force of gravity; in these cases they are essential for controlling or preventing those movements that are the opposite of their own prime mover actions. This may be appreciated from the simplified schematic representation of the main muscle groups around the hip (see Fig. 17-19).

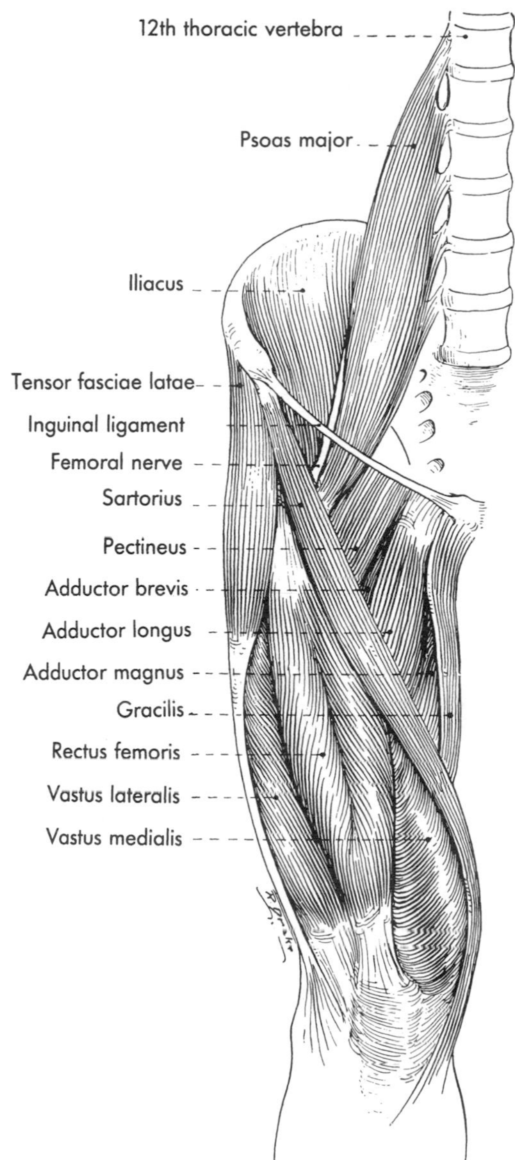

FIGURE 17-22.
An anterior view of the muscles associated with the hip region.

Flexors. Several muscles with primary actions other than hip flexion are actually capable of flexing this joint because a vector component of their line of pull crosses the hip anteriorly. However, such muscles become important in hip flexion only when the chief flexors of the hip are weak or paralyzed. The chief flexors are the **iliacus** and the **psoas major** muscles, which cross the hip anteriorly (see Fig. 17-22) and insert on the lesser trochanter. Because they insert by a common tendon (see Fig. 17-6D), they are often spoken of as the *iliopsoas*. The iliacus originates from the pelvic surface of the ilium (see Fig. 17-3C) and can move only the hip joint. The same is true, in essence, of the psoas, despite that it is attached to the last thoracic and all lumbar vertebrae. Its ineffectiveness as a vertebral flexor is considered in Chapter 12. The two muscles produce hip flexion whether the trunk or the legs are stabilized. A low level of electrical activity is present in them during relaxed standing as they assist the iliofemoral ligament in counterbalancing the force of gravity.

The **rectus femoris** (see Fig. 17-22) forms one of the four heads of the quadriceps femoris, the chief extensor muscle of the knee. It is the only head that crosses the hip and is quite effective as a hip flexor, especially when the knee is also flexed. The pectineus, sartorius, and all the hip adductors can also contribute to hip flexion.

The spinal cord segments chiefly concerned with hip flexion are L-2 and L-3 (see Table 13-1), and they are distributed to these muscles by the lumbar plexus. Owing to the developmental rotation of the limb, as well as the variety of muscles involved, the nerves to hip flexors do not conform as clearly to the basic plan of limb innervation as the nerves supplying flexors of the shoulder (see Chap. 13 and 14). The psoas major is innervated directly by anterior rami L-1, L-2, and L-3; L-2 and L-3 fibers reach the iliacus, pectineus, and sartorius by the femoral nerve, which also supplies the extensors of the knee. The adductors are innervated by the obturator nerve, formed by the anterior divisions of the lumbar plexus.

The strength of the chief hip flexors is tested by opposing the movement in a seated subject whose legs are hanging over the edge of the table or chair. The examiner should apply resistance to the distal end of the femur as the subject flexes one hip after the other, exerting maximum effort.

Extensors. Hip extensors include the gluteus maximus and the hamstring muscles. Mention has been made of their relative role in producing extension of the hip (see under Gluteal Region).

As described in the next chapter, the hamstrings make up the muscle mass of the posterior compartment of the thigh (in other words, the ham). They insert below the knee and are flexors of that joint. When their distal attachment is fixed, however, the hamstrings exert force on the pelvis. They cause extension of the hip because their line of pull on the ischial tuberosity, to which they are attached proximally, is posterior to the hip joint. Which one of the joints moves depends on the balance of other stabilizing factors. The hamstrings are more active as hip extensors during ambulation than the gluteus maximus. They are supplied by segments L-5, S-1, and S-2 through the tibial part of the sciatic nerve.

Abductors. The main abductors of the hip are the **gluteus medius** and **gluteus minimus** (see Figs. 17-11 and 17-12). The tensor fasciae latae and the piriformis also exert abduction force on the femur. The actions of these muscles are described in an earlier section (see under Gluteal Region). The role of the gluteus medius and minimus in stabilizing the pelvis is further explained by the simple stick diagrams in Figure 17-19C through E. The other abductors are too weak to compensate for paralysis of these two gluteal muscles: To maintain balance, the subject so affected lurches the trunk sharply to the side of paralysis to place most of the body weight directly over the stance leg (see Fig. 17-19E). This cancels out the need for the abduction force required to keep the pelvis level, which is several times that of the gravitational force of the body (see Fig. 17-19D).

Adductors. The adductors occupy the medial compartment of the thigh (see Figs. 18-10 and 18-18). Why the hip is endowed with such a large and powerful adductor musculature is a matter of conjecture, as the use of these muscles as prime movers is rather limited. They do, however, participate in postural reflexes during ambulation: they stabilize the pelvis on the femora during the phase of the gait cycle when both feet are on the ground (double support), and they apparently stabilize the femur when the knee is forcefully flexed or extended. During these efforts, their contraction becomes palpable.

The group includes the **adductor longus** and **brevis** (see Fig. 17-22), and the **adductor magnus** (see Figs. 18-10 and 18-18). They arise in continuity from the body of the pubis and the conjoint ramus (see Fig. 17-3C), and fan out laterally to insert into the linea aspera (see Fig. 17-6D). They are all supplied by the obturator nerve (L-2, L-3, and L-4). Other muscles with adductor action, but much less functional significance, include the gracilis, pectineus, and some small muscles around the hip with some adductor capabilities (see Chap. 18). Contracture of the adductors produces abnormalities of gait and posture and results in an apparent shortening of the affected leg (see Fig.17-19F and G).

The power of the adductors is assessed clinically by trying to force the extended legs apart while the subject attempts to keep the thighs together.

Rotators. The short rotators of the hip are discussed with the gluteal region (**piriformis**, **obturator internus**, **gemelli**, and **quadratus femoris**). All these muscles rotate the femur laterally, and there is no corresponding group of medial rotators. Moreover, several other muscles also rotate laterally (**obturator externus** and **gluteus maximus** and **medius**). Precisely which muscles contribute to medial rotation, a fairly powerful movement, is still a matter of dispute. The anterior fibers of the **gluteus medius** and **minimus** are undoubtedly involved and, according to electromyographic evidence, so are the **adductors**, despite that analysis of their attachments and line of pull intuitively predicts lateral rather than medial rotation.

The role of the **iliopsoas**, if any, in rotation at the hip is enigmatic. This muscle has been championed as both a medial and a lateral rotator, even though electromyography has failed to provide evidence of significant participation in either of these movements. A role in lateral rotation is suggested by observation of patients in whom the *femoral neck is fractured*; in these patients the iliopsoas does produce lateral rotation of the femoral shaft. It is evident on physical examination by the lateral deviation of the foot in the supine subject when the extended legs are resting on the supporting surface, a sign recognized as diagnostic of the lesion.

FUNCTIONAL EVALUATION

Throughout life, the hip is the joint most frequently affected by disease. Its clinical evaluation consists of the systematic testing of the functional integrity of the structures in the gluteal and hip regions. Earlier sections of this chapter deal with the palpation of bony points, the testing of ranges of movement and muscle action as the anatomy of various structures is discussed. The purpose of this section is to link together some of these procedures, just as they are linked in a physical examination, and provide a summary of the functional evaluation of the hip joint and the role it plays in ambulation and in the maintenance of posture. Some clinical examples have already been introduced (femoral fracture, slipping and avascular necrosis of the femoral epiphysis, muscle weakness or paralysis, congenital dislocation of the hip, contractures); others are mentioned in the following because the diagnostic maneuvers for their detection can be understood by applying the anatomic information presented in the earlier sections of this chapter.

Symptoms

Pain and a limp are the chief complaints indicative of functional disturbances in the hip. Although the hip of the weight-bearing leg is subjected to compression forces that are several times greater than the weight of the body (see Fig. 17-19D), there is no awareness of this compression because articular cartilage lacks innervation. The underlying bone, however, does receive somatic pain afferents, as do the joint capsule, its ligaments, and the synovial membrane. The hip becomes painful when articular cartilage is eroded, subjecting the bone to compression, or when the capsule and ligaments are put under undue tension owing to the distension of the joint cavity or to excessive mechanical forces. The latter, if sufficiently strong, can lead to tears. Thinning of the cartilage is associated with aging and may become excessive in osteoarthritis (also known as degenerative joint disease). Its chief presenting symptom is pain exacerbated by weight-bearing. Bone infection (osteomyelitis) within the femoral head or neck, as well as inflammation of the synovial membrane and capsule owing to various causative agents of arthritis, also present as a painful hip, not only because exudate distends the joint, but also because of the inflammation of the respective tissues. Pain in these conditions also tends to increase as weight is put on the joint. Consequent sparing of the joint is manifest as a limp, and may be associated with postural adjustments that minimize the forces acting at the hip (see, for instance, Fig.17-19E). A limp that is not associated with pain results from mechanical abnormalities (e.g., shortened leg, muscle paralysis, or contracture).

Hip pain is usually felt in the groin and may be referred to the medial side of the thigh (in the cutaneous area of distribution of the obturator nerve, which innervates the hip; see Fig. 18-21). Because of the overlapping innervation of the hip and the knee (see Chap. 18), hip pathology may present as pain in the knee without any complaints in the hip region. To complicate matters further, groin pain may be due to femoral or inguinal hernia, to inflamed inguinal lymph nodes, or to a psoas abscess, rather than to hip pathology per se. Such pain can be misdiagnosed as originating in the hip, particularly since, in each case, the pain may be worse during walking. Pain may also be referred to the hip region from a number of distant structures because the pain afferents from these structures reach the same spinal cord segments as those from the hip joint (e.g., lumbar spine, sacroiliac joints, or pelvic organs). Such referred pain is usually felt in the gluteal region and radiates down the back of the thigh, especially if it is of nerve root origin. Ischemia of the gluteal muscles may produce pain in the buttock during walking (intermittent claudication); this is due to blockage of the internal iliac arteries in the pelvis from which originate the superior and inferior gluteal arteries that supply the gluteal muscles.

Physical Examination

Inspection, palpation, testing of active and passive ranges of movement, and testing of muscle strength are supplemented by some diagnostic tests that evaluate anatomic integrity in the gluteal and hip regions.

Inspection. In addition to inspecting the bony and soft tissue contours of the gluteal and hip regions themselves, clinical evaluation of the hip joint must include observation of the gait (see Chap. 18), curvatures of the spine (see Figs. 12-35 and 12-36), and the orientation of the bony pelvis (see Fig. 17-5). The subject should be observed from the front, back, and side in the static anatomic position as well as during movements. Inequalities in stride length, lurching of the trunk, as well as a limp, call for the testing of specific anatomic structures. Scoliotic, lordotic, and kyphotic curves of the spine, or deviation of the entire trunk to one or the other side may be secondary to fixed pelvic deformity or to hip pain. Tilts of the pelvis must be assessed by observing the alignment of the iliac spines and pubic tubercles (see Fig. 17-5), as well as the flattening or exaggeration of the normal lumbar curvature (see Fig. 12-35). The posture of the legs should be noted in relaxed standing with reference to the positions adopted not only by the hip but also by the knee and the foot. Are any of the joints flexed or hyperextended? Is the entire sole of each foot in contact with the ground? Are the legs wide apart; is there any crossover? Are both feet and both patellae facing symmetrically forward? Are the two gluteal folds symmetric? In infants, is there symmetry of the skin folds that are normally present in the thighs and groin? Any deviation from the normal may reflect abnormalities of the femur or the hip joint. Local swelling, redness, scars, or open wounds in the gluteal or hip region invite special investigation.

Palpation. All bony points available for palpation should be felt and the two sides compared. These include the iliac crests with their spines, the pubic crests and tubercles, the greater trochanters, and the ischial tuberosities. Areas of swelling, tenderness, or regions of increase in skin temperature should be defined in terms of anatomic structures. Soft tissues of the inguinal region and femoral triangle should be included in the examination, feeling for lymph nodes and the pulsation of the femoral artery half way between the anterior superior iliac spine and the symphysis pubis (see Chap. 18). Deep to the artery is the iliopsoas and the hip joint. A swelling in this region, inferior to the inguinal ligament, is likely to be a psoas abscess, rather than a distended hip joint. A *psoas abscess* is a sequela of tuberculous or other suppurative lesions of lumbar vertebrae. Pus tracks down from these lesions to the thigh within the fascial covering of the psoas major. Psoas abscess is seen in those populations in whom tuberculosis is prevalent. It must be distinguished from inguinal and femoral hernias (see Chap. 26) and from inguinal lymphadenopathy.

Ranges of Movement. The normal ranges of movement are described earlier in the chapter. It is important to test the active and passive ranges of hip flexion, extension, abduction, adduction, and medial and lateral rotation in both the flexed and extended position of the hip. Before testing for contractures, it is best to assure that the pelvis lies square on the examination table, allowing the legs to adopt the position dictated by any existing contracture. The Thomas test should be performed to rule out hip flexion contracture (see Fig. 17-20).

Muscle Strength. The various muscle groups should be tested as described earlier. The Trendelenburg test is an important maneuver for assessing the functional efficiency of the abductors. Understanding of its anatomic basis, however, should make it clear that a positive Trendelenburg test may result from other conditions besides abductor weakness. Dislocation of the hip, for example, or coxa vara, or a femoral neck fracture that has not united, could all yield a positive result. These conditions either approximate the greater trochanter to the iliac crest (thus approximating the origin and insertion of the chief abductors) or disturb the stability of the fulcrum for the femoral head. All these factors result, in effect, in the inefficiency of hip abductors.

Leg Length Measurements. A limp, particularly one that is not associated with pain, or abnormal resting posture at the hip, knee, or ankle, call for assessing the length of the two legs. The supine position is the best for measuring any discrepancy between the length of the two legs. Ideally, the distance should be recorded between the head of the femur and the sole of the foot. Since the head of the femur cannot be palpated, the anterior superior iliac spine is, by custom, taken as the superior reference point; instead of the sole of the foot, the precisely identifiable medial malleolus of the tibia (see Fig. 18-2) is chosen as the inferior reference point (Fig. 17-23). This distance is known as **true leg length.** It is important to be aware, however, that "true leg length" will vary for the same leg, depending on its position in the abduction–adduction plane. This is because the anterior superior iliac spine is located *lateral* to the femoral head. Adduction of the leg increases true leg length and abduction decreases it. Therefore, the two legs must be placed in a comparable position relative to the pelvis; that is, if there is a fixed adduction deformity of the leg (see Fig. 17-19F and G), the other hip must be adducted to the same angle before true leg length on the two sides can be meaningfully compared.

Shortening may be due to a short tibia or femur, to dislocation of the hip, or to coxa vara. The length of the femora may be compared by measurements between the tip of the greater trochanter and the femoral condyles. The same can be done for the tibia, using the tibial condyles and the medial malleolus as reference points. In cases of dislocation or femoral neck deformity, the relation of the tip of the greater trochanter to other bony points of the pelvis will be distorted. There are several tests for detecting such deformity, although the diagnosis must be based chiefly on radiographic examination.

With the patient lying in the lateral position, the tip of the greater trochanter normally falls along or below the line that connects the ischial tuberosity and the anterior superior iliac spine (Nélaton's line). Dislocation and coxa vara displace the trochanter upward. Similarly, the medial extension of a line that connects the tip of the trochanter to the anterior superior iliac spine of its own side normally intersects a similar line from the opposite side in the median plane

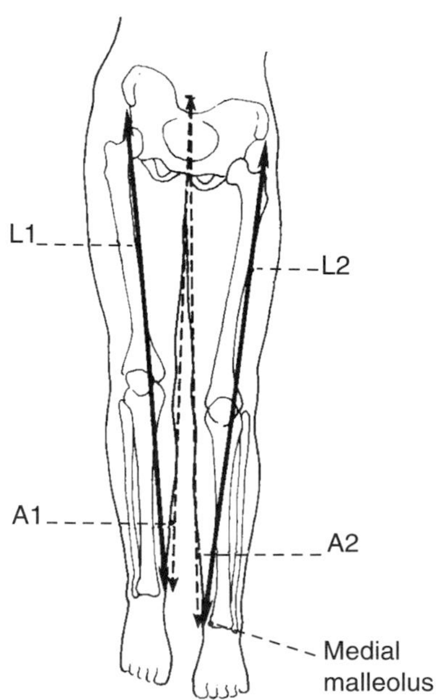

FIGURE *17-23.*
Points of reference in measuring true (*L*) and apparent (*A*) leg lengths. In the case illustrated the right leg appears shorter because of a pelvic tilt ($A_1 < A_2$), but true lengths are equal ($L_1 = L_2$).

and above the umbilicus (Schoemaker's line). A simple diagrammatic sketch can readily demonstrate that displacement of one or both trochanters in relation to the anterior superior iliac spine distorts this relation.

If true leg length is found to be equal by measurement of a subject in whom one leg appears shorter in the standing position, it is important to measure **apparent leg length**. For this measurement the legs of a supine subject must be placed parallel to one another and in line with the trunk. The inferior reference point remains the medial malleolus, but superiorly the measurement is taken from the umbilicus or from the xiphisternal junction (see Fig. 17-23). An inequality in apparent leg length is evidence for the existence of a fixed lateral pelvic tilt.

RECOMMENDED READINGS

Akita K, Sakamoto H, Sato T. Innervation of the anteromedial muscle bundles of the gluteus medius. J Anat 1993; 182: 433.

Basmajian JV, Greenlaw RK. Electromyography of iliacus and psoas with inserted fine-wire electrodes. Anat Rec 1968; 160: 310.

Basmajian JV, DeLuca CJ. Lower limb. In: Muscles alive: their functions revealed by electromyography. 5th ed. Baltimore: Williams & Wilkins, 1985.

Bakland O, Hansen JH. The axial sacroiliac joint. Anat Clin 1984; 6: 29.

Bos JC, Stoeckart R, Klooswijk AIJ, van Linge B, Bahadoer R. The surgical anatomy of the superior gluteal nerve and anatomical radiologic bases of the direct lateral approach to the hip. Surg Radiol Anat 1994; 16: 253.

Bowen V, Cassidy JD. Macroscopic and microscopic anatomy of the sacroiliac joint from embryonic life until the eighth decade. Spine 1981; 6: 620.

Chandler SB. The iliopsoas bursa in man. Anat Rec 1934; 58: 235.

Crock HV. A revision of the anatomy of the arteries supplying the upper end of the human femur. J Anat 1965; 99: 77.

Gardner E. The innervation of the hip joint. Anat Rec 1948; 101: 353.

Haymaker W, Woodhall B. Peripheral nerve injuries: principles of diagnosis. 2nd ed. Philadelphia: WB Saunders, 1953.

Hollinshead WH. Anatomy for surgeons: vol 3, the back and limbs. 3rd ed. Philadelphia: Harper & Row, 1982.

Hoppenfeld S. Physical examination of the spine and extremities. New York: Appleton-Century-Crofts, 1976.

Hoppenfeld S. Orthopaedic neurology: a diagnostic guide to neurologic levels. JB Philadelphia: Lippincott, 1977.

Inman VT. Functional aspects of the abductor muscles of the hip. J Bone Joint Surg 1947; 29: 607.

Kaplan EB. The iliotibial tract: clinical and morphological significance. J Bone Joint Surg 1958; 40A: 817.

MacConaill MA, Basmajian JV. Hip, thigh and leg. In: Muscles and movements: a basis for human kinesiology. Baltimore: Williams & Wilkins, 1969.

Roberts WH. The locking mechanisms of the hip joint. Anat Rec 1963; 147: 321.

Woodburne RT. The accessory obturator nerve and the innervation of the pectineus muscle. Anat Rec 1960; 136: 367.

Hollinshead's Textbook of Anatomy, by Cornelius Rosse and Penelope Gaddum-Rosse.
Lippincott-Raven Publishers, Philadelphia, © 1997.

CHAPTER 18

The Free Lower Limb: Thigh, Leg, and Foot

The thigh, leg, and foot are the segments of the free lower limb. The free lower limb is an extension of the gluteal and hip regions: there is both anatomic and functional continuity between the pelvic girdle and the free limb, as there is between regions and segments of the free limb itself. The hip, knee, and ankle joints that link the pelvic girdle and the segments of the free limb to one another are crossed from one region to the next, not only by muscles and tendons that move these joints, but also by nerves and vessels.

The thigh, leg, and foot are built on the same basic plan as the arm, forearm, and hand (see Chap. 14). Although morphologically equivalent structures are readily recognized in the upper and lower limbs, differences in terms of developmental rotation and functional requirements are reflected by notable anatomic differences. Nevertheless, much is gained by making reference to the simpler organization of the upper limb when explaining the seemingly more complex anatomy of corresponding segments of the lower limb.

The thigh of *Homo sapiens* is distinguished from the arm by its massive musculature, a reflection of the bipedal mode of existence. The function of this muscle mass is to extend the knees, raising the body into the upright posture, and to balance, on the tibial condyles, the femora and the pelvis which support the rest of the body. Unlike the elbow, the knee is a weight-bearing joint and, while allowing movement, it converts the lower limb into a solid pillar in the fully extended position, relying for stability on only its ligaments. In all other positions, however, muscle power is required to maintain balance at the knee during both standing and locomotion. The position of the preaxial and postaxial bones of the leg, the limb's intermediate segment, is fixed in relation to one another, and movements equivalent to pronation and supination are not possible between the tibia and fibula (see Fig. 14-4). The foot functions both as a dynamic platform for supporting the body and as a segmented lever that enhances the propulsive forces transmitted to it by the musculature of the more proximal limb segments. The anatomy of the ankle joint is adapted to these functional requirements, rather than to enhancing freedom of movement for the distal segment, as occurs with the wrist joint. Therefore, only flexion and extension are possible at the ankle joint, and the side-to-side adjustments of the foot to uneven ground, which mimic pronation and supination, are accommodated by joints of the tarsus. These adjustments constitute the movements of inversion and eversion of the foot. Although the terms supination and pronation, as well as abduction and adduction, are used to describe elements of inversion and eversion, these movements cannot be produced independently, as they can in the upper limb, and they do not correspond to movements of the hand.

Differences in the degrees of freedom for movement between the bones of the intermediate and distal segments of the upper and lower limbs are reflected in the organization of muscle groups in the forearm and leg. An understanding of the anatomic similarities and differences between the upper and lower limbs is critical for diagnosing and treating disability, and for restoring the anatomy necessary for meeting their respective functional needs.

The chapter begins with a general orientation that provides the background for the more detailed regional anatomy of the free lower limb, segment by segment. It concludes with a description of the integrated movements responsible for the gait cycle.

GENERAL ORIENTATION

Parts and Regions

The **thigh**, or *femoral region*, built around the femur, is the proximal segment of the free limb. The intermediate segment, called the **leg** or *crus*, is built around the tibia and fibula and is joined to the thigh by the **knee region** or *genus*. The **ankle** or *talocrural region* links the leg to the terminal segment of the limb, the **foot** or *pes*. Like the wrist, the ankle region has its own skeletal frame made up of seven tarsal bones, and represents the proximal subsegment of the foot. The backward-projecting **heel** (*calx* or *regio calcanea*) is distinguished from the remainder of this region, generally referred to as the **tarsus**. Five metatarsal bones form the **metatarsus**. Like the hand, the foot terminates distally in five *digits*, called the **toes**. The first toe is the *hallux*, or **big toe**, and the fifth one is the **little toe** or *digitus minimus*. In anatomic and clinical descriptions of the lower limb, all the Latin versions of the names are used extensively as roots of various terms. The section on the foot introduces a further classification into the regions of the hindfoot, midfoot, and forefoot.

Except for the foot, the lower limb's shape is more or less cylindrical. Nevertheless, as in the upper limb, it is customary to define and speak of anterior and posterior surfaces and medial and lateral borders in each limb segment. In applying these terms, however, it is important to be aware of the reversed relations that come about in the lower limb, compared with the upper one, as a consequence of its rotation and extension during development (see Chap. 14). Whereas the anterior surfaces of upper limb segments are their flexor surfaces, and they lie over corresponding flexor compartments, the flexor surfaces and flexor compartments of the thigh and leg face posteriorly. Flexion of the knee approximates the posterior surfaces of the thigh and leg (the latter commonly called the **calf**). The **popliteal region** and popliteal fossa (corresponding to the cubital fossa) face posteriorly. The prominence of the knee, known as the **patellar region**, is anterior, rather than posterior, as is the equivalent prominence (olecranon) of the elbow. Moreover, unlike the hand, the foot assumes a position at right angles to the leg. The **sole of the foot** (*planta pedis*), corresponding to the palm of the hand, faces downward and the **dorsum of the foot** upward. Therefore, flexion of the foot (at the ankle joint) is often qualified as **plantar flexion**, and extension of the foot, which approximates the dorsum to the anterior (extensor) surface of the leg, as **dorsiflexion**. These last two terms are confusing, take no account of the anatomic and functional compartmentalization of limb segments, and are inconsistent with the naming of movements at the knee; nevertheless, they remain in extensive use.

Differences between the upper and lower limb in the naming of surfaces are also reflected in the borders. The lateral border of the upper limb is its preaxial border and, in its intermediate and distal segments, is designated the radial border. The **preaxial border** of the lower limb corresponds to its *medial border* and, in the leg and foot, is referred to as the *tibial border*. The *lateral* or *fibular border* corresponds to the **postaxial border** of the limb.

Skeleton and Bony Landmarks

The skeleton of the free lower limb consists of the femur, patella, tibia and fibula, tarsal and metatarsal bones, and the phalanges. Because an understanding of the hip requires knowledge of the femur, most of its anatomy is described in the previous chapter (see Fig. 17-6). The articular surfaces of its condyles are examined in detail in the section on the knee joint, but the palpable points of its lower end are discussed in this section along with those of the other bones in the knee region.

Patella

The patella, or knee cap, is a sesamoid bone formed in the stout tendon of the extensor musculature of the knee, known as the quadriceps (Fig. 18-1). It is the largest such bone in the body. Its rather flat, more or less round shape is readily discerned by palpation, because the patella is largely subcutaneous. Its normal position on the femur, in front of the articular facet that spans the gap between the medial and lateral condyles, is higher than is often appreciated (see Fig. 18-1*A*). Its broadly rounded superior margin is designated as its **base**; its inferior margin presents a blunt **apex**. The bone on the **anterior surface** and sides is rough for the attachment of tendon fibers and is perforated by numerous vascular foramina that lead to the cancellous bone within the compact bony shell. Except for that of the apex, the **posterior surface** of the patella is smooth and is covered by articular cartilage. The articular facets that come in contact with the medial and lateral condyles of the femur are distinct, and are demarcated by a vertical, smooth ridge (see Fig. 18-1*C*). The patella interrupts the continuity of the quadriceps tendon fibers, except for a few that continue over its anterior surface. Below the patella, the quadriceps tendon is still an integral

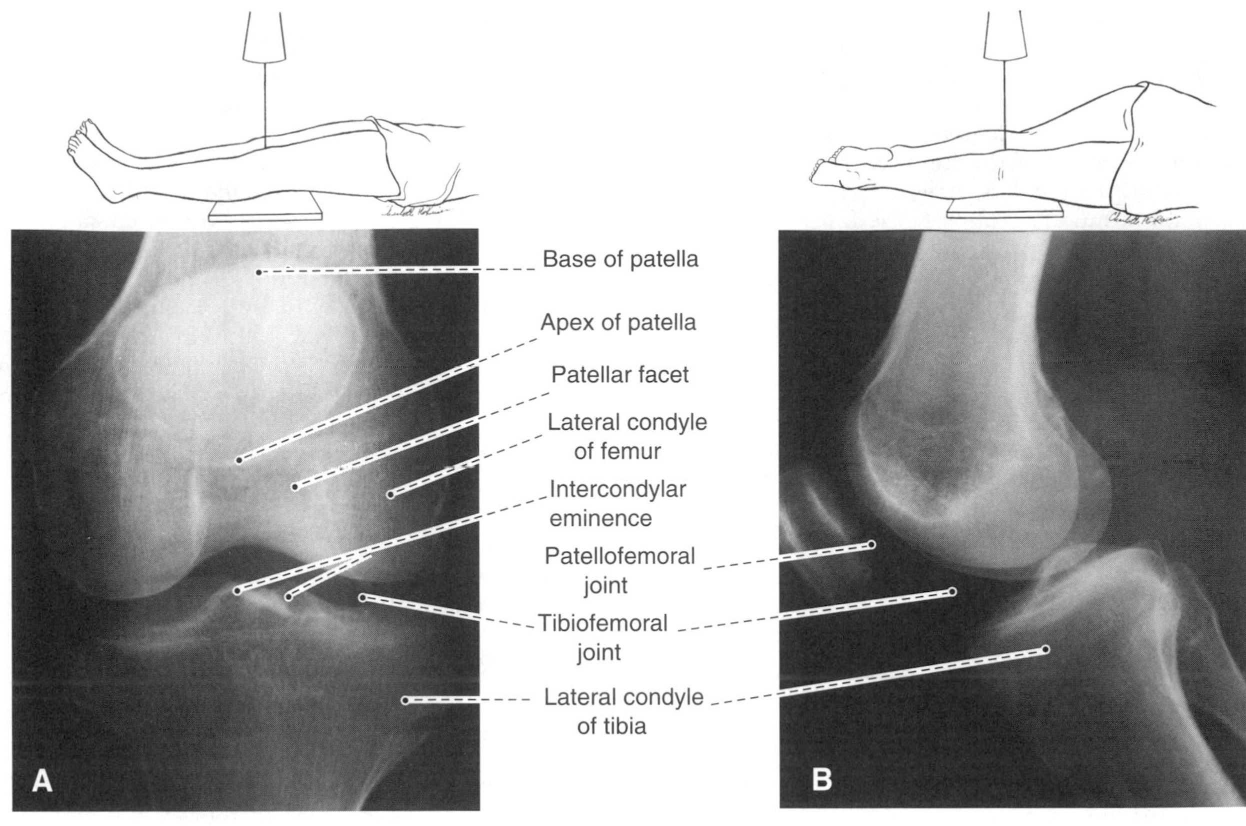

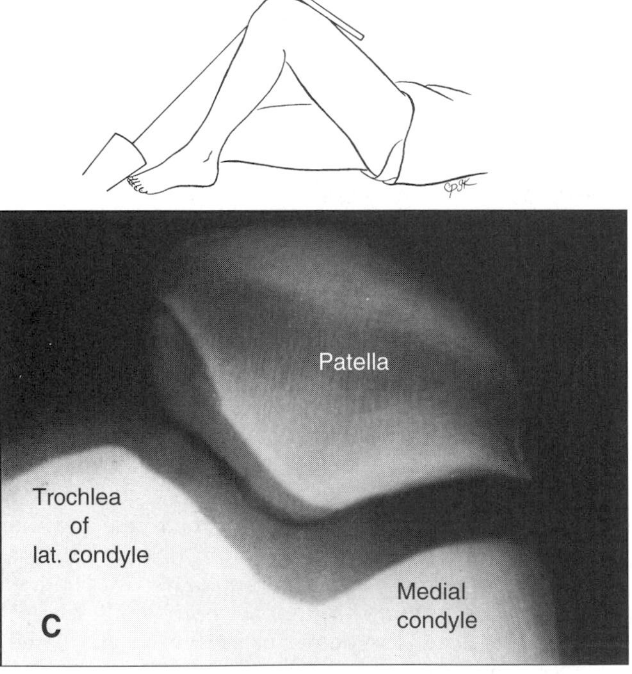

FIGURE *18-1.*
X-ray films of the patella, lower end of the femur, and upper end of the tibia: (A) anterior view, (B) lateral view, (C) a view into the patellofemoral joint. The sketches illustrate the positions of the limb, the x-ray beam, and the x-ray film. (Courtesy of Dr. Rosalind H. Troupin.)

part of the extensor mechanism of the knee, but receives a separate name: the **patellar ligament** (*ligamentum patellae*).

> **Injuries.** The patella affords additional leverage to the quadriceps muscle during extension at the knee by holding the tendon forward and acting as a pulley. Because of the forces to which it is subjected, articular cartilage on its posterior surface is predisposed to injury. Roughening and fibrillation of the cartillage leads to degeneration (**chondromalacia of the patella**), which gives rise to pain in the knee, often becoming worse during long periods of sitting with knees bent. **Fractures** of the patella usually result from direct violence and the bone may shatter into many pieces, necessitating its complete removal. Because the quadriceps is thereby deprived of a mechanical advantage, the knee is left with some weakness and disability.

Tibia and Fibula

The tibia is the preaxial bone of the leg, located on the medial side; the fibula, lateral to it, is the postaxial bone (Fig. 18-2): Each is a long bone, the **shaft** or **body** of which terminates in expanded epiphyses. The proximal epiphysis, or expanded upper end, of the tibia is made up of two **condyles**; the upper end of the fibula forms its **head**. The distal epiphysis of each bone is smaller and extends inferiorly as a stout process, called the **malleolus**. The lateral and medial condyles of the tibia articulate with corresponding condyles of the femur at the knee joint. The fibula, on the other hand, is excluded from the knee joint; its head forms a separate synovial joint with the lateral condyle of the tibia, the **tibiofibular joint**. The lower ends of the tibia and fibula are secured to one another by a strong fibrous joint, the **tibiofibular syndesmosis**. Here, both bones articulate with one of the tarsal bones, the talus, forming the ankle, or **talocrural joint**. The articular facets that cover the inferior surface of the tibia and the sides of the two malleoli that face each other, together form a mortiselike socket into which fits the talus (Fig. 18-3).

The **crural interosseous membrane** stretches between the shafts of the tibia and fibula. It is similar to the interosseous membrane of the forearm. Gaps exists in the membrane superiorly and inferiorly to allow the passage of blood vessels between posterior and anterior compartments of the leg. Although, strictly speaking, the membrane is a fibrous joint, its main function is to provide areas for muscle attachments.

> There may be **congenital absence** of either the fibula or the tibia. The entire bone, or only a part of it, may fail to develop. Of all the long bones of the limbs, the fibula is most frequently defective. When the lower end of either the tibia or the fibula is missing, the ankle joint is malformed: the sole of the foot is turned toward the side of the defect. Such defects are often associated with absences of toes, tarsals, or metatarsals.

Tibia. The **upper end** of the tibia consists of its expanded medial and lateral condyles, an intercondylar region and the tibial tuberosity (see Figs. 18-1, 18-2, and 18-4). An articular facet on the upper surface of each condyle is covered by articular cartilage, and the pair of facets, together with the nonarticular intercondylar region, make up what is often called the **tibial plateau**. Both **condylar articular facets** are oval and slightly concave, the medial more so than the lateral. The posterior lip of the lateral facet is smooth and extends slightly onto the posterior surface of the condyle. The semilunar cartilages (menisci) of the knee joint rest on the facets (see Fig. 18-40) so that direct contact with the femoral condyles occurs only in the central region.

The intercondylar regionof the plateau consists of an **anterior** and a **posterior intercondylar area**, to which the menisci and intra-articular ligaments of the knee joint attach (Fig. 18-4). These rough areas are separated by the smoother **intercondylar eminence**, bare of any attachments. The **medial and lateral intercondylar tubercles**, sometimes called *spines*, project from the center of the intercondylar eminence.

The margin of the tibial plateau is rather sharply defined laterally and medially. Well below the margin is located the **fibular articular surface** on the posterolateral surface of the lateral condyle. A groove marks the medial condyle just below its margin and accommodates attachments of the joint capsule and muscles. Posteriorly, the intercondylar area leads to the smooth popliteal surface of the metaphysis. The anterior intercondylar area slopes gradually to the anterior surface of the epiphysis and leads to the rugged **tibial tuberosity**, located between the two condyles as they blend with the tibial shaft (see Fig. 18 2*A*). The patellar ligament attaches to the rough inferior part of the tuberosity; a bursa lies against its smooth upper half.

The **body** or **shaft** of the tibia is triangular in cross section, presenting anterior, medial, and interosseous **borders** and medial, lateral, and posterior **surfaces**. The anterior border begins at the prominent tibial tuberosity and remains well marked on the upper two thirds of the bone. It separates the lateral from the medial surface. The latter is subcutaneous and, unlike the other surfaces, is bare of muscle attachments. Posteriorly, the oblique soleal line, properly called the *line of the soleus muscle*, demarcates the upper popliteal portion from the rest of the posterior surface (see Fig. 18-2*B*).

The **distal epiphysis** is only slightly expanded and appears asymmetric because of the **medial malleolus**, which projects from it inferiorly. The **inferior articular facet** occupies the distal surface of the epiphysis and the **malleolar articular facet** the lateral surface of the malleolus; both facets contact the talus (see Fig. 18-3). On the lateral aspect of the epiphysis, the **fibular notch** accommodates the fibula. Rough areas mark the attachments of strong ligaments both in the fibular notch and on the nonarticular parts of the lateral surface of the medial malleolus. These ligaments, examined later, constitute and reinforce the tibiofibular syndesmosis. Behind the malleolus is the *malleolar sulcus*, around which tendons pass from the posterior side of the leg to the plantar aspect of the foot.

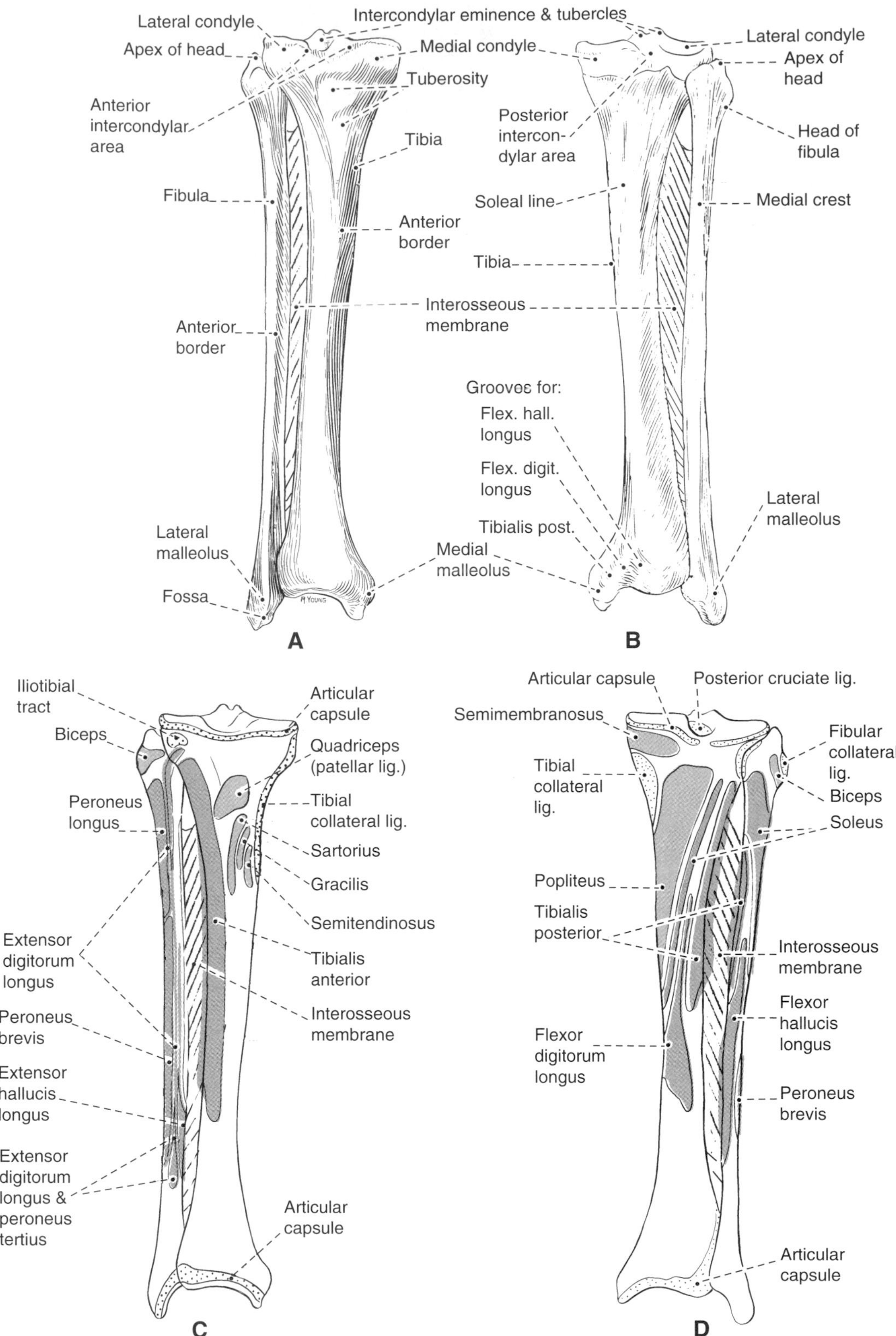

FIGURE *18-2.*
(A) Anterior and (B) posterior views of the tibia and fibula; (C and D) the muscular and ligamentous attachments to their surfaces: Muscle origins are shown in *red*, insertions in *blue*.

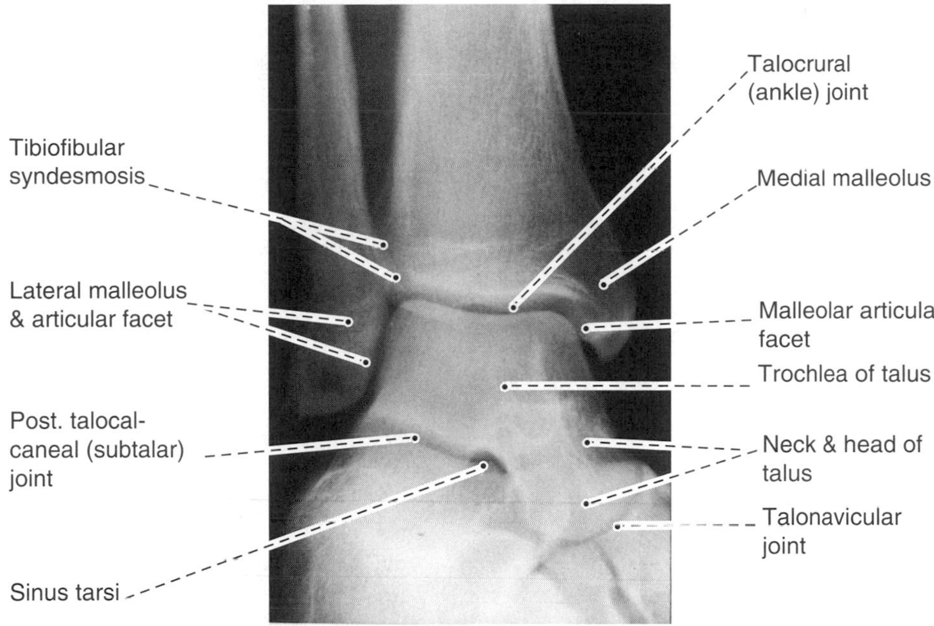

FIGURE 18-3.
The lower ends of the tibia and fibula and their articulation with the talus (talocrural or ankle joint) seen in a radiograph. (Courtesy of Dr. Rosalind H. Troupin.)

Fibula. The expanded upper end of the fibula, the **head**, presents a pointed **apex** (sometimes called the styloid process) and an articular facet for its joint with the tibia (see Fig. 18-2*A* and *B*). The narrower **neck** continues into the long slender **body**, which has anterior, interosseous, and posterior **borders** and medial, lateral, and posterior **surfaces**. All are surrounded by muscles and merit no further description. The expanded lower end of the fibula is the **lateral malleolus**. It bears a facet on its medial side for articulation with the talus (see Fig. 18-3). Behind and below it is a roughened *fossa* for the attachment of the *posterior talofibular ligament*. A groove on the posterior surface of the bone accommodates tendons.

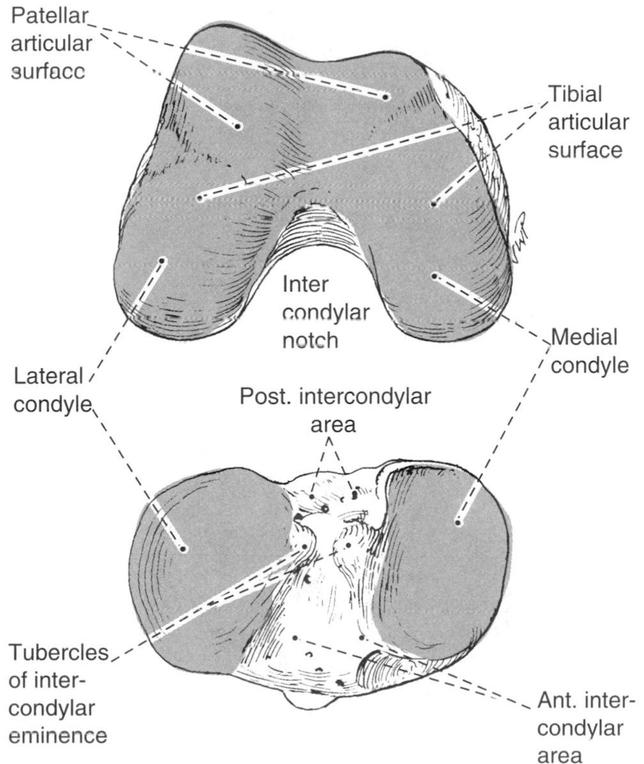

FIGURE 18-4.
Articular surfaces of the femur (above) and tibia (below). The areas covered with articular cartilage are *blue*. Note the grooves on the lateral and medial condyles of the femur that separate its tibial and patellar articular surfaces.

Bony Landmarks

Palpable bony points are important landmarks for establishing an anatomic diagnosis of many disorders in the knee and ankle regions. They are equally important for orientation when learning the anatomy of the lower limb.

The **patella** is prominent in the extended knee. When the extensors of the knee are relaxed, the relatively flat patellofemoral articular surfaces (see Fig. 18-1) permit manual, side-to-side displacement of the patella. However, the patella becomes fixed when the knee extensors contract or when the knee is flexed. Isometric contraction of the quadriceps in an extended knee throws into prominence the stout quadriceps tendon as well as the patellar ligament. In the relaxed knee, the relatively high position of the patella may be confirmed by palpation: its apex is at least 1 cm proximal to the tibial plateau, a position verifiable by reference to x-ray films of the knee (see Fig. 18-1*A*).

Palpable points of the **lower end of the femur** and **upper end of the tibia** are best examined with the knee flexed. Running the hand down the medial side of the thigh, the first bony point reached is the **adductor tubercle** on the femur's medial condyle (see Fig. 17-6*A*). Proceeding farther distally, first the **medial epicondyle** and then the articular margin of the medial condyle are reached. The latter is separated by a narrow gap from the articular margin of the tibia's medial condyle. The **articular margins** on both bones may be traced with precision anteriorly. The femoral articular margin leads anteriorly to the patella, and that of the tibia to the ligamentum patellae and the tibial tuberosity. The space between the diverging anterior margins of the two medial condyles is occupied by tissue of soft consistency. This is an intra-articular fat pad, to be described in the section on the knee joint (see Figs. 18-34 and 18-38). The fat pad is also palpable on the lateral side of the ligamentum patellae between the diverging margins of the two lateral condyles. In the depth of these spaces the **menisci** may be identified by firm, deep palpation. The edges of these semilunar cartilages may be felt slipping in and out between the tibial and femoral articular margins as the tibia is rotated medially and laterally, while keeping the knee bent. The menisci are palpable along each side of the joint, though they cannot be discerned as distinct structures along the joint line. Should they be injured, pain will be elicited by such palpation. From the sides of the joint, the articular margins on both the tibia and the fibula can be traced posteriorly for some distance, until the contents of the popliteal fossa preclude further palpation.

The **head of the fibula** is visible and palpable posterolaterally on the lateral condyle of the tibia. Just above it, across the joint line, the **lateral epicondyle** is palpable as a tubercle on the femoral condyle. In addition to its head, the upper and lower thirds of the fibula are directly palpable. The **lateral malleolus** is especially obvious.

Anteriorly, the **tibial tuberosity** is both visible and palpable. The skin slides readily over it, as it does over the patella, owing to underlying bursae (see Fig. 18-34). Below the tuberosity, the subcutaneous **anterior border** and the **medial surface of the tibia** form the *shin* of the leg and are readily traceable all the way down to the medial malleolus. The tip of the medial malleolus is at a higher level than the lateral malleolus (see Fig. 18-3).

Ossification. The ossification of the **femur** is discussed in Chapter 17 (see Fig. 17-7*A*). The epiphysis at its lower end is visible in Figure 18-5, along with the ossification centers and epiphyseal cartilages of the tibia, fibula and patella. The **tibia and fibula** develop from primary ossification centers for the bodies, which appear in each bone during early fetal life. The proximal epiphysis for the tibia usually appears during the ninth prenatal month and gives rise not only to the condyles, but also to the tibial tuberosity; the center for the lower end usually appears during the first year. By the end of the first year, there is a secondary center at the lower ends of both the tibia and the fibula, but the one in the fibular head appears later (Fig. 18-5C). Thus both bones ossify from three centers. A separate center may appear for the tibial tuberosity at 10 to 12 years of age; more often, however, this is an extension of the center for the proximal epiphysis. Its appearance has been attributed to the pull of the quadriceps on the collagen fibers that penetrate the cartilage from the tendon. The epiphyses join the shaft of each bone between the ages of 15 and 19 years.

Tarsal Bones

The tarsus is the proximal region of the foot, built around a set of seven short bones. Their arrangement into proximal and distal rows is not as clear as that of the corresponding carpal bones (Fig. 18-6). Only one of them, the **talus**, articulates with the tibia and fibula (see Figs. 18-3

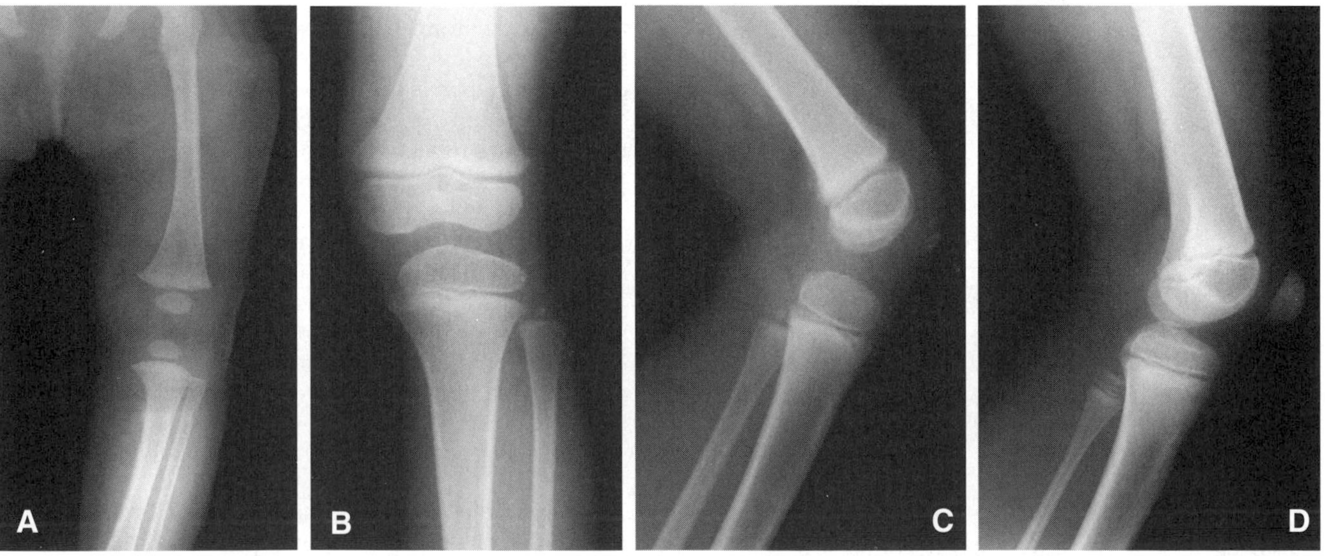

FIGURE *18-5.*
Ossification around the knee: (A) 4 months of age; epiphyses for the lower end of the femur and upper end of the tibia are present; (B and C) anterior and lateral views of the same knee at 3 years of age; the epiphysis for the head of the fibula and the ossification center for the patella have appeared; (D) 6 years of age; epiphyses have enlarged, but have not yet fused. (Courtesy of Dr. Eric L. Effmann.)

and 18-6). The talus rests on the upper surface of the **calcaneus**, a large part of which projects posteriorly as the *heel*. These two bones incorporate the primitive skeletal elements that, in the upper limb, form the four proximal bones of the carpus. There are three separate joints between them: the anterior, middle, and posterior *talocalcaneal joints*.

The four bones of the distal row, articulating with the metatarsal bones, are the **medial**, **intermediate**, and **lateral cuneiform bones** and, most lateral of all, the **cuboid bone**. The last tarsal bone, the **navicular**, is interposed between the talus and the three cuneiforms. The talus, therefore, articulates with the navicular (talonavicular joint) as well as with the calcaneus and the tibia and fibula. The cuneiforms, in addition to articulating with the navicular (cuneonavicular joints) and the metatarsals (cuneometatarsal joints) also articulate with each other (intercuneiform joints). The cuboid articulates with the calcaneus proximally (calcaneocuboid joint), the lateral two metatarsals distally (metatarsocuboid joints), and with the lateral cuneiform (cuneocuboid joint). It should be evident that all these joints, described in a later section, are readily named according to the bones that form them. The following section describes the anatomic features of the tarsal bones, to which reference is made when soft tissues are discussed.

Talus. The talus has a **body**, which articulates inferiorly with the calcaneus; a **head**, which articulates with the navicular and is joined to the body by the **neck**; and a **trochlea** which surmounts the body and forms the distal articular surface in the ankle joint. Thus, much of the talus is covered by articular facets. The nonarticular regions are marked by tubercles, processes, grooves and vascular foramina.

Inferiorly, the talus has three articular facets for the calcaneus: posterior, middle, and anterior. The latter two are continuous with one another and extend, without interruption in the articular cartilage, onto the head of the talus (see Fig. 18-63). A deep groove, the **sulcus tali**, separates the posterior and middle calcaneal facets. When the talus is in place on the calcaneus, the sulcus roofs over a similar groove on the calcaneus (*sulcus calcanei*), thus forming the **tarsal canal**. The canal begins laterally as the **sinus tarsi**, a wide opening bounded by the talar neck and the calcaneus (see Fig. 18-6*D*). The trochlea of the talus (*trochlea tali*) transmits the weight of the body to all the other weight-bearing bones of the foot. It presents medial and lateral articular surfaces for the malleoli and a superior articular surface for the distal end of the tibia; they are all continuous with one another (see Fig. 18-6*A*, *D* and *E*).

There are two processes on the talus. The **lateral process** is a rough projection below the lateral articular surface of the trochlea; it serves for the attachment of a lateral ligament at the ankle. The **posterior process** projects backward from below the posterior margin of the trochlea's superior articular facet. It is divided by a groove into a *medial* and a *lateral tubercle*. The groove (*sulcus*) houses the tendon of the flexor hallucis longus muscle.

Calcaneus. Largest of the tarsals, the calcaneus (*os calcis*) forms an irregular block of bone (see Fig. 18-6). Its upper surface has three articular facets for corresponding facets on the talus. The posterior facet is separated from the middle and anterior ones by the **sulcus calcanei** (see Fig. 18-63). The middle facet is on a stout process of the calcaneus which bears the descriptive name of **sustentaculum tali**. Posteriorly, the rest of the superior surface belongs to the heel, as do the posterior and much of the inferior surfaces. The *tendo calcaneus* (Achilles tendon) attaches to the rough lower half of the posterior surface. At the back end of the inferior surface is the downward-projecting **tuber calcanei** (*calcanean tuberosity*), which bears rounded *medial* and *lateral tuberal processes* that support the weight upon the heel. The sustentaculum tali projects from the medial surface; at its base is the *groove for the flexor hallucis longus tendon*. The lateral surface of the calcaneus is relatively featureless, presenting only a small projection, the *peroneal trochlea*, with a slight groove behind it for the tendon of the peroneus longus. The anterior surface of the bone is occupied by an articular facet for the cuboid bone.

The Smaller Tarsal Bones. The **navicular bone**, so named because of its fancied resemblance to a boat, presents a concave proximal articular surface for accommodation of the head of the talus and a convex distal one for the three cuneiform bones (see Fig. 18-6). Medially and inferiorly is the rough **tuberosity**, to which a major portion of the tibialis posterior tendon attaches.

The **cuboid bone** presents proximally an articular surface for the calcaneus and distally, one each for the fourth and fifth metatarsals. On the upper posterior part of its medial border is a facet for the lateral cuneiform. The ridge on the lateral and inferior surfaces of the bone is its *tuberosity*, delimited anteriorly by the *sulcus for the tendon of the peroneus longus muscle*. The tuberosity may present a smooth articular facet for a sesamoid bone that frequently lies in the tendon of the peroneus longus.

Of the three **cuneiform bones**, the medial is the largest. Its lower surface is broader than its upper one, and its medial surface is rounded. This bone presents articular surfaces for the navicular, the first and second metatarsals, and the intermediate cuneiform. The contiguous areas of the cuneiforms not occupied by articular surfaces are rough for the attachment of heavy interosseous ligaments.

The intermediate cuneiform is the smallest, and both it and the lateral cuneiform have broad dorsal surfaces and narrow plantar ones. The intermediate cuneiform has articular surfaces for the navicular, the second metatarsal, and the medial and lateral cuneiforms. The lateral cuneiform articulates with the navicular, the intermediate cuneiform, the cuboid, the third metatarsal and, to a small extent, the second and fourth metatarsals.

No muscles insert on the dorsal aspect of any tarsal bone, but the tibialis anterior and posterior both insert in part into the plantar surfaces of several tarsals.

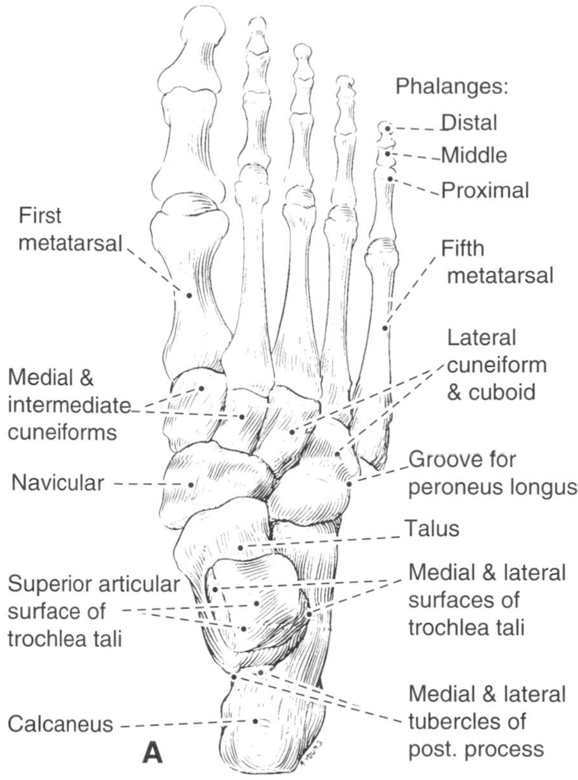

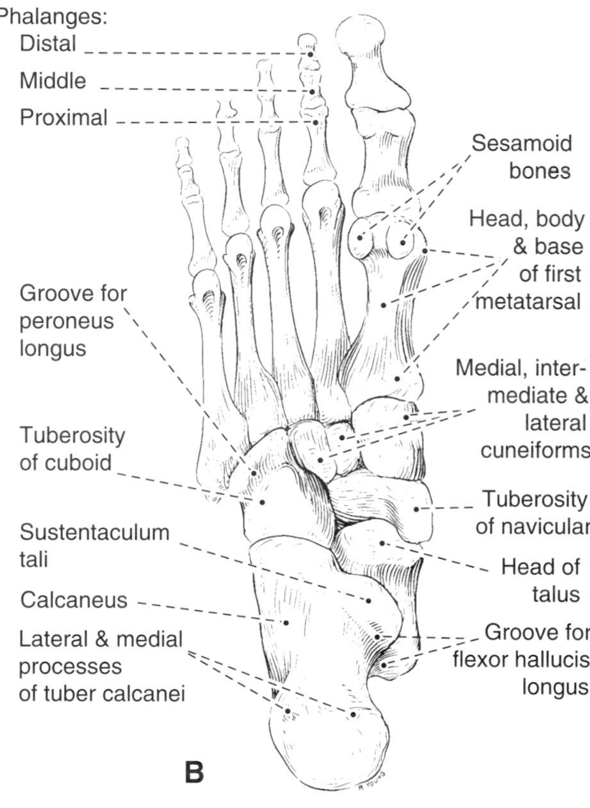

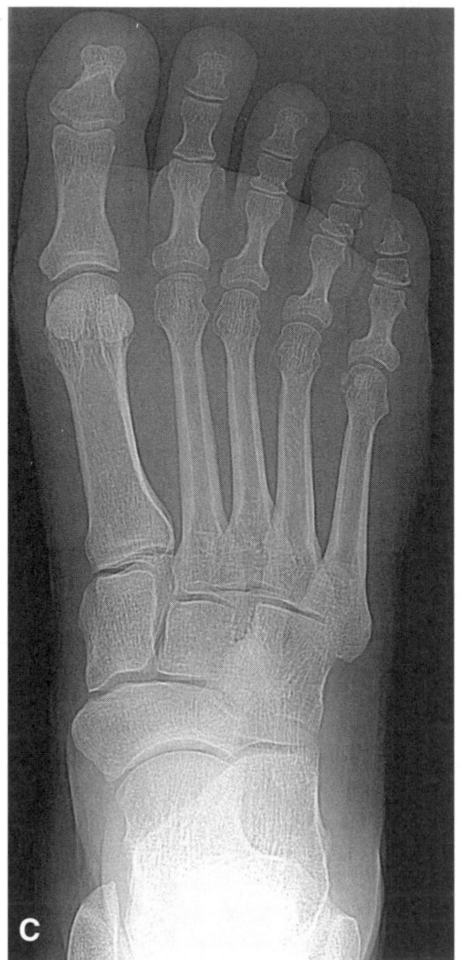

FIGURE *18-6.*
Skeletal anatomy of the foot: (A) dorsal view; (B) plantar view; (C) a radiograph in the same orientation as panel A (D) lateral and (E) medial views; (F) a radiograph in the same orientation. (Panels C and F, courtesy of Dr. Thurman Gillespy III.)

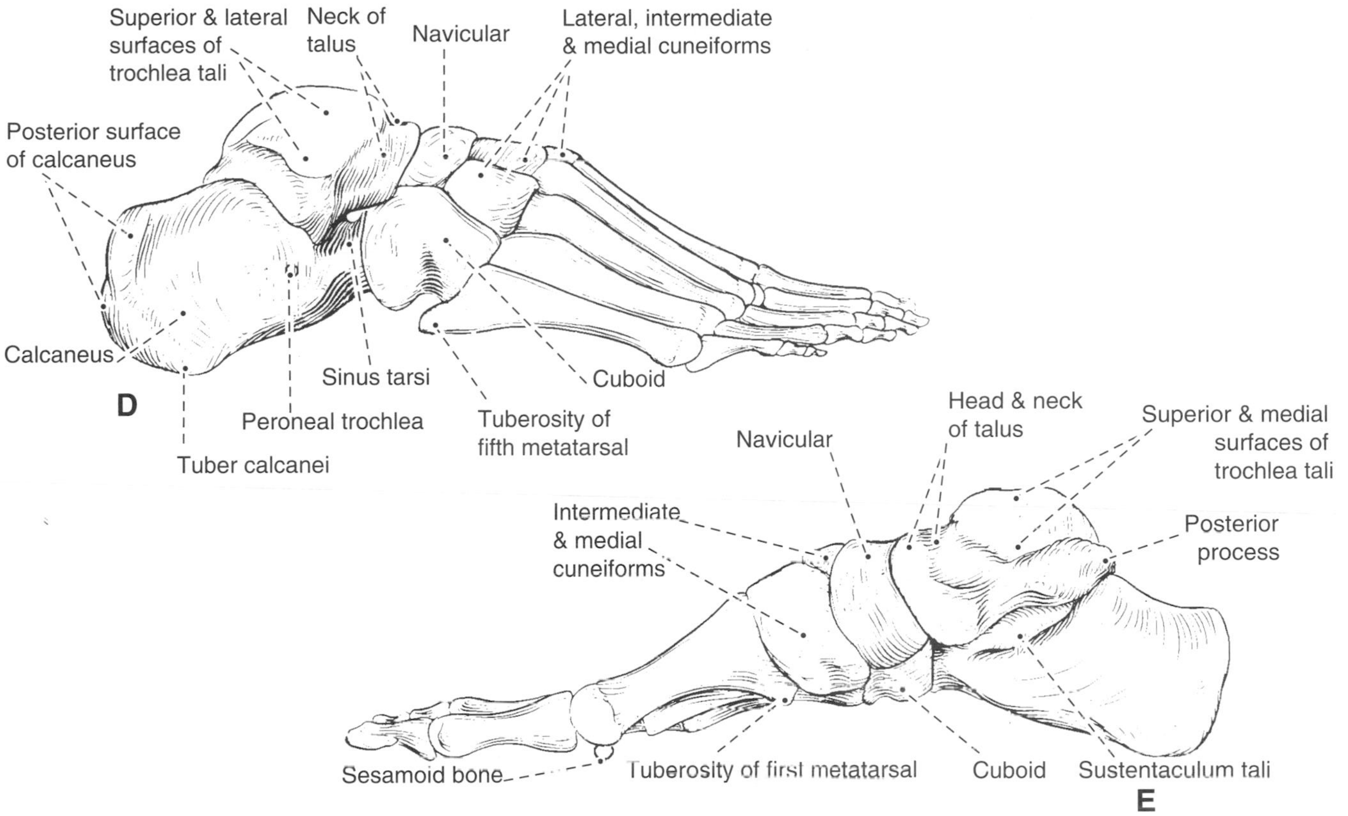

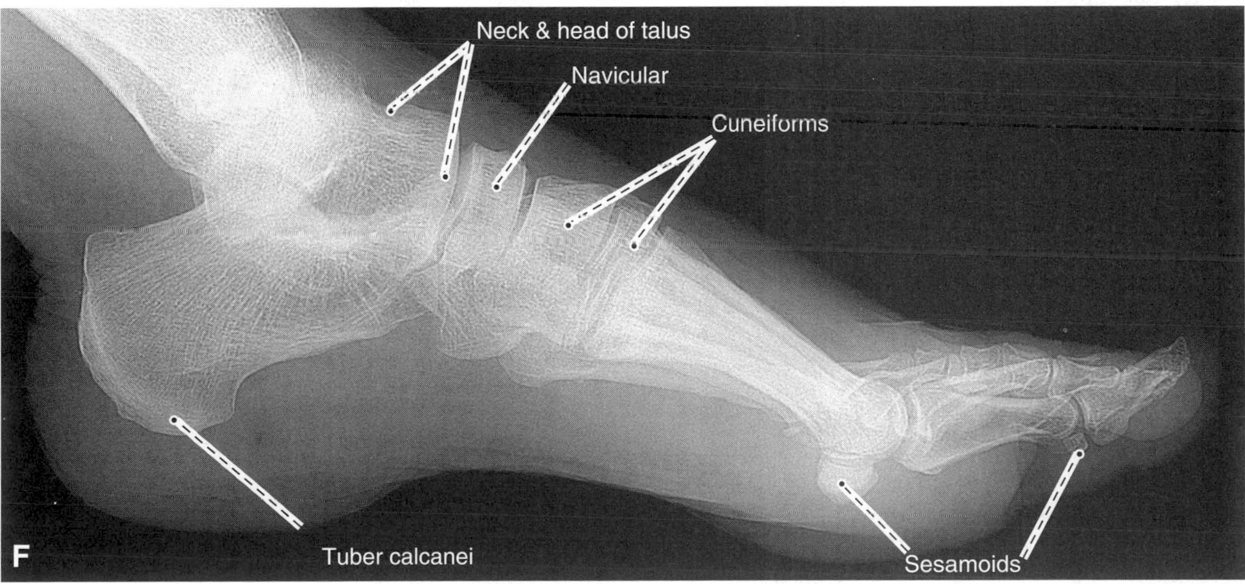

FIGURE *18-6. Continued*

Metatarsals and Phalanges

The metatarsals comprise the intermediate segment, and the phalanges the distal segment, of the skeleton of the foot (see Fig. 18-6). Their arrangement corresponds closely to that in the equivalent segments of the hand. Each bone has a body or shaft, a proximal base and a distal head. (In some of the phalanges, however, the shaft is too short to discern). The metatarsal bone of the hallux is more robust, although somewhat shorter, than those aligned in the other so-called rays of the foot. The big toe, like the thumb in the hand, has two rather than three phalanges. They are more substantial than those of the other toes. Two sesamoid bones articulate with the plantar aspect of the head of the first metatarsal and take a major share in transmitting force to the ground. Some of the anatomic features of the metatarsals and phalanges are discussed in the following, because further reference to them is made in subsequent sections.

The **bases** of all metatarsals bear articular surfaces for the tarsals with which they articulate in the tarsometatarsal joints. The base of the second metatarsal is inset among the cuneiform bones and articulates with all three of them. There is no joint between the first and second metatarsals, but the bases of the others bear articular facets on their sides for articulation through the intermetatarsal joints with their neighbors. The base of the first metatarsal has a *tuberosity* on its plantar surface for the attachment of the peroneus longus tendon. The **heads** of the metatarsals are covered distally, but not on their sides, by cartilage for articulation with the phalanges at the metatarsophalangeal joints.

The bases and heads of the **phalanges** are covered with articular cartilage and form the *interphalangeal joints*. The facet on each base is concave or saddle-shaped; that on the head is shaped like a pulley. The distal phalanx of the big toe is large, but the others are tiny pieces of bone. There is a *tuberosity* on the plantar surface at the distal end of each terminal phalanx.

Palpation of Bones of the Foot

Both **malleoli** are subcutaneous and their contours can be readily explored by palpation. The malleoli conceal much of the **talus**, which is hardly accessible to palpation. Only its neck can be palpated, just anterior to the fibular malleolus, especially when the foot is plantar-flexed and inverted. It does not yield to pressure, demonstrating the close fit of the talus between the malleoli. The bulk of the **calcaneus** represents the backward projecting heel, the surfaces of which can be explored by palpation. The calcanean tuberosity offers resistance to deep pressure on the plantar surface of the heel, and it is possible to discern its lateral and medial processes, especially when one or both are tender. Two other points are useful landmarks on the calcaneus: 1) Just lateral to the talar neck, the upper surface of the calcaneus is palpable through the soft tissues of the dorsum of the foot. The bony depression filled by the soft tissues is the **sinus tarsi**, the lateral aperture of the tarsal canal. 2) A finger breadth below the tip of the medial malleolus, the **sustentaculum tali** can be identified as a buttress projecting medially from the calcaneus.

The **navicular** is identifiable by its tuberosity, which is 3.5 cm anterior to the medial malleolus, on level with the sustentaculum tali. In the interval between the sustentaculum and the navicular is the **spring ligament**; the talus is in contact with all these structures (see Figs. 18-61*A* and 18-63). The **cuneiforms** are in line with the three medial rays of the foot, but they cannot be discerned separately by palpation. The **cuboid** is in line with the lateral two metatarsals and is palpable immediately proximal to the prominent *tuberosity of the fifth metatarsal* that overlaps the cuboid as it projects backward from its base (see Fig. 18-6).

Through the thickness of the foot, all metatarsals and phalanges can be grasped between finger and thumb. The so-called ball of the big toe is made up of the metatarsal head and the two sesamoid bones. It is hard to discern them separately. A major difference between the hand and foot is that the metatarsal bone of the big toe is not independent and does not enjoy the freedom of movement with which the thumb is endowed.

Ossification of Bones of the Foot

Each **tarsal bone** typically develops from a single center of ossification; the exception is the calcaneus, which has a small epiphysis at its posterior end as well. The calcaneus begins to ossify during the sixth fetal month, and the talus during the seventh month; they are the only tarsal bones that show ossification at birth. A center for the cuboid appears shortly after birth, and those for the other tarsals during the first 3 to 4 years.

The **metatarsals** and the **phalanges**, like the corresponding bones of the hand, each have a center for the body, but only one epiphysis; this is at the distal end of each metatarsal except the first, which, like all the phalanges, has its epiphysis at its base. The primary centers of ossification appear during the seventh to tenth weeks of fetal life, and the secondary centers during the second and third years. Epiphyseal fusion occurs between the ages of 14 and 19 years. Centers of ossification for the **sesamoids** of the big toe develop between the ages of 10 and 12 years.

Congenital Anomalies. Congenital absence of bones in the foot is mentioned earlier in connection with abnormalities of the tibia and fibula. As in the carpus, congenital fusion may occur between two tarsal bones, and there may be accessory bones. Approximately 30 different **accessory tarsal bones** have been described; the incidence of some sort of accessory bone is much higher in the tarsus than it is in the wrist. A separate tuberosity of the fifth metatarsal is called the *os vesalianum;* a separate lateral tubercle of the posterior process of the talus is called the *os trigonum*. The latter may be the result of fracture, rather than a congenital anomaly. Accessory sesamoids at the interphalangeal joints of the toes are relatively common. (see Fig. 18-6*F*).

Muscle Groups and Fascial Compartments

This section provides an overview of the functional grouping and topographic compartmentalization of the muscles of the free lower limb. More detailed descriptions of individual muscles are found in the various sections devoted to the regions of the limb. Like the upper limb, the lower limb is ensheathed in deep fascia, from which septa extend inward, many of them attaching to bone. They compartmentalize the musculature in all the segments of the limb.

Muscle Groups

The developmental rotation of the lower limb, mentioned earlier and discussed in Chapter 14, distorts the primitive organizational pattern of the limb bud (see Fig. 14-5). Primordia of the flexor musculature that begin their development in the ventral compartment of the limb bud become relocated posteriorly, whereas the extensor muscles of the dorsal compartment come to lie anteriorly. Consequently, flexor muscles of the knee, known collectively as the hamstrings, occupy the posterior compartment of the thigh, whereas the quadriceps, the extensor muscle mass of the knee, is located anteriorly (see Fig. 18-10). Medially, the thigh accommodates the bulky adductor musculature of the hip; the abductors for this joint are confined to the gluteal region. Muscles in the posterior compartment are innervated predominantly by the tibial component of the sciatic nerve, and those in the medial compartment by the obturator nerve. Both of these nerves are formed by anterior divisions of the roots of the limb plexus. Muscles of the anterior compartment are served by the femoral nerve.

Developmental rotation changes the positions of the flexor and extensor muscles below the knee, as well as above it. Thus the flexors of the ankle joint make up much of the muscle bulk of the calf, whereas the extensors (dorsiflexors) occupy the anterior compartment of the leg (see Fig. 18-23). Some of the muscles located on the medial side of the leg also invert the foot, whereas the prime movers of eversion, the peroneal muscles, occupy their own compartment on the lateral aspect of the leg. There is no counterpart for this compartment in the forearm. Like the forearm, the leg contains the extrinsic flexors and extensors of the digits, including distinct muscles for the hallux. Thus there is a flexor digitorum longus and a flexor hallucis longus deep in the posterior compartment, and an extensor digitorum longus and extensor hallucis longus in the anterior compartment. Extrinsic or long abductors are lacking for the big toe, since it is not possible to abduct this digit actively. Likewise, equivalents of pronators and supinators cannot be readily identified.

Muscles in the posterior compartment of the leg receive their innervation from the tibial nerve, and those in the anterior compartment from the deep division of the common fibular nerve. The everters in the lateral compartment are supplied by the superficial division of the same nerve.

There is a second set of digital flexors and extensors, just as there is in the upper limb. However, in contrast with the upper limb, these muscles are located in the terminal segment (the foot), rather than the intermediate segment (leg). They make up the flexor digitorum brevis in the sole of the foot, which corresponds to the flexor digitorum supeficialis in the upper limb, and the extensor digitorum brevis on the dorsum of the foot, corresponding to the second set of digital extensors in the upper limb (extensors pollicis longus, indicis, and digiti minimi). Other intrinsic muscles of the foot are the equivalents of those in the hand and are grouped and compartmentalized in the sole in a similar manner. They even bear similar names, despite the fact that several of the actions suggested by their names are largely wanting in the foot (e.g., abductor digiti minimi, adductor hallucis). Muscles in the sole of the foot are supplied by the medial and lateral plantar nerves (terminal branches of the tibial nerve), which correspond to the median and ulnar nerves.

Fascias

Superficial Fascia. The superficial fascia of the thigh and leg, composed of loose areolar tissue, contains a variable amount of fat. Cutaneous nerves and vessels, including some large superficial veins, run in it. Where the limb joins the inguinal region, the fascia is differentiated into two distinct layers: a *superficial fatty layer* and a *deep membranous layer*, the latter resembling deep fascia. Both fatty and membranous layers are continuous with corresponding layers in the anterior abdominal wall (see Fig. 23-2C).

Over the knee and the patellar tendon, the fascia is largely devoid of fat and forms the *subcutaneous prepatellar* and *infrapatellar bursae* (see Fig. 18-34). On the dorsum of the foot, the fascia is thin and loose, but in the sole, it shows specializations which are described in the section on the foot.

Deep Fascia. The deep fascia of the lower limb extends like a stocking from the gluteal, hip, and inguinal regions through the thigh and leg into the foot. The attachments that secure it proximally to the pelvic girdle are described in Chapter 17. Known over the thigh as the **fascia lata**, and over the leg as the **crural fascia**, it continues onto the dorsum and sole of the foot, and invests the toes as well. Around the knee and ankle and over the tibia, the deep fascia fuses with the periosteum of the subcutaneous bones. The intermuscular septa that compartmentalize the thigh, leg, and foot may be considered an inward extensions of the deep fascia. In addition to segregating the functional muscle groups topographically (see Figs. 18-10, 18-23, and 18-46), the fascia and its septa provide surfaces for muscle attachments and play an important role in aiding venous return from the lower limb. Owing to the relative inelasticity of the deep fascia, muscle contraction generates pressure within the fascial compartments which compresses the veins, in effect pumping blood out of them. Valves within the veins ensure that the flow is directed upward.

The **fascia lata** extends from the inguinal ligament, the conjoint ramus of the coxal bone, the ischial tuberosity, and the lower borders of the gluteus maximus and tensor fasciae latae to the knee. Directly below the medial third of the inguinal ligament, the fascia lata presents an apparent deficiency, called the **saphenous opening** (*hiatus*; see Figs. 18-8 and 18-16). On its lateral side the opening has a sharp crescentic edge, the *falciform* (sickle-shaped) *margin*, which tapers off above and below as the *superior* and *inferior cornua* (horns). The part of the membranous layer of the superficial fascia that roofs over the opening is called the *cribriform* (sievelike) *fascia* because it is perforated by several small vessels, as well as a large one. The latter is the *great saphenous vein*, after which the hiatus is named.

The arrangement of the fascia lata at the saphenous opening is perhaps best explained as follows: If the fascia lata were imagined to be wider than the circumference of the thigh, one way of making it fit would be by making a vertical slit in the fascia and tucking one cut end under the other. If the lateral flap is the more superficial one and is anchored to the pubic tubercle, and the medial flap is tucked deep and secured to the anterior superior iliac spine, then the lateral flap would correspond to the so-called *superior cornu of the falciform margin* and the beginning of the medial flap to the *inferior cornu*. Superiorly, both flaps attach along the inguinal ligament.

The fascia lata is thinnest medially. Laterally, it is reinforced by longitudinally running tendon fibers that are actually derived from the insertions of the tensor fasciae latae and the gluteus maximus muscles into the fascia. The strong band thus formed is the **iliotibial tract** (see Fig. 17-10). Below, the tract attaches to the anterior part of the lateral tibial condyle (see Fig. 18-2C). Some of its fibers blend with the capsule of the knee joint (as do other parts of the fascia lata). The iliotibial tract exerts a stabilizing function on both the hip and the knee, and is discussed further in sections dealing with those joints.

The **crural fascia** is attached around the knee to all the bony prominences. Posteriorly, its blending with the fascia lata of the thigh forms the *popliteal fascia*, which roofs over the popliteal fossa. Below the knee, the crural fascia encircles the leg, blending with the periosteum of the subcutaneous portion of the tibia (see Fig. 18-23). Some muscles of the anterior and peroneal compartments arise from its deep surface.

Close to the ankle, the crural fascia is thickened by transverse fibers that form **retinacula** about the tendons crossing the ankle. There are five retinacula around the ankle (see Fig. 18-45): anteriorly are the *superior* and *inferior extensor retinacula*; posteromedially is the *flexor retinaculum*; and posterolaterally are the *superior and inferior peroneal retinacula*. These retinacula are described in the section dealing with the ankle region.

Intermuscular Septa. The fascia lata forms two, and the crural fascia three, intermuscular septa. In the distal two-thirds of the thigh, the fascia lata sends a **medial** and a **lateral intermuscular septum** to the linea aspera of the femur (see Fig. 18-10). The lateral septum separates the knee extensors from the hamstrings, and the medial septum separates the hip adductors from the knee extensors. For much of its length, the iliotibial tract is anchored to the femur by the lateral intermuscular septum.

On the lateral side of the leg, the crural fascia gives rise to two intermuscular septa that attach to the fibula (see Fig. 18-23). The **anterior intermuscular septum** separates the lateral compartment, containing the peroneal muscles, from the anterior compartment that contains the extensors of the ankle and extrinsic extensors of the toes; the **posterior intermuscular septum** separates the peroneal muscles from the muscles of the calf in the posterior compartment. The posterior compartment is subdivided by a transverse intermuscular septum, the *deep transverse fascia of the leg*, which passes across the calf from one side to the other and separates the superficial muscles from the deep ones.

The fascias and compartments of the foot are described in a subsequent section.

Cutaneous Nerves and Vessels

The cutaneous nerves and vessels arborize in the superficial fascia and are best studied throughout the limb before structures located beneath the deep fascia are dissected region by region.

Nerves

The cutaneous innervation of the gluteal, hip, and inguinal regions is provided chiefly by nerves that supply the skin of the trunk (see Chap. 17; Fig. 18-7). Beyond the root of the limb, the skin is supplied by branches of the lumbosacral plexus. These cutaneous nerves distribute somatic afferents from L-1 to S-2 spinal ganglia and cord segments to dermatomal areas of the lower limb (see Figs. 13-24, 13-25, and 18-7). The main cutaneous nerves of the thigh are often described with the adjective *femoral* (even if not derived from the femoral nerve), and they are named according to their anatomic location as *anterior, lateral*, and *posterior femoral cutaneous nerves*. Alternative names, used interchangeably, are *anterior, lateral*, and *posterior cutaneous nerves of the thigh*. In the leg, cutaneous nerves have various names: *saphenous, fibular* (peroneal), and *sural*, the latter pertaining to the calf of the leg in Latin. The sensory innervation of the foot and toes corresponds overall to that of the hand and fingers, and is provided by *dorsal* and *plantar digital nerves*.

Thigh. In the thigh the chief cutaneous nerves are derived from the femoral nerve or directly from the lumbosacral plexus (see Fig. 18-7). There are usually two or three **anterior femoral cutaneous nerves** (*anterior cutaneous nerves of the thigh*); all are branches of the femoral nerve. (They are sometimes distinguished by naming them *intermediate* and *medial femoral cutaneous branches*). They pierce the deep fascia at various levels and supply

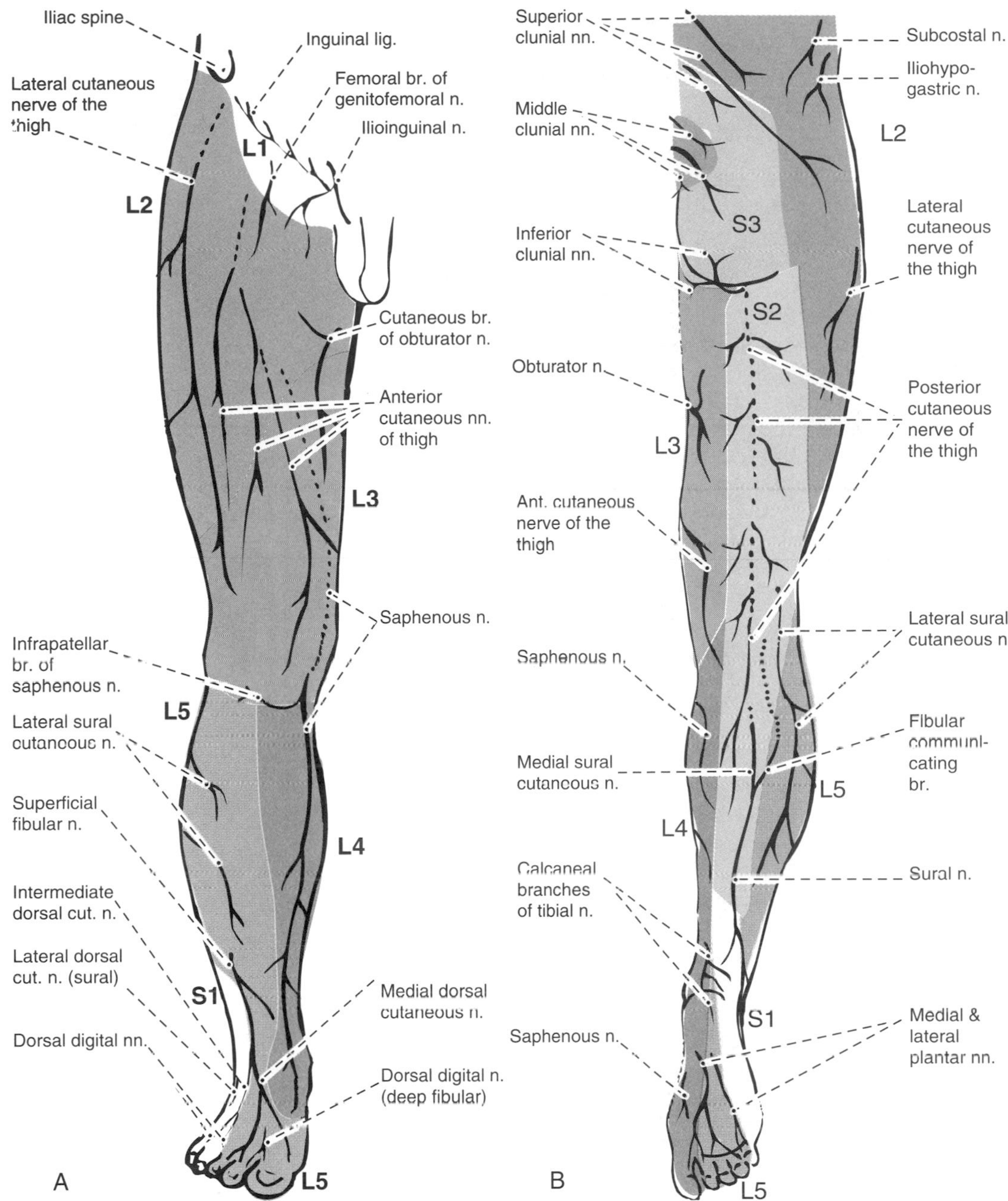

FIGURE *18-7.*
Cutaneous nerves of the lower limb, superimposed on the dermatomes: (A) anterior view; (B) posterior view.

anterior and anteromedial skin as far as the knee (L-2 and L-3). The **lateral femoral cutaneous nerve** (*lateral cutaneous nerve of the thigh*), derived directly from the lumbar plexus (see Fig. 17-9), appears just below the anterior superior iliac spine and supplies anterolateral skin as far as the knee (L-2 and L-3). The femoral branch of the **genitofemoral nerve** (also derived directly from the lumbar plexus) enters the thigh on the femoral artery and supplies a variable area of skin below the inguinal ligament (L-1 and L-2). The **ilioinguinal nerve**, a branch of the lumbar plexus, supplies the same dermatomal areas more medially. Lower down, the medial side of the thigh is supplied by the rather variable **cutaneous branch of the obturator nerve** (L-3).

The **posterior femoral cutaneous nerve** (*posterior cutaneous nerve of the thigh*), given off by the sacral plexus, enters the thigh as it emerges from beneath the gluteus maximus, and descends along the posterior midline of the thigh under the deep fascia (see Fig. 18-7*B*). It sends branches through the fascia to the skin of the posterior aspect of the thigh (S-2). Its main stem comes through the deep fascia near the popliteal fossa and continues some distance down the posterior aspect of the calf. It supplies a strip of skin along the midline of the calf, in continuity with that of the thigh, sometimes for as much as two-thirds of the leg.

Leg and Foot. The cutaneous nerves of the leg and foot are derived chiefly from the tibial and common fibular nerves, but with a substantial contribution from the femoral nerve as well.

The **saphenous nerve**, the longest branch of the femoral nerve, descends along the medial side of the thigh without supplying any skin (see Fig. 18-7*A*). It becomes subcutaneous above the medial side of the knee. After giving off an *infrapatellar branch* that curves forward to supply the anteromedial part of the leg below the knee, the nerve runs downward with the great saphenous vein and gives off a series of medial cutaneous branches (L-4). Passing in front of the medial malleolus, it continues forward along the medial side of the foot about as far as the metatarsophalangeal joint of the big toe, and supplies the overlying skin (L-4).

The terminal part of the **superficial fibular nerve** becomes cutaneous as it emerges at the lower third of the anterolateral side of the leg. It gives off twigs to the leg and continues onto the foot to supply much of its dorsum, dividing into two **dorsal cutaneous nerves** as it does so (L-5). Its medial branch (*medial dorsal cutaneous nerve*) is distributed to the medial side of the big toe and to the adjacent sides of the second and third toes. Its lateral branch (*intermediate dorsal cutaneous nerve*) usually divides into two **dorsal digital** branches that supply the adjacent sides of the third, fourth, and fifth toes.

The **lateral sural cutaneous nerve** (*lateral cutaneous nerve of the calf*) arises from the common fibular nerve above the knee and pierces the popliteal fascia. It runs down the posterolateral aspect of the calf, giving off branches to the lateral side of the leg (L-5).

The **medial sural cutaneous nerve** arises from the tibial nerve in the popliteal fossa, and runs downward in the groove between the two heads of the most superficial muscle of the calf (gastrocnemius). It penetrates the deep fascia at the middle of the leg and is soon joined by a **fibular communicating branch** given off by the common fibular nerve. The nerve formed by their union, the **sural nerve**, is distributed down the posterolateral side of the leg (L-5 and S-1). It passes behind the lateral malleolus and then onto the dorsal aspect of the foot, where it assumes the name **lateral dorsal cutaneous nerve** (S-1). The latter may supply only the lateral side of the little toe or may spread medially to anastomose with, or take over some of the territory supplied by, the intermediate dorsal cutaneous nerve. Although the *deep fibular nerve* is predominantly muscular in its distribution, its terminal branch emerges on the foot and divides into **dorsal digital nerves** for the adjacent sides of the first and second toes (L-5).

The plantar surface of the foot is supplied by the medial and lateral plantar nerves, the terminal branches of the tibial nerve in the foot. The **lateral plantar nerve** supplies a strip of skin corresponding to one and one-half toes (S-1); the **medial plantar nerve** innervates skin corresponding to three and one-half toes (L-5). The region of the heel is supplied by branches given off by the tibial nerve (calcaneal branches) before it divides into the plantar nerves (L-4, L-5, and S-1).

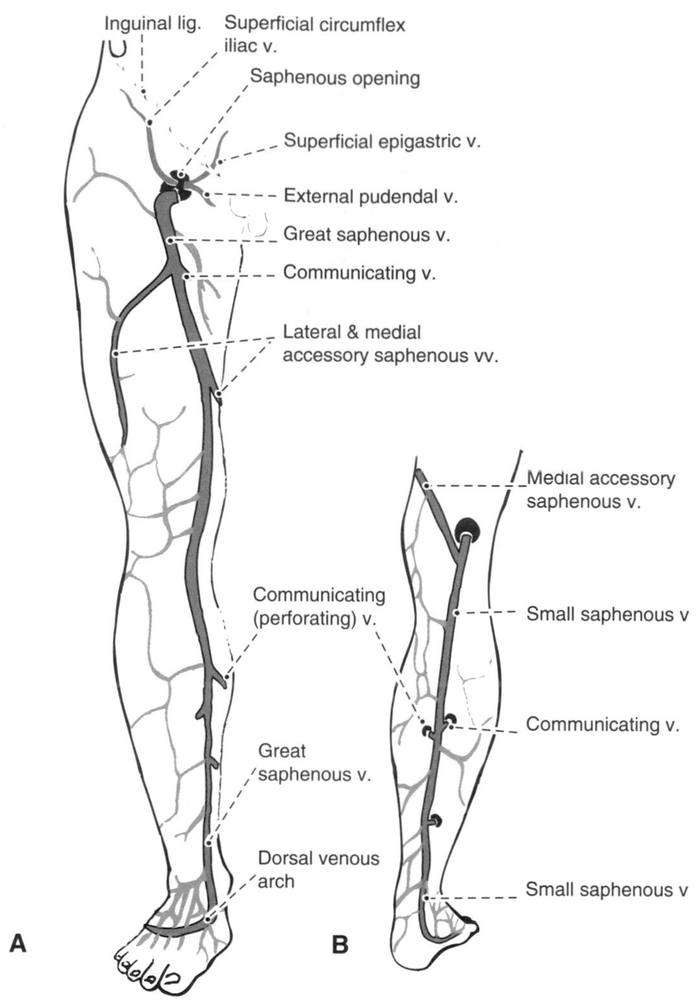

FIGURE *18-8.*
Superficial veins of the lower limb.

There is a good deal of variation in the amount of skin supplied by individual cutaneous nerves, particularly in the leg and foot. The dermatomal areas, however, are more constant. The assignment of dermatomes to the distribution territories of the various nerves in Figure 18-7, however, is an approximation.

Arteries

Arteries that run in the superficial fascia and supply the skin are branches of the main arterial trunks in respective segments of the limb (see Fig. 14-9). Only in the upper part of the front of the thigh are they of sufficient size to deserve mention; here several of them can be traced by dissection.

Small branches of the femoral artery emerge through the saphenous hiatus or penetrate the fascia lata close to it. Three of the named branches may arise separately or by a common stem. The **superficial circumflex iliac artery** runs upward and laterally toward the anterior superior iliac spine; the **superficial epigastric artery** runs upward and medially toward the umbilicus; and the **external pudendal artery** runs medially toward the external genitalia.

Veins

The general pattern of limb veins is discussed in Chapter 14 (see Fig. 14-10). Superficial veins of the lower limb are large vessels that return a significant amount of blood to the popliteal and femoral veins. Along their course, particularly in the leg, they are interconnected with the deep veins through *communicating veins* (known also as perforating veins, or "perforators"). Superficial, communicating, and deep veins contain valves. The valves in the superficial veins direct the flow upward and break up the long column of blood into smaller segments; those in the communicating veins direct the flow toward the deep veins. Disruption of this pattern increases venous pressure in the superficial veins leading to not only varicosities, but also to swelling (edema), ulceration of the skin, and other abnormalities (see later discussion).

The veins begin in the foot. Those of the plantar surface are small and embedded in tough connective tissue. They drain into the subcutaneous **dorsal venous plexus** (*dorsal venous network*) either directly, around the borders of the foot, or by way of deep veins in the sole, which are connected to the dorsal plexus by veins passing between the metatarsals. The dorsal plexus is composed of relatively large veins. It is established by the meeting of *dorsal digital veins* to form *metatarsal veins* which, in turn, anastomose to form a **dorsal venous arch** (Fig. 18-8). The great and small saphenous veins ascend from this arch; they correspond to the preaxial and postaxial veins of the limb, respectively (see Fig. 14-10).

The **great** (*long*) **saphenous vein** takes origin from the medial side of the arch (see Fig. 18-8). Starting anterior to the medial malleolus, it passes upward along the medial side of the leg, accompanied by the saphenous nerve. In its ascent the vein receives tributaries from all surfaces of the leg, some of them connecting it to the small saphenous vein. Communicating veins pass from it and its tributaries to the deep veins of the leg. Skirting the medial side of the knee, the great saphenous vein continues upward along the medial side of the thigh and terminates in the femoral vein, having passed through the cribriform fascia and the saphenous hiatus of the fascia lata.

Tributaries of the great saphenous vein include the veins that correspond to the cutaneous arteries of the inguinal region; these are the **superficial circumflex iliac, superficial epigastric**, and **external pudendal veins**. The great saphenous also receives tributaries from the sides of the thigh. Although variable, they usually include the **lateral** and **medial accessory saphenous veins**. The latter connects with the small saphenous vein (see following).

The **small** (*short*) **saphenous vein** begins at the lateral side of the dorsal venous arch and ascends behind the lateral malleolus (see Fig. 18-8). It passes almost straight up the middle of the calf, penetrates the crural or popliteal fascias, and terminates in the popliteal vein. In its course it receives tributaries from the posterior surface of the leg and gives off communications to the great saphenous vein and to the deep veins. Before it enters the popliteal vein, it sends a communicating branch around the medial side of the thigh to the great saphenous vein. Sometimes the entire small saphenous takes this course.

Venous Return. As mentioned in connection with the deep fascia of the lower limb, the mechanical force responsible for making blood flow upwards in the veins of the leg is generated by the contraction of muscles within their respective osseofascial compartments. In addition to increasing pressure within the compartments, the contracting muscles compress segments of the deep veins located between them. Because the venous valves prevent backflow, the stream is directed upward. Even though the movements of respiration create a pressure gradient facilitating venous return to the heart, blood will tend to stagnate in the veins of a leg in which muscles remain silent. Therefore, the danger exists in individuals who are immobilized that blood will clot in the leg veins (deep leg venous thrombosis). This may set up some inflammation in the veins (thrombophlebitis) and may also lead to pulmonary embolism. The latter condition results when a loosened clot is carried through the heart into a branch of the pulmonary artery and produces an infarct of the lung (pulmonary infarction).

Varicose Veins. When there is interference with the mechanisms of venous return, superficial veins become visibly dilated and tortuous. Quite gross distension is possible because the superficial fascia in which these veins are embedded provides little support. The factors that predispose to this condition remain unknown. Usually, however, varicose veins are associated with incompetent valves in some or all of the perforating veins. When the valves no longer function, the normal direction of blood flow isreversed: muscle contraction pumps blood from the deep veins into the superficial veins.

Lymphatics and Lymph Nodes

As in the upper limb, extracellular fluid is returned to the venous system by sets of deep and superficial lymphatic vessels. The **deep lymphatic vessels**, relatively few in number, follow the blood vessels as the latter run through the compartments of the limb. **Superficial lymphatic vessels** are far more numerous and run in the superficial fascia. Relatively few lymphatic vessels terminate in **popliteal lymph nodes** located deep in the popliteal fossa; the majority ascend to the groin and end in groups of deep and superficial **inguinal lymph nodes** (Fig. 18-9).

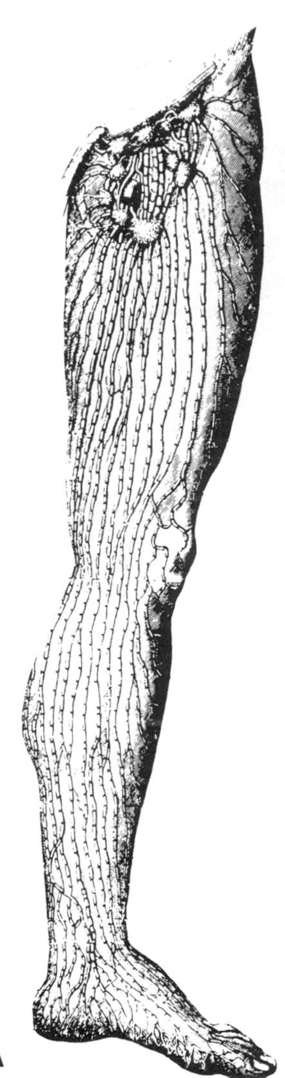

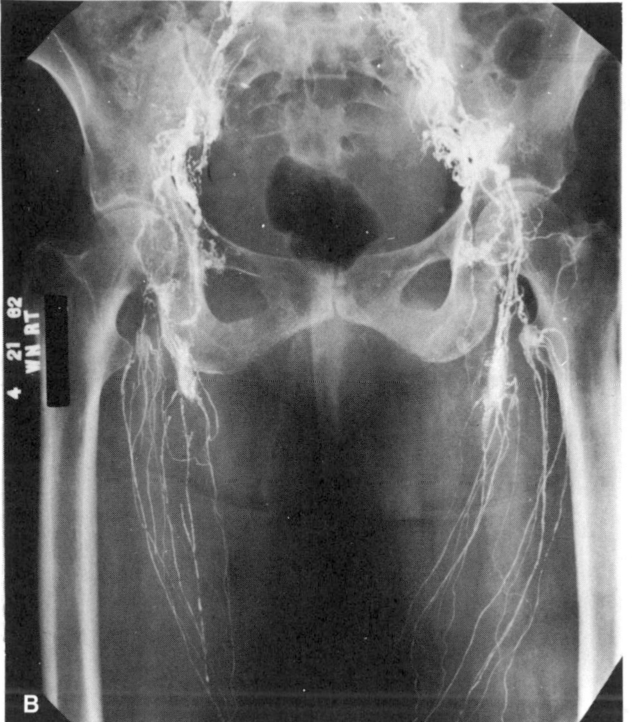

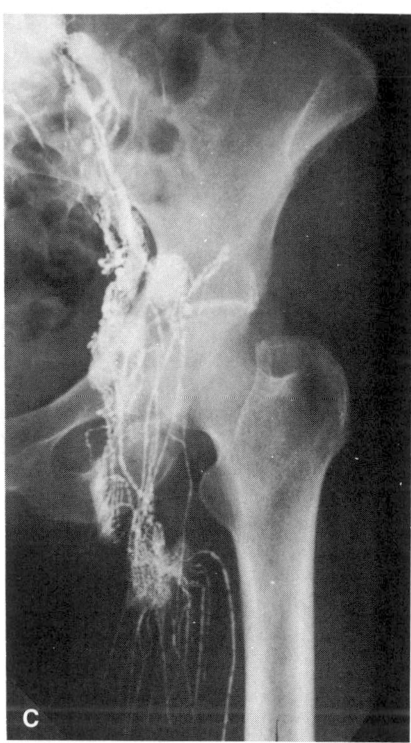

FIGURE *18-9.*
Superficial lymphatics of the lower limb: (A) drawing of a preparation of superficial lymphatic vessels coursing in the superficial fascia; (B and C) lymphangiograms showing opacified lymphatics, superficial inguinal lymph nodes, and their drainage into iliac nodes. (Panels B and C courtesy of Dr. W. E. Miller.)

A rich lymphatic plexus pervades the dermis and superficial fascia of the foot. Many superficial lymphatics ascend in the subcutaneous fascia of all surfaces of the leg and thigh. The largest vessels are usually found along the great saphenous vein, anterior to the medial malleolus. These may be cannulated for the injection of a radiopaque contrast medium to produce a lymphangiogram (see Fig. 18-9). Since lymphatic vessels are hard to find, it is usually necessary to inject a vital dye into the skin between the toes; the dye is carried from the cutaneous lymphatic plexus into the larger vessels, thereby aiding their identification. The technique of injecting various materials into the skin, subcutaneous tissues, and larger lymphatic vessels was used by anatomists in the 18th and 19th centuries to reveal the anatomy of lymphatics in different parts of the body. Figure 18-9*A* is based on such anatomic preparations, some of which are preserved to this day in anatomy museums.

Lymphatics from the lateral side of the foot and those along the back of the leg tend to converge on the small saphenous vein. Some of them penetrate the deep fascia with the vein and end deep in the popliteal fossa in one or two popliteal lymph nodes. The majority, however, continue uninterrupted to the inguinal nodes, as do all lymphatics from the medial side of the foot and leg (see Fig. 18-9*A*).

Inguinal Nodes. There are two main groups of lymph nodes in the inguinal region. The **deep inguinal nodes** are few and lie along the femoral vein deep to the fascia lata. The **superficial inguinal nodes** are in the superficial fascia around the saphenous hiatus. They vary in number from 12 to 20; some may be too small to be recognized in a dissection.

The superficial nodes tend to be arranged in two ill-defined subgroups: those lying parallel to the inguinal ligament, and those that lie along the upper end of the great saphenous vein. The latter group receives virtually all the lymph from the lower limb, whereas the former drains the anterior and posterior surfaces of the trunk below the level of the umbilicus, the gluteal region, the gluteal cleft, and the perineum, including the lower part of the anal canal, the vagina, and all of the external genitalia in both genders, with the exception of the testes (see Chap. 28).

The superficial inguinal lymph nodes are drained by

efferent lymphatics, some of which end in the deep inguinal lymph nodes. Most of them, however, pass deep to the inguinal ligament into the abdomen to end in external iliac nodes along the external iliac vessels. These nodes also receive efferents from the deep inguinal nodes.

Inguinal Lymphadenopathy. Because of the large drainage territory of inguinal lymph nodes, their enlargement calls for meticulous physical examination. Apart from distinguishing true inguinal lymphadenopathy (enlargement of lymph nodes) from other lumps in the groin, it is necessary to scrutinize all areas and regions that are drained by the nodes. Attention should be paid to the spaces between the toes (e.g., athlete's foot), the surfaces of the entire lower limb, the umbilicus, the natal cleft, anal canal, vagina, and external genitalia. Inflammatory lesions usually cause tenderness in the nodes. Lymph node enlargement caused by metastases from melanomas and carcinomas may not cause tenderness. Enlarged inguinal nodes may also signify generalized neoplastic disease of the immune system.

THE THIGH

The femur does not separate the thigh as clearly into a flexor and an extensor compartment (Fig. 18-10), as the humerus and intermuscular septa do in the arm (see Fig. 16-10). The extensor muscles (vastus medialis, lateralis, and intermedius) almost completely surround the femur as they arise from it, leaving only the linea aspera, a narrow strip of bone posteriorly, for the attachment of other muscles. Of the hamstring muscles in the posterior compartment, only the relatively small short head of the biceps femoris originates on the femur; the others arise from the ischial tuberosity and descend to insert around the knee. More bulky than these knee flexors are the adductors of the hip, the homologues of which, in the arm, are represented only by the insignificant coracobrachialis. They occupy a large medial part of the posterior compartment, an area that is often referred to as the adductor compartment, even though no septum intervenes between the flexor and adductor muscles.

There being no equivalent of the axilla, the main vessels of the limb (the femoral artery and vein) pass through a shallow, triangular, intermuscular space, the *femoral triangle*, as they emerge from beneath the inguinal ligament. They continue down the medial side of the thigh in an intermuscular tunnel (*adductor*, or subsartorial, *canal*), which runs between the extensor and adductor muscles and is roofed over by the sartorius muscle (see Figs. 17-22, 18-10, and 18-14). The femoral and obturator nerves are represented in the extensor and adductor compartments, respectively, only by their branches (see Figs. 18-13*C* and 18-21*C,D*). The sciatic nerve approaches the popliteal fossa sandwiched between the hamstrings and the adductor muscles. Its tibial component distributes branches to the muscles that originate from the ischial tuberosity (see Fig. 18-17). The other portion of the sciatic, the common fibular nerve, is destined primarily for muscles and skin below the knee.

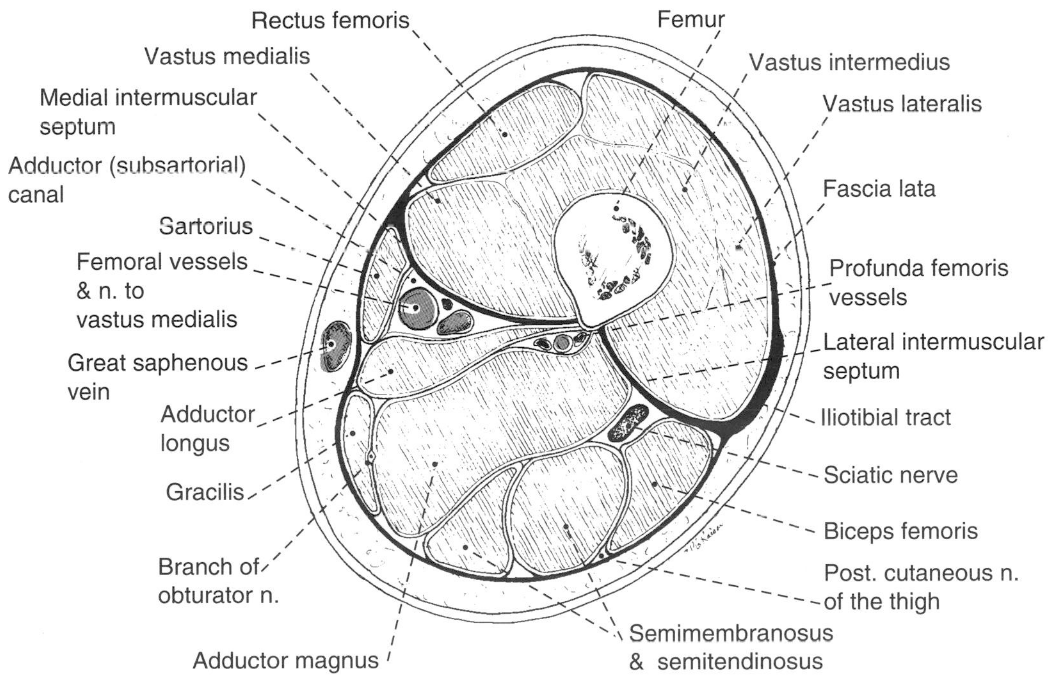

FIGURE *18-10.*
A transverse section through the middle third of the thigh, drawn to show schematically the division of the musculature into compartments and to illustrate the position of the main nerves and vessels. The thickness of the fascia lata, intermuscular septa, and iliotibial tract is exaggerated.

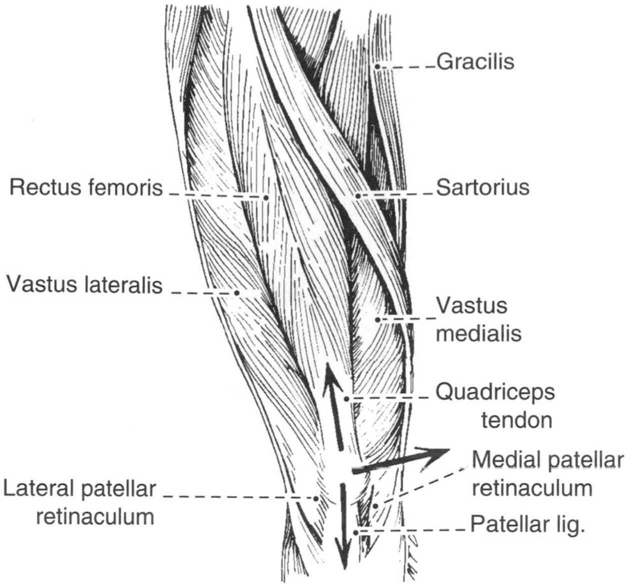

FIGURE *18-11.*
The quadriceps: The rectus femoris conceals the vastus intermedius. Note the insertion of some fleshy fibers of the vastus medialis into the medial side of the patella, which helps balance the pull on the patella by the quadriceps tendon and the patellar ligament. *Arrows* indicated directions of pull.

Anterior Compartment

Muscles

The large **quadriceps femoris** dominates the anterior compartment of the thigh. Its four constituent heads are the **rectus femoris, vastus medialis, vastus lateralis,** and **vastus intermedius** (see Figs. 17-22 and 18-11 through 18-13). A long strap muscle, the **sartorius**, spans the distance between the anterior superior iliac spine and the medial side of the tibia, across the front of the quadriceps. Among other muscles that are sometimes included in this group are the tensor fasciae latae, the iliopsoas, and the pectineus; the first two are described with the gluteal and hip regions in the previous chapter as well as in Chapter 25, and the pectineus, later with the adductor muscles.

Quadriceps Femoris. The quadriceps is the bulky extensor muscle complex of the knee. Its four heads arise independently and blend into the common, stout **quadriceps tendon**, through which they insert into the base of the patella (Fig. 18-11). The action of the quadriceps is exerted on the knee through the **patellar ligament** (*ligamentum patellae*), which attaches the apex of the patella to the tibial tuberosity. The rectus femoris is the most prominent, anterior member of the complex; the vastus intermedius is deep to it and covers most of the shaft of the femur; the medial and lateral vasti conceal the underlying vastus intermedius on respective sides of the thigh (see Fig. 18-11).

The **rectus femoris** arises from the ilium by two separate heads, both of which are tendinous: a *straight head* attached to the anterior inferior iliac spine and a *reflected head* to a point just above the margin of the acetabulum (see Fig. 17-3C). After combining with one another, the tendons of origin give rise to a bulky, fusiform muscle belly that terminates in the central and superficial component of the quadriceps tendon. Because the rectus femoris slants medially from its origin to its insertion, the force it transmits to the patella would tend, if unopposed, to dislocate the patella laterally (see Fig. 18-11). It is the only member of the quadriceps complex that acts on the hip as well as the knee (see Chap. 17).

The **vastus lateralis** covers the entire lateral aspect of the thigh and extends onto its anterior and posterior aspects. Because it is separated from most of the lateral surface of the femur by the underlying vastus intermedius, it arises mainly from the posterior aspect of the femur. Its attachment begins along the lower border of the greater trochanter and continues downward along the lateral lip of the linea aspera (see Fig. 17-6*B* and *D*). Some of its fibers take origin from the lateral intermuscular septum and the partial septum between it and the vastus intermedius (see Fig. 18-10). Most of the muscle inserts into the tendon of the rectus femoris, adding to its bulk to form the quadriceps tendon. Some fleshy fasciculi reach the upper and lateral border of the patella. Aponeurotic expansions from

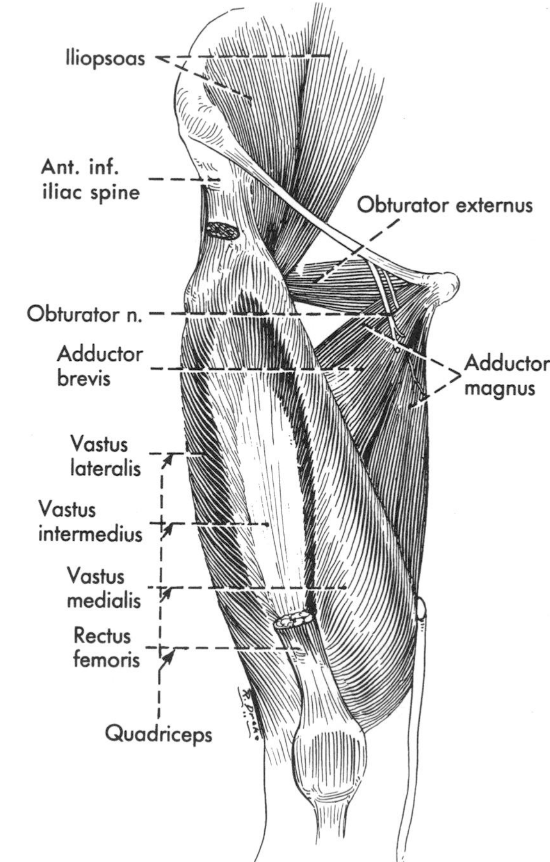

FIGURE *18-12.*
The three vastus muscles with the rectus femoris removed. Some of the deeper-lying adductor muscles on the medial side of the thigh are also illustrated.

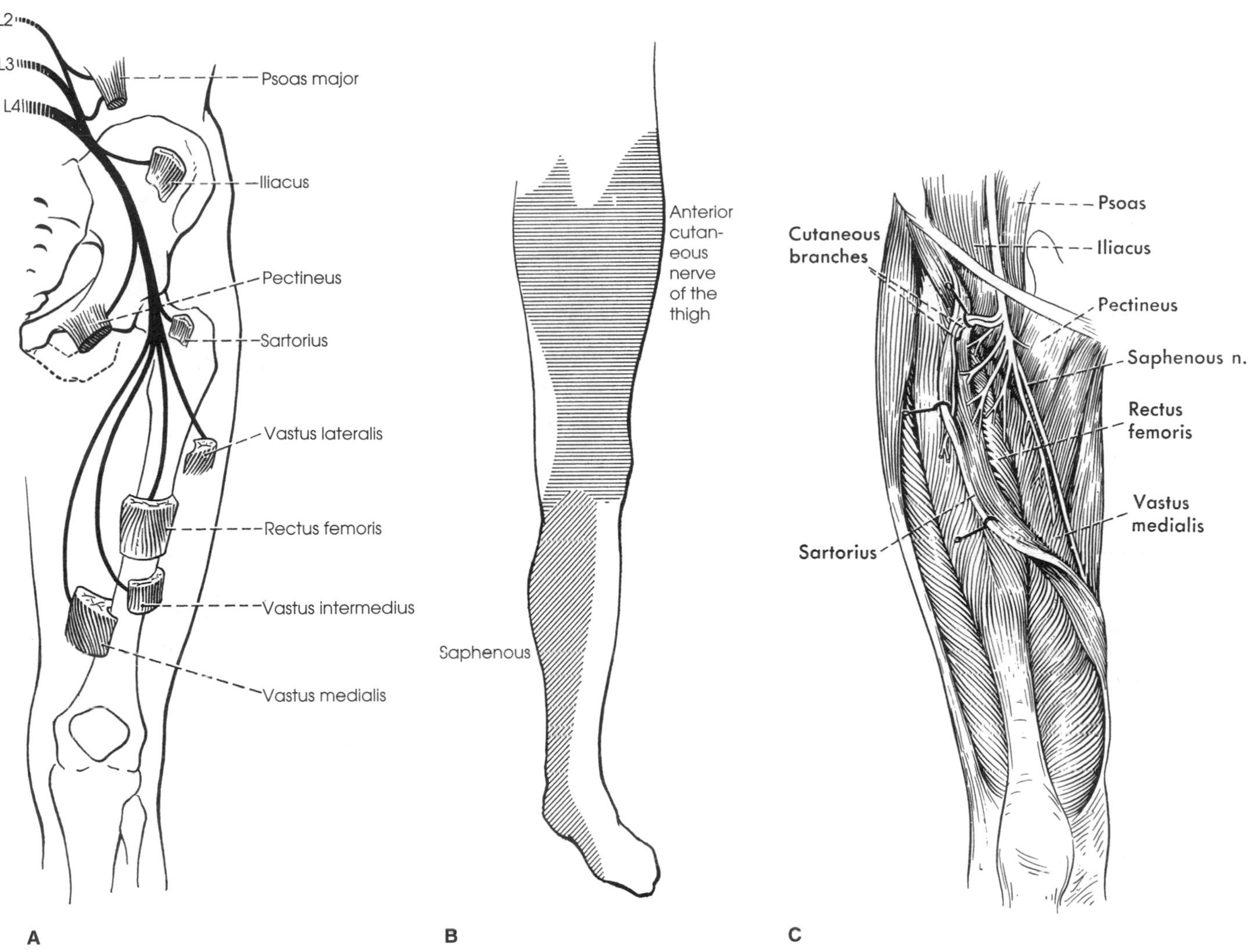

FIGURE *18-13.*
Distribution and course of the femoral nerve: (A) muscular distribution; (B) cutaneous distribution; (C) relation of the branches in the thigh.

the latter fibers blend with other connective tissue to help form the *lateral patellar retinaculum*, which makes up a part of the knee joint capsule (see Fig. 18-11).

The **vastus medialis** is largely separated from the front and medial side of the femur by the vastus intermedius (see Fig. 18-10). It arises from the lower portion of the intertrochanteric line, the medial lip of the linea aspera (see Fig. 17-6*B* and *D*), and the medial intermuscular septum, and inserts into the medial border of the quadriceps tendon. A substantial number of its inferior fibers insert directly into the medial side of the patella. In a muscular subject, the latter part of the muscle forms a definite bulge on the medial side of the knee cap. These fibers stabilize the patella, counterbalancing that force vector of the rectus femoris that tends to displace the patella laterally (see Fig. 18-11). Like the vastus lateralis, the vastus medialis contributes to the knee joint capsule through aponeurotic fibers that help to form the *medial patellar retinaculum*.

The **vastus intermedius** arises from the extensive smooth surface of the femoral shaft that extends from one lip of the linea aspera to the other, and also from the lateral intermuscular septum (see Fig. 17-6*C* and *D*). It is covered by the rectus femoris and the other two vasti. Above, deep fascia resembling a septum separates the lateral and medial vasti from it but, as the three vasti approach the knee, their muscle bellies fuse with each other (Fig. 18-12). The vastus intermedius inserts into the posterior surface of the upper border of the patella through tendon fibers that make up the deep part of the quadriceps tendon.

Deep to the inferior part of the vastus intermedius is a slender muscle composed of one or more small muscle bundles, the **articularis genus**. It is often considered a part of the vastus intermedius. It arises from the front of the femur, a hand's breadth above its condyles (see Fig. 17-6C), and inserts into the suprapatellar bursa, a fold of synovial membrane that extends upward from the knee joint, deep to the quadriceps tendon (see Fig. 18-34).

Innervation. The quadriceps is innervated by branches of the femoral nerve (Fig. 18-13). The segments involved are L-2, L-3, and L-4 (chiefly L-4). An elicitation of the knee jerk tests the integrity of these segments (see Table 13-1 and Fig. 13-23) as well as the femoral nerve and the muscles.

Each component of the quadriceps receives one or more branches from the femoral nerve. The vastus intermedius often receives extensions of nerves to the vastus medialis and lateralis, in addition to its own nerve. The articularis genus is supplied by the continuation of the branch to the vastus intermedius.

Action. The four heads of the quadriceps, acting in unison through the quadriceps tendon, the patella, and the ligamentum patellae, extend the tibia on the femur. The quadriceps is the only muscle that can actively extend the leg. As such, it is tonically contracted whenever full extension of the knee is maintained with the foot off the ground. By contrast, when the fully extended knee supports the body weight, the quadriceps is completely relaxed. It is reflexly recruited, however, as soon as the weight-bearing knee flexes. Its contraction is readily palpable not only during rising from a seated position (knee extension) but also during the reverse act, which is accompanied by progressive knee flexion. Indeed, it is a critical muscle for stabilizing the weight-bearing knee in any position other than full extension.

The quadriceps is best demonstrated by opposing knee extension, with the subject seated on the edge of an examination table. The strength of the muscle can be built up by lifting weights with the foot. An athlete can lift one-third of his or her body weight through 90°.

Sartorius. The sartorius arises from the anterior superior iliac spine (see Fig. 17-3C) and inserts on the upper medial surface of the tibial shaft, close to the insertions of two other slender muscles of the thigh, the gracilis and the semitendinosus (see Fig. 18-2C). The straplike belly of the muscle crosses the thigh as it curves downward toward the medial side of the knee (see Figs. 17-22, 18-11, and 18-14). Its insertion is separated from that of the other muscles by the *anserine bursa*.

Because the sartorius crosses both the hip and the knee, it can affect both joints. It has a flexor action on both the hip and knee and can also contribute to lateral rotation of both the tibia and femur, as well as abduction of the femur. Compared with other larger muscles that produce these actions, however, its contribution is negligible. Acting together with other muscles that originate on the pelvic girdle and insert on the tibia, it probably helps in balancing the pelvis. It received its name (*sartor*; Latin for tailor) because it assists in putting the leg into a position adopted by a tailor when he or she, sitting cross-legged, supports a garment on one thigh, placing the lateral malleolus on the opposite knee.

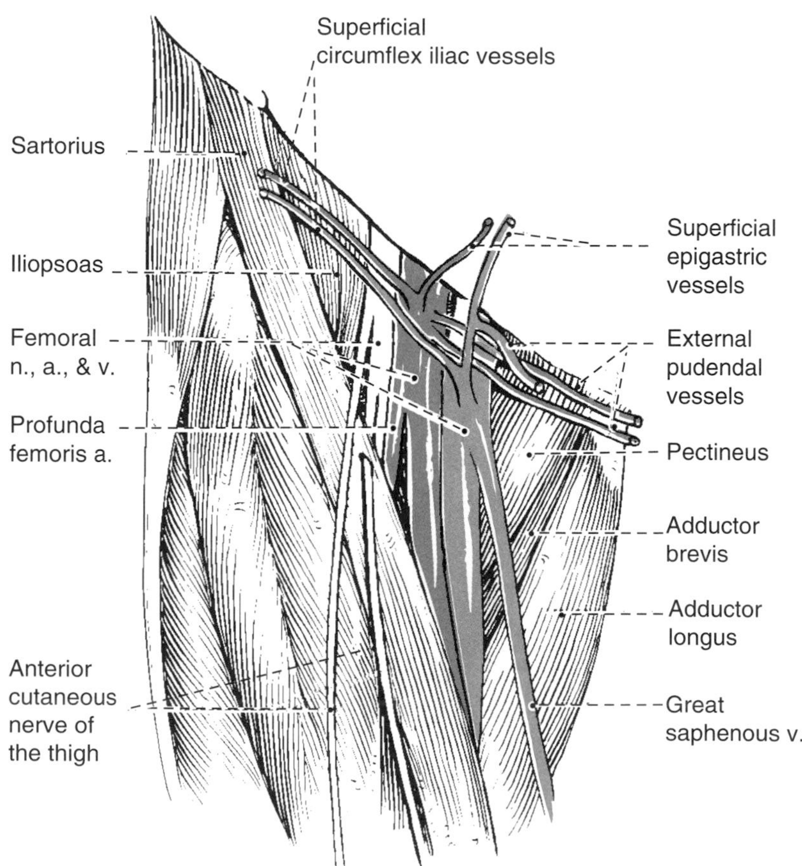

FIGURE *18-14.*
The femoral triangle and its contents.

The sartorius is a useful topographic landmark because it forms the lateral boundary of the femoral triangle (Fig. 18-14) and roofs over the adductor canal (see Fig. 18-10). It receives two branches from the femoral nerve and is frequently pierced by cutaneous branches of that nerve.

Femoral Nerve

The femoral nerve innervates all muscles in the anterior compartment of the thigh and supplies the skin covering the front of the thigh and the medial side of the leg and foot (see Fig. 18-13). Clinically it can be evaluated by eliciting the knee jerk, testing the power of knee extension, and examining cutaneous sensitivity over the medial malleolus.

Formed by the posterior divisions of L-2, L-3, and L-4 roots of the lumbar plexus (see Fig. 17-9), the femoral nerve descends on the posterior abdominal wall between the psoas major and iliacus muscles before it enters the thigh behind the inguinal ligament. Here the nerve lies on the surface of the iliopsoas muscle; medial to it is the femoral artery (see Figs. 18-14 and 26-17). It has a very short course in the upper part of the femoral triangle, before breaking up into a number of muscular, cutaneous, and articular branches.

The **muscular branches** of the femoral nerve include two branches to the *sartorius*, two to the *rectus femoris*, and at least one branch to each of the *three vastus muscles*. Some fibers from the nerves to the vastus lateralis and the vastus medialis continue into the vastus intermedius, and the nerve of the vastus intermedius continues into the articularis genus. Usually, as soon as it enters the femoral triangle, the femoral nerve also gives a branch to the *pectineus*, the most proximal adductor muscle of the thigh. Muscular branches of the femoral nerve contain fibers mainly from L-3 and L-4 roots of the plexus.

The **cutaneous branches** of the femoral nerve are described earlier (see General Orientation). These are the *anterior femoral cutaneous nerves* and the *saphenous nerve* (see Figs. 18-7 and 18-13). One or more of these may send a branch Into the sartorius, and others pass through the muscle. The saphenous nerve descends in the adductor canal sheltered by the sartorius. The cutaneous branches convey predominantly L-2, L-3, and L-4 fibers to the skin (see Fig. 18-7).

The femoral nerve gives **articular branches** to the hip and knee joints. *Nerves to the hip joint* may arise directly from the femoral nerve or from one of its muscular branches. *Nerves to the knee joint* are given off by the nerves to the vasti.

Femoral Vessels

The femoral artery is the chief artery of the lower limb (see Fig. 14-9). It is the direct continuation of the external iliac artery, the vessel changing its name as it passes deep to the inguinal ligament. After entering the popliteal fossa, the artery becomes known as the popliteal artery. The femoral vein, which accompanies the femoral artery, commences inferiorly as the popliteal vein and continues superiorly as the external iliac vein. The musculature of the thigh is supplied predominantly by the deep branch of the femoral artery (*profunda femoris artery*); the femoral artery itself passes through the thigh to serve primarily the leg and foot. The same is true for the femoral vein and its tributary, the *profunda femoris vein*.

Femoral Artery. The femoral artery enters the femoral triangle midway between the symphysis pubis and the anterior superior iliac spine (see Fig. 18-14). It emerges from underneath the inguinal ligament, which forms the base of the triangle, and leaves at the triangle's apex, which is formed at the meeting point of the sartorius and adductor longus. Here it enters the adductor (subsartorial) canal. Just above the adductor tubercle of the femur, the artery inclines posteriorly and enters the popliteal fossa passing through a hiatus in the tendinous attachment of the adductor magnus to the femur. (Fig. 18-15)

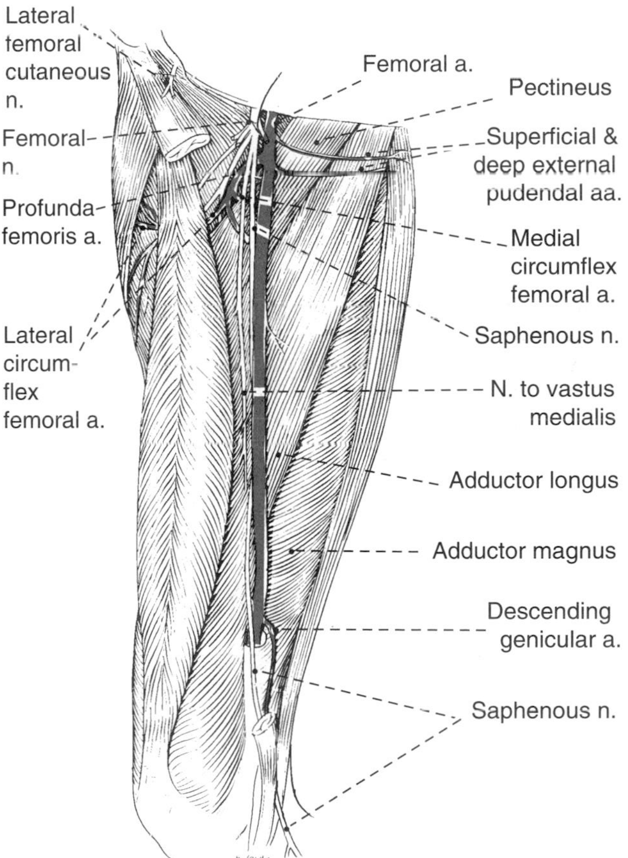

FIGURE *18-15.*
The course of the femoral artery in the right thigh after the sartorius muscle and the fascia covering the adductor canal have been removed.

Relations. The changing relation between the femoral artery and the femoral vein as they descend through the femoral triangle and the adductor canal is a reflection of the developmental rotation of the limb. Starting out in a medial position at the triangle's base, the vein winds behind the artery as the two vessels approach the triangle's apex (see Fig. 18-14). This relation is retained throughout the adductor canal, in which the artery and vein run toward the medial condyle of the femur (Fig. 18-15).

In its descent from the midinguinal point to the adductor hiatus, the artery lies on the pectineus, adductor longus, and the lower part of the adductor magnus (see Fig. 18-15). Its pulsations may be felt through the fascial roof of the femoral triangle as the artery is compressed against the pectineus. In the adductor canal, the vastus medialis and sartorius are its anterior relations (see Fig. 18-10). In the femoral triangle, the femoral nerve is lateral to the artery. Two of the femoral nerve's branches, the saphenous and the branch to the vastus medialis, accompany the femoral artery in the adductor canal (see Fig. 18-15).

Branches. The femoral artery has several small superficial and muscular branches, as well as two large branches, the *profunda femoris* and *descending genicular arteries*.

The *superficial circumflex iliac, superficial epigastric*, and *external pudendal arteries* are given off by the femoral artery in the femoral triangle for the supply of the superficial tissues of the groin and the external genitalia (see Figs. 18-14 and 18-15). Other small branches given off in the adductor canal supply the neighboring muscles.

The **profunda femoris artery** (*deep femoral artery*) is the largest and most important branch. It arises from the posterolateral side of the femoral artery in the femoral triangle and provides the chief source of blood for the thigh musculature. Clinicians sometimes refer to the femoral artery above the origin of this vessel as the *common femoral artery*, and to the continuation of the main vessel below this branch as the *superficial femoral artery*.

The profunda femoris artery passes posterolaterally in the femoral triangle, then curves behind the femoral artery and enters the posterior compartment by passing between the pectineus and adductor longus (see Fig. 18-15). Its course and most of its branches are described in a later section (see Fig. 18-19). Before it leaves the femoral triangle, the deep femoral artery gives off two of its largest branches, the **lateral** and **medial circumflex femoral arteries**. They participate in the circumtrochanteric and cruciate anastomoses, and send branches as far down as the knee (**descending branch of the lateral circumflex**).

The **lateral circumflex femoral artery** typically arises from the lateral side of the upper end of the profunda, but in some 15% or so of instances it is given off by the femoral above the profunda. It runs laterally across the front of the iliopsoas muscle, between the branches of the femoral nerve, to pass behind the sartorius and rectus femoris muscles. Here it divides into an *ascending*, a *descending*, and a *transverse branch*. They all supply adjacent muscles and anastomose with other arteries. The *ascending branch* runs laterally and upward, deep to the rectus femoris and the tensor fasciae latae, to anastomose with branches of the superior gluteal vessels. It also gives branches to the femur. The *descending branch* (which sometimes arises separately from the femoral or from the profunda) runs downward behind the rectus femoris and gives branches into the vastus lateralis and intermedius muscles. Above the knee, it anastomoses through the vasti with perforating branches of the profunda femoris and also with branches of the genicular vessels. Thus it contributes to the collateral circulation around the knee joint (see Fig. 18-43). The *transverse branch* of the lateral circumflex artery passes through the vastus lateralis and participates in the formation of what is called the *cruciate anastomosis* in the buttock (see Chap. 17).

The **medial circumflex femoral artery** arises from the medial side of the profunda (sometimes, directly from the femoral artery) and turns posteriorly between the iliopsoas and pectineus muscles. It gives off muscular branches and an *acetabular branch* that anastomoses with the posterior branch of the obturator artery and helps that vessel supply tissues in the acetabular fossa. The *artery of the ligament of the femoral head* is the continuation of one or the other vessel. The circumflex artery divides into a *superficial* and a *deep branch*; the latter divides into an *ascending* and a *transverse branch*, both of which enter the buttock in relation to the quadratus femoris muscle (see Fig. 17-12). The ascending branch heads toward the trochanteric fossa to anastomose with branches of the gluteal vessels, whereas the transverse branch contributes to the cruciate anastomosis.

Close to the lower end of the adductor canal, the femoral artery gives off its last named branch, the **descending genicular artery**, which divides into *articular* and *saphenous branches*. The former enters into the anastomosis near the knee (see Fig. 18-43), and the latter supplies the muscles on the medial side of the knee and sends twigs to the overlying skin.

Intermittent Claudication. The femoral artery and its branches are frequently affected by atherosclerosis. Atheroma may seriously limit, or completely block, blood flow. The resulting ischemia in the muscles, especially during exercise, manifests itself by pain. The pain develops during walking and is rapidly relieved by rest. The condition is known as intermittent claudication (*claudicatio*; Latin for limping).

If the profunda femoris artery is blocked, pain develops in the thigh muscles during walking. Blockage of the femoral artery distal to the origin of the profunda leads to intermittent claudication in the calf. If the artery is blocked more proximally, symptoms develop in the calf sooner than in the thigh, because blood finds its way from other vessels to the thigh muscles through the extensive anastomoses established by the circumflex femoral arteries.

Femoral Vein. The course and tributaries of the femoral vein correspond to the course and branches of the femoral artery. The vein receives numerous muscular tributaries and, in the femoral triangle, the **profunda femoris vein** and the **great saphenous vein** empty into it. Both *circumflex femoral veins* typically enter the femoral vein instead of the deep femoral vein, but otherwise the deep femoral artery and vein are quite similar.

Anatomic Relations

A description of anatomic relations in the femoral triangle, femoral sheath, and adductor canal provides a useful summary of the structures in the anterior compartment of the thigh.

Femoral Triangle. The triangle is an intermuscular space in the proximal part of the anterior compartment of the thigh (see Fig. 18-14). The sides and floor of the triangle are formed by muscles, its roof by the fascia lata. The base of the triangle is the *inguinal ligament*. The lateral border, composed of the *sartorius*, meets the medial border, formed by the *adductor longus*, at the triangle's apex. The floor is formed by the *iliopsoas* laterally and the *pectineus* medially, which slope toward each other forming a sulcus. The femoral artery and vein occupy this sulcus from the base of the triangle to its apex. In addition to these vessels, which are enclosed in their own fascial sleeve called the *femoral sheath*, the triangle also contains the femoral nerve and its branches, the profunda femoris artery and vein, the circumflex femoral vessels, and the deep inguinal lymph nodes. The relations of the artery, vein and nerve to one another are described earlier (see under Femoral Artery).

The saphenous opening is located in the roof of the triangle and the vessels that pass through the cribriform fascia have a short passage within the triangle. These include the great saphenous vein, the superficial circumflex iliac, superficial epigastric and external pudendal vessels, and efferent lymphatics from the superficial to the deep inguinal lymph nodes.

Femoral Sheath. The femoral sheath is a sleeve formed around the proximal parts of the femoral artery and vein by extensions of fascial laminae that line the abdominal cavity. The clinical significance of the femoral sheath is its association with femoral hernias, which are discussed in Chapter 26 (see Figs. 26-17 and 26-18). The sheath is formed as if the femoral vessels had dragged a diverticulum of the fascial lining of the abdomen with them into the femoral triangle.

The sheath begins posterior to the inguinal ligament within the abdomen. The anterior layer of the sheath is formed by an extension of transversalis fascia, which covers the inner surface of the abdominal wall muscles; its posterior lamina is an extension of the fascia on the abdominal surface of the iliopsoas (see Fig. 26-17). Thus formed, the femoral sheath fuses with the adventitia of the femoral vessels 3 to 4 cm below the inguinal ligament.

The space enclosed by the sheath is divided into three compartments by two septa that pass between its anterior and posterior walls (Fig. 18-16): the *lateral compartment* contains the femoral artery and the femoral branch of the genitofemoral nerve (which pierces the anterior wall of the sheath to become subcutaneous); the *intermediate compartment* contains the femoral vein; the *medial compartment* shorter than the other two, contains only a slight amount of loose connective tissue and one or two lymphatic vessels and nodes discussed later. The latter compartment is known as the **femoral canal**. It forms a potential space into which the femoral vein can expand when it transmits an increased amount of blood during muscular activity in the lower limb.

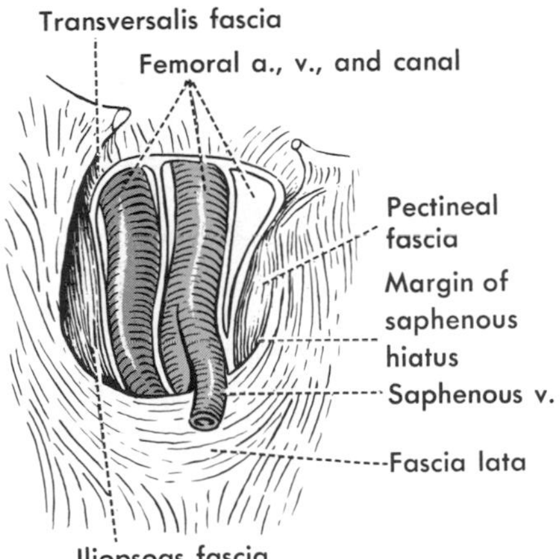

FIGURE *18-16.*
The three compartments of the femoral sheath as seen on the *right side* opened from the *front*. The cribriform fascia has been removed.

Femoral Hernia. In cases of femoral hernia, abdominal contents protrude into the femoral canal (see Fig. 26-16). As the hernia expands, it dilates the femoral canal and the femoral sheath. Emerging through the saphenous opening, it also expands the cribriform fascia. The descent of the hernia into the thigh is prevented by the attachment of the membranous layer of the superficial fascia to the fascia lata below the inferior margin of the saphenous hiatus.

Adductor Canal. Known alsoas the *subsartorial canal*, this intermuscular passage transmits the femoral vessels toward the region of the knee. The adductor canal is located between the quadriceps and the adductor muscles (see Fig. 18-10). It commences at the apex of the femoral triangle and terminates above the medial condyle of the femur at the adductor hiatus. The posterior wall of the canal is formed, for the most part, by the adductor longus, and its anterior wall by the vastus medialis. As its alternative name implies, it is roofed over by the sartorius. Deep to the sartorius, however, there is a definite lamina of fascia that connects the medial intermuscular septum to the deep fascia of the adductor muscles and intervenes between the sartorius and the contents of the canal (see Fig. 18-10).

In addition to the femoral artery and vein, the canal transmits the saphenous nerve and the nerve to the vastus medialis.

Posterior Compartment

The posterior compartment of the thigh, separated from the anterior by the lateral and medial intermuscular septa, encloses the hamstring muscles (flexors of the knee) and the adductor muscles of the hip. The nerves associated with these muscles are the tibial and obturator nerves, respectively, both derived from the anterior divisions of the lumbosacral plexus. The tibial nerve is united by connective tissue to the common fibular nerve, and the branches it gives off appear as branches of the sciatic nerve; the obturator nerve (like the femoral nerve) is represented by only its branches in the thigh. The entire compartment is served by branches and tributaries of the profunda femoris vessels.

Muscles

Hamstring Muscles. The hamstring muscles include the biceps femoris, the semitendinosus, the semimembranosus, and the posterior (ischial) component of the adductor magnus (Fig. 18-17). All these muscles attach proximally to the ischial tuberosity; before reaching their distal attachments, all but the adductor magnus cross the knee joint. The latter muscle, therefore, has no action on the knee, but the biceps, semimembranosus, and semitendinosus flex that joint. The extensor action of these muscles on the hip joint is considered in the previous chapter.

As the hamstring muscles approach the knee, they diverge to enclose the popliteal fossa between them. Only the biceps femoris passes to the lateral side; the semimembranosus, semitendinosus, and adductor magnus are medial. The tendons of insertion around the knee are associated with a number of bursae.

As its name implies, the **biceps femoris** has two heads, a long and a short head. The *long head* arises from the ischial tuberosity with the semitendinosus (see Fig. 17-3C). The *short head* arises from the lateral lip of the linea aspera and the lateral intermuscular septum (see Fig. 17-6*D*). The two heads unite in the lower third of the thigh, and their tendon of insertion crosses the posterolateral aspect of the knee joint to attach to the head of the fibula (Fig 18-2*C* and *D*). Just before it attaches, the tendon splits to let through the fibular collateral ligament, and also sends some fascial extensions to the lateral tibial condyle and the deep fascia of the leg.

The **semitendinosus**, a slender muscle, arises from the ischial tuberosity from a tendon that it shares with the long head of the biceps femoris (see Fig. 17-3C). Its muscle belly is usually interrupted by a tendinous partition. As it passes downward it diverges medially and gives rise to another tendon, which crosses behind the knee joint and then curves forward to insert in association with the sartorius and gracilis into the medial aspect of the body of the tibia just below the medial condyle (see Fig. 18-2C). The *anserine bursa* separates the tendons of these muscles. Like most of the tendons around the knee, that of the semitendinosus gives off fibrous expansions that blend with the fascia of the leg.

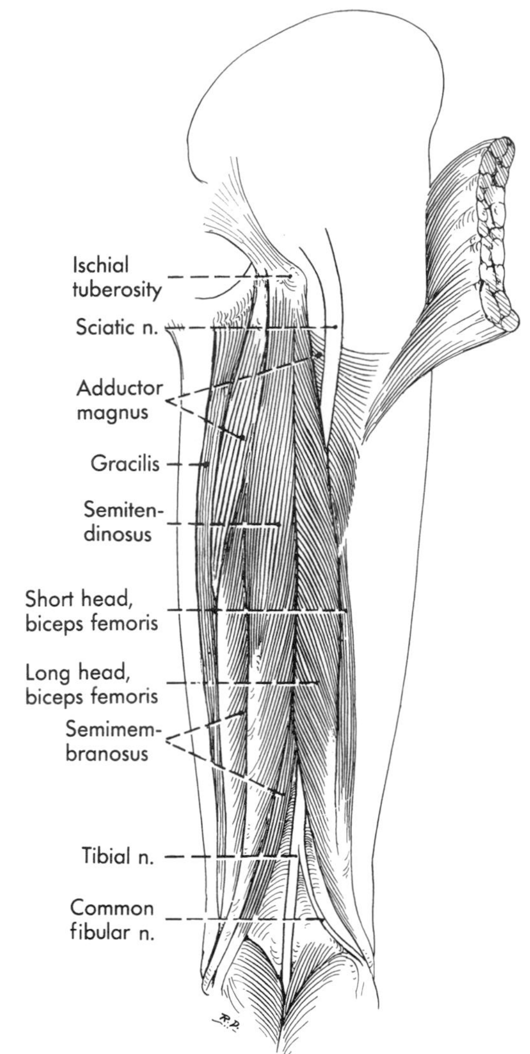

FIGURE *18-17.*
The posterior (hamstring) muscles of the right thigh: The gracilis, also shown here, belongs to the adductor group.

The **semimembranosus** is tendinous at both its origin and its insertion. Its tendon of origin, attached to the lower portion of the ischial tuberosity (see Fig. 17-3C), is long and flat (resembling a membrane). It passes downward deep to the semitendinosus and, at the middle of the thigh, gives rise to muscle fibers. The muscle, in turn, is replaced by a rounded tendon that inserts into the posteromedial side of the medial tibial condyle. The tendon gives off a heavy lateral expansion into the knee joint capsule, forming much of the substance of the *oblique popliteal ligament* (see Fig. 18-36). Fascial expansions from the tendon also reinforce the medial patellar retinaculum and blend with fascia over the popliteus muscle in the depth of the popliteal fossa. A *bursa* intervenes between the tendon of the semimembranosus and the edge of the medial condyle, and another separates it from the medial head of the gastrocnemius.

The **posterior** (*ischial*) **component of the adductor magnus** resembles the flexors of the knee on the medial side of the thigh in every respect except that its tendon does not cross the knee joint, but rather, inserts on the lower end of the femur (chiefly the adductor tubercle; see following). In various other vertebrate species, the tendon of this muscle does indeed cross the knee joint, just as those of the hamstrings, and inserts into the tibia; in humans, the tendon appears to have "retreated," as it were, to a more proximal insertion on the femur. In its place, a strong band of connective tissue, the *tibial collateral ligament*, continues on to the tibia (see Figs. 18-36 and 18-37). This ligament is believed to be a vestigial remnant of the distal part of the tendon which, in some other vertebrates, crosses the knee joint. The muscle is described in the next section together with its pubic or anterior component.

Innervation. All muscles in the posterior compartment of the thigh, including the ischial part of the adductor magnus, receive one or more branches from the tibial component of the sciatic nerve. There are usually two nerves each to the semitendinosus, the somimembranosus and sometimes also to the long head of the biceps. Reminiscent of the branch supplied by the radial nerve to the brachialis, the short head of the biceps femoris is innervated by the common fibular component of the sciatic nerve, rather than its tibial component. The spinal cord segments represented in these branches are predominantly L-5 and S-1 (see Fig. 13-23), with some L-4 and S-2 fibers supplementing the branches to some of the muscles.

Adductor Muscles. The adductor musculature of the thigh occupies the medial part of the posterior compartment, which is often called the adductor compartment. In addition to the adductor brevis, adductor longus, and adductor magnus, this group includes the obturator externus, the pectineus and the gracilis (Fig. 18-18). They are innervated by the obturator nerve, except for the pectineus, which is often supplied by the femoral nerve.

Most of these muscles have already been encountered in this chapter or in the previous one (in which their actions at the hip joint are discussed). The obturator externus is the deepest and most proximal muscle. The pectineus is in the floor of the femoral triangle. The adductor brevis, longus, and magnus fan out from their pubic attachments to the linea aspera; through the part of the adductor magnus that originates from the ischial tuberosity, they blend with the hamstring muscles. The gracilis is the only member of the group that crosses the knee joint.

The **obturator externus** is at poor mechanical advantage for adducting the thigh (see Fig. 18-18*A* and *B*). Located at the proximal limit of the adductor compartment (see Fig. 18-12), it arises from the external surface of the obturator membrane and from adjacent surfaces of the pubis and ischium (see Fig. 17-3C). It forms a twisted cone as its fibers converge to insert into the trochanteric fossa. It is adjacent to the inferior part of the hip joint capsule as it twists to gain the back of the femur. It produces lateral rotation rather than adduction at the hip. The muscle is concealed from view in the femoral triangle by the iliopsoas and pectineus.

The **pectineus muscle** (see Fig. 18-18*C* and *D*) lies just medial to the iliopsoas and forms the medial part of the floor of the femoral triangle (Fig. 18-19). It arises from the pecten of the pubis and the bone anterior to the pecten, and inserts on the pectineal line, the proximal extension of the linea aspera (see Figs. 17-6*B* and *D* and 18-18*D*).

The **adductor brevis** (see Fig. 18-18*A* and *B*) is the distal neighbor of the pectineus, and is largely posterior to the adductor longus. It arises from the body and inferior ramus of the pubis and expands in a triangular fashion as it approaches its insertion on the upper part of the linea aspera (see Fig. 17-6*D*).

The **adductor longus** (see Figs. 18-18*C* and *D* and 18-19) is the most anterior member of the adductor group. It arises by a strong tendon from the front of the body of the pubis, just below the pubic tubercle, and expands to insert on the linea aspera. The muscle forms much of the posterior wall of the *adductor canal*. The femoral ("superficial femoral") vessels pass downward on its anterior surface (see Fig. 18-15), and *deep femoral vessels* pass behind it, lying on the adductor brevis and the adductor magnus (see Fig. 18-19).

The **adductor magnus**, the largest and most posterior member of the adductor group (see Figs. 18-18*E* and *F* and 18-19), is a composite muscle consisting of distinct anterior (pubic) and posterior (ischial) parts that have fused with each other. The *anterior (pubic) component of the adductor magnus* arises from the inferior ramus of the pubis and the ramus of the ischium, and fans out to insert along the length of the medial lip of the linea aspera (see Fig. 18-18*E* and *F*). The most superior fibers arising anteriorly run almost horizontally to the upper end of the linea aspera, whereas those arising further along the conjoint ramus run in increasingly oblique directions to attach in continuity along the linea. In its morphology and innervation, the anterior component of the muscle is a bona fide member of the adductor musculature.

The *posterior (ischial) component of the adductor magnus* is composed of vertical fibers that originate on the ischial tuberosity and insert on the adductor tubercle and medial supracondylar ridge of the femur (see Fig. 17-6*A*). Except for its action, this component of the muscle resembles the hamstring muscles. The vertical fibers are inseparable from the anterior component of the muscle and form the medial margin of the adductor magnus. Close to its insertion, the posterior component becomes tendinous. Just above the tubercle, there is a gap in the tendon's attachment to the supracondylar ridge; the gap is the **tendinous** (*adductor*) **hiatus**. As the femoral vessels pass through the hiatus from the adductor canal to the popliteal fossa, they become known as popliteal vessels. Much smaller gaps in the attachment of the anterior component of the muscle to the linea aspera allow the perforating branches of the deep femoral vessels to reach the posterior compartment (see Figs. 18-19 and 18-22).

The **gracilis** is a long, slender muscle lying superficially along the medial side of the thigh (see Fig. 18-18*E* and *F*). It arises from the body and inferior ramus of the pubis and inserts into the medial surface of the upper end of the tibia below the medial condyle. Below the knee, its tendon curves forward and expands before it attaches to the bone close to the insertions of the sartorius and semi-

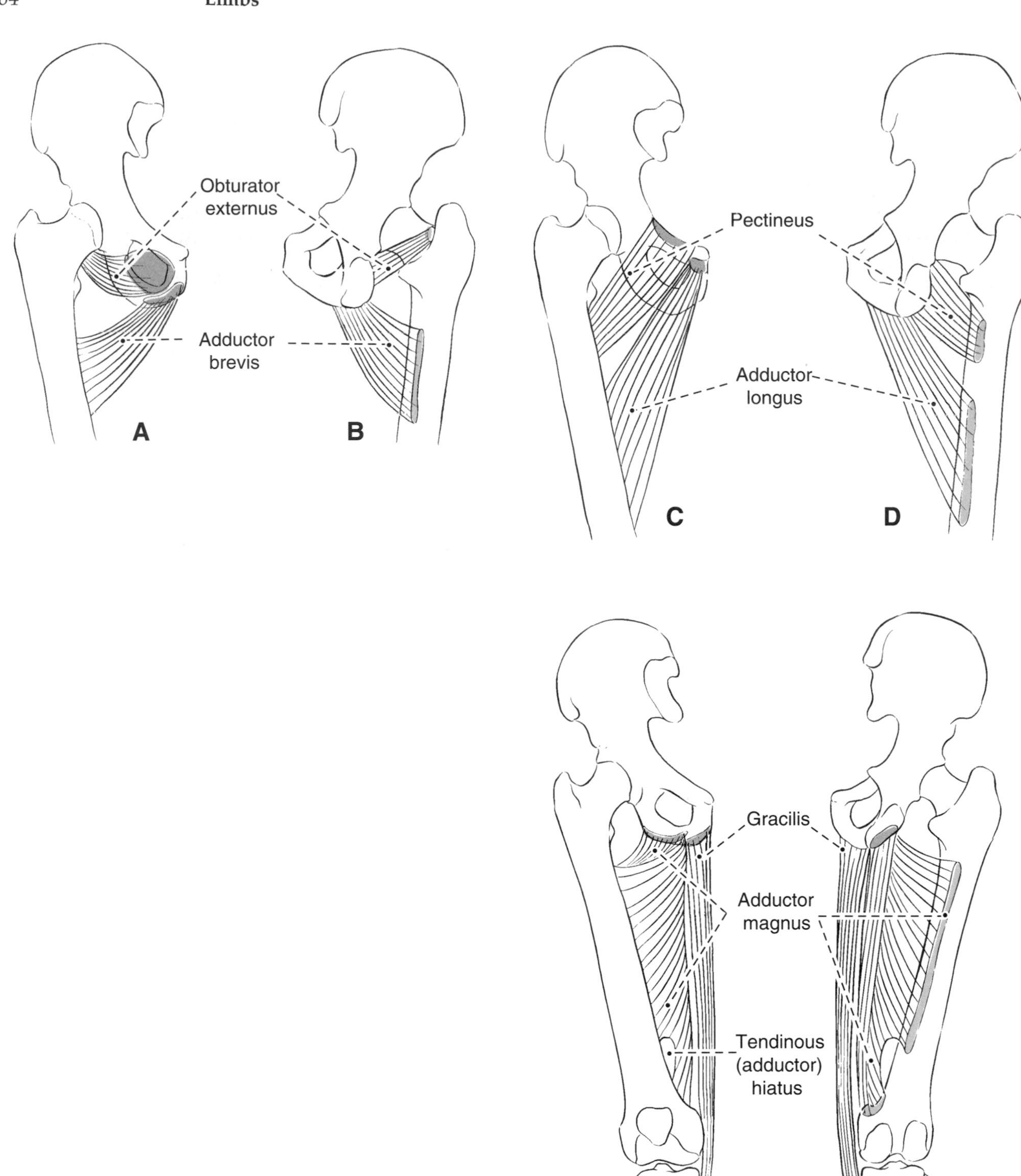

FIGURE *18-18.*
The adductor muscles of the thigh: (A, C, and E) anterior views; (B, D, and F) posterior views. Sites of origin are shown in *red*, insertions in *blue*.

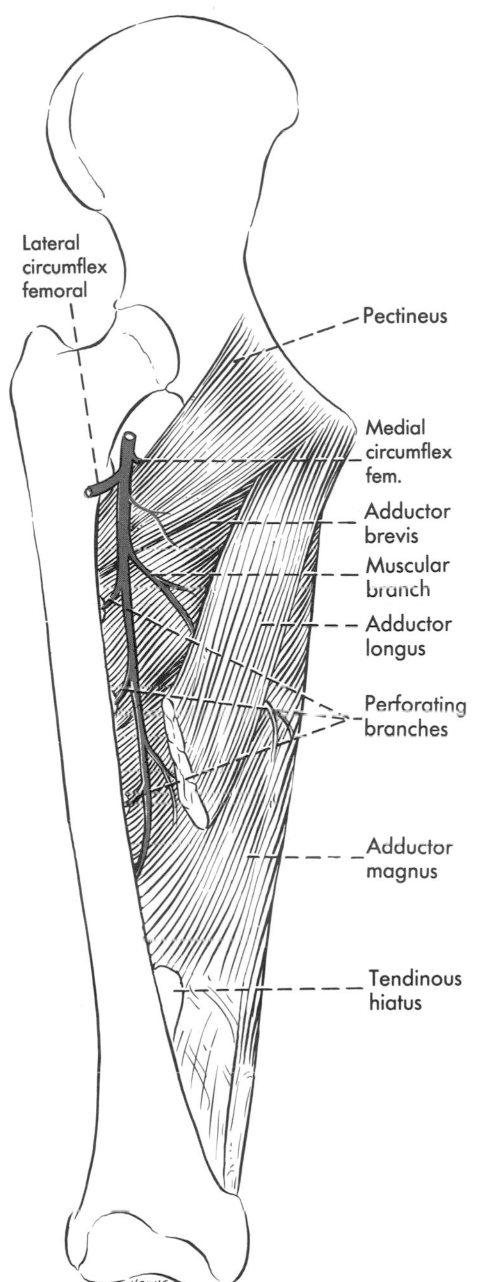

FIGURE *18-19.*
The profunda femoris (deep femoral) artery and the muscles related to it.

tendinosus. The expanded tendons of these three muscles are sometimes referred to as the *pes anserinus*, named after their fanciful resemblance to the foot of a goose. The lobulated *bursa anserina* intervenes between the three tendons.

Variations. The anterior upper part of the adductor magnus may form a separate, relatively distinct muscle, which is then called the **adductor minimus**. Occasionally there may be some fusion between the adductor brevis and longus, or between these and the pectineus.

Innervation. The main nerve supply for the adductor muscles is provided by the obturator nerve (see Fig. 18-21). The nerve gives branches to the obturator externus, adductor brevis and longus, and the gracilis (from its anterior division), and to the anterior (pubic) component of the adductor magnus (from its posterior division). The segments represented in these branches are predominantly L-3 and L-4. The pectineus muscle is only rarely supplied entirely by the obturator nerve, although it often receives a branch from it; usually, the muscle is innervated by a branch of the femoral nerve. The ischial (posterior) component of the adductor magnus is supplied by the tibial half of the sciatic nerve.

Actions. With the exception of the ischial part of the adductor magnus, which is an extensor of the hip joint, all muscles in the adductor group run in a more or less medial to lateral direction and, therefore, produce adduction of the thigh. Because the pubic attachments of these muscles are anterior to their femoral attachments, they also flex the hip. The adductor brevis, longus, and the pubic part of the adductor magnus are most effective in adduction, whereas the pectineus is the most effective flexor in the group. Because the gracilis crosses the knee as well as the hip, it can flex the knee as well as adduct and flex the hip. It also rotates both the tibia and the femur medially.

The other muscles in the adductor group also impart a rotational force vector to the femur, for they insert posterior to the long axis of the bone. The direction of the rotation, however, remains controversial. The obturator externus contributes to lateral rotation, but the direction of rotation produced by the other muscles may vary, depending on whether they act on a limb that is weight-bearing or one that is off the ground. Some electromyographic studies of these muscles report activity in them during lateral rotation, others during medical rotation. The importance of the adductors in relation to hip movements, posture, and ambulation is discussed in the preceding chapter.

Nerves

Sciatic Nerve. The sciatic nerve is a composite nerve in that two major terminal branches of the sacral plexus are united within it by connective tissue. Of these two components, the tibial nerve is largely medial and the common fibular nerve is largely lateral.

Course. The sciatic nerve begins its course through the thigh in the buttock, located deep to the gluteus maximus, half way between the ischial tuberosity and the greater trochanter (see Chap. 17). From this point it runs straight down within the posterior compartment and terminates when its two components separate from one another in the popliteal fossa (Fig. 18-20). There is no major artery that follows a similar course for the chief blood

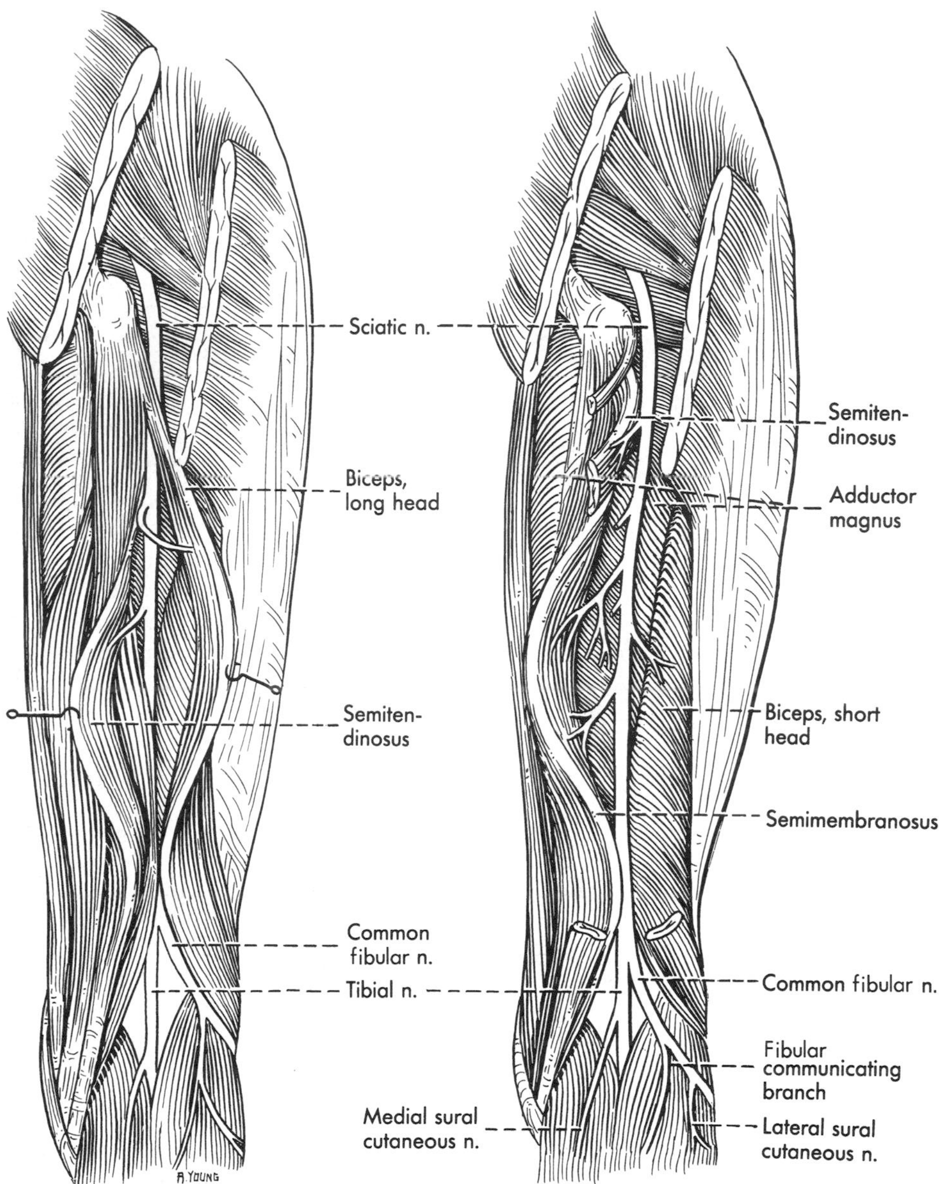

FIGURE *18-20.*
Course and branches of the sciatic nerve in the thigh. Note that its only lateral branch is to the short head of the biceps.

supply to the posterior aspect of the thigh is through branches of the anteriorly placed deep femoral artery. The minor artery associated with the nerve (*arteria comitans nervi ischiadici*) is of developmental interest only, as it represents the axial artery of the limb bud (see Chap. 14).

While still hidden by the gluteus maximus, the nerve disappears deep to the combined origin of the long head of the biceps and the semitendinosus muscle (see Fig. 18-20). Sheltered thereafter by the semimembranosus, the sciatic nerve descends on the posterior surface of the adductor magnus and the short head of the biceps. It usually divides into its terminal branches as soon as it reaches the popliteal fossa. Variations in the level of this division are described in the previous chapter.

Branches. Several branches are given off from the medial side of the sciatic nerve and only one from its lateral side (see Fig. 18-20). The latter, derived from the common fibular nerve, enters the short head of the biceps femoris. The medial branches, all derived from the tibial nerve, enter the other hamstring muscles, including the long head of the biceps and the ischial part of the adductor magnus.

The **common fibular** (*common peroneal*) **nerve** diverges laterally from the sciatic nerve and follows the lower edge of the biceps toward the head of the fibula. The **tibial nerve** continues almost straight down the middle of the popliteal fossa, gradually passing posterior to the popliteal vessels.

Obturator Nerve. The obturator nerve supplies all the adductor muscles of the thigh and an area of skin on the medial side of the thigh (Fig. 18-21). It also sends articular branches to both the hip and the knee joint.

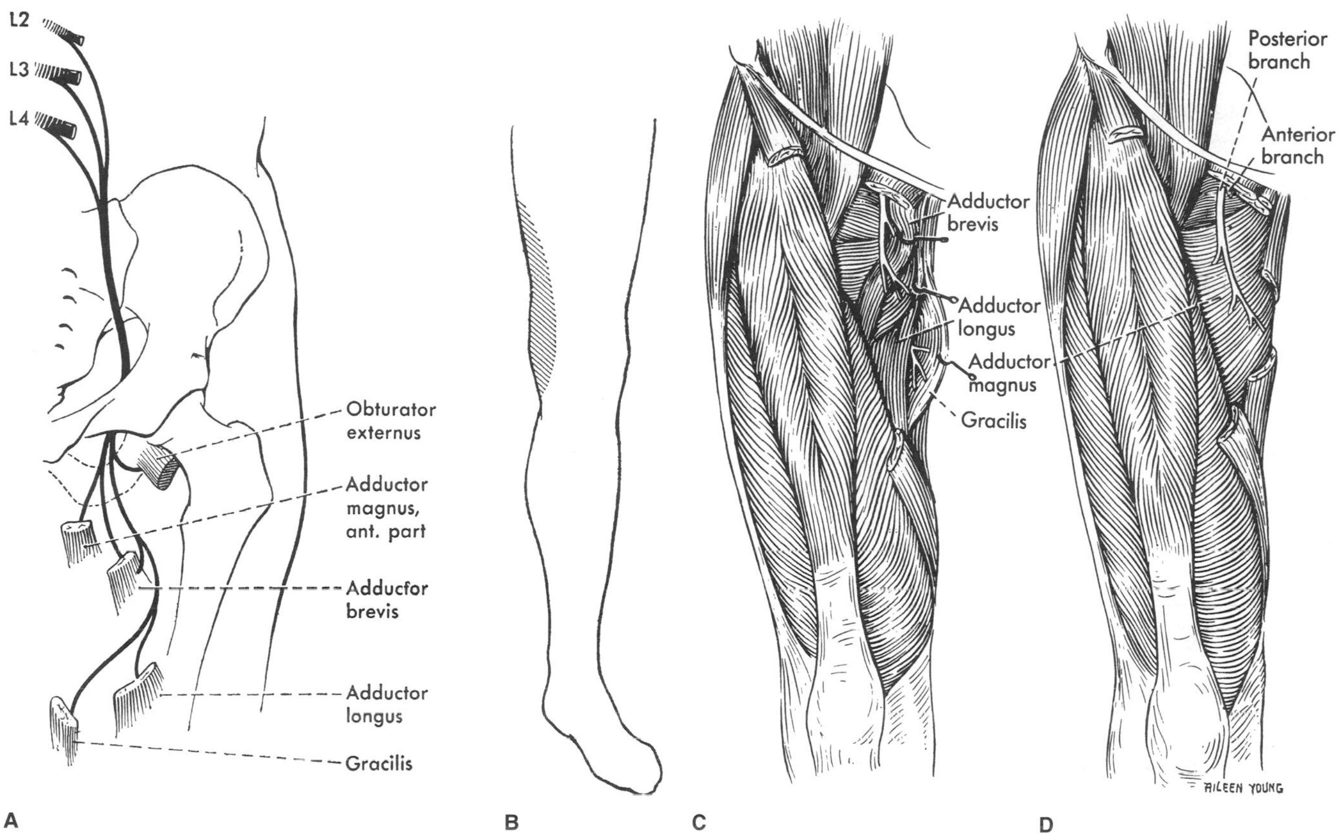

FIGURE *18-21.*
Distribution of the obturator nerve: (A) to muscles (the occasional branch to the pectineus is omitted); (B) to skin. The course and relations of (C) the anterior branch and (D) posterior branch of the obturator nerve are also shown.

Formed by the anterior divisions of L-2, L-3, and L-4 roots of the lumbar plexus (see Fig. 17-9), the obturator nerve diverges from the femoral nerve in the substance of the psoas major muscle. Surfacing on the medial side of the psoas, it crosses the ala of the sacrum and passes along the lateral pelvic wall to the obturator canal (see Figs 25-2 and 27-11). While in the canal, the nerve supplies the obturator externus and the hip joint, and then splits into an *anterior* and a *posterior branch* (or *division*). Both branches enter the thigh behind the pectineus muscle, sometimes passing through the obturator externus, and are separated from one another by the adductor brevis (see Fig. 18-21C).

The *anterior branch* (see Fig. 18-21*C*) runs down on the anterior surface of the adductor brevis and gives off branches to this muscle and the adductor longus, and ends in the gracilis. It also gives rise to the *cutaneous branch* to the medial side of the thigh.

The *posterior branch* runs behind the adductor brevis and longus, on the anterior surface of the adductor magnus (see Fig. 18-21*D*). It distributes its branches to the anterior or pubic part of the adductor magnus. It may supply the adductor brevis as well, which may be innervated by either or both divisions of the obturator nerve. The posterior branch also gives rise to an *articular branch to the knee joint* that descends along the femoral artery.

Accessory Obturator Nerve. In about 10% of lower limbs, there is an accessory obturator nerve. The nerve is not aptly named, because in its course and distribution it resembles the femoral, rather than the obturator nerve. When present, the accessory obturator nerve is a branch of the lumbar plexus, formed by fibers from L-2 and L-3, or the L-3 and L-4 roots of the plexus, at the point where the femoral and obturator nerves separate from each other. The nerve follows the course of the femoral nerve, entering the thigh deep to the inguinal ligament on the surface of the pectineus muscle. It innervates the pectineus muscle and sends an articular branch to the hip joint. It frequently communicates with the obturator nerve, but only rarely does it take over the supply of some of the muscles served by the obturator nerve.

Vessels

Profunda Femoris Artery. The origin and course of the deep femoral artery are described in the section dealing with the anterior compartment of the thigh. After it has given off its circumflex femoral branches in the femoral triangle, the profunda femoris artery runs down behind the main femoral vessels on the surface of the pectineus and adductor brevis muscles (see Fig. 18-19). Reaching the upper margin of the adductor longus, it passes behind that muscle and comes to lie directly on the front of the adductor magnus. The artery dispenses branches to muscles of the adductor group, and from its lateral side gives off a set of **perforating branches**. These vessels are so named because they pass through the tendinous insertions of the adductor muscles and thus make their way into the posterior compartment (Fig. 18-22). As a rule there are four perforating branches, including the terminal branch of the deep femoral artery. The usual pattern is for the first two perforating vessels to penetrate the adductor brevis and the upper segment of the adductor magnus, and for the last two branches, including the terminal branch, to perforate the adductor magnus only.

The perforating branches provide the chief blood supply to the posterior muscles. However, the *inferior gluteal artery* gives twigs to the upper ends of the muscles attaching to the ischial tuberosity, and the *transverse branch of the medial circumflex femoral artery* also contributes.

The **profunda femoris vein** corresponds to the artery and its tributaries accompany the arterial branches. The vein terminates in the femoral vein.

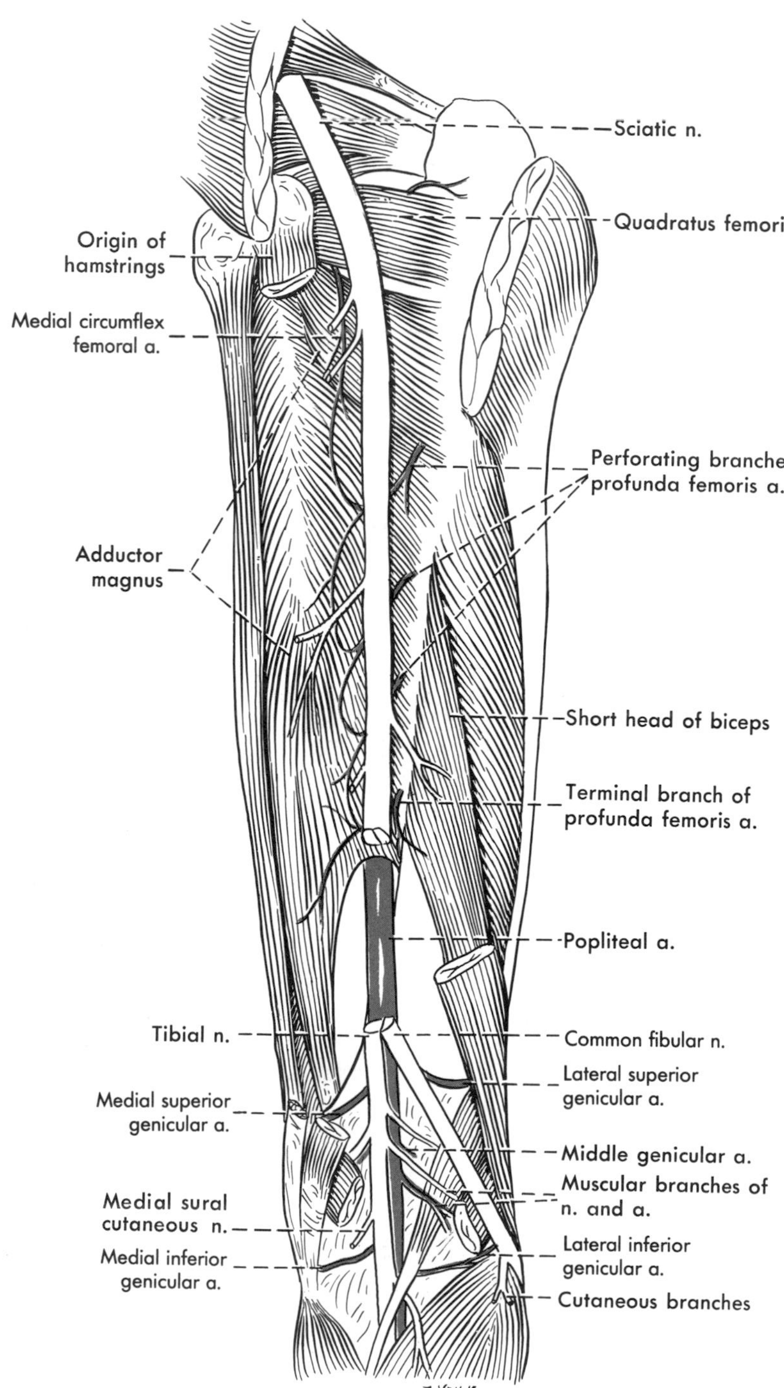

FIGURE *18-22.*
The popliteal fossa and nerves and arteries of the posterior compartment of the thigh. Not all branches of the sciatic nerve are shown. The popliteal vein and a section of the sciatic nerve have been removed to show the course of the popliteal artery through the adductor (tendinous) hiatus.

Obturator Vessels. The obturator artery arises in the pelvis from the internal iliac artery (see Figs. 27-8 and 27-9), and the accompanying vein enters the internal iliac vein. They do not contribute to any significant extent to the blood supply of the limb.

The vessels accompany the obturator nerve in the pelvis and, as they emerge through the obturator canal, divide into anterior and posterior branches. Instead of continuing down into the thigh, they encircle the obturator foramen, supplying the obturator externus muscle and the adjacent bone. The posterior branch of the obturator artery gives rise to an acetabular branch, which enters the acetabular notch, anastomoses with the acetabular branch of the medial circumflex femoral artery and supplies tissue in the acetabular fossa. The small artery of the ligament of the head of the femur arises more often from the posterior branch of the obturator artery than from the medial circumflex femoral.

Lymphatics. There are relatively few deep lymphatics in the thigh, which drain lymph from all tissues deep to the fascia lata. Drainage is upward along the femoral artery and its branches. The lymphatics end in one to three **deep inguinal lymph nodes** that lie on the medial side of the femoral vein near the inguinal ligament. The highest and largest of these nodes is located in the femoral canal and receives lymph from the glans penis or clitoris, directly or through superficial inguinal nodes. The deep inguinal nodes drain along the femoral vessels into the external iliac nodes.

THE POPLITEAL FOSSA

The popliteal fossa is a rhomboidal intermuscular space located behind the knee joint, in the adjoining posterior compartments of the thigh and the leg; in other words, in the popliteal region. Largely filled by fat, the fossa transmits the major nerves and blood vessels between the thigh and the leg. Although several structures that form its boundaries are described fully in a subsequent section, the fossa is best considered here because it is a region of transition into the leg. Its extent can be appreciated only after the popliteal fascia has been reflected, and the muscles that form its boundaries separated.

Boundaries

Proximally, the lateral boundary of the fossa is formed by the biceps femoris, and the medial boundary by the semitendinosus and semitendinosus (see Fig. 18-17). The lower borders are formed by the large superficial muscle of the calf, the gastrocnemius, the two heads of which arise from the medial and lateral epicondyles of the femur and converge toward each other in the calf (see Fig. 18-24). The fossa is roofed over by the popliteal fascia; in its floor are the popliteal surface of the femur, the knee joint capsule, and the popliteus muscle, which covers the back of the upper end of the tibia (see Fig. 18-25).

Contents

Deepest in the popliteal fossa is the popliteal artery (see Fig. 18-22); the popliteal vein is directly posterior to it, and the tibial nerve is posterior to the vein. These three structures, as well as the common fibular nerve, all give off a number of branches or receive tributaries while in the fossa. Embedded in popliteal fat are the popliteal lymph nodes and lymphatics.

Popliteal Artery

The popliteal artery commences at the adductor hiatus as the continuation of the femoral artery and terminates by dividing into *anterior and posterior tibial arteries* after it has left the fossa. It descends through the middle of the popliteal fossa anterior to the popliteal vein and gives off sets of *genicular arteries* for the supply of the knee joint as well as a number of muscular branches. The genicular and muscular arteries participate in an extensive circumarticular anastomosis described with the knee joint (see Fig. 18-43). Although these anastomotic channels are quite extensive, they are rarely adequate when sudden occlusion of the popliteal artery occurs. In such cases, gangrene of the foot and leg usually ensues. Gradual occlusion, as in the case of atheroma, may allow for some enlargement of the anastomotic vessels.

Branches. A pair of **superior genicular arteries,** *medial and lateral,* run around the lower end of the femur. Similarly a pair of **inferior genicular arteries,** *medial and lateral,* encircle the upper end of the tibia (see Figs. 18-22 and 18-43). A single **middle genicular artery** passes anteriorly to enter the joint capsule and is distributed to structures within the joint. The largest muscular branches of the popliteal artery are the **sural arteries,** given off just before the artery terminates. They are paired vessels that are the chief source of blood for the gastrocnemius and soleus muscles.

Popliteal Vein

Formed by the union of anterior and posterior tibial veins, the popliteal vein ascends along the popliteal artery, lying superficial (posterior) to it. Passing through the adductor hiatus, it becomes the femoral vein. There is some variability in the pattern of formation of the popliteal vein, and in the distribution of its tributaries. Usually, however, the pattern resembles that of the popliteal artery and its branches. One unique feature is the presence of the small saphenous vein, which drains into the popliteal vein at approximately the midpoint of the popliteal fossa. Occasionally, the lower end of the popliteal vein is doubled, or the vein divides into two vessels proximally. One of these veins joins the femoral vein and the other, the profunda femoris vein.

Nerves

The *sciatic nerve* usually reaches the popliteal fossa and divides into the *tibial and common fibular nerves* in the upper part of the fossa, lying posterolateral to the popliteal vessels. The common fibular nerve diverges laterally to pass around the lateral side of the leg, whereas the larger tibial nerve descends almost straight down through the fossa (see Fig. 18-22). Tibial nerve and popliteal vessels together pass deep to the converging heads of the gastrocnemius muscle.

Branches. Usually the **common fibular nerve** gives off two **cutaneous branches** (the *fibular communicating branch* and the *lateral sural cutaneous nerve*; see Fig. 18-7) before it leaves the fossa. It does not innervate any muscles until it divides in the leg. The **tibial nerve** has one cutaneous and several muscular branches, as well as an articular branch to the knee joint. The cutaneous branch is the **medial sural cutaneous nerve** (see Fig. 18-7), and the **muscular branches** are for the calf muscles that arise from the femur.

Popliteal Lymph Nodes

These few small nodes receive both superficial and deep lymphatics. The superficial lymphatics accompany the small saphenous vein and drain lymph from the lateral side of the foot and the back of the leg. The deep ones run with the anterior and posterior tibial arteries and drain the deep tissues of the leg and the foot. Efferents from the popliteal nodes course along the popliteal and femoral arteries to the deep inguinal nodes.

THE LEG

The compartments of the leg are mentioned in an earlier section (see General Orientation), including the muscle groups they contain and the nerves that supply them. Figure 18-23 shows the topographic arrangement. Understanding of individual muscles in the various compartments will be facilitated by first considering their functional grouping relative to their actions at the ankle joint and the joints of the foot. In these considerations reference should be made to Figures 18-23 to 18-26 and 18-30.

Functional Grouping of Muscles

The flexors of the ankle and the digits occupy the posterior compartment or the calf, and the extensors are located in the anterior compartment (see Fig. 18-23). A lateral compartment contains the peroneal muscles. Each of these compartments is supplied by its own nerve; the tibial nerve serves the flexor compartment, the deep fibular nerve the extensors, and the superficial fibular nerve the peroneal muscles.

Prime Movers of the Ankle

Corresponding to the radial (preaxial) and ulnar (postaxial) flexors and extensors of the wrist, there are, in the appropriate compartments, a pair of primary plantar flexors and a pair of dorsiflexors for the ankle.

The **plantar flexors** include the two heads of the **gastrocnemius**, which are functional analogues of the two wrist flexors (Fig. 18-24). The **soleus**, lying deep to the gastrocnemius, corresponds morphologically to the flexor digitorum superficialis in the forearm and, like that muscle, originates from both bones in the limb's intermediate segment. However, the soleus does not reach the sole of the foot, for its path is interrupted by the backward projecting heel: Therefore, it inserts, together with the gastrocnemius, through the massive **calcaneal** or **Achilles tendon** into the posterior surface of the calcaneus. Acting together as the **triceps surae**, the three muscle bellies represent the most important element in providing the impetus for propulsion.

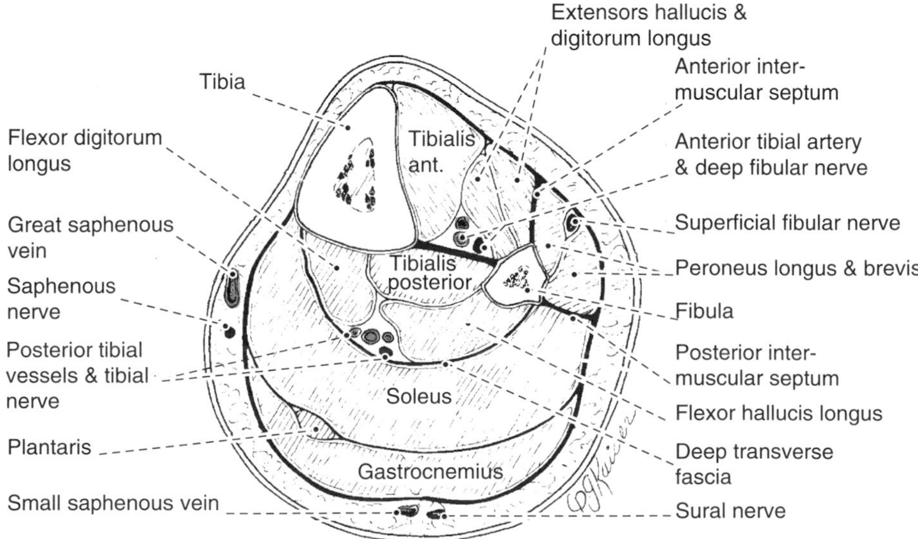

FIGURE *18-23.* **Transverse section through the middle third of the leg to show its compartments.**

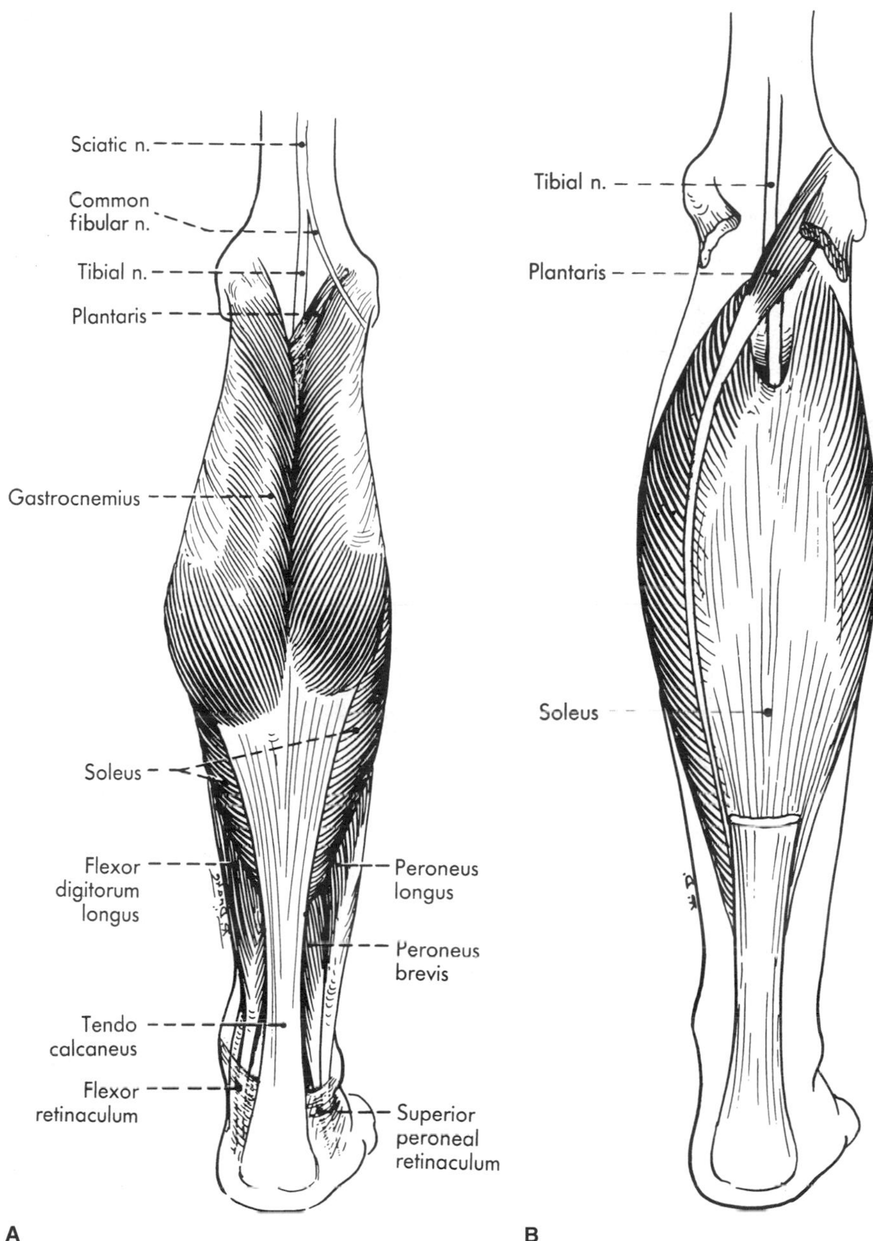

FIGURE *18-24.*
Muscles of the calf: (A) after removal of the crural fascia; (B) after removal of the gastrocnemius.

The **plantaris** resembles the palmaris longus, but its tendon is not continuous with the plantar aponeurosis because the muscle, like the soleus, is "captured" by the heel (see Fig. 18-24). Other muscles that pass behind the axis of the ankle joint can also plantar flex the foot. However, because they do not make use of the heel as a lever arm, they are less powerful and less effective. Of these, the most important is the **tibialis posterior** (Fig. 18-25).

The primary **dorsiflexors** of the ankle on the preaxial and postaxial borders of the leg are the **tibialis anterior** and the **peroneus tertius** (see Fig. 18-30). The latter muscle is badly misnamed because it is in the extensor, rather than the peroneal, compartment and functions primarily as an extensor.

Extrinsic Prime Movers of the Toes

Because the superficial digital flexor represented by the soleus does not reach the digits, there is only one common extrinsic digital flexor in the calf, the **flexor digitorum longus** (see Fig. 18-25). It corresponds to the flexor digitorum profundus in the forearm. As in the forearm, the flexor of the first digit, here the **flexor hallucis longus**, is a separate muscle. The corresponding extensors are the

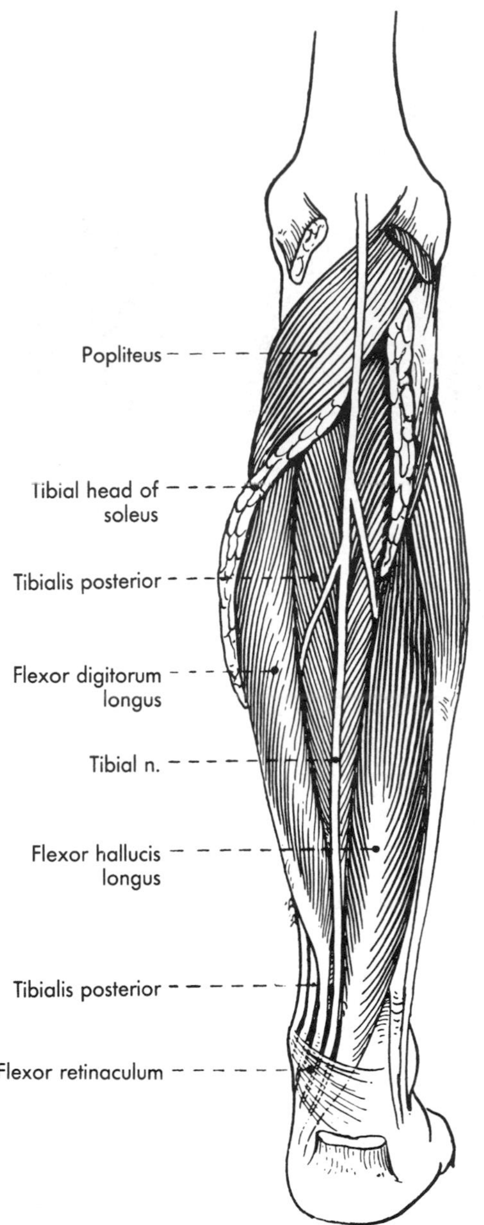

FIGURE *18-25.*
Deep muscles of the calf.

extensor digitorum longus and **extensor hallucis longus,** both located deep in the anterior compartment (see Fig. 18-30).

Invertors and Evertors

Eversion is a movement peculiar to the foot and is produced by the **peroneus longus and brevis** muscles (see Fig. 18-30). The peroneus tertius, a dorsiflexor of the ankle, can assist in eversion because its line of pull is also lateral to the subtalar axis. The principal **invertor** of the foot is the **tibialis posterior,** but it is substantially assisted by the **tibialis anterior.** The tibialis posterior is the deepest muscle in the flexor compartment; its anterior counterpart is superficially located in the anterior compartment (see Figs. 18-23 and 18-30).

Posterior Compartment

The posterior compartment of the leg constitutes the calf. Its boundaries are the posterior surfaces of the tibia, fibula, and crural interosseous membrane; the posterior intermuscular septum and the crural fascia (deep fascia), spanning the posterior surface of the leg. The muscles of the calf are divided into a superficial and a deep group by a transverse intermuscular septum, the *deep transverse fascia* (see Fig. 18-23). The deeper muscles of the calf arise from the upper part of this fascia, whereas the lower part is thickened at the ankle to form the flexor retinaculum. In addition to muscles, the posterior compartment contains the tibial nerve and the posterior tibial vessels. They and their branches run between the superficial and deep group of muscles.

Superficial Muscles

The superficial muscles include two large muscles, the gastrocnemius and soleus, and the small plantaris (see Fig. 18-24).

The **gastrocnemius** is the superficial member of the triceps surae. It arises by medial and lateral heads from just above the medial and lateral femoral condyles (see Fig. 17-6). The junction of the two heads forms the prominent upper muscular mass of the calf. Approximately halfway down the leg, the muscle gives rise to a tendon that receives on its deep surface the insertion of the soleus muscle as well. This combined tendon, called the **tendo calcaneus** or *Achilles tendon,* inserts on the lower part of the posterior surface of the calcaneus. Deep to each head of the gastrocnemius there is usually a bursa; the medial one may communicate with the cavity of the knee joint and the bursa of the semimembranosus tendon. A bursa also intervenes between the calcaneus tendon and the upper part of the posterior surface of the calcaneus.

The **soleus** forms the deeper component of the triceps surae (see Fig. 18-24). It arises from the upper part of the fibula and from the soleal line on the tibia (see Fig. 18-2*B* and *D*). A tendinous arch (*arcus tendineus*) unites the two so-called heads of origin. The upper part of the muscle is largely covered by the gastrocnemius; below the middle of the leg, however, the soleus is broader than the tendon of the gastrocnemius and, therefore, is visible on either side of it. The muscle fibers insert into the anterior surface of the tendo calcaneus. As the latter runs toward the heel, it twists laterally so that the part associated with the gastrocnemius inserts largely laterally, and the part belonging to the soleus inserts more medially. This twisting is of importance when tendon-lengthening procedures are carried out, which are sometimes necessary to correct different types of abnormalities.

The slender **plantaris** muscle arises from the femur just above the origin of the lateral head of the gastrocnemius (see Fig. 17-6). It runs downward, partly covered by the gastrocnemius, to cross posterior to the tibial nerve and popliteal vessels and lie between the gastrocnemius and soleus muscles. Its muscular belly is short, commonly not more than 5 to 10 cm. Its long, slender tendon usually inserts into the calcaneus medial or anteromedial to the tendo calcaneus; sometimes, however, it may blend with it.

Innervation. The **tibial nerve** supplies the gastrocnemius and the soleus through several branches with fibers derived from S-1 and S-2 spinal nerves (see Table 13-1). The plantaris receives a small twig from the tibial nerve that often arises in common with the branch to the lateral head of the gastrocnemius.

Action. The triceps surae is the chief **plantar flexor** at the ankle. Although the deep calf muscles and the peroneus longus and brevis are in appropriate anatomic positions to be flexors, their smaller bulk and lack of leverage make them far less effective than the triceps. Its power can be tested by opposing plantar flexion, or better, by observing elevation of the heel during an attempt to stand on "tiptoe." If a subject, instructed to hop up and down on his or her toes with one foot, lands flat-footed, weakness of the triceps surae must be suspected. The ankle jerk objectively tests the integrity of the muscle and the nervous pathways.

Paralysis of the triceps surae, or rupture of the calcaneus tendon, make walking difficult, and the patient is usually unable to rise onto the toes. Similarly, contracture of the triceps surae maintains the foot in plantar flexion, a position known as *talipes equinus*. This is a form of clubfoot in which the heel does not contact the ground and weight is borne on the "toes," as it is in a horse's foot.

Deep Muscles

The deep muscle group includes the popliteus, the flexor digitorum longus, the flexor hallucis longus, and the tibialis posterior (see Fig. 18-25). The popliteus lies in the upper part of the leg; the other three parallel each other along the leg and send their tendons into the foot, passing behind the medial malleolus. All receive one or more branches from the tibial nerve. The spinal cord segments are predominantly L-5 and S-1.

The **popliteus muscle** (Fig. 18-26) forms the lower part of the floor of the popliteal fossa. Its femoral attachment to the lateral surface of the lateral condyle is enclosed within the fibrous capsule of the knee joint. Inside the joint capsule, the muscle also has a tendinous attachment to the lateral meniscus of the knee (see Fig. 18-37*C*) and is tethered to the arcuate popliteal ligament of the capsule (see Fig. 18-36) as it leaves the joint. The popliteus expands into a somewhat triangular muscle that slants medially to attach to the posterior surface of the tibia above the soleal line (see Figs. 18-2*D* and 18-26). Within the knee joint the muscle lies between the synovial membrane and the fibrous capsule. A diverticulum of the joint's synovial membrane forms a bursa, the *subpopliteal recess*, between the muscle and the surface of the tibia.

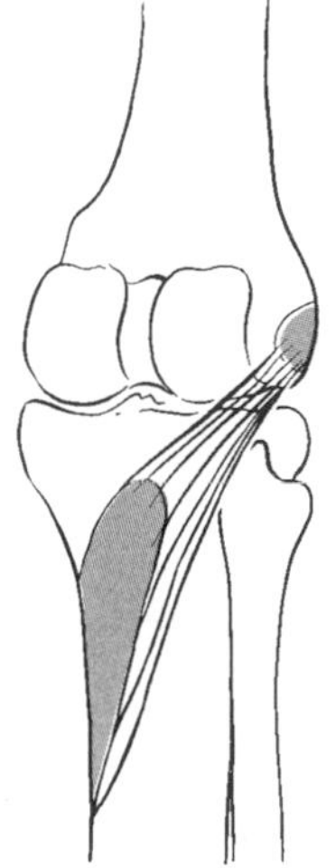

FIGURE *18-26.*
Schematic representation of the popliteus muscle with its attachments.

The *tibial nerve* supplies the popliteus with a branch that usually curves around the lower border of the muscle and enters its deep surface. The popliteus is a weak flexor of the knee and resists anterior displacement of the femur on the tibia when weight is supported by a partially flexed knee. Its rotatory action on the knee is more important, however; it medially rotates the tibia ifthe leg is off the ground or, in a weight-bearing leg, it laterally rotates the femur, acting from its tibial attachment as its origin. The significance of this action becomes apparent in the analysis of knee movements described in the section on the knee joint.

The **flexor digitorum longus** arises from much of the middle part of the posterior surface of the tibia (see Fig. 18-2*D*), and from the deep transverse fascia. It terminates in a tendon some distance above the ankle (see Fig. 18-25). In the sole of the foot, the tendon divides into four slips that insert on the distal phalanges of the four lateral toes. The muscle's action is analogous to that of the flexor digitorum profundus in the hand; as its name implies, it flexes the lateral four toes at the distal interphalangeal joints. In the lower part of the leg, the tendon of the flexor digitorum longus joins company with those of the tibialis posterior and flexor hallucis longus. The three tendons enter the foot behind the medial malleolus, passing deep to the flexor retinaculum (see Figs. 18-25 and 18-45*B*). Their relations around the ankle and in the foot are examined in subsequent sections.

Most fibers of the **flexor hallucis longus** arise from the posterior surface of the fibula (see Fig. 18-2); some take origin from the covering fascia and adjacent fascial septa. The muscle crosses from the lateral to the medial side of the leg, and its tendon enters the foot with that of the flexor digitorum longus and tibialis posterior (see Fig. 18-25). It inserts on the distal phalanx of the big toe. It flexes the interphalangeal joint of the big toe and, as explained in the section on the foot, contributes to maintaining the dynamic architecture of the foot.

The **tibialis posterior** lies between the flexor hallucis longus and the flexor digitorum longus and is partly overlapped by both (see Fig. 18-25). It arises from the posterior surface of the interosseous membrane and from adjacent surfaces of the tibia and fibula (see Fig.18-2*D*). Its tendon passes into the plantar surface of the foot and inserts into a number of bones. Attachment sites include the tuberosity of the navicular bone (the chief attachment), the plantar surfaces of the three cuneiforms, the bases of the second, third, and fourth metatarsals, and the cuboid bone.

In the leg, the tibialis posterior passes medially and forward, crossing deep to the flexor digitorum longus as its tendon nears the ankle to occupy the most anterior position of the three tendons that proceed into the foot deep to the flexor retinaculum. In addition to providing the primary force for inversion, the tibialis posterior is also a weak flexor of the ankle, as are the two long flexors of the toes.

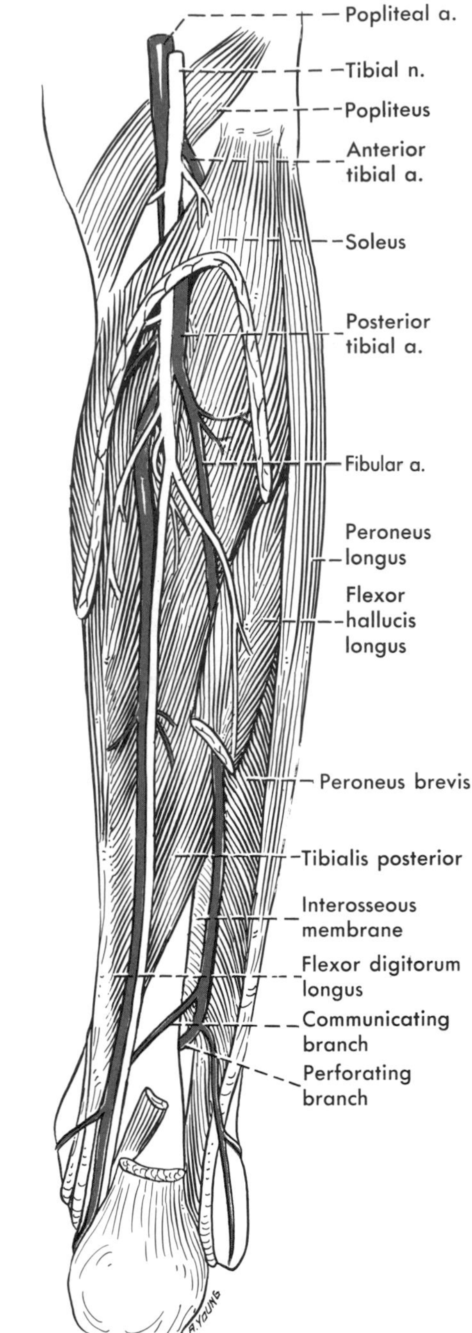

FIGURE *18-27.*
Nerves and arteries of the calf.

Nerves and Vessels

The tibial nerve and popliteal artery enter the posterior compartment of the leg by passing across the posterior surface of the popliteus and deep to the tendinous arch of the soleus (Fig. 18-27). The popliteal artery ends at the lower border of the popliteus muscle by dividing into anterior and posterior tibial arteries. Formed by tributaries that correspond to these arteries, the popliteal vein ascends from here to the popliteal fossa, sandwiched between the nerve and the artery. The posterior tibial artery accompanies the tibial nerve down the leg between the superficial and deep calf muscles. They both give off branches as they approach the medial side of the ankle to enter the sole of the foot, where each divides into medial and lateral plantar branches.

Tibial Nerve. Formed by the anterior divisions of L-4, L-5, S-1, S-2, and S-3 roots of the sacral plexus, the tibial nerve descends through the thigh as the medial component of the sciatic nerve. Entering the popliteal fossa it continues vertically after the common fibular component of the sciatic nerve has deviated laterally (see Fig. 18-22). Throughout its course it distributes branches to muscles in the flexor compartments of the thigh and leg and, through its terminal branches (medial and lateral plantar nerves), to muscles in the sole of the foot (Fig. 18-28). Compared with this extensive muscular distribution, its cutaneous distribution is relatively small. It gives articular branches to the knee and ankle joints; joints of the foot receive twigs from its terminal branches.

Before it leaves the popliteal fossa, the tibial nerve gives off one or more *branches to the knee joint*, as well as the *medial sural cutaneous nerve* to the skin of the leg and foot (see Fig. 18-7). In the lower part of the fossa, it gives off branches to *both heads of the gastrocnemius* and to the *plantaris*. The nerve leaves the fossa along the popliteal vessels between the two heads of the gastrocnemius. It sends a branch into the superficial surface of the soleus and then disappears deep into that muscle, usually supplying it with a second branch from the deep side. It also supplies the *popliteus*. It then courses down the leg on the posterior surface of the tibialis posterior, giving off a variable number of branches to the remaining *deep muscles of the calf*. At the ankle the tibial nerve, together with the posterior tibial vessels, enters a special compartment in the

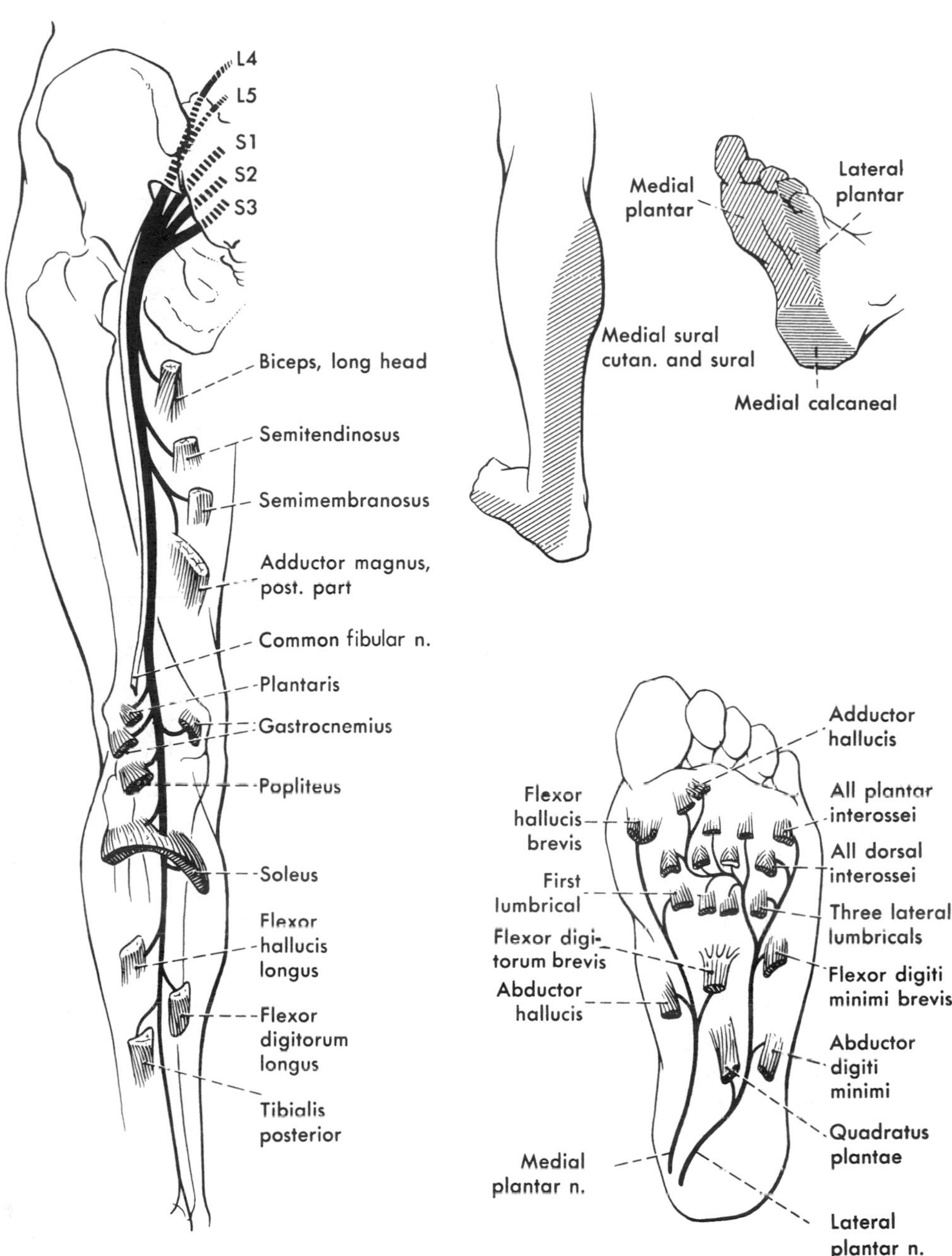

FIGURE 18-28. **Muscular and cutaneous distribution of the tibial nerve.**

flexor retinaculum, situated between the flexor hallucis longus and the flexor digitorum longus.

As it passes onto the plantar surface of the foot, it gives off *medial calcaneal branches* and divides into medial and lateral plantar nerves.

Posterior Tibial Artery. The artery arises as a terminal branch of the popliteal artery at the lower border of the popliteus (Fig. 18-29; and see Fig. 18-27) and courses downward with the tibial nerve on the tibialis posterior muscle. It divides into medial and lateral plantar branches as it reaches the plantar surface of the foot. A little below its origin, it gives off a large branch called the **fibular** (*peroneal*) **artery**, from which much of the blood supply of the posterior and lateral compartments is derived. Smaller, named branches of the posterior tibial artery include a *nutrient artery to the tibia*, and near the ankle, *medial malleolar* and *calcaneal* branches. The *circumflex fibular artery* may also arise from the posterior tibial artery near its origin or, alternatively, from the anterior tibial or the popliteal artery. The posterior tibial also gives off a several unnamed branches to muscles.

The **circumflex fibular artery** leaves the posterior compartment by piercing the soleus, and winds around the neck of the fibula to supply the peroneal muscles (see Fig. 18-29). The **fibular** (*peroneal*) **artery** may actually be larger than the continuation of the posterior tibial. Originating from the lateral aspect of that vessel in the upper

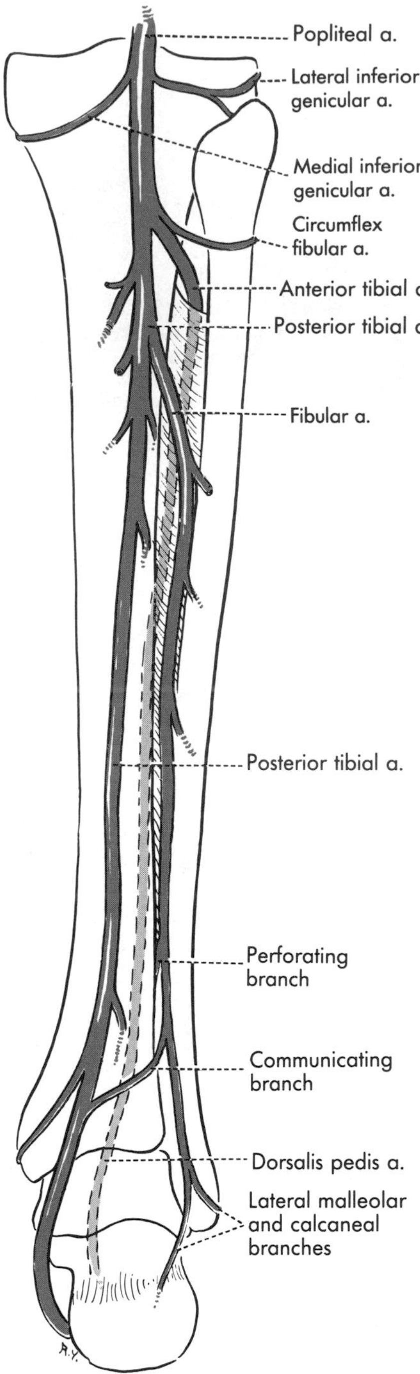

FIGURE *18-29.*
Diagram of the arteries of the leg; posterior view.

part of the leg, it passes laterally across the surface of the tibialis posterior muscle to lie between the interosseous membrane and the fibula under cover of, or in the substance of, the flexor hallucis longus muscle. It gives off muscular branches, some of which pass through the interosseous membrane to help supply anterior muscles, and a *nutrient artery to the fibula*. Some distance above the ankle, the fibular artery sends a *perforating branch* through the interosseous membrane to reach the lateral aspect of the leg and dorsum of the foot. The perforating branch gives off *lateral calcaneal* and *malleolar branches*, and sometimes gives rise to the *dorsalis pedis artery*. Above or below the origin of its perforating branch, the fibular artery is linked to the posterior tibial artery by a *communicating branch* (see Figs. 18-27 and 18-29). When the posterior tibial artery is small or deficient in the lower part of the leg, it is the communicating branch of the fibular artery that continues into the foot as the plantar arteries.

Most of the arteries of the leg are accompanied by **paired veins**. These unite in several different patterns and terminate in the popliteal vein. **Deep lymphatics** in the calf accompany the posterior tibial and fibular vessels and end in the **popliteal nodes**.

Anterior and Lateral Compartments

The medial side of the front of the leg is occupied by the subcutaneous medial surface of the tibial shaft. The muscles of the front of the leg are located on the lateral side and, except for a subcutaneous area above the lateral malleolus, cover the shaft of the fibula (see Fig. 18-23). They are separated into an anterior and a lateral compartment by the anterior intermuscular septum. The anterior compartment contains the tibialis anterior, extensor digitorum longus, extensor hallucis longus, and peroneus tertius muscles; the lateral compartment accommodates the peroneus longus and brevis muscles. The tendons of all of these cross the ankle joint to insert on the bones of the foot. They are retained around the ankle by retinacula.

The common fibular nerve enters the lateral compartment, where it divides into its deep and superficial branches. The latter descends in the lateral compartment, supplying the muscles within it, and becomes cutaneous in the lower third of the leg; the deep fibular nerve enters the anterior compartment, supplies its muscles and has a negligible cutaneous distribution. The anterior tibial artery parallels the deep fibular nerve on the front of the leg and furnishes the chief blood supply to the area, but branches of the posterior arteries penetrate the interosseous membrane and provide an additional supply to both fascial compartments in the front of the leg.

Muscles

Anterior Compartment. The **tibialis anterior** is the most bulky muscle in the front of the leg (Fig. 18-30; see Fig. 18-23). It arises from the lateral surface of the tibia and the interosseous membrane (see Fig. 18-2C), the crural fascia in the upper part of the leg, and from an intermuscular septum between it and the extensor digitorum longus. Its strong tendon crosses the ankle joint anterior to the medial malleolus and passes across the medial side of the dorsum of the foot to insert into the medial and lower surfaces of the medial cuneiform bone and into the base of the first metatarsal. The tendon may be split, each half attaching to one of these points. The deep fibular nerve and

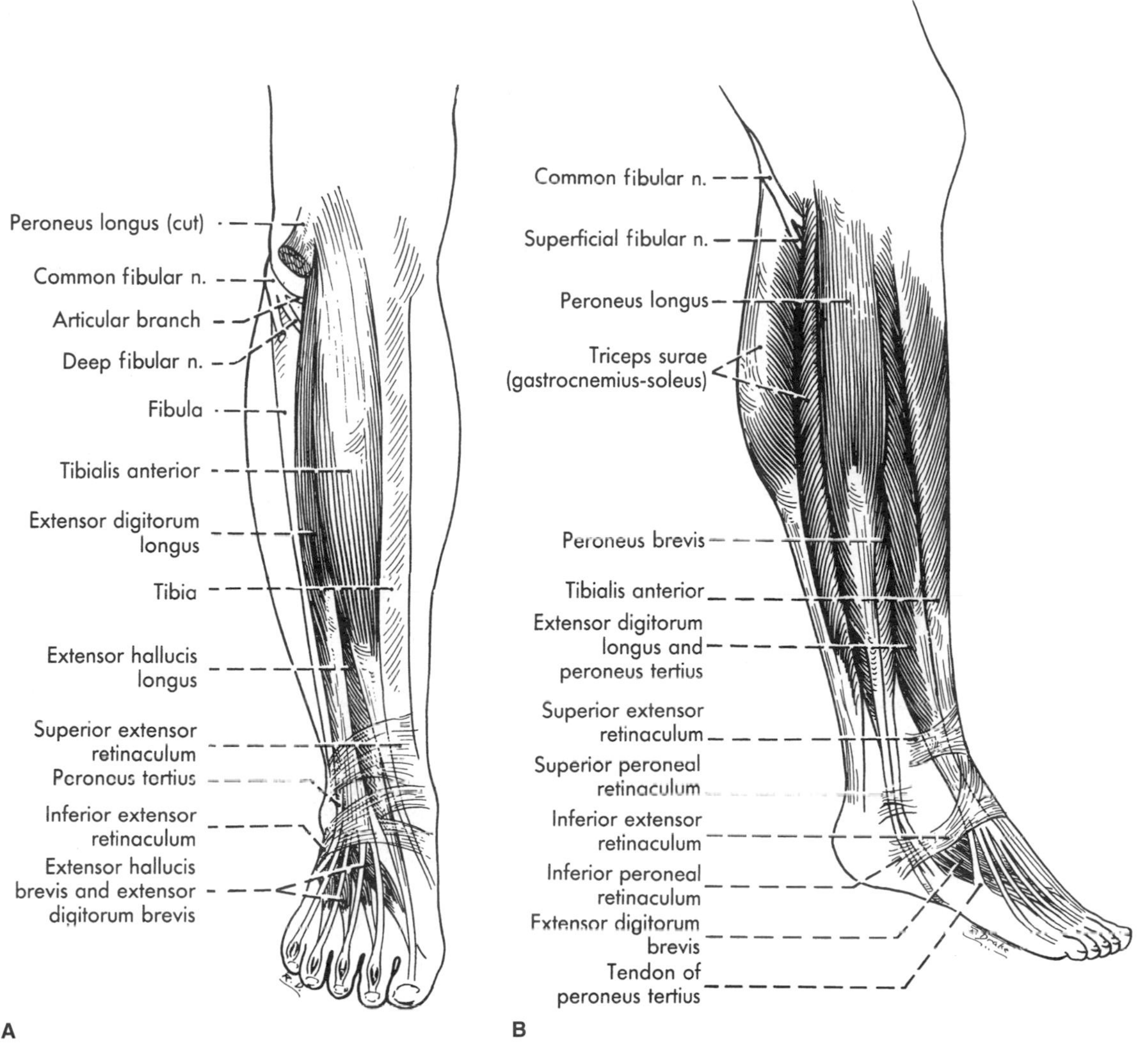

FIGURE *18-30.*
(A) Anterior muscles of the leg; (B) muscles of the lateral or peroneal compartment in relation to the anterior and posterior musculature.

the anterior tibial artery lie deep to the muscle on its lateral side (see Fig. 18-23).

The **extensor digitorum longus** and **peroneus tertius** are continuous at their origin (see Fig. 18-2*C*), and their joint muscle bellies give rise to a single tendon (see Fig. 18-30*B*). The extensor digitorum longus arises mostly from the anterior surface of the fibula (see Fig. 18-2*C*) but also has attachments to the lateral condyle of the tibia, the interosseous membrane, and an intermuscular septum that it shares with the tibialis anterior. The peroneus tertius arises from the fibula and the anterior intermuscular septum. As soon as the combined tendon of the two muscles crosses the ankle, it splits into its component parts: the tendon of the peroneus tertius diverges laterally to insert into the dorsal surface of the base of the fifth metatarsal bone, and that of the extensor digitorum longus divides into four individual tendons for the four lateral toes. Like the extensor tendons on the fingers, they form dorsal digital expansions that are joined by other muscles.

The upper part of the **extensor hallucis longus** is largely covered by the tibialis anterior and the extensor digitorum longus (Fig. 18-30*A*). It arises from the anterior surface of the fibula and the adjacent interosseous membrane (Fig. 18-2*C*), emerges between the two covering muscles, and inserts upon the distal phalanx of the big toe, sometimes sending a slip to the proximal phalanx.

Innervation. The *deep fibular nerve* gives off multiple branches to each of the muscles in the anterior compartment. (Some branches may also come from the common fibular nerve). The segmental innervation is from L-4 and L-5 (see Table 13-1) with some contribution from S-1.

Actions. The common action of all these muscles is to *dorsiflex the foot,* although with varying strength. The tibialis anterior is a particularly important dorsiflexor, as well as an invertor. The extensor digitorum longus extends the four lateral toes, but since the interphalangeal joints of these toes are usually held in flexion by the more powerful flexors, its chief action on the toes is hyperextension at the metatarsophalangeal joints (see Fig. 18-70). The extensor hallucis longus is primarily an extensor of the big toe and is the weakest dorsiflexor of the foot. It can also assist in inversion. The extensor digitorum longus and the peroneus tertius work together to dorsiflex and evert the foot. The muscles can be tested by opposing dorsiflexion. The tendons will become prominent on the dorsum of the foot. The tendon of the tibialis anterior is the first prominent tendon anterior to the medial malleolus.

Lateral Compartment. The **peroneus longus** arises from the lateral surface of the upper third of the fibula and from the adjacent deep fascia and intermuscular septa. The common fibular nerve runs deep to it just below the fibular head (see Fig. 18-30). The muscle gives rise to a tendon halfway down the leg, which joins that of the more deeply lying peroneus brevis. Both tendons pass behind the lateral malleolus deep to the peroneal retinacula. The tendon of the peroneus longus enters the lateral side of the foot, passing in a groove on the plantar surface of the cuboid bone. It crosses to the medial side of the sole and inserts into the medial cuneiform and the base of the first metatarsal bone. In its course across the sole, it is invested in a tendon sheath which may be continuous with the one beneath the peroneal retinacula. The tendon may contain a sesamoid bone where it crosses the surface of the tuberosity of the cuboid. The role of the muscle in maintaining the dynamic architecture of the foot is discussed in a subsequent section.

The **peroneus brevis** arises from the lower lateral surface of the fibula and from the adjacent intermuscular septa. It is located deep to the peroneus longus. After passing behind the lateral malleolus, its tendon curves forward onto the dorsum of the foot and inserts on the dorsolateral surface of the base of the fifth metatarsal.

Innervation and Action. Predominantly L-5 and S-1 fibers are distributed to the two peroneal muscles by the superficial fibular nerve as it passes between them. The chief action of both muscles is to evert the foot. They are also weak plantar flexors.

Nerves and Vessels

Common, Deep, and Superficial Fibular Nerves. The muscles in the anterior and lateral compartments of the leg, as well as those on the dorsum of the foot, are innervated from posterior divisions of the sacral plexus. The common fibular nerve gathers these fibers and conveys them, as the lateral component of the sciatic nerve, to the popliteal fossa (Fig. 18-31). Only one branch is given off in the thigh, to the short head of the biceps femoris (see Figs. 18-22 and 18-31). Two more are given off in the popliteal fossa (fibular communicating branch and lateral sural cutaneous nerve), both of which supply skin on the posterolateral aspect of the leg (see Figs. 18-7 and 18-31). The nerve leaves the popliteal fossa by crossing the lateral head of the gastrocnemius and becomes subcutaneous as it skirts the neck of the fibula. Here it can be easily rolled against the bone (and also easily injured). It then penetrates the posterior intermuscular septum and the upper fasciculi of the peroneus longus to enter the lateral compartment, where it immediately divides to form the superficial and deep fibular nerves (Fig. 18-32).

The **superficial fibular nerve** descends in the lateral compartment (see Fig. 18-32), at first between the peroneus longus and the fibula and then between the peroneus longus and brevis. After supplying both muscles, it emerges between them to supply skin of the lower part of the leg and the dorsum of the foot (see Fig. 18-31).

The **deep fibular nerve** runs forward around the fibula, deep to the peroneus longus, and immediately enters the anterior compartment. After passing deep to the extensor digitorum longus, it turns inferiorly and runs down on the interosseous membrane alongside the anterior tibial artery (Fig. 18-33). Initially located between the extensor digitorum longus and the tibialis anterior, it comes to lie between the extensor hallucis longus and the tibialis anterior. Close to the ankle it emerges, along with the anterior tibial artery, between the tendons of the extensor digitorum and hallucis longus muscles. Having dispensed all its muscular fibers, it terminates as two dorsal digital nerves that supply adjacent sides of the big and second toes (see Fig. 18-7).

The deep fibular nerve gives off two branches while in the lateral compartment: a *branch to the peroneus longus muscle* and a *recurrent branch* that runs upward to innervate the knee joint. Descending in the anterior compartment, it gives off a series of muscular branches that vary in number and position; several may arise by a common stem (see Figs. 18-31 and 18-33).

Vessels. The blood supply of the anterior and lateral compartments is provided by the anterior tibial artery and vein, supplemented by branches of the posterior tibial and fibular vessels, which penetrate the interosseous membrane or the intermuscular septa. There is no major vessel in the lateral compartment.

The **anterior tibial artery** originates in the posterior compartment as a terminal branch of the popliteal artery. It enters the anterior compartment through the gap at the upper end of the interosseous membrane (see Figs. 18-29 and 18-33). Lying against the interosseous membrane, the artery descends along the medial side of the anterior tibial nerve. Some distance above the ankle it crosses behind the nerve to appear on its lateral side as they pass deep to the extensor retinacula at the ankle (see Figs. 18-33 and 18-47). The vessel becomes known as the **dorsalis pedis artery** as it crosses the ankle joint.

The anterior tibial artery gives off several named

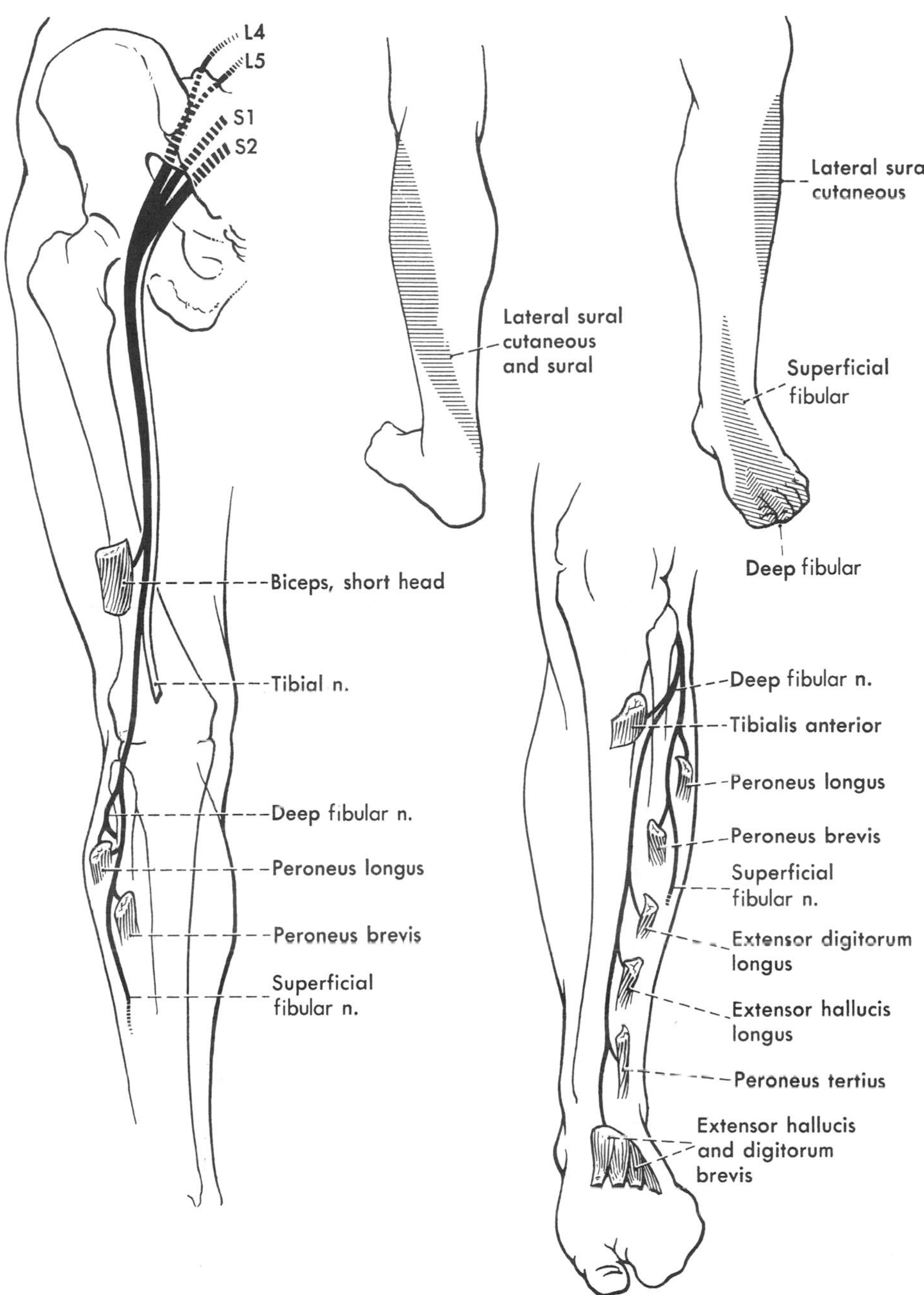

FIGURE *18-31.*
Muscular and cutaneous distribution of the common fibular (common peroneal) nerve.

branches and a number of unnamed ones. Among the first is the *anterior tibial recurrent artery,* which runs upward to enter into the anastomosis around the knee joint (see Fig. 18-43). As the anterior tibial descends, it gives off branches to the surrounding muscles and also small branches that penetrate the membrane to help supply the deep muscles of the calf. Its last branches are usually the *medial and lateral anterior malleolar arteries,* although these may arise from the dorsalis pedis artery. In about 3.5% of limbs, the anterior tibial artery either fails to reach the foot or is reduced to a very slender stem by the time it does so.

Paired **anterior tibial veins** are formed by the confluence of tributaries that correspond to the arterial branches. The veins pass through the gap above the margin of the interosseous membrane and help to form the popliteal vein.

The only vessel of any size related to the lateral compartment is the **circumflex fibular artery** (see Fig. 18-29). As noted earlier, this artery typically arises from the posterior tibial and rounds the lateral surface of the fibula a little below the fibular nerve to end in the peroneal muscles.

A few **deep lymphatics** accompany the anterior tibial vessels. There may be a tiny *anterior tibial lymph node* at the upper end of the interosseous membrane. It receives some of the deep lymphatic vessels but the majority end in popliteal nodes.

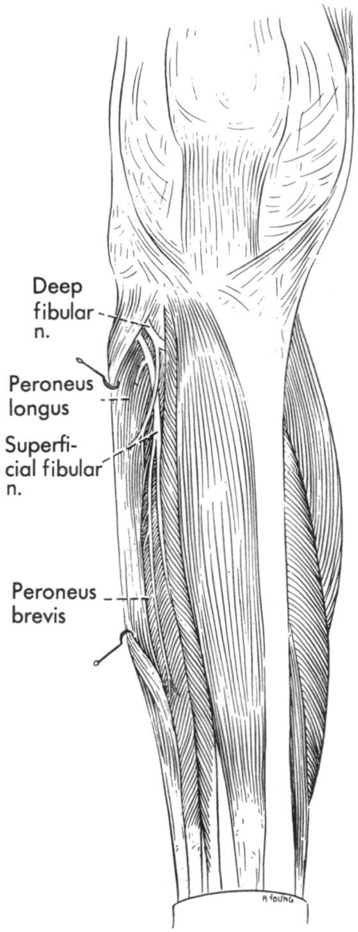

FIGURE *18-32.*
Nerves of the lateral compartment of the leg.

THE KNEE JOINT

The knee is the largest joint in the body. Its anatomy and mechanics are quite complex. Normal function and its derangement can be appreciated only by knowing the anatomy of all its constituent structures. Most knee disorders encountered in clinical practice result from injury and the structures subject to injury are accessible by palpation or can be tested clinically. Therefore, it should be possible to make an anatomic diagnosis in practically all knee injuries.

The knee joint consists of two articulations that are closely integrated (Fig. 18-34). The distal end of the femur articulates with the tibia at the **tibiofemoral joint**, and with the patella at the **patellofemoral joint** (see Fig. 18-1). The fibula is excluded from the knee joint (see Fig. 14-4*A*) and articulates independently with the lateral condyle of the tibia at the **tibiofibular joint**.

Anatomy of the Joint

The knee is a compound synovial joint that functions as a hinge. However, in addition to flexion and extension produced by the rolling of the tibiofemoral articular surfaces on one another, tibiofemoral gliding or translation also take place. In the knee the latter movements are more pronounced, and contribute more to the flexion–extension range, than in any other hinge joint. This gliding is responsible for the constantly changing position of the hinge axis and also for a significant degree of tibiofemoral rotation. The up-and-down gliding of the patella on its sellar articular surface (see Fig. 18-1C) is integrated with tibiofemoral flexion and extension, and needs no further discussion. The tibiofemoral articulation, on the other hand, has to be understood in some detail.

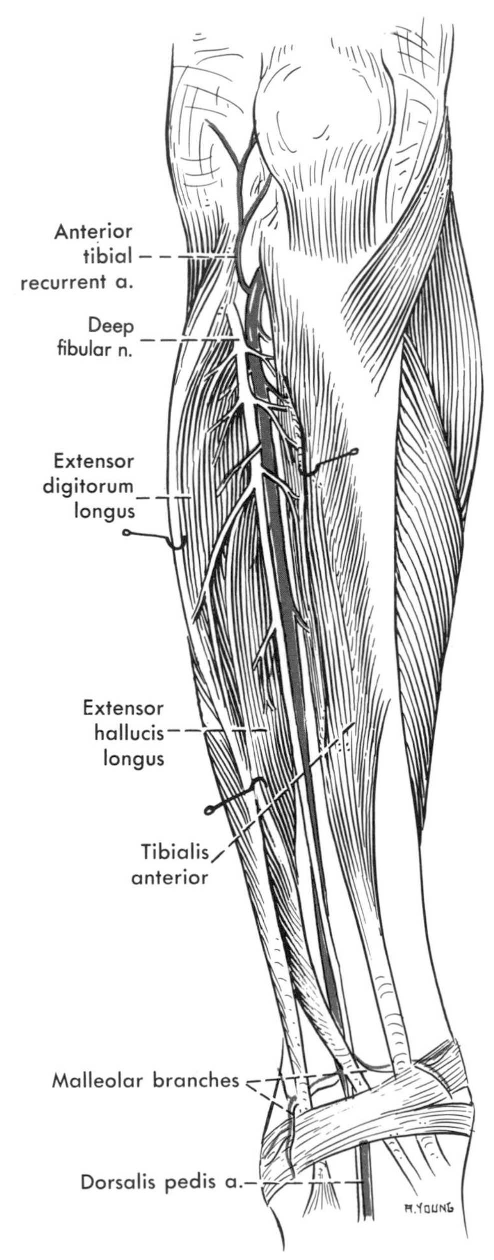

FIGURE *18-33.*
The deep fibular nerve and the anterior tibial artery.

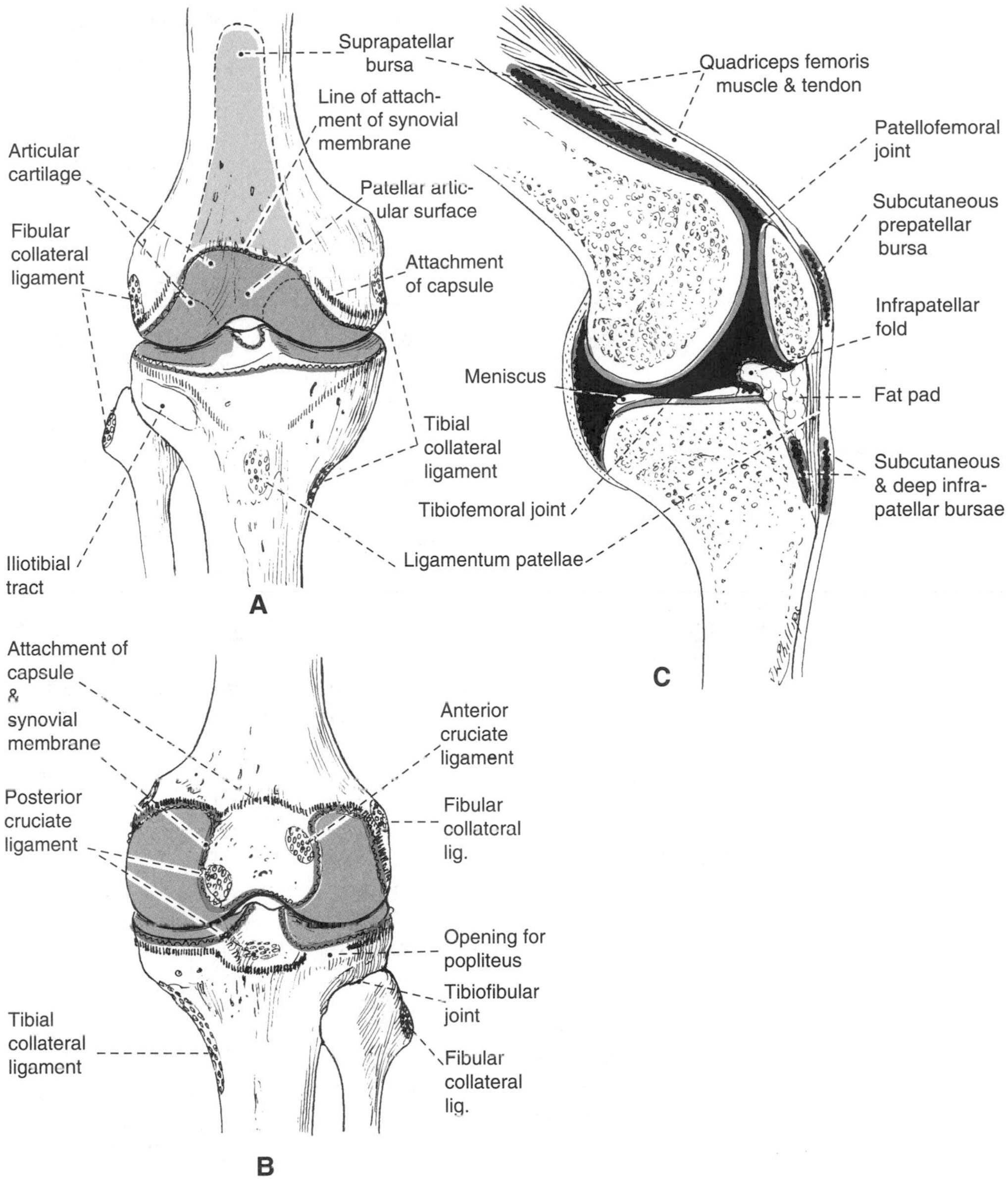

FIGURE *18-34.*
The anatomy of the knee joint, showing the attachments of the capsule, synovial membrane, ligaments, and menisci: (A) anterior view; (B) posterior view; (C) sagittal section cut to one side of the midline. The attachment of the capsule is indicated with a *dashed black line*; that of the synovial membrane with a *red line*. Cavities filled with synovial fluid are shown in *black* in panel C.

Articular Surfaces

Interposed between the medial and lateral condyles is a pair of semilunar cartilages or menisci that prevent direct contact between the circumferences of the tibial and femoral articular facets (see Fig. 18-40). Nevertheless, the configuration of these surfaces is a determining factor as far as movements are concerned.

Viewed from behind, the two femoral condyles are seen to be separated from one another by a depression, the **intercondylar fossa** (see Figs. 17-6*B* and 18-34*B*). The fossa is shown to advantage in x-ray films of the slightly flexed knee (Fig. 18-35; and see Fig. 18-20), or in "end-on" views of the femur (see Fig. 18-4), when it appears as a deep indentation, thus giving rise to its alternative name of *intercondylar notch*. The presence of the notch makes the femur's articular surface somewhat U-shaped. The two limbs of the U (on the condyles) become united anteriorly. The conjoined anterior portion accommodates the patella, whereas the limbs of the U, including their rounded, posterior ends, articulate with the menisci and the tibia. On each femoral condyle, the tibial and patellar surfaces are

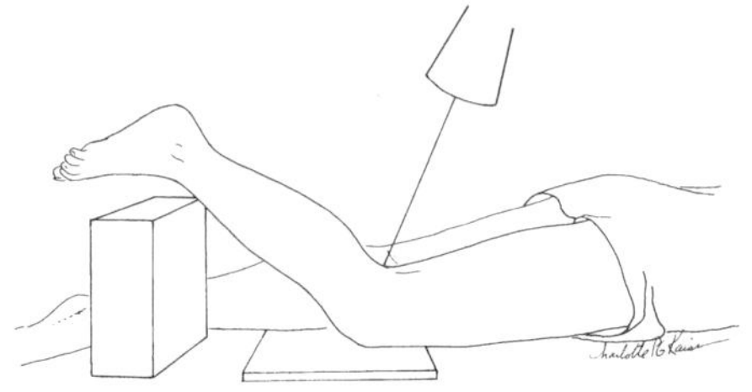

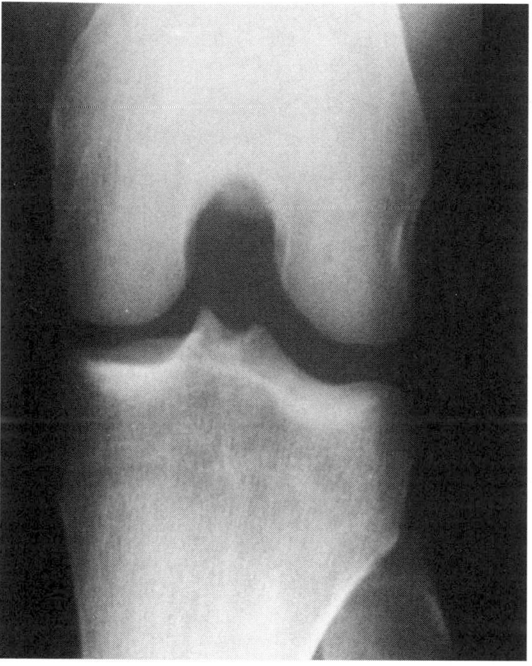

FIGURE *18-35.*
Radiologic anatomy of the knee joint. The radiograph was taken to optimally reveal the condylar articular surfaces, the nonarticular femoral intercondylar notch and the tibial intercondylar eminence. The femoral articular surfaces are convex from side to side, whereas the tibial surfaces are slightly concave. The menisci and articular cartilage are invisible; the apex of the patella can just he made out in the intercondylar notch. The fibula is some distance below the tibiofemoral joint line. (Courtesy of Dr. Rosalind H. Troupin.)

separated by a shallow, but distinct groove, better marked on the cartilage than on the bone (see Fig. 18-4). The patellar surface is larger on the lateral condyle, and protrudes farther anteriorly than it does on the medial condyle. This lateral prominence, well seen when the bone is viewed end on (see Fig. 18-4), has no official anatomic name, but is called the **trochlea** by clinicians. In view of the role it plays in stabilizing the patella, it deserves such distinction. Although the medial condyle appears smaller for lack of a "trochlea," its tibial articular surface is actually greater than that of the lateral condyle. The importance of the unequal articular surfaces of the condyles becomes clear in the discussion of the close-packed position of the knee.

On the tibia, the **intercondylar eminence** is interposed between the two condylar articular facets (see Figs. 18-1, 18-2*A*, and 18-35). The two facets upon which the menisci rest are entirely separate from one another (see see Figs. 18-4 and 18-39). Posteriorly, articular cartilage extends over the smooth lip of the lateral condyle, but otherwise the articular surfaces are confined to the tibial plateau.

Capsule and Its Ligaments

Unlike that of most synovial joints, the capsule of the knee does not form a closed fibrous sleeve around the joint. The typical arrangement is present only medially and laterally, where the thin fibrous capsule bridges the joint space between femoral and tibial articular margins. Even here, this simple arrangement is complicated by the capsule's attachment to the circumference of the menisci. Portions of the capsule above and below their meniscal attachments are known as the **coronary ligaments** (Fig. 18-36). These "ligaments" are thin and loose and permit the necessary sliding and twisting of the menisci during joint movement. On the lateral femoral condyle, the fossa in which the tendon of the popliteus is attached (see Fig. 18-26) is enclosed within the capsule, as is part of the muscle itself (see Fig. 18-36).

Posteriorly, the capsular attachment does not follow the articular margins. On the femur it continues from one condyle to the other, enclosing the intercondylar notch within the capsule (see Fig. 18-34*B*). On the tibia, the posterior line of capsular attachment is interrupted at one point; the gap thus formed provides a hiatus for the exit of the popliteus muscle (see Figs. 18-34*B* and 18-36). The

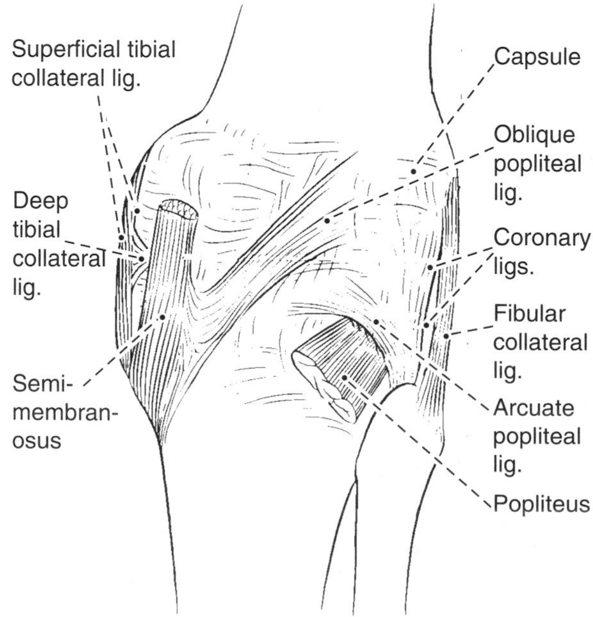

FIGURE *18-36.*
Posterior view of the capsule of the knee joint.

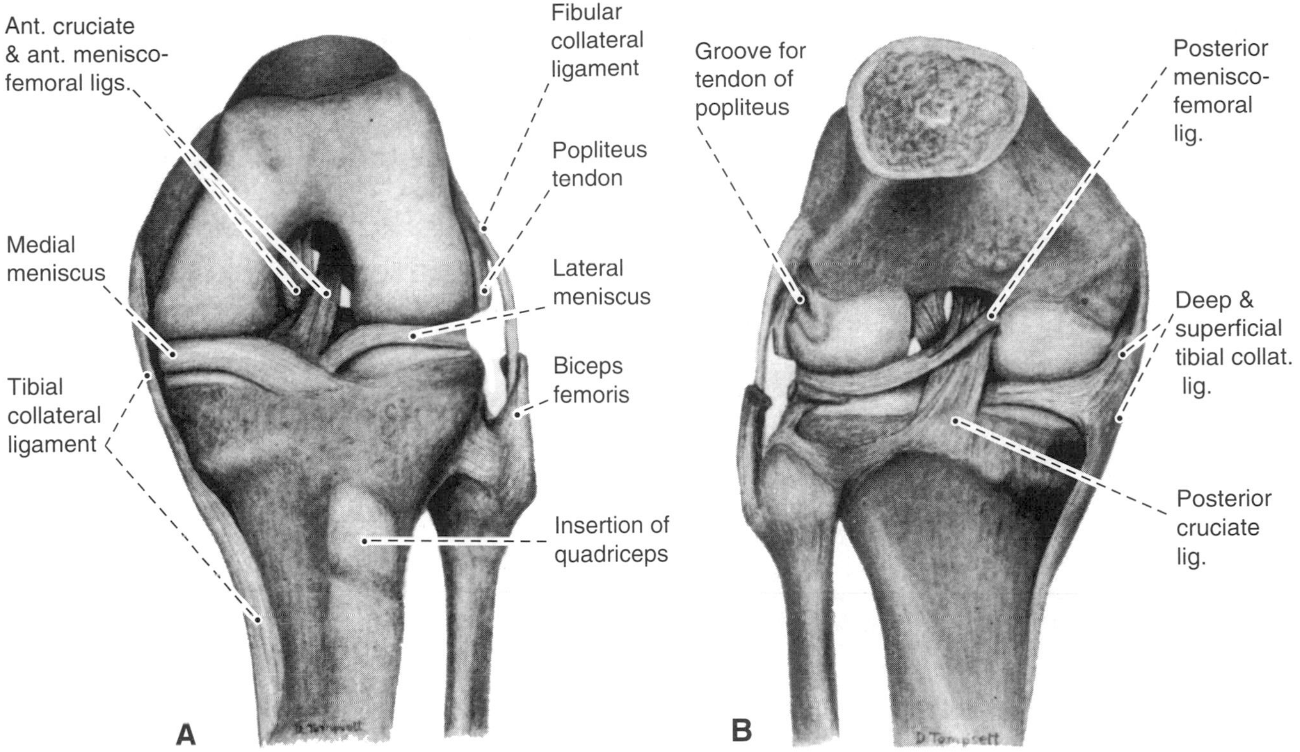

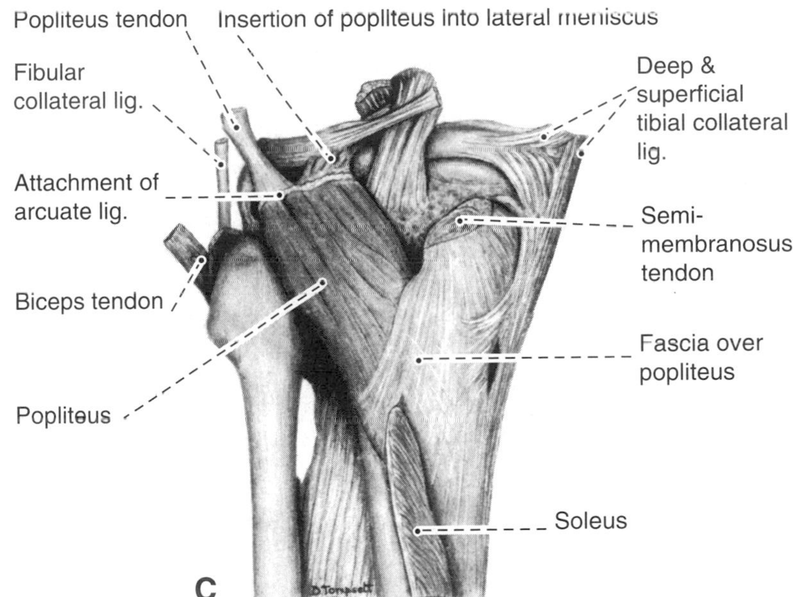

FIGURE *18-37.*
Dissections to show the interior of the knee joint, drawn from specimens in the Anatomy Museum of the Royal College of Surgeons of England: (A) anterior view; (B and C) posterior views. (Adapted from McMinn RMH, ed. Last's anatomy, regional and applied. 8th ed. New York: Churchill Livingstone, 1990.)

edge of the capsule, which arches over the muscle, is known as the **arcuate popliteal ligament**.

Anteriorly, the capsular attachment line is also deficient, there being a gap on the front of both the femur and tibia (see Fig. 18-34*A*). The deficiency is closed by the quadriceps tendon, the patella, and the ligamentum patellae. The fibrous capsule fuses on each side with these structures, enclosing within the joint a large, irregular space that is mostly filled with intra-articular fat (see Figs. 18-34C and 18-38). The capsule is substantially reinforced on each side of the patella and ligamentum patellae by tendinous fibers derived from the quadriceps: instead of inserting into the patella, they join the ligamentum patellae directly. These aponeurotic expansions fuse with the capsule and are known as the medial and lateral **patellar retinacula** (see Fig. 18-11).

The capsule is reinforced at the back, as well as on the sides (see Fig. 18-36). Posteriorly the reinforcement is derived largely from a tendinous expansion of the semimembranosus and is known as the **oblique popliteal**

ligament. The lateral and medial reinforcements are intrinsic to the capsule and represent the **deep** or **capsular components** *of the tibial and fibular collateral ligaments.*

Accessory Ligaments

The major ligaments of the knee are independent of its capsule. One pair, the proper tibial and fibular collateral ligaments, are outside and the other pair, the cruciate ligaments, are inside the joint (Fig. 18-37).

The **tibial** (*medial*) **collateral ligament** is a broad, flat band extending from the medial epicondyle of the femur to the tibia, about 10 cm below the joint line. It has a deep component to it which, as mentioned earlier, forms one of the intrinsic capsular ligaments (see Figs. 18-36 and 18-37C). By this capsular component, the medial meniscus is tethered to the tibial collateral ligament proper.

The **fibular** (*lateral*) **collateral ligament** is cordlike and runs between the lateral femoral epicondyle and the apex of the fibula. It probably represents the vestige of the attachment of the peroneus longus to the femur. Unlike its counterpart on the medial side, it has no connection with either the deep, capsular portion of the fibular collateral ligament or with the lateral meniscus. Both tibial and fibular collateral ligaments become taut in full extension, but their chief function is to provide side-to-side stability to the knee joint.

The **cruciate ligaments** inside the joint run in a crisscross fashion between the tibia and the femur (Fig. 18-38; see Fig. 18-37). Their main function is to prevent anteroposterior displacement of the two bones upon one another. In full extension both cruciate ligaments are tight, and they also impart side-to-side stability to the knee. The ligaments are named in accordance with their *tibial* attachments. The **anterior cruciate ligament** is attached to the *anterior* part of the intercondylar eminence (Fig. 18-39) and passes backward into the intercondylar notch to attach far posteriorly to the lateral condyle of the femur. The **posterior cruciate ligament** is attached to the *posterior* part of the intercondylar eminence (see Fig. 18-39) and passes forward in the intercondylar notch to attach to the medial condyle of the femur.

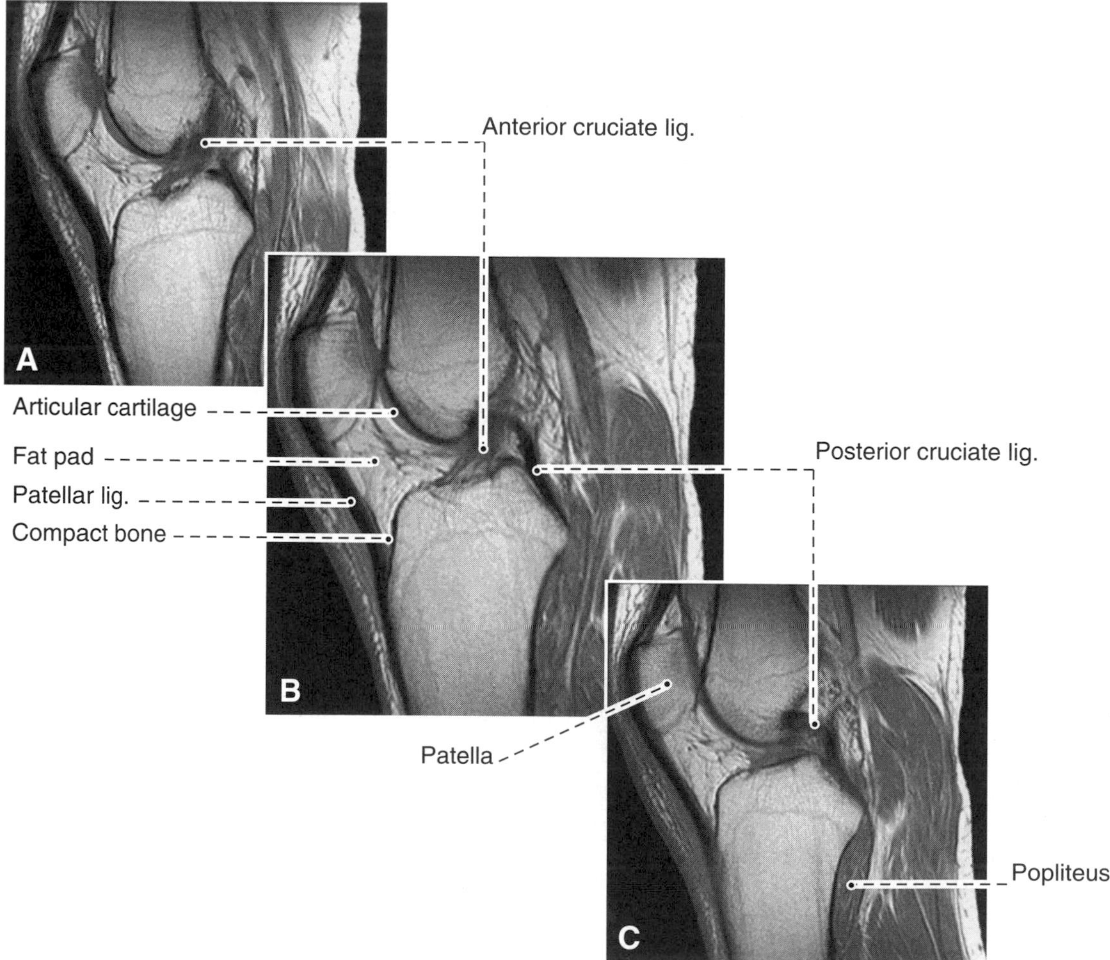

FIGURE *18-38.*
Successive magnetic resonance imaging (MRI) scans of the knee joint obtained in sagittal planes. (Courtesy of Dr. Thurman Gillespy III.)

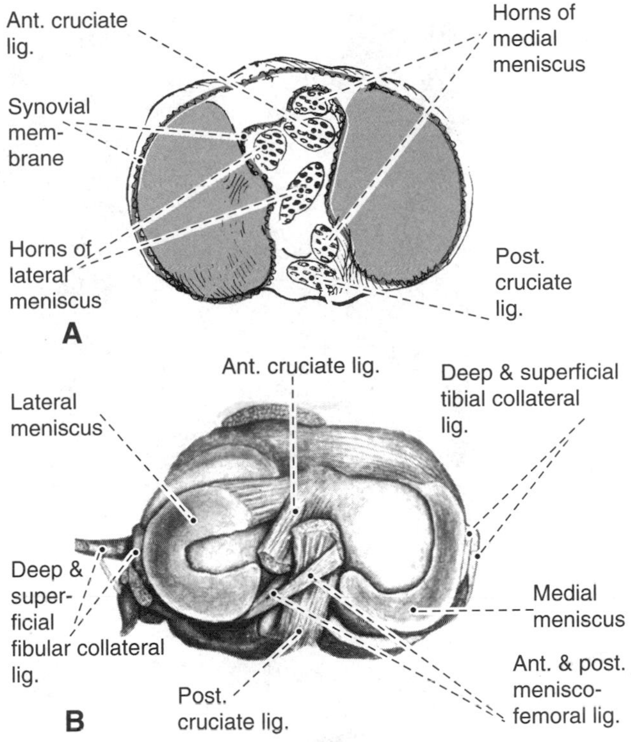

FIGURE *18-39.*
The menisci: (A) bony attachments of structures on the tibial plateau; (B) the menisci and associated ligaments, drawn from a specimen in the Anatomy Museum of the Royal College of Surgeons of England. (B, adapted from McMinn RMH, ed. Last's anatomy, regional and applied. 8th ed. New York: Churchill Livingstone, 1990.)

Menisci

The menisci are two fibrocartilaginous, semilunar-shaped wedges that partially divide the joint cavity and deepen the shallow articular facets of the tibia (Fig. 18-40; see Fig. 18-39*B*). Their concave inner margins are very much thinner than their convex peripheral rims that fuse with the inner surface of the capsule. The upper and lower surfaces of the menisci are in contact with the articular cartilage of the femoral and tibial condyles, respectively, and both surfaces are moistened by synovial fluid. Both menisci are anchored by their anterior and posterior horns to the intercondylar eminence (see Fig. 18-39*A*). The lateral meniscus also gains attachment posteriorly to the medial condyle of the femur by the **meniscofemoral ligaments** (see Figs. 18-37*B* and 18-39). Therefore, the movements of the lateral meniscus are guided by the movements of the femur. Its mobility is enhanced by the **popliteus muscle**, which gives a muscle slip to the meniscus as it passes out of the joint (see Fig. 18-37*C*). The muscle can pull the meniscus backward over the smooth edge of the lateral tibial condyle, which is covered with articular cartilage. The medial meniscus is more fixed and is more widely open than the lateral meniscus. The tibial collateral ligament attached to it at the joint line is partly responsible for its restricted mobility (see Fig. 18-37*B*).

The menisci are penetrated by nerves derived from the capsular plexus, but they are avascular, except for their most peripheral zones, which are fused with the capsule. When a meniscus is torn, there is pain, but no intra-articular hemorrhage. Owing to their avascularity, they do not heal. A torn meniscus (see Fig. 18-40) has to be resected; as a rule, a new one regenerates as an ingrowth from the capsular connective tissue.

Synovial Membrane

The attachment of the synovial membrane follows closely the articular margins (see Figs. 18-34 and 18-39*A*). Synovium lines the capsule and covers all intra-articular structures except the menisci. The cruciate ligaments, the popliteus muscle, and a large fat pad behind the ligamentum patellae are therefore intracapsular, but extrasynovial.

The **infrapatellar fat pad** fills the space between the ligamentum patellae and the anterior intercondylar area of the tibia (see Figs. 18-34 and 18-38). The synovial membrane isdraped over the fat pad, and is raised up into an **infrapatellar fold**. This fold is attached anteriorly to the lower margin of the patella (see Fig. 18-34*C*). From this relatively wide attachment at the front of the synovial cavity, the fold narrows down and reaches backward in the midline across the cavity, deep into the intercondylar notch; it makes its posterior attachment in the apex of the notch, on the margin of the femoral articular surface. The fold thus forms a crescentic ridge in the midline (not seen in Fig. 18-34*C* because that section is cut to one side of the midline). The two limbs of the U-shaped synovial cavity communicate with each other over the ridge. Anteriorly, the extrasynovial space behind the ligamentum patellae is filled by the fat pad, and posteriorly, between the limbs of the U, the extrasynovial space within the capsule is occupied by the cruciate ligaments, which fill the intercondylar notch.

Bursae

Several bursae are associated with the knee joint. At the anterior conjoined portion of the cavity, the synovial membrane sweeps upward from its femoral attachment to cover the anterior surface of the femur (see Fig. 18-34*C*). At a hand's breadth above the patella, the synovial membrane reflects forward onto the posterior surface of the quadriceps tendon and attaches to the superior margin of the patella. The large cul-de-sac created in this fashion is the **suprapatellar bursa** or **pouch** (Fig. 18-41). The suprapatellar bursa apparently develops as a separate synovial cavity independent of the joint, but the septum separating the two cavities breaks down sometime after birth, or probably when the child begins to walk.

Posteriorly, a much smaller extension of the synovial cavity is interposed in the form of a bursa between the popliteus muscle and the tibia as that muscle exits from the joint. This is the **subpopliteal recess** or bursa (see Fig. 18-41).

There are numerous other bursae around the knee which normally do not communicate with the joint, although quite often some of them may do so. The bursae

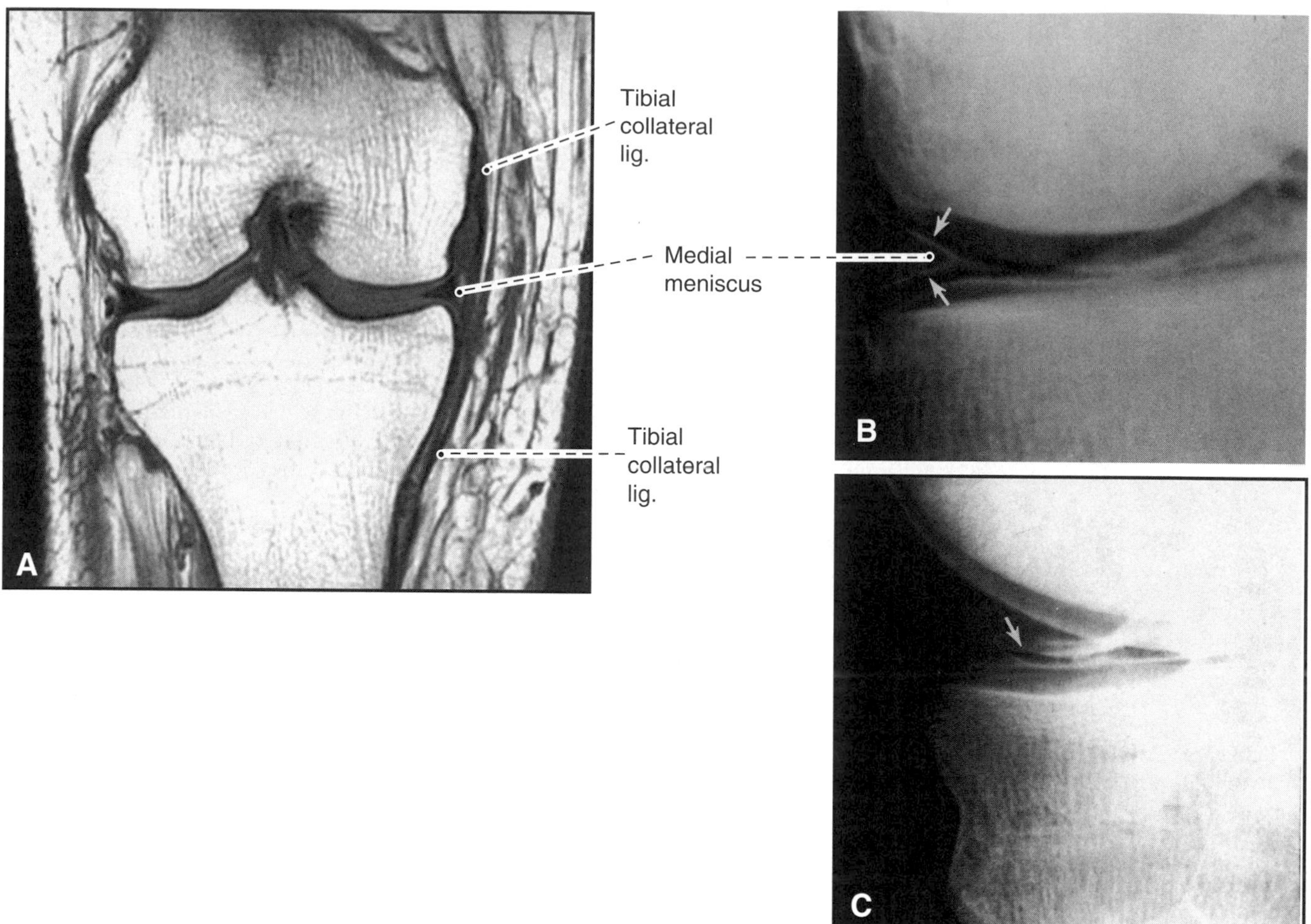

FIGURE *18-40.*
Radiologic anatomy of the menisci and associated structures: (A) coronal MRI scan of the knee joint; (B and C) arthrograms of the knee; iodinated contrast material has been injected into the knee joint after sterile preparation and infiltration of a local anesthetic. In panel B, the normal triangular cross-sectional profile of the medial meniscus is outlined by the radiolucent air in the joint cavity (*arrows*). Panel C shows a torn medial meniscus with air and contrast medium within the fissure of the tear (*arrow*). (A, courtesy of Dr. Thurman Gillespy III; B and C, courtesy of Dr. Rosalind H. Troupin.)

are clinically important in the differential diagnosis of swellings at the knee. Several are associated with the patella and the patellar ligament (see Fig. 18-34*C*). The **subcutaneous prepatellar bursa** lies between the skin and the patella. The **subcutaneous** and **deep infrapatellar bursae** lie superficial and deep, respectively, to the ligamentum patellae. Both of the subcutaneous bursae are susceptible to injury and may become distended and inflamed. Such a condition affecting the prepatellar bursa has been called *housemaid's knee*, whereas inflammation of the infrapatellar bursa has been termed *clergyman's knee*.

Posteriorly, there are bursae associated with muscle attachments around the knee (semimembranous, medial, and lateral heads of the gastrocnemius). There is a bursa around the fibular collateral ligament separating it from the biceps tendon and the joint capsule. A bursa also lines the pocket between the free anterior part of the tibial collateral ligament and the capsule. As mentioned earlier, a complicated bursa intervenes between the tendons of insertion of the semitendinosus, sartorius, and gracilis (bursa anserina).

Effusions into the Knee

In the normal extended knee, the patella is in contact with the femur and depressions are visible on either side of the patella. A large effusion in the joint obliterates these depressions and elevates the patella. The elevation can be confirmed by ballottement of the patella against the femoral condyles (Fig. 18-42*A*). Moderate effusions may not be sufficient to elevate the patella. However, if fluid is first displaced from the suprapatellar bursa and the side of the joint cavity by compression, elevation of the patella will occur and may be confirmed by ballottement (see Fig. 18-42*B* and

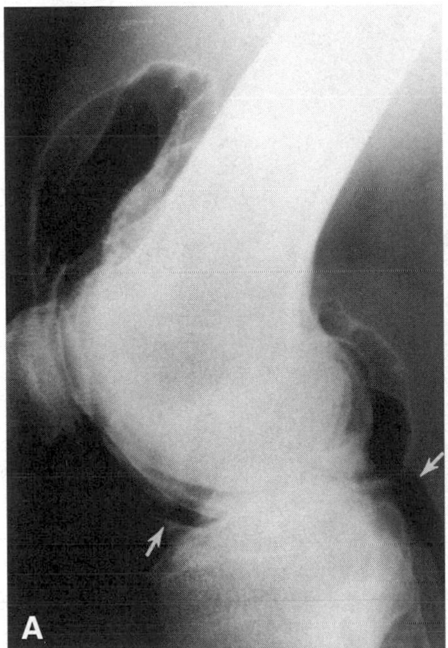

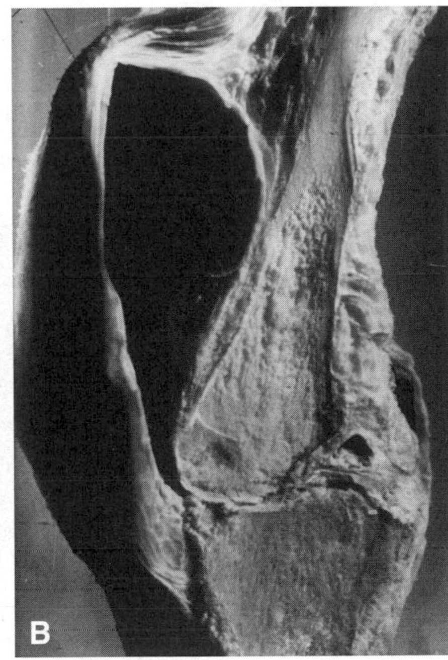

FIGURE *18-41.*
The synovial cavity and bursae associated with the knee joint: (A) A pneumoarthrogram of the normal knee. Introduction of a small amount of contrast medium, which sticks to the surface of the synovium, was followed by injection of about 20 cc of air into the synovial cavity. The extent of the synovial membrane is outlined. Note the spacious suprapatellar bursa and the posterior extent of the two limbs of the U-shaped cavity, the profiles of which overlap in this projection. Part of the infrapatellar fold is visible (*anterior arrow*). The popliteus bursa is filled with air and is revealed as a radiolucency (*posterior arrow*). (B) A specimen from the Anatomy Museum of the Royal College of Surgeons of England, showing in a sagittal section (cut to one side of the patella) a distended suprapatellar bursa. The knee shows degenerative changes with some degree of ankylosis.

C). Even this maneuver will not elevate the patella in small effusions. In such cases, the fluid must be milked into the depression on one side of the patella; then the effusion may be demonstrated by transmission of the fluid or a fluid impulse by percussion from one side of the patella to the other.

Blood and Nerve Supply

An arterial anastomosis is formed around the knee which is fed chiefly by genicular branches of the popliteal artery (Fig. 18-43). The paired superior and inferior **genicular arteries** skirt the femoral and tibial condyles and supply the bones as well as the joint. Their anastomosis is reinforced by descending and ascending genicular branches derived from the femoral and anterior tibial arteries, respectively. An unpaired middle genicular branch of the popliteal artery supplies mainly the contents of the intercondylar notch.

The knee joint is supplied by several nerves, some of which innervate the hip joint as well. This explains why pain is so readily referred from a diseased hip to the knee. The general rule is that the nerves that supply the prime movers of a joint also innervate that joint. Accordingly, the femoral nerve supplies the knee by its branches to the vasti and by the saphenous nerve; one or more large branches are contributed to the knee by the tibial nerve, the chief nerve of the flexors. In addition, both the obturator and fibular nerves send articular branches to the knee joint.

Movements

Flexion of the knee is normally limited by contact between the calf and the thigh. In full extension, the angle between the tibia and femur is slightly greater than 180° in women, and slightly less than 180° in men.

In full flexion, the rounded articular surfaces on the posterior aspects of the femoral condyles are in contact with the tibial plateau and the menisci. In this position the articular surfaces are maximally incongruent and permit a wide range of accessory movements as well as active rotation of the tibia. As the tibia is extended, more and more anterior parts of the femoral articular surfaces come in contact with the tibia and the menisci. Because the curvature of the two femoral condyles is neither equal nor circular, the resultant movement is a composite of the tibia's sliding and rolling (see Fig. 5-13) on the femoral condyles in a forward direction. This takes place when the knee is extended with the foot off the ground. During weight bearing, the tibia is stabilized and the femur rolls on it in a forward direction. Concomitant with the forward roll, the femur has to slide backward on the tibia to maintain contact and achieve increasing congruence between the articular surfaces.

Maximum stability of the knee is attained in full extension because close packing of the joint is obtained in this position (see Chap. 5). The chief requirement of close pack is maximal congruence of the articular surfaces. Because the articular facet for the tibia does not extend as far forward on the lateral as on the medial femoral condyle (see Fig. 18-4), congruence is attained sooner between the lateral condyles than between the medial condyles. When the lateral condyles are close-packed, the tibia and femur are in a straight line, and the anterior edge of the lateral meniscus has reached the groove on the femoral condyle that marks the boundary between the tibial and patellar articular surfaces. This is not so on the medial side. To bring the edge of the medial meniscus to the anterior limit of the tibial articular surface of the femoral condyle, either the tibia or the femur has to rotate. If the femur is stabilized, the tibia will spin and slide in a lateral direction; if the tibia is stabilized, the femur will spin and slide medially. This element of rotation during the final phase of knee extension is essential for close-packing or *locking* the knee. In the locked position no accessory movements are permitted, nor is there any possibility for active rotation of the tibia. The capsule and all ligaments of the joint are maximally taut and the knee is converted into a solid pillar.

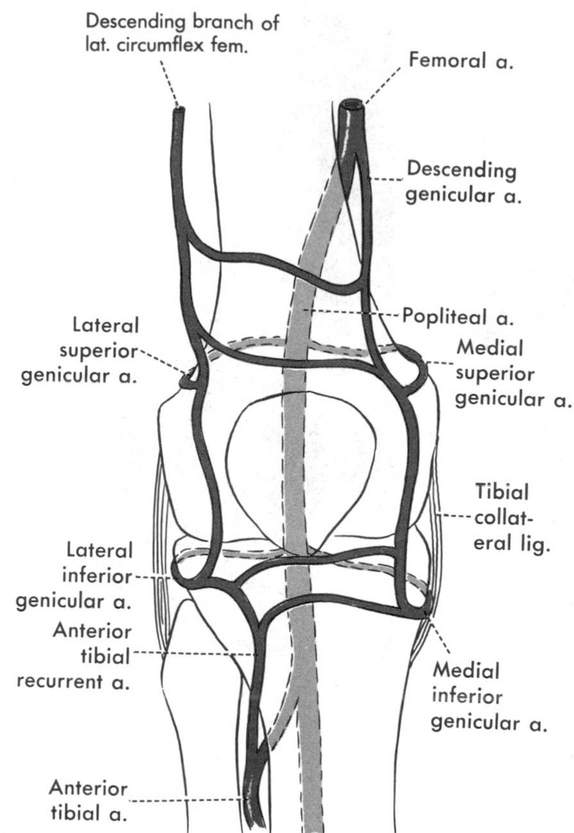

FIGURE *18-43.*
Diagram of the arteries that form an anastomosis around the knee joint and supply it; anterior view.

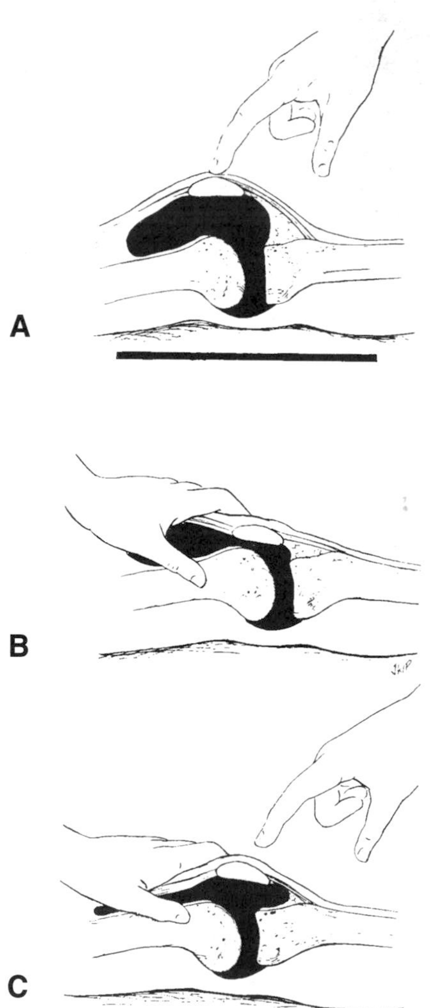

FIGURE *18-42.*
Effusion into the knee joint and its detection: (A) ballottement of the patella, in a large effusion into the joint; (B and C) when there is moderate effusion, fluid from the suprapatellar bursa has to be displaced before ballottement of the patella can be performed.

The rotation associated with extension is *conjunct rotation*, the inevitable outcome of extension determined by the shape of the articular surfaces. No rotator muscles are called into action to effect the required tibial or femoral spin. The conjunct rotation is produced by the knee extensors, muscles that are incapable of rotating the femur or the tibia actively and independent of extension.

Before flexion can begin, the knee has to be *unlocked* by reversing the conjunct rotation of extension. For this, a specific force is required, which is furnished by the popliteus muscle. The latter can medially rotate the tibia or laterally rotate the femur, depending on which bone is stabilized. The rotation restores the joint into loose pack, and flexion or active rotation may proceed.

The menisci play a passive but important role in movements of the knee. The flexion–extension component of movement takes place mainly between the femoral condyles and the menisci, the latter adapting their shapes to the curvature of the advancing femoral condyles. The rotational component of the movement occurs chiefly between the menisci and the tibia, the menisci moving with the femur.

Muscles

The bulk of the thigh musculature consists of the prime movers of the knee (see Fig. 18-10) which, in addition to producing knee flexion and extension, are important in stabilizing the joint when it is in loose pack. A number of thigh muscles capable of exerting force across the knee can also move the hip (rectus femoris, hamstrings, sartorius, gracilis and, with the iliotibial tract, the gluteus maximus and tensor fasciae latae). These muscles evidently play a role in coordinating movement between the two joints and recruiting appropriate muscles, by postural reflexes, for stabilizing the joints and balancing the trunk at the hip and knee.

The quadriceps is the only **extensor** muscle of the knee. Other muscles can assist in knee extension by their actions at the hip and ankle joints: the gluteus maximus, for example, extends the hip joint, and the soleus and gastrocnemius flex the ankle joint, and by so doing these muscles resist flexion of the knee. In a weight-bearing limb, knee flexion cannot occur without simultaneous flexion at the hip and dorsiflexion at the ankle.

The **flexors** of the knee include several muscles: the semimembranosus, semitendinosus, short head of the biceps, and gracilis are the best flexors, the sartorius a weaker one. The popliteus is said to be a weak flexor, assisting flexion more by rotating the femur on the tibia, or vice versa, than by its direct pull in flexion. The gastrocnemius, because it crosses behind the knee joint, flexes this joint when the limb is not supporting weight. The long head of the biceps, although assisting flexion, relaxes while knee flexion is still being completed by other muscles.

In the loose-packed position of the knee, the tibia can be **rotated** medially and laterally which swings the foot medially and laterally when the knee is bent. With the knee locked, the rotation occurs at the hip. Medial rotation of the tibia or the femur is produced by the semimembranosus, semitendinosus, sartorius, and gracilis, whereas the biceps femoris and popliteus are lateral rotators.

Stability of the Knee Joint

Joint stability is crucial for the function of the knee. Because bony factors of stability are negligible in this joint, the integrity of ligaments and muscles is indispensable.

In relaxed standing the force of gravity maintains the knee in extension (see Figs. 17-2 and 18-72). In this position the joint is dependent on its ligaments for stability. The reinforced posterior part of the capsule and the anterior cruciate ligament are the chief factors in checking hyperextension, but the tension in all ligaments is increased in this extended position. The functional evaluation of ligamentous integrity is described later in this section.

As soon as the weight-bearing knee is flexed, muscles are called into action to stabilize the joint. Even a few degrees of flexion are accompanied by contraction of the quadriceps. A powerful quadriceps can maintain stability in the knee despite considerable laxity of ligaments. Wasting or weakness of this muscle results in instability of the knee, described by the patient as a feeling of insecurity or the knee "giving way."

Stabilization of the patella is a crucial factor in the quadriceps mechanism. Because the femoral shaft articulates with the tibia at an angle, the pull of the quadriceps tends to displace the patella laterally. Lateral displacement of the patella is prevented by 1) the prominent trochlea of the lateral femoral condyle (see Figs. 18-1*C* and 18-4) and 2) the attachment of the vastus medialis into the medial border of the patella (see Fig. 18-11).

In the flexed position of the weight-bearing knee, the femoral condyles have a tendency to slip forward on the tibial plateau (see Fig. 18-1*B*). The popliteus, together with the posterior cruciate ligament, oppose this tendency. Especially important is the **iliotibial tract** which is attached to the anterior surface of the lateral tibial condyle (see Figs. 17-10 and 18-34) and transmits force to the knee from the gluteus maximus and tensor fasciae latae. This stout tendonlike band becomes prominent when weight is borne on the flexed knee. The pelvis with the femur is balanced on the sloping tibial plateau by the gluteus maximus and tensor fasciae latae by the iliotibial tract.

Injuries to the Knee

Injuries of the knee are common, the most frequently damaged structures being ligaments and menisci. Ligaments are torn when an external force is applied to the knee. Which ligament bears the brunt of such an impact depends on the direction of the force. Injury of the menisci, on the other hand, usually results from forces generated within the limb.

The **tibial collateral ligament** is most frequently injured by a force applied to the outer (lateral) side of the joint while the foot is weight-bearing. If the knee is extended in such an injury, the anterior cruciate ligament is also tightened and, if sufficient force is imparted, it may rupture. In a rupture of the tibial collateral ligament, the medial meniscus may lose its attachment and become displaced into the joint cavity. Isolated injury may also occur in the **anterior** or the **posterior cruciate ligaments** from hyperextension force when the foot is fixed to the ground. In these injuries the posterior capsule is also torn. In children and adolescents, the result may be avulsion of a piece of bone on the anterior part of the intercondylar eminence, to which the cruciate ligament is attached, rather than ligament rupture.

Meniscus injuries occur when a meniscus gets caught between the tibial and femoral condyles in a weight-bearing limb when the knee is bent.

During extension, tension is first built up in the anterior cruciate ligament, which then guides the rotation of the femur. When movement occurs suddenly while the limb is weight-bearing, a meniscus gets caught between the condyles, and a tear results (see Fig. 18-40C). The lateral meniscus, owing to its controlled mobility, enjoys a much greater degree of protection than the medial meniscus, and it is seldom damaged. Although there are a number of physical signs produced by different types of tears, the most useful sign of a torn meniscus in the acute state is accurately localized tenderness over the injured meniscus, between the femoral and tibial articular margins.

Functional Evaluation of the Knee

Rather than to provide a comprehensive description, the purpose of this section is to illustrate that familiarity with the anatomy of the knee enables a physician to localize injury or disease to particular anatomic structures, based on the complaints of a patient and the history of an injury. The physical examination of the knee is a systematic evaluation of the function of the structures that constitute the joint.

Symptoms. Knowledge of the innervation of the knee explains how, in addition to local causes, **pain** may be referred to the normal knee from compressed lumbar spinal nerves or, more commonly, from a diseased hip. Knee movement may exaggerate the pain in both instances because it may stretch the compressed nerve roots, or because hip movement is associated with most habitual movements of the knee. **Weakness** and wasting of the quadriceps predispose to a feeling of insecurity or to an actual giving way of the knee. This complaint is usually a sequela of a knee injury, which has been treated with prolonged immobilization. There may be a tendency for the patella to subluxate or dislocate. **Clicks** occur commonly in many normal joints, and there is no pain associated with them. The sounds are generated in the patellofemoral joint or by the movement of the menisci. Painful grating or clicking sounds indicate degenerative joint disease or a damaged meniscus.

Physical Examination. Systematic inspection, palpation, testing of passive and active ranges of movement, and assessment of muscle strength and joint stability, constitute the physical examination. It is, in fact, a survey of the anatomic components of the knee region, and the relation of the joint to other segments of the limb. Testing of muscles and ranges of movement are discussed in earlier sections of this chapter.

Inspection. In the anatomic position, inspection of the subject in anterior and side views should verify the alignment of the femur with the tibia, the patella with the foot, the levels of the two patellae and popliteal skin creases, the lack of any flexion at the joint when the soles of both feet are in contact with the ground, symmetry of soft-tissue contours, particularly that of the patellar fibers of the vastus medialis, as well as the presence or absence of swellings and red areas of the skin.

Malalignments include *knock-knee* (*genu valgum*) and *bowlegs* (*genu varum*), normal in mild degrees in children and usually corrected by normal growth. Growth plate injuries and malunion of fractures, however, may lead to permanent deformities. *Hyperextension* deformity (*genu recurvatum*) results from muscle imbalance, growth abnormalities, or unhealed ligamentous injuries. All these deformities distort the mechanics of the joint, displace the normal relation of the line of gravitational force relative to the knee, and predispose to degenerative joint disease. The knees should also be inspected during walking, paying attention to the phases of the gait cycle described at the end of this chapter.

Palpation. Unless there are contraindications, all accessible anatomic structures should be palpated, noting tenderness, swelling, or breach in continuity. **Bony landmarks** around the knee are discussed with the bones (see General Orientation). In addition to the palpable bony features, the quadriceps tendon, the ligamentum patellae, and the tendons of the hamstrings are useful landmarks on either side of the popliteal fossa, especially if the muscles are isometrically contracted with the knee in the flexed position. The tendon of the biceps attached to the head of the fibula and, on the medial side, the overlapping tendons of the semitendinosus and semimembranosus can be distinguished.

Both **patellar** and **femoral surfaces** of the patellofemoral joint may be examined if the patella is manually displaced laterally or medially, while the quadriceps is kept relaxed. The edges of the **menisci** should be palpated along the joint line, starting anteriorly on either side of the patellar ligament. Tenderness is suggestive of meniscal tear. Such tenderness can be distinguished from that due to partial tear in the collateral ligaments. The anterior edge of the **tibial collateral ligament** is not discernible, but it does not extend further forward than a vertical line drawn down from the adductor tubercle. The **fibular collateral ligament** is lax in the flexed knee but adduction of the tibia in this position will tighten it. Sufficient adduction (varus) force will be applied to the knee by resting the flexed leg on the opposite knee. The ligament can then be felt as a tense cord above the head of the fibula. The thickness of the **synovial membrane** can be assessed by feeling the tissues over the relaxed knee above and below the patella. Hypertrophied synovium in a rheumatoid joint has a characteristic, thickened, doughy texture. The identity of localized swellings (e.g., of the bursae associated with the patella and patellar ligament: see Fig. 18-34C) may be determined by palpation based on knowledge of the landmarks. The contents of the popliteal fossa should be palpated while the knee is bent.

Stability. Each of the collateral and cruciate ligaments can be tested. In assessing ligamentous integrity, the muscles must be relaxed. To test the collateral ligaments the knee must be slightly flexed. This eliminates the stabilizing effect of the cruciate ligaments on the extended knee. The tibial collateral ligament is tested by grasping the subject's ankle with one hand and using the other hand as a fulcrum at the knee. Abduction force is applied at the ankle, attempting to produce a valgus deformity of the knee. The lateral collateral ligament is tested by attempting to produce a varus deformity (Fig. 18-44*A* and *B*). Complete tear of the ligaments results in

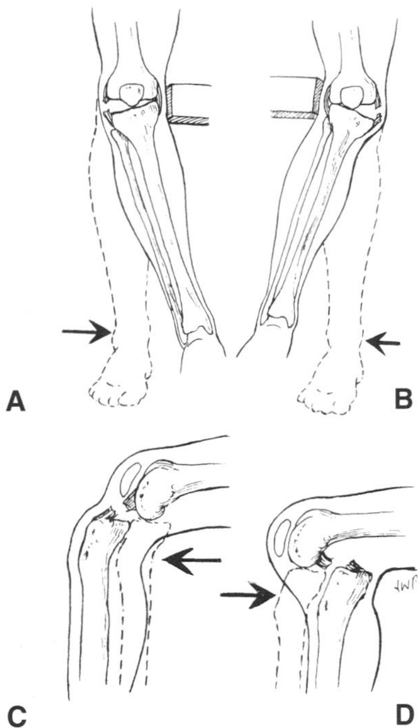

FIGURE 18-44.
Testing for ligamentous injuries of the knee: (A and B) collateral ligaments; (C and D) anterior and posterior cruciate ligaments.

separation of the femoral and tibial articular margins. Incomplete tear produces pain confirmed by tenderness over the ligament.

The anterior cruciate ligament is tested by attempting to displace the tibia anteriorly on the femur with the knee flexed to about 90° and the foot stabilized. The proximal end of the tibia is grasped and pulled forward. If the anterior cruciate ligament is torn, a forward displacement of the tibia will occur (drawer sign). Integrity of the posterior cruciate ligament is tested in an identical manner by posterior displacement of the tibia (see Fig. 18-44*C* and *D*).

THE ANKLE

Connecting the leg and the foot, the ankle transmits the tendons of those muscles that act as prime movers at the ankle joint and the joints of the foot, as well as the major nerves and vessels of the foot. The prominent landmarks in this region are the medial and lateral malleoli and the tendo calcaneus, all of which are subcutaneous. The soft tissues of the ankle are best described in reference to these landmarks and to the fascial bands, called retinacula, that retain the tendons in position and prevent their bowstringing around the ankle joint when the muscle bellies contract.

Retinacula

The retinacula at the ankle, like those at the wrist, are reinforcements in the deep fascia and consist predominantly of transverse collagen fiber bundles. Altogether, there are five of them (Fig. 18-45): anteriorly the superior and inferior extensor retinacula; behind the medial malleolus is the flexor retinaculum; and behind the lateral malleolus are the superior and inferior peroneal retinacula.

The **superior extensor retinaculum** is poorly defined and is represented by a few additional transverse fibers in the crural fascia that stretch between the tibia and the fibula (see Fig. 18-45*A*). The **inferior extensor retinaculum** is more complex. It arises from the lateral side and upper surface of the calcaneus (in the sinus tarsi; see Fig. 18-6*D*). As it crosses the front of the ankle, it divides into an upper and a lower limb. The upper limb attaches to the medial malleolus, and the lower one blends with the fascia on the medial side of the sole of the foot. The tendons crossing the front of the ankle run through compartments in the retinaculum, where they are invested in synovial *tendon sheaths*. One sheath encloses the tendon of the tibialis anterior, another that of the extensor hallucis, longus, and a third the tendons of the extensor digitorum longus and peroneus tertius. There are no such sheaths or compartments beneath the superior retinaculum.

The deep fibular nerve and anterior tibial artery emerge between the tendons of the extensor hallucis longus and extensor digitorum longus, deep to the inferior extensor retinaculum, and occupying their own compartment (see Fig. 18-47). Distal to the retinaculum, the artery becomes known as the dorsalis pedis artery.

The **flexor retinaculum** runs between the medial malleolus and the calcaneus (see Fig. 18-45*B*). The space deep to the retinaculum is divided by three septa into four compartments: in the most anterior one is the tendon of the tibialis posterior, and in the next the flexor digitorum longus tendon; the third compartment contains the tibial nerve and posterior tibial vessels; the most posterior one is occupied by the tendon of the flexor hallucis longus. Each of the three tendons passing through the flexor retinaculum is invested in a *tendon sheath* that begins a little above the retinaculum and may extend a short distance into the plantar surface of the foot.

The **superior peroneal retinaculum** extends from the lateral malleolus to the calcaneus (see Fig. 18-45C). Deep to it run the tendons of the peroneus longus and brevis, enclosed in a common *tendon sheath*. The **inferior peroneal retinaculum** is attached at both ends to the calcaneus, and its upper end blends with the stem of the inferior extensor retinaculum. From its deep surface, it sends a septum to the calcaneus that divides the common sheath and separates the two peroneal tendons. The synovial sheath around the peroneus brevis stops above the lateral border of the foot. That of the peroneus longus travels farther, and may continue into the sole of the foot.

Relations

The order of structures across the front of the ankle, beginning on the medial side, is as follows. The first tendon in front of the medial malleolus is that of the tibialis anterior. It is rendered prominent by dorsiflexing and inverting the foot. Next to it is the tendon of the extensor hallu-

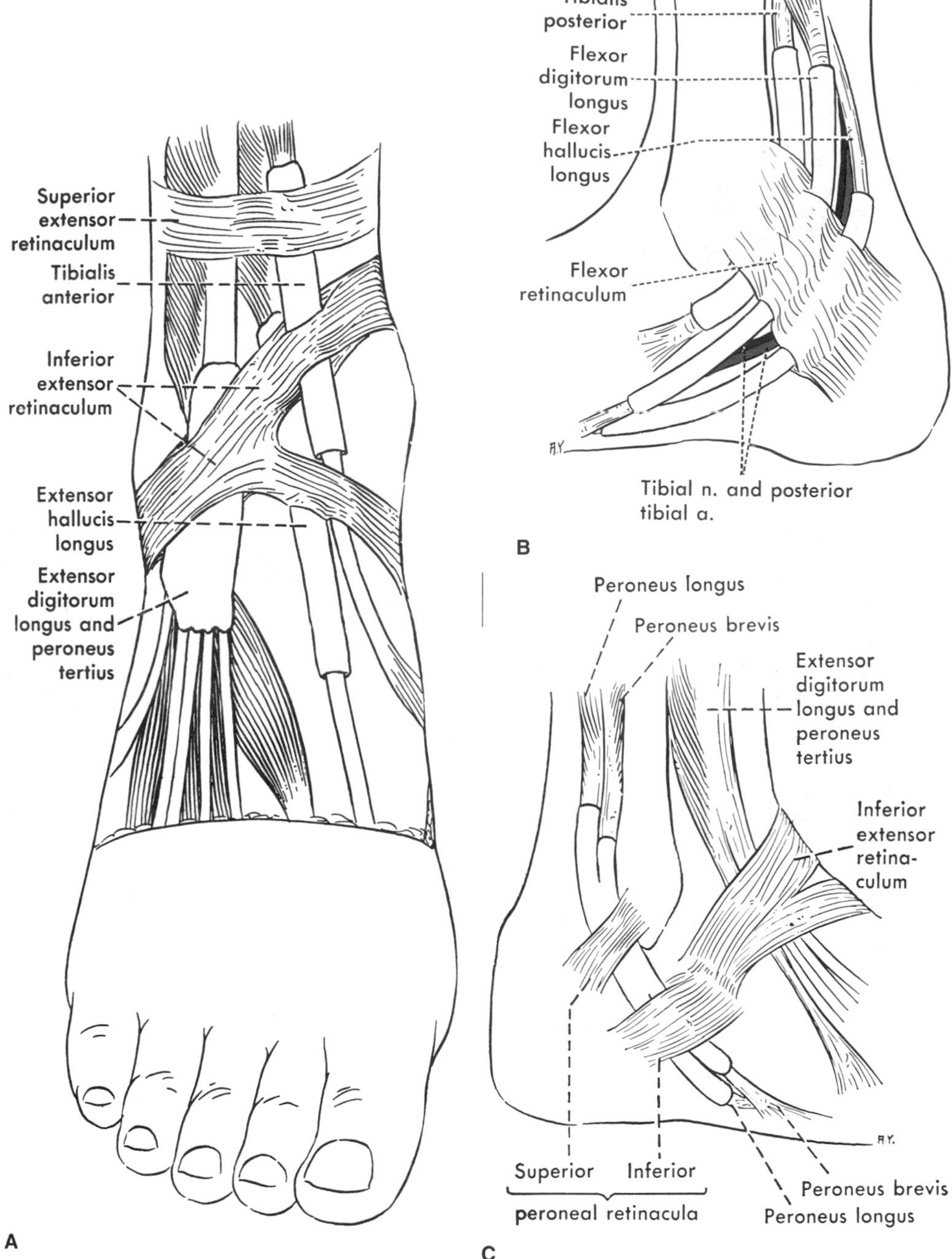

FIGURE *18-45.*
Retinacula and anatomic relations in the ankle region: (A) anterior view; (B) medial view; (C) lateral view. The tendons running beneath the retinacula are invested in synovial tendon sheaths.

cis longus, readily identifiable when the big toe is extended. Lateral to it, the pulsations of the dorsalis pedis artery are palpable. Lateral to the artery, but not palpable, is the deep fibular nerve. In front of the lateral malleolus, the tendons of the extensor digitorum longus can be identified when the toes are extended. Eversion of the foot helps to distinguish the tendon of the peroneus tertius, in front of the lateral malleolus.

The structures passing behind the medial malleolus, deep to the flexor retinaculum, are less readily discernible by palpation. Their order is dictated by the contents of the four compartments of the retinaculum, described earlier. The pulsations of the posterior tibial artery are palpable and often visible.

Eversion of the foot throws into prominence the peroneal tendons located posteroinferiorly to the lateral malleolus; that of the brevis is anterior to that of the longus.

THE FOOT

Although it retains the same basic pentadactyl morphology, greater anatomic differences distinguish the terminal segment of the lower limb of *Homo sapiens* from the corresponding segment of the upper limb, than in any other primate or mammal. The anatomy of the foot is more characteristic of the human species

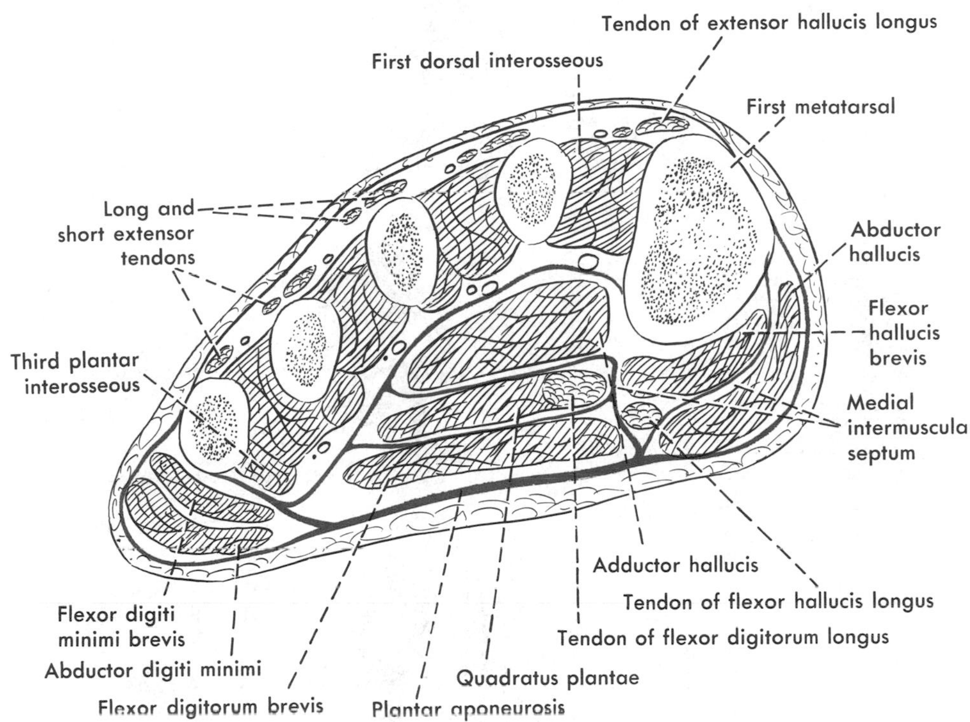

FIGURE *18-46.* **Schematic cross section through the foot showing fascial septa and muscle layers.**

than the anatomy of the hand. The erect bipedal habit accounts for these differences. Despite the differences, the anatomy of the foot is profitably explained in terms of the simpler, basic anatomy of the hand.

The introductory section of this chapter (General Orientation) describes the skeletal anatomy of the foot and introduces its joints, fascias, and superficial nerves and vessels. Figure 18-46 shows that the general arrangement of extrinsic and intrinsic muscles on the dorsal and plantar aspects of the foot conforms to that in the hand, as do its fascial spaces, nerves, and blood vessels. Except for one muscle (quadratus plantae) all structures can be readily comprehended in the figure because of their close correspondence to equivalent structures in the hand. The simpler anatomy of the dorsum is discussed before the more complex plantar aspect of the foot.

Dorsum of the Foot

The rather sparse superficial fascia of the dorsum of the foot contains dorsal digital nerves and vessels. The thin fascia of the dorsum is continuous above with the inferior extensor retinaculum and blends on the sides with the plantar fascia. Deep to it are located the tendons of the long digital extensors, the extensor digitorum brevis and extensor hallucis brevis (intrinsic muscles of the foot) and their tendons, and nerves and vessels that supply the muscles as well as the skin (Fig. 18-47).

Muscles

The tendons of the long (extrinsic) extensors of the toes proceed from the inferior extensor retinaculum to their insertions on the toes. Tendons of the extensor digitorum longus to the second, third, and fourth toes are joined by corresponding tendons of the extensor digitorum brevis (see Fig. 18-47). The **extensor digital expansions** thus formed, like those of the fingers, are joined by tendons of the lumbrical muscles and some aponeurotic fibers from the interossei. Over the proximal phalanx, each tendon complex divides into three bands: the middle band inserts on the middle phalanx, and the two lateral bands come together and insert on the distal phalanx in a manner resembling that in the fingers (see Figs. 16-58 and 16-59).

The **extensor digitorum brevis** muscle arises from an anterolateral part of the upper surface of the calcaneus (just lateral to the sinus tarsi) and from the deep surface of the inferior extensor retinaculum. The muscle splits into four small bellies, one for each of the four medial toes, each terminating in a tendon. The largest and most medial belly separates early from the main muscle mass and is given a separate name: **extensor hallucis brevis.** Its tendon goes to the proximal phalanx of the big toe. The tendons of the three remaining bellies go toward the second, third, and fourth toes. At approximately the level of the heads of the metatarsals, each joins the corresponding long extensor tendon and inserts with it upon the middle and distal phalanges. A tendon may also pass to the little toe.

The extensor hallucis brevis and extensor digitorum brevis are supplied by the *deep fibular nerve.* The former muscle extends the proximal phalanx of the big toe and the latter aids the extensor digitorum longus in extending the other toes. The action of the short extensors differs from that of the long ones in that they can effect digital extension without concomitant dorsiflexion of the foot.

Nerves and Vessels

Nerves. Both superficial and deep fibular nerves terminate in dorsal digital nerves on the dorsum of the foot (see Fig. 18-7*A*). The deep nerve also has muscular and articular branches.

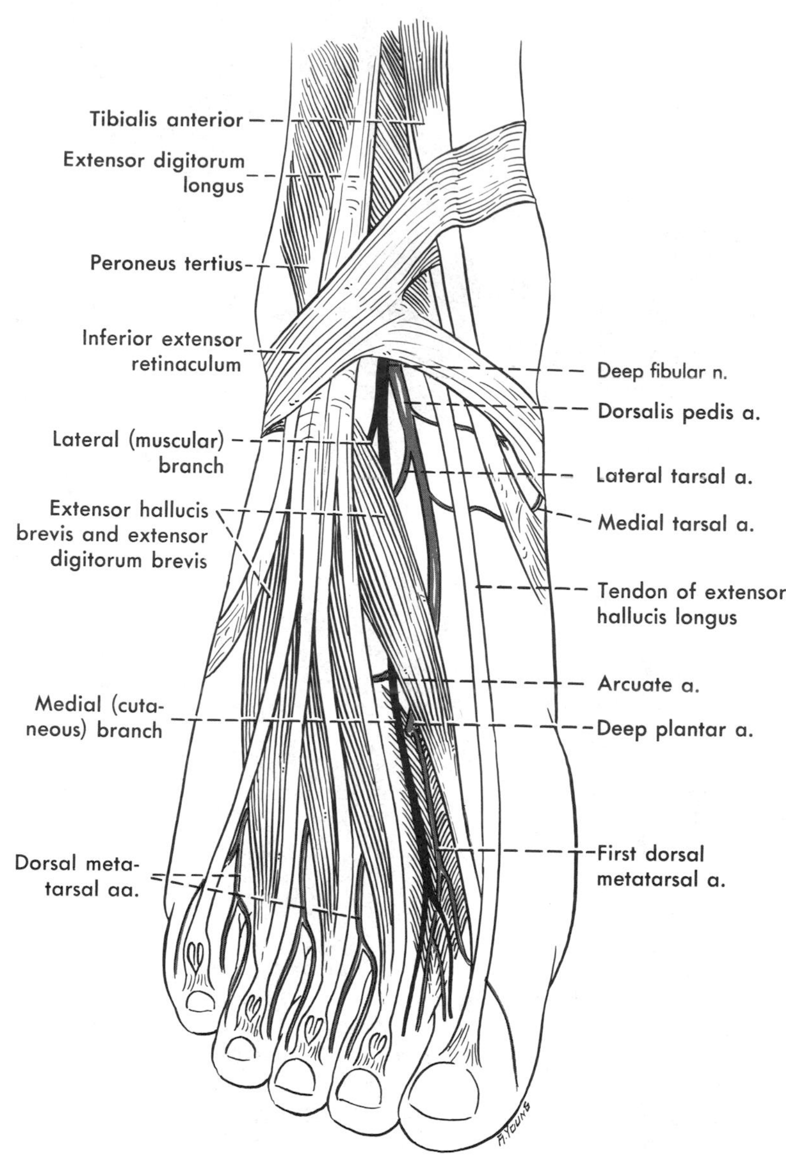

FIGURE *18-47.*
The deep fibular nerve in the foot and the dorsalis pedis artery.

The **superficial fibular nerve** enters the dorsum in the superficial fascia. Its branches and territory of supply are described in an earlier section on the cutaneous nerves.

The **deep fibular nerve** emerges on the dorsum between the tendons of the extensor hallucis longus and the extensor digitorum longus (see Fig. 18-47). As it runs distally deep to the extensor hallucis brevis, it gives off a *lateral branch* that in part goes to the short extensor muscles and in part spreads over the dorsal surface of the foot to supply the intertarsal joints. The remainder of the deep fibular nerve divides into two *dorsal digital nerves* for the adjacent sides of the first and second toes.

Arteries. The chief artery of the dorsum is the **dorsalis pedis artery** (see Fig. 18-47). Its mode of origin and distribution may vary. Most often the continuation of the anterior tibial, it enters the foot under the inferior extensor retinaculum and runs distally toward the interspace between the first and second toes. It ends by dividing into two branches. The larger branch is the **deep plantar artery** that disappears between the two heads of the first dorsal interosseous muscle into the sole of the foot (a course similar to that of the radial artery). The smaller branch is the **arcuate artery**, which runs transversely across the dorsum and provides most of the **dorsal metatarsal arteries**. (The first dorsal metatarsal usually arises separately, as a branch of the dorsalis pedis just before the origin of the deep plantar artery). The dorsal metatarsal arteries receive communications from the plantar arch and the plantar metatarsal arteries, and end as tiny **dorsal digital arteries**.

In its course, the dorsalis pedis gives off *medial and lateral tarsal arteries* (Fig. 18-48). The lateral tarsal tends to anastomose with the arcuate artery. There may also be anastomoses between the lateral tarsal, the lateral malleolar, and the perforating branch of the fibular artery. The varying development of these anastomoses and of the dorsalis pedis accounts for most of the variations in the arterial pattern. When the anterior

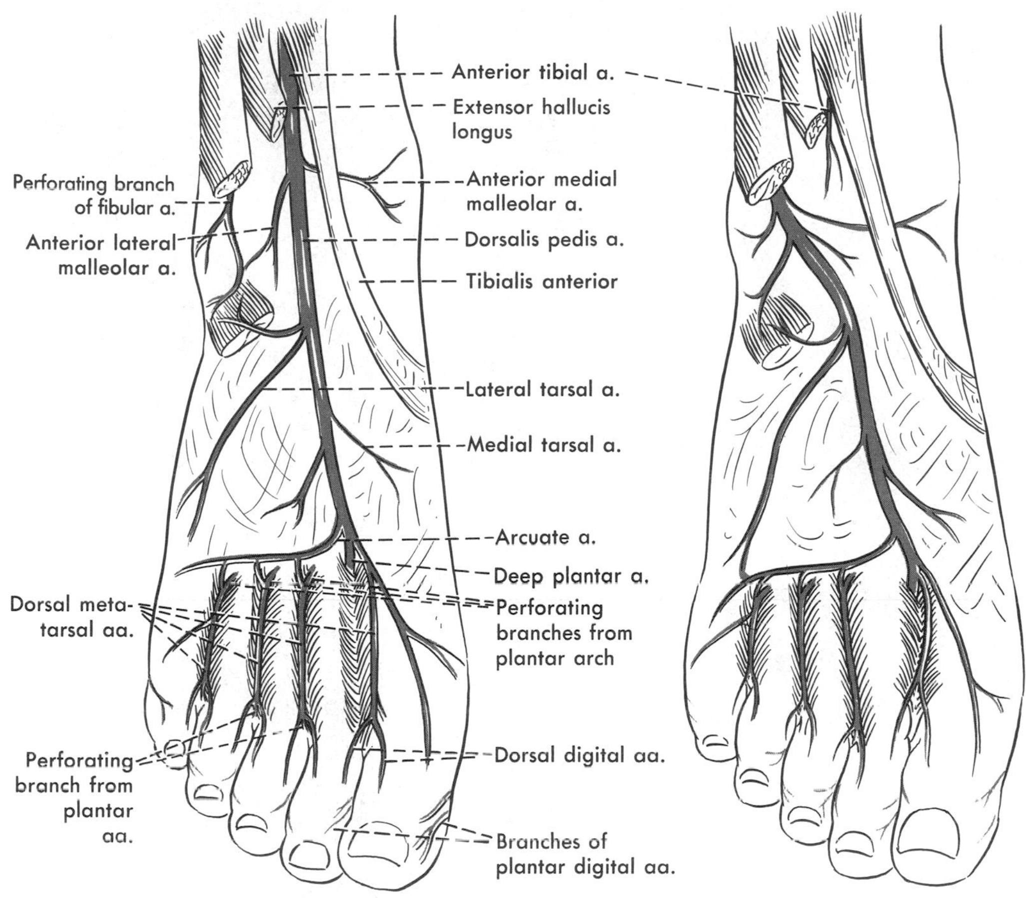

FIGURE *18-48.*
Two patterns of the arteries on the dorsum of the foot; in the second, the dorsalis pedis arises from the perforating branch of the fibular artery.

tibial artery fails to reach the foot, the dorsalis pedis artery is derived from the *perforating branch of the fibular artery* (see Figs. 18-29 and 18-48). The linkup is established through anastomotic connections. Similarly, if the arcuate artery is small or missing, the dorsal metatarsal branches that it usually gives off may be supplied by the lateral tarsal artery.

The **perforating branch of the fibular artery** passes through a gap in the lower part of the interosseous membrane (see Fig. 18-29) and descends under cover of the extensor digitorum longus and peroneus tertius. It usually anastomoses with the anterior lateral malleolar branch of the tibialis anterior artery and, with this, contributes to the blood supply of the lateral side of the foot.

Plantar Aspect of the Foot

The general arrangement and layering of structures in the sole of the foot is shown in Figure 18-46. Deep to the specialized superficial fascia is the plantar aponeurosis and, deep to that, the digital flexors. This arrangement corresponds to that in the hand. However, in the hand, the digital flexors are represented only by two sets of tendons, their muscle bellies being confined to the forearm. In the foot, the equivalent of one of these flexors, the flexor digitorum superficialis, is an intrinsic muscle, the flexor digitorum brevis. The tendons of the flexor digitorum longus, corresponding to the profundus in the hand, are associated not only with the lumbricals (as in the hand), but also with an additional intrinsic muscle, the quadratus plantae. This muscle is actually the only structure in Figure 18-46 that has no equivalent in the hand. The deepest structures are the plantar and dorsal interossei and, as in the hand, adjacent to their plantar aspects is the adductor of the first digit, in this case the adductor hallucis. The intrinsic muscles of the first and fifth digits are located on the medial and lateral borders of the foot, corresponding to the thenar and hypothenar muscles, respectively. They are surrounded by extensions of the deep fascia and plantar aponeurosis, which create septa and define potential spaces within the sole. In the central compartment, transverse laminae of the deep fascia help to delineate four muscle layers.

Plantar Fascias and Plantar Aponeurosis

The **superficial fascia** forms a tough and thick padding over the sole. Strong retinacula cutis (skin ligaments) tether the skin to the underlying plantar aponeurosis. They are particularly well developed over the metatarsal

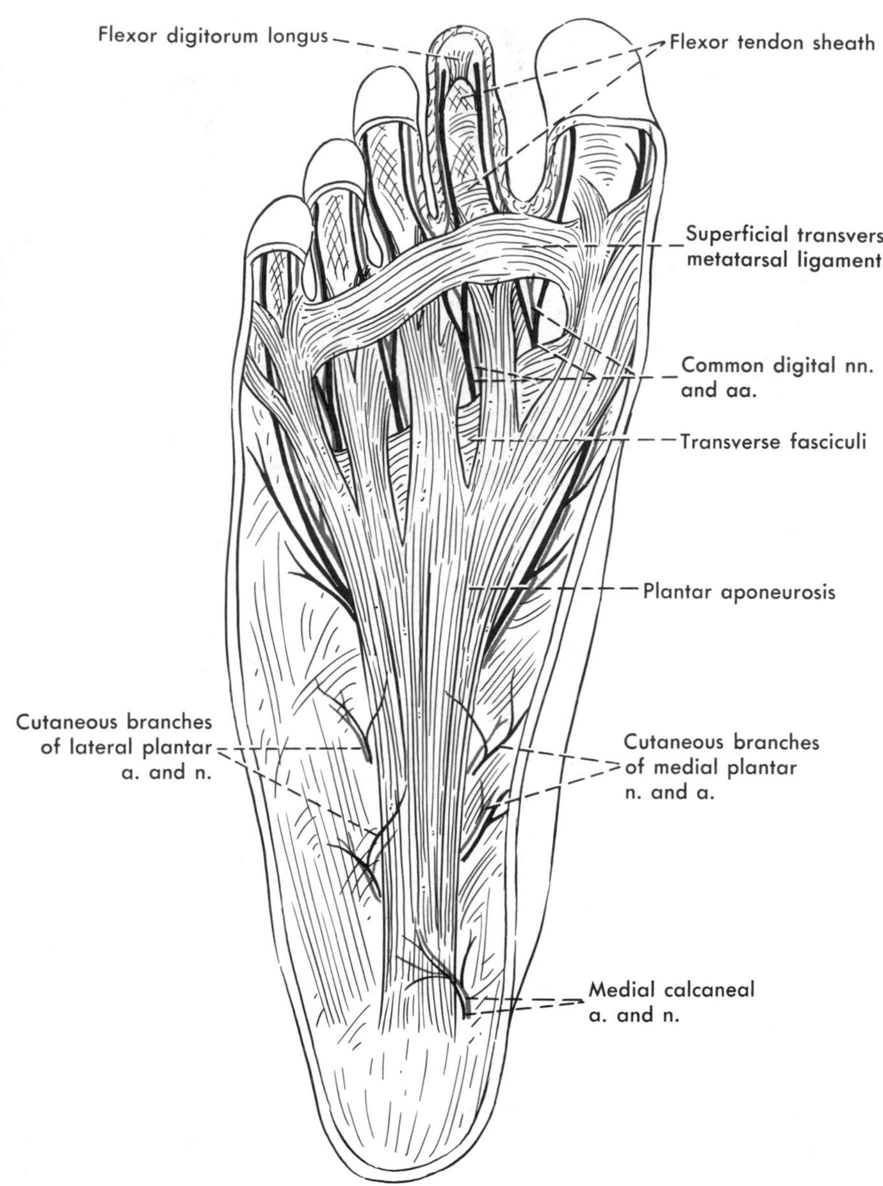

FIGURE *18-49.*
The plantar aponeurosis and superficial nerves and arteries of the plantar surface of the foot.

heads and fix the skin, allowing the necessary sliding of structures deep to the aponeurosis during extension and flexion of the toes when weight is borne over the ball of the foot. Lobulated fat fills the spaces between the retinacula cutis and provides padding over weight-bearing areas of the sole and over the terminal phalanges.

The **deep fascia** of the foot closely resembles that of the hand. There is a central **plantar aponeurosis** that extends forward and divides into digitations for the toes (Fig. 18-49). It is attached proximally to the calcaneus. Its digitations, united at first by transverse fasciculi, split to pass around the flexor tendon sheaths of the digits. Some fibers blend with the sheaths, others continue on to attach to the deep transverse metatarsal ligaments and the bases of the proximal phalanges (see Fig. 18-66).

During the gait cycle (discussed at the end of this chapter), the movement of the skin over the ball of the foot is integrated with the movement of the toes by the digitations of the aponeurosis and by its superficial fibers that attach to the dermis. The fibrous sheets of the toes, the digitations of the aponeurosis and the skin ligaments become taut when the toes are extended, as happens at push-off (see Fig. 18-73). In this manner the aponeurosis and skin become fixed over the ball of the foot. But when the metatarsal heads first contact the ground, just before weight transfer to the forefoot, the toes are in the neutral position, the digitations and skin ligaments are lax, and this permits the skin to slide freely over the metatarsal heads.

Close to the heads of the metatarsals, the digitations of the plantar aponeurosis are crossed superficially by the **superficial transverse metatarsal ligament** (see Fig. 18-49). The digital nerves and vessels appear between the digitations of the aponeurosis and pass distally deep to (above) the superficial transverse metatarsal ligament.

Intermuscular septa spring from the medial and lateral edges of the aponeurosis and demarcate the intrinsic muscles of the first and fifth digits from a more central compartment (see Fig. 18-46). These septa pass dorsally and are usually described as dividing the foot into three compartments: lateral, intermediate, and medial.

The **lateral septum** attaches over the tarsal bones proximally, and to the fifth metatarsal distally, and thus delineates a compartment for the muscles of the little toe. The **medial intermuscular septum** is more complicated. It has been described as dividing into medial and lateral leaflets as it is traced dorsally. The medial leaflet turns in a medial direction and passes deep to the abductor hallucis to attach to the first metatarsal; the lateral leaflet takes a more straightforward course dorsally, and is soon joined by fascial septa running transversely in the foot (see Fig. 18-46). The transverse septa define the muscle layers in the intermediate compartment. The spaces in this compartment extend proximally into the posterior compartment of the leg. Dyes injected into the fascial spaces containing the tendons of the flexor digitorum longus and flexor hallucis longus spread along these tendons to the deep compartment of the leg (a route infections can also follow), but dye injected into any of the other spaces remains confined to the sole of the foot.

Over the ball of the foot additional sagittal septa connect the plantar aponeurosis to the fascia that covers the interosseous muscles and to the deep transverse metatarsal ligament (see Fig. 18-66), located between the heads of the metatarsals. In this manner, tunnels are created that transmit the flexor tendons, lumbricals, and some of the digital nerves. Cushions of connective tissue sprouting from these septa and fat pads protect the tendons, muscles, and nerves from compression (Fig. 18-50). The compression is greatest in the ball of the foot during the heel-off to toe-off phases of the gait cycle (see Fig. 18-73).

Superficial Nerves and Vessels

Except for its medial and lateral borders, the sole of the foot is furnished with cutaneous nerves by the **medial and lateral plantar nerves**. As they proceed toward the toes from their point of entry inferior to the medial malleolus, they give off branches that reach the skin along the borders of the plantar aponeurosis (Fig. 18-51; see Fig. 18-49). The nerves run in the fascial plane dorsal to the aponeurosis, and are revealed only after the latter has been reflected. The general pattern of branching is for each nerve to divide into *common plantar digital branches*, which in turn divide into *proper plantar digital nerves*. Branches of the lateral and medial plantar arteries accompany the cutaneous nerves.

The **plantar digital nerves** and **vessels** emerge between slips of the plantar aponeurosis or deep fascia to become subcutaneous close to the bases of the digits (see Fig. 18-49). Of the digital nerves, those to the medial three and one-half toes are usually supplied by the medial plantar nerve, and those to the lateral one and one-half toes by the lateral plantar nerve, a distribution similar to that of median and ulnar nerves in the hand. Frequently, the lateral plantar nerve gives off a branch that joins the branch of the medial plantar nerve to the interspace between the third and fourth toes; a similar connection between the ul-

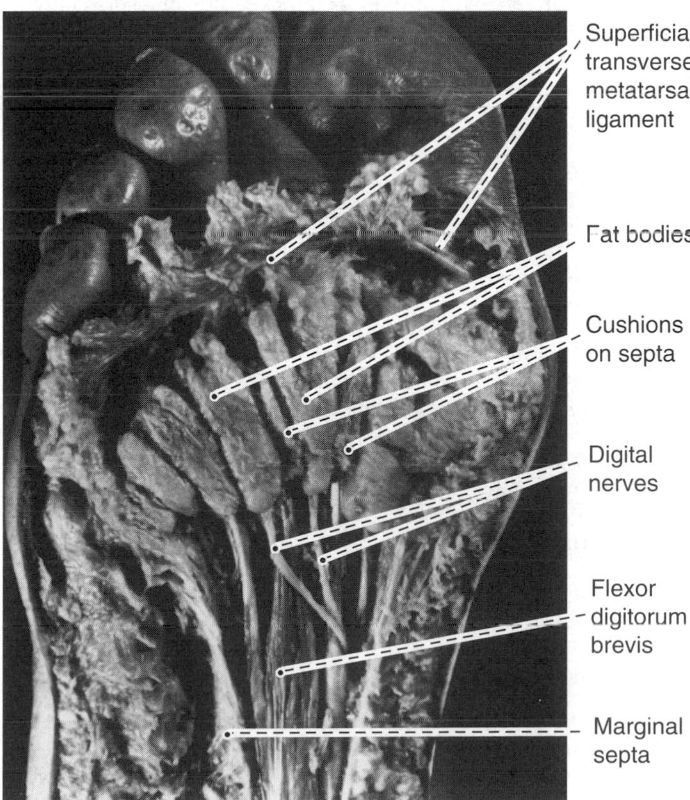

FIGURE 18-50.
Dissection of the sole of the foot with specializations of its fascia. The plantar aponeurosis has been removed. (Boysen-Möller F, Flagsted KE. Plantar aponeurosis and internal architecture of the ball of the first. J Anat 1976;121:599; with permission.)

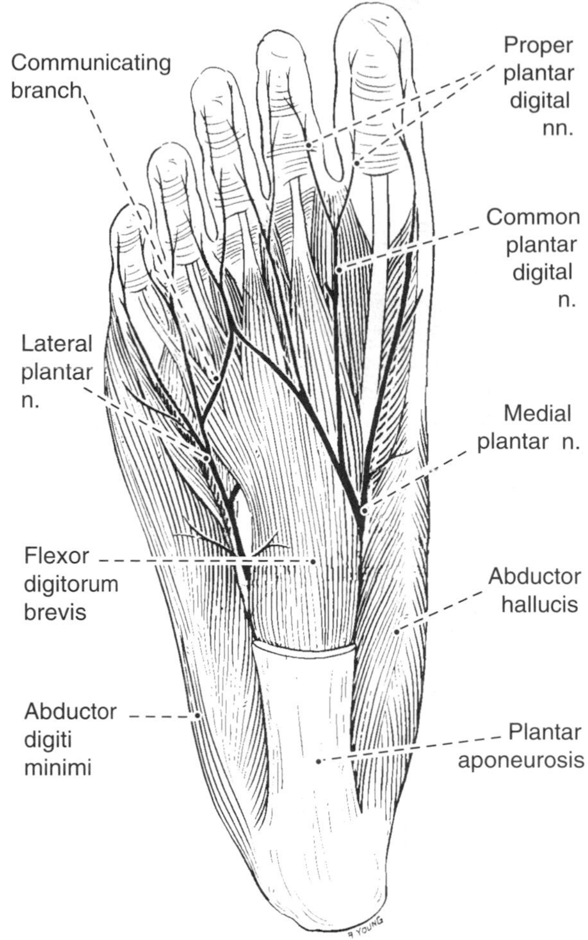

FIGURE *18-51.*
The digital nerves and the first layer of muscles in the sole of the foot shown after removal of the plantar aponeurosis.

nar and median nerves of the hand is also common. The **plantar digital arteries** are formed primarily by metatarsal arteries.

Muscles

A summary of the general grouping of muscles in analogy with the palm of the hand is helpful before describing the muscles of each layer, an approach that is profitably taken in a dissection.

Intrinsic muscles for the first and fifth toes include a superficially placed **abductor** and, deep to it, a **short flexor** for each. This arrangement corresponds closely to that for the first and fifth digits in the hand. Opponens muscles, however, are lacking in the foot and have probably merged with the short flexors. The **flexor hallucis brevis** consists of two heads; so does the **adductor hallucis**, which resembles the adductor of the thumb. The tendons of the short muscles of the hallux fuse on the lateral and medial sides of the metatarsal head and each fused tendon contains a sesamoid bone before it attaches to the proximal phalanx. The metatarsal head actually rests on the two sesamoid bones when the ball of the big toe contacts the ground (see Fig. 18-6*F*).

The deepest muscle layer of the sole consists of the **dorsal and plantar interossei** (see Fig. 18-46). Plantar to them, in the intermediate compartment, is the oblique head of the adductor hallucis and, in the next layer, the **tendons of the flexor digitorum longus** and **flexor hallucis longus**, both extrinsic muscles of the foot. Associated with the tendons of the extrinsic digital flexor are the **lumbrical muscles** and a small muscle, the **quadratus plantae**. The **flexor digitorum brevis**, the most superficial muscle in the intermediate compartment, provides the second set of flexor tendons for the lateral four toes.

Superficial Layer. Located deep to the plantar aponeurosis, the superficial layer consists of the flexor digitorum brevis centrally, the abductor hallucis medially, and the abductor digiti minimi laterally (see Figs. 18-46 and 18-51). All three arise primarily from the calcaneus, but also take origin from the intermuscular septa and other adjacent fascial layers.

The **abductor hallucis** arises from the medial process of the tuber calcanei (see Fig. 18-6*B*) and from the lower border of the flexor retinaculum. It inserts into the proximal phalanx of the big toe, on the medial side of its base. Before its insertion, it unites with the medial tendon of the flexor hallucis brevis, the combined tendon having also some insertion into the medial sesamoid bone of the big toe.

The **flexor digitorum brevis** also arises mainly from the medial process of the tuber calcanei. It gives rise to four tendons that proceed toward the four lateral toes. These tendons lie immediately below (superficial to) the tendons of the flexor digitorum longus. As they reach the level of the metatarsal heads, the short and long tendons for each toe acquire a digital tendon sheath that invests them with synovial membrane. The sheaths are essentially similar to the digital sheaths of the fingers and line the corresponding *fibrous flexor sheaths* (see Fig 16-36). There is no continuity between the synovial tendon sheaths of any of the toes and the sheaths that invest the tendons under the flexor retinaculum. Within the digital tendon sheaths, the tendons of the flexor digitorum brevis split to allow the long flexor tendons to pass through to the distal phalanges; the slips then interchange fibers dorsal to the long tendons and insert on the middle phalanges. The long flexor tendons have short *vincula* over the distal interphalangeal joints, and the short flexor tendons have short vincula over the proximal interphalangeal joints, essentially similar to those in the hand (see Fig. 16-36); long vincula, also present, vary considerably.

The lateral muscle of this group, the **abductor digiti minimi**, arises from the calcaneus and adjacent fascia and inserts on the lateral side of the proximal phalanx of the little toe. Some of its lateral fibers may attach to the tuberosity of the fifth metatarsal and constitute an accessory muscle, the **abductor ossis metatarsi quinti**.

Innervation. Both the abductor hallucis and flexor digitorum brevis are supplied by the *medial plantar nerve*, which corresponds to the median nerve in the hand. The

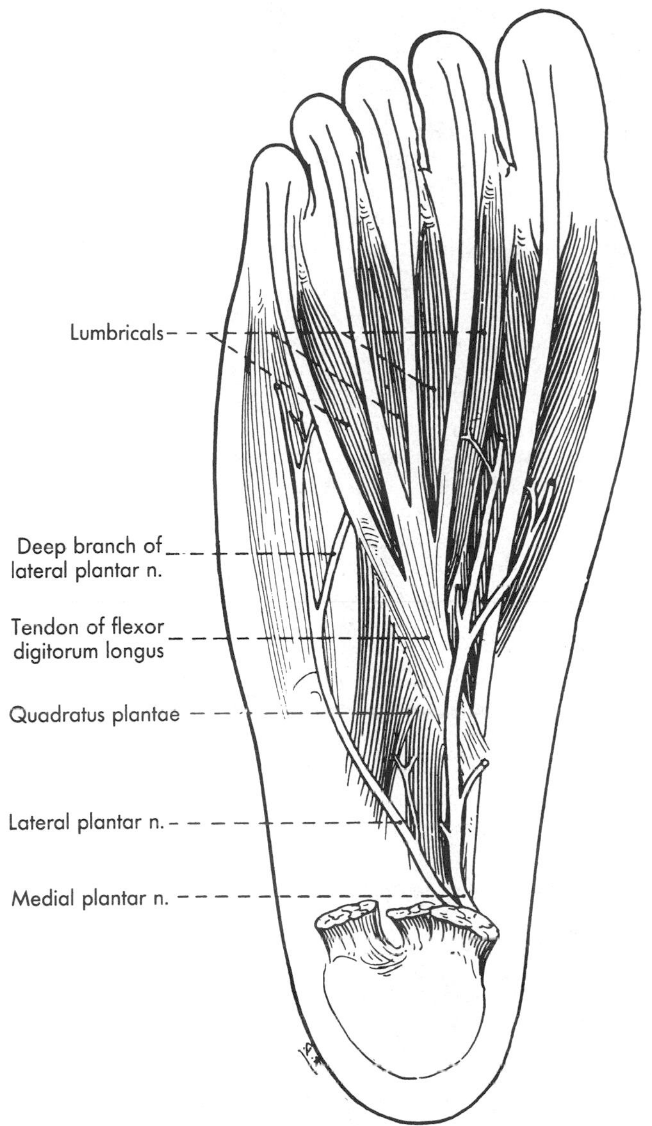

FIGURE *18-52.*
The second layer of plantar muscles and the long flexor tendons in the foot.

abductor digiti minimi and the abductor of the fifth metatarsal, if present, are supplied by the *lateral plantar nerve.*

Second Layer. The second layer of plantar structures consists of the long flexor tendons and their associated muscles (Fig. 18-52). It contains the tendon of the flexor digitorum longus, the quadratus plantae, four lumbrical muscles, and the tendon of the flexor hallucis longus.

The tendon of the **flexor digitorum longus** rounds the ankle anterior to that of the flexor hallucis longus and crosses superficial (inferior) to that tendon in the foot. It usually receives a tendinous slip from the flexor hallucis longus and, as it divides into its four tendons, it receives the insertion of the quadratus plantae muscle. Distally it gives origin to the lumbricals.

The **quadratus plantae** (accessory flexor) muscle arises by two heads from the medial and lateral sides of the plantar surface of the calcaneus, and inserts into the lateral edge of the tendon of the flexor digitorum longus (see Fig. 18-52). No equivalent of the quadratus plantae is found in the hand. Its role in the foot is to modify the effects of the flexor digitorum longus; as this muscle's tendon enters the sole on the medial side, its line of pull is oblique across the foot, tending to abduct the toes in reference to the second digit (the axis of which represents the axis of the foot), as well as to flex them. The quadratus plantae corrects for this obliquity.

The **lumbrical muscles** arise from the tendons of the flexor digitorum longus, just as those in the hand arise from the profundus. The first (most medial) lumbrical arises from the medial side of the tendon to the second toe, but each of the other three lumbricals arises from both the tendons between which it lies. As they run forward to the medial sides of the four lateral toes, they pass below the *deep transverse metatarsal ligaments* (see Fig. 18-66) and then turn dorsally to join the dorsal digital expansions.

The tendon of the **flexor hallucis longus** brings with it into the foot the flexor tendon sheath that surrounds it as it lies deep to the flexor retinaculum (see Fig. 18-45*B*), The sheath usually stops just before the tendon crosses that of the flexor digitorum longus. The two tendon sheaths sometimes communicate here. The tendon of the flexor hallucis longus usually gives a slip to the tendon of the flexor digitorum longus and then runs forward on the flexor hallucis brevis to enter a digital tendon sheath, which invests it almost to its insertion on the distal phalanx of the big toe.

Innervation. The muscle bellies of the long extrinsic digital flexors are supplied by the tibial nerve in the calf. The quadratus plantae receives a branch from the *lateral planter nerve* as this crosses its superficial surface (see Fig. 18-52). The first lumbrical is supplied by a branch from the medial plantar nerve, and the other three lumbricals by twigs from the *deep branch of the lateral plantar nerve*, a pattern that accords with the innervation of the palmar lumbricals.

Third Layer. The third layer consists of three muscles, the flexor hallucis brevis, the adductor hallucis, and the flexor digiti minimi brevis (Fig. 18-53).

The **flexor hallucis brevis** arises by tendinous fibers from the cuboid and lateral cuneiform bones. The muscular belly divides distally into two parts: the *medial part* blends with the insertion of the abductor hallucis, sharing with it the medial sesamoid of the big toe, and inserts on the medial side of the base of the proximal phalanx; the *lateral part* blends with the two heads of the adductor hallucis, sharing with them the lateral sesamoid, and inserts on the lateral side of the base of the proximal phalanx.

The **adductor hallucis** consists of an oblique and a transverse head (like the correspondingly named muscle in hand). The *oblique head* is usually the larger and arises from the bases of the 2nd to 4th metatarsal bones and from the long plantar ligament (see Fig. 18-66). The *transverse head* usually has no bony origin. It arises from a variable number of the plantar and deep transverse metatarsal ligaments associated with the

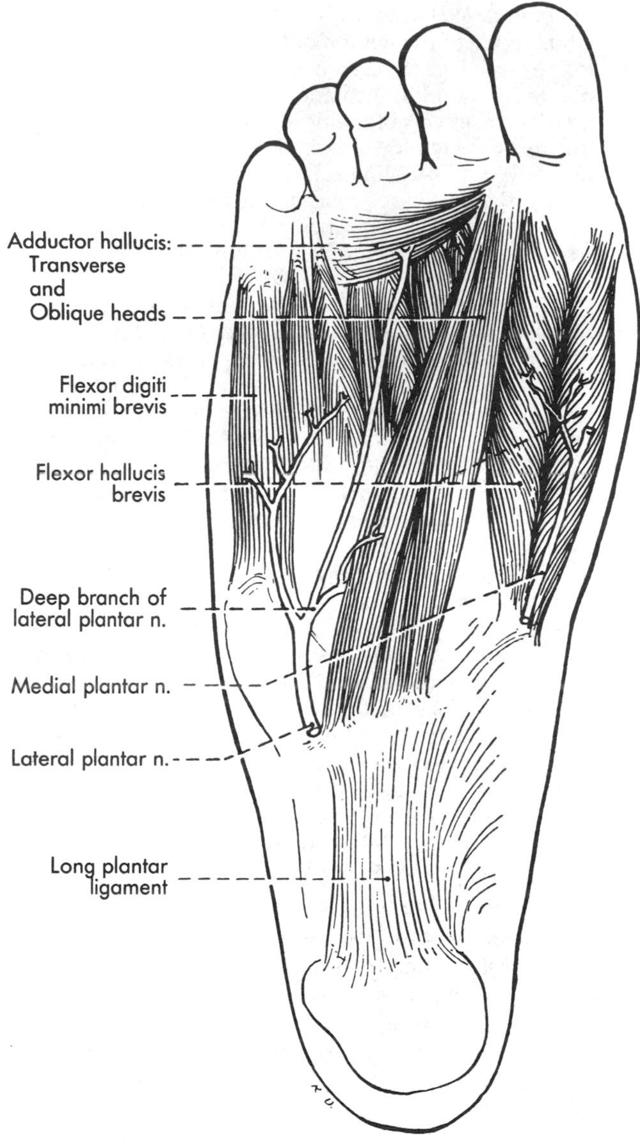

FIGURE *18-53.*
The third layer of plantar muscles.

second to the fifth toes. The two heads converge; as they join, they also blend with them the lateral tendon of the flexor hallucis brevis, sharing the lateral sesamoid with it. The common tendon inserts on the lateral side of the base of the proximal phalanx of the big toe.

The **flexor digiti minimi brevis** arises from the base of the fifth metatarsal bone and from the long plantar ligament as this covers the tendon of the peroneus longus. It inserts into the plantar surface of the base of the proximal phalanx of the little toe. Its tendon of insertion usually blends laterally with that of the abductor digiti minimi and often sends a slip to the extensor tendon of the little toe.

Innervation. The flexor hallucis brevis receives a branch from the *medial plantar nerve* as this nerve runs forward on it. Each head of the adductor hallucis receives a nerve from the *deep branch of the lateral plantar nerve*, as does the flexor digiti minimi (see Fig. 18-53).

Fourth Layer. The fourth layer consists of three plantar and four dorsal interosseous muscles (Fig. 18-54). As in the hand, both plantar and dorsal interossei are visible from the plantar aspect of the foot; the dorsal interossei can also be seen on the dorsum of the foot, filling the spaces between the metatarsal bones.

Like the interossei of the hand, each plantar interosseous arises from a single bone, the metatarsal of the toe with which it is associated. Each dorsal interosseous arises from the two metatarsals between which it lies. The plantar interossei are associated with the three lateral toes: each arises from the medial surface of the metatarsal and inserts on the medial side of the base of the proximal phalanx of the same digit (see Fig. 18-54). The first two dorsal interossei attach to the second toe, one on each side, and the third and fourth attach to the lateral sides of the third and fourth toes, respectively. Thus, in theory, the plantar and dorsal interossei are positioned to adduct and abduct, respectively, the toes in relation to the second digit (which represents the axis of the foot). In reality, however, such movements are not possible in the foot

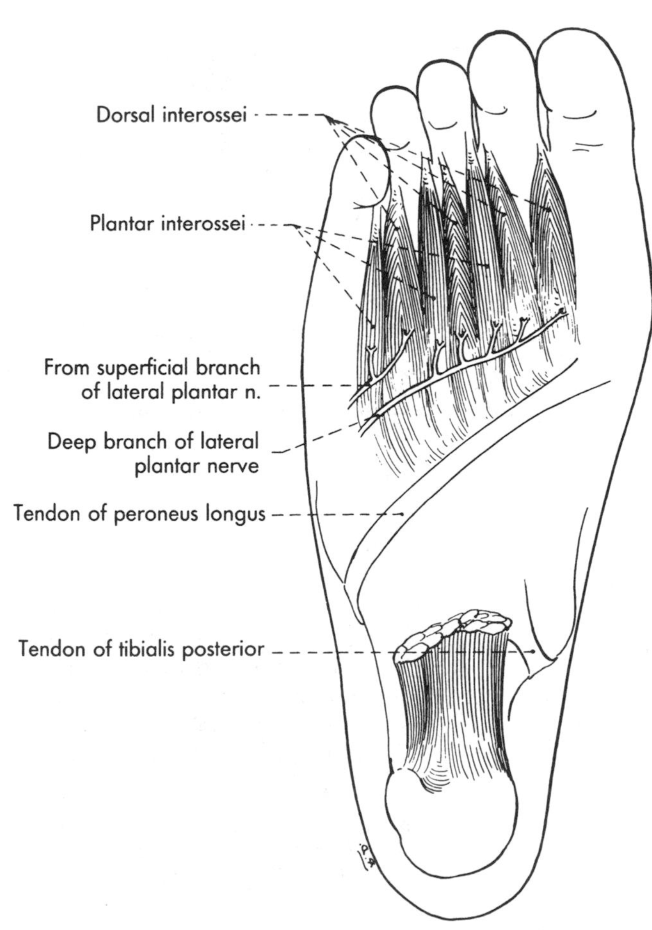

FIGURE *18-54.*
The interossei of the foot.

as they are in the hand. A minor anatomic difference between the interossei of hand and foot is that those of the foot contribute little or nothing to the dorsal digital expansions of the toes. As they cross the metatarsophalangeal joints, the interossei are separated from the lumbrical muscles by the *deep transverse metatarsal ligaments* (see Fig. 18-66); they pass dorsal to these ligaments.

All the interossei are innervated by the *lateral plantar nerve*, which crosses their plantar surfaces in company with the plantar arch.

Actions. Although the names of some of the intrinsic muscles of the first and fifth toes may imply abduction and adduction, such movements are not possible to any appreciable extent for these digits. All these muscles contribute to flexion of the metatarsophalangeal joints. Flexion is effected at the distal interphalangeal joints by the long extrinsic flexors and at the middle interphalangeal joints by the short digital flexor. The resting tone of these muscles keeps the lateral four toes in flexion at the interphalangeal joints, whereas the metatarsophalangeal joints at rest are kept in extension. By simultaneously flexing the metatarsophalangeal joints and extending the interphalangeal joints, the interossei and lumbricals transfer some of the weight from the metatarsal heads to the toes. Their strength can be gauged by observing a slight elevation of the metatarsal heads when the subject presses on the ground firmly with all the toes, while keeping the heel in contact with the ground. Paralysis of the intrinsic muscles of the foot leads to distortion of its arches, discussed further in the section on deformities of the foot.

Nerves and Vessels

Plantar Nerves. The medial and lateral plantar nerves correspond in their course and distribution to the median and ulnar nerves, respectively, of the hand. They are the terminal branches of the tibial nerve.

Where the tibial nerve lies deep to the flexor retinaculum, it gives off *medial calcaneal branches* to the medial side and plantar surface of the heel and divides into medial and lateral plantar nerves. These enter the sole close together and in company with the correspondingly named arteries. They lie dorsal (deep) to the abductor hallucis. The medial plantar nerve runs forward deep to the abductor (Fig. 18-55*A*), and the lateral plantar nerve runs laterally, passing between the flexor digitorum brevis and the quadratus plantae, and then turns forward (see Fig. 18-55*B*).

Under cover of the abductor hallucis, the **medial plantar nerve** gives off a branch into this muscle, one to the flexor digitorum brevis (see Fig. 18-55*A*) and branches to the skin of the sole (see Figs. 18-28 and 18-49). As it emerges between the abductor hallucis and the flexor digitorum brevis, it divides into four terminal **plantar digital nerves** (see Fig. 18-51). The most medial of these is a proper digital branch for the medial side of the big toe; it also supplies the flexor hallucis brevis and twigs to the sole of the foot before reaching the toe. The second branch is the *common digital branch* to the adjacent sides of the big and second toes; it gives a branch to the first lumbrical muscle and subsequently divides into proper digital nerves. The remaining two lateral branches are also common digital nerves and divide into proper digital nerves for the adjacent sides of the second, third, and fourth toes. The most lateral of these nerves may receive a communication from the lateral plantar nerve.

As it passes laterally and forward between the flexor digitorum brevis and the quadratus plantae, the **lateral plantar nerve** gives off a branch into the latter muscle and another that supplies the abductor digiti minimi (see Figs. 18-52 and 18-55*B*). It ends by dividing, close to the base of the fifth metatarsal bone, into deep and superficial branches. The latter has both muscular and cutaneous branches, whereas the deep branch serves only muscles and joints.

Before becoming cutaneous, the **superficial branch** of the lateral plantar nerve supplies the flexor digiti minimi and sometimes the third plantar and fourth dorsal interossei (see Fig. 18-55*B*). Then it emerges between the flexor digitorum brevis and the abductor digiti minimi to divide into two **plantar digital branches**, a proper one for the free side of the fifth toe and a common one for the adjacent sides of the fourth and fifth toes (see Fig. 18-51). The latter, which may communicate with the adjacent common digital branch of the medial plantar nerve, divides into proper digital nerves for adjacent sides of the fourth and fifth toes.

The **deep branch** of the lateral plantar nerve runs medially with the plantar arch across the proximal ends of the interossei and deep to the oblique head of the adductor hallucis. In this course, it gives off muscular branches to all the interossei (except when the third plantar and fourth dorsal muscles are supplied by the superficial branch), to the lateral three lumbricals, and to both heads of the adductor hallucis (see Figs. 18-53, 18-54, and 18-55*B*). It also gives articular branches to most of the joints in the foot.

Plantar Arteries and Plantar Arch. The medial and lateral plantar arteries are terminal branches of the posterior tibial artery. The lateral plantar artery forms the plantar arch, which links up with the dorsalis pedis artery, chiefly through the first intermetatarsal space. Numerous perforating branches also connect the plantar arch and its branches to the arteries on the dorsum. Corresponding veins accompany the arteries and their branches.

The division of the **posterior tibial artery** and its accompanying **veins** into medial and lateral plantar vessels takes place beneath the flexor retinaculum (Fig. 18-56). These enter the foot under cover of the abductor hallucis and in company with the medial and lateral plantar nerves. The medial plantar vessels and nerves then run forward, and the lateral ones diverge laterally to pass above (deep to) the flexor digitorum brevis.

The **medial plantar artery** has a rather insignificant deep branch and a larger superficial branch (see Fig. 18-56). The deep branch passes into the intrinsic muscles of the big toe, among which it lies. The superficial branch

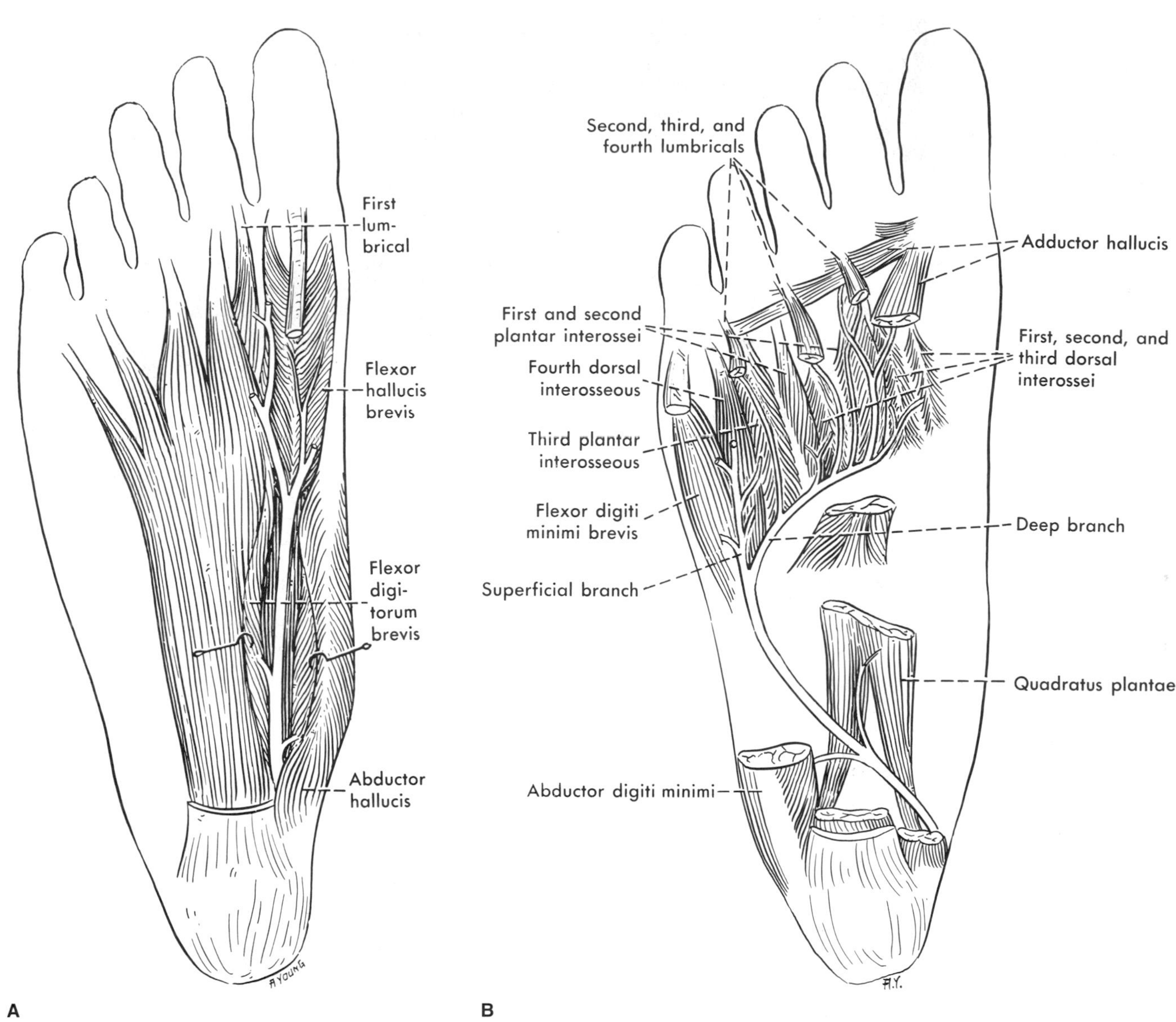

FIGURE *18-55.*
The muscular distribution of (A) the medial plantar nerve and (B) the lateral plantar nerve.

gives twigs to the cutaneous surface of the medial side of the foot (see Fig. 18-49) and continues along the free side of the big toe. It also gives rise to tiny *digital arteries* that run distally and laterally across the lower surface of the flexor digitorum brevis to join the plantar metatarsal arteries and, thus, supplement arterial input to the proper digital arteries (see Fig. 18-56).

The **lateral plantar artery** is larger than the medial and passes obliquely forward and laterally across the foot, crossing between the flexor digitorum brevis and the quadratus plantae. It then runs forward with the lateral plantar nerve between the flexor digitorum brevis and the abductor digiti minimi, giving off twigs to muscles and skin of the lateral side of the foot (see Fig. 18-49) and *digital arteries* to the lateral one and one-half toes. It ends by turning medially across the foot, on the proximal ends of the interossei, as the plantar arch (see Fig. 18-56).

The **plantar arch** is completed by the *deep plantar branch of the dorsalis pedis artery* (see Figs. 18-48 and 18-56), which links up with the lateral plantar artery through an anastomosis established between the first two metatarsals. As the arch crosses the foot, it gives off four **plantar metatarsal arteries** that run forward on the interossei. These are joined by the small digital arteries given off by the superficial branch of the medial plantar artery. Thus reinforced, the short terminal segment of each plantar metatarsal artery assumes the name of **common plantar digital artery**; it soon divides into **proper plantar digital arteries** for the adjacent toes. Two sets of **perforating branches**, one from the plantar arch and the other, more distally, from the ends of the plantar metatarsal arteries, pass dorsally to join the dorsal metatarsal arteries and, thus, shunt blood to the dorsum of the foot. The perforating branches of the plantar arch

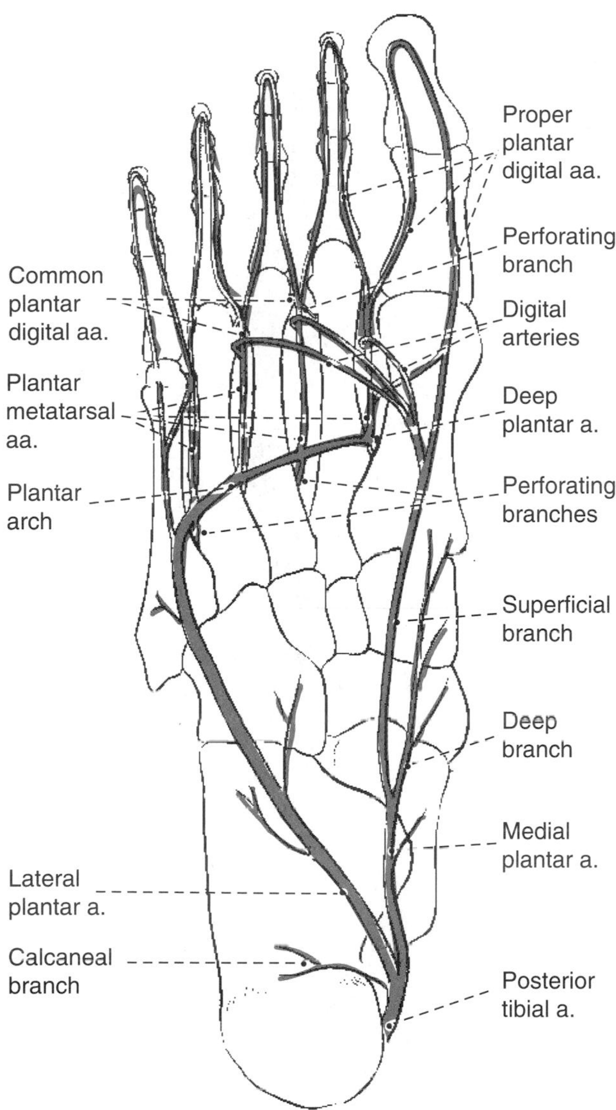

FIGURE *18-56.*
Diagram of the plantar arteries.

are sometimes the chief source of blood to the dorsal arteries.

The **plantar digital veins** drain into metatarsal veins, which join the **plantar venous arch**. This drains alongside the medial and lateral plantar arteries to join the posterior tibial veins. Much of the venous blood, however, is shunted from the sole of the foot into the *dorsal venous arch* through numerous perforating veins.

JOINTS OF THE ANKLE AND FOOT

The ankle or talocrural joint is the articulation between the leg and the foot. Because its anatomic and functional integrity depends on the distal articulation between the tibia and fibula, this section includes the tibiofibular articulations. The foot itself contains numerous joints of different types at which a variety of movements are possible. The joints can be classified as the intertarsal joints, tarsometatarsal joints, intermetatarsal joints, and metatarsophalangeal and interphalangeal joints. Individual joints in these groups are named according to their position or according to the bones that they unite. Before describing individual joints, however, it is helpful to define segments in the foot skeleton, and clarify the various movements possible in the foot. For understanding the dynamic mechanisms of the foot, not only the joints but the ligaments and intrinsic and extrinsic muscles have to be taken into consideration. The architecture and dynamic behavior of the foot will, therefore, be discussed at the end of this section.

Segments and Movements of the Foot

In clinical contexts it is customary and expedient to refer to segments of the foot, rather than to individual bones, when describing movements and deformities. The segments are the forefoot, midfoot, and hindfoot. These terms, omitted from the anatomic nomenclature, are largely self-explanatory and are used rather loosely. The **hindfoot** consists of the talus and calcaneus, and the **forefoot** is made up of the metatarsals and phalanges. The navicular, cuboid, and cuneiforms comprise the **midfoot**. During the stance phase of ambulation (see Fig. 18-73), body weight is transferred from the hindfoot to the forefoot. In this process the midfoot and the forefoot become converted into a rigid lever as the propulsive force is imparted to the ground at push-off. The greatest amount of intrinsic foot movement takes place between the hindfoot and midfoot. The intertarsal joints involved are the talonavicular (with some contribution from the calcaneus) and calcaneocuboid joints. Together, they are spoken of as the **transverse tarsal** *midtarsal*) **joint**.

In the neutral or anatomic position, the foot makes an angle of somewhat less than 90° with the tibia (see Fig. 17-2). **Plantar flexion** increases, and **dorsiflexion** decreases, this angle. The motions occur principally at the ankle joint, the axis passing through the tips of the two malleoli. Owing to the different levels of these two bony points, however, the axis slopes backward, downward, and laterally. Because of this deviation from the horizontal, the foot also deviates from the sagittal plane during plantar flexion and dorsiflexion. Plantar flexion is associated with some **toeing in** and dorsiflexion with **toeing out**. Toeing in and out may also be produced by tibial rotation or fixed tibial torsion, but not by abduction–adduction at the ankle. The talocrural joint permits only flexion and extension.

Inversion and eversion which turn the sole of the foot inward and outward, entail side-to-side rotation of the foot. This motion takes place at the subtalar and transverse tarsal joints, the most important intertarsal joints. The movement takes place around an axis that is roughly anteroposterior, but deviates somewhat from the sagittal plane. Both the heel and the forefoot participate in these movements. During inversion and eversion the heel devi-

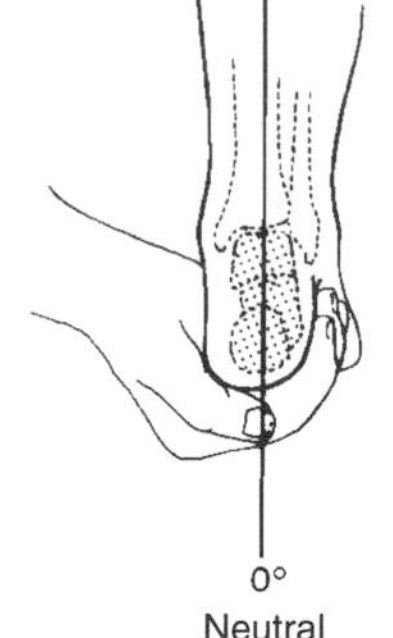

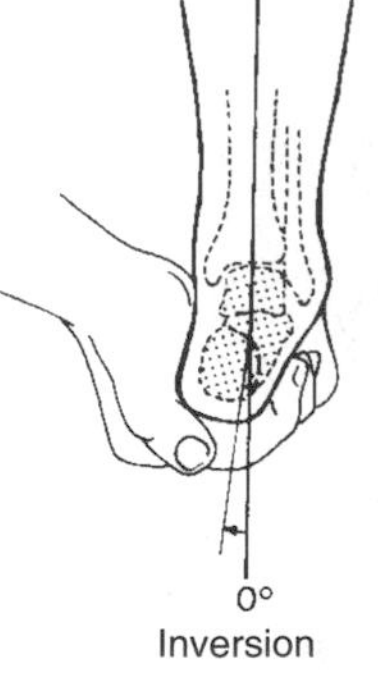

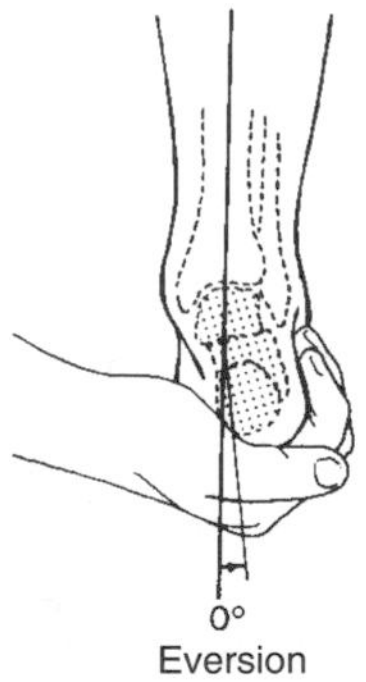

FIGURE *18-57.*
Inversion **and** ***eversion*** **of the heel: In the** ***neutral*** **position, the vertical axis of the heel is aligned with the longitudinal axis of the tibia. (Joint motion, methods of measuring and recording. Chicago: American Academy of Orthopaedic Surgeons, 1965.)**

ates medially and laterally from its neutral position, that is, one in which the calcaneus is vertically aligned with the midline of the tibia (Fig. 18-57). The deviation of the forefoot is gauged by the line of the second metatarsal in relation to the tibia (Fig. 18-58).

Because the axis of inversion and eversion is not strictly in the sagittal plane, in addition to the rotation movement, the forefoot is **adducted** during inversion and **abducted** during eversion (see Fig. 18-58). These movements occur chiefly at the transverse tarsal joint. Active abduction or adduction of the forefoot, independently of inversion and eversion, is not possible. What appear to be abduction and adduction of the whole foot, especially when the heel is used as a fulcrum, are due to tibial or femoral rotation.

Yet another pair of movements is associated with inversion and eversion. These movements are **supination** and **pronation**. In contrast to the radioulnar movements designated by the same terms in the forearm, supination and pronation of the foot are the result of displacement of the metatarsals in relation to one another. The movements involve the transverse tarsal joint and joints distal to it. The foot cannot be actively pronated and supinated independently of inversion and eversion. In the neutral position, the heads of the metatarsals are in the same horizontal plane (in contact with the ground). Supination (associated with inversion) elevates the head of the first metatarsal and depresses the head of the fifth. Pronation (associated with eversion) has the opposite effect. In other words, supination and pronation entail twisting of the forefoot.

Although the first time around it is simplest to consider these movements with the foot off the ground, it is more important to understand them in the planted, weight-bearing foot and in the gait cycle. Instead of producing toeing in and toeing out, the obliquity of the ankle axis imposes rotation on the tibia as it travels over the talus in plantar and dorsiflexion when the foot is fixed. Standing on a sloping surface with the feet parallel, one foot higher than the other, requires inversion of the lower and eversion of the upper foot. Standing on a wedge, placed under the metatarsal heads from the medial side, puts the forefoot into supination. Putting the wedge under the metatarsals from the lateral side pronates the foot.

Tibiofibular and Talocrural Articulations

Tibiofibular Joints

The tibia and fibula are united to one another at their distal ends by the strong tibiofibular syndesmosis, along their shafts by the crural interosseous membrane, and at their proximal ends by the rather insignificant tibiofibular joint.

The proximal and distal tibiofibular articulations differ radically from the corresponding radioulnar joints, which permit pronation and supination of the hand. Movement of any significant degree is prevented between the tibia and the fibula by the **tibiofibular syndesmosis**. This is the only syndesmosis in the entire appendicular skeleton. Its function is to fix the distal end of the fibula in a groove on the lateral aspect of the tibia; this fibrous joint

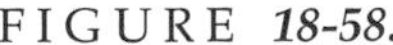
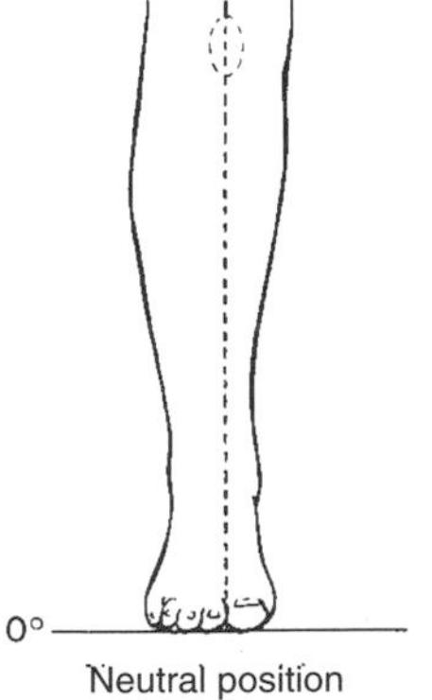

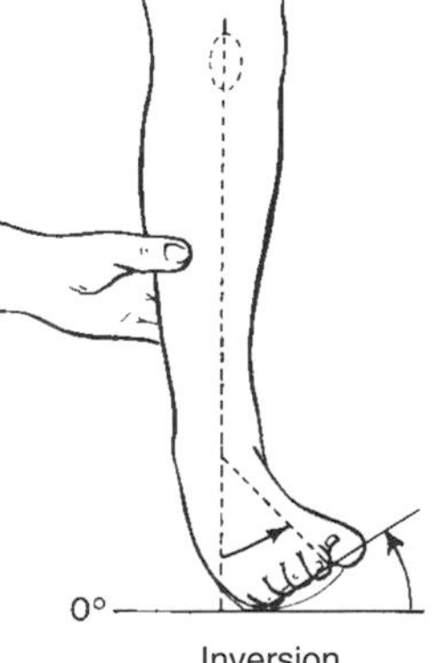

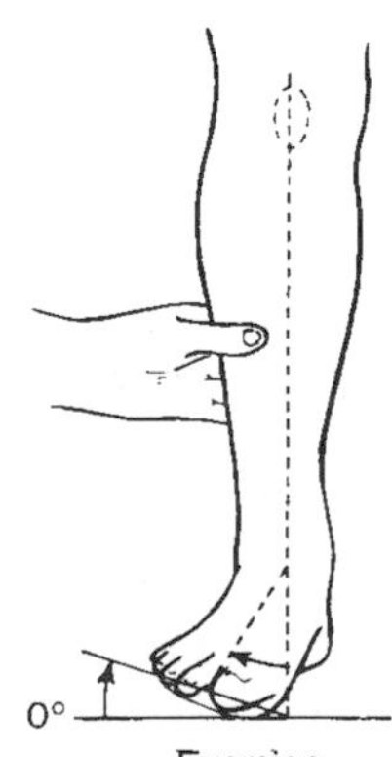

FIGURE *18-58.*
Inversion **and** ***eversion*** **of the forefoot. In the** ***neutral*** **position the line of the second metatarsal is aligned with the midline of the tibia. Inversion is associated with adduction, and eversion with abduction, of the foot. (Joint motion, methods of measuring and recording. Chicago: American Academy of Orthopaedic Surgeons, 1965.)**

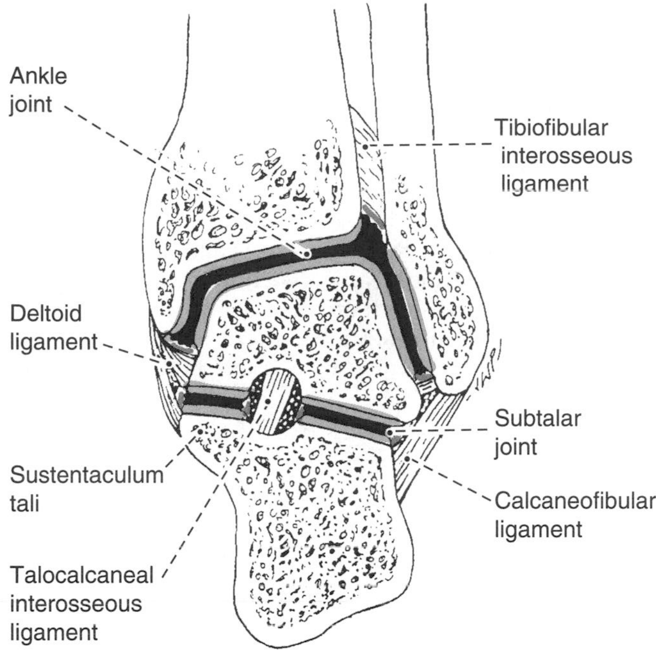

FIGURE *18-59.*
A schematic diagram of a coronal section through the ankle joint showing the tibiofibular syndesmosis, the ankle joint with its collateral ligaments, and the subtalar joint with the talocalcaneal interosseous ligament.

is essential for the integrity of the ankle joint. The fibrous tissue that bridges the narrow gap between the two bones for a distance of 3.5 cm is the **tibiofibular interosseous ligament** (not named in *Nomina Anatomica*). Its short, strong fibers run from the tibia to the fibula and stop just short of the ankle joint (Fig. 18-59). Distinct from the crural interosseous membrane and much stronger, the interosseous ligament is the key structure in preventing separation of the two bones by forces applied to the lateral malleolus by the talus and the calcaneus. When these forces are excessive (in an eversion injury, for example), the fibula will break proximal to the ligament rather than the ligament rupture. The tibiofibular syndesmosis is reinforced by ligaments placed superficially on the front and back of the joint, the **anterior** and **posterior tibiofibular ligaments**. Being thinner and weaker than the interosseous ligament, they tear more easily.

The interosseous ligament acts as a fulcrum between two lever arms. Minor rotational displacements of the malleolus, the short arm of the lever, are magnified at the proximal end of the fibula. Here, the **tibiofibular joint** is a synovial joint. Its flat surfaces and thin capsule accommodate a greater amplitude of movement than does the syndesmosis. The small and oval articular facets of the joint are located on the head of the fibula and lateral condyle of the tibia. The joint cavity is separate from the knee joint, but it may communicate with it through the popliteus bursa.

Talocrural Joint

The ankle or talocrural joint is a synovial articulation of the hinge variety between the talus and the distal ends of the tibia and fibula.

Articular Surfaces. The talar articular facet is the **trochlea**, which is convex superiorly in an anteroposterior direction (see Fig. 18-6) and becomes relatively flat where it extends down on each side of the talus to articulate with the malleoli (see Figs. 18-3 and 18-59). The trochlea resembles more closely a tangential slice of a truncated cone than a slice of a cylinder (Fig. 18-60). As the apex of the imaginary cone points medially, the medial malleolar facet is smaller than the lateral one. Correspondingly, the medial curvature of the trochlea has a smaller radius than its lateral curvature.

The tibiofibular or crural socket into which the trochlea is received is customarily described as a mortise. A cast of it would duplicate all contours of the trochlea. There is better congruence between the articular surfaces here than in any other joint. A good fit is maintained through the whole range of plantar flexion and dorsiflexion, and in no position does the mortise permit any lateral

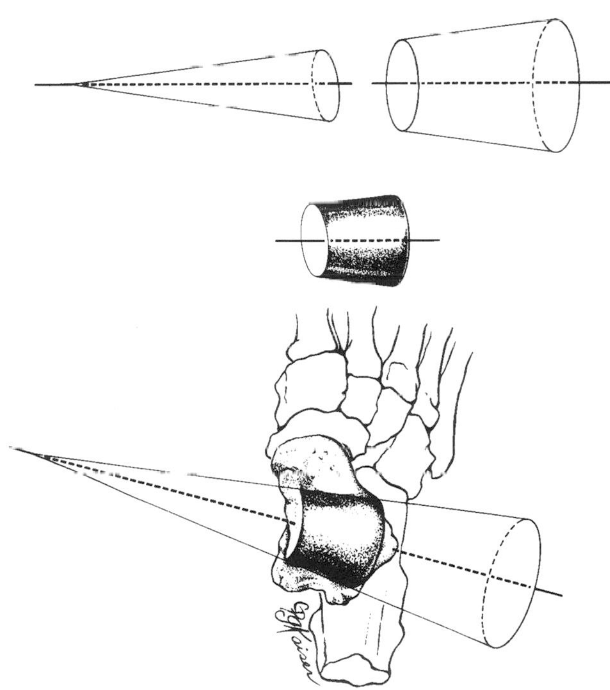

FIGURE *18-60.*
Schematic representation of the trochlea of the talus: The trochlear articular surface resembles a segment of a *truncated cone*, the apex of which points medially and forward. Therefore, the articular surface for the medial malleolus is smaller than that for the lateral malleolus and, accordingly, medial and lateral curvatures of the trochlea have different radii. Note also that medial and lateral facets of the truncated cone are cut at different angles. The axis of the cone coincides with the axis of the talocrural joint. (Adapted from Inman VT. The joints of the ankle, Baltimore: William & Wilkins, 1976.)

play or accessory movement. That such is true has been proved, contradicting the widely held opinion that the talus is loose in plantar flexion and tight in dorsiflexion. The distance between the malleoli does not increase when the ankle is dorsiflexed, although a small amount of lateral rotation of the fibular malleolus may be permitted by the obliquity of the tibiofibular interosseous ligament. Rigid surgical fixation of the tibiofibular syndesmosis by screws or other means does not limit the range of dorsiflexion.

The obliquity of the joint axis discussed earlier and the conical shape of the talocrural articular surfaces fully explain the mechanisms of ankle flexion and extension and also account for most of the toeing in and toeing out associated with these movements.

Ligaments. The thin fibrous capsule that surrounds the joint is reinforced on both sides by collateral ligaments. They are attached to the tips of the malleoli, and each has components that span not only the ankle joint but the talocalcaneal joints as well (Fig. 18-61). By virtue of their calcaneal attachments, these bands stabilize both the ankle and talocalcaneal joints and play a role in integrating motion between them.

The **medial collateral ligament** is known as the **deltoid ligament** because it fans out in a delta shape

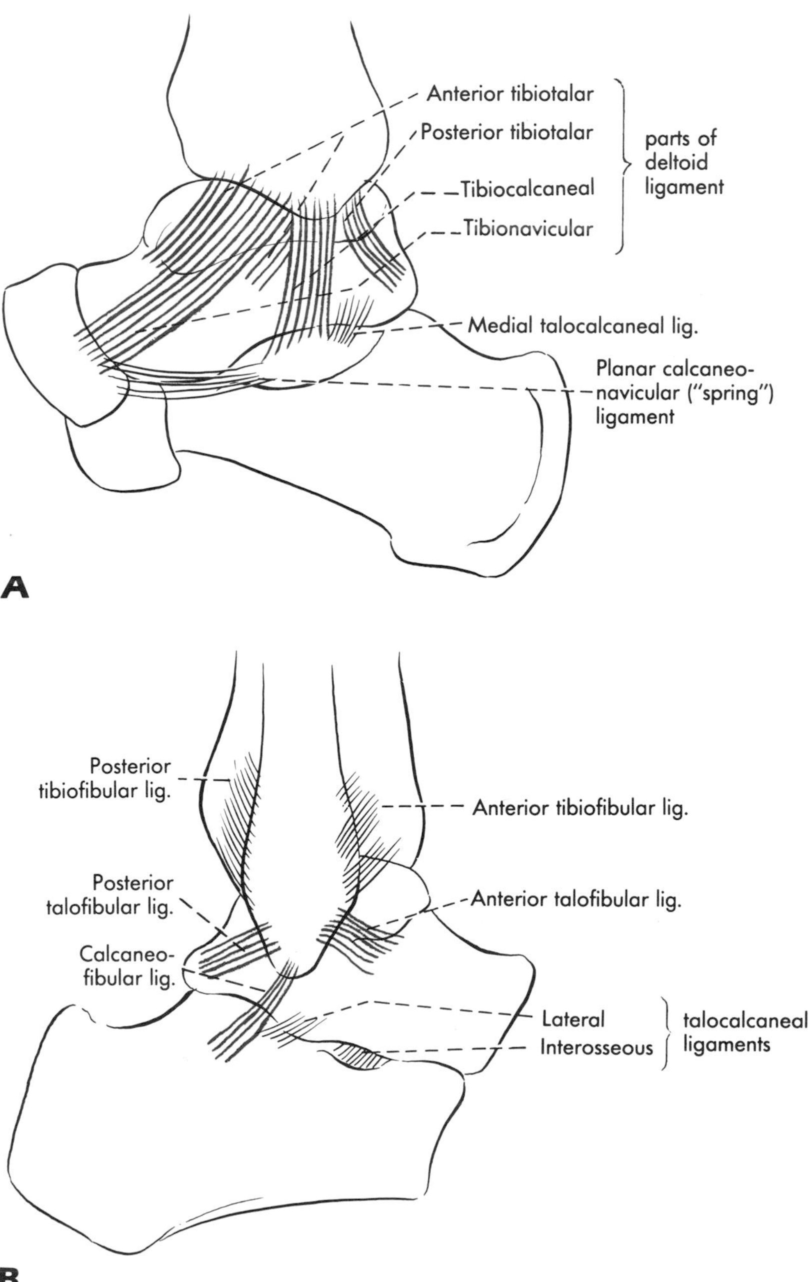

FIGURE *18-61.*
The ligaments of the ankle, seen (A) from the medial side and (B) from the lateral side. The ligaments of the talocrural joint are *red*; others are *black*.

from the margins of the tibial malleolus, and attaches in continuity from the navicular in front to the calcaneus and talus behind (see Fig. 18-61*A*). The ligament is robust and consists of deep and superficial portions. The deep fibers (*anterior tibiotalar ligament*) attach to the nonarticular medial surface of the talus overhung by the malleolus (see Fig. 18-59). The superficial portion is made up of the longer and thinner *tibionavicular, tibiocalcaneal*, and *posterior tibiotalar* fibers that merge with one another. Some fibers also attach to the spring ligament, filling in the gap between the navicular and the sustentaculum tali.

The **lateral collateral ligament** consists of three discrete bands (see Fig. 18-61*B*): the *anterior* and *posterior talofibular ligaments*, counterparts of similar fibers on the medial side, and the much longer, cordlike **calcaneofibular ligament** that passes from the tip of the malleolus downward and backward.

The collateral ligaments give side-to-side stability to the ankle. Plantar flexion is limited by the anterior talofibular and tibiotalar ligaments and dorsiflexion by the posterior counterparts. Tibiocalcaneal and calcaneofibular ligaments also stabilize the talocalcaneal joints. The collateral ligaments are the ligaments of the ankle that are prone to rupture in inversion and eversion injuries. In such injuries the malleoli may also fracture. The medial malleolus is particularly susceptible in that regard; some injuries result in avulsion of the malleolus, rather than rupture of the deltoid ligament.

Prime Movers. The triceps surae (gastrocnemius and soleus) is the only good functional **plantar flexor** at the talocrural joint. Even this, because of its short leverage arm, is at a disadvantage and must exert a pull of about 45 kg (100 lb) to generate a pressure of 22.7 kg (50 lb) on the ball of the foot. The other plantar flexors include the negligible plantaris, the flexor hallucis longus, flexor digitorum longus, and peroneus longus. Even when working together, these muscles are weak plantar flexors: their combined pull is only about 5% of that of the triceps.

The chief **dorsiflexors** of the foot are the tibialis anterior and the extensor digitorum longus and associated peroneus tertius. The extensor hallucis longus contracts only weakly in dorsiflexion of the foot; when the tibialis anterior is paralyzed, however, it contracts strongly and dorsiflexes both the foot and the big toe.

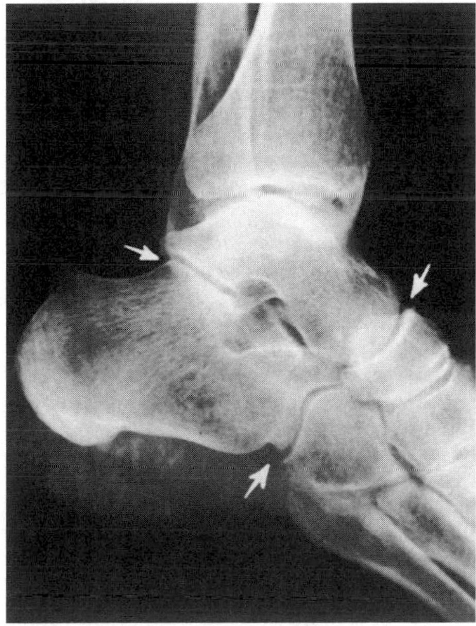

FIGURE *18-62.*
A radiograph of the foot to show intertarsal joints. The *posterior arrow* indicates the subtalar joint; the *two arrows anteriorly* indicate the transverse tarsal joint. (Courtesy of Dr. D. G. Pugh.)

Joints of the Foot

Of the joints of the hindfoot, two intertarsal joints deserve detailed description, namely, the subtalar and transverse tarsal joints. Joints of the midfoot and forefoot are treated rather summarily, placing emphasis on those ligaments that are not mentioned in connection with the subtalar and transverse tarsal joints.

Subtalar and Transverse Tarsal Joints

The *subtalar joint* is the intertarsal joint between the reciprocal articular surfaces of the talus and calcaneus at the back (Fig. 18-62); hence, its descriptive name: posterior talocalcaneal joint. The *transverse tarsal joint* is actually made up of two intertarsal joints: the simple calcaneocuboid joint laterally and the more complex talocalcaneonavicular joint medially (see Fig. 18-62). Inversion and eversion movements take place around the talus and involve synchronously both the subtalar and transverse tarsal joints. The subtalar joint, functioning as a link between the talus and the calcaneus, permits inversion and eversion of the heel (see Fig. 18-57). The transverse tarsal joint functions as a link between the hindfoot and the midfoot, and its movements account chiefly for inversion and eversion of the forefoot (see Fig. 18-58). Independent movements are not possible in any of these joints.

Articular Surfaces. Figure 18-63 shows the articular surfaces associated with the subtalar and transverse tarsal joints. The talus has been lifted off the calcaneus and turned over. Of the reciprocal articular facets on the inferior surface of the talus and superior surface of the calcaneus, the posterior pair form the **posterior talocalcaneal joint**; this articulation is also known as the **subtalar joint**. The remaining reciprocal facets on the talus and calcaneus, together with the large facets on the talar head and the navicular, form a complex articulation known as the **talocalcaneonavicular joint**. The talar head and the anterior and middle facets on the neck make up the proximal, ball-shaped articular surface; the distal "socket" is a composite made up of the navicular, the upper surface of the sustentaculum tali and the small calcaneal facet anterior to it, and a strong ligament that connects the sustentacu-

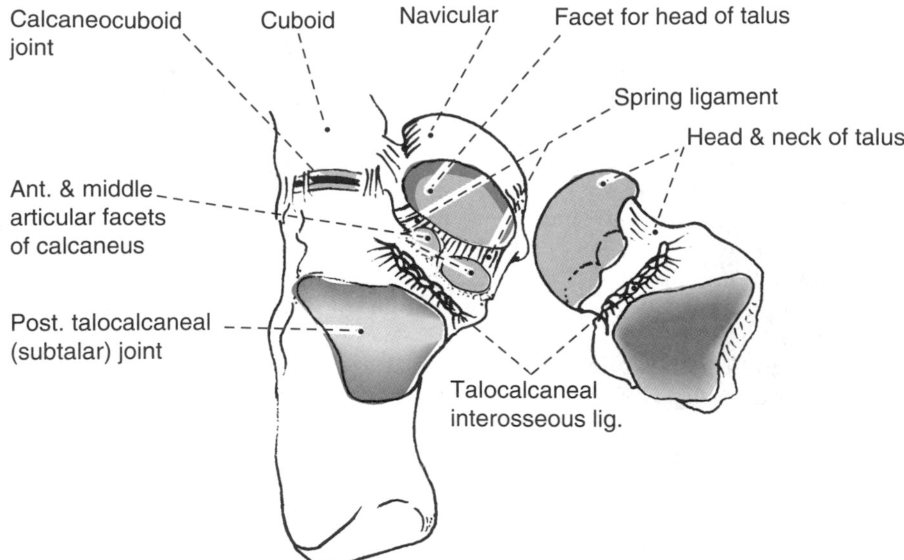

FIGURE *18-63.*
Articular surfaces of the subtalar and the talocalcaneonavicular joints of the left foot. The talocalcaneal interosseous ligament has been cut and the talus turned to the right, revealing its inferior surface.

lum tali to the navicular, known as the **spring ligament** (*plantar calcaneonavicular ligament*; see Figs. 18-61*A*, 18-63, and 18-66). The complex joint thus formed is the medial component of the **transverse tarsal joint**; the lateral component, the calcaneocuboid joint, is simple and has relatively plane facets.

Movements. In the **subtalar joint**, the concave talar and convex calcaneal articular facets move in relation to one another like two members around a mitered hinge (Fig. 18-64), the axis of which inclines backward, downward, and laterally. Rotation of the horizontal member is evident as inversion–eversion, whereas rotation of the vertical member is evident as tibial rotation. The latter is an important component of movement at the ankle, the mechanisms of which are beyond the scope of the present discussion. The subtalar joint is a determinative joint of the foot and influences movement at both the medial and the lateral components of the transverse tarsal joint.

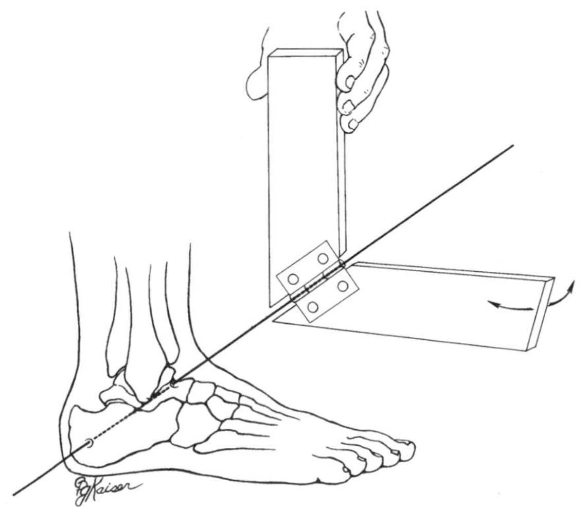

FIGURE *18-64.*
The subtalar joint compared with a mitered hinge: The axis of the joint and the hinge are indicated. Swinging of the horizontal member of the hinge in medial and lateral directions mimics inversion and eversion of the calcaneus, respectively. (Adapted from Inman VT. The joints of the ankle. Baltimore: William & Wilkins, 1976.)

The functional integration of calcaneal movements at the subtalar joint with movements of the midfoot becomes self-evident as soon as it is appreciated that the **spring ligament** unites the calcaneus (hindfoot) and the navicular (midfoot) into the socket of the talocalcaneonavicular joint (see Fig. 18-63). Movements at the calcaneocuboid joint, the lateral portion of the transverse tarsal articulation, are an inevitable outcome of calcaneal movements and of the lack of appreciable independent movement within the midfoot. Figure 18-65 explains how the transverse tarsal joint adds a pivotal element to midfoot movements in inversion and eversion.

Eversion of the heel and the associated pronation of the foot render the transverse tarsal joint particularly mobile, permitting passive flexion, extension, abduction, adduction, and rotation between the hindfoot and forefoot. However, inversion of the heel and the associated supination of the forefoot apparently locks the transverse tarsal joint, because all movements between the hindfoot and forefoot now become restricted. In the gait cycle, elevation of the heel off the ground (heel-off) is associated with heel inversion and the transverse tarsal joint becomes close-packed, converting a pliable foot into a rigid lever.

Ligaments. The subtalar joint and lateral and medial components of the transverse tarsal joint are enclosed by independent fibrous capsules lined by synovial membrane. The **spring** (*plantar calcaneonavicular*) **ligament** is critical for the integrity of the socket of the talocalcaneonavicular joint (see Fig. 18-63; Fig. 18-66). It supports the head of the talus and prevents it from being driven downward between the calcaneus and the navicular. The **collateral ligaments of the ankle**, through their tibiocal-

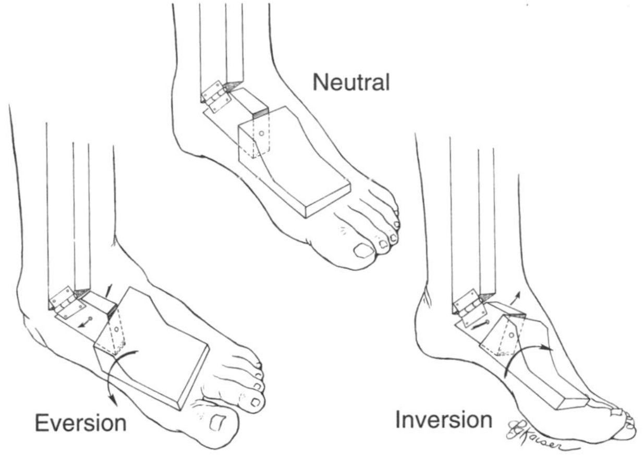

FIGURE *18-65.*
Schematic representation of the movements of the forefoot in *inversion* and *eversion*. The horizontal member of the mitered hinge represents the calcaneus, which moves as explained in Figure 18-64. The midfoot and forefoot skeleton is represented by a stylized block, which is linked to the hindfoot by the transverse tarsal joint. Pivoting of the block on the hindfoot in medial and lateral directions increases the range of eversion and inversion in this model. Associated movements of adduction and abduction are disregarded. (Adapted from Inman VT, Mann RA. In: Inman VT, ed. DuVries' surgery of the foot. 3rd ed. St Louis, Mosby, 1972.)

caneal and calcaneofibular components (see Figs. 18-59 and 18-61), assist in retaining the talus on the calcaneus, but the strongest ligament with this function is the **talocalcaneal interosseous ligament** (see Figs. 18-59 and 18-63). It occupies the tarsal canal (and, therefore, is sometimes called the *ligament of the tarsal canal*) and separates the subtalar from the talocalcaneonavicular joints, reinforcing both. The calcaneocuboid joint is supported inferiorly by the **short plantar** (*calcaneocuboid*) **ligament** and the **long plantar ligament** (see Fig. 18-66). The latter is the more superficial, and extends from the calcaneus to the bases of the metatarsals. It forms the floor for the sulcus of the tendon of the peroneus longus on the cuboid bone, converting it into a tunnel. The short plantar ligament is in the roof of the tunnel. Both the short and long plantar ligaments, the peroneus tendon, as well as the spring ligament, are important in maintaining the arches of the foot (see Fig. 18-69).

A number of weaker ligaments interconnect the talus, calcaneus, navicular, and cuboid on both the dorsal and plantar aspects of the foot; most are illustrated diagrammatically in Figures 18-66 and 18-67.

The **cervical ligament**, located lateral to the talocalcaneal interosseous ligament in the sinus tarsi, is attached to the neck of the talus and the upper surface of the calcaneus. More anteriorly in the sinus, one limb of the **bifurcate ligament** runs between the calcaneus and the navicular (*dorsal calcaneonavicular ligament*, of much less consequence than its plantar counterpart, the spring ligament) and the other limb between the calcaneus and cuboid (*dorsal calcaneocuboid ligament*). The plantar counterpart of the latter (*plantar calcaneocuboid ligament*) is the important short plantar ligament.

Prime Movers. The most effective **invertors** are the tibialis anterior and posterior. Concomitantly, they also produce adduction and supination of the forefoot. The flexor hallucis longus and flexor digitorum longus can exert a supinator action on the forefoot, particularly when opposition to this movement has to be overcome or when the chief invertors are paralyzed. The triceps surae, in plantar flexing the foot, inverts the heel and adducts the forefoot.

The most effective **evertors** are the peroneus longus, brevis, and tertius, with the lateral part of the extensor digitorum longus providing assistance.

In movements of the foot, the invertors and evertors usually act together in combinations that permit pure plantar flexion or pure dorsiflexion. Thus, the tendency of the triceps surae to invert is counteracted during plantar flexion by the tendency of the peroneus longus to evert. In dorsiflexion, the tendency of the tibialis anterior to invert is counteracted by the tendency of the peroneus tertius and lateral part of the extensor digitorum longus to evert.

Joints of the Midfoot and Forefoot

Intertarsal joints distal to the transverse tarsal articulation possess more or less plane surfaces, as do the **tarsometatarsal joints** (see Fig. 18-6). Numerous *plantar and dorsal interosseous ligaments* secure the bones to one another and reinforce the capsules of these synovial joints (see Fig. 18-66; Fig. 18-67). The anatomy of the **metatarsophalangeal joints** resembles that of the metacarpophalangeal joints in the hand. Between the metatarsal heads the **deep transverse metatarsal ligament** connects the thick *plantar ligaments* or plates of these joints (see Fig. 18-66). Some fibers of the ligaments also attach to the bases of the proximal phalanges and the metatarsal heads. At these joints, the range of extension exceeds that of flexion. The anatomy of the **interphalangeal joints** corresponds to that in the hand.

The intertarsal joints of the midfoot typically share a single synovial cavity. The relatively large **cuneonavicular joint**, between the navicular bone and the three cuneiforms, is continuous with the *intercuneiform joints* between the cuneiform bones. It usually extends between the third cuneiform and the cuboid as well, although sometimes the cuneocuboid joint is separate. The three cuneiforms are connected anteriorly by two *interosseous intercuneiform ligaments*, and the lateral cuneiform and the cuboid are connected by the *interosseous cuneocuboid ligament*.

There are typically three separate cavities for the **tarsometatarsal joints**: a medial cavity for the first metatarsal, an intermediate for the second and third metatarsals, and a lateral cavity for the fourth and fifth metatarsals. They are separated from each other by *interosseous cuneometatarsal ligaments*. These joints

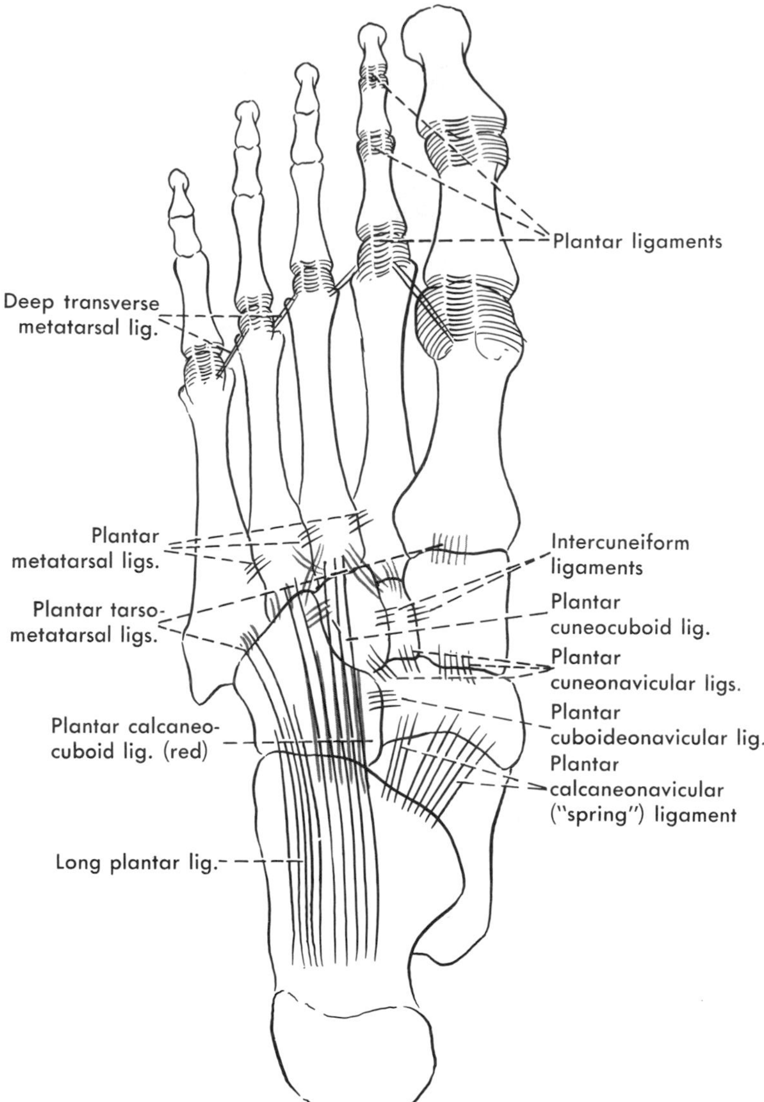

FIGURE *18-66.*
Diagram of the plantar ligaments of the ankle and foot; tarsometatarsal ligaments and the deep-lying calcaneocuboid and cuneocuboid are *red*.

extend a little distance proximally between the cuneiforms and between the lateral cuneiform and the cuboid; the intermediate joint often communicates, between the intermediate and medial cuneiforms, with the cuneonavicular joint. Otherwise, they are separated from this joint by interosseous intercuneiform ligaments. In the four lateral rays of the foot, the tarsometatarsal joint cavities extend forward between the bases of the metatarsals to become continuous with the cavities of the **intermetatarsal joints**. These are sealed distally by *metatarsal interosseous ligaments*, which may extend proximally to subdivide the joint cavities into dorsal and ventral parts. Usually, there is no joint cavity between the first and second metatarsals. The two bones are united by a large metatarsal interosseous ligament.

The capsule of each **metatarsophalangeal** and **interphalangeal joint** is thickened by a concave plate, the *plantar ligament* (see Fig. 18-66). To the edges of this ligament attach the fibrous digital sheaths as well as the lateral part of the fibrous capsule of the joint. The sides of the capsules are reinforced by *collateral ligaments*. On the dorsal aspect, the dorsal digital expansion largely replaces the fibrous capsule. The plantar ligament of the metatarsophalangeal joint of the big toe contains the two sesamoid bones of this joint. Other ligaments may contain similar bones as well.

Prime Movers. Movement of the toes is simple. Although the big toe can be extended while the others are flexed, the reverse cannot be done, nor can the other toes be moved independently. Prolonged training, however, can enhance these movements considerably.

Extension (*dorsiflexion*) at the metatarsophalangeal joints is carried out by both the long and the short extensors of the toes. Because the metatarsals slope downward from their bases to their heads, the toes are typically somewhat dorsiflexed relative to the long axes of the metatarsals during normal standing. The higher the heel of a shoe, the more dorsiflexed the toes become. An increase in dorsiflexion at the metatarsophalangeal joints produces, in turn, more plantar flexion at the interphalangeal joints because the

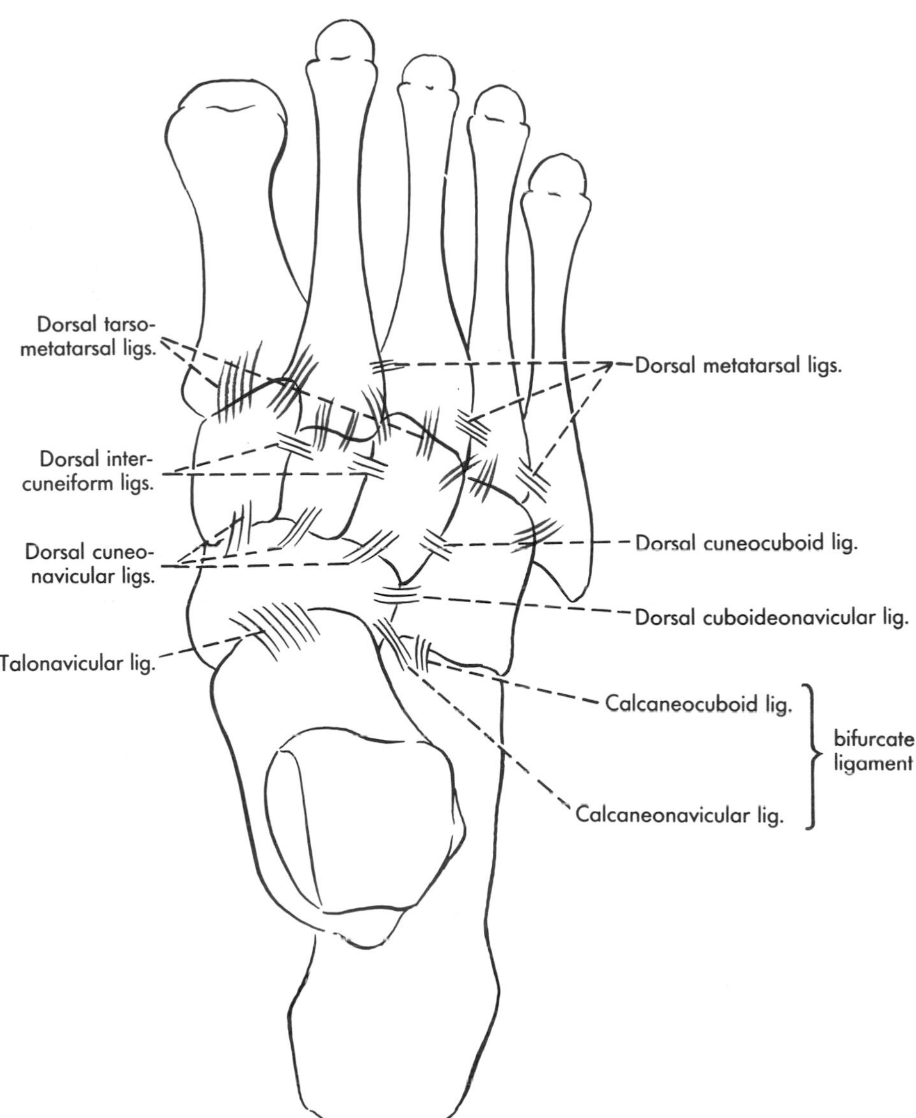

FIGURE 18-67.
Diagram of the dorsal ligaments of the ankle and foot; tarsometatarsal ligaments are *red*.

passive pull of the long flexors overcomes the action of the extensors of these joints. Clawing of the toes is the result. Because of the passive pull of the long flexors, the extensor digitorum longus further hyperextends the metatarsophalangeal joints instead of extending the interphalangeal joints (see Fig. 18-70). The lumbricals, and to a less extent the interossei, are potential extensors of the interphalangeal joints.

Flexion of the interphalangeal joints is brought about by the flexor digitorum longus, the quadratus plantae, the flexor digitorum brevis, and the flexor hallucis longus. The flexor digitorum longus and flexor hallucis longus act strongly only on the distal phalanges. The quadratus assists the flexor digitorum longus and helps overcome the medial pull of its tendon. When the long extensor is electrically stimulated, the toes are not only flexed but also rotated so that the tips are turned medially. When the quadratus plantae is stimulated as well, however, the rotation element of the movement is cancelled out. The flexor digitorum brevis is said to flex the middle phalanges forcefully and the proximal ones weakly.

Flexion of the metatarsophalangeal joints is brought about by all the interossei, the lumbricals, the short flexors and abductors of the big and little toes, and the adductor of the big toe. As these joints are flexed, the interphalangeal joints tend to extend, largely as a result of the passive pull of the long extensor tendons.

Architecture of the Foot

Arches

The skeletal pieces of the foot are so shaped that, when they are held together, they form a twisted plate (Fig. 18-68). The anterior edge of the plate, represented by the metatarsal heads, is horizontal and is in contact with the ground. The posterior edge of the plate is vertical and coincides with the vertical axis of the heel. The edges on the sides of such a twisted plate, of necessity, describe arcs, one more pronounced than the other. In the foot, the

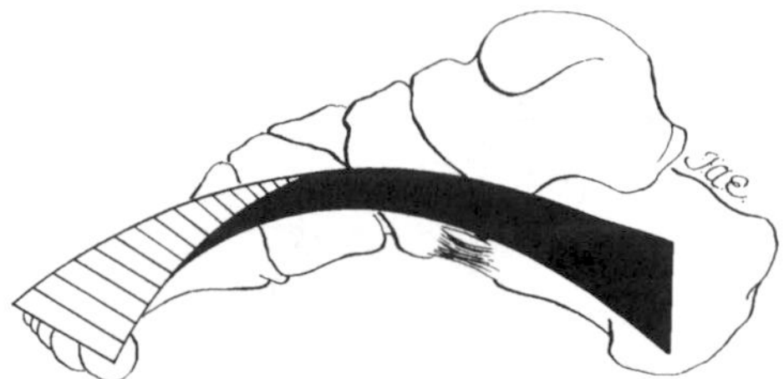

FIGURE *18-68.*
The osseoligamentous framework of the foot represented as a twisted plate. (Adapted from MacConnaill MA, Basmajian JV. Muscles and movements. Baltimore: Williams & Wilkins, 1969.)

lower arc is lateral and the higher arc is medial. In a long foot these arcs are less pronounced than in a short foot.

Intrinsic movements between the bones of the foot tend to increase or decrease the degree of twist in the osseoligamentous plate. Standing with the feet wide apart untwists the foot; this is the result of inversion and supination. Standing with the feet together increases the twist, and standing with crossed legs maximally exaggerates it. In the latter position, the feet are everted and pronated. The medial and lateral arcs in the twisted foot are clearly recognizable as arches. By comparison, an untwisted foot appears flat. Inspection of the footprint with the feet wide apart, together, or crossed over confirms this observation.

Traditionally, the foot has been described as an arched structure, the two feet placed side by side resembling a dome. In such a description, a **transverse arch** of the largest span is said to be present across the bases of the metatarsals. In each foot, a **medial** and a **lateral longitudinal arch** are also recognized. The anterior pillar of the medial arch is taken to be the medial three metatarsals, the cuneiforms, and the navicular; the posterior pillar is represented by the calcaneus. The lateral arch consists anteriorly of the lateral two metatarsals and the cuboid and, posteriorly, of the calcaneus.

The medial arch is surmounted by the talus, which transmits most of the body weight to the two pillars by the subtalar and talocalcaneonavicular joints. A part of this force is transmitted to the lateral arch by the subtalar joint. These terms retain their usefulness, but the dynamic concept of a twisted plate is closer to reality than the architectural units of a rigid edifice.

Maintenance of Foot Architecture. The shape of the bones themselves is responsible for the existence of the twisted plate and, consequently, also for the arches. The maintenance of foot architecture, however, depends on the structures that hold the bones together and provide joint stability in the resting, weight-bearing, and striding foot. Ligaments play the chief role. They are so positioned that they not only retain the bones in alignment, but permit changes in the degree of the twist. Ligaments alone are responsible for maintaining the arcs in the twisted plate of the relaxed foot and also in the weight-bearing static foot. The medial and lateral arches of the foot will be maintained without recruiting any muscles, intrinsic or extrinsic, when up to 181 kg (400 lb) of weight are applied to the knees of seated subjects.

The more important ligaments are shown schematically in Figure 18-69. The plantar calcaneonavicular or **spring ligament** ties together the anterior and posterior pillars of the medial arch. The **long plantar ligament** runs from the calcaneus to the cuboid and to the bases of the lateral metatarsals, reinforcing the lateral arch. The **short plantar ligament**, deep to it, plays a similar role, but other ligaments are also important. The **plantar aponeurosis** spans the distance between the anterior edge of the twisted plate and the lower end of its vertical posterior edge (see Figs. 18-49 and 18-69).

As soon as the distribution of weight within the foot skeleton is shifted by movement, muscles are recruited. These include both extrinsic and intrinsic muscles. Of the extrinsic muscles, the **tibialis posterior** and **peroneus longus** are the most important. After heel strike in the gait cycle (see Fig. 18-73), the lateral part of the forefoot makes first contact with the ground (the foot is inverted and supinated). Then, as the weight is transferred to the ball of the big toe, the foot increasingly pronates and everts. The **tibialis posterior** and **peroneus longus** work in concert during the stance phase, when weight is being transferred to the forefoot, and control the shift of the forefoot from supination into pronation. Both muscles also help stabilize the leg on the dynamic foot. Contraction of the long digital flexors stabilizes the toes when the body weight is borne only on one foot. The intrinsic flexors contribute to this function. The abductors and short flexors are in an ideal location for stabilizing and supporting the medial and lateral arches. They relieve the ligaments of undue strain in the loaded, moving foot. The plantar aponeurosis becomes tensed by dorsiflexion of the toes and this also

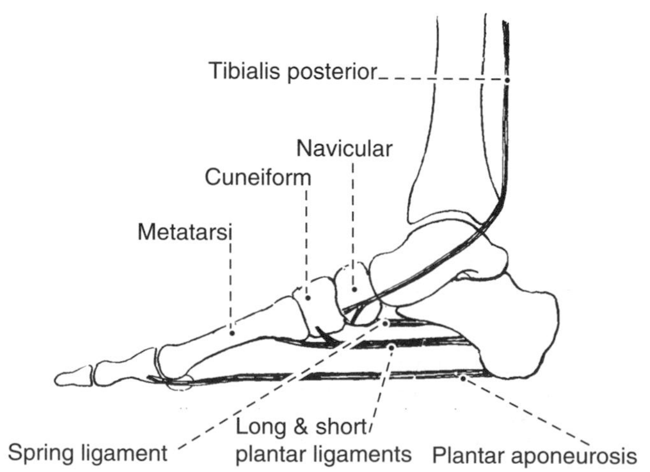

FIGURE *18-69.*
Schematic representation of the most important structures responsible for maintaining the longitudinal arches of the foot. For simplicity's sake, all ligaments are shown in the same sagittal plane and are seen from the medial side.

supports and increases the arches, especially after the heel has been lifted off the ground.

Foot Deformities

In those societies in which shoes are worn, nearly 50% of the population suffers from some structural abnormality of the feet. A minor proportion of deformities is due to congenital causes, the early diagnosis of which is important for preventing permanent disability. After introducing the types of deformities, some examples are briefly discussed, highlighting the anatomic factors responsible for them.

The causes of many deformities remain unknown. Skeletal defects are less common than muscular imbalance. Although the architecture of the foot is primarily maintained by its ligaments, muscle imbalance due to spasticity, weakness, or paralysis invariably leads to foot deformity because the ligaments eventually yield to the unbalanced deforming forces. Deformities that are initially supple may eventually become fixed owing to contracture of the muscles or abnormal bony development during growth. Congenital and acquired deformities may be altered during the growth period. However, treatment of foot deformities must not be neglected after the growth period, even if the cause of the deformity is incurable, because the tendency remains for the bones and the soft tissues to adapt to the deforming forces. Without treatment, the deformity is likely to become worse.

Types of Deformity. Typical deformities of the foot are described by well-accepted terms. In a so-called **equinus** deformity the foot points downward and is fixed in the position of plantar flexion. In a **calcaneus** deformity the heel points downward and the foot is fixed in dorsiflexion. In **varus** the entire foot deviates toward the midline of the body at a number of joints distal to the ankle joint (inversion, adduction, supination); in **valgus** deformity the foot deviates in a direction opposite to the varus (eversion, abduction, pronation). In **pes planus** (flatfoot) the arches are flattened, whereas in **pes cavus** they are exaggerated. The various deformities often occur in combination. An example of a complex deformity is clubfoot.

Clubfoot. Although, in general, usage of this term means a deformed foot, in medical practice the term clubfoot (*talipes* in Latin) has come to be restricted to the most common type of *congenital foot deformity*, **talipes equinovarus**. The foot is in equinus (plantar flexed), often owing to underdevelopment or contracture of the calf muscles. The forefoot is also inverted, adducted, and supinated, owing in many cases to underdevelopment of the peroneal muscles. The heel is also inverted. With such a deformity the child will bear the body weight on the base and shaft of the fifth metatarsal. In cases of bilateral deformity, the possibility of spina bifida, with associated spinal cord anomalies, should be examined. The deformity will become permanent because of the misshapen tarsal bones unless treatment is instituted.

Flatfoot. As explained earlier, untwisting of the osseoligamentous plate reduces or eliminates the arches. There are no defined criteria for distinguishing a pathologic from a normal flatfoot. Only one out of a thousand people with flat feet develops symptoms. A flexible flat foot need not be considered abnormal. When such a subject stands on the toes, the medial longitudinal arch is restored in the foot through the windlass action of the plantar aponeurosis and the contraction of the long and short toe flexors. In a fixed or rigid flat foot this is not so. Rigid flatfoot may result from congenital fusion of the tarsal bones or from spasticity or contracture in the peroneal or other muscles.

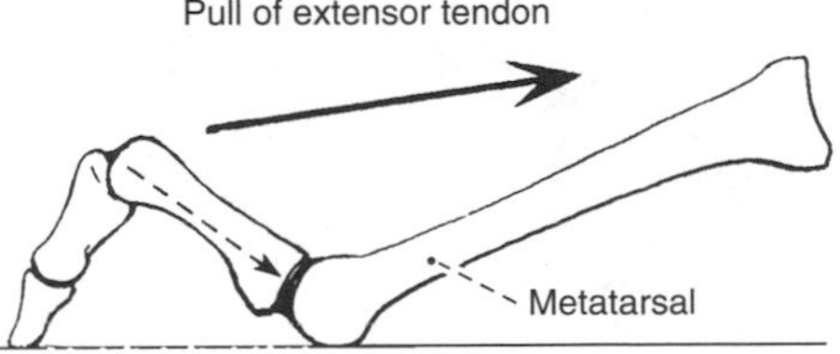

FIGURE *18-70.*
Mechanism of metatarsalgia caused by displaced tendons of the toes. The *solid arrow* indicates the direction of pull not only of the extensor digitorum, but also of the displaced intrinsic muscles and the flexor digitorum.

Pes Cavus. Abnormally high arches are either due to congenital causes or to muscle imbalance, usually resulting from neurologic disorders. Exaggeration of the arches compromises the foot more than flattening of its arches. Pes cavus is usually associated with clawing of the toes (Fig. 18-70). This deformity excludes the toes from taking their normal share of weight off the metatarsal heads. The metatarsophalangeal joints are hyperextended and the unopposed pull, or later the contracture, of the digital extensors depresses the metatarsal heads by the force vector transmitted along the hyperextended proximal phalanx (see Fig. 18-70). If the interossei are intact, their displaced tendons in relation to the metatarsophalangeal joint axis will have a similar effect. In addition to the body weight, these excessive forces provide the explanation for the hard, extensive callosities over the ball of the foot that are usually associated with pes cavus, and also for the pain (metatarsalgia) experienced over the metatarsal heads.

Hallux Valgus. As much as one-third of the shoe-wearing population exhibits some lateral deviation of the big toe at the metatarsophalangeal joint. Wearing shoes with high heels and pointed toes is undoubtedly the most important cause in the majority of cases.

Lateral (valgus) deviation of the big toe is almost always associated with medial deviation of its metatarsal which renders its head medially prominent (Fig. 18-71). Friction and trauma lead to hypertrophy, distension and inflammation of a subcutaneous bursa overlying the medial side of the metatarsal head. This soft-tissue swelling is the **bunion**, but sometimes the complex of bony deformities is also included under this name.

THE GAIT CYCLE*

Throughout sections of this chapter, as well as in discussions of the hip, references have been made to the location of the center of mass and gravity's line of force relative to

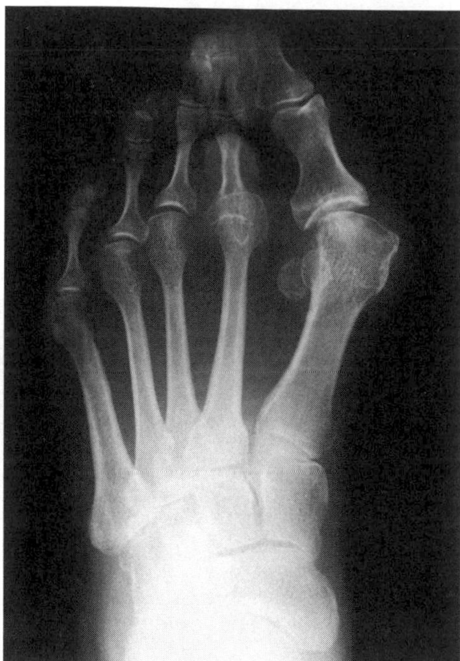

FIGURE 18-71.
Hallux valgus deformity: Note that in addition to the valgus deformity at the first metatarsophalangeal joint, there is pronounced metatarsus varus. The metatarsal head is hypertrophied and rotated medially, and the sesamoid bones are displaced laterally into the first intermetatarsal space. The latter is partly due to the rotation of the metatarsal along its long axis, and partly to the displaced line of force exerted by the intrinsic muscles of the hallux. (Courtesy of Dr. Rosalind H. Troupin.)

the joints between different limb segments (see Fig. 17-2). This section extends such considerations from the position of relaxed standing to ambulation, and serves as a summary of the functional anatomy of the lower limb.

Figure 18-72 schematically summarizes the forces required to counterbalance gravity in relaxed standing. At the hip and knee joints these forces are provided by the tension of ligaments. Muscular energy is expended only by the triceps surae to balance the ankle joint. Flexion of the hip and knee joints while they are weight-bearing displaces the gravity force line and recruits other muscle groups to maintain the upright posture during ambulation. Ambulation is the type of locomotion by which the body is translated on a surface from one point to another. The synchronized and rhythmically recurring movements of the various limb segments and joints during ambulation constitute the gait cycle, in which specific phases can be defined.

* This section has been prepared under the guidance of Dr. Walter Stolov, professor and chairman of the Department of Rehabilitation Medicine at the University of Washington. The preparation of the figures and the text would not have been possible without his contribution.

Phases of the Gait Cycle

The gait cycle can be divided into two major phases: **stance phase**, when the foot is on the ground, and **swing phase** when the foot is in the air (Fig. 18-73). Stance phase is subdivided according to the posture of the foot. The first event is **heel strike** (HS), when the heel first touches the ground. Then the midfoot makes contact with the ground, followed by the forefoot; **foot-flat** (FF) is attained as soon as the entire foot is on the ground. The body then moves forward over the planted foot, shifting the center of gravity forward until **heel-off** (HO) occurs. The final event of the stance phase is **toe-off** (TO). **Midstance** (MST) is the period during which all of the foot is in contact with the ground, that is, from FF until HO. The last portion of the stance phase, HO to TO, constitutes a phase called **push-off**, during which most of the propulsive force is exerted. Swing phase begins with TO and ends with HS. During its first part the limb is accelerated, changing at **midswing** (MSW) to deceleration, which results in HS. The cycles of the two limbs overlap for a time

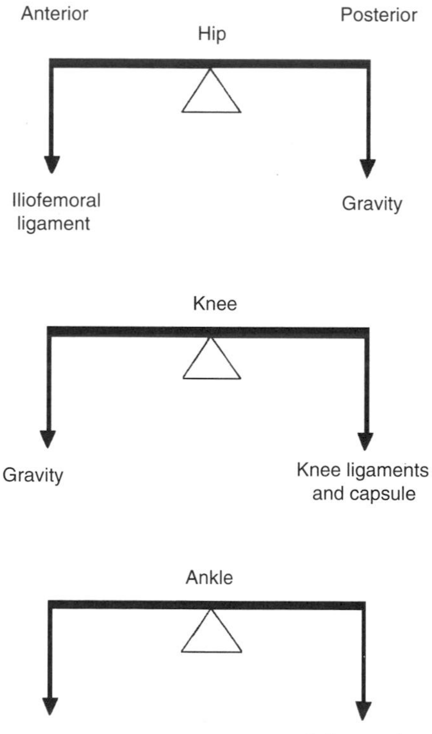

FIGURE 18-72.
Schematic representation of forces acting to maintain balance in relaxed standing: (*Hip*) Iliofemoral ligament anteriorly balances the force of gravity posteriorly. No active muscle contraction is required. (*Knee*) Ligaments and capsule provide the restraining force posteriorly that balances the gravitational force anteriorly. No active muscle contraction is required. (*Ankle*) Gravitational force anteriorly is balanced by the contraction of the gastrocnemius and soleus posteriorly. (Courtesy of Dr. Walter C. Stolov.)

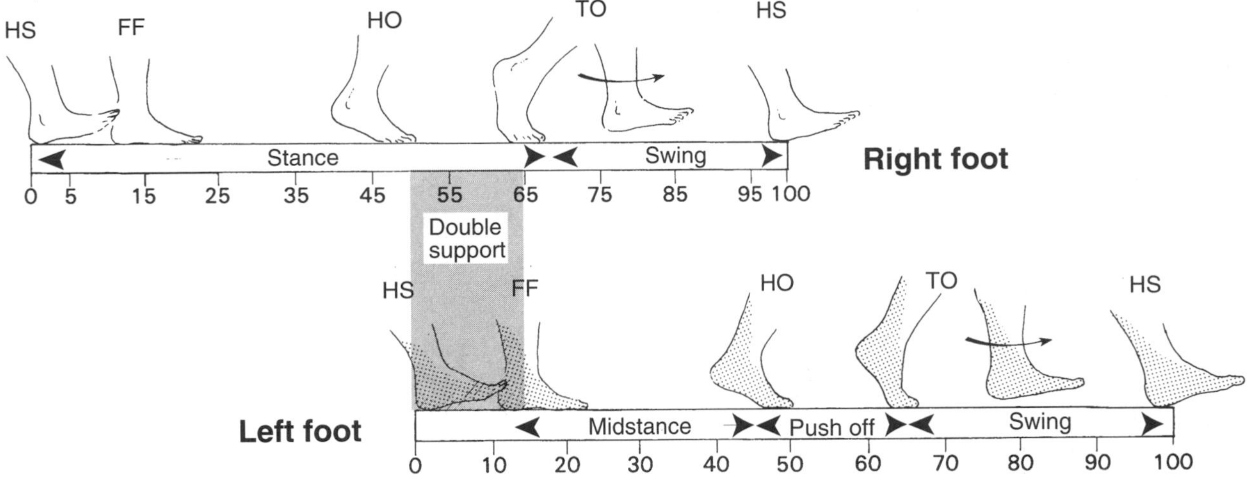

FIGURE 18-73.
The phases of the gait cycle shown on the same time axis for *right* and *left* legs. For abbreviations see text. (Courtesy of Dr. Walter C. Stolov.)

during stance phase. This is the period of **double support** (DS), which extends from HS of one limb to TO off the other (see Fig. 18-73). The duration of DS decreases with the speed of walking. *Running* is defined as ambulation in which no DS exists.

Center of Mass Oscillations

Were the body translated on wheels, rather than on two legs, its center of mass would move along a line parallel to the surface, which would entail a minimum expenditure of energy. Bipedal ambulation, however, is associated with oscillations of the center of mass both in the vertical and in the horizontal plane (Fig. 18-74), requiring additional energy expenditure. Vertical movements of the center of mass can be eliminated by keeping the hips and knees flexed while walking. However, more energy needs to be expended by hip and knee extensors, to prevent these joints from collapsing under the force of the gravity, than is needed to elevate the body's center of mass during ambulation. Normal ambulation is a compromise between the energy required for elevating the center of mass

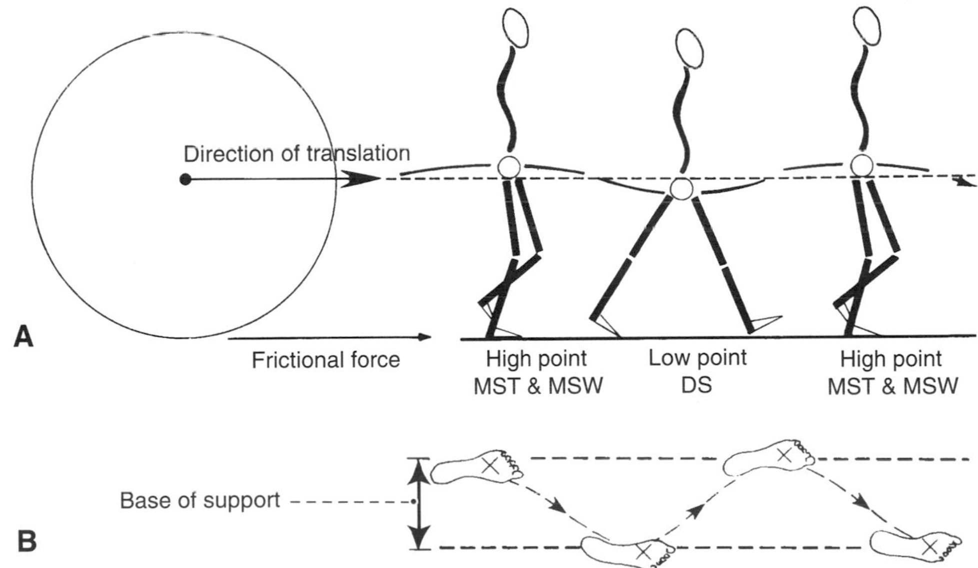

FIGURE 18-74.
Oscillations of the center of mass during ambulation: (A) Schematic comparison of the progression of a wheel and normal bipedal ambulation. In the latter, the center of mass describes a *sinusoidal curve*, whereas the wheel's center of mass is translated parallel to the ground. (B) Horizonal oscillations of the body's center of mass (lateral trunk sway) as the body is alternately supported on each stance leg. The extent of the sway is determined by the base of support, which is the distance between the two heels as they cross each other (10–20 cm). (Courtesy of Dr. Walter C. Stolov.)

and the energy needed to maintain the hips and knees flexed. The resulting sinusoidal oscillations of the body's center of mass need to be correlated with the phases of the gait cycle to understand the muscle groups that come into action during normal ambulation and the muscle actions that compensate for gait abnormalities.

The center of mass reaches its high point during MST and its low point during DS (see Fig. 18-74*A*). During MST, the high point is reduced by allowing: 1) a downward tilt of the pelvis of about 4° to 5° on the side of the swing leg, and 2) approximately 15° of flexion at both the hip and the knee. The first is controlled by the contraction of the hip abductors of the stance leg (see Fig. 17-19*C* and *D*) and the second, by the contraction of hip and knee extensors. In addition, the amount by which the center of mass is allowed to fall during DS is reduced by the rotation of the pelvis. The anterior superior iliac spine on the side of the leg reaching HS is anterior to that of the contralateral leg (Fig. 18-75). The center of mass remains higher, and the stride length is longer, when pelvic rotation is allowed to occur than when it is voluntarily (or pathologically) prevented from occurring.

Swinging of the arms is coordinated with pelvic rotation (see Fig. 18-75). Although it does not affect center of mass oscillations, it imparts an angular momentum to the thoracic spine that is the reverse of the angular momentum in the lumbar spine that results from pelvic rotation.

Bringing the gravitational force line over the stance leg with each step requires **lateral sway**, or side-to-side oscillations of the center of mass (see Fig. 18-74*B*). The total amplitude of lateral sway is about 5 cm. Its extent is determined by the size of the **base support**, which is the distance between the heels at midswing.

Joint Movements and Muscle Actions

During the gait cycle muscle contraction serves three purposes: 1) to accelerate or decelerate the advancing limb; 2) to counterbalance the force of gravity; and 3) to counterbalance forces imparted by the ground to the limb. In the latter two instances the movement produced by the force at a joint (flexion, for example) will be counterbalanced or controlled by muscles that oppose that movement (extensors, in the case of flexion). These muscles will contract even while they elongate (eccentric contraction). Without frictional force between the foot and the ground, walking becomes difficult or impossible, as demonstrated by attempts to walk on ice. Movements and muscle actions are discussed with reference to stages of the gait cycle.

Heel Strike to Foot-Flat. In the first part of the stance phase, the hip is flexed, the knee extended and the ankle is in neutral position as the heel strikes the ground. The reactive force from the ground generates further flexion of the hip and initiates flexion of the knee and plantar flexion of the foot, which continues until FF. Contraction of the extensor musculature of all these joints is required to prevent collapse of the limb under the body weight. These muscles include the gluteus maximus and hamstrings at the hip, the quadriceps (which absorbs the jarring of HS) and the tibialis anterior with the extensor digitorum longus and hallucis longus, which control plantar flexion, thus preventing slapping of the foot on the ground.

Foot-Flat to Midstance. After reaching FF, the body moves forward on the planted foot to reach MST, eliminating plantar flexion and hip flexion and, consequently, also the contraction of hip and ankle extensors. Quadriceps activity, however, continues to maintain the knee in 15° of flexion as it comes to support the weight of the body. At MST the opposite leg is in swing phase and hip abductors of the stance leg (gluteus medius and minimus) are called into action to control pelvic tilt. As the momentum of the body forces the foot into dorsiflexion, the triceps surae contracts to counterbalance this force. Lateral rotation of the stance leg and the pelvis begin as the opposite limb advances. The rotation continues until TO.

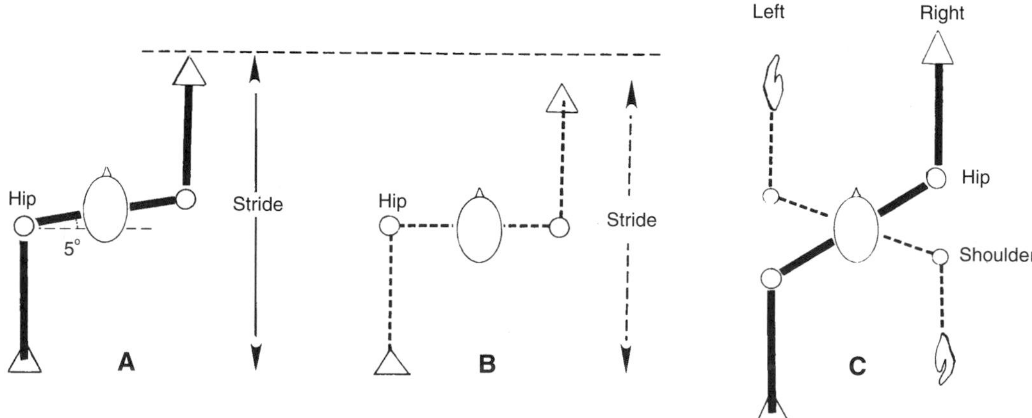

FIGURE *18-75.*
Stride length and arm swing during ambulation: (A) Stride length with pelvic rotation and (B) without pelvic rotation, when the same degree of hip flexion and hip extension occurs in each case. (C) Arm swing coordinates with leg advance. Forward arm swing matches contralateral leg advance. (Courtesy of Dr. Walter C. Stolov.)

Midstance to Heel-off. Continued forward momentum displaces gravity's line of force anteriorly, generating a reactive force from the ground, which extends the hip and knee without any activity from their extensor muscles. Quadriceps contraction ceases, and the iliopsoas is recruited to counterbalance the extension force at the hip. The ground reaction force shifts from the heel to the metatarsal heads and contraction of the plantar flexors peaks, lifting the heel off the ground and providing the force required for propulsion. Contraction of the gastrocnemius prevents the knee from reaching full extension. The hip abductors of the stance leg remain active until the opposite leg becomes planted.

Heel-off to Toe-off. Representing push-off, this is the last period of the stance phase and coincides with double support as the opposite heel strikes the ground. The plantar flexors exert their main thrust on the metatarsal heads and the reactive force transmitted from them flexes the knee. The foot moves from a dorsiflexed position at the commencement of HO to marked plantar flexion at TO. Continued action of the iliopsoas, assisted by the adductors, flexes the hip in anticipation of the swing phase. The hip abductors become silent as the toe is lifted.

Toe-off to Midswing. During this first period of the swing phase, hip flexors provide the acceleration force to the thigh, letting the knee continue its flexion passively. Flexion of these joints shortens the swinging leg, and the foot is also dorsiflexed to clear the ground. Medial rotation begins to reverse the lateral rotation attained in the stance phase and continues into the commencement of the next stance phase.

Midswing to Heel Strike. Contraction of the hamstrings decelerates the thigh, and the knee is rapidly extended, mainly as a result of pendulum action, which is controlled by the increasing tone of the hamstrings. The knee is fully extended as the heel strikes the ground. Heel strike is the only point in the gait cycle where the knee attains full extension.

Neural Control

Table 18-1 summarizes the activity of the main muscle groups during different phases of the gait cycle. Smooth coordination of these groups requires postulation of controlling mechanisms in the central nervous system. There is both experimental and clinical evidence for the existence of a pair of genetically determined, so-called **pattern generators** for the lower limbs in the lumbar spinal cord and for the upper limbs in the cervical cord. They are postulated to be programmed for turning on appropriate groups of motor neurons for flexor and extensor muscles in a pattern that results in coordinated gait. Linked to one another by interneuronal connections, the limb pattern generators are believed to be controlled by a central command system located in the midbrain. The pattern generators are influenced by input from specific receptors located in the joints (particularly the hip) and by various spinal reflexes.

TABLE *18-1* **Activity of Muscle Groups During Phases of the Gait Cycle**

Muscles	Gait Cycle Action*
Quadriceps	HS to MST TO to MSW
Gluteus maximus	HS to MST
Gluteus medius and minimus	HS to TO
Tibialis anterior and peroneals	HS to FF TO to HS
Gastrocnemius and soleus	MST to TO
Iliopsoas and adductors	TO to MSW
Hamstrings	MSW to HS

* See text for abbreviations.

Gait Abnormalities

There are five classes of problems that give rise to characteristic patterns of abnormal gait: 1) pain, 2) muscle weakness, 3) reduced range of passive joint movement (e.g., contractures), 4) central nervous system disturbances, and 5) functional inhibition. Diagnosis depends on meticulous observation of the gait in front, back, and side views, supplemented by confirmatory physical examination. Description of the abnormal gait patterns and the routine for observing them is beyond the purpose of this account. A brief mention of antalgic gait, however, may be instructive.

Antalgic gait is a pattern adopted to minimize pain. The characteristics of the pattern vary according to the location of the pain, but some common features apply to all. Heel strike is eliminated to avoid jarring. Stance phase on the affected side is shortened with a corresponding reduction in the swing of the opposite leg, which accounts for a shorter stride length. Reference has been made to hip pain and its gait abnormalities in Chapter 17. Midline vertebral pain, unilateral back pain, knee pain, or even pain in the metatarsophalangeal joint of the big toe produce characteristic variants of antalgic gait, which can be explained by an understanding of the phases of the gait cycle.

RECOMMENDED READINGS

Bardeen CR. Development and variation of the nerves and the musculature of the inferior extremity and of the neighboring regions of the trunk in man. Am J Anat 1907; 6: 259.

Basmajian JV, DeLuca CJ. Muscles alive: their functions revealed by electromyography. 5th ed. Baltimore: Williams & Wilkins, 1985.

Bojsen-Møller F, Flagstad KE. Plantar aponeurosis and internal architecture of the ball of the foot. J Anat 1976; 121: 599.

Brasseur JL, Luzzati A, Lazennec JY, Guérin-Surville H, Roger B, Grenier P. Ultrasono-anatomy of the ankle ligaments. Surg Radiol Anat 1994; 16: 87.

Bundens WP, Bergan JJ, Halasz NA, Murray J, Drehobi M. The superficial femoral vein: a potentially lethal misnomer. JAMA 1995; 274: 1296.

Cahill DR. The anatomy and function of the contents of the human tarsal sinus and canal. Anat Rec 1965; 153: 1.

Cailliet R. Knee pain and disability. Philadelphia: FA Davis, 1973.

Cailliet R. Foot and ankle pain. Philadelphia: FA Davis, 1968.

Connell J. Popliteal vein entrapment. Br J Surg 1978; 65: 351.

Fuss FK. Anatomy of the cruciate ligaments and their function in extension and flexion of the human knee joint. Am J Anat 1989; 184: 165.

Gardner E. The innervation of the knee joint. Anat Rec 1948; 101: 109.

Gülman B, Kopuz C, Yazici M, Karaismailoglu N. Morphological variants of the suprapatellar septum: an anatomical study in neonatal cadavers. Surg Radiol Anat 1994; 16: 363.

Hallsy JE. The muscular variations in the human foot. A quantitative study. General results of the study: 1. Muscles of the inner border of the foot and the dorsum of the great toe. Am J Anat 1930; 45: 411.

Hamada N, Ikuta Y, Ikeda A. Arteriographic study of the arterial supply of the foot in one hundred cadaver feet. Acta Anat 1994; 151: 198.

Hassine D, Feron J-M, Henry-Feugeas M-C, Schouman-Clæs E, Guérin-Surville H, Frija G. The meniscofemoral ligaments: magnetic resonance imaging and anatomic correlations. Surg Radiol Anat 1992; 14: 59.

Haymaker W, Woodhall B. Peripheral nerve injuries: principles of diagnosis. 2nd ed. Philadelphia: WB Saunders, 1953.

Heller L, Langman J. The menisco-femoral ligaments of the human knee. J Bone Joint Surg Br 1964; 46B: 307.

Hollinshead WH. Anatomy for surgeons: vol 3, the back and limbs. 3rd ed. Philadelphia: Harper & Row, 1982.

Hoppenfeld S. Physical examination of the spine and extremities. New York: Appleton-Century-Crofts, 1976.

Horwitz MT. Normal anatomy and variations of the peripheral nerves of the leg and foot: application in operations for vascular diseases; study of one hundred specimens. Arch Surg 1938; 36: 626.

Huene DB, Bunnell WP. Operative anatomy of nerves encountered in the lateral approach to the distal part of the fibula. J Bone Joint Surg Am 1995; 77A: 1021.

Inman VT. The joints of the ankle. Baltimore: Williams & Wilkins, 1976.

Kamel R, Sakla FB. Anatomical compartments of the sole of the human foot. Anat Rec 1960; 140: 57.

Kinmonth JB, Simeone FA. Motor innervation of large arteries with particular reference to the lower limb. Br J Surg 1942; 39: 333.

Kjaer I. Skeletal maturation of the human fetus assessed radiographically on the basis of ossification sequences in the hand and foot. Am J Phys Anthropol 1974; 40: 2577.

Kubik S, Manestar M. Topographic relationship of the ventromedial lymphatic bundle and the superficial inguinal nodes to the subcutaneous veins. Clin Anat 1995; 8: 25.

Last RJ. Some anatomical details of the knee joint. J Bone Joint Surg Br 1948; 30B: 683.

Lieb FJ, Perry J. Quadriceps function: an electromyographic study under isometric conditions. J Bone Joint Surg Am 1971; 53A: 749.

Lovejoy JF Jr, Harden TP. Popliteus muscle in man. Anat Rec 1971; 169: 727.

Lovell AGH, Tanner HH. Synovial membranes, with special reference to those related to the tendons of the foot and ankle. J Anat Physiol 1908; 42: 415.

Mackenzie R, Logan BM, Shah NJ, Keene GS, Dixon AK. Direct anatomical–MRI correlation: the knee. Surg Radiol Anat 1994; 16: 183.

Manchot C. The cutaneous arteries of the human body. New York: Springer-Verlag, 1983.

Mann R, Inman VT. Phasic activity of intrinsic muscles of the foot. J Bone Joint Surg Am 1964; 46A: 469.

Mann RA. The great toe. Orthop Clin North Am 1989; 20: 519.

Mann RA, Coughlin MJ. Hallux valgus: etiology, anatomy, treatment and surgical considerations. Clin Orthop 1981; 157: 31.

Mauro MA, Jacques PC, Moore M. The popliteal artery and its branches: embryologic basis of normal and variant anatomy. Am J Roentgenol 1988; 150: 435.

Procter P, Paul JP. Ankle joint biomechanics. J Biomech 1982; 15: 627.

Rasmussen O. Stability of the ankle joint: analysis of the function and traumatology of the ankle ligaments. Acta Orthop Scand 1985; suppl 211.

Ratiu P, Conley D, Rosse C. The digital anatomist: interactive atlas of the knee (CD-ROM). Seattle: University of Washington School of Medicine, 1995.

Rauschning W, Glenn WW. The knee: MR-imaging,arthroscopy and anatomy correlations (videodisc). Bethesda, MD: American Academy of Orthopedic Surgeons and National Library of Medicine, 1986.

Rosset E, Hartung O, Brunet C, et al. Popliteal artery entrapment syndrome: anatomic and embryologic bases, diagnostic and therapeutic considerations following a series of 15 cases with a review of the literature. Surg Radiol Anat 1995; 17: 161.

Sarrafian SK. Anatomy of the foot and ankle. Philadelphia: JB Lippincott, 1993.

Saunders JBDeCM, Inman VT, Eberhart HD. The major determinants in normal and pathological gait. J Bone Joint Surg Am 1953; 35A: 543.

Sherman RS. Varicose veins: anatomy, re-evaluation of Trendelenburg tests, and operative procedure. Surg Clin North Am 1964; 44: 1369.

Siegler S, Chen J, Schneck CD. The three-dimensional kinematics and flexibility characteristics of the human ankle and subtalar joints—part 1: kinematics. J Biomech Eng 1988; 110: 364.

Silver RL, de la Garza J, Rang M. The myth of muscle balance: a study of relative strengths and excursions of normal muscles about the foot and ankle. J Bone Joint Surg Br 1985; 67B: 432.

Staubesand J, Hackländer A. Topography of the perforating veins on the medial side of the leg (Cockett's veins). Clin Anat 1995; 8: 399.

Stolov WC. Normal and pathologic ambulation. In: Rosse C, Clawson DK. The musculoskeletal system in health and disease. Hagerstown: Harper & Row, 1980.

Strobel M, Stedtfeld HW. Diagnostic evaluation of the knee. Berlin: Springer, 1990.

PART V

THORAX

Hollinshead's Textbook of Anatomy, by Cornelius Rosse and Penelope Gaddum-Rosse.
Lippincott-Raven Publishers, Philadelphia, © 1997.

CHAPTER 19

The Thorax in General

The thorax is the upper part of the trunk, distinguished from the abdomen by the presence of the **rib cage**. This resilient, expandable, skeletal frame is constructed of the *sternum*, the *ribs*, and the *costal cartilages* and is supported on the vertebral column, which forms the posterior wall of the **thoracic cavity**, enclosed within the rib cage. The central organs of respiration and circulation are housed within the thoracic cavity. The ribs also provide protection for some major abdominal organs.

The **thoracic wall** consists of the thoracic skeleton and associated soft tissues. Integrity of the wall is necessary for generating the subatmospheric pressure within the thoracic cavity that causes air to be sucked into the lungs during respiration.

A broad median septum, known as the **mediastinum**, partitions the thoracic cavity and separates the two hollow spaces that are filled by the right and left lungs (Fig. 19-1). The bulk of the mediastinum is made up of the **heart** enclosed in the **pericardial sac** and of the major pulmonary and systemic veins and arteries. The **trachea** and **esophagus** enter the mediastinum from the neck through the **superior thoracic aperture**. This relatively small opening between the first pair of ribs also transmits the great arteries and veins of the head, the neck, and the upper limbs. The **inferior thoracic aperture** is wide and irregular; through it, the abdominal cavity protrudes high into the chest. Abdominal and thoracic viscera are separated from one another, however, by the **diaphragm**, a musculotendinous sheet that is attached to the inner margins of the inferior thoracic aperture. The diaphragm bulges up into the chest like a dome and varies its height by rhythmic contraction and relaxation. This pistonlike action is an important factor in respiratory movements and usually contributes twice as much to pressure and capacity changes in the thorax as the movements of the ribs. The lungs follow the excursions of the thoracic walls because their surface is held apposed to the inner aspects of the walls by the **pleura**. The pleura is a serous membrane, the parietal layer of which lines the two hollow spaces on either side of the mediastinum, whereas its visceral layer invests the expandable lungs. Thus, the thorax not only contains and protects the central organs of respiration and circulation, but its mechanisms also produce pressure changes necessary for respiration and for venous return to the heart.

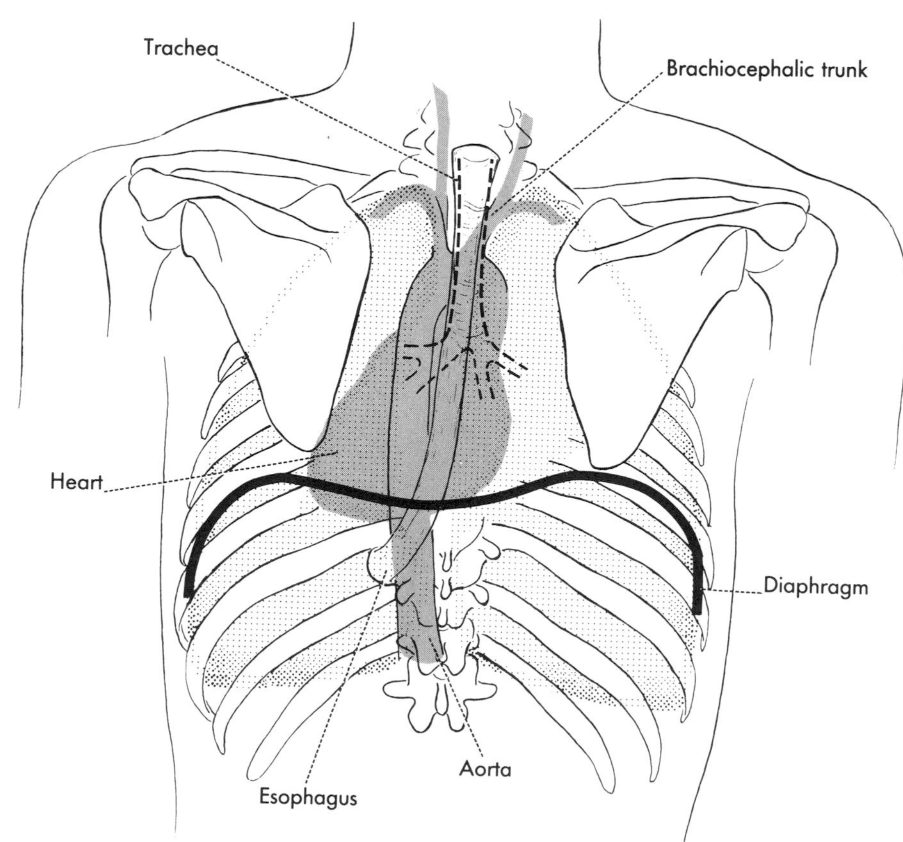

FIGURE *19-1.*
The thorax seen from behind. The bulky shoulders obscure a relatively small rib cage; the diaphragm rises high up into the chest. The pleural cavities, which extend over the posterior surface of the domes of the diaphragm, are indicated by *stippled areas*: the heart and great arteries in the mediastinum are shown in *pink*.

THE THORACIC WALL

Between the outer covering of skin and the inner pleural lining, the walls of the thoracic cavity are made up of more or less concentric layers of muscles and fascia that are supported by the thoracic skeleton (Fig. 19-2). The nerves, blood vessels, and lymphatics of the body wall pass among these layers, serving not only the thoracic wall, but also a major part of the abdominal wall. Practically all clinical information pertaining to the thoracic viscera, and to some of the major abdominal viscera, has to be obtained by eliciting physical signs across the thoracic wall, which is possible only by knowing skeletal landmarks and the functional anatomy of the thorax.

The thoracic cage supports the bones and muscles of the pectoral girdle. The square shoulders and the bulky girdle musculature obscure the relatively small thoracic cage (see Fig. 19-1). Except for a median strip of the sternum and the tips of the thoracic vertebral spines, the thoracic skeleton is largely covered by muscles that belong to the upper limb or the vertebral column. The more important of these are the pectoral muscles and the serratus anterior anterolaterally, the trapezius and latissimus dorsi posterolaterally, and, lying deep to the latter two, the erector spinae in the back (see Fig. 19-2). Supplied by nerves other than those serving the true body wall, these muscles anatomically are not considered a component of the thoracic wall. Nevertheless, surgical and clinical access to the thoracic cavity is possible only through them. The lower part of the rib cage is covered anteriorly by the rectus abdominis and the external oblique muscles of the abdominal wall.

The female breast covers a large area of the anterior chest wall. Its adipose tissue merges with the superficial fascia along the periphery of the organ (see Fig. 19-2). During palpation and percussion of the chest, the breast can readily be pushed out of the way owing to its relatively free mobility: it can be moved around on the underlying muscles (see Chap. 15). Posteriorly, the scapula and its associated muscles prevent direct access to much of the chest (see Fig. 19-2). However, to obviate this disadvantage in examining the lungs, the scapula may be moved out of the way by abduction of the arm and protraction of the shoulder.

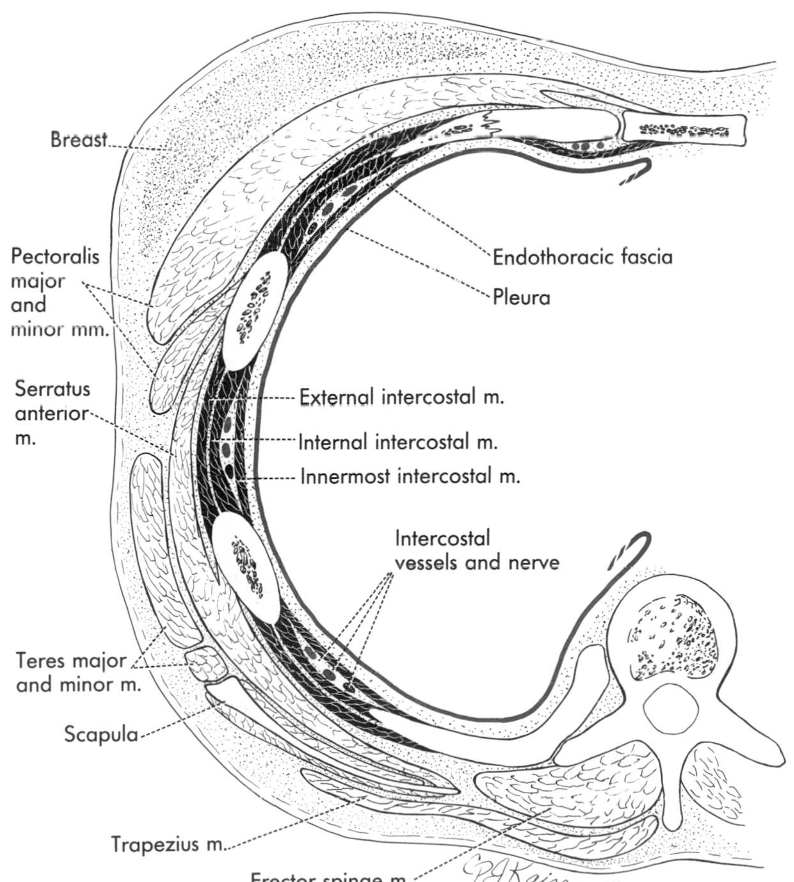

FIGURE *19-2.*
Layers of the thoracic wall. The muscle layers of the thoracic wall proper are *black*; The muscles in *white* belong to the pectoral girdle.

The Thoracic Skeleton

The rib cage and the thoracic vertebral column form an irregularly shaped, truncated cone (Fig. 19-3). The cone is flattened anteroposteriorly, a peculiarly human characteristic. Ten of the 12 pairs of ribs form loops or arches between respective vertebrae and the sternum, whereas the last two pairs of ribs float free anteriorly (**floating ribs**). All ribs slant downward from their vertebral attachment, and this slant tends to become slightly more pronounced the more inferiorly the ribs lie. Because the sternum anteriorly is much shorter than the length of the thoracic spine and because of the downward tilt of the shafts of the ribs, the anterior segment of each costochondral loop slants upward so that the costal cartilages may articulate with the sternum. The upward slant of the cartilages becomes gradually steeper below the fourth rib, and the seventh is the last cartilage to reach the sternum directly. The eight, ninth, and tenth costal cartilages terminate short of the sternum and articulate with their proximal neighbor. In this manner, the **costal margin** is formed on each side. The right and left costal margins together form the **costal arch.** Between the costal margins in the *infrasternal angle* is the epigastrium, the uppermost region of the abdomen.

It follows from the foregoing description that 1) the **superior thoracic aperture** is small; its plane slopes downward and forward; its boundaries are the first thoracic vertebra, the first pair of ribs with their cartilages, and the superior margin of the manubrium sterni; and 2) the **inferior thoracic aperture** is large and irregular; it is formed by the 12th thoracic vertebra, the 12th pair of ribs, and the costal arch made up of costal cartilages ten to seven.

It can be readily appreciated that the thoracic cage is made both resilient and compressible by its architecture. Use is made of this property in the application of external cardiac massage during resuscitation. The costochondral loops permit rhythmic compression of the heart between the sternum and the vertebral column sufficient to effect some rhythmic pumping of blood, even though the heart itself is quiescent.

Movement of the skeletal pieces is required for respiration, and these movements are mediated by several joints. The bony shaft of each rib is directly united to its cartilage (**costochondral synchondrosis**); each typical costochondral loop articulates with the thoracic spine through two synovial joints (**costovertebral joints**), and another synovial joint joins it directly or indirectly to the sternum (**sternocostal** and **interchondral joints**). The first rib is an exception in that its cartilage is directly united to the manubrium, which ensures stability in the frame of the superior aperture. In addition, the three component pieces of the sternum can move in relation to one another at the **manubriosternal** and **xiphisternal joints**.

The Sternum

The sternum, or breast bone, forms the anteromedian portion of the thoracic wall (see Fig. 19-3). It is an elongated, flat bone. Its interior, filled with cancellous bone, contains hematopoietic bone marrow throughout life and has been the site for clinical bone marrow biopsies. Up to puberty the sternum consists of six segments or **sternebrae** held together by hyaline cartilage. The central four sternebrae

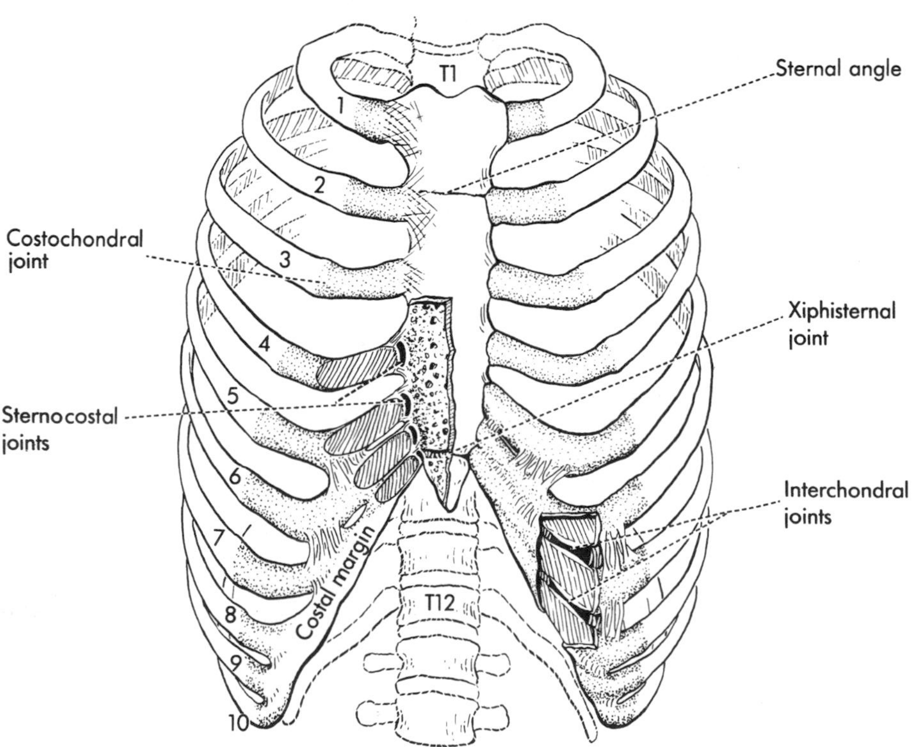

FIGURE *19-3.*
Anterior view of the skeleton of the thorax. Part of the sternum and costal cartilages has been cut away to reveal some of the joints.

fuse between years 14 and 21 to form the **body** (*corpus*) of the sternum; however, the superior and inferior segments remain independent as the **manubrium sterni** and the small **xiphoid** (sword-shaped) **process**, respectively. Two cartilaginous joints hold together these three parts of the sternum and permit some changes in angulation between them. This movement at the manubriosternal joint accommodates for the respiratory excursions of the ribs, which are of different lengths. In later life, however, the cartilage of the sternal joints tends to disappear, and both joints may ossify.

All three parts of the sternum are palpable. The superior margin of the manubrium forms the **jugular notch**, which can be felt between the two clavicles. It lies on one level with the second thoracic vertebra. The manubriosternal joint is palpable as the **sternal angle**, a smooth ridge produced by the angulation of the bones and their slightly everted articular edges. The sternal angle is level with the second costal cartilages and with the lower border of the fourth thoracic vertebra. The body of the sternum is flat, and from its lower edge, the xiphoid process inclines backward. During youth, much of the process consists of cartilage and can be moved passively until its bony center has expanded and fused to the body of the sternum. Palpation of the xiphoid process in the apex of the infrasternal angle causes some discomfort; therefore, the xiphisternal junction is a more convenient landmark. Level with the xiphisternal junction is the sixth pair of costal cartilages and the tenth thoracic vertebra. The projection of the thoracic vertebrae on the sternum is telescoped, owing to the anterior concavity of the thoracic vertebral column.

On either side of the jugular notch, the manubrium receives the sternal end of the clavicles in a shallow concave facet, thus forming the **sternoclavicular joints**. On the sides of the sternum are the *costal incisures*, or notches, for articulation with the ribs. Those for the first ribs lie on the sides of the manubrium: those for the second lie at the manubriosternal junction. The costal notches for the third, fourth, fifth, and sixth ribs lie on the sides of the body; that for the seventh rib, the lowest to articulate with the sternum, lies at the junction of body and xiphoid process.

Ossification. The sternum ossifies from several centers that form independently of the ribs. Usually, there is a single center for the manubrium and a single one for the uppermost part of the body; each of the remaining three segments that contribute to the body may have a single or a paired center of ossification. A single center is typical for the xiphoid process. The centers, except for that of the xiphoid, which appears during the third year of life, arise (from above downward) during the late prenatal period. Fusion of the parts of the body begins below and extends upward, being completed at age 21.

The Ribs

There are 12 pairs of ribs (*costae*), of which the upper seven are called **true ribs** because they form complete loops between the vertebrae and the sternum, whereas the lower five, which fail to reach the sternum, are considered the **false ribs**. The ribs are long, thin, curved bones, segmentally arranged and separated by **intercostal spaces**. Anteriorly, each rib terminates in a bar of hyaline cartilage, the **costal cartilage**, which, until it ossifies partially in old age, contributes significantly to the springiness and mobility of the rib cage. The posterior portion of the rib, made of cancellous bone, is much longer and itself has several named parts: the **head**, which abuts against the vertebral column; the relatively short **neck**; and the **body**, which has a definite bend in it known as the **costal angle** (Fig. 19-4).

Typical Ribs. The **head** has an upper and lower articular facet divided by a *crest* for articulation with two adjacent vertebrae in a costovertebral joint. The upper border of the narrower **neck** also displays a *crest* for the attachment of ligaments (costotransverse ligaments). The neck ends laterally at the *tubercle*, a knuckle-shaped enlargement on the outer or posterior surface of the rib. The tubercle bears an oval, convex facet for articulation with the transverse process of the similarly numbered vertebra (costotransverse joint). Lateral to the facet is a small rough area to which the lateral costotransverse ligament is attached.

The tubercle marks the junction of the neck and body of the rib. The **body** soon turns rather sharply forward at the *costal angle* and slants downward as well as forward, reaching its lowest point just before it becomes cartilaginous. The body is twisted as well as bent and its external surface generally turns to face slightly upward, conforming to the overall cone shape of the thorax (Fig 19-5, rib 3). The anterior end of the bony rib receives the costal cartilage in a definite pit or fossa.

The upper border of the rib is smooth and rounded, whereas the lower border projects downward as a sharp lip, most pronounced posterolaterally (see Fig. 19-4). This lip shelters the *costal groove* on the internal surface of the rib in which the intercostal vessels and nerves are located.

Although ribs may **fracture** under direct violence at any point, the most frequent fractures are due to compression forces on the thorax, and these occur just anterior to the costal angle, the weakest point of the rib. The broken end tends to spring outward; however, a direct force may drive it inward, causing hemorrhage or injury to the lung, which predisposes to pneumothorax. Even though rib fractures usually heal without any splinting, a fractured costal cartilage may cause pain for a long time because the reparative capacity of cartilage is poor. Fractured cartilage heals eventually by fibrosis.

Atypical Ribs. The foregoing anatomic descriptions apply to all the ribs, with the exception of the first two and the last three pairs, which are to some degree atypical. The **first rib** is the most highly curved and is particularly broad (see Fig. 19-5). Its inner margin forms the boundary of the superior thoracic aperture, and its surfaces face primarily upward and downward. The subclavian artery exiting from the thorax marks the upper surface of the rib by a *sul-*

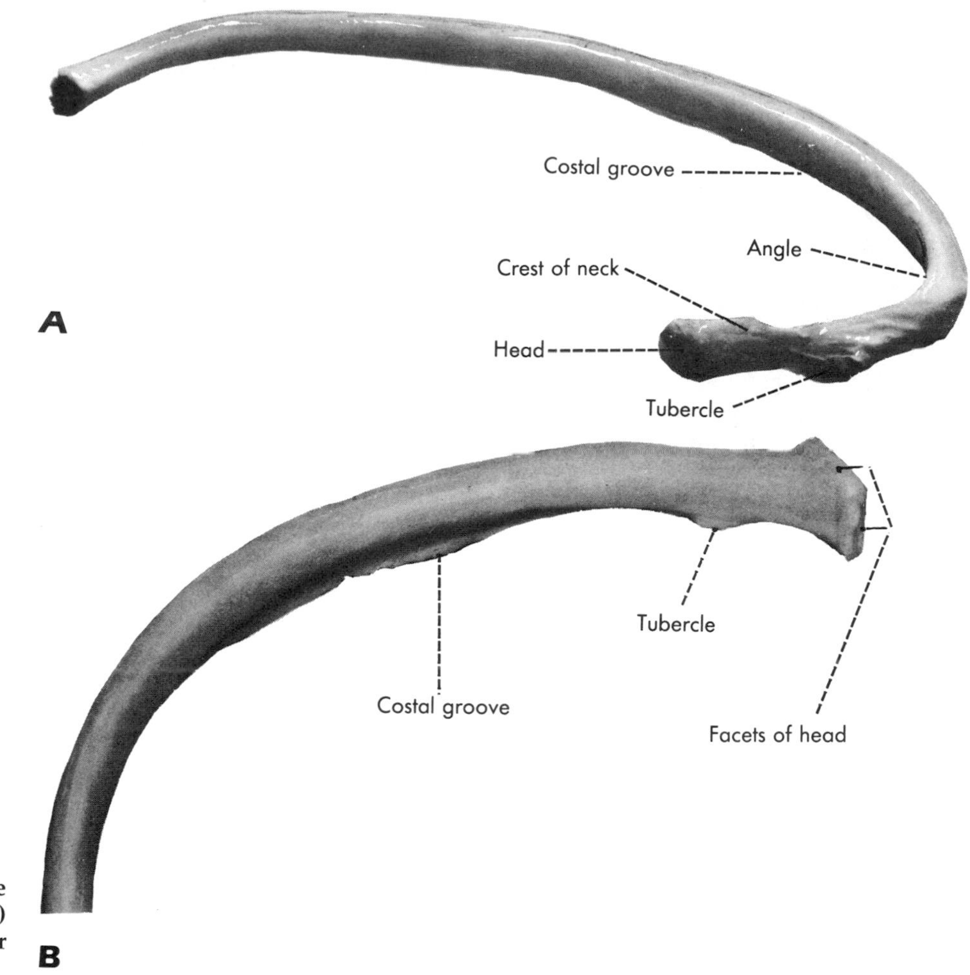

FIGURE 19-4.
The fifth right rib showing the features of a typical rib: (A) viewed from the back; (B) inner aspect of the vertebral end.

cus, as does the subclavian vein, which enters the aperture anterior to the artery. The two sulci are separated by a small eminence, *the tubercle of the anterior scalene muscle.* The head of the first rib bears a single articular facet, for it articulates only with the first thoracic vertebra. The **second rib** is similar in shape to the first, but larger, and its head has two facets (one each for the first and second thoracic vertebrae). It is distinguished by a broad, rough eminence, the *tuberosity of the serratus anterior muscle.* Usually the heads of the 10th, 11th, and 12th ribs each articulate only with their own vertebra, and the latter two have no tubercles or angles and do not articulate with the transverse processes.

Variations. Ribs are present as separate bones only in the thoracic region; however, vertebrae in all regions of the spine have costal elements associated with them. Those associated with cervical and lumbar vertebrae typically fuse with their transverse processes and become parts of them. In some cases a costal element associated with either a seventh cervical or a first lumbar vertebra develops as a rib instead of fusing with the transverse process. The incidence of **cervical rib** has been said to be between 0.5% and 1%. Cervical ribs are sometimes associated with signs of pressure on the brachial plexus or subclavian vessels (see Chap. 15); lumbar ribs have no clinical significance except that identification of vertebral levels may be inaccurate when the ribs are counted from below. The same confusion may arise when the 12th pair of ribs is missing, or they are so short that they are not palpable. There is said to be a tendency in humans toward the reduction of the 12th rib. According to one survey, in more than one-fourth of cases the rib was less than 5 cm long.

Counting of Ribs. The ribs form important landmarks to thoracic and abdominal viscera. In most individuals, all ribs are palpable, although the first is rather inaccessible because of the overlying clavicle. Reference points for counting are the sternal angle, which identifies the second rib, and the xiphisternal junction, on level with which is the sixth rib. The vertebral border of the scapula, when the arm is fully abducted, roughly corresponds in the back to this rib. The seventh costal cartilages form the apex of the infrasternal angle, and the tenth cartilages are palpable as the most inferior points of the rib cage along the costal margins.

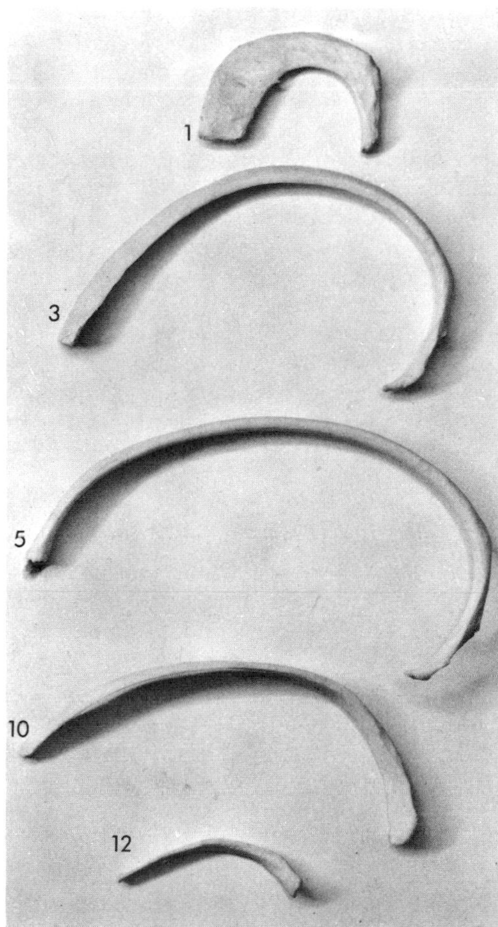

FIGURE 19-5.
The 1st, 3rd, 5th, 10th, and 12th right ribs seen from above.

Ossification. Most of the ribs are ossified from four centers: a primary center for the body and three epiphyseal centers, of which one is for the head and two are for the tubercle. The 11th and 12th ribs, however, have no separate centers for tubercles. Ossification of the body begins early in fetal life; the epiphyseal centers appear between the ages of 16 and 20 years and unite at about 25 years.

Joints and Movements of the Ribs

During inspiration, reduction of intrathoracic pressure is brought about by increases in the anteroposterior, lateral, and vertical diameters of the thoracic cavity. The vertical increase is due to diaphragmatic movement, whereas the anteroposterior and lateral increases depend on movements of the ribs. Most ribs articulate with the vertebral column at two joints: the *joint of the head of the rib* between the head of the rib and the vertebral bodies, and the *costotransverse joint*, between the tubercle and the transverse process (Fig. 19-6). Both joints are synovial; they are known collectively as the **costovertebral joints**.

When the head of a rib articulates with two vertebral bodies, the cavity of the joint is divided by a ligament attaching the crest of the head to the intervertebral disk. Although the articular capsule is simple, it is thickened anteriorly by a **radiate ligament**, the three components of which anchor the head to the intervertebral disk and to the bodies above and below the disk.

The **costotransverse joints** have small synovial cavities that are surrounded by lax articular capsules. The joints are strengthened by three **costotransverse ligaments** (see Fig. 19-6). These extend between the crest of the rib neck and the transverse process above the rib (superior ligament), between the posterior aspect of the rib neck and its own transverse process (the costotransverse ligament proper), and between the tip of the transverse process and the rough part of the costal tubercle (lateral costotransverse ligament).

The reciprocally shaped articular facets on the tubercle and transverse process determine the type of movement a rib is capable of and whether this movement increases either the anteroposterior or lateral diameter of the thorax. The tubercular facets of the upper ribs are ac-

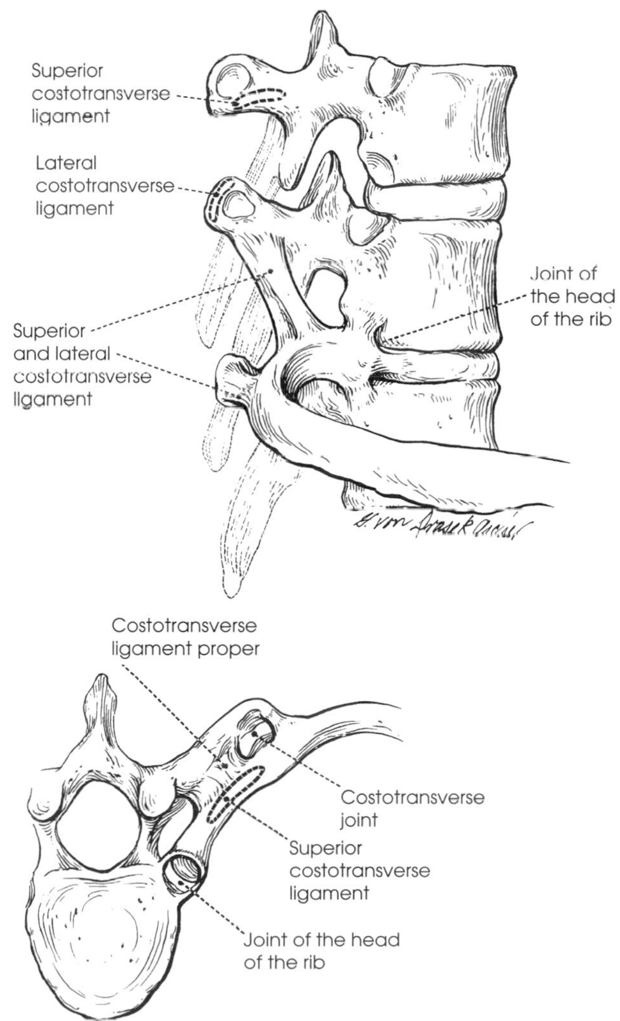

FIGURE 19-6.
Costovertebral joints with their associated ligaments.

commodated in deep, cup-shaped sockets on the transverse processes. The tubercle, therefore, is compelled to roll in this fixed socket along an axis that connects the joint of the rib head and the costotransverse joint (Fig. 19-7*A*). No sliding (or translation) of the tubercle is permitted.

Slight movement at these joints will be greatly amplified at the anterior end of the rib that will be raised when the tubercle, and the neck with it, rotates downward. This movement has been likened to that of a *pump handle*. The thrust is transmitted along the costal cartilages to the sternum, which becomes not only bodily elevated but also pushed forward, increasing the anteroposterior thoracic diameter. The pump-handle movement of the upper ribs is readily confirmed by laying the hands over the pectoralis major and watching them rise and fall with inspiration and expiration. Such a movement is absent over the back where the relatively fixed rib neck is permitted to roll only. Nor is the pump-handle movement demonstrable over the lower ribs. The tubercular facets of these ribs, and the articular facets of their transverse processes, are plane or flat. When the rib moves here, the tubercle rides up and down on the transverse process. Each rib, therefore, hinges on an axis that joins the joint of the rib head to the appropriate sternocostal or intercostal joint (see Fig. 19-7*B*). Elevation of the rib will raise the entire costochondral loop as a *bucket handle* is lifted on its hinges from the side of the bucket. The lateral thoracic diameter between elevated costochondral loops will be greater than that of the same loops when they are dependent. This bucket-handle type of movement can be verified by placing the hands on the sides of the lower part of the chest. The movement will be equally pronounced whether viewed from the front or the back.

The **sternochondral** and **interchondral joints** are involved in these movements, and deformation of the costal cartilages contributes to their amplitude. The lax capsules of the interchondral joints permit some sliding of the cartilages on one another, which contributes to the visible elongation of the costal margins during inspiration and to the widening of the infrasternal angle. Limitation of rib movements because of pain or arthritic involvement of the joints of the ribs may impair respiratory function.

Muscles and Fascia

Ventrolateral to the vertebral column and the paraspinal musculature, the muscles of the body wall are arranged in three layers: external, internal, and innermost. In the embryo, these muscles arise on each side as ventral extensions from the myotomes and meet each other along the ventral midline. These myotomal cells segregate into three layers; however, their ventral edges remain unsplit and form two parallel, longitudinal muscle masses, the

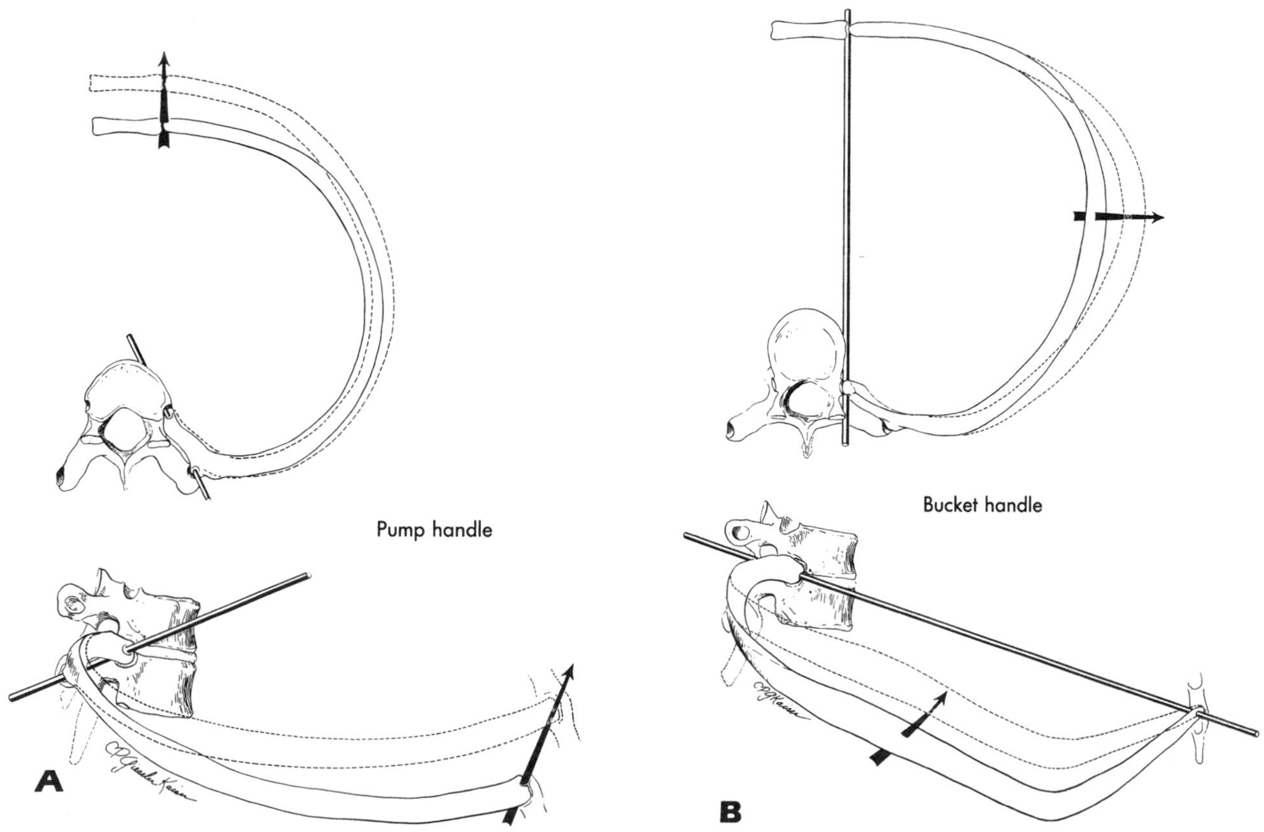

FIGURE *19-7.*
(A) Pump handle and (B) bucket handle type movements of the ribs during respiration. The axes of the movements are indicated by solid bars.

rectus muscles. In the thoracic region, the three muscle layers derived from one myotome are separated by a rib from the muscles derived from the next myotome. These are the *intercostal muscles*, and their segmental origin remains evident throughout life. Over the abdomen, on the other hand, the consecutive myotomes fuse, although, here too, the muscles retain a segmental pattern of innervation and blood supply. The rectus muscle, well developed only over the abdomen, disappears over the thorax, except in 0.5% of individuals in whom it persists as the *sternalis*. The body wall mesoderm (*somatopleur*), into which the myotomal cells migrate, provides the fascial coverings of the muscles, the lining of the body wall (endothoracic fascia and parietal pleura, or endoabdominal fascia and parietal peritoneum) and superficial fascia. From it also develop the blood vessels and lymphatics of the body wall; however, the segmental nerves grow into the body wall from the spinal cord.

Intercostal Muscles

There are 11 pairs of intercostal spaces and each contains an external, an internal, and an innermost intercostal muscle. All three are thin sheets of muscle in which fibers run from one rib to the next and, although none of them spans an intercostal space from vertebra to sternum, owing to their overlap they completely seal the spaces.

Each **external intercostal muscle** begins posteriorly, just lateral to the tubercle of the rib, and extends anteriorly, slightly past the costochondral junction (Fig. 19-8). Beyond this, up to the sternum, the muscle is represented in the upper intercostal spaces by the *external intercostal membrane*. In the lower intercostal spaces, the muscular fibers of the external intercostals merge with the external oblique muscle of the anterior abdominal wall as the external oblique takes its origin from the ribs. The fibers of the external intercostals slant downward and forward from one rib to the next, and the fibers of the external oblique conform to this direction.

The **internal intercostal muscles** have a different slant; their fibers run upward and forward from the upper border of one rib to the lower border of the next above. These muscles reach the sternum anteriorly (Fig. 19-9*A*) (they are visible through the external intercostal membrane, Fig. 19-8*A*). Posteriorly, they extend only about as far as the costal angles (see Fig. 19-9*B*). Medial to the angles, they are represented by *internal intercostal membranes*. The lower internal intercostal muscles merge with the internal oblique muscle of the abdomen.

The **innermost intercostal muscles** (*intercostales intimi*) lie internal to the internal intercostals. They are less well developed than the other two intercostal muscles, occupy chiefly the middle part of the length of each intercostal space, and are best distinguished by the fact that they are separated from the internal intercostals by the intercostal nerves and vessels.

The innermost muscle layer in the thorax has vestigial muscles in addition to the innermost intercostals (see Fig 19-9). The **subcostal muscles** are variable fiber bundles, placed posteriorly, that span two to three intercostal spaces. The **transversus thoracis** is a thin layer of muscle, the fibers of which fan out from the posterior surface of the lower part of the sternum to the neighboring costal cartilages. These two muscles, together with the innermost intercostals, are said to be equivalent to the transversus muscle of the abdomen. The peripheral fibers of the **diaphragm** are derived also from the same muscle layer; other parts of the diaphragm have different origins. The diaphragm is discussed in Chapter 25.

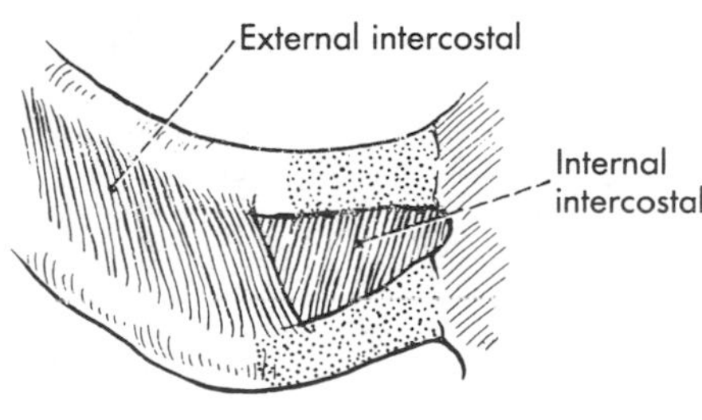

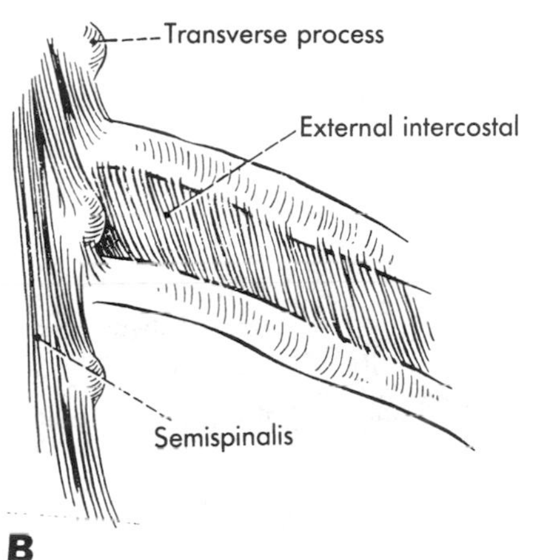

FIGURE *19-8.*
(A) Anterior and (B) posterior ends of an intercostal space seen from the outside. In panel A, the external intercostal membrane, covering the internal intercostal muscle, is treated as if it were transparent; in panel B, some of the overlying back muscles have been cut away.

All the muscles of the thoracic wall are innervated by the associated intercostal nerves. Their chief function is to move the ribs, although there remains some controversy about their specific action. Their attachments and the direction of their fibers tend to suggest that both internal and external intercostal muscles could elevate the ribs if their proximal attachment is considered as their point of origin and that both sets of muscles could depress the ribs if the inferior point of attachment is considered the origin. Electromyographic studies in humans tend to confirm Galen's original teaching—that, at least in some of the intercostal spaces, the external intercostals are active in inspiration and the internal intercostals, in expiration. Other studies suggest that both sets are active in forced in-

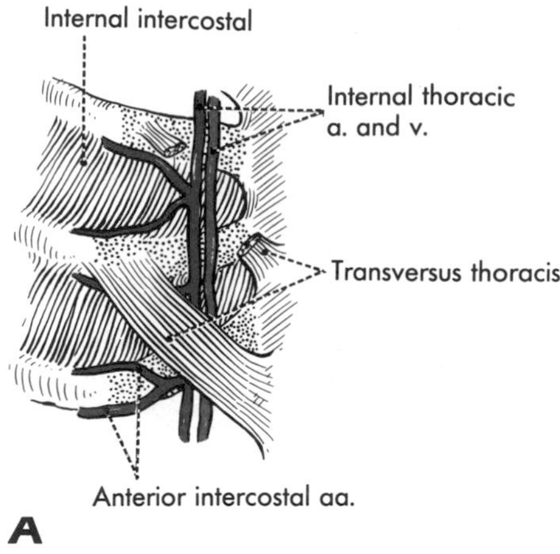

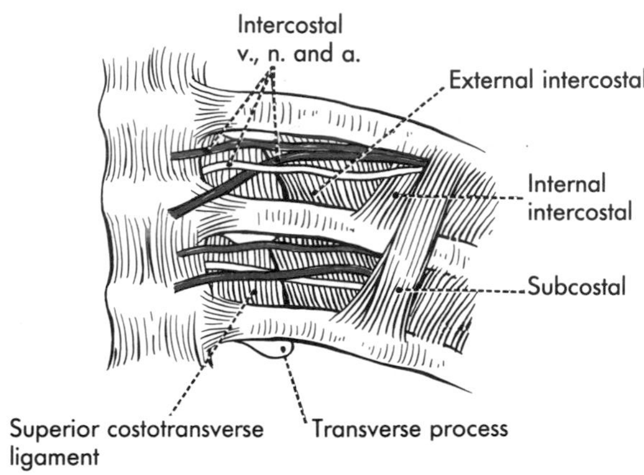

FIGURE *19-9.*
(A) Anterior and (B) posterior ends of the intercostal space seen from the inside of the thorax. The innermost intercostal muscles lie further laterally and are not visible in either panel A or B. In panel B, the internal intercostal membrane, covering the external intercostal, is treated as if it were transparent. Sympathetic ganglia and collateral branches of vessels and nerves have been omitted for clarity.

spiration and expiration. Intercostal muscles also contract during phonation, blowing, and sucking. When muscles of an intercostal space are paralyzed in a spare individual, paradoxical respiratory movement may be observed over that space. The tissues of the space will be sucked in during inspiration and blown out during expiration.

Fascias

The special feature of the **superficial fascia** over the thorax is the breast (see Chap. 15; Fig. 19-2). The **deep fascia** is thin and inseparable from the epimysium of the muscles that cover the rib cage, except posteriorly, where it is thick and specialized over the erector spinae as the **thoracolumbar fascia** (see Fig. 12-31). The internal aspect of the thoracic wall is lined by a hardly perceptible amount of loose connective tissue called the **endothoracic fascia**, which also covers the thoracic surface of the diaphragm (see Fig. 19-2). The function of the fascia is to fix the parietal pleura to the thoracic walls and the diaphragm so that the parietal pleura moves with these during respiratory movements. The only place where the endothoracic fascia appears as a distinct layer is over the lateral portions of the superior thoracic aperture. Here the fascia forms the **suprapleural membrane** that limits bulging of the lung into the neck. The parietal pleura (and the lung with it) projects above the level of the first rib as the **cupula** (little dome) and is supported there by the suprapleural membrane, which is likewise dome shaped, and its highest point is fixed to the transverse process of the seventh cervical vertebra.

Innervation of the Thoracic Wall

The body wall is innervated by the anterior rami of T-1 to T-12 spinal nerves. T-1 to T-11 are the *intercostal nerves*, and T-12, analogous with them, is known as the *subcostal nerve*. These are somatic nerves and provide the motor and sensory supply to all layers of the body wall, but do not innervate the girdle musculature attached to the rib cage, even though some of their branches pass through these muscles to the skin. With the following two exceptions, thoracic anterior rami supply the skin over the entire trunk as far down as the inguinal region.

1. Over the paravertebral area of the back, the skin is supplied by the posterior rami of the corresponding spinal nerves, which also innervate the erector spinae.
2. Anteriorly, as far down as the sternal angle, the skin is innervated by supraclavicular nerves, anterior rami of C-4 and C-5 (see Figs. 13-24 and 13-25).

Somatic efferent fibers in the intercostal nerves supply segmentally all the intercostal and subcostal muscles, the transversus thoracis, all three muscle layers of the abdominal wall, and the rectus abdominis. The same nerves conduct proprioceptive impulses from these muscles and also from the peripheral portions of the diaphragm, derived from the body wall. In addition to visceral afferents from the lung (see Chap. 20), these somatic afferents are probably also involved in maintaining reflexly the rhythmic movements of respiration. The intercostal nerves conduct pain and other exteroceptive sensations from the skin, breast, ribs, costal cartilages, and sternum and also from the parietal pleura that lines the thoracic wall and covers the *periphery* of the diaphragm. They are also sensory to the parietal peritoneum lining the entire abdominal wall and the *periphery* of the diaphragm. The pleura and peritoneum that cover central regions of the diaphragm are innervated by the phrenic nerves derived from cervical segments of the cord (predominantly C-4). Branches of the intercostal nerves contain sympathetic fibers that are motor to the smooth muscle of the blood vessels in the body wall and of hair follicles, and to sweat glands in the skin.

Intercostal Nerves

The basic anatomy of intercostal nerves has already been described as an example of a "typical" spinal nerve (see Chaps. 7 and 13; Figs. 7-3 and 13-22). The second through the sixth intercostal nerves are confined to the thorax, but the 7th to 11th intercostals and the subcostal nerve continue into the abdominal wall.

The first intercostal nerve represents only a small part of the anterior ramus of the first thoracic nerve; the major part of this ramus joins the brachial plexus. A typical intercostal nerve continues the direction of the spinal nerve as it emerges from its intervertebral foramen. After the posterior ramus has been given off, the intercostal nerve runs, at first, outside the pleura, more or less in the middle of the intercostal space, across the internal surface of the internal intercostal membrane (Fig. 19 9*B*). A sympathetic ganglion is suspended from each nerve in this position. Close to the angle of the rib, the nerve enters the fascial space between the internal intercostal and the innermost intercostal muscles and also attains the shelter of the costal groove, where it accompanies the intercostal vessels. The nerve lies below the vein and the artery. As it continues forward it gives off muscular branches and a **lateral cutaneous branch** (Fig. 19-10).

The upper six nerves follow the curve of the ribs and costal cartilages toward the sternum and terminate as **anterior cutaneous branches** that pierce the internal intercostal muscles, the external intercostal membrane, and the pectoralis major. Nerves 7 through 11 leave their intercostal space by crossing the internal surface of the costal margin and continue their course anteriorly between the internal oblique and transversus abdominis. The subcostal nerve running along the lower border of the 12th rib enters this fascial space without having to cross the costal margin. The termination of these nerves is discussed with the anterior abdominal wall.

Blood Supply of the Thoracic Wall

The thoracic wall is supplied chiefly by intercostal arteries and is drained by intercostal veins. These vessels are found in each intercostal space running in the costal groove just above the respective intercostal nerves (see Fig. 19-9*B*). Their course and branches closely conform to those of the nerve. Superficial structures over the thorax are served, in addition, by branches of the axillary and subclavian arteries and veins (see Chap. 15). These vessels anastomose in the superficial fascia with branches of the intercostal vessels.

Intercostal Arteries

In each intercostal space there are two sets of intercostal arteries, posterior and anterior, that anastomose with one another (see Fig. 19-10). The **posterior intercostal arteries** of all but the first two spaces are branches of the descending thoracic aorta, which lies in the mediastinum on the left side of the vertebral column. Consequently, arteries on the right are longer than those on the left because they cross over the vertebrae, passing posterior to all other structures to reach the intercostal spaces on the right side. The arteries of the first two spaces arise from a common stem (the *supreme intercostal artery*) given off by the *costocervical branch* of the subclavian artery in the root of the neck. The arteries of the upper six spaces terminate by anastomosing with the anterior intercostal arteries of the

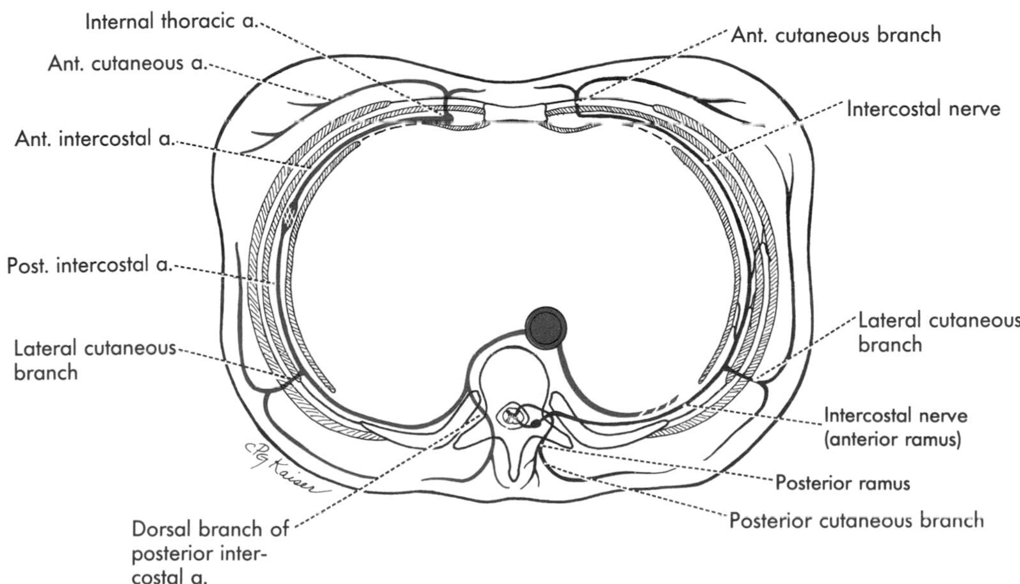

FIGURE *19-10.*
The course and branches of an intercostal artery and an intercostal nerve shown in a schematic transverse section of the thorax, viewed from below.

same space; those of the lower spaces and the **subcostal artery**, continue to the abdominal wall, as do the corresponding nerves.

Each posterior intercostal artery dispenses muscular branches (the largest of which, called the **collateral branch**, runs along the upper border of the rib below the space; it is accompanied sometimes by a similar branch of the nerve), a **lateral cutaneous branch**, and a **dorsal branch** that passes posteriorly with the posterior ramus of the corresponding spinal nerve. This branch supplies the back muscles and the skin and contributes to the supply of the contents of the vertebral canal through a *spinal branch* that enters the intervertebral foramen.

The **anterior intercostal arteries** are branches of the *internal thoracic artery*, a rather slender vessel that runs down on each side of the sternum parallel with its margin and crosses the inner surface of the costal cartilages (see Figs. 19-9; and 19-11). The anterior intercostal arteries are much smaller than their posterior counterparts and are somewhat variable. As a rule, they run along the lower border of each costal cartilage in the same fascial plane of the body wall as the posterior arteries. In the lower five spaces, similar branches come off the *musculophrenic artery*, one of the terminal branches of the internal thoracic, and anastomose with branches of the posterior intercostal artery, rather than with the vessel itself, as occurs in the upper spaces.

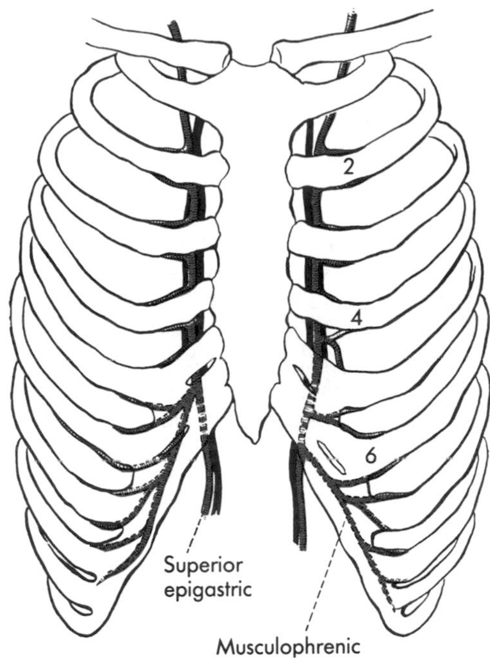

FIGURE *19-11.*
The course of the internal thoracic vessels: The anterior intercostal branches, usually two in each space, are not labeled. The artery is *red*, and the accompanying veins are *black*.

The Internal Thoracic Artery

The internal thoracic artery is given off by the subclavian artery at the base of the neck as that vessel arches over the suprapleural membrane. It descends behind the subclavian vein and the first rib. Its general course from this point is illustrated in Figure 19-11. The internal thoracic artery, like the intercostal vessels, runs in the neuromuscular plane of the thorax; that is, anterior to the transversus thoracis and on the internal surface of the costal cartilages and the internal intercostal muscles. Behind the sixth cartilage, it divides into its two terminal branches, the **musculophrenic** and the **superior epigastric arteries**. The former has been described; the latter descends into the abdominal wall to anastomose with the inferior epigastric artery. Apart from the anterior intercostal arteries, the internal thoracic artery gives branches to the mediastinum, the thymus, the pericardium (pericardiacophrenic artery), the sternum, and some *perforating branches*. The perforating branches pass to the skin with the anterior cutaneous branches of the intercostal nerves and, in the second, third, and fourth intercostal spaces, contribute to the supply of the breast; these vessels enlarge during lactation.

Veins

All arteries described in the foregoing and their branches are accompanied by veins designated by identical names. The veins anastomose in the same manner as the arteries. The **posterior intercostal veins** terminate in the *azygos* or *hemiazygos veins*, which run along the bodies of the vertebrae (see Chap. 22). The veins of the upper two spaces drain into the *brachiocephalic vein*, as do the *internal thoracic veins*, which receive the **anterior intercostal veins**.

Anastomoses

The intercostal and internal thoracic vessels participate in an important anastomotic system. Should the descending aorta or one of the venae cavae become obstructed, this anastomosis provides alternative channels for arterial and venous blood flow. The internal thoracic vessels are the superior segment of a longitudinal, ventral anastomotic chain that links the subclavian artery and brachiocephalic vein to the external iliac vessels. The intercostal vessels connect this chain to the descending aorta and azygos system of veins. In addition, in the superficial tissues of the thorax, branches of the axillary and subclavian arteries anastomose with the intercostal arteries, providing a possible conduit for blood flow from the subclavian system to the descending aorta. Should there be an obstruction between the arch of the aorta and the descending aorta, as there is in coarctation of the aorta, this anastomosis assumes a great importance (see Chap. 22). In such cases the circumscapular and intercostal arteries greatly enlarge: the former visibly pulsate around the scapula, and the latter may erode the ribs, as evidenced on x-ray films by notches along their inferior edges.

Lymphatic Drainage

Lymphatics of the superficial tissues of the thorax, including the breast, drain primarily into **axillary lymph nodes**; some, however, follow the perforating branches of the internal thoracic vessels and terminate in **parasternal lymph nodes**. The parasternal lymph nodes are irregularly placed along the internal thoracic vessels and collect lymph from the medial half of the breast, the anterior portion of the chest wall, and the anterior mediastinum. Lymphatics running with the posterior intercostal vessels terminate in **intercostal lymph nodes**, which lie along the azygos and hemiazygos veins in the posterior mediastinum. They drain lymph from the deep tissues of the chest wall; superficial tissues from the back drain to the axillary nodes.

THE THORACIC CAVITY

Developmental Considerations

In an early embryo, as the developing thoracic walls approximate each other ventrally, they enclose 1) a portion of the foregut, which develops into the esophagus; 2) the primitive heart tube, which has assumed a position ventral to the foregut; and 3) the rostral horseshoe-shaped portion of the intraembryonic celom, which is lined by a continuous layer of mesothelium (Fig. 19-12*A*). The more caudal portion of the celom, which will form the future peritoneal cavity, will be closed off from the thoracic part by the **pleuroperitoneal membranes**. These membranes later become incorporated into the diaphragm.

The heart soon sinks into the ventral portion of the celom, the future **pericardial cavity** (see Fig. 19-12*B*). Dorsolaterally, the lungs, budding off the foregut, bulge more and more into what will become the **pleural cavity**, without breaking the mesothelial lining of the cavity (see Fig. 19-12*C*). The pericardial cavity becomes partitioned off from the pleural cavities by bilateral septa derived from the inner mesoderm of the embryonic thoracic wall. This septum, the **pleuropericardial membrane**, is raised up and drawn across the body cavity on each side by a major vein (common cardinal vein), which drains the body wall and empties into the heart (see Fig. 19-12*C*, and *D*). This partition consists of "embryonic endothoracic fascia" and will develop into the **fibrous pericardium**. The mesothelial lining of the common body cavity in the thorax is thus separated into three independent blind sacs: two **pleural sacs** and the **serous pericardial sac** (Fig. 19-12*E*). Moreover, the definitive topography of viscera in the thoracic cavity is now established: between the two pleural sacs, is the *mediastinum*, an irregular, broad, median partition of the thoracic cavity, which for practical purposes, includes all the contents of the thoracic cavity except the lungs themselves.

The developing lungs covered with a layer of mesothelium, now designated as **visceral** or **pulmonary pleura**, grow more and more into the pleural cavity. Eventually, their pulmonary mesothelial surface will contact the **parietal pleura**, the outer wall of the sac, which is draped over the thoracic wall and the fibrous pericardium (Fig. 19-13). Parietal and visceral layers of the pleural sacs remain continuous with one another around the **root of the lung**, the pedicle that contains the pulmonary vessels and bronchi and attaches the lung to the mediastinum. The pleural cavity is thus reduced to a mere slit, which contains nothing except enough serous fluid to moisten the adjacent mesothelial surfaces. This should be borne in mind even though it is customary to speak of the lungs as if they were occupying the pleural cavity. In truth each lung is outside its pleural sac.

The anterior edge of the growing lung pushes the pleura before it and peels off the fibrous pericardium more and more from the chest wall until the serous pericardial sac, with the heart in it, becomes completely enclosed in the fibrous bag (see Figs. 19-12*E* and 19-13). This permits the two pleural sacs to approximate each other in front of the fibrous pericardium. However, they will not fuse with each other. The arrangement of pleural and pericardial sacs is shown in Figure 19-13. The serous pericardium, consisting of parietal and visceral layers, is enclosed by the fibrous pericardium in the same manner as the body wall encloses the pleural sacs. The greater part of the thoracic cavity comes to be occupied by the lungs. The boundaries and interior of this cavity are best described by considering the parietal pleura and the pleural cavity. Discussion of the lungs themselves and the contents of the mediastinum is deferred to subsequent chapters.

The Pleura and Pleural Cavities

The surfaces of the pleura that face into the pleural cavity are covered by mesothelium. This delicate squamous epithelium is strengthened on its abluminal surface by a substantial connective tissue membrane, an integral part of the pleura, which is sufficiently thick to support blood vessels, lymphatics, and nerves. It can be cut and sewn. The pleura can be peeled off the lung, but, because it tears readily, only with difficulty. It is easier to separate it from endothoracic fascia, especially over the fibrous pericardium, where the endothoracic fascia is sparse or laden with fat. In a dissection, it is possible to lift off the anterior thoracic wall, after the ribs and intercostal muscles have been cut, without opening the pleural sacs. This requires gently burrowing in the plane of the endothoracic fascia and pushing the pleura away from the wall as the wall is being lifted. It is instructive to inspect the pleural sacs from their exterior and to feel between finger and thumb the reflection of the lining off the walls onto the mediastinum or the diaphragm (Fig. 19-14).

Parietal Pleura

The parietal pleura is divided into several named regions according to the structures it covers. The **costal pleura** lines the thoracic wall and forms the anterior, lateral, and posterior walls of the pleural cavity. Superiorly, it is con-

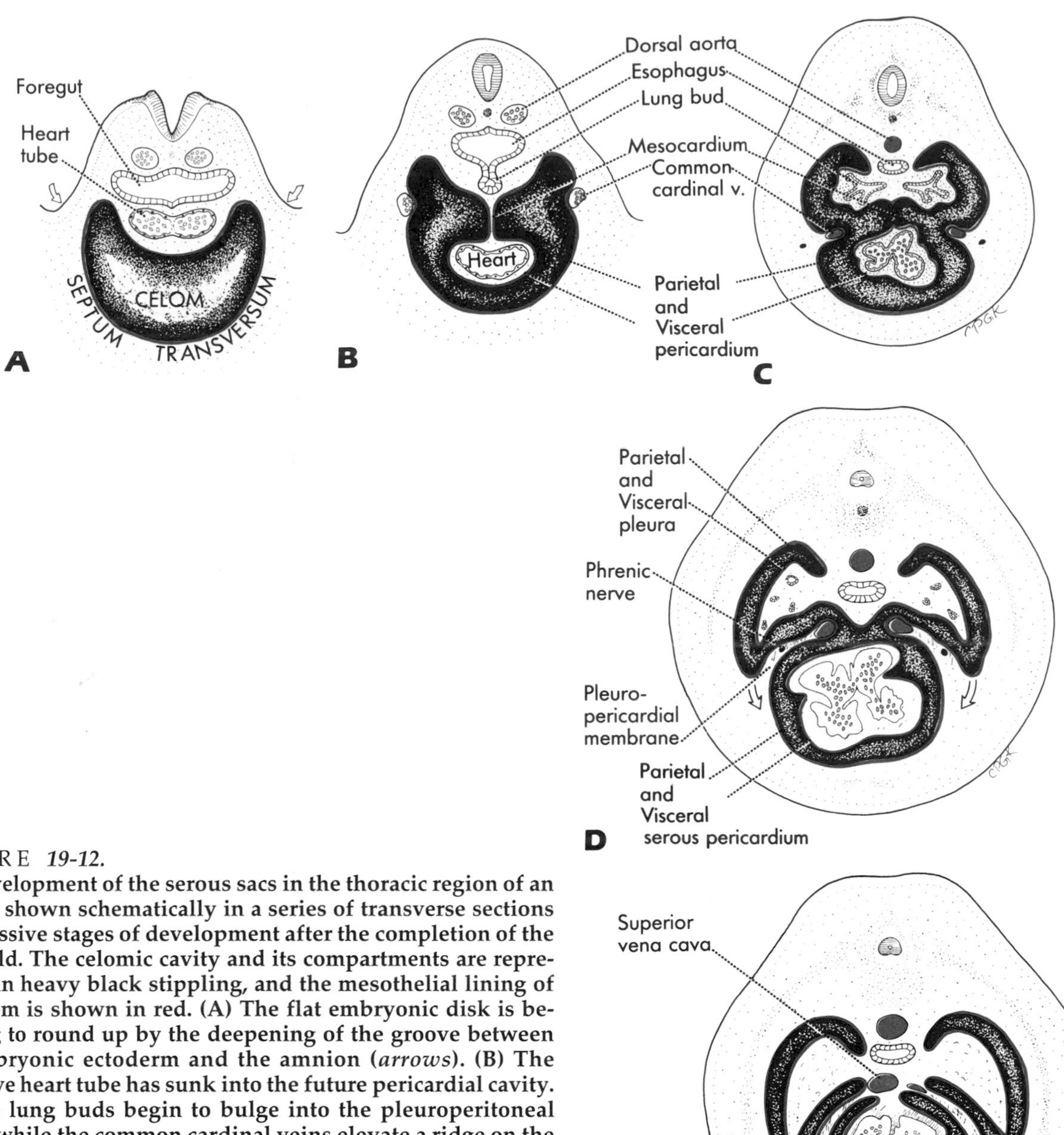

FIGURE *19-12.*
The development of the serous sacs in the thoracic region of an embryo shown schematically in a series of transverse sections at successive stages of development after the completion of the head fold. The celomic cavity and its compartments are represented in heavy black stippling, and the mesothelial lining of the celom is shown in red. (A) The flat embryonic disk is beginning to round up by the deepening of the groove between the embryonic ectoderm and the amnion (*arrows*). (B) The primitive heart tube has sunk into the future pericardial cavity. (C) The lung buds begin to bulge into the pleuroperitoneal canals, while the common cardinal veins elevate a ridge on the lateral wall of the celom that will become the pleuropericardial membranes. (D) After the pleuropericardial membranes are well formed, the pleural cavities expand anteriorly (*arrows*). (E) The formation of the fibrous pericardium completes the separation of the pericardial cavity from the pleural sacs, which continue their expansion anteriorly.

tinuous with the **cupula of the pleura**, which rises above the level of the first rib, and, inferiorly, it reflects to become the **diaphragmatic pleura**, forming the floor of the pleural and thoracic cavities. The **mediastinal pleura** is continuous anteriorly and posteriorly with the costal pleura and inferiorly with the diaphragmatic pleura. In front of the root of each lung, the phrenic nerve and the accompanying pericardiacophrenic vessels lie between the pleura and the pericardium, often surrounded by an appreciable quantity of fat. Behind the pericardial sac, the mediastinal pleura surrounds the root of the lung and, like a wide sleeve, invests it. The sleeve is very short. It is here that the parietal pleura becomes visceral pleura as the sleeve doubles back on itself, reflecting onto the lungs where the root of the lung enters the *pulmonary hilum* (see Figs. 19-17, and 20-3). The wide pleural sleeve around the lung root and hilum is redundant inferiorly and, viewed from within the pulmonary cavity, hangs down as a pleural fold. This fold of pleura is the **pulmonary ligament**. After the lung is removed from the pleural cavity, the cut

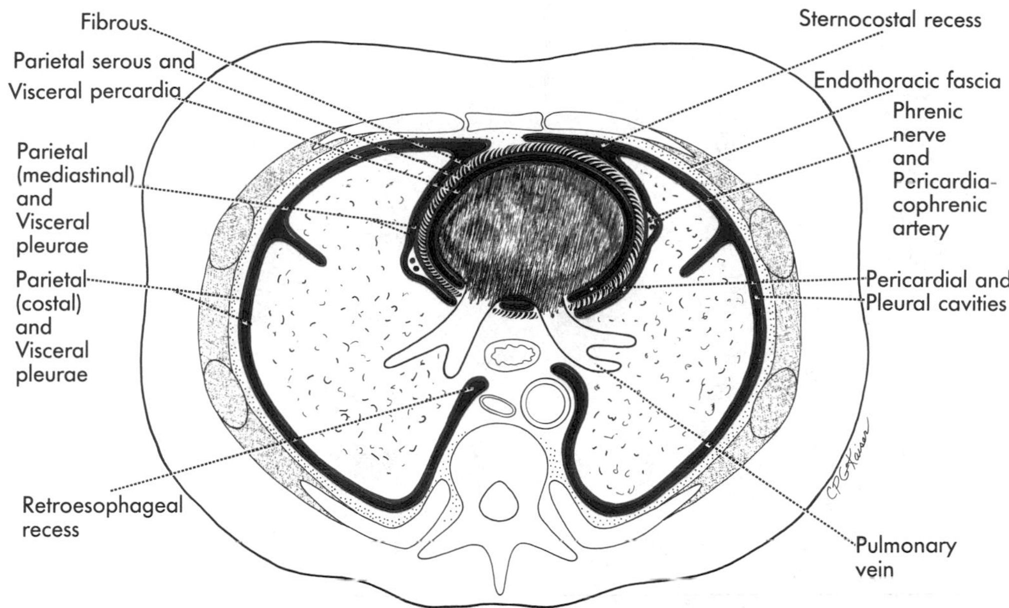

FIGURE *19-13.*
The arrangement of the pleural and pericardial sacs shown in a schematic transverse section of the thorax. The serous cavities are *black*, and the serous membranes are *red*.

profiles of the two layers of the pulmonary ligament are visible, both on the lung (see Fig. 20-3) and on the mediastinal pleura (see Figs. 22-3 and 22-4).

Lines of Pleural Reflection. The sharp lines of reflection, where costal pleura becomes continuous with mediastinal or diaphragmatic pleura, are important because they limit the pleural cavities. These lines can be mapped on the surface of the chest in relation to bony landmarks.

The anterior lines of reflection of the parietal pleura are shown in Figure 19-15. Between the pleural cupulae, the two pleural sacs are far apart, but converge as they are traced down toward the sternal angle where the right and the left pleural sacs come in contact with each other. The right pleura then continues downward close to the midline of the sternum. At the lower end of this bone, it swings outward and then turns down along the seventh costal cartilage. In contrast, the anterior reflection of the left pleura typically begins to diverge laterally at about the level of the fourth rib and is usually lateral to the sternum at the level of the fifth and sixth interspaces. Thereafter, it follows the seventh costal cartilage. The deviation of the left pleura is known as the *cardiac notch*. If the notch is marked enough, it leaves sufficient room between the pleura and sternum to introduce a needle into the pericardial sac without penetrating the pleural cavity. Pericardial fluid can be obtained by inserting a needle into the fifth or sixth intercostal space close to the edge of the sternum. Even if the notch is small, the danger of contaminating the pleural sac with infected pericardial fluid is lessened because the enlarged pericardial sac tends to push the pleura laterally.

Inferiorly, the pleural reflection line does not quite coincide with the costal margin. Leaving the seventh costal cartilage, the pleura crosses the eighth rib in the midclavicular line and the tenth rib in the midaxillary line. The pleura usually reaches its lowest point at about the middle of the 11th rib and then runs posteriorly almost horizontally, swinging slightly upward as it approaches the 12th thoracic vertebra (Fig. 19-16).

The fact that the lower edge of the pleura, posteriorly, may run below the tip of a short 12th rib matters when posterior incisions, such as those for an approach to the kidney, are made. Normally, the incision is far enough lateral (because of the back muscles) to reach the 12th rib before reaching the pleura. When the 12th rib is particularly short, however, carrying the incision to this rib, or mistaking the 11th for a normal 12th, would involve opening the pleural cavity.

The posterior line of reflection between the costal and the mediastinal pleura is usually rounded, rather than sharp, therefore. It is shown as lying either anterior to the tips of the transverse processes or immediately on each side of the vertebral bodies. However, the right pleura particularly, and the left to a smaller extent, may extend anterior to the vertebral bodies, so that sometimes the two pleural sacs almost touch on the front of the vertebral column. If they actually do so, they lie in front of the aorta, the azygos and hemiazygos veins, and the thoracic duct. These pleural pockets are located behind the esophagus and are known as the **retroesophageal recesses** (see Fig. 19-13).

Nerve and Blood Supply. The parietal pleura shares the nerve and blood supply of the structures that the different parts cover. The costal pleura is supplied by intercostal nerves and vessels, as is the peripheral part of the diaphragmatic pleura. The phrenic nerve supplies the

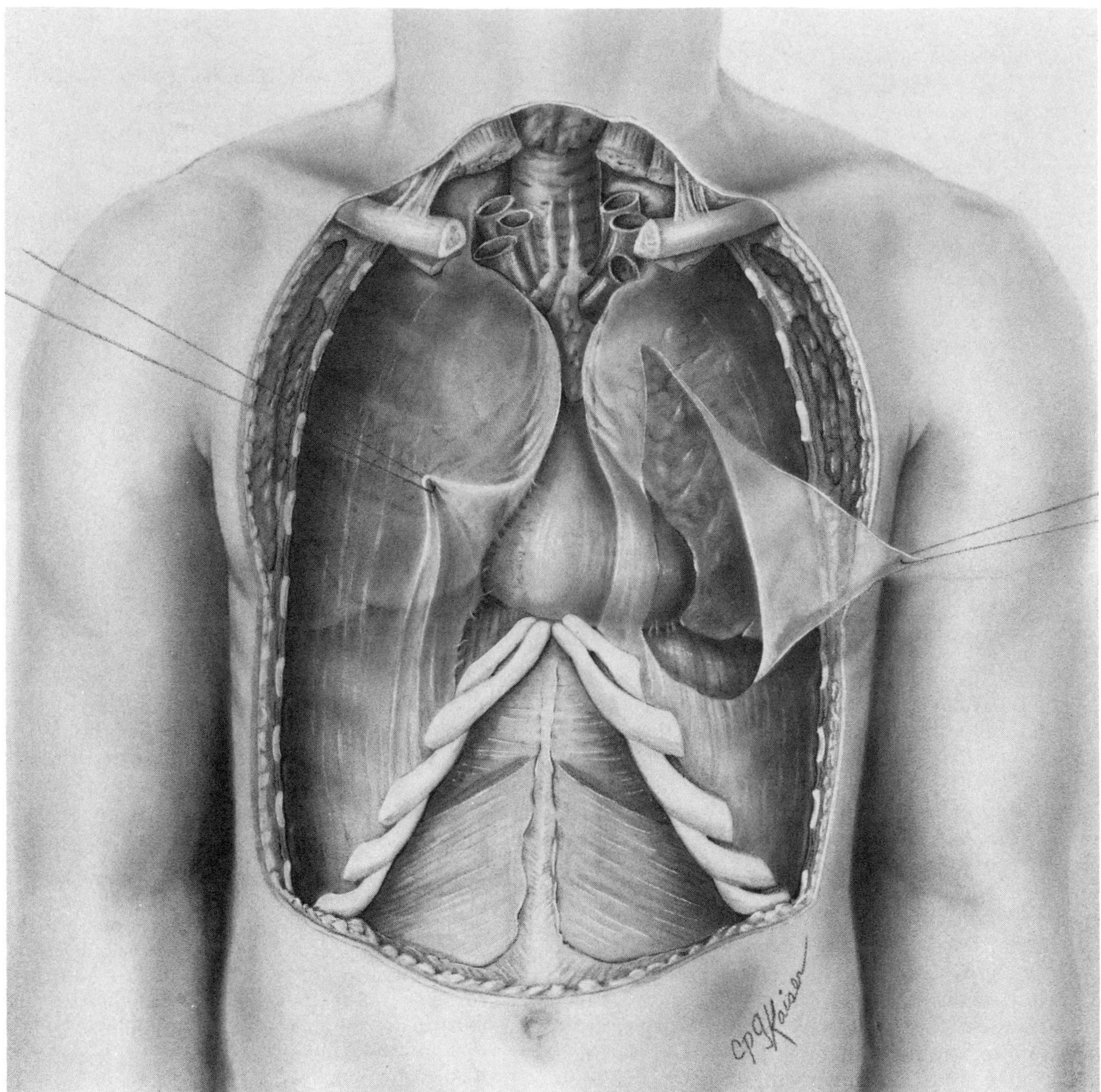

FIGURE *19-14.*
A dissection of the thorax to show the arrangement of the pleural sacs. The anterior chest wall has been lifted off, the right pleural sac has been elevated from the pericardial sac and the diaphragm, and an opening has been cut in the parietal pleura on the *left side* to reveal the lung covered with visceral pleura.

major, central portion of the diaphragmatic pleura and also the entire mediastinal pleura. The pain of pleurisy (pleural inflammation or irritation) is mediated along somatic afferent pathways in these nerves. By contrast, visceral pleura, supplied by autonomic nerves of the lung, is insensitive to pain stimuli.

Inflammation caused by infection, irritation, emboli, or neoplasms in segments of the lung causes hyperemia of the overlying pleura, which leads to exudate formation. When the inflammation spreads across the pleural cavity and involves the parietal pleura (or when the parietal pleura is primarily inflamed owing to viral infections, for instance), respiratory movements become painful because somatic pain afferents are excited. Sufficient exudate sooner or later separates the pleural layers and minimizes mechanical irritation. Resolution of the inflammation usually leaves adhesions between parietal and visceral pleura, and these, as a rule, are painless.

Visceral Pleura and Pleural Recesses

The **visceral pleura** (also commonly called **pulmonary pleura**) is tightly attached to the outer surface of each lung and dips into the fissures of the lung (see Fig. 19-13). In the fissures, the pulmonary pleura is in contact with itself,

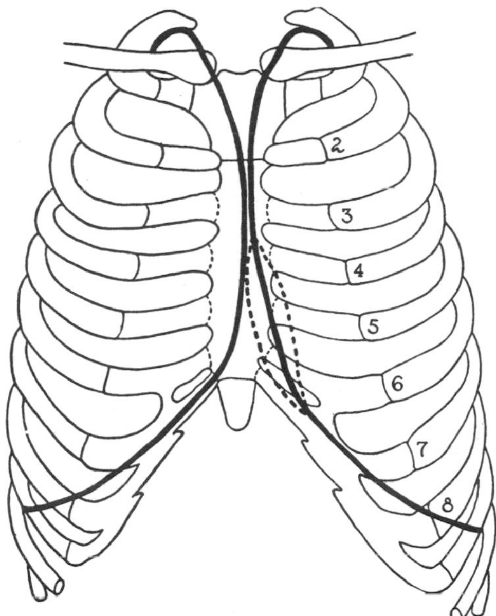

FIGURE *19-15.*
Relations of the pleural reflections to the anterior thoracic wall. The two *broken lines* on the left pleural boundary indicate variations in the cardiac notch; within these lay 70% of Woodburne's cases. The *solid line* between the broken lines represents the mean found in this series. (Redrawn from Woodburne RT; Anat Rec 1947;97:197.)

whereas over the surfaces of the lung, it touches the parietal pleura. However, only during deep inspiration is all of the parietal pleura (practically speaking) in contact with visceral pleura. In expiration and during quiet breathing, recesses exist in the pleural cavity. In these recesses, parietal pleura is in contact with parietal pleura, and the lung peels them apart as it expands into the recesses during inspiration. The pleural recesses are deepest inferiorly, where the costal pleura leaves the inner aspect of the rib cage and, in an acute angle, sweeps up onto the superior surface of the diaphragm, thus creating the **costodiaphragmatic recess** (Fig. 19-17; and see Fig. 19-14). Smaller recesses exist behind the sternum, where costal pleura doubles back on itself to become mediastinal pleura, so creating the **sternocostal recesses** (see Fig. 19-13). Much more shallow **retroesophageal recesses** exist where mediastinal pleura continues into costal pleura.

In quiet breathing, the inferior edge of the lungs remains about two ribs higher posterolaterally than that of the pleura (see Fig. 20-2). The surface projection of the inferior pulmonary edge is at the sixth rib in the midclavicular line, at the eighth rib in the midaxillary line, and at the tenth thoracic vertebra in the back. Thus, it is possible to thrust a large needle or a small trocar and cannula through the eighth intercostal space in the axilla and obtain a biopsy of the liver without injuring the lung, while transgressing the body wall, the pleural cavity, the diaphragm, and the peritoneal cavity.

No pleural recesses exist superiorly, and the lungs fit snugly into the pleural cavity (see Fig. 19-17).

MOVEMENTS OF RESPIRATION

The basis for the voluntary movements of respiration are the mechanical forces generated in the chest wall that are transmitted to the lung across the pleural cavity. Contrary to many accounts of respiratory movements, which explain the adherence of visceral and parietal pleurae to one another by surface tension—similar to the adherence of two wet glass plates—surface force of attraction plays no part in the mechanics of respiratory movements. The forces acting across the pleural cavity are such that under normal circumstances both fluid and gas tend to be absorbed from the pleural cavity, thereby leaving the lung and the chest wall in apposition, as it were, by default.

Actually, a force is always present that, rather than keeping them together, tends to pull the pleural surfaces apart. Even at the end of a normal expiration, the pressure within the pleural cavity is 5 cm H_2O below atmospheric pressure. This subatmospheric pleural pressure—often referred to as "negative" pressure—is due to retractive forces that perpetually stretch the chest wall and the lung to such an extent that they tend to pull away from each other. The lung is stretched or distended by atmospheric pressure in the alveoli, while atmospheric pressure compresses the chest wall externally. When a thoracotomy is performed, the lung collapses and the cut ends of the ribs spring outward. The lung can be made to collapse further if the pressure in the airways is lowered below the atmospheric pressure while the chest is open. In the intact chest, it is the force of recoil in the stretched elastic tissues of the lung and chest wall that is constantly pulling them apart, thereby generating the

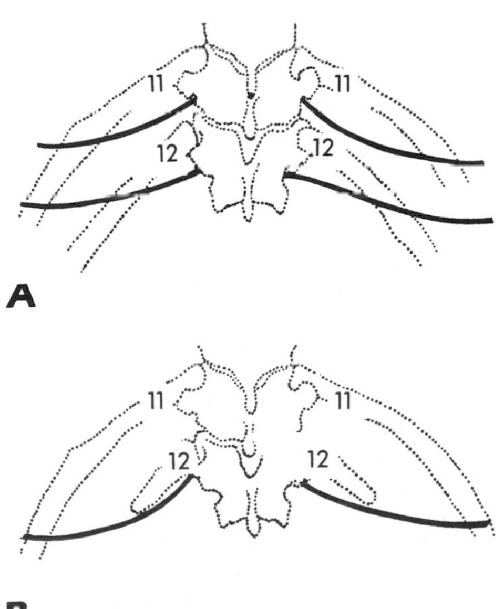

FIGURE *19-16.*
The lower boundary of the pleura: (A) the extremes of the posterior pleural reflections in Melinkoff's series: (B) the usual relation of the pleura when the 12th rib is rudimentary (Adapted from Melinkoff A. Arch Klin Chir 1923;23:133.)

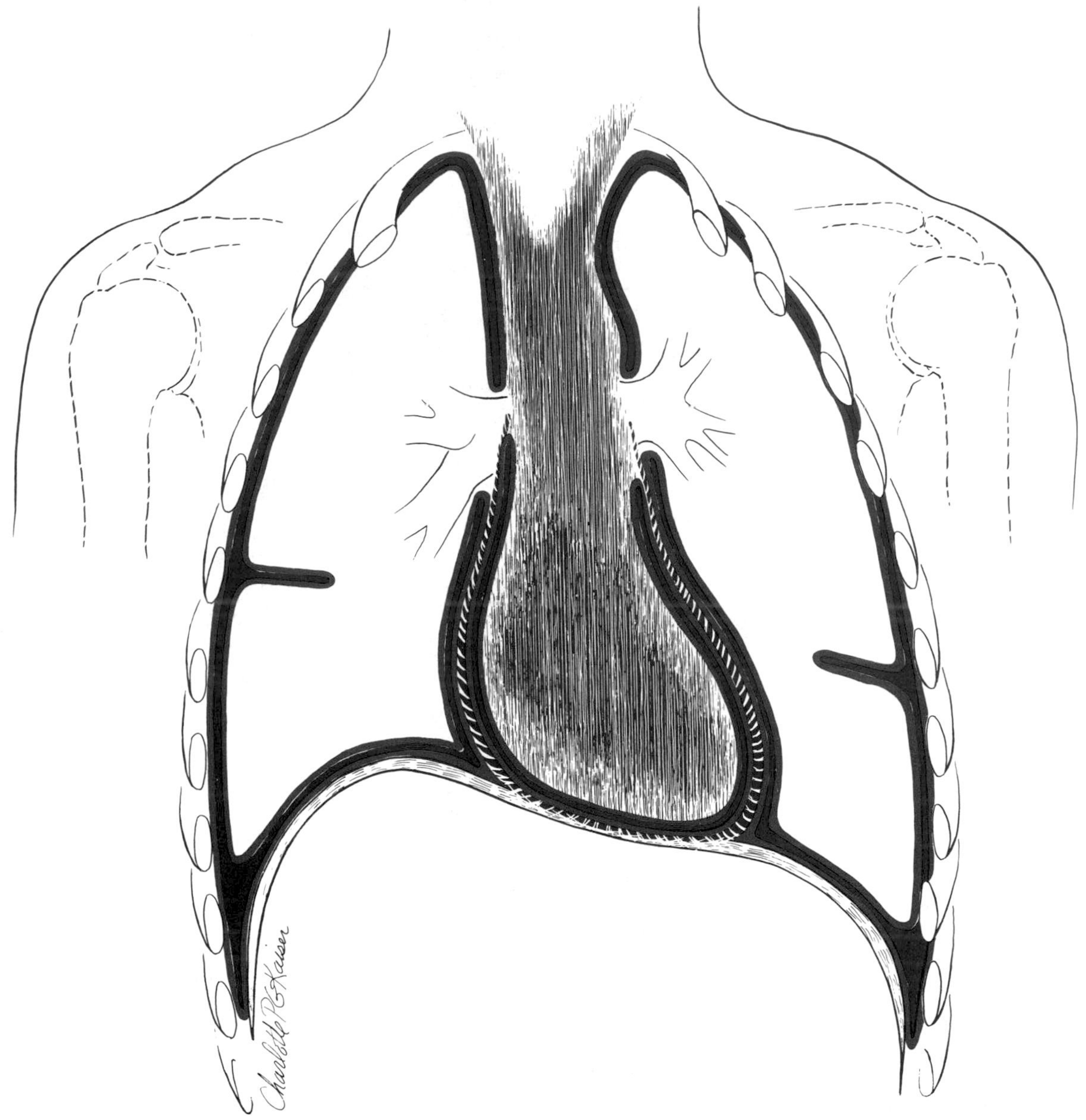

FIGURE *19-17.*
The relation of the pleural and pericardial sacs shown in a schematic coronal section of the thorax. Note the costodiaphragmatic recesses. The serous cavities are *black*, and the serous membranes are *red*. The fibrous pericardium is shown as a heavy dashed line, which blends the central component (tendon) of the diaphragm.

subatmospheric pleural pressure, whereas atmospheric pressure acting on the outside of the wall and on the inside of the lung is the force that keeps them together.

The balance of hydrostatic and colloid osmotic pressures in the capillaries of the visceral and parietal pleurae is such that subatmospheric pleural pressure creates a small, but definite, pressure gradient, which causes a continuous movement of fluid across the pleural cavity from the systemic capillaries to the pulmonary capillaries of the visceral pleura. This pleural fluid lubricates the pleural surfaces and facilitates their movement on one another. If the pulmonary capillary pressure becomes elevated, the visceral pleura will no longer be able to absorb the transudate, and fluid will accumulate in the pleural cavity. A rise in the protein concentration of pleural fluid, itself, will lead to the same outcome. The subatmospheric pleural pressure may cause some movement of air across the alveolar walls and the visceral pleura into the pleural cavity. The air will be absorbed promptly by the capillaries of the parietal pleura because the partial pressure of blood gases in the systemic venous capillaries is much lower than intrapleural pressure. Thus, physiologic conditions prevent the accumulation of both air and fluid between the pleural layers. Therefore, as long as the muscles of respiration can overcome the resistance to air entry into the lungs, the lungs and the chest wall will not separate and will move in unison. When the lung cannot expand with the chest wall because of airway obstruction, expansion of the chest wall causes a further fall in intrapleural pressure, which leads to augmented exudation of fluid from the pleural capillaries. Thus, the space between the collapsed lung and the chest wall will always be filled with exudate as long as the surface of the lung and wall are intact.

The role of the ribs in increasing the anteroposterior and transverse diameters of the thorax by their pump-handle and bucket-handle type movements has been discussed earlier (see Fig. 19-7). Two-thirds of the increase in thoracic capacity is due to diaphragmatic movements. This is so, even in those individuals in whom costal breathing is quite pronounced. The domes of the diaphragm rise from the margins of the inferior thoracic aperture as high as the fourth intercostal space on the right and the fifth space on the left. In normal, quiet breathing, rhythmic contraction of the peripherally placed muscle fibers produces an up-and-down movement of the domes without much change in their curvature. A deep inspiration calls for maximal excursion of the ribs and causes the domes to flatten as well. The inferior thoracic aperture becomes fixed by the contraction of the abdominal muscles, especially the quadratus lumborum, providing a firm base for diaphragmatic contraction. With the descent of the diaphragm, abdominal viscera are compressed, and the mediastinum is elongated. Powerful diaphragmatic contraction also elevates the lower ribs because the fibers of the diaphragm run upward from the costal arch. Diaphragmatic contraction contributes to the bucket-handle movement of the ribs.

Accessory muscles are also recruited in an increased inspiratory effort. These are the scalene muscles and the sternomastoids, which elevate the superior thoracic aperture (and the entire rib cage with it), and the muscles of the pectoral girdle, which act from their humeral insertion and elevate the ribs if the arms are fixed. Consequently, patients in respiratory distress lean on their elbows to immobilize their humeri, and they prefer the sitting to the supine position because their abdominal contents do not bulge so much into the chest.

In normal breathing, expiration is largely passive, owing to the elastic recoil of lungs and rib cage and the relaxation of the diaphragm. The abdominal muscles play an important role in forced expiration. They fix the margins of the inferior thoracic aperture so that the intercostal and subcostal muscles can depress the ribs. More important, however, by raising intra-abdominal pressure they push the abdominal contents into the chest, which is permitted by the relaxed diaphragm. These contractions are spasmodic in violent expiratory efforts such as coughing and sneezing, but are more refined and controlled during phonation. They may also play some role in the course of normal respiration.

RECOMMENDED READINGS

Basmajian JV, DeLuca CJ. Muscles of respiration. In: Muscles alive: their functions revealed by electromyography. 5th ed. Baltimore: Williams & Wilkins, 1985.

Baue AE. Chest wall, pleura, lungs and diaphragm. In: Davis JK, ed. Clinical surgery. St. Louis: CV Mosby, 1987.

Campbell EJM, Agostoni E, Davis JN. The respiratory muscles: mechanics and neural control. 2nd ed. London: Lloyd-Luke, 1970.

Chudnoff J, Shapiro H. Two cases of complete situs inversus. Anat Rec 1939;74:189.

Conley DM, Rosse C. The digital anatomist: interactive atlas of thoracic viscera (CD-ROM). Seattle: University of Washington School of Medicine, 1996.

David PR, Troup JDG. Human thoracic diameters at rest and during activity. J Anat 1966;100:397.

Dwinnell FL Jr. Studies on the nerve endings of the visceral pleura. Am J Anat 1966;118:217.

Farkas GA, DeCramer M, Rochester DF, DeTroyer A. Contractile properties of intercostal muscles and their functional significance. J Appl Physiol 1985;59:528.

Gray DJ, Gardner ED. The human sternochondral joints. Anat Rec 1943;87:235.

Hollinshead WH. Anatomy for surgeons: vol 2, the thorax, abdomen, and pelvis. 2nd ed. New York: Harper & Row, 1971.

Jackson CM. On the developmental topography of the thoracic and abdominal viscera. Anat Rec 1909;3:361.

Kubik S. Surgical anatomy of the thorax. Philadelphia: WB Saunders, 1970.

Lachman E. A comparison of the posterior boundaries of the lungs and pleura as demonstrated on the cadaver and on the roentgenogram of the living. Anat Rec 1942;83:521.

McLoud TC, Flower CDR. Imaging the pleura: sonography, CT and MR imaging. Am J Roentgenol 1991;156:1145.

Morrissey BM, Bisset RAL. The right inferior lung margin: anatomy and clinical implication. Br J Radiol 1993;66:503.

Munro RR, Adams, C. Electromyography of the intercostal muscles in connected speech. Electromyography 1971;11:365.

Peters RM. The mechanical basis of respiration. Boston: Little, Brown, 1969.

Scatarige JC, Hamper UM, Shet S, Allen HA. Parasternal sonography of the internal mammary vessels: technique, normal anatomy, and lymphadenopathy. Radiology 1989;172:453.

Hollinshead's Textbook of Anatomy, by Cornelius Rosse and Penelope Gaddum-Rosse.
Lippincott-Raven Publishers, Philadelphia, © 1997.

CHAPTER 20

The Lungs

The lungs are paired organs specialized for the exchange of gases between atmospheric air and the blood. Their essential tissue is a squamous epithelium, a single attenuated layer of cells that forms the walls of minute spaces, the **alveoli**, and intervenes between capillaries of the pulmonary circulation and the air contained in the alveoli. The alveoli are connected to the exterior by a branching system of tubes, the **bronchial tree**, and remain filled with air even during expiration; they account for the greatest volume of the lungs by far. When the lung is normally distended with air, the chest sounds hollow to percussion, and the lungs remain afloat if immersed in water. If air has never entered the lungs, as in a stillbirth, the solid, glandlike lung tissue sinks in water. The bronchi and blood vessels constitute, by comparison, a small amount of tissue in the interior of this delicate, air-filled sponge, and when the alveoli collapse, the lung or one of its lobes or segments shrinks to a size many times smaller than that of its normally inflated state.

DEVELOPMENTAL CONSIDERATIONS

The tracheobronchial tree develops as a ventral diverticulum of the foregut that elongates and undergoes repeated buddings, yielding about 20 generations of endodermal tubes on both the right and the left side. These buddings entrap splanchnic mesoderm of the embryonic mediastinum. This branching establishes the anatomic pattern of the airways, the most distal of which are the alveolar sacs and the most proximal, the right and left principal bronchi. All but the main bronchi become embedded in the substance of the growing lungs. The surfaces of the lungs come to be delineated and defined by the visceral pleura as the developing lungs contact the embryonic pleural sacs, indent them, and expand with them into the thoracic cavity (see Chap. 19; Fig. 19-12). From the mesoderm entrapped among the future airways, smooth muscle and cartilage differentiate for the support of the bronchial epithelial lining. The pulmonary arterial and venous capillary beds and larger vessels, which hook up proximally with the arterial and venous ends of the developing heart, are also derived from the same mesoderm.

The internal anatomy of the lungs conforms to a segmental pattern laid down during development by the budding of the bronchi. The **bronchopulmonary segments** are the anatomic units of the lung. Clinical evaluation, as well as surgical resection, of diseased portions of the lungs relies on the anatomy of bronchopulmonary segmentation. Before dealing with the bronchial tree and the bronchopulmonary segments, the external anatomy of the lungs is discussed.

EXTERNAL ANATOMY OF THE LUNGS

The pliable lungs have assumed the shape of the space available to them on each side of the mediastinum in the thoracic cavity (Fig. 20-1). When they are removed from the chest in the fresh or the fixed state, each lung is roughly conical, presenting a tapered upper end, the **apex**, and a broad **base**. On each lung there are three external surfaces (costal, diaphragmatic, and medial) separated from each other by **borders** or margins (anterior and inferior). All surfaces are completely covered in visceral pleura, which unites with the mediastinal parietal pleura around the **root of the lung**. The root of the lung is a relatively narrow pedicle that suspends the lung from the mediastinum in the pleural cavity and enters its substance at the **pulmonary hilum**. **Fissures** divide the lungs into **lobes**. Typically, the left lung is divided by the **oblique fissure** into an upper and a lower lobe, whereas the right lung is divided into upper, lower, and middle lobes by the **oblique** and **horizontal fissures**. In the depths of the fissures, visceral pleura covers the *interlobar surfaces*, where it is in contact with itself; over all other surfaces visceral pleura is in contact with parietal pleura.

Even though the pleural sacs intervene between the lung and all other intrathoracic structures, several of these structures in contact with the lung through the pleura leave impressions on the pulmonary surfaces that are perceptible in the fixed, but not in the fresh, lung.

Surfaces and Borders

The **apex** fits into the cupula of the pleura and, in the lateral portions of the superior thoracic aperture, rises into the base of the neck 3 cm above the medial third of the clavicle. It is level with the spine of the first thoracic vertebra. The medial surface of the right apex is in contact with the esophagus and the trachea, whereas on the left, branches of the arch of the aorta (common carotid and left subclavian arteries) separate the lung from the trachea. The coarse tracheal breath sounds are, therefore, transmitted to the right apex but not to the left. The subclavian arteries and veins arch over both lungs in the superior thoracic aperture, making their impressions on the lungs.

The **costal surface** is convex and extends from the vertebrae to the sternum. The **diaphragmatic surface** is concave and it is separated from the costal and medial surfaces by a sharp **inferior border**, which extends into the costodiaphragmatic recesses. On the right side, the resonant percussion note obtained over the lungs is gradually replaced by dullness as the inferior pulmonary border is approached. This is due to the presence of the solid liver under the right dome of the diaphragm. On the left, the inferior border cannot be mapped out by percussion

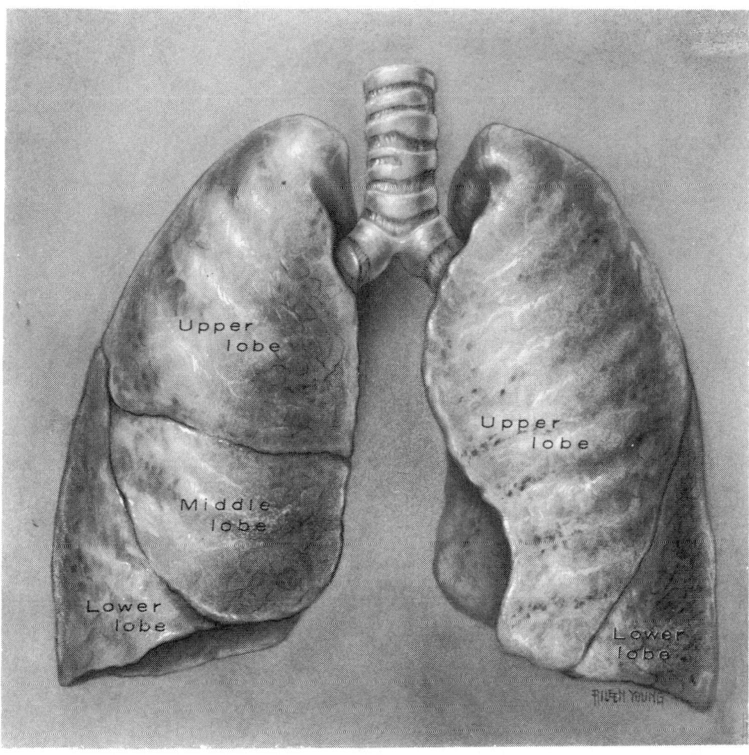

FIGURE *20-1.*
Anterior view of the lungs and the lower end of the trachea.

because the fundus of the stomach under the left dome of the diaphragm is full of air and yields a resonant percussion note, like the lung itself. The surface projection of the inferior border of the lung, in relation to the pleural reflection lines is mentioned in the previous chapter and is illustrated in Figure 20-2.

The sharp **anterior margin** occupies the sternocostal recesses and separates costal and medial surfaces of the lung. On the left, the margin is indented by the heart, creating the *cardiac notch* (see Fig. 20-1). The small tonguelike process of the lung that projects below the notch is the *lingula* (Fig. 20-3*B*). It is part of the left upper lobe. On the **medial surface**, anterior to the hilum of the lung, the *cardiac impression* is created by the right atrium and a larger impression is created by the left ventricle, on the respective sides (see Fig. 20-3). Behind the hilum, the right lung is grooved by the esophagus and the left lung is grooved by the descending aorta. Medial and costal surfaces merge with one another posteriorly, and here the lung is related to the vertebral bodies. The arch of the aorta makes an impression on the left lung as it passes above the hilum, and the azygos vein grooves the right lung as it arches over its hilum.

The Hilum

The hilum is a somewhat wedge-shaped area at which the structures that form the root of the lung enter and leave the organ (see Fig. 20-3). Most posterior in the upper part of each hilum is the bronchus; in front of it are the pulmonary artery and, in an even more anterior plane, the superior pulmonary vein. The inferior pulmonary vein is below the bronchus and occupies the space between the leaves of the *pulmonary ligament*. Usually, two bronchi are severed at the right hilum when the entire lung is removed; these are the upper lobe bronchus and the interlobar portion of the main bronchus. In the left hilum, only one bronchus is severed. The pulmonary artery is located above, rather than directly in front of, the left bronchus.

The hilum also transmits the bronchial vessels, pulmonary nerve plexuses, and lymphatics. Several bronchopulmonary lymph nodes are also located in it. The **pulmonary ligament**, the inferiorly redundant part of the pleural sleeve that surrounds the root of the lung, provides the dead space in which the root of the lung may move up and down during respiratory movements as diaphragmatic contractions pull down and release the mediastinum.

Lobes and Fissures

As the lung grows, the spaces or fissures that separate individual bronchopulmonary buds or segments become obliterated except along two planes, evident in the fully developed lungs as the oblique and horizontal fissures. Although the right lung has three lobes and the left only two, the bronchopulmonary segments in right and left lungs correspond. Both anatomically and clinically, what is of significance is the underlying pattern of bronchopulmonary segmentation; the division into lobes is inconsequential. Nevertheless, the concept of lobes, and the position of fissures, is useful in locating the bronchopulmonary segments.

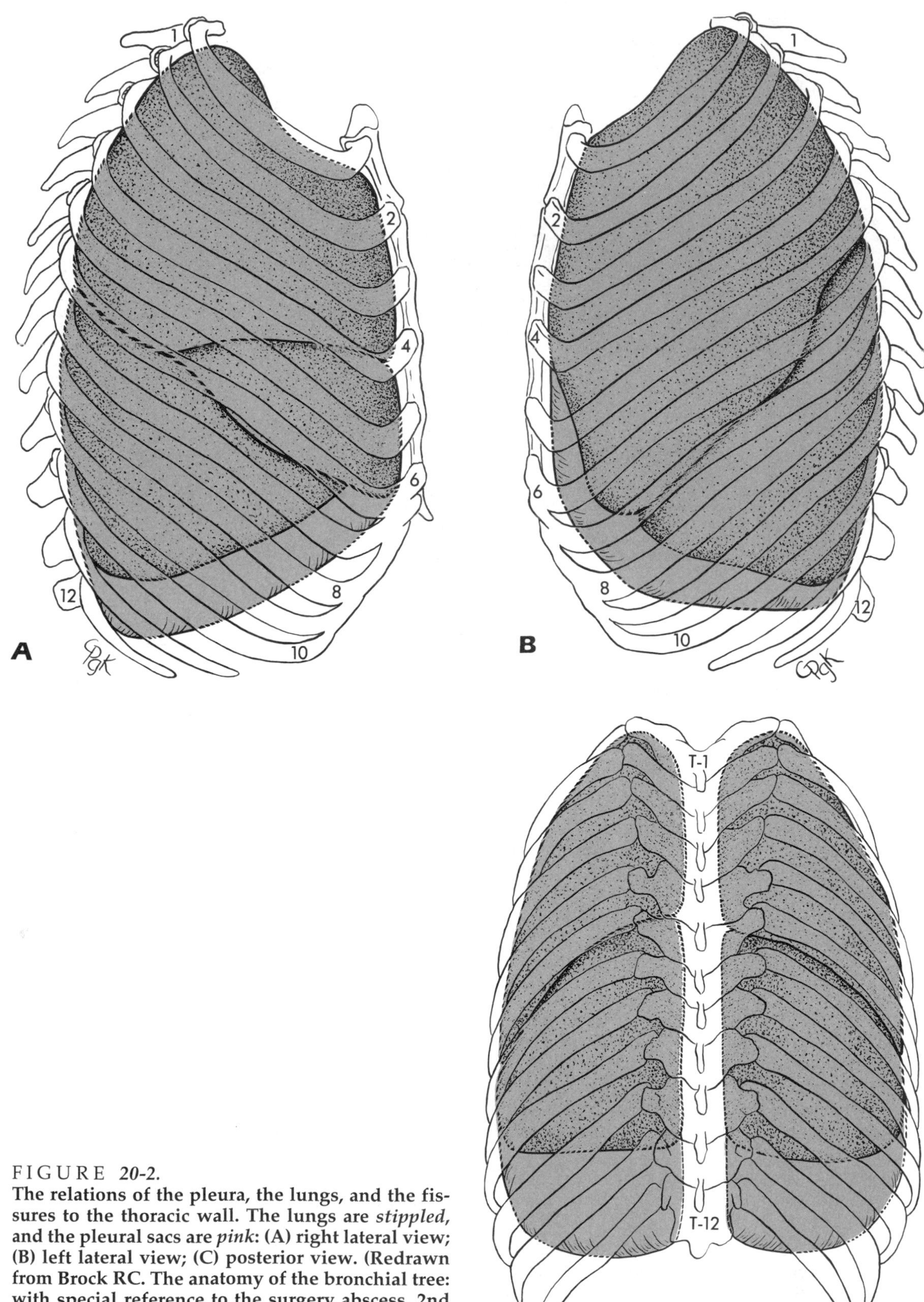

FIGURE *20-2.*
The relations of the pleura, the lungs, and the fissures to the thoracic wall. The lungs are *stippled*, and the pleural sacs are *pink*: (A) right lateral view; (B) left lateral view; (C) posterior view. (Redrawn from Brock RC. The anatomy of the bronchial tree: with special reference to the surgery abscess. 2nd ed. London, Oxford University Press, 1954.)

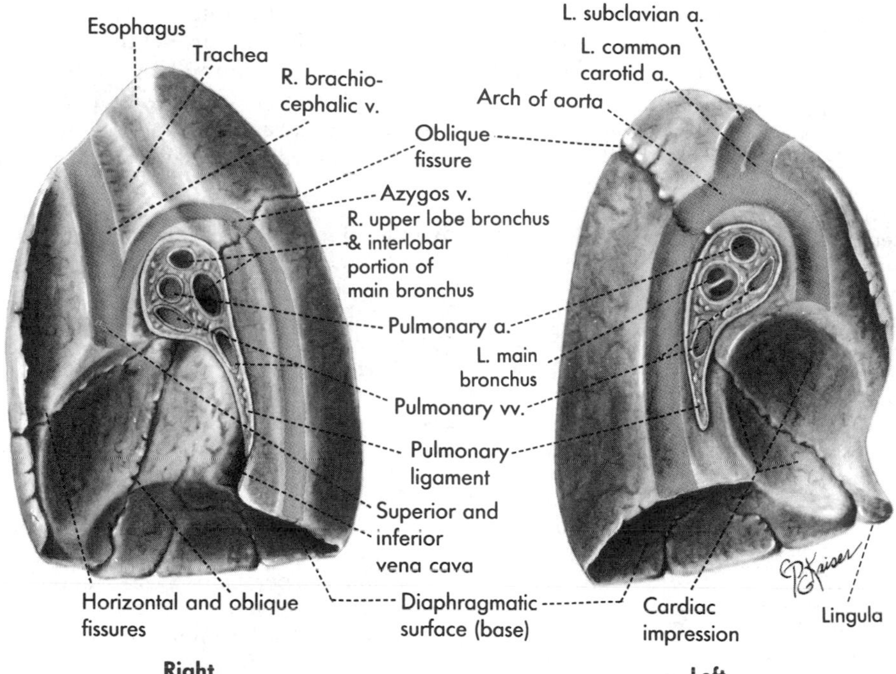

FIGURE *20-3.*
The mediastinal surface of the right and left lungs.

The fissures facilitate the movements of the lobes in relation to one another, which accommodates the greater distention and movement of the lower lobes during respiration. The lung may be divided completely by the fissures, and the lobes remain held together only at the hilum by the bronchi and pulmonary vessels. However, more often than not the fissures are incomplete or may be absent altogether, as they are between the majority of bronchopulmonary segments.

Both lungs are sliced across from their costal and mediastinal surfaces by an **oblique fissure**. This fissure cuts the vertebral border of the lung at a variable distance below the apex. However, the level of the fourth or fifth thoracic spine is an adequately accurate guide to it for mapping the fissures on the surface of the chest. The plane of the oblique fissure slopes forward and downward to intersect the diaphragmatic surface just behind the anteroinferior border of the lung. The surface projection of the fissure follows roughly the sixth rib (or the vertebral border of the abducted and protracted scapula) and intersects the inferior border of the lung at the anterior axillary line (see Fig. 20-2). On the left, the fissure is somewhat lower and corresponds more closely to the seventh rib in front of the midaxillary line.

In the right lung, a **horizontal fissure** separates two bronchopulmonary segments into the **middle lobe**, the equivalents of which, on the left, remain attached to the upper lobe. The horizontal fissure commences in the oblique fissure as it crosses the midaxillary line and intersects the anterior border of the lung on level with the fourth costal cartilage (see Fig. 20-2). The middle lobe is between the horizontal and oblique fissures.

Owing to the forward and downward slope of the oblique fissure, the left and right upper lobes and the middle lobe are anterior, as well as superior, to the lower lobes. Upper and middle lobes project to the anterior chest wall, where they are available for clinical evaluation, whereas none of the inferior lobe is accessible anteriorly. The converse is true from the posterior view. The pulmonary projections posteriorly are dominated by the lower lobes; little of the upper lobes are available for examination in the back.

Sometimes, especially in the infant, fissures of varying depth can be seen in abnormal locations on the lung, delimiting anomalous lobes. Usually, the anomalous "lobes" correspond to the normal bronchopulmonary segments. The most striking abnormalities of lobation are the occurrence of a "middle lobe" in the left lung (about 8%) and the very rare *azygos lobe* in the right, produced by the azygos vein's cutting into the pleura and the apex of the lung.

INTERNAL ANATOMY OF THE LUNGS

The Bronchial Tree

The budding of the lung diverticulum, which lays down the pattern of the bronchial tree, does not progress in a strictly dichotomous fashion. Therefore, asymmetric branching and trifurcation of the bronchi normally occur. Knowledge of the arrangement of the first three or four generations of bronchi has anatomic and clinical significance. The bronchi provide the framework of the lung parenchyma, and the major branches of the pulmonary arteries and veins conform to the bronchial tree in a definable manner. Not only resection of parts of the lung, but also interpretation of clinical and radiologic findings, have to rely on the internal anatomy of the lung.

The **bronchi** are hollow tubes kept patent by incomplete rings or plates of hyaline cartilage. They are lined by respiratory, pseudostratified, ciliated epithelium, which is rich in goblet cells. The cilia beat toward the trachea. The submucosa contains serous and mucous glands, which open into the lumen. A large amount of elastic tissue is present in the submucosa, which permits elongation and retraction of the bronchi with the respiratory movements. At the termination of the bronchi, the elastic tissue fans out into the interalveolar connective tissue septa of the lung. Within the confines of the cartilage plates, the bronchi are encircled by smooth muscle fibers arranged in two helical strands. The muscle is under neural control and is also sensitive to such stimulants in the circulation as histamine, serotonin, and norepinephrine.

The Trachea and Principal and Lobar Bronchi

The larynx is a highly specialized sphincter located at the branching point of the alimentary and respiratory tracts (see Chap. 34). The **trachea** is the distal continuation of the larynx and it descends through the neck into the thorax, lying anterior to the esophagus. Its relations in the neck and mediastinum are described in Chapters 29 and 22, respectively. The trachea bifurcates into the **right** and **left principal bronchi**, and from each of these primary bronchi originate the secondary or **lobar bronchi**. On the right, the *superior lobar bronchus* branches off from the principal bronchus before the latter enters the hilum. The remaining main stem, sometimes called the *interlobar bronchus*, gives off, more distally, the *middle lobe bronchus*, which runs forward and downward. The main or interlobar bronchus becomes the *bronchus of the inferior lobe*.

The left principal bronchus gives off the *superior lobar bronchus* as soon as it has entered the hilum, and the remaining main stem becomes the bronchus of the inferior lobe. The counterpart of the middle lobe bronchus on the left is the *lingular bronchus*, which forms the lower division of the left upper lobe bronchus. It serves the lingula, which corresponds to the middle lobe on the right. Only the upper division of the superior lobe bronchus is equivalent to the right superior lobar bronchus. The bronchial tree is illustrated in Figure 20-4 and shows the first three or four generations of bronchi.

The division of the trachea into principal bronchi takes place behind the ascending aorta, to the right of, and below, the arch of the aorta. The bifurcation lies in the cadaver at about the level of the sternal angle (lower border of the fourth thoracic vertebra); however, in x-ray films of living persons, it is much lower, usually at the level of the seventh thoracic vertebra. It is marked internally by a ridge, the *carina*, that separates the openings of the two principal bronchi.

The **right principal bronchus** is wider than the left one and leaves the trachea at an angle of about 25°. It passes downward and laterally behind the superior vena cava and reaches the hilum of the lung after a course of only about 2.5 cm. The **left principal bronchus** is slightly smaller in diameter than the right one and almost twice as long (some 4 to 5 cm). It leaves the trachea at an angle of about 45° and passes below the arch of the aorta and the left pulmonary artery on its way to the hilum of the left lung.

A foreign body inhaled into the trachea is much more likely to lodge in the right bronchus because this is more directly in line with the trachea and because it is of larger caliber than the left main bronchus. The left bronchus, in spite of its greater length, is more difficult to handle surgically than the right one because of its vascular relations. Both bronchi are mobile and pliable, however, and can be easily manipulated and moved by a bronchoscope.

Bronchoscopy. The bronchoscope is a telescope with a built-in light source that can be passed into the bronchi through the larynx and the trachea. Bronchoscopy is usually performed under general anesthesia, although it can be done in a conscious individual if the pharyngeal, laryngeal, and tracheal mucosae are anesthetized. It provides direct inspection of the interior of the bronchi. Foreign bodies may be located, grasped by forceps, and removed from the lung through the bronchoscope. The scope is also used for obtaining biopsies of bronchial lesions and bronchial washings in which exfoliated neoplastic cells may be identified.

Segmental Bronchi

The third generation of bronchi serve wedge-shaped districts of the lung that are defined as the bronchopulmonary segments. These tertiary bronchi are designated, therefore, as the *segmental bronchi*. The basic branching pattern is found on the right and is only slightly modified on the left. There are ten segmental bronchi on each side, and they are designated by names identical with those of the bronchopulmonary segments they serve. The bronchi and the segments are numbered in definite sequence starting at the apex (see Fig. 20-4).

The right superior lobar bronchus divides into three segmental bronchi: the **apical** (1), **posterior** (2), and **anterior** (3). The middle lobe bronchus bifurcates into the **lateral** (4) and **medial** (5) segmental bronchi. The remaining five segmental bronchi are branches of the inferior lobar bronchus. The first of these, the **superior** (6), arises high on the posterior wall of the main stem and serves the apical area of the lower lobe. The other four are called basal bronchi because they distribute to the base of the lung. They are named according to their anatomic positions: **medial basal** (7), **anterior basal** (8), **lateral basal** (9), and **posterior basal** (10).

On the left, the apical and posterior bronchi spring by a common stem, the **apicoposterior bronchus**, from the upper division of the superior lobe bronchus, which also yields the anterior bronchus. The two bronchi derived from the inferior division (lingular bronchus) are called **superior** and **inferior lingular** (4 and 5, respectively),

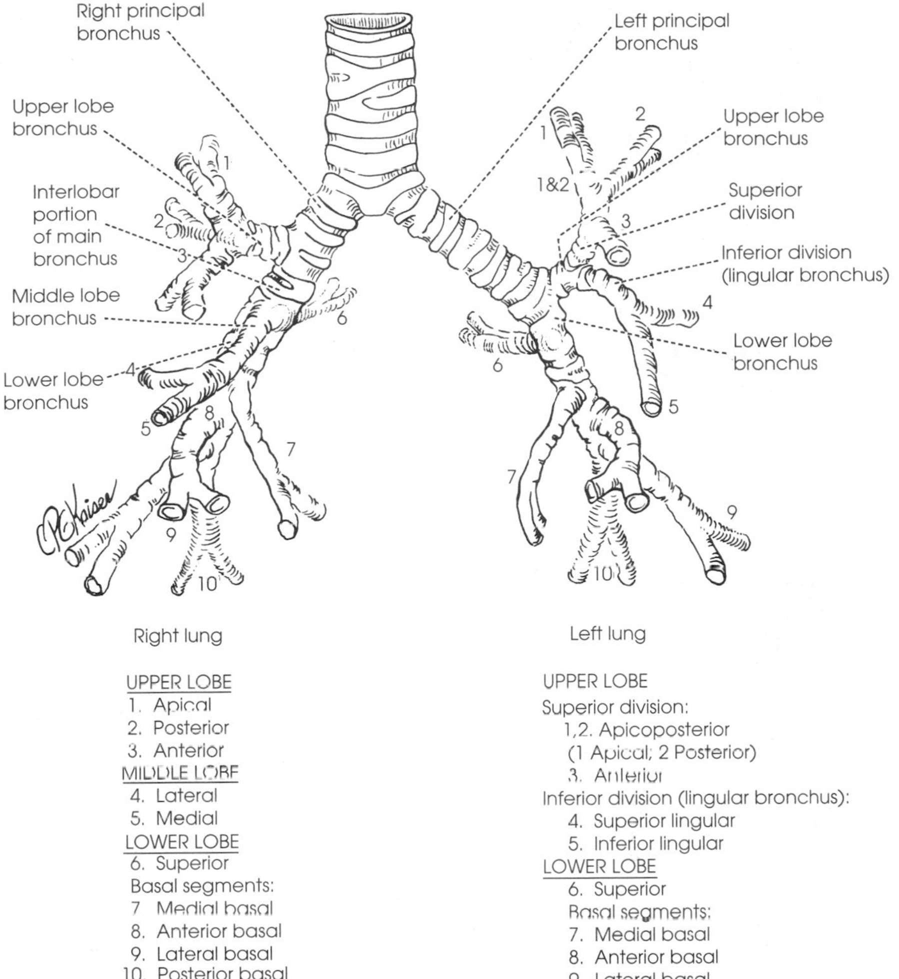

FIGURE *20-4.*
The tracheobronchial tree, with the segmental bronchi identified.

rather than lateral and medial bronchi as on the right. The segmental bronchi in the left lower lobe are identical with those on the right, including the presence of the left medial basal bronchus, which was erroneously omitted from earlier descriptions.

Variations. The branching pattern described in the foregoing section is the *ideal* pattern, which serves as reference for variations that are chiefly the concern of pulmonary specialists. No two lungs are exactly alike. Many variations in the pattern of the bronchi have been described. Two segmental bronchi that usually arise separately may share a common stem as the apical and posterior bronchi on the left usually do. Additional bronchi may arise from the main stem and distribute to a segment that already has its regular bronchus. A common variation of this type is a *subsuperior bronchus*, which distributes to a zone between the superior and posterior basal segments. A portion of a segment may receive a subsegmental bronchus from a neighboring segment.

Bronchoscopy. It is possible to inspect the orifices of the segmental bronchi by bronchoscopy (discussed in the previous section); some even admit the bronchoscope. The directions in which the orifices of the various bronchi face are, therefore, of importance to the bronchoscopist; so is the sequence in which the orifices are encountered by the advancing bronchoscope.

Bronchograms. Although the bronchi are normally not visible on a plain film, they can be demonstrated radiographically by coating their mucosa with a radiopaque substance. The segmental and subsegmental bronchi can be identified on such a film (Fig. 20-5).

The Respiratory Portion of the Bronchial Tree

Beyond the segmental bronchi, approximately ten more generations of bronchi are produced, the most distal of which are approximately 1 mm in diameter. All these tubes retain the basic structure described earlier in this section. The next two to three generations of airways are the **bronchioles**, which lack cartilage, but otherwise are similar to the smallest bronchi (Fig. 20-6). The most distal of the bronchioles, the **terminal bronchiole**, forms the stem of the respiratory unit of the lung,

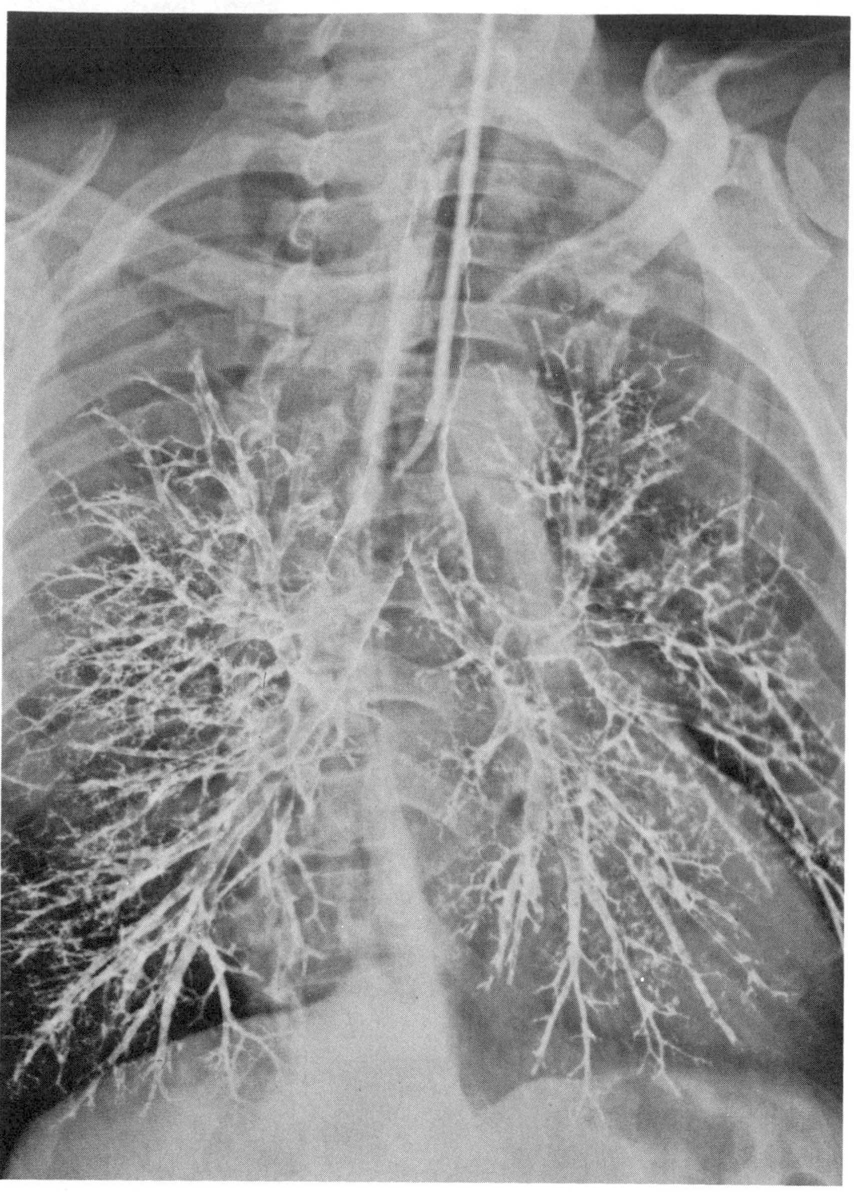

FIGURE 20-5.
A bronchogram of a cadaver chest in which both principal bronchi and most of the segmental bronchi are visualized. (Courtesy of the late Dr. E. Allen Boyden.)

known as the **acinus**, or lobule. As the name implies, the acinus is reminiscent of a bunch of berries, representing the alveoli. Each acinus contains over 3000 alveoli, and there are nearly 100,000 acini in the lung.

Within the acinus, each terminal bronchiole branches into several **respiratory bronchioles**. These are the most proximal respiratory passages through which gas exchange can take place. Their muscular walls are studded with a few alveoli (see Fig. 20-6). The respiratory bronchioles give rise to the **alveolar ducts**, which lead into the **alveolar sacs**. The walls of the ducts and sacs are devoid of muscle and are densely crowded with alveoli. Alveolar sacs intricately interlock with their neighbors, including those of neighboring acini, and entrap between them the pulmonary capillary bed. In these most peripheral respiratory passages, the walls consist almost exclusively of the attenuated squamous epithelium of the alveolar wall, supported on a basement membrane. The sparse connective tissue in the interalveolar septa contains elastic fibers and supports the capillaries on the surface of the alveoli.

Blood Vessels and Lymphatics of the Lungs

The lung has two circulations, the pulmonary and the bronchial. The latter is part of the systemic circulation and carries blood for the nutrition of the bronchi and the connective tissue of the lung. The bronchial arteries are insignificant in size by comparison with the pulmonary arteries, which convey as much blood for gas exchange to the lungs per unit time as the aorta delivers to the entire body. Four pulmonary veins return the same volume of oxygenated blood to the left atrium; the small bronchial veins drain into the azygos and hemiazygos systems.

The pulmonary arteries end ultimately in dense capillary networks around the alveolar sacs, and the confluence of the venules that arise from these capillaries forms pulmonary veins. The capillary bed fed by the bronchial arteries is in the walls of the bronchi and in the connective tissue of the lung. Anastomoses do exist between the bronchial and pulmonary systems at the capillary level and also between some larger, precapillary branches of the bronchial and pulmonary arteries.

Because the aortic pressure is normally much higher than the pulmonary arterial pressure, the bronchial arteries deliver to the pulmonary capillaries a small amount of blood that is already oxygenated. These connections become important when there is chronic interference with the pulmonary arterial circulation. In such instances, the bronchial arteries, and their connections to the pulmonary arteries, may become very much enlarged and, in certain cases, may account for much of the arterial circulation of the lung.

The Pulmonary Arteries

The common stem of the right and left pulmonary arteries is the **pulmonary trunk** (Fig. 20-7). The trunk arises from the right ventricle and has its entire course within the pericardial sac. Its anatomy is described with that of the heart in the next chapter.

The bifurcation of the pulmonary trunk takes place on the left of the ascending aorta in the concavity of the aortic arch. The **left pulmonary artery** immediately leaves the pericardial sac. Just outside the pericardial sac, it is connected to the arch of the aorta by the *ligamentum arteriosum*, the fibrous remains of the *ductus arteriosus*, which in the fetus served as a shunt between the two vessels. The **right pulmonary artery** is longer than the left, and much of it is covered by serous pericardium. It runs horizontally behind the ascending aorta and superior vena cava before it leaves the pericardial sac in the concavity of the arch of the aorta. The artery emerges from the sac posterior to the superior vena cava.

Soon after leaving the pericardial sac, both right and left pulmonary arteries arch over the principal bronchi as they enter the hilum of the lung. Thereafter, both arteries descend, lying deep in the interlobar fissures lateral to the bronchi. The left pulmonary artery crosses the left principal bronchus and, at the hilum, is superior to it, whereas the right pulmonary artery crosses the interlobar portion of the right bronchus, having given off a major branch to the upper lobe (*truncus anterior*) before it enters the hilum. The branches of the pulmonary artery closely follow the segmental bronchi and receive names and numbers to correspond with the bronchi (see Fig. 20-7). These segmental arteries can be approached and dissected in the depth of the interlobar fissures. Peripheral branches of the segmental pulmonary arteries are not strictly confined to their own bronchopulmonary segments and tend to enter neighboring segments.

The foregoing description emphasizes the basic branching pattern of the pulmonary artery. There are numerous deviations from this pattern; however, these are the concern of the thoracic surgeon. On the right, the upper lobe receives two arteries in addition to the

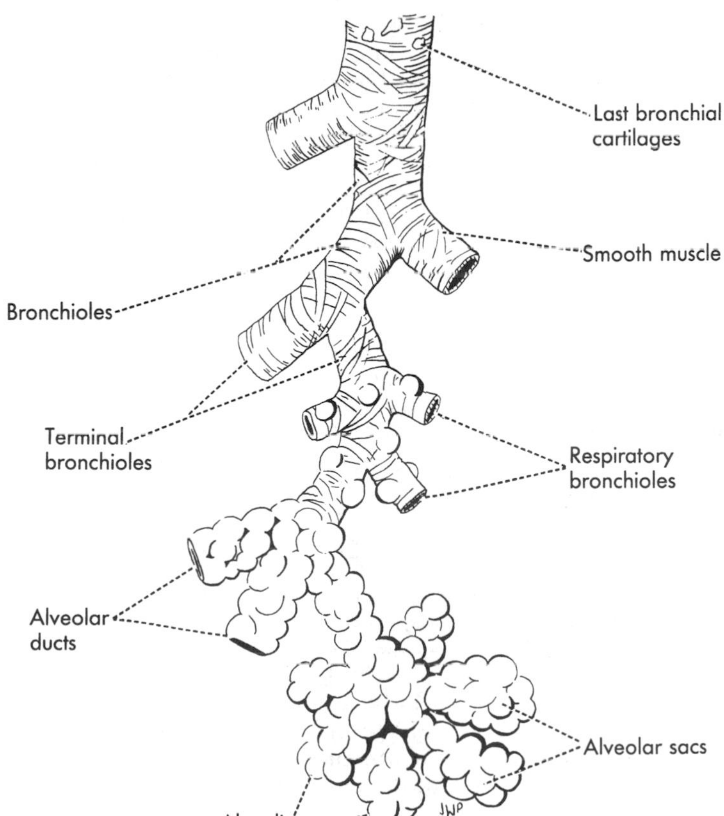

FIGURE *20-6.*
The respiratory portion of the bronchial tree. (Courtesy of the late Dr. E. Allen Boyden.)

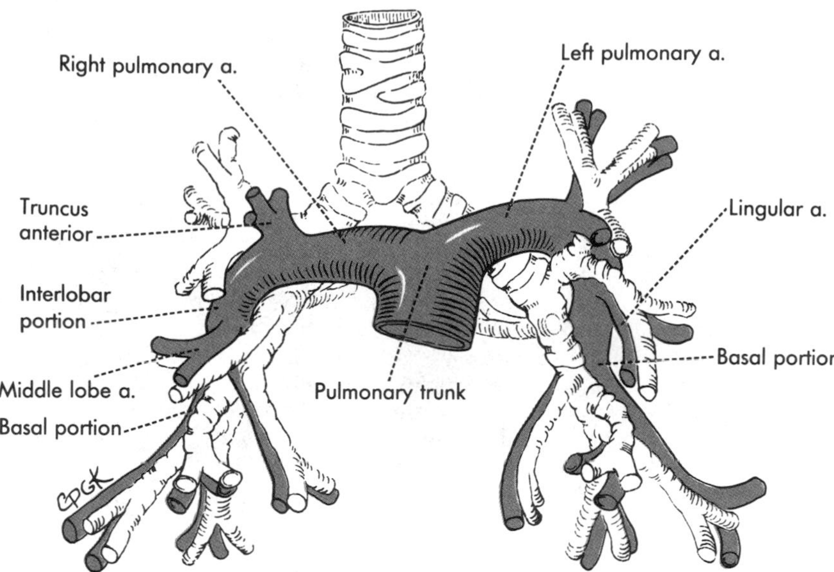

FIGURE 20-7.
The pulmonary arteries and their branches related to the bronchial tree.

three segmental branches of the upper lobe artery (*truncus anterior*). These additional arteries ascend to the posterior and anterior segments from the interlobar portion of the artery. The left pulmonary artery, as a rule, has no truncus anterior. The left upper lobe receives as many as four to seven independent arteries, given off from the main trunk mostly in the interlobar fissure. This renders resection of the left upper lobe, or parts of it, particularly difficult.

Anomalous pulmonary arteries sometimes arise from the aorta or its major branches at the base of the neck. The most common origin for such a vessel is from the descending aorta in the thorax; however, they may arise even in the abdomen and reenter the thorax. The abnormal arteries from the descending aorta enter the lungs through the pulmonary ligament. They may supply an otherwise normal segment of lung; often the tissue they supply is abnormal and eventually must be removed by operation.

The Pulmonary Veins

A superior and an inferior pulmonary vein passes from the hilum of each lung to the left atrium (Fig. 20-8). The superior pulmonary veins collect blood from the right upper and middle lobes and from the left upper lobe. On both sides, the inferior veins drain the lower lobes. The primary tributaries of the pulmonary veins are related to given bronchopulmonary segments and are named and numbered according to the segmental bronchi. Typically, a pulmonary vein from each segment has two major tributaries. One of these passes along the bronchus and the pulmonary artery within the segment (*intrasegmental branch*), whereas the other runs along the inferior border of the segment (*infrasegmental branch*). The infrasegmental branches drain blood from neighboring segments, except when the intersegmental planes face into the fissures or onto the diaphragmatic surface of the lung. Here, and also in the substance of the lung, infrasegmental veins help demarcate the boundaries of the segments and serve as guides in the dissection and resection of the segments.

The pattern of union of the segmental veins is such that, on the right, the veins of the three upper lobe segments form a large vein, the *upper lobar vein*, which receives the *middle lobe vein*, and the two form the right superior pulmonary vein. The same is true on the left, the *lingular vein* substituting for the middle lobe vein. On both sides, the inferior pulmonary veins are formed by the confluence of two large veins, the *superior vein* and the *common basal vein*. The latter collects all the veins of the basal bronchopulmonary segments.

The left pulmonary veins empty closer together than do the right ones and about 25% of the time unite to open together instead of separately into the left atrium. The two right pulmonary veins usually terminate some distance apart and rarely fuse before entering the atrium. A more striking variation is the presence of three veins, one from each lobe.

The pattern of pulmonary veins shows even more variation than that of the arteries. Truly *anomalous pulmonary veins* sometimes occur. For example, one or more pulmonary veins instead of emptying into the left atrium will join the superior vena cava or its tributaries. Otherwise, they may empty directly or indirectly into the *right atrium*. Anomalous pulmonary veins may join the azygos system or esophageal veins as the venous plexuses of the lung buds connect to veins that surround the primitive gut. The drainage of pulmonary veins into systemic veins overloads the right side of the heart. Also, because oxygenated blood must be delivered to the left side of the heart if it is to be circulated to the body as a whole, the condition is incompatible with life unless the anomalous return is only partial or an intracardiac defect allows blood to be shunted from the right to the left side.

The Bronchial Arteries and Veins

The small bronchial arteries usually arise from the thoracic portion of the descending aorta, either directly or from a right intercostal artery at about the level of the tracheal bifurcation. They are rather easily broken in the dissecting laboratory when the lungs are mobilized for study. There may be only one bronchial artery to each lung, although multiple vessels are common. The bronchial arteries also arise fairly frequently from the arch of the aorta; sometimes one arises from a subclavian artery in the base of the neck. The bronchial arteries usually give off branches to the esophagus and then follow the bronchi into the lung, branching and rebranching with these as they supply the bronchi themselves and the adjacent connective tissue. The bronchial arteries send their branches along the interalveolar connective tissue septa to the pulmonary pleura.

The small **bronchial veins** unite along the bronchi to form a single vein that leaves the hilum and empties on the right side into the azygos vein and on the left into the hemiazygos system. Many of the bronchial veins end within the lungs in the tributaries of the pulmonary veins. The bronchial veins, therefore, return to the systemic veins somewhat less blood than the bronchial arteries deliver to the lung.

Lymphatics

Plexuses of lymphatic capillaries pervade the visceral pleura, the submucosa, and wall of the bronchi; the interalveolar septa, and other connective tissue planes of the lungs; and the walls of the larger blood vessels. Lymph flow participates in clearing exudate from the alveoli and the pleural cavity. Inhaled minute particulate matter, such as dust and carbon particles, are also conveyed by lymphatics and filtered out by the lymph nodes. The black appearance of smokers' lungs is due to carbon particles deposited in pulmonary lymphatics and lymph nodes. Lymphatics are the primary route of spread for bronchogenic carcinoma. Lymph nodes are always involved in tuberculosis of the lung. The calcification of the nodes induced by tuberculosis will be a permanent radiographic reminder of the disease after the primary infection has been resolved.

Lymph from all the lymphatic plexuses of the lung is drained toward the hilum by lymphatic vessels that follow the bronchi. The lymph flow is interrupted by numerous lymph nodes, many of which are situated at the forking points of the bronchi. The nodes may become sufficiently enlarged to compress the bronchi and produce collapse of segments or even lobes (atelectasis; middle lobe syndrome). Enlarged hilar lymph nodes produce a characteristic shadow on x-ray film.

The most peripheral nodes embedded in the substance of the lung are the **pulmonary nodes** (Fig. 20-9). These send their efferent lymphatics to the **bronchopulmonary nodes** situated at the hilum. Several groups of **tracheobronchial nodes**, located around the bifurcation of the trachea, receive the lymph from the hila and also from several mediastinal structures, including the heart. The largest of these nodes, the **paratracheal nodes**, lie more proximally along each side of the trachea. The efferents of the paratracheal nodes unite with the parasternal lymphatics to form the *bronchomediastinal lymph trunks*. These are the chief drainage vessels of the thoracic viscera, and they empty independently on each side of the neck in the angle of junction between the subclavian and internal jugular veins. The left trunk may join the thoracic duct, and the right trunk, the right lymph duct.

Lymphatics from each lung drain chiefly to tracheobronchial and paratracheal nodes on the homolateral side. Some, but not all, of the lymphatics from the left lower lobe drain to the right side of the trachea.

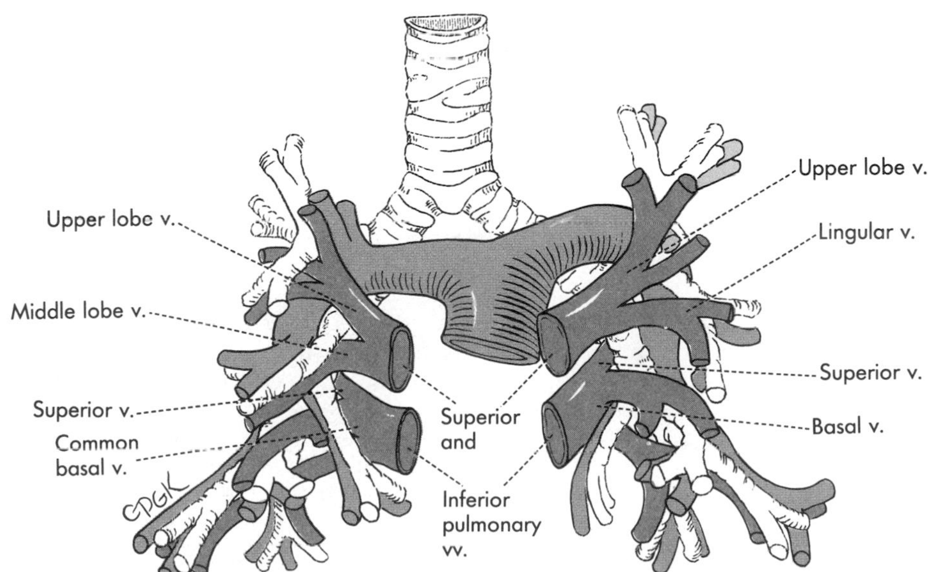

FIGURE *20-8.*
The pulmonary veins and their branches related to the pulmonary arteries and the bronchial tree.

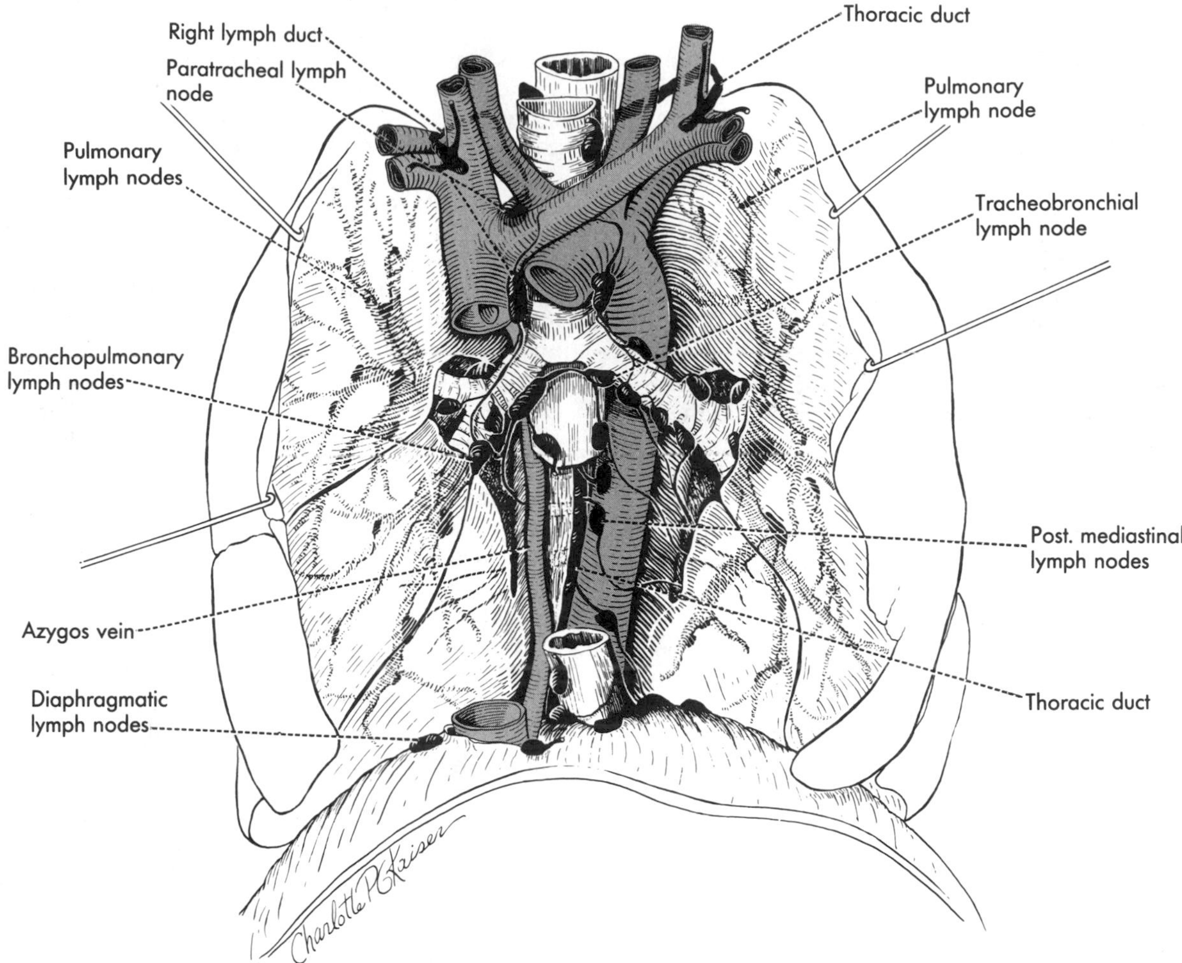

FIGURE *20-9.*
Lymph nodes and lymphatics of the lungs.

When visceral pleura adheres to parietal pleura owing to inflammatory or neoplastic processes, lymph from the lungs may drain with the lymphatics of the parietal pleura to the axillary, parasternal, or intercostal nodes, thus explaining the presence of carbon particles or tumor metastases in these nodes (see Chap. 19).

Nerve Supply of the Lung

Each lung is supplied by visceral efferent and visceral afferent nerve fibers through the **pulmonary plexuses**. How these fibers reach the pulmonary plexus from the sympathetic trunks and the vagi is described in Chapters 7 and 22. The pulmonary plexuses enter the hilum of the lung on the surface of the bronchi and the pulmonary arteries as extensions of the *cardiac plexus*, which lies in front of the tracheal bifurcation. **Visceral efferents** are contributed to the pulmonary plexuses by the **vagus** and **thoracic sympathetic ganglia**. The sympathetic fibers in the plexus are postganglionic and the vagal fibers are preganglionic. The latter relay in small parasympathetic ganglia that are located in the peribronchial plexuses, extensions of the pulmonary plexus. **Visceral afferents** from the lung have been demonstrated only in the vagus, and their cell bodies are in the superior and inferior vagal ganglia.

The **vagus** is motor to bronchial and bronchiolar smooth muscle and produces bronchoconstriction. The vagus apparently does not innervate smooth muscle in the wall of the pulmonary vessels. **Sympathetic visceral efferents** are motor to the bronchial glands and also produce vasoconstriction of pulmonary blood vessels. It is doubtful whether such fibers terminate on bronchiolar muscles, although it is well established that sympathomimetic drugs produce bronchodilation.

Afferents from the lung are concerned with innervation of the bronchial mucosa, sensing stretch in the alveoli, the interalveolar septa, and the pleura; monitoring pressure in the pulmonary veins; and mediating pain sensation. As stated earlier, all these impulses, including pain, travel in the vagus. They are concerned with the afferent limb of such reflexes as the cough reflex and the stretch reflex, which regulates respiration.

In summary, the anatomic evidence supported by

studies on the human bronchial tree indicates that the vagus furnishes the great majority, if not all, of the afferent fibers to the lung, and that it is also the constrictor of the bronchi. The sympathetic, on the other hand, is the vasoconstrictor and also furnishes secretomotor fibers to the glands of the bronchial tree.

ANATOMIC RELATIONS IN THE ROOT OF THE LUNGS

All the structures that constitute the root of the lung have been dealt with individually in previous sections of this chapter. The relation of these structures to one another matters because they provide principal clues to the dissection of the internal anatomy of the lungs, and they are the landmarks during the resection of the lobes and segments (Figs. 20-10 and 20-11).

The roots of the lungs are posterior to the upper part of the pericardial sac. The trachea bifurcates behind and slightly above the sac, and the principal bronchi are anchored to the heart by major blood vessels that arch over the bronchi in the obtuse angles made by the trachea and each principal bronchus (see Fig. 20-10). The lower end of the trachea is displaced slightly to the right of the midline by the arch of the aorta, which occupies the angle between the trachea and the left bronchus. Before the left bronchus enters the lung, the left pulmonary artery ascends over its anterior surface and crosses it just distal to the arch of the aorta. Thus, two major blood vessels, the aorta and the left pulmonary artery, come to rest of the superior surface of the left principal bronchus. On the right, only the azygos vein occupies the angle between the trachea and the bronchus because the right pulmonary artery crosses the interlobar portion of the bronchus distal to the origin of the superior lobe bronchus. The azygos vein terminates in the superior vena cava before the latter enters the pericardial sac anterior to the root of the lung.

Immediately anterior to the principal bronchi are the pulmonary arteries (see Fig. 20-3). The left one ascends across its bronchus, whereas the right pulmonary artery passes slightly below its bronchus before it bends across it in the hilum.

The superior pulmonary vein is the most anterior structure, and the inferior pulmonary vein the most inferior structure, in the root of the lung (see Fig. 20-11). Thus, on both sides, the principal order of structures in an anteroposterior direction is vein, artery, bronchus. This order is reversed if the hilum is approached from the back. The inferior pulmonary veins lie below the bronchus on both sides, and below them is the pulmonary ligament into which they can expand. The inferior veins become visible in an anterior approach to the hilum only if, in addition to the anterior margins of the lungs, the middle lobe or the lingula is retracted. On the right side, the superior pulmonary vein passes behind the superior vena cava and the inferior pulmonary vein passes behind the right atrium before they pierce the pericardial sac over the left atrium. They terminate in this chamber, having prac-

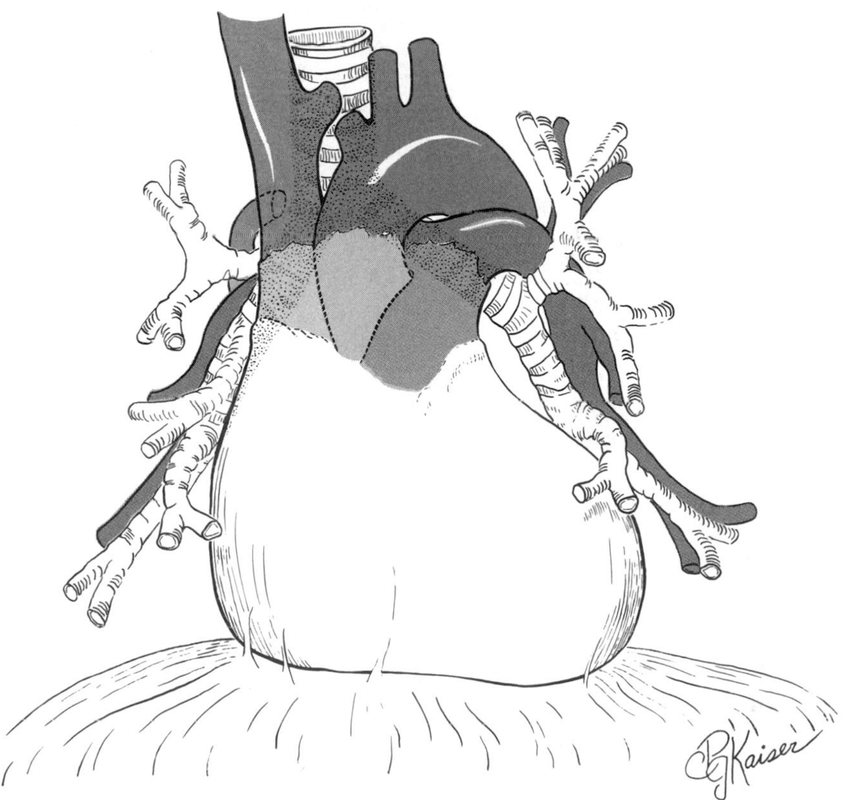

FIGURE *20-10.*
The relation of the great arteries and great veins to the principal bronchi.

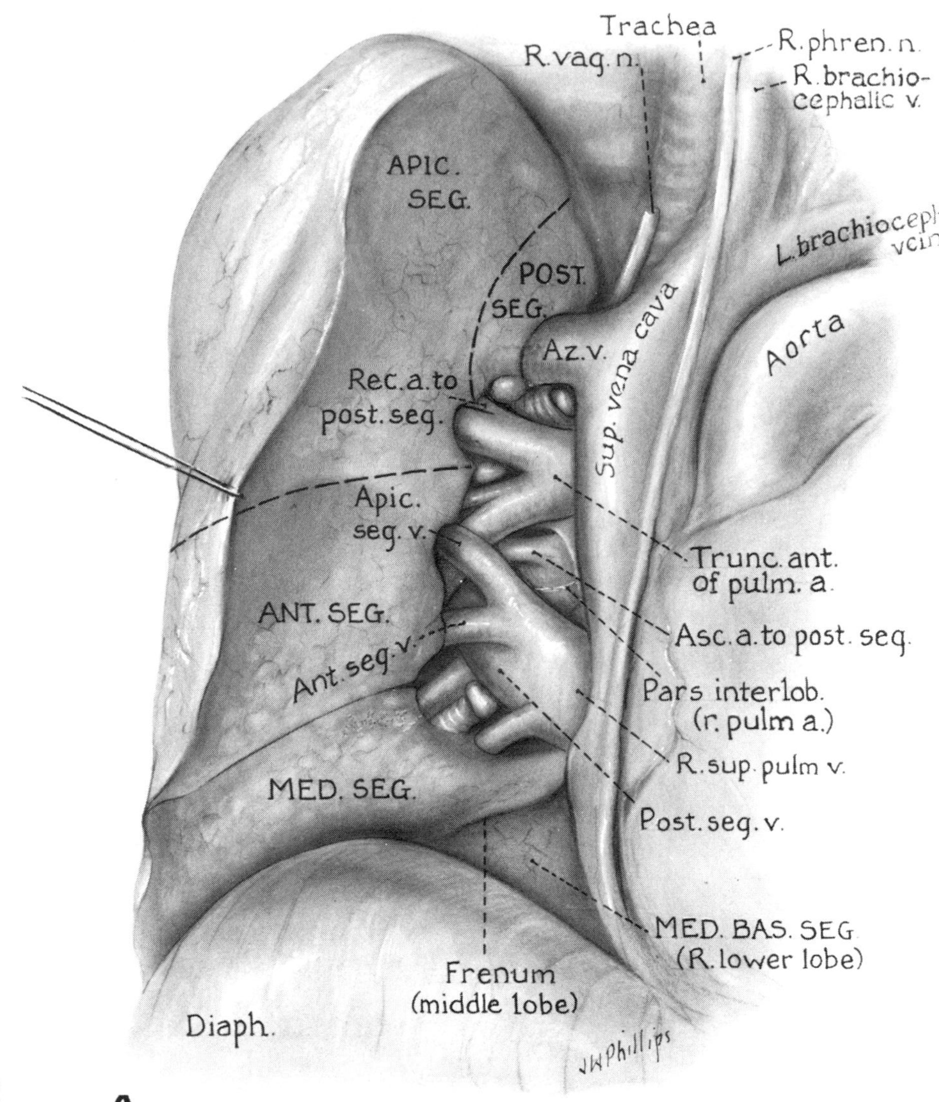

FIGURE *20-11.*
Anatomic relations in the root of the (A) right and *(continued)*

tically no intrapericardial course. The left veins are shorter and are related to the lateral part of the left atrium anteriorly before they enter it.

The posterior relations of the lung roots differ on the two sides. The tracheal bifurcation and the left bronchus rest on the esophagus. More laterally, the left bronchus crosses the descending aorta, and so does the left inferior pulmonary vein at a lower level. The right inferior pulmonary vein crosses the esophagus.

On the posterior surface of the bronchi are located the delicate bronchial vessels. The vagi pass behind the hila, where they contribute numerous twigs to the bronchi and the pulmonary plexuses. Right and left vagus nerves commingle with each other behind the tracheal bifurcation, forming the *esophageal plexus*. The phrenic nerves run down on the pericardial sac and are located anterior to the hila (see Fig. 20-11). The right phrenic nerve is close to the lung root as it passes from the surface of the superior vena cava onto the pericardium. The left nerve is some distance from the lung root, being pushed forward by the left ventricle.

THE BRONCHOPULMONARY SEGMENTS AND THEIR CLINICAL IMPORTANCE

A bronchopulmonary segment is a bronchovascular unit of the lung (Fig. 20-12). Each segment is pyramidal in shape, is aerated by a segmental bronchus, and is served principally by a segmental branch of the pulmonary artery and a segmental pulmonary vein. Some branches of a segmental pulmonary artery do, however, enter neighboring segments, and one of the branches of a segmental pulmonary vein runs in connective tissue between neighboring segments. Thus, the bronchopulmonary segments can be conceived of as the anatomic bronchovascular units of the lungs.

If suitably prepared dyes of contrasting color are injected into the orifices of the segmental bronchi so that the most peripheral branches of the bronchial tree become filled with the dye all the way to the visceral

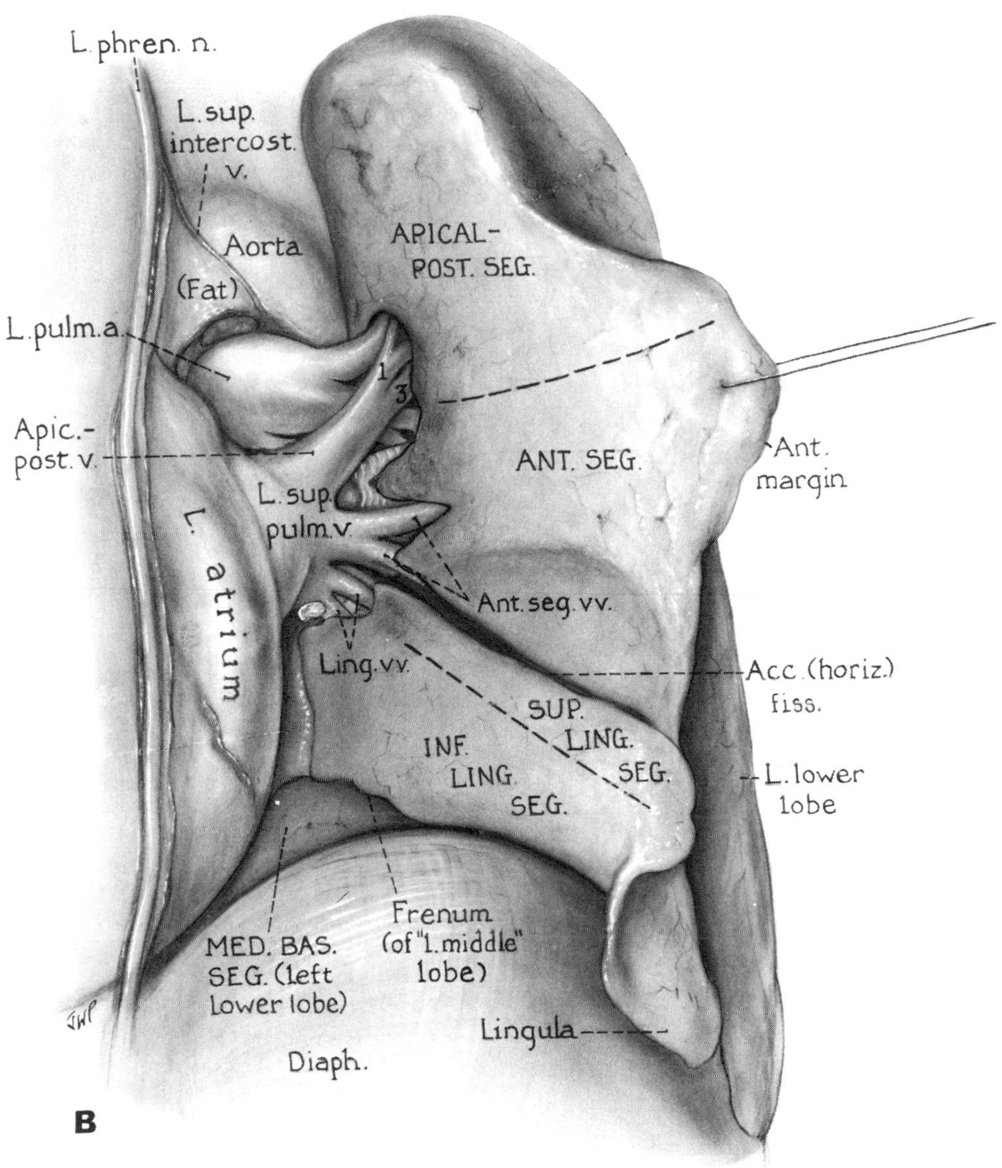

FIGURE *20-11.* *(Continued)*
(B) left lungs seen in an anterior approach to the hila. (Boyden EA. The segmental anatomy of the lungs. In: Myers IA, ed. Diseases of the chest including the heart. Springfield IL: Charles C Thomas, 1959.)

pleura, the bronchopulmonary segments will be sharply demarcated on the surface of the lung without any mixing of colors at the boundaries of the segments. Also, if a segmental bronchus, artery, and vein are cut and clamped close to the hilum, and if traction is applied to this triad of structures, the wedge-shaped segment may be stripped away from its neighbors by blunt dissection with a gauze sponge in the intersegmental planes; no blood vessels or bronchi of any size need be severed.

There are ten bronchopulmonary segments in each lung. Their segmental bronchi have already been described and named in the section on the bronchial tree (see Fig. 20-4). The bronchopulmonary segments, as they appear on the surfaces of the lungs, are shown in Figure 20-13.

The right upper lobe consists of the **apical, posterior**, and **anterior segments**, identifiable on the costal and medial surfaces of the lung. The middle lobe has two segments, **lateral** and **medial**. Both are present on the costal surface: only the medial projects onto the mediastinal surface. On the left, all five segments are incorporated into the superior lobe. However, the segments corresponding to the lateral and medial segments of the right lung are called **superior** and **inferior lingular** on the left. Both lingular segments project onto the costal and medial sur-

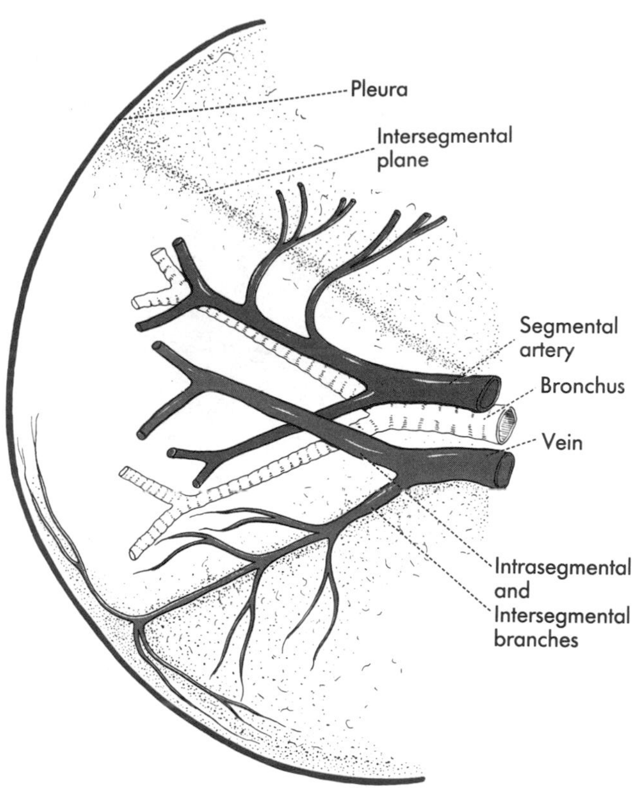

FIGURE *20-12.*
A schematic representation of a bronchopulmonary segment, the bronchovascular unit of the lung.

faces. Each of the two lower lobes consists of five segments, and these receive corresponding names on the two sides. The apex of each inferior lobe is occupied by the **superior segment**, and the base of the lobes is shared by the **medial basal, anterior basal, lateral basal**, and **posterior basal segments**. All the basal segments project onto the costal surface except the medial basal. The superior, the medial basal, and the posterior basal segments are present on the medial surface of the lungs.

The segments that rest on the diaphragm include all the basal segments plus the medial segment of the middle lobe and the inferior lingular segment of the left upper lobe (see Fig. 20-13C).

The projection of these segments to the chest wall is shown in Figure 20-14. The segments can be mapped if the position of the fissures and the borders of the lungs described earlier in this chapter are known. This map of the bronchopulmonary segments should be borne in mind when air entry into the lungs is clinically evaluated and when the lungs are examined by x-ray films. There is considerable superimposition of various segments because of the sloping plane of the oblique fissure. Some of the segments superimposed can be examined individually in the axilla. The same principle applies to radiologic examination of the segments (Fig. 20-15). Posteroanterior and lateral exposures are required to locate a segment accurately. In a physical examination, it should be remembered that anteriorly the lung fields are dominated by segments of the upper and middle lobes and posteriorly they are dominated by segments of the lower lobes.

Some diseases, such as bronchopneumonia, lung abscess, bronchiectasis, and pulmonary infarction, affect the lung in a segmental pattern. Identification of the diseased segment is important because *postural drainage* may need to be employed to aid removal of infected exudate, mucus, or pus from the involved segments. The patient has to be positioned in such a way that the segment to be drained is uppermost so that gravity can aid the discharge of the bronchial contents into the main bronchus. For this, it is necessary to know the position of the segment and the direction of the segmental bronchus. Rhythmic and forceful percussion of the chest wall over the diseased segment facilitates dislodgement of bronchial contents.

Segmental resection may be indicated for lung abscess, bronchiectasis, and for benign, and some malignant neoplasms, if they are diagnosed sufficiently early. After the removal of one or more segments, or of a lobe, the remaining lung will expand to fill the entire pleural cavity.

Physical Examination of the Lungs

Physical examination of the lung essentially evaluates their functional anatomy. The physical signs employed rely on the fact that the lung is filled with air and that the air moves in and out of the lung with each respiratory cycle.

Inspection of the movements of respiration over the thorax and the abdomen gives information about air entry into the lungs. Asymmetric movement, or the lack of movement, suggests that air is not moving in and out of a substantial portion of the lung, or that there is some interference with the mechanisms of respiratory movements (paralysis, rib fracture).

The normal chest sounds hollow when percussed. Loss of a resonant percussion note over a segment or segments indicates that the portion of the lung is collapsed, filled with fluid, or solidified. Fluid in the pleural cavity also yields a dull percussion note, whereas a large amount of air in the pleural cavity will sound hyperresonant when percussed.

The movement of air in and out of the respiratory passages generates the *breath sounds*, best heard with a stethoscope. Over the lung fields the sounds are fine and are heard only during inspiration when the alveolar sacs are being distended. These are the *vesicular breath sounds*. In the trachea and the larger bronchi, much more coarse sounds are generated by the movement of air. These sounds are audible during inspiration and expiration and are known as *bronchial breath sounds*. They can be heard over the trachea, but not over the lung fields in a normal chest. However, when a portion of the lung solidifies, it transmits the bronchial breath sounds to the chest wall.

Normally, the sliding of the visceral pleura on the parietal pleura is inaudible. However, if one or both of the pleural surfaces become roughened by inflammation, a *pleural rub*, which is present during both inspiration and expiration, will be heard.

Added to an understanding of pulmonary anatomy, these physical signs permit the diagnosis of whether or not air is moving normally in and out of all bronchopulmonary segments, and if some segments

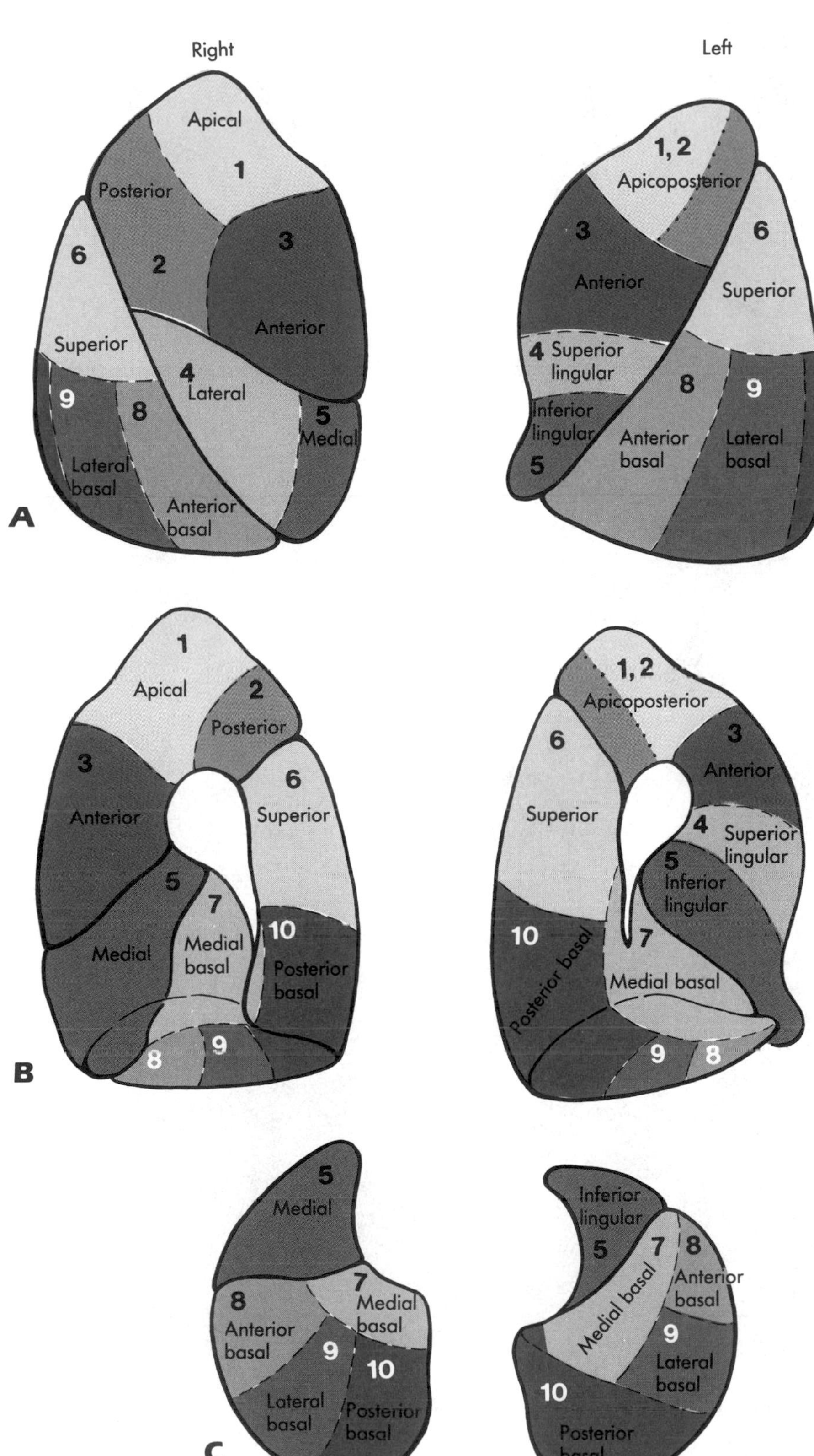

FIGURE *20-13.*
The bronchopulmonary segments as seen on the surface of the lungs after segmental bronchi have been injected with dyes of various colors: (A) lateral surface; (B) medial surface; (C) base or diaphragmatic surface. (Adapted from Boyden EA: The segmental anatomy of the lungs. New York: McGraw-Hill, 1955.)

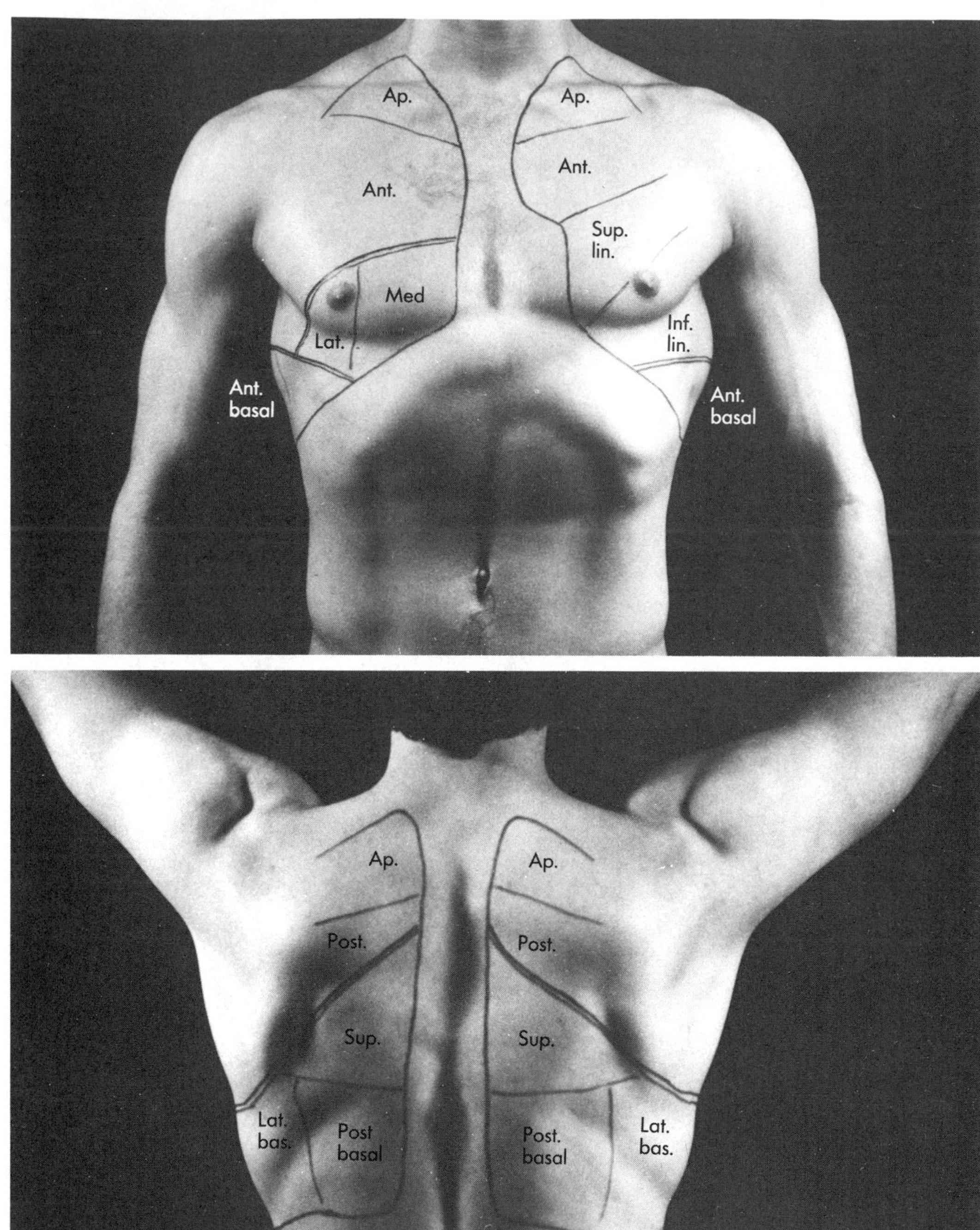

FIGURE *20-14.*
Projection of the bronchopulmonary segments to the surface of the chest.

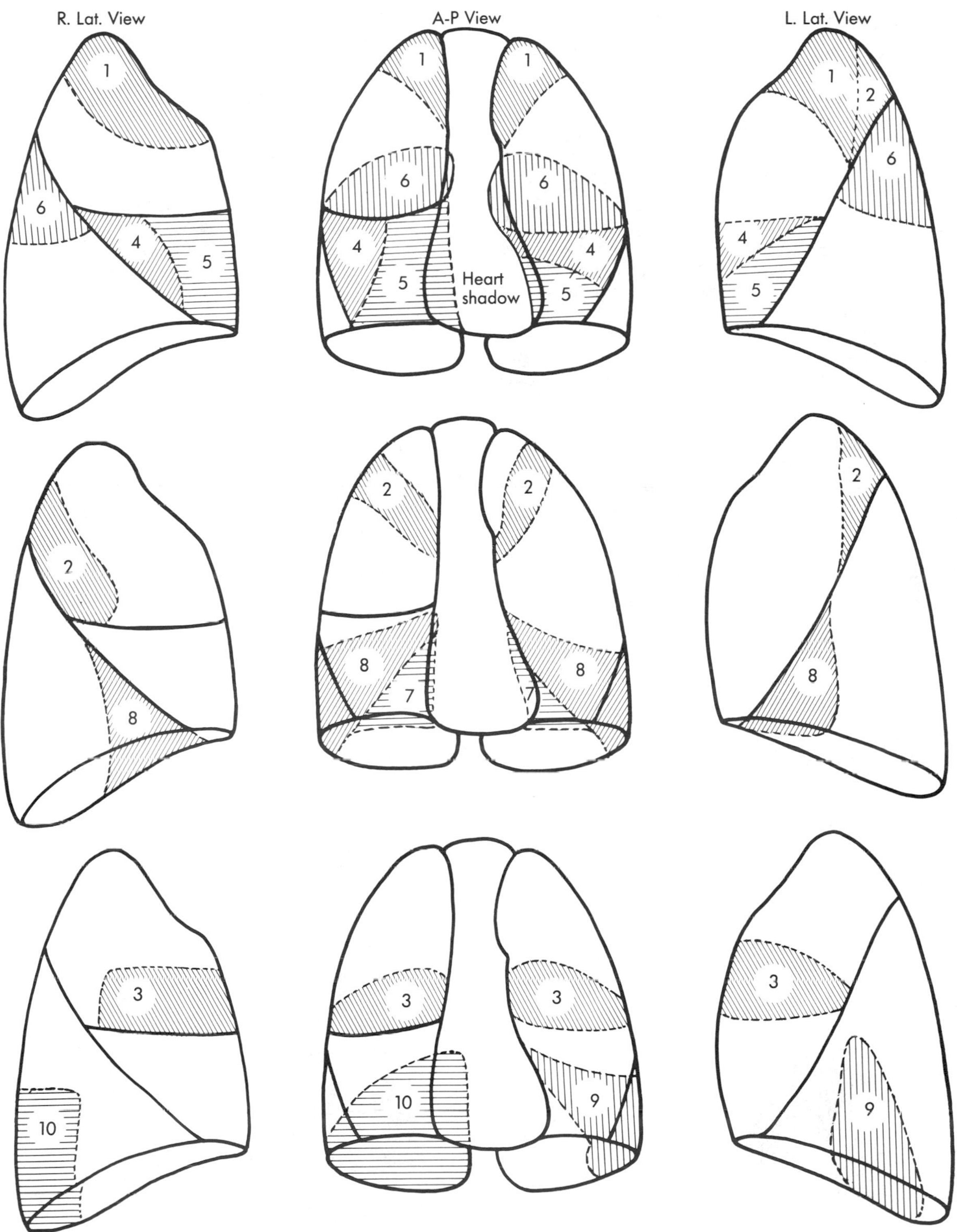

FIGURE *20-15.*
Diagrams illustrating the shadows of the lung segments on x-ray film. Consolidation or disease confined to individual segments create characteristic shadows that can be identified by combined lateral and anteroposterior views. (*Upper row*) shadows of the apical (*1*), lateral (*4*), medial (*5*), and superior (*6*) segments; (*middle row*) posterior (*2*), medial basal (*7*), and anterior basal (*8*) segments; (*lower row*) anterior (*3*), lateral basal (*9*), and posterior basal (*10*) segments. (Adapted from Boyden EA. The segmental anatomy of the lungs. In: Myers JA, ed. Diseases of the chest including the heart. Springfield IL: Charles C Thomas, 1959.)

are not aerated, the basic cause of the condition can be deduced.

Radiologic Examination

The lung parenchyma absorbs so little of the x-rays that pass through it that, for practical purposes, the lungs appear as transparent to x-rays as air. On a plain chest x-ray film, the mediastinal structures create a definite shadow that contrasts with the bilateral radiolucent lung fields (Fig. 20-16). The bronchi are invisible, but the major branches of the pulmonary arteries and veins create linear shadows radiating from the hilum. Occasionally, the fissures can be identified because the small amount of pleural fluid trapped between the lobes absorbs more x-rays than the lung itself. When air is absorbed from a segment or when segments become filled with fluid or solidify, they create a shadow on the film (see Fig. 20-15). The same is true of cysts, neoplasms, and enlarged lymph nodes.

DEVELOPMENT OF THE LUNGS

In the preceding section of this chapter, repeated reference was made to the development of the lungs because the anatomy of this organ, as of any other, is most readily understood through its development. The development of the lung is divided into five periods: the embryonic, pseudoglandular, canalicular, terminal sac, and neonatal periods. The establishment of the internal gross anatomy of the lung takes place during the first two of these periods; the subsequent three phases are concerned chiefly with the differentiation and elaboration of the terminal respiratory passages for increasingly efficient gas exchange.

The **embryonic period** is the period of budding and takes place during the fourth to seventh weeks of gestation. The primordium of the lung arises as the laryngotracheal diverticulum on the ventral aspect of the foregut at the lower end of the pharynx (see Fig. 22-5). The diverticulum soon divides into right and left lung buds, which are essentially two endodermal sacs. The stalk of the lung buds (the trachea) elongates and separates from the esophagus as lobar buds appear on the two lung sacs. These, in turn, give rise by division to the bronchi of the future bronchopulmonary segments. The buds of the bronchopulmonary segments bulge on the surface of the pleura, giving it a mulberry appearance. By the end of the seventh week, growth has proceeded to several generations of subsegmental bronchi. The embryonic period ends with the closure of the pleuroperitoneal canals. During this period, branches of the pulmonary arteries and veins become associated with the bronchi. These vessels arise from the splanchnic mesoderm entrapped by the bronchial buds. Centrally, the arteries hook up with the sixth aortic arch, and the pulmonary veins, with the left atrium. All anatomic anomalies of the lung become established during this earliest of developmental stages. The bronchial arteries grow into the lungs during the next stage of development.

The **pseudoglandular period** (8th to 16th weeks) is the principal growth period of the bronchi, and the requisite number of divisions in each segment are established all the way to the future respiratory bronchioles and alveolar ducts. The prolific growth by epithelial budding gives the lung a glandular appearance from which the period receives its name. The next phase is the differentiation period of the future respiratory epithelium and is called **canalicular** because the cuboidal epithelium in the region of the

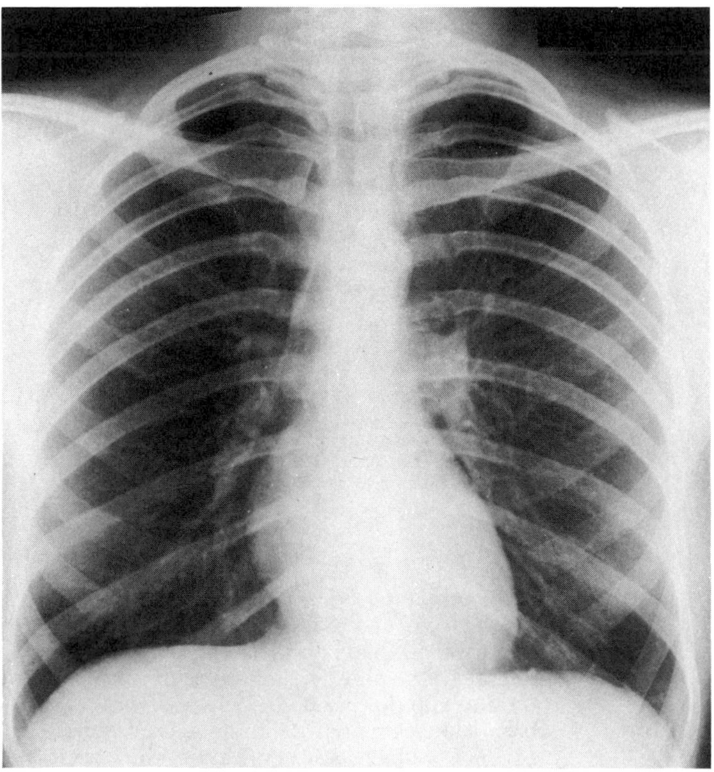

FIGURE *20-16.*
An anteroposterior view of the thorax: The indistinct shadows in the lungs are caused by the pulmonary vessels. (Courtesy of Dr. D. G. Pugh.)

future alveolar sacs becomes invaded or "*canalized*" by pulmonary capillaries. Over the capillary loops, the epithelium becomes stretched and acquires the squamous character of the alveolar lining. Toward the end of this period, which lasts from the 17th to the 26th week, some of the alveolar cells begin to secrete *surfactant*, which enables the fetus, if prematurely born, to breathe. During the next phase, called the **terminal sac period**, which lasts up to birth, the regions of the alveolar ducts grow and expand, forming thin-walled sacs that as yet lack true alveoli. The full-term fetus is born without alveoli. Alveolar development gets under way during the **neonatal period** and continues up to the age of 12 years. A rapid increase in alveoli occurs up to 6 months of age and proceeds at the slower rate thereafter. The peripheral respiratory zone grows by elongation, and the respiratory surface is increased by the appearance of alveoli within the expanding acini. The number of alveoli increases during the first 8 years from 24 million terminal saccules to 280 million alveoli (296 million in the adult), and the air tissue interface increases from 2.8 to 32 m^2 during the same period. It is 75 m^2 in the adult.

RECOMMENDED READINGS

Auer J. The development of the human pulmonary vein and its major variations. Anat Rec 1948;101:581.

Bloomer WE, Liebow AA, Hales MR. Surgical anatomy of the bronchovascular segments. Springfield IL: Charles C Thomas, 1960.

Boyden EA. Development of the human lung. In: Brennemann's practice of pediatrics, vol 4. Hagerstown: Harper & Row, 1975.

Boyden EA. Segmental anatomy of the lungs: a study of the patterns of the segmental bronchi and related pulmonary vessels. New York: McGraw-Hill, 1955.

Boyden EA. The pulmonary artery and its branches. In: Luisada AA, ed. Cardiology. An encyclopedia of the cardiovascular system, sponsored by The American College of Cardiology, vol 1. New York: McGraw-Hill, 1959.

Carles J, Clerc F, Dubrez J, Couraud L, Drouillard J, Videau J. The bronchial arteries: anatomic study and application to lung transplantation. Surg Radiol Anat 1995;17:293.

Conley D, Rosse C. The digital anatomist: interactive atlas of thoracic viscera (CD-ROM). Seattle: University of Washington School of Medicine, 1996.

Fishman AP, Hecht HH, ed. The pulmonary circulation and interstitial space. Chicago: University of Chicago Press, 1969.

Hollinshead WH. Anatomy for surgeons: vol 2, the thorax, abdomen, and pelvis. 2nd ed. New York: Harper & Row, 1971.

Jackson CL, Huber JF. Correlated applied anatomy of the bronchial tree and lungs with a system of nomenclature. Dis Chest 1943;9:319.

Jardin M, Rémy J. Segmental bronchovascular anatomy of the lower lobes. Am J Roentgenol 1986;147:453.

Larsell O, Dow RS. The innervation of the human lung. Am J Anat 1933;52:125.

Lodge T. Anatomy of blood vessels of the human lung as applied to chest radiology. Br J Radiol 1946;19:1.

Morton DR, Klassen KP, Curtis GM. The clinical physiology of the human bronchi: II. The effect of vagus section upon pain of tracheobronchial origin. Surgery 1951;30:800.

Murray JF. The normal lung. 2nd ed. Philadelphia: WB Saunders, 1986.

Nagaishi C. Functional anatomy and histology of the lung. Baltimore: University Park Press, 1972.

O'Rahilly R, Boyden EA. The timing and sequence of events in the development of the human respiratory system during the embryonic period proper. Z Anat Entwicklunggesch 1973;141:237.

Pump KK. Distribution of bronchial arteries in the human lung. Chest 1972;62:447.

Riquet M, Manac'h D, Dupont P, Dujon A, Hidden G, Debesse B. Anatomic basis of lymphatic spread of lung carcinoma to the mediastinum: anatomo-clinical correlations. Surg Radiol Anat 1994;16:229.

Ross JS, O'Donovan BP, Paushter DM. Tracheobronchial tree and pulmonary arteries: MR imaging using electronic axial rotation. Radiology 1986;160:839.

Thurlbeck WM. Structure of the lungs. Int Rev Cytol 1977;14:1.

Yamashita H. Roentgenologic anatomy of the lung. Stuttgart: Thieme, 1978.

Hollinshead's Textbook of Anatomy, by Cornelius Rosse and Penelope Gaddum-Rosse.
Lippincott-Raven Publishers, Philadelphia, © 1997.

CHAPTER 21

The Pericardium, The Heart, and the Great Vessels*

*Sections of this chapter relating to congenital anomalies of the heart and fetal circulation were written in collaboration with Dr. Lore Tenckhoff, Cardiologist and Director of Cardiac Ultrasound, Children's Orthopedic Hospital and Medical Center, Seattle, Washington, and Clinical Professor of Pediatrics and Radiology, The University of Washington, Seattle, Washington.

Basic features of the heart, and the circulation through it, are outlined in Chapter 8. After the eighth week of embryonic development, the human heart consists of four chambers: the right and left atria and the right and left ventricles. The right and left sides of the heart become completely partitioned off from one another at birth, and on each side, blood can flow only from the atrium to the respective ventricle. The superior and inferior venae cavae return venous blood from the systemic circulation into the right atrium, and this blood is then propelled by the right ventricle through the pulmonary trunk to the lungs. Oxygenated blood from the lungs is returned by the pulmonary veins to the left atrium and is then ejected into the systemic circulation by the left ventricle through the aorta. The heart has its own blood supply: the coronary arteries and the cardiac veins. Cardiac nerves modify the rate and strength of the heart beat and also conduct visceral afferent impulses.

The heart is surrounded by its own serous cavity, the *pericardial cavity*, which is a potential space between visceral and parietal layers of the *serous pericardium*. The serous pericardial sac itself is surrounded by the *fibrous pericardium*, a substantial, dense connective tissue membrane (see Figs. 19-13 and 19-17). In addition to the heart, the pericardium encloses the roots of the major systemic and pulmonary blood vessels. The pericardium and its contents occupy the middle mediastinum. An understanding of the anatomic arrangement of the pericardium and the structures enclosed by it is aided by a preliminary consideration of development.

Developmental Considerations

The Primitive Heart Tube. The heart develops as two parallel, thin-walled endothelial tubes, which, with the establishment of the head fold of the embryo, come to lie ventral to the foregut and dorsal to the future pericardial cavity. The pericardial cavity at this stage of development forms the ventromedian portion of the intraembryonic celom (see Fig. 19-12*A*). Side-to-side fusion of the two heart tubes proceeds as they sink into the pericardial cavity, acquiring a lamina of celomic mesothelial covering, the *epicardium*, or *visceral pericardium*, on their outer surface (see Fig. 19-12*B*).

Differential growth defines five segments of the heart tube, which, from a rostral to caudal direction, receive the following names: (1) **truncus arteriosus,** (2) **bulbus cordis,** (3) **primitive ventricle,** (4) **primitive atrium,** (5) **sinus venosus** (Fig. 21-1*A* and *B*). At the rostral end, the **aortic sac** appears as a continuation of the truncus, and six pairs of **aortic arches** that arise from this sac skirt around the foregut and link the truncus to the bilateral *dorsal aortae* (see Fig. 21-1*A* and *B*). At the caudal end, the sinus venosus receives three pairs of veins, which deliver blood to the heart from three sources: the two *umbilical veins* from the placenta, two *vitelline veins* from the yolk sac and the gut, and two *common cardinal veins* that drain blood from the body of the embryo (see Figs. 21-1*A* and 21-22). By the completion of development, the truncus arteriosus will have given rise to the pulmonary trunk and the ascending aorta, the bulbus cordis to the major part of the anatomic right ventricle, and the primitive ventricle to the major part of the anatomic left ventricle. The right half of the primitive atrium and the sinus venosus become incorporated into the anatomic right atrium. The anatomic left atrium is formed from the left side of the primitive atrium and from the primitive common pulmonary vein that enters the embryonic atrium directly, rather than through the sinus venosus.

The Pericardium. Soon after the heart tube sinks into the celom, the pericardial cavity becomes partitioned

FIGURE *21-1.*
A highly schematic representation of the primitive heart tube and the pericardial cavity: (A) the heart tube is seen from its ventral aspect and (B) from its left lateral aspect. The left and right horns of the sinus venosus (*SV*), with their tributaries, are embedded in the septum transversum (*shaded area*), and the aortic arches, given off by the truncus arteriosus (*TA*), skirt around the foregut to form the paired dorsal aortae. At this stage, only the first two pairs of aortic arches have formed. Later other pairs will develop and the aortic sac (*AS*) will become identifiable as a dilation on the rostral of the truncus. (C) The heart tube is seen suspended in the primitive pericardial cavity. A large window has been cut in the wall of the cavity that is formed by the parietal layer of the serous pericardium. The serous pericardium is shown as a *pink* membrane that covers the heart tube and is continuous with the parietal serous pericardium through the *mesocardium* and through reflections at the arterial and venous ends of the heart. The mesocardium is in the process of being broken down, thus creating the transverse sinus (*TS*) in the pericardial cavity. Caudally, the pericardial cavity continues into the *pericardiopleural* canal, which is being pinched off from the pericardial cavity by the common cardinal veins (see also Fig. 19-12). (D) The heart is shown in a section at the stage of development when the bulbus (*B*) has fused with the ventricle (*V*) and the atria (*A*) have been drawn out of the septum transversum. The continuity of the epicardium with the parietal serous pericardium can be traced now only around the truncus arteriosus and the sinus venosus.

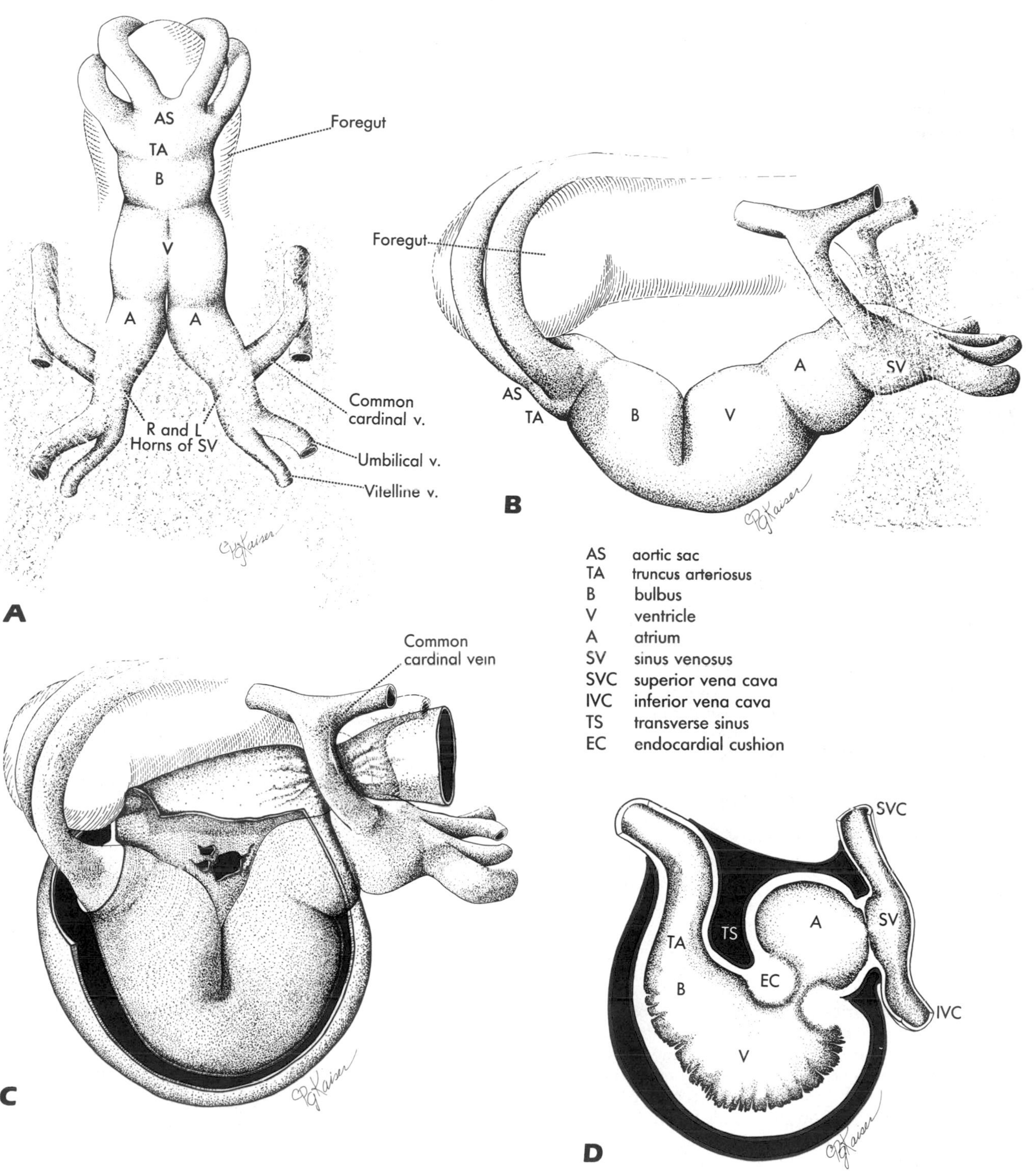
AS
TA
B
V
A
A
Foregut
Common cardinal v.
R and L Horns of SV
Umbilical v.
Vitelline v.
A
Foregut
AS
TA
B
V
A
SV
B
AS aortic sac
TA truncus arteriosus
B bulbus
V ventricle
A atrium
SV sinus venosus
SVC superior vena cava
IVC inferior vena cava
TS transverse sinus
EC endocardial cushion
Common cardinal vein
C
SVC
TS
A
SV
TA
EC
B
IVC
V
D

off from the future pleural cavity (pleuropericardial canal) by the development of the *pleuropericardial membranes* (see Fig. 19-12*D*). It is explained in Chapter 19, in connection with the development of divisions in the thoracic cavity, how this membrane is lifted off and dissected away from the inner mesodermal lamina of the body wall. The pleuropericardial membrane differentiates into the **fibrous pericardium** and separates the ventromedian pericardial cavity of the embryo from the dorsolateral pleural cavities. The parietal **serous pericardium** (in essence, the celomic mesothelium) lines the deep aspect of the fibrous pericardium, forms the walls of the pericardial cavity, and is continuous with the epicardium (visceral serous pericardium). An understanding of this continuity will help to explain the gross anatomy of the pericardial cavity and the existence of its sinuses.

After the dorsal mesocardium disappears (see Figs. 19-12*C* and 21-1*C*), the heart tube is suspended in the pericardial cavity only at its arterial and venous ends. The epicardium is continuous with the parietal serous pericardium around the truncus arteriosus as the truncus leaves the cavity rostrally and around the sinus venosus as this enters the cavity from the substance of the septum transversum (Fig. 21-1*D*). Thus, there is a serous pericardial sleeve around the arterial end of the heart and another around its venous end, just as there is a pleural sleeve around the root of the lung.

The heart tube grows at a faster pace than the pericardial cavity and, as a consequence, the heart buckles, or loops, creating on the dorsal aspect a sharp infolding between the bulbus and the ventricle (see Fig. 21-1*B*). This looping of the heart tube approximates its arterial end to its venous end, an event accentuated by the emergence of the atria from the septum transversum into the pericardial cavity (see Fig. 21-1*D*). Only a narrow channel of communication remains between the right and left portions of the pericardial cavity across the dorsal aspect of the heart where originally the mesocardium was located. This channel, limited anteriorly by the truncus and posteriorly by atria, is the future *transverse sinus* of the pericardial cavity (see Fig. 21-1*D*).

The truncus arteriosus will become divided into two major arteries: the ascending aorta and the pulmonary trunk. However, the pericardium around them will not split, and the two great arteries remain enclosed in a single pericardial sleeve. The same is true at the venous end, although the developmental changes that occur within that sleeve are more complex. Most of the sinus venosus becomes incorporated into the right atrium; therefore, its tributaries will come to be enclosed by the pericardial sleeve. The three pairs of veins (umbilical, vitelline, and common cardinal) that drained into the primitive sinus venosus become radically modified, and by the completion of development, only two large veins, derived from the original six, enter the pericardial cavity (see Fig. 21-1*D*). These two are the superior and inferior venae cavae. In addition, four pulmonary veins, not represented among the primitive tributaries of the sinus venosus, gain access to the left atrium through the pericardial sleeve. Thus, the six veins that enter the fully developed atria are enclosed by this common sleeve around the venous end of the heart, but these veins are not analogous with the six primitive tributaries of the sinus venosus. With the growth of the atria, the orifices of these veins are drawn away from one another, and the venous pericardial sleeve becomes distorted in a ʃ shape. The cul-de-sac between the limbs of the ʃ is known as the *oblique sinus* of the pericardial cavity (see Fig. 21-3).

Establishment of Definitive Cardiac Anatomy. The basic anatomy of the heart is established early. The looping of the heart tube displaces the bulbus not only only ventrally (see Fig. 21-1*B* and *C*), but also to the right (not shown in Fig. 21-1, because it is a side view). This so-called dextro loop (or *d* loop) places the bulbus to the right side of the primitive ventricle where the bulbus will develop into the definitive right ventricle. At this stage of development the flange of the bulboventricular septum partially separates the future right and left ventricles from one another (see Fig. 21-1*C*); however, this separation is temporary because the bulboventricular septum soon becomes absorbed (see Fig. 21-1*D*), which creates a single ventricle that will have to be divided by the development of the definitive interventricular septum.

The atria enlarge; the right atrium incorporates much of the sinus venosus, and the left takes up the primitive, common pulmonary veins and its primary tributaries. Two external features result from the atrial enlargements: 1) a deep groove develops between the atria and ventricle, known as the *coronary sulcus*; 2) the most ventral extensions of the atria, the right and left *auricles*, expand to embrace anteriorly the developing ascending aorta and pulmonary trunk. The single atrioventricular canal, through which the common atrium communicates with the primitive ventricle, will be divided into right and left channels by the fusion of a dorsal and a ventral *endocardial cushion* (see Fig. 21-1*D*). These cushions contribute to the formation of the atrioventricular valves. The development of the interatrial and interventricular septa completes the division of the heart into four chambers. These septa are marked on the exterior by shallow sulci, but the development of the septa is best discussed at the end of this chapter when embryonic equivalents of the gross structures can be defined.

THE PERICARDIAL SAC

The pericardium is a fibrous sac that surrounds the heart and the roots of the great arteries and veins as they leave or enter the heart. The outer lamina of the sac, composed of dense connective tissue, is the *fibrous pericardium*. To the inner aspect of the fibrous pericardium is closely bound the *parietal lamina of the serous pericardium*, which lines the fibrous sac and reflects onto the surface of the heart around the roots of the great vessels. Beyond these reflections, the serous membrane is known as the *visceral lamina of the serous pericardium* or the *epicardium*. Between visceral and parietal laminae of the serous pericardium is the *pericardial cavity*, which is completely closed and contains nothing but sufficient fluid to moisten the opposing surfaces of the serous pericardial sac. The function of the serous sac is to lubricate the moving surfaces of the heart, whereas the outer fibrous sac retains the heart in position within the thoracic cavity and limits its distention (Fig. 21-2).

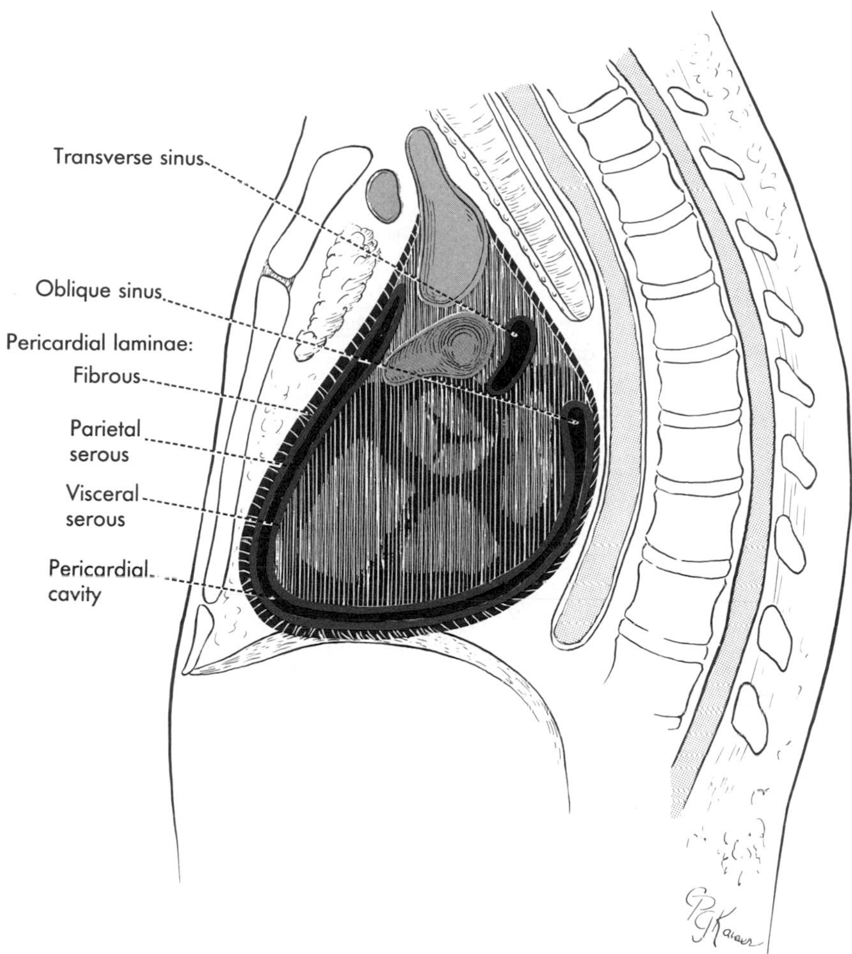

FIGURE 21-2.
A schematic representation of the pericardial sac seen in a sagittal section of the thorax: The serous pericardium is shown as a *heavy red line* (its thickness relative to the scale of other structures is much exaggerated), and the pericardial cavity enclosed within the serous sac is *solid black* (see also Figs. 19-13 and 19-17). The ascending aorta is *pink*; the pulmonary trunk, *purple*; and the left brachiocephalic vein, *blue*.

The Fibrous Pericardium

Similar to a cone-shaped bag, the fibrous pericardium rests with its base on the diaphragm, and its narrow opening is sealed superiorly around the superior vena cava, the ascending aorta, and the pulmonary arteries (see Figs. 19-17 and 21-2). The base of the bag is pierced on the right by the inferior vena cava and posteriorly by the four pulmonary veins, which enter it independently.

The pericardium is fixed in the thoracic cavity because the base of the fibrous bag is inseparably fused to the anterior portion of the central tendon of the diaphragm; both structures in this region are derived from the septum transversum. Elsewhere, the pericardium is attached to the tendon by loose connective tissue. Behind the sternal angle, the fibrous pericardium blends imperceptibly with the adventitia of the superior vena cava, ascending aorta, right and left pulmonary arteries, and ligamentum arteriosum. This fusion of the connective tissues closes the pericardial sac superiorly. The anterior surface of the pericardium is attached to the sternum by two rather poorly defined and variable *sternopericardial ligaments*, which may be demonstrable in the region of the manubriosternal and xiphisternal junctions. The pretracheal fascia, which descends into the mediastinum from the neck, fuses with the anterior surface of the pericardium. Posteriorly, membranous connective tissue attaches the pericardium to the tracheal bifurcation and the principal bronchi.

With the descent of the diaphragm during inspiration, the pericardial sac is pulled downward and becomes elongated; this forces the heart into a more vertical position (see Fig. 21-19). Ascent of the diaphragm during expiration relaxes the pericardium allowing the sac to bulge laterally and the heart to become more horizontal. These movements are evident on x-ray films as alterations in the cardiac silhouette because the heart adapts its shape to the inelastic pericardial sac (see Fig. 21-19). The fibrous pericardium consists chiefly of dense interlacing collagen bundles and some elastic tissue in its deeper layers.

The pericardial sac with its contents comprises the *middle mediastinum*. The anterior mediastinum is in front of the sac and the posterior mediastinum behind it. The pericardium is overlapped and largely obscured anteriorly by the two pleural sacs and the anterior edges of the lungs, which occupy the sternocostal recesses (see Fig. 19-13). Where the two pleural sacs deviate from one another, the pericardium is in contact with the posterior surface of the sternum and the fourth and fifth left costal cartilages (see Fig. 19-14). Before adolescence, the thymus intervenes between the pericardium and the pleural sacs or the sternum, but in the adult there is little demonstrable thymic tissue in the anterior mediastinum. On each side, mediastinal pleura is draped over the lateral surface of the pericardium, with the phrenic nerve and the pericardiacophrenic vessels sandwiched between pleura and pericardium (see Fig. 19-13). The nerve and vessels are embedded in variable amounts of areolar or adipose tissue. Posteriorly, the pericardium is in contact with the esophagus, the descending thoracic aorta, and, more superiorly, both principal bronchi. On each side of these structures, the pleural sacs contact the posterior aspect of the pericardium. Occasionally, a small *infracardiac bursa* is present behind the pericardium just above the diaphragm. The bursa is a remnant of the embryonic *pneumatoenteric recess*.

The Serous Pericardium and Pericardial Cavity

A cut made in the pericardium opens the pericardial cavity because the parietal lamina of the serous pericardium is closely adherent to the fibrous pericardium. The visceral lamina or **epicardium** is more loosely bound to the myocardium. The loose subepicardial connective tissue may contain a good deal of fat, especially along the blood vessels. The glistening surface of the serous pericardium is covered by a single layer of mesothelium. The mesothelium is supported by a delicate, transparent connective tissue membrane in which blood vessels, lymphatics, and nerves arborize.

The heart is completely invested in epicardium except for a posterior, narrow, and irregular area that is between the entrances of the two venae cavae and the four pulmonary veins into the atria (Fig. 21-3). Here the atrial myocardium is in contact with the fibrous pericardium. This "bare area" exists because there is an uninterrupted line of reflection between the epicardium and parietal pericardium, which encloses all six veins in a single, short, and highly distorted pericardial sleeve (see Fig. 21-3). How this arrangement came about is explained earlier in this chapter, under Developmental Considerations. Of the six veins, only the superior vena cava has a significant intrapericardial portion, but it is not free in the cavity as are the ascending aorta and the pulmonary trunk. Only in the front and on its sides is the vena cava covered by serous pericardium over a length of 3.5 cm above the right atrium. Posteriorly, the vena cava contacts fibrous pericardium and the right pulmonary artery.

The superior vena cava is derived from the *right common cardinal vein* of the embryo; its left counterpart, the left common cardinal vein, normally atrophies. Sometimes the obliterated fibrous vestige of the left common cardinal vein is identifiable on the posterior wall of the pericardial cavity. It elevates a slight fold in the parietal pericardium between the left pulmonary artery and the left superior pulmonary vein. This fibrous vestige, called the *ligament of the left superior vena cava*, continues into the oblique vein of the left atrium, which drains into the coronary sinus. Sometimes both left and right common cardinal veins persist as left and right venae cavae, or the left vena cava may develop and the vessel on the right atrophy.

The ascending aorta and pulmonary trunk may be grasped within the pericardial cavity. The two vessels can be enclosed by a ligature, or by finger and thumb, if the index finger is inserted from the left side behind the pulmonary trunk (as shown by the horizontal arrow in Fig. 21-3). This is possible because the two great arteries are enclosed by a common pericardial sleeve as explained earlier under Developmental Considerations. Anteriorly, this pericardial sleeve reflects forward from the aorta and pulmonary trunk to line the fibrous pericardium at about the level of the sternal angle where the fibrous pericardium fuses with the adventitia of these vessels (see Fig. 21-2). Posteriorly, the epicardial sleeve reflects off the aorta and pulmonary trunk in a backward and downward direction to line the portion of the pericardial cavity into which the index finger was inserted in the foregoing exercise (see Figs. 21-2 and 21-3). This space is called the **transverse sinus** of the pericardium. The transverse sinus is a passage from the left to the right side of the pericardial cavity (see Fig. 21-1). It is behind the great arteries. In its posterior wall, covered by serous pericardium, runs the right pulmonary artery (as it passes to the right within the concavity of the arch of the aorta); the floor of the transverse sinus is formed by the left atrium. The superior vena cava (representing the venous end of the heart; see Fig. 21-1*D*) is posterior to the sinus as the sinus opens into the main pericardial cavity to the right of the ascending aorta (see Fig. 21-3).

The pericardial cavity has a second sinus called the **oblique sinus,** which is a *cul-de-sac* rather than a passage. The oblique sinus may be explored by elevating the apex of the heart and sliding the fingers behind the left ventricle and left atrium. The oblique sinus is limited superiorly and on each side by the distorted, ʃ-shaped pericardial sleeve and the six major veins enclosed within it, as described earlier (see Fig. 21-3). The oblique sinus is behind the left atrium, and its posterior wall is formed by the double layer of parietal and fibrous pericardium.

The pericardium surrounds the heart loosely, but the capacity of the pericardial cavity is small, usually about 300 mL. If there is gradual cardiac enlargement, or if fluids slowly accumulate in the pericardial cavity, the sac will accommodate to the enlargement by gradual distention. Sudden filling of the sac with blood or exudate (*cardiac tamponade*) will embarrass the action of the heart by interfering with the expansion of the atria, necessary for receiving incoming blood. The condition may be fatal. As a result of chronic pericarditis, the pericardium may become greatly thickened and adherent to the heart (*constrictive pericarditis*), and this also restricts the filling of the heart. The pericardium in these cases must be dissected away.

The most striking **congenital defect** of the pericardium results from failure of the fibrous pericardium to develop. This leaves the pleural and pericardial cavities in continuity as they are in the early embryonic stages (see Fig. 19-12). The total absence of the pericardium does not interfere with the action of the heart. In less severe cases, there is a communication between the pericardial and (usually the left) pleural cavities. This may cause problems if part of the heart herniates through the defect.

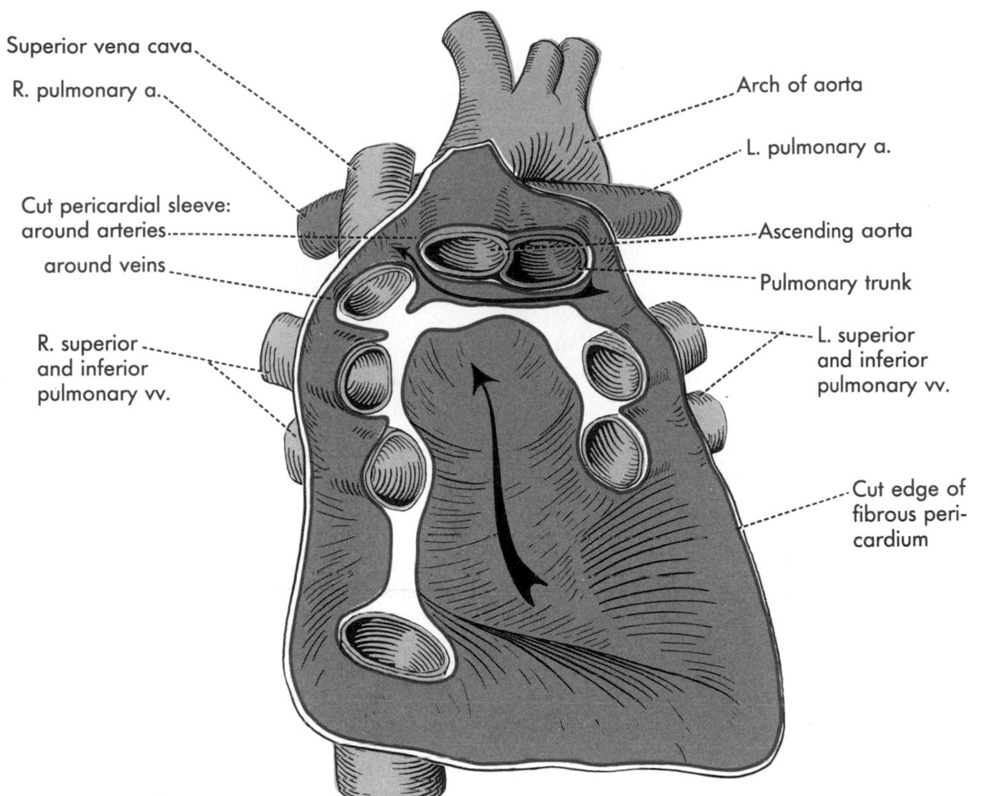

FIGURE *21-3.* **The posterior wall of the pericardial sac after the heart has been removed by severing its continuity with the great arteries and veins and by cutting the two pericardial sleeves that surround the arteries and veins. The parietal serous pericardium is *pink*; the fibrous pericardium is *white*; the *horizontal arrow* is in the transverse sinus; the *vertical arrow* is in the oblique sinus of the pericardium.**

Innervation and Blood Supply

Pericardial pain is mediated by *somatic afferents* distributed to the fibrous and parietal laminae of the pericardium by the **phrenic nerves.** The epicardium, supplied by autonomic nerves from the coronary plexuses, is insensitive to pain. Pericardial pain is felt behind the sternum and is usually due to inflammation of the pericardium caused by viral or bacterial infections or by neoplastic involvement.

The epicardium shares its blood supply with the myocardium, whereas the fibrous and parietal laminae of the pericardium are supplied by small twigs from the internal thoracic vessels, from the pericardiacophrenic vessels (themselves branches of the internal thoracic), from the aorta, from bronchial arteries, and from arteries of the diaphragm.

THE HEART

The heart is the central organ of the cardiovascular or circulatory system. Its name in Latin is *cor* and in Greek, *kardia*. Both names serve as roots for adjectives commonly used in describing the anatomy of the heart. The walls that enclose the hollow, four-chambered interior of the heart are thick and contractile and consist of three definable layers. The thickest of these is the middle or muscular layer, the **myocardium,** covered on the heart's exterior by the **epicardium,** and lined on the interior by the **endocardium.** The endocardium consists of endothelium supported by some delicate underlying connective tissue, and it is continuous with the tunica intima of the blood vessels entering and leaving the heart.

External Anatomy

External Form

The heart somewhat resembles a short cone (Fig. 21-4) and is described as having a base and an apex as well as surfaces and borders. The borders or margins are poorly defined on the heart itself (as one might expect from its essentially conical shape), but are useful in describing the radiologic anatomy of the heart. The division of the heart into four chambers is indicated on its surface by the coronary and interventricular sulci, which are useful landmarks for relating the chambers to external features.

Base and Apex. The **base** of the heart faces posteriorly and is made up largely of the **left atrium** and a more narrow portion of the right atrium (Fig. 21-5). Owing to the obliquity of the interatrial septum, the left atrium lies behind, rather than to the left, of the right atrium. A variable shallow groove situated to the right of the right pulmonary veins may indicate the position of the oblique interatrial septum.

All the great veins enter the base of the heart and fix it posteriorly to the pericardial wall. Between the entrances of the great veins into the atria, the base of the

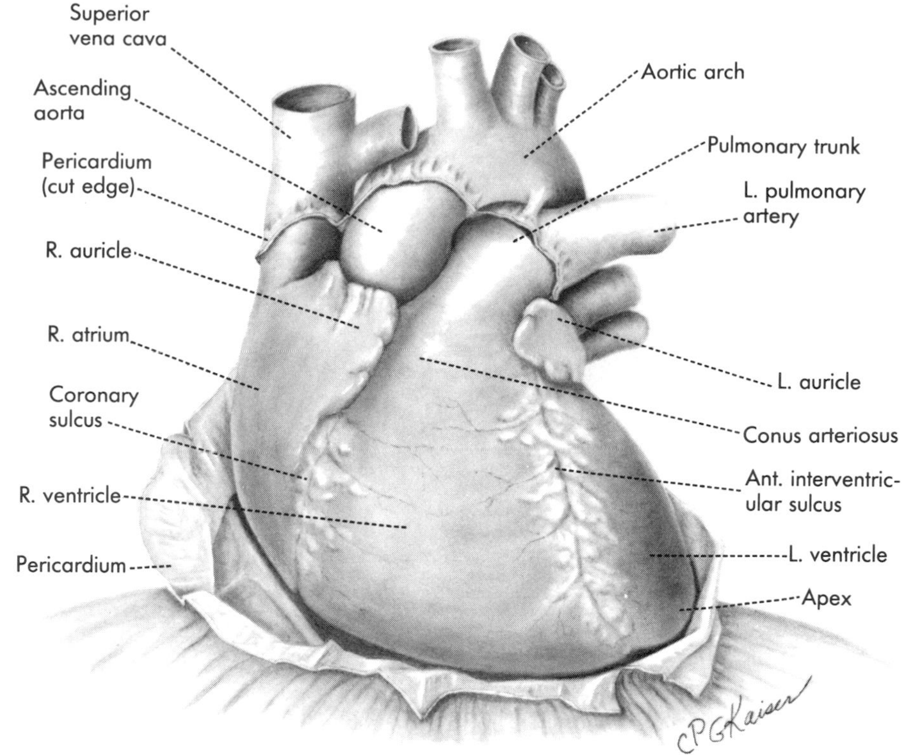

FIGURE *21-4.*
Anterior view of the heart: The pericardial sac has been cut open and reflected toward the diaphragm, on which the heart is resting.

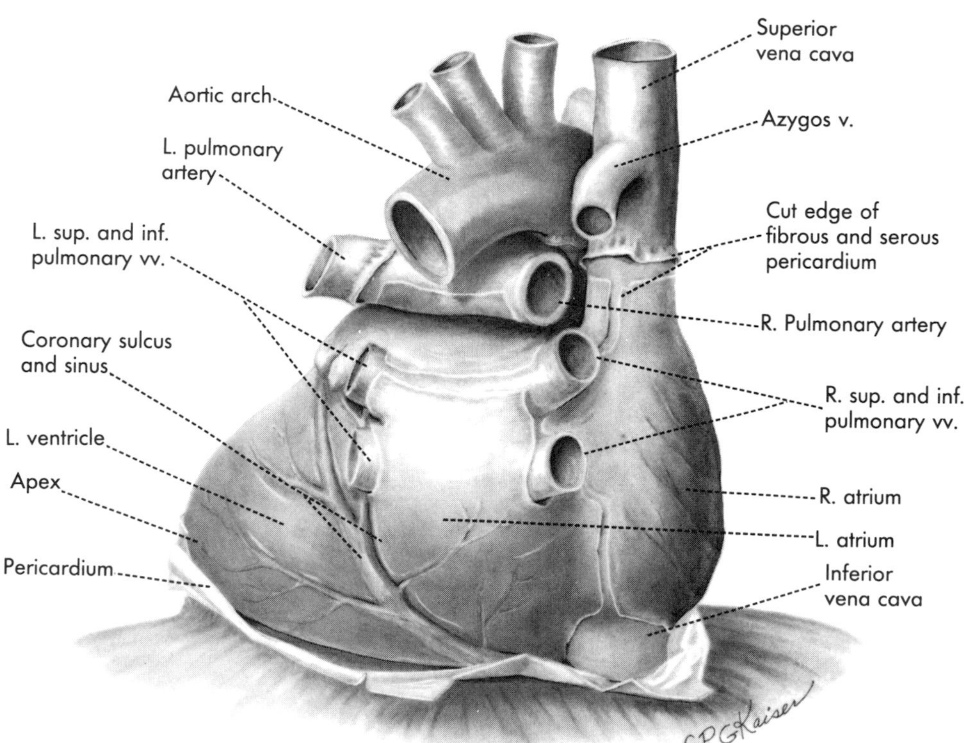

FIGURE *21-5.*
Posterior view of the heart retained in the same position as shown Figure 21-4.

heart forms the anterior wall of the oblique pericardial sinus.

From the base, the heart projects forward to terminate in the blunt **apex.** The apex of the heart points downward and toward the left as well as forward. It is formed by the left ventricle.

Surfaces. In addition to the base, four surfaces are described on the heart. These are the diaphragmatic or inferior, the sternocostal or anterior, and the left and right surfaces. The **diaphragmatic surface,** formed largely by the **left ventricle** and a more narrow portion of the **right ventricle,** extends from the base to the apex, faces inferiorly, and rests on the diaphragm (Fig. 21-6). A large vein, the *coronary sinus,* lodged in the coronary sulcus, separates this surface from the base. The *posterior interventricular sulcus,* occupied by an artery and vein, runs from the coronary sulcus toward the apex, and it demarcates the ventricles from one another.

The **sternocostal surface** faces anteriorly and is dominated by the right ventricle, with the right atrium visible to the right and the left ventricle visible to the left (see Fig. 21-4). Superiorly on the right, the superior vena cava leads into the **right atrium.** The free upper border of the atrium projects in front of the vena cava and extends anteriorly as the right auricle. The **auricle,** a flaplike, muscular pouch, overlaps the ascending aorta and obscures the superior portion of the coronary sulcus. The *coronary sulcus* separates the right atrium from the ventricle and runs from the root of the aorta toward the inferior vena cava (see Figs. 21-4 and 21-6). The inferior vena cava is at the right inferior corner of the sternocostal surface, but is not visible from the front view. The sulcus turns posteriorly at the right inferior corner of the heart and in the back separates the base of the heart from its inferior surface. Along the inferior border of the sternocostal surface, the **right ventricle** extends from the coronary sulcus almost to the apex of the heart and is in contact with the diaphragm. Superiorly, the right ventricle tapers toward the origin of the pulmonary trunk, and this funnel-shaped portion forms the **conus arteriosus** or **infundibulum.** The infundibulum continues into the pulmonary trunk. At its root, the pulmonary trunk interrupts the continuity of the coronary sulcus. But for this interruption, the sulcus encircles the heart between the atria and the ventricles. It is identifiable to the left of the pulmonary trunk where the **left auricle** overlies the pulmonary trunk. The *anterior interventricular sulcus,* occupied by an artery and one or two veins, descends from here toward the apex and marks the position of the interventricular septum. The interventricular septum sometimes creates a slight notch (*incisura*) just to the right of the apex. The coronary sulcus proceeds to the left from the pulmonary trunk and soon turns posteriorly, where it separates the left atrium from the left ventricle.

Both the **left** and the **right surfaces** of the heart face the lungs, but only the left is described, sometimes, as the **pulmonary surface.** Both are broad and convex; the right surface consists entirely of the right atrium, and the left, of the left ventricle, with the left auricle just above.

Margins or Borders. One may speak of the right, left, and inferior margins of the heart, although currently, official anatomic terminology recognizes only a right margin (*margo dexter*). Truly, the right and left margins correspond to the right and left surfaces. Only along the inferior border of the heart is there a relatively sharp edge between the sternocostal and diaphragmatic surfaces of the right ventricle to warrant calling it a margin.

In a posteroanterior **chest x-ray film,** the cardiovascular shadow presents definite borders on the right and

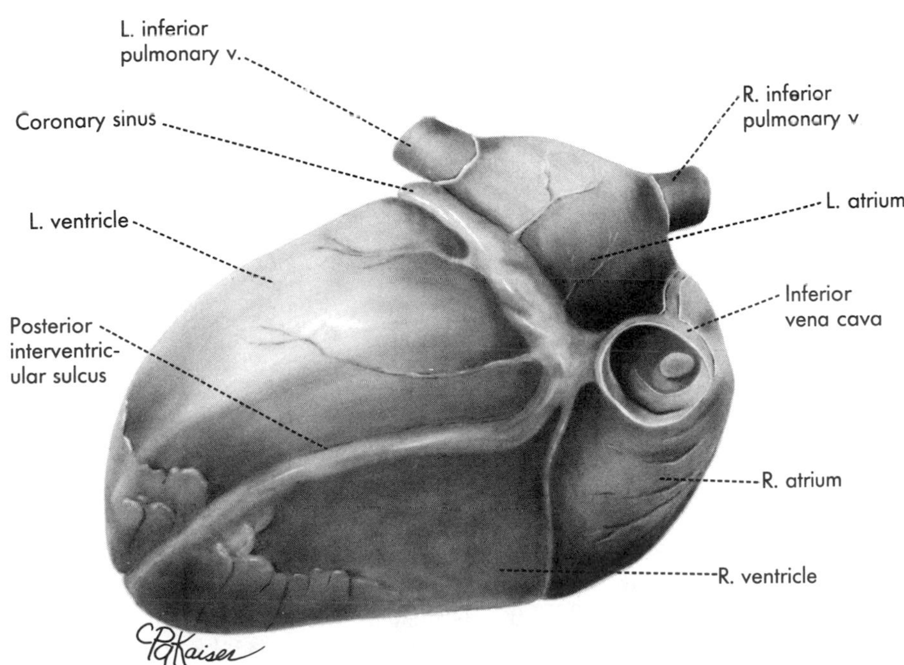

FIGURE *21-6.*
The inferior, or diaphragmatic, surface of the heart.

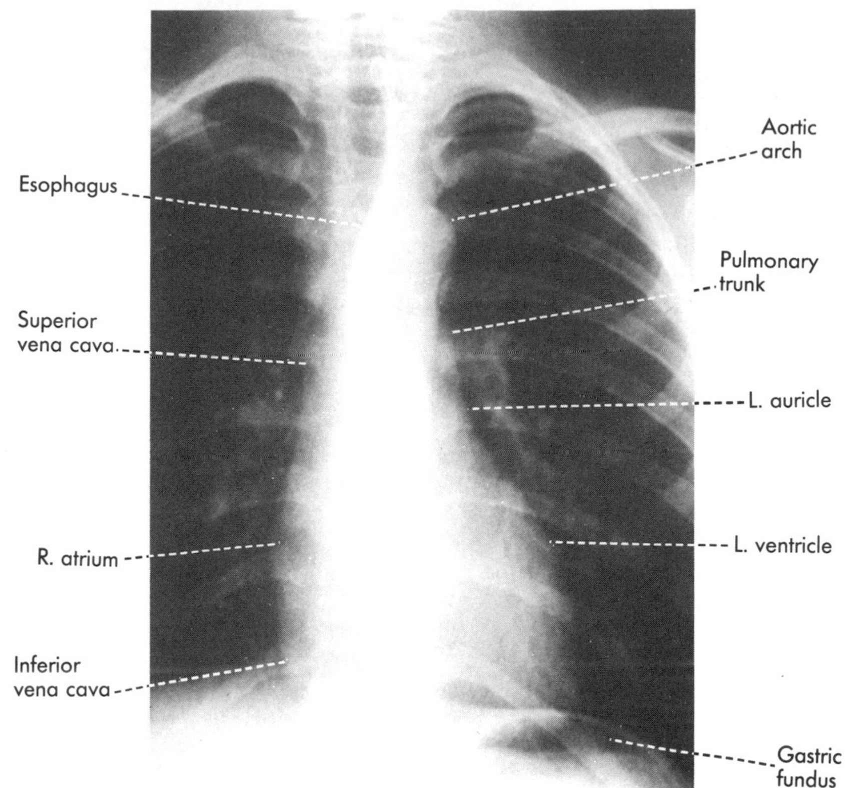

FIGURE *21-7.*
A posteroanterior chest radiograph of a young man. The esophagus contains some barium, and the fundus of the stomach contains some gas.

left as it abuts the radiolucent lung field (Fig. 21-7). The inferior border is largely obscured by the liver because the heart rests on the forward slope of the diaphragm. Knowledge of the structures that constitute the borders of the cardiac silhouette is of diagnostic importance in determining the enlargement of various chambers.

On a posteroanterior x-ray film the **right border** consists, from above downward, of the superior vena cava, right atrium, and inferior vena cava. The **left border** is made up of the arch of the aorta, pulmonary trunk, left auricle, and left ventricle. The right ventricle and, at the apex, the left ventricle, constitute the inferior border. Often the apex may be difficult to identify radiographically.

Radiologic examination of the heart includes lateral and oblique projections, the detailed description of which is beyond our present purpose. In the right and left lateral views, the cardiovascular shadow is made up anteriorly of the right ventricle and its conus arteriosus and posteriorly of the left atrium.

Relations

The relation of the cardiac chambers to one another is discussed with the surface projection and physical examination of the heart. Through the pericardium, the various chambers are related to a number of organs.

The **right atrium** is related anteriorly and laterally to the mediastinal surface of the right lung. Posterior to most of the right atrium is the left atrium. On the right, the right inferior pulmonary vein courses behind the right atrium (the superior vein is behind the superior vena cava). The sternocostal surface of the **right ventricle** is separated from the chest wall by the pericardium, the pleural sacs, and the areolar tissue in the anterior mediastinum. The **left atrium,** on the base of the heart, is in contact with the esophagus through the oblique sinus and the pericardium. When the atrium is enlarged, it displaces the esophagus, which is demonstrable radiographically by a barium swallow. Over the roof of the left atrium arch the pulmonary trunk and the ascending aorta. The transverse sinus intervenes between the atrium and these vessels. The **left ventricle** is related to the mediastinal surface of the left lung; the inferior surface of the ventricle is related, through the diaphragm, to the left lobe of the liver and the fundus of the stomach.

Internal Anatomy

The Cardiac Chambers

The Right Atrium. Situated on the right surface of the heart, this quadrangular chamber receives blood into its upper posterior corner from the superior vena cava, whereas the inferior vena cava and the coronary sinus open into its lower posterior corner (Fig. 21-8). From the atrium, the blood is emptied into the right ventricle through the *right atrioventricular ostium* that faces forward and medially. The ostium is guarded by the right atrioventricular or *tricuspid valve,* which will be described from its ventricular surface.

The interior of the atrium is partially divided into two main parts by the **crista terminalis,** a smooth muscular

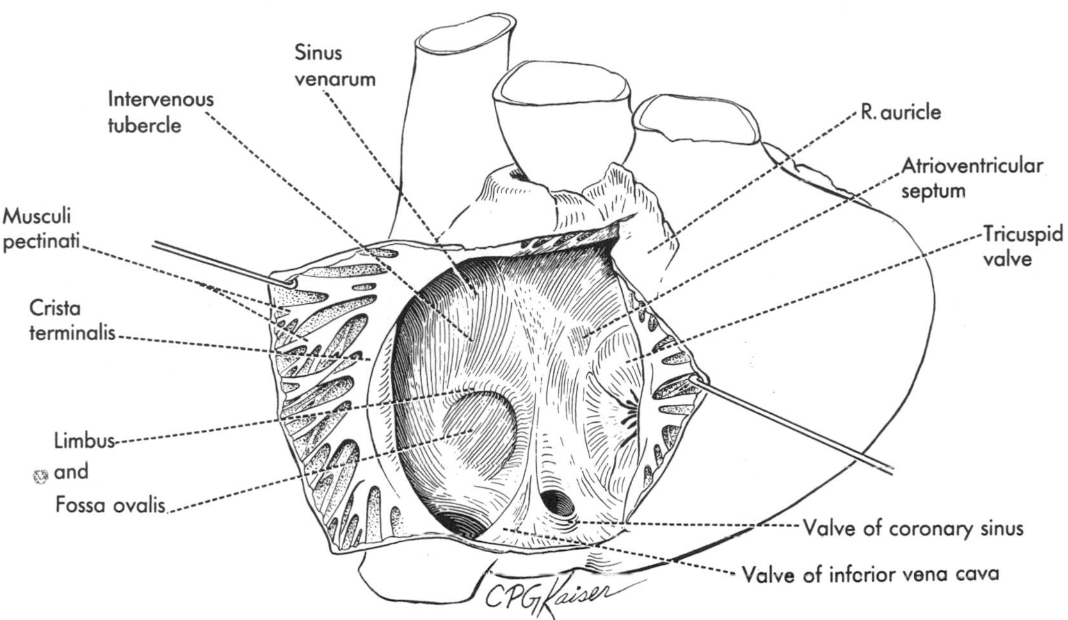

FIGURE *21-8.*
The interior of the right atrium seen from the right side. The view is toward the interatrial septum.

ridge that commences on the roof of the atrium just in front of the opening of the superior vena cava and extends down on the lateral wall of the chamber to the anterior lip of the inferior vena cava. The cavity posterior to the crista terminalis is the **sinus venarum (sinus venarum cavarum),** into which the two venae cavae open. The anterior half of the chamber that includes the **right auricle** is sometimes spoken of as the **atrium proper.** The walls of the sinus venarum are smooth, as is the surface of the interatrial septum, which separates the sinus from the left atrium. By contrast, the walls of the anterior half of the chamber, including the auricle, are ridged by the **musculi pectinati,** which fan out, comblike, from the crista terminalis. Only this anterior half corresponds to the primitive atrium of the embryonic heart; the sinus venarum represents the right horn of the sinus venosus, which had merged with the embryonic right atrium during development. In fact, the crista terminalis and the so-called *valve of the inferior vena cava,* a rudimentary endothelial flap on the anterior lip of the vessel, are derived from one of the valves that guarded the opening of the sinus venosus into the right atrium (see Fig. 21-23). Medial to the opening of the inferior vena cava is the *ostium of the coronary sinus* bordered by a small fold, the rudimentary *valve of the coronary sinus,* also derived from the valve of the sinus venosus.

The **interatrial septum** faces both forward and to the right, for the left atrium lies, in part, behind the right atrium as well as to its left (see Fig. 21-11). There is a depression in the septum just above the orifice of the inferior vena cava (see Fig. 21-8). This is the **fossa ovalis,** and its prominent margin is the **limbus fossae ovalis.**

The fossa marks the location of the *foramen ovale,* an aperture through which the blood flows from the right to the left atrium before birth. The floor of the fossa is formed by the *septum primum* of the embryonic heart, which seals the foramen after birth. A small opening may remain patent superiorly in the foramen throughout life and is of no functional consequence. The limbus corresponds to the margin of the foramen ovale formed by the lower edge of the *septum secundum.* These septa are described later in the section on the development of the heart.

On the posterior wall of the sinus venarum, between the two caval openings, is a smooth eminence, the *intervenous tubercle,* which, before birth, may assist in separating the two streams of blood that enter the atrium from the two venae cavae. The tubercle may direct the stream from the superior vena cava chiefly toward the right ventricle and the stream from the inferior vena cava chiefly toward the left atrium through the foramen ovale. Several small openings, the foramina of the smallest cardiac veins (*venae cardiacae minimae*), are scattered about the wall of the right atrium. Similar venous openings are found in all other chambers as well.

The Right Ventricle. Blood flows into the right ventricle from the right atrium in a horizontal and forward direction because the right ventricle is situated in front, as well as to the left, of the right atrioventricular opening. The cavity of the right ventricle extends almost to the apex of the heart and projects onto most of the sternocostal surface and along the anterior edge of the diaphragmatic surface. In cross section, the cavity is C-shaped (Fig. 21-9). Blood is received from the right atrium into the posterior limb of the C; the anterior limb leads superiorly into the **conus arteriosus** or **infundibulum,** which is the outflow tract of the ventricle (see Fig. 21-4). Inflow and outflow tracts are demarcated by a smooth muscular crest, the

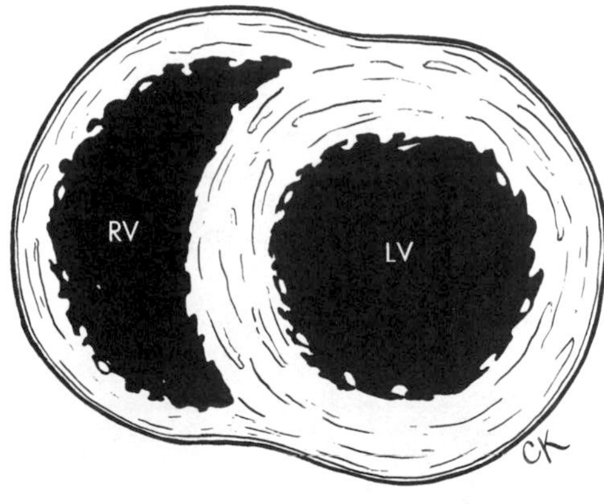

FIGURE *21-9.*
A schematic representation of a cross section of the ventricles (*seen from below*) to illustrate the shape of their lumina and the difference in the thickness of their wall.

crista supraventricularis, that partially divides the interior of the ventricle into two portions (Fig. 21-10). Above, the funnel-shaped infundibulum, or conus, leads into the pulmonary trunk through the *pulmonary orifice.*

The walls of the conus arteriosus are smooth, whereas the surface of the myocardium in the inflow part of the ventricle has prominent fleshy ridges, the **trabeculae carneae.** These trabeculae give rise to columnlike or nipplelike projections called *papillary muscles.*

At least one of the trabeculae carneae is elevated into a free band that forms a bridge between the interventricular septum and the anterior wall close to the apex of the ventricle. This is the *septomarginal trabecula,* formerly known as the moderator band; along it runs a branch of the atrioventricular bundle, part of the conducting system of the heart, to be described later. There are usually three sets of **papillary muscles,** anterior, posterior, and septal, named according to the location of their bases. From the apex of each papillary muscle several tendonlike fibrous cords, known as **chordae tendineae,** extend to the cusps of the atrioventricular valve. The largest and most constant is the anterior papillary muscle; the septal muscle is tiny, or may even be absent, and the chordae tendineae spring directly from the septum. There may be one to three posterior muscles and some chordae tendineae may, in addition, attach directly to the ventricular wall. The papillary muscles and chordae tendineae prevent the cusps of the valve from being everted into the atrium by the pressure developed in the contracting ventricle. This pressure closes the valve, and as the size of the ventricle decreases during contraction, the papillary muscles also contract so that they maintain tension on the cusps.

The **right atrioventricular valve** is also known as the **tricuspid valve** because in some hearts it consists of three cusps or leaflets. More often than not, however, there are only two cusps, and, in the literal sense, the use of the term *tricuspid* is not always apt. The bases of the cusps are secured to the fibrous ring that surrounds the atrioventricular ostium (see Fig. 21-13). The chordae tendineae attach to the ventricular surface of the cusps, and when the valve is opened, the three scalloped edges of the cusps project into the ventricle. Close to their bases, the cusps are continuous with one another along lines known to clinicians as *commissures.* The three cusps are named according to their position: anterior, posterior, and septal. Each receives chordae tendineae from two papillary muscles. The cusps consist of dense fibrous tissue covered by endocardium, and only along their bases are some blood vessels found in their substance.

The *orifice of the pulmonary trunk* is closed by the **pulmonary valve,** which consists of three semilunar *valvules,* or cusps (Fig. 21-11; and see Fig. 21-10). Each cusp is formed by the reduplication of endothelium with little fibrous tissue between the layers, and each resembles a distended vest pocket, projecting with its free edge upward into the lumen of the pulmonary trunk. At the middle of the free edge of each valvule is a thickening, the *nodule,* and the thin margin on each side of the nodule is the *lunula.* In the "pocket" of each valvule is a *sinus* or dilation of the pulmonary trunk, and the valvules attach along the curved inferior margin of each sinus. After blood is ejected from the right ventricle, the nodules and lunules of each valvule are forced together tightly by the pressure of blood in the pulmonary trunk, causing distention of the pulmonary sinuses. The pulmonary valve thus prevents regurgitation of blood into the ventricle. Two of the cusps of the pulmonary valve are anterior, and one is posterior. The official naming of the cusps is confusing, however, because it is based on the fetal position of the heart before it completes its rotation. Accordingly, the *Nomina Anatomica* recognizes one anterior valvule, one left valvule, and one right valvule (see Fig. 21-11).

The Left Atrium. Similar to the right atrium, the interior of the left atrium is divided into two portions, although there is no definite line of demarcation here. The posterior half of the chamber, into which the four pulmonary veins empty, has smooth walls and may be designated as the inflow part of the chamber; this part of the atrium is derived from the proximal portions of the embryonic pulmonary veins, the walls of which were incorporated into the atrium during development. The anterior portion is continuous with the **left auricle,** has *musculi pectinati* on its wall, and is derived from the embryonic atrium. The interatrial septum forms part of the anterior wall of the left atrium (see Fig. 21-11). The thin area on the septum is the *valvule of the foramen ovale,* visible in the right atrium as the floor of the fossa ovalis. In the fetus, it functioned as a valve, for blood coming into the right atrium could push it aside and enter the left atrium, but blood attempting to pass in the opposite direction would force it against the rather rigid rim of the foramen. In approximately 20% of adults, the original free edge of the valvule is incompletely fused, so that the tip of a small probe or a catheter can be passed between the atria.

The Left Ventricle. The left ventricle lies to the front of the left atrium, and blood flows toward its apex from the left atrioventricular orifice, chiefly in a forward direction. The myocardium is thickest in the wall of this chamber, which occupies the rounded lateral surface of the

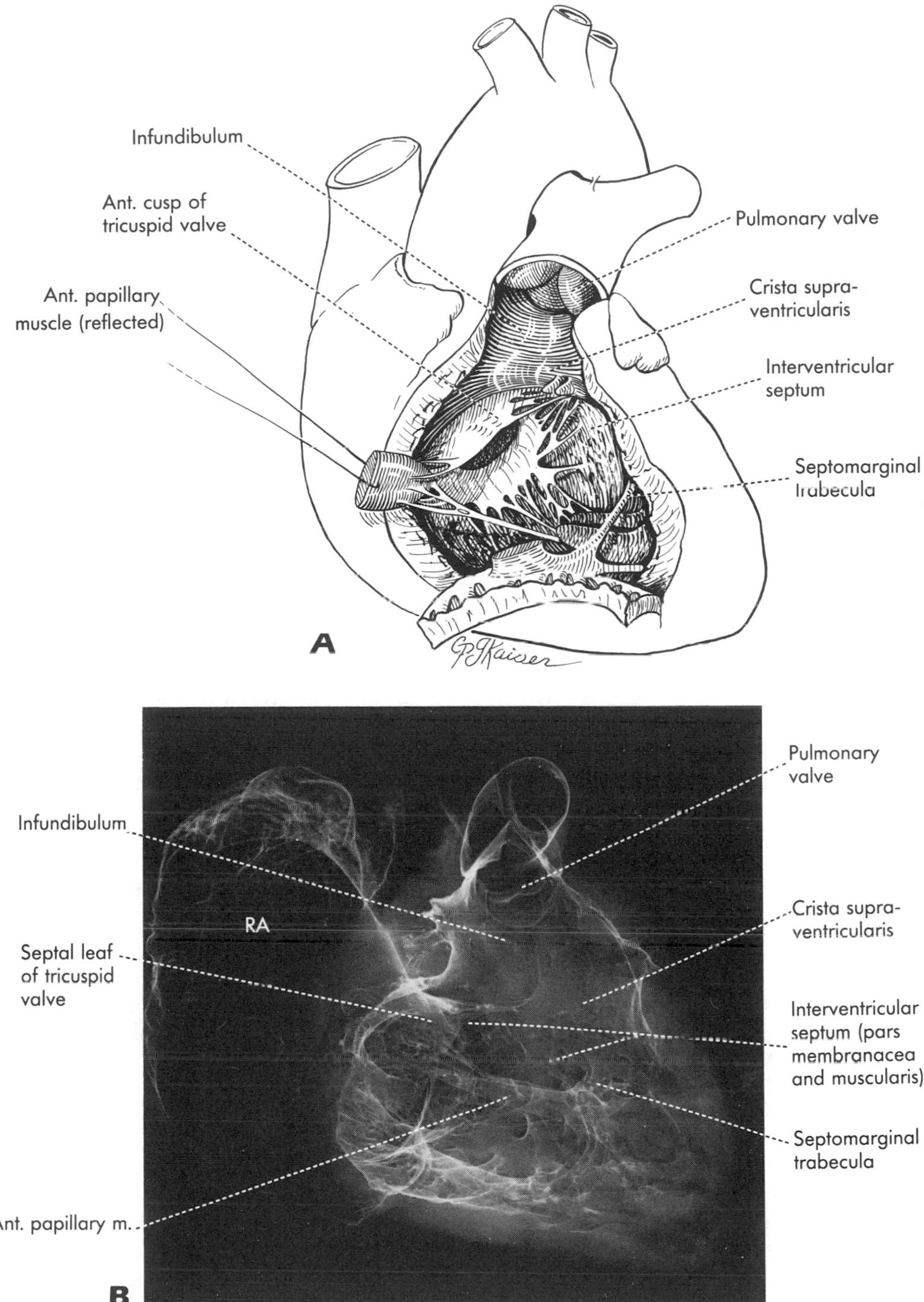

FIGURE *21-10.*
The interior of the right ventricle: (A) The drawing of a dissection, corresponds to (B) radiograph that was obtained after the heart was fixed, its walls impregnated with wax, and the interior of the right ventricle dusted with barium powder. The crista supraventricularis separates the inflow part of the ventricle from the infundibulum, or conus arteriosus. Note the great distance between the septal leaf of the tricuspid valve and the pulmonary valve. *RA*, right atrium. (Panel B was prepared and kindly provided by Dr. Lore Tenckhoff).

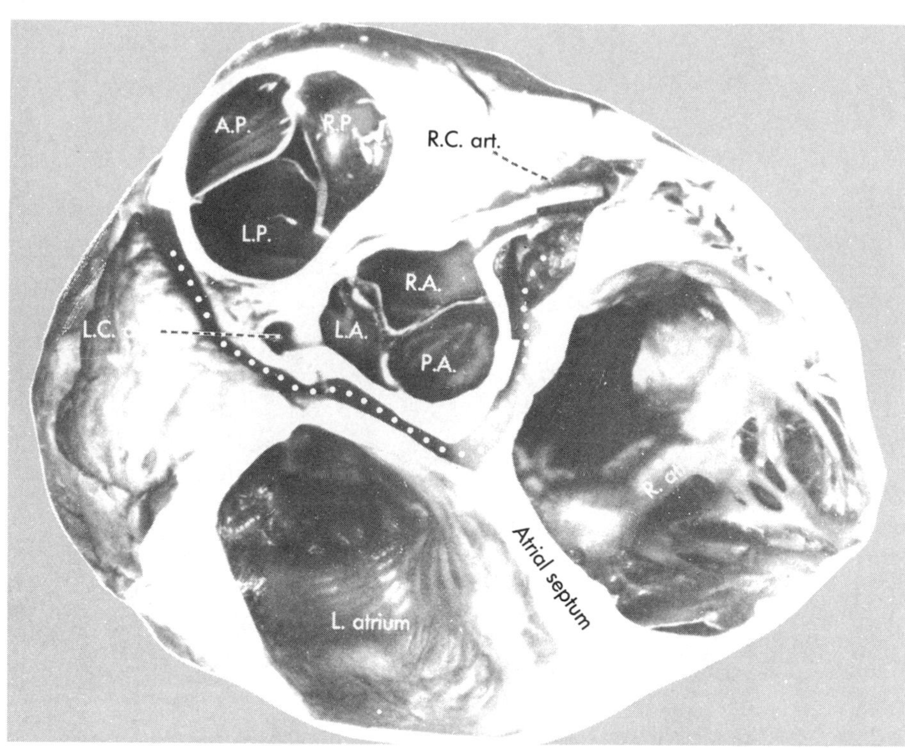

FIGURE *21-11.*
Photograph of a heart cut obliquely across the pulmonary trunk, the aorta, and the two atria. The aorta is cut just above the level of the origin of the two coronary arteries (*RC art* and *LC art*), and the three valvules of the aortic valve are visible: left (*LA*), right (*RA*), and posterior (*PA*). Anterior to the aorta is the pulmonary trunk, closed off from the right ventricle by the anterior (*AP*), right (*RP*), and left (*LP*) cusps of the pulmonary valve. The transverse sinus of the pericardium (indicated by a *white dotted line*) separates the pulmonary trunk and the aorta from the atria. Two cusps of the mitral valve and one cusp of the tricuspid valve are visible through the left and right atria. Note the obliquity of the interatrial septum. (Modified from Edwards JE, Burchell HB. Thorax 1957;12:123.)

heart, including the apex and most of the inferior surface. The cavity of the left ventricle is conical, and the outline of its cross section is nearly circular (see Fig. 21-9). Inflow and outflow tracts are not as clearly demarcated in the left ventricle as in those of the right. The trabeculae carneae in the left ventricle are fine and delicate in contrast with the coarse trabeculae in the right ventricle. The septal wall is smooth and leads superiorly toward the aortic orifice. This outflow tract, designated as the **aortic vestibule,** corresponds to the conus arteriosus (infundibulum) on the right, which lies directly anterior to it, and like the conus is derived from the embryonic bulbus cordis (Fig. 21-12).

Because the right ventricle lies largely in front of the left ventricle, the **interventricular septum** forms the anterior and right-hand wall of the left ventricle. Its thick part is the *pars muscularis.* Above, close to the atrioventricular orifices, the septum is thin and membranous; this is the *pars membranacea* (see Fig. 21-12). A tiny part of the pars membranacea lies above the attachment of the septal cusp of the tricuspid valve and thus between the cavities of the left ventricle and right atrium; this is the *atrioventricular septum* (see Fig. 21-8).

The *left atrioventricular ostium* opens into the posterior and right side of the upper part of the left ventricle (see Fig. 21-12). The ostium is protected by the *left atrioventricular valve,* which has two cusps. The two cusps are reminiscent of a bishop's miter; hence, the valve is also known as the **mitral valve.** Its cusps are anterior and posterior (Fig. 21-13). Attached to the free edges of the cusps are *chordae tendineae,* which originate in *papillary muscles.* There are usually only two papillary muscles in the left ventricle, an anterior and a posterior (either may show some duplication), and the chordae tendineae of each go to both cusps of the mitral valve.

Behind the infundibulum of the right ventricle, the aortic vestibule gives rise to the aorta. The aortic orifice is closed by the **aortic valve,** which resembles the pulmonary valve in every respect. These two valves are often referred to as the **semilunar valves,** a name that aptly describes the shape of their valvules. The three valvules, or cusps, harbor in their "pockets" the three *aortic sinuses.* The sinuses and the cusps are named right, left, and posterior (see Fig. 21-11), and from the right and left sinuses originate the right and left coronary arteries, respectively (see Fig. 21-13). The posterior sinus and valvule are designated as the noncoronary sinus and cusp.

Structure of the Myocardium

The cardiac muscle fibers are arranged in somewhat indistinct bundles that attach to the heavy fibrous connective tissue sometimes referred to as the **skeleton of the heart.** This connective tissue forms the foundation to which the valves—pulmonary, aortic, and atrioventricular—as well as the myocardial fiber bundles are attached. The four **fibrous rings** (*annuli fibrosi*) that support the four sets of valves are fused to one another (see Fig. 21-13).

The connective tissue between the aortic ring and the two atrioventricular rings shows two localized thickening, the *fibrous trigones.* The upper, membranous part of the interventricular septum (pars membranacea) blends with the connective tissue between the aortic ring and the right atrioventricular ring. The fibrous skeleton of the heart separates the musculature of the atria from that of the ventricles. Atrial bundles attach to the upper borders of the rings, and ventricular bundles attach to the lower borders. The two sets of muscle are

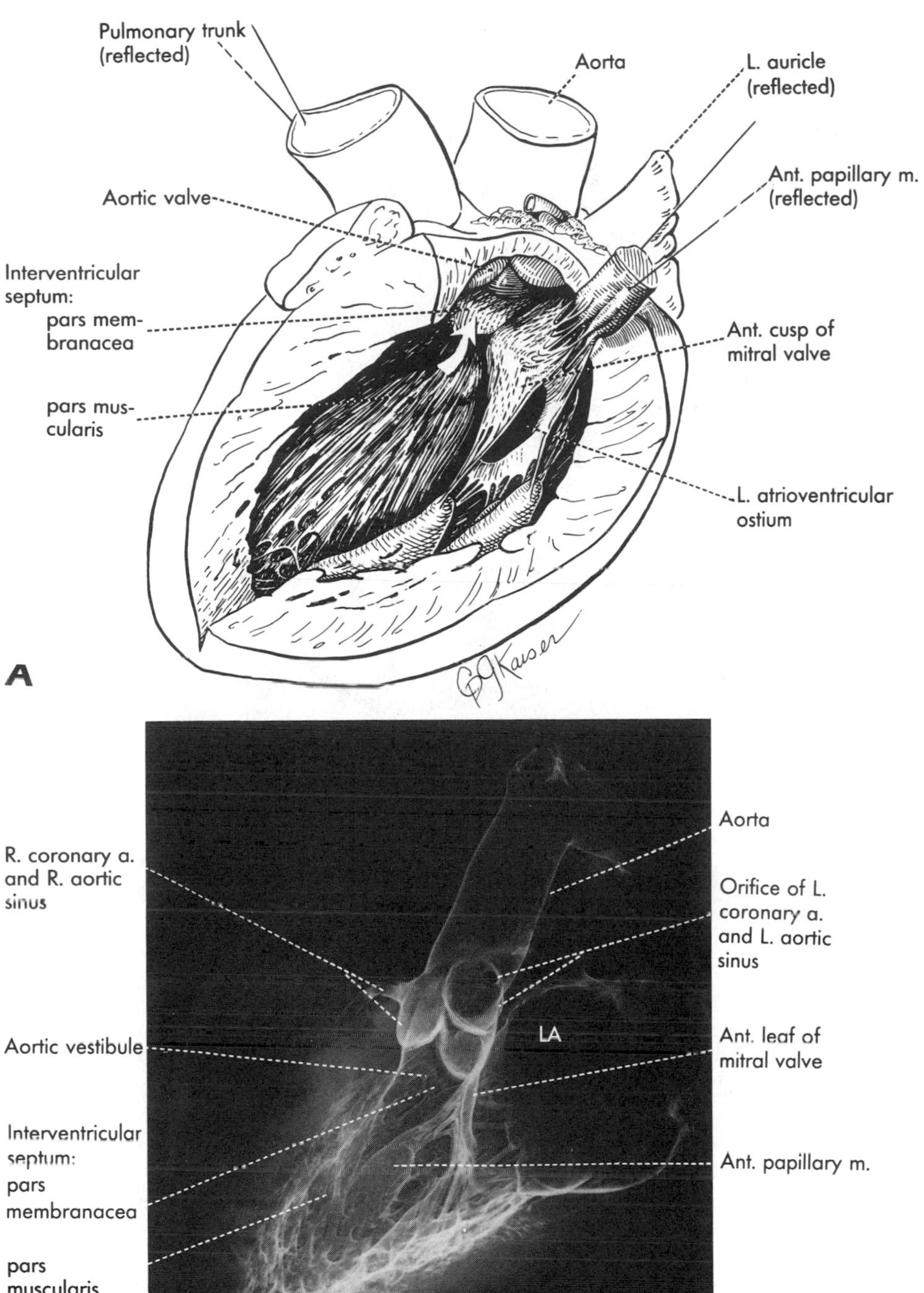

FIGURE *21-12.*
The interior of the left ventricle: (A) a schematic dissection, the wall on the left side of the ventricle has been cut away; (B), radiograph of a heart prepared as explained in the legend of Figure 21-10. The interior of the left ventricle, left atrium (*LA*), and aorta have been dusted with barium powder. Note the proximity of the anterior cusp of the mitral valve to the aortic valve. The outflow tract of the left ventricle (aortic vestibule) is indicated in panel A by a *white arrow*. (B prepared and kindly provided by Dr. Lore Tenckhoff.)

united only by a specialized conducting bundle, the atrioventricular bundle (described under The Innervation and the Conducting System of the Heart). This bundle differs histologically from regular cardiac muscle, and it penetrates the fibrous partition.

The numerous fiber bundles of the atria are usually grouped into two systems, superficial and deep. The superficial fibers tend to run transversely across both atria and originate chiefly around the superior vena cava. Some of the deep fibers are annular and surround the several venous openings into the atria or circle the auricles. Other bundles originate from the atrioventricular fibrous ring, loop around one atrium and contribute to the interatrial septum, and then attach again to the atrioventricular ring.

Sheets of myocardial fibers encircle the ventricular chambers in a rather complex manner reminiscent of the windings of a turban. The information contained in Figure 21-14 about their anatomy is more than adequate for the purpose of this chapter.

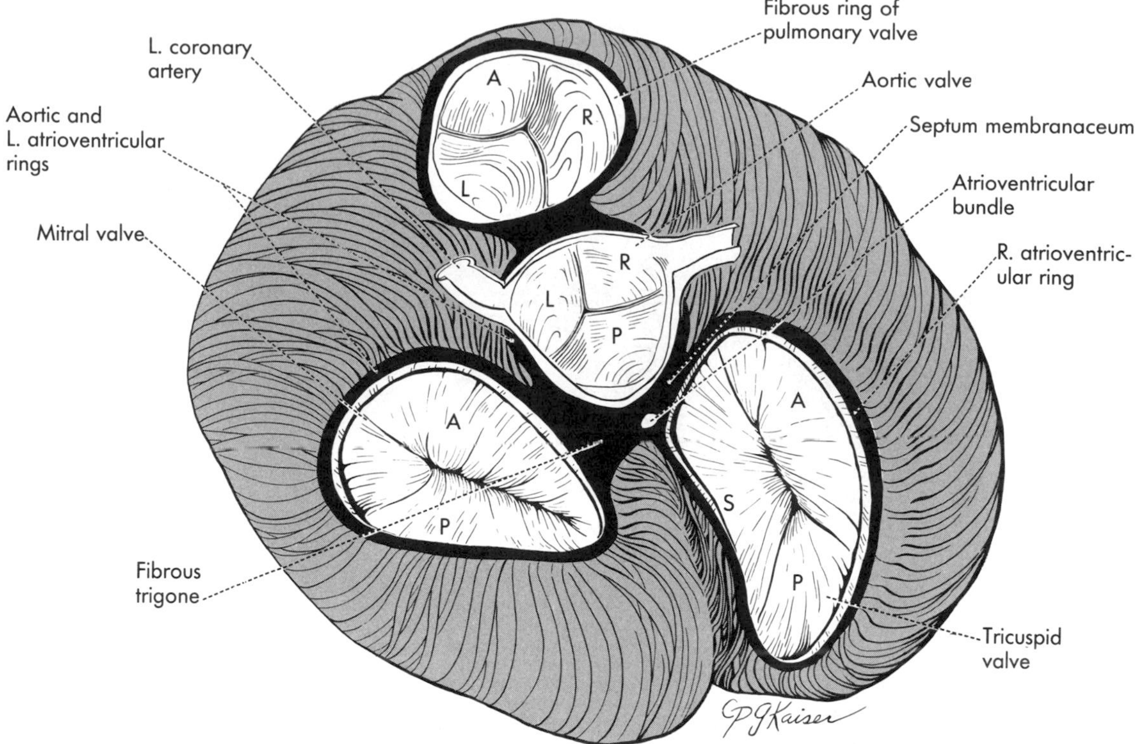

FIGURE *21-13.*
The fibrous skeleton of the heart (*solid black*). The orientation of the heart is similar to that shown in Figure 21-11, but the atria have been dissected away. The ventricular muscle fibers can be seen to radiate away from their attachment to the fibrous rings that support the valves. The cusps or valvules of the various valves are identified (*A*, anterior; *P*, posterior; *R*, right; *L*, left; *S*, septal).

Blood Supply

The arteries that supply the heart are the coronary arteries; the veins of the heart are known as the cardiac veins (venae cordis).

Coronary Arteries

The right and left coronary arteries arise from the aorta just above its origin from the left ventricle while the aorta is still behind the pulmonary trunk (Fig. 21-15). The **right coronary artery** originates from the right aortic sinus and passes to the right, behind the pulmonary trunk, to run downward in the coronary sulcus between the right atrium and the right ventricle. Then it turns posteriorly around the inferior margin of the heart and continues in the coronary sulcus, supplying throughout its course the right ventricle and the right atrium. The largest branch of the right coronary artery is the *posterior interventricular branch,* which runs forward in the posterior interventricular sulcus toward the apex and supplies the diaphragmatic surface of both ventricles and approximately the posterior one-third of the interventricular septum. Smaller named branches include the *marginal artery* and those that are given off to the *sinuatrial* and *atrioventricular nodes* and to the *conus arteriosus.*

The **left coronary artery** arises from the left aortic sinus (see Fig. 21-15). Shortly after its origin, usually while it is still behind the pulmonary trunk, the artery bifurcates into an anterior interventricular and a circumflex branch. The *anterior interventricular branch* skirts the left margin of the pulmonary trunk and descends toward the apex in the anterior interventricular sulcus. It gives branches to both ventricles, including the conus arteriosus, and to most of the interventricular septum. The *circumflex branch* runs toward the left in the coronary sulcus, first between the left auricle and left ventricle, and then it circles to the posterior aspect of the heart. It usually does not reach the posterior interventricular sulcus, but when it does, it may give rise to the posterior interventricular artery. The biggest branch of the circumflex artery, called the *posterior left ventricular branch,* supplies the diaphragmatic surface of the left ventricle. Other named branches of the circumflex artery include a *marginal,* an *intermediate,* and occasionally a *sinuatrial* and an *atrioventricular* artery.

In summary, the right coronary artery typically supplies the right ventricle, the posterior part of the left ventricle and the interventricular septum, the right atrium, and the interatrial septum, including the sinuatrial and atrioventricular nodes (parts of the conducting system of the heart). The left coronary artery regularly supplies most of the left ventricle and left atrium, and its anterior

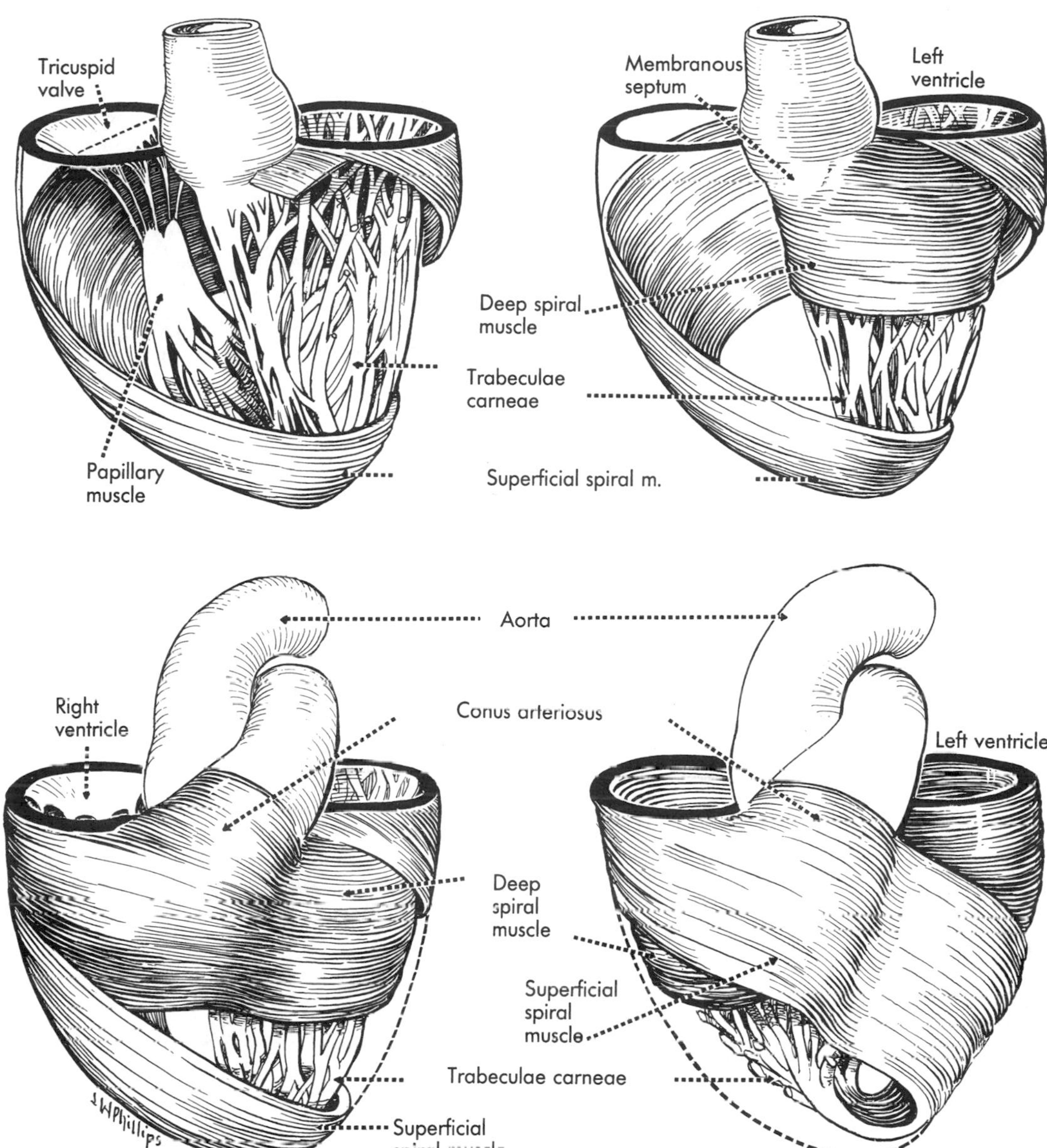

FIGURE *21-14.*
Some myocardial fiber bundles of the ventricles. Superficial spiral bundles arise principally from the atrioventricular fibrous rings and form a vortex at the apex. On the inside of the ventricles, these fibers emerge from the vortex as trabeculae carneae or papillary muscles and spiral back toward the atrioventricular orifices. The deep spiral bundles are also attached to the fibrous rings; some encircle one, others both, of the ventricles. Although this anatomic arrangement could not be confirmed in canine and porcine hearts, it appears to be correct for the human heart. (After Robb JS, Robb RC. Am Heart J 1942;23:455; Rushmer RF. Structure and function of the cardiovascular system. 2nd ed. Philadelphia WB Saunders 1976;178).

interventricular branch is the chief source of blood to the interventricular septum. This territory of supply includes the atrioventricular bundle and its branches (parts of the conducting system of the heart) as they lie in the septum. The left coronary artery may help supply, or may be the sole supply, of the sinuatrial and atrioventricular nodes.

Variations. The distribution of the smaller branches of the coronary arteries is not constant, and the branching of the larger vessels may deviate from the pattern described in the foregoing. Both interventricular branches may arise from the left coronary artery, or the anterior interventricular branch may be double. Occasionally, the two coronary arteries arise by a common stem, or the circumflex branch originates separately from the anterior interventricular branch. Either vessel may be abnormally placed on the aorta. Of more concern is the origin of a coronary artery from

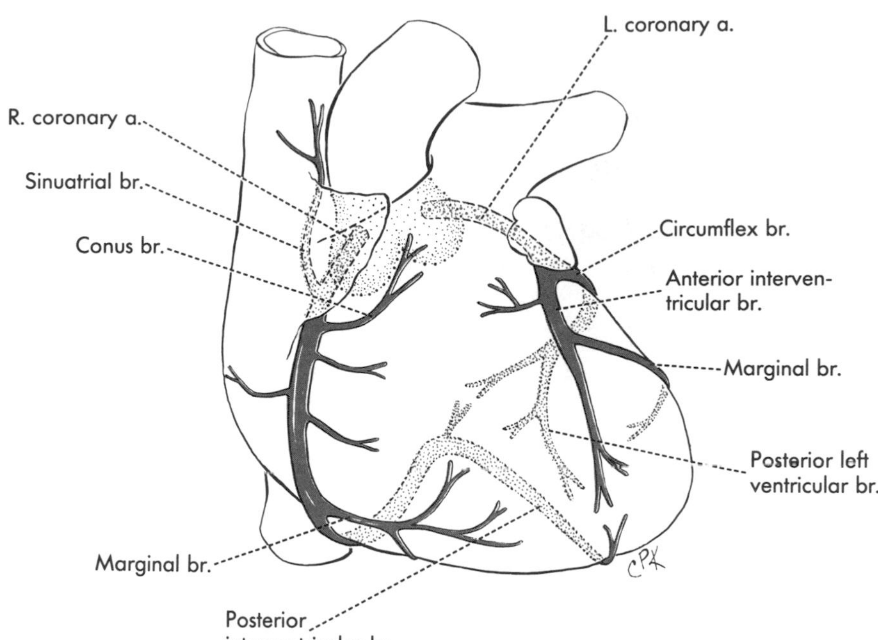

FIGURE *21-15.*
The coronary arteries shown from an anterior view of the heart.

the pulmonary trunk, because such a vessel cannot provide oxygenated blood to the heart.

Myocardial Infarction and Intercoronary Anastomoses. The constant rhythmic activity of cardiac muscle makes the heart particularly dependent on a good blood supply. The density of capillaries in cardiac muscle is more than 80 times that in skeletal muscle. The coronary arteries are not end arteries. The myocardium of the normal human heart contains abundant arteriolar anastomotic channels that range in diameter from 20 to 200 μm. Some of these anastomoses connect various branches of one coronary artery; others are intercoronary anastomoses. Despite their considerable size, the anastomoses possess only a thin wall and, in healthy hearts, cannot be demonstrated by arteriography because they are too small or apparently nonfunctional. However, when a major vessel is obstructed in the coronary circulation, blood will flow through the existing collateral vessels, owing to the pressure gradient created between the vessels that the anastomotic channel connects. The lumen of a major vessel has to be reduced by 90% before the collateral vessels open up. The time required for the opening up of these anastomoses is not exactly known. Once flow through the collateral vessels is established, they become elongated and tortuous and may dilate 1 to 2 mm in diameter. The location of these collaterals has been studied by coronary angiography, and knowledge of their functional status matters in considering indications for coronary arterial surgery.

Gradual narrowing of the coronary arteries by *atheroma* leads to myocardial ischemia, which gives rise to characteristic chest pains (*angina pectoris*). When occlusion is advanced or complete, depending on the size and location of the affected artery, a varying amount of cardiac muscle becomes devitalized. The damage caused may vary from death of a small amount of muscle compatible with fibrous repair and scarring of the myocardium to such disruption of cardiac function that the "heart attack" is immediately fatal.

The number and size of anastomoses may increase with age in the coronary circulation, especially when there is progressive arterial narrowing. Many of these anastomoses develop in subepicardial fat and may reroute sufficient blood to the ischemic myocardium to prevent an infarct from occurring or may reduce its size. Meticulous medical care following a nonfatal infarct often allows nature the necessary time to establish a collateral circulation.

Early surgical attempts to augment the coronary circulation included the creation of adhesions between the epicardium and such vascular structures as the greater omentum or the lung, which were approximated and affixed to the heart through an opening made through the pericardium. These procedures have been abandoned in favor of more direct methods such as the *coronary bypass* operation. A localized obstruction is bypassed with a vein graft that extends from the aorta to the portion of the coronary artery distal to the obstruction.

Cardiac Veins

Most of the venous blood is collected from the myocardium by veins that parallel the arteries (Fig. 21-16). These cardiac veins terminate in the coronary sinus, a large vein that empties into the right atrium. The rest of the blood in the coronary circulation is returned from the myocardium by small veins that open directly into the four chambers of the heart.

The **great cardiac vein** lies in the anterior interventricular sulcus and drains upward alongside the anterior interventricular branch of the left coronary artery. As it reaches the coronary sulcus, it turns to the left to run along the circumflex branch of the artery. The great cardiac vein becomes continuous with the coronary sinus at the point where the *oblique vein of the left atrium* enters it. As the **coronary sinus** continues to the right in the coronary sulcus, it is usually covered partially by superficial

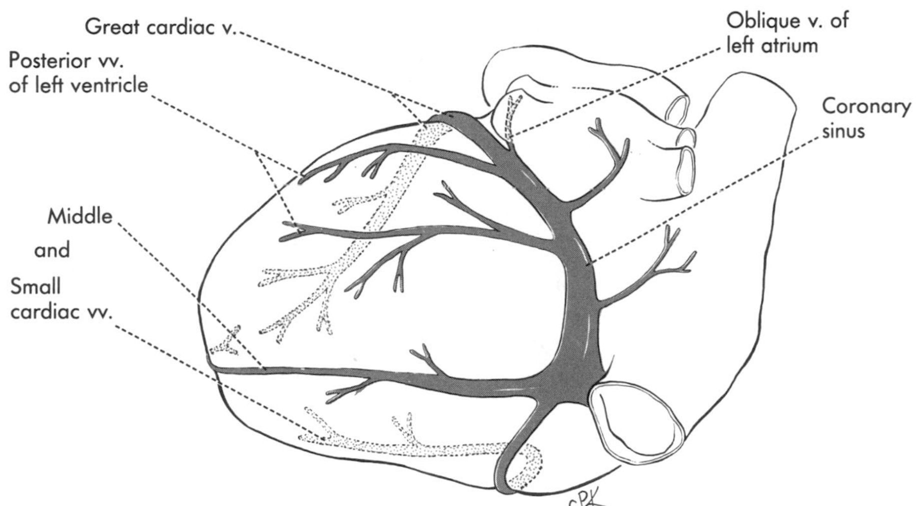

FIGURE 21-16.
The cardiac veins shown from a posterior view of the heart.

muscle fibers of the atrium. It ends in the posterior wall of the right atrium and, fairly close to its ending, receives the middle and small cardiac veins. The **middle cardiac vein** runs in the posterior interventricular sulcus, and the **small cardiac vein** runs in the coronary sulcus along the right coronary artery. The **posterior veins of the left ventricle** drain the diaphragmatic surface of the ventricle and enter the coronary sinus soon after the sinus has been formed.

The *coronary sinus* represents the left horn of the embryonic sinus venosus (see Fig. 21-22); the right horn became incorporated into the right atrium. The **oblique vein of the left atrium** is invisible or very small, but is of interest because it is the remnant of the embryonic left common cardinal vein. When the vein is of any size, a remnant of the left superior vena cava can also usually be identified.

In addition to the tributaries of the coronary sinus, there are several small **anterior cardiac veins** that arise on the anterior surface of the right ventricle and pass across the coronary sulcus to penetrate directly the anterior wall of the right atrium. Finally, although not visible by dissection, there are, in the muscular walls of the heart, minute veins, the **least cardiac veins** (*venae cardiacae minimae*), that empty into the cardiac chambers. These small venous orifices are said to be most numerous in the right atrium and least numerous in the left ventricle.

Lymphatic Drainage

The lymphatics of the heart form networks adjacent to the endocardium and the epicardium. The efferent vessels drain along the coronary arteries and empty into lymph nodes associated with the lower end of the trachea (tracheobronchial nodes; see Fig. 20-9).

The Innervation and the Conducting System of the Heart

A number of cardiac nerves derived from both the sympathetic and parasympathetic components of the autonomic nervous system commingle in the cardiac plexus, located in front of the tracheal bifurcation (Fig. 21-17). Offshoots of this plexus innervate the lungs (pulmonary plexuses described in the previous chapter) and the heart. These nerves reach the heart along the coronary arteries

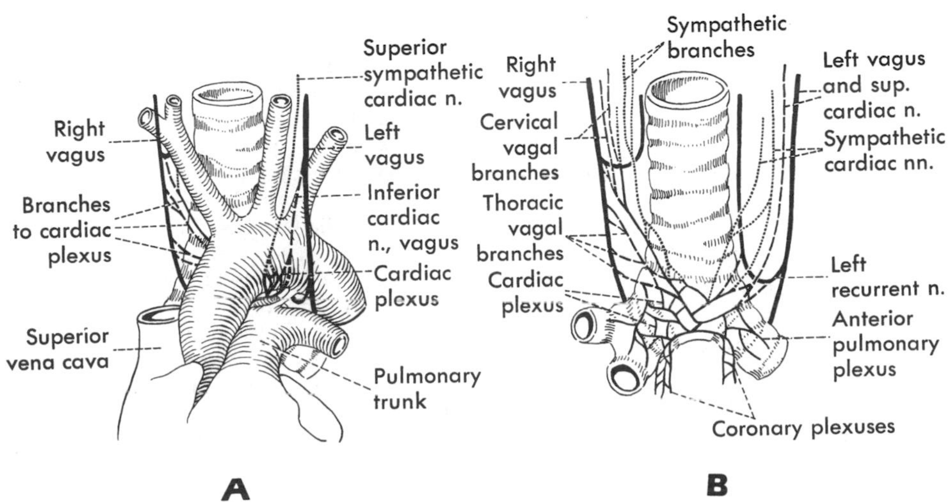

FIGURE 21-17.
Cardiac nerves and the cardiac plexus: (A) the aorta and pulmonary trunk left *in situ*; (B) the vessels removed to expose the bifurcation of the trachea. Cardiac branches of the vagi are shown in *broken lines*, and cardiac branches of the cervical sympathetic ganglia are shown in *dotted lines*. The thoracic cardiac nerves, medial branches of the upper thoracic sympathetic ganglia, are not shown.

and serve to modify the rate and strength of the heart beat; they are not responsible for initiating or maintaining it. The atria and ventricles contract in orderly sequence before nerves contact the embryonic heart, and the same is true when the transplanted heart is severed from its nervous connections. This automatic rhythmicity is largely generated by an intrinsic "pacemaker" known as the sinuatrial node, from which impulses spread to the rest of the myocardium. The node is the first component of the heart's so-called conducting system, an anatomically discrete network of myocardial tissue specialized for rapid conduction. Efferent nervous impulses primarily influence the pacemaker and coronary blood flow, whereas afferent impulses are concerned with reflex adjustments of the heart beat, circulation, and respiration, and they also mediate cardiac pain.

The Cardiac Plexus

This diffuse network of delicate nerves extends from in front of the trachea to the arch of the aorta, the pulmonary trunk, and the ligamentum arteriosum, which connects the two vessels (see Fig. 21-17).

The **parasympathetic** input to the plexus is provided by the two vagi, whereas the **sympathetic** input comes from the sympathetic trunks (see Chap. 7). Two long, slender branches (or groups of branches) arise from each vagus in the neck: the superior and inferior *cervical cardiac branches*. A variable number of shorter nerves are also given off in the thorax, either from the vagal trunks or from their recurrent laryngeal branches (*thoracic cardiac branches*). Sympathetic cardiac branches likewise arise in both the neck and the thorax. The high origin of the major cardiac nerves is a reminder of the location of the developing heart, opposite cervical segments, when it first received its nerve supply (see Chap. 7). Each sympathetic trunk in the neck gives off three cardiac branches: the superior, middle, and inferior *cervical cardiac nerves*. They arise from the superior cervical, middle cervical, and cervicothoracic (stellate) ganglion, respectively. The small and delicate *thoracic cardiac nerves* are given off from the upper four or five ganglia of the thoracic sympathetic trunk.

Efferent vagal fibers that enter the cardiac plexus are preganglionic axons of neurons located in vagal nuclei of the brain stem. They synapse in minute *cardiac ganglia* found in the plexus or in the walls of the atria. Vagal stimulation slows the heart beat and constricts the coronary arteries.

Sympathetic efferents that enter the plexus are postganglionic. The corresponding preganglionic neurons are in the intermediolateral cell column of the first four or five thoracic cord segments, and their axons relay in ganglia of the sympathetic trunk from which the cardiac nerves issue. Sympathetic efferents increase the rapidity and strength of the heart beat and dilate the coronary vessels.

Both vagal and sympathetic nerve fibers reach the heart by the two **coronary plexuses** given off from the cardiac plexus. The nerves are distributed along the coronary vessels chiefly to the atria, the sinuatrial node, and other components of the conducting system, which are said to have a particularly rich innervation. Although numerous nerve endings have been described, the nature of the contact between nerve fibers and cardiac muscle remains unknown.

All vagal fibers to the heart can be blocked only by interruption of the individual cardiac branches of both vagi, or by interruption of the vagal trunks above the level of origin of all their cardiac branches. This is also true of the sympathetic innervation to the heart: the cervical portion of the sympathetic trunk receives no preganglionic fibers from cervical nerves, for its preganglionic fibers ascend from the upper part of the thoracic portion of the trunk (see Chap. 7). Therefore, removal of the upper thoracic portion of the trunk over a distance of about five segments will interrupt not only the origins of the thoracic cardiac nerves, but also the preganglionic fibers that synapse in sympathetic ganglia located in the neck.

Visceral afferents from the heart join the major part of the cardiac plexus and then pass along the sympathetic and vagal cardiac branches. The vagal afferents are concerned with cardiac reflexes, whereas afferents in the sympathetic cardiac nerves conduct pain sensation from the heart.

The vagal afferent impulses originate in various types of interoceptors that sense changes in tension or pressure (baroreceptors) or in the carbon dioxide or oxygen content of blood (chemoreceptors). Baroreceptors are located in the wall of the great veins as they enter the heart and help regulate the cardiac output according to the amount of filling in these veins; others are in the wall of the arch of the aorta or its branches at the base of the neck where they sense changes in blood pressure and set in operation the reflexes that adjust it. Chemoreceptors (variably called aortic or para-aortic bodies, glomus aorticum, and glomus pulmonale) are located on the outside of the great vessels, primarily between the ascending aorta and the pulmonary trunk, and initiate respiratory and cardiac reflexes in response to lowered oxygen tension in aortic blood.

Whereas cardiac afferents in the sympathetic nerves may also be involved in reflexes, it is important to realize that sympathetic cardiac nerves are the sole conductors of *pain from the heart*. From the sympathetic trunks, all pain afferents eventually enter the posterior roots of the upper four or five thoracic nerves, the same segments that give rise to preganglionic cardiac efferents. The afferent fibers in the cardiac branches of cervical sympathetic ganglia descend in the sympathetic trunks to the upper thoracic segments and join the pain fibers that enter the T1 to T5 chain ganglia through the thoracic cardiac nerves. Thus, bilateral destruction of the upper five segments of the thoracic sympathetic trunks can be expected to interrupt the entire pathway for pain from the heart and, indeed, has been shown to abolish entirely the pain typically associated with coronary arterial disease and with aneurysms of the arch of the aorta. Because afferent fibers concerned with cardiac pain terminate in the posterior horns of the same cord segments as somatic afferents contained in upper thoracic spinal nerves, the pain of *angina pectoris* usually is interpreted by the patient as being localized along the ulnar border of the upper limb (dermatomes supplied by T-1 and T-2) and the upper part of the thorax (dermatomes T-2 through T-5). The pain is caused by myocardial ischemia and is sensed by pain receptors in the heart, but it is **referred** to somatic structures supplied from the same cord segments as the heart.

The Conducting System

The conducting system of the heart consists of the sinuatrial node, the atrioventricular node, the internodal fasciculi, and the atrioventricular bundle or fasciculus. The latter divides into a left and a right bundle branch, or crura (Fig. 21-18). In each ventricle, these branches, or crura, terminate in a subendocardial plexus of so-called Purkinje fibers, which become continuous with ventricular myocardial fibers. All these components of the conducting system are specially differentiated cardiac muscle fibers, separated from ordinary myocardium by delicate envelopes of connective tissue. In the human heart, the conducting system is hard to demonstrate by dissection and is best identified by serial histologic sections, whereas in ungulates, the atrioventricular bundle and its branches are macroscopically visible and may be displayed by dissection or by injection of their connective tissue sheath with India ink. Histologic differences between conducting tissue and ordinary myocardium are likewise less marked in the human than in some animals.

The **sinuatrial (SA) node** is a crescent-shaped structure, 5 to 8 mm in length, that occupies the whole thickness of the wall of the right atrium. It is located on the anterior lip of the superior vena caval orifice near the top of the crista terminalis. It functions as the pacemaker.

The **atrioventricular (AV) node** is oval and slightly smaller than the sinuatrial node. The node lies in the substance of the interatrial septum, resting on the fibrous atrioventricular ring, close to the attachment of the septal cusp of the tricuspid valve. Within the septum, the node extends forward from the opening of the coronary sinus, and its cells continue anteriorly into the atrioventricular bundle, which connects the node to the ventricles (see Fig. 21-13).

The atrioventricular node is also connected to the sinuatrial node by three delicate fiber bundles of conducting tissue. These **internodal fasciculi** or **tracts,** although clearly definable anatomically, are of doubtful significance in the conduction of impulses from the sinuatrial to the atrioventricular node. According to physiologic studies, impulses generated in the pacemaker spread to the atrioventricular node uniformly through the atrial myocardium; the internodal fasciculi (as well as the interatrial fasciculus, a fourth bundle that leaves the sinuatrial node) do not appear to be involved in activating the atrioventricular node.

The activation of the ventricles is achieved through the **atrioventricular (AV) bundle.** Disruption or block of the bundle dissociates the beat of the ventricles from that of the atria and is responsible for clinically well-defined cardiac arrhythmias. The atrioventricular bundle is a fasciculus of conducting tissue that has the thickness of a wooden matchstick. It commences as the forward continuation of the atrioventricular node. The bundle passes through a hole in the fibrous tissue separating the atria from the ventricles (see Fig. 21-13); it is the only connection between the myocardium of the atria and the ventricles. On the ventricular side, the bundle runs downward and forward, skirting the posterior margin of the membranous part of the interventricular septum, and soon branches into a right and a left crus. The two **crura (bundle branches)** straddle the upper border of the muscular part of the interventricular septum. Each crus descends toward the apex under the endocardium of the septum. Knowledge of these relations matters in the surgical repair of interventricular septal defects.

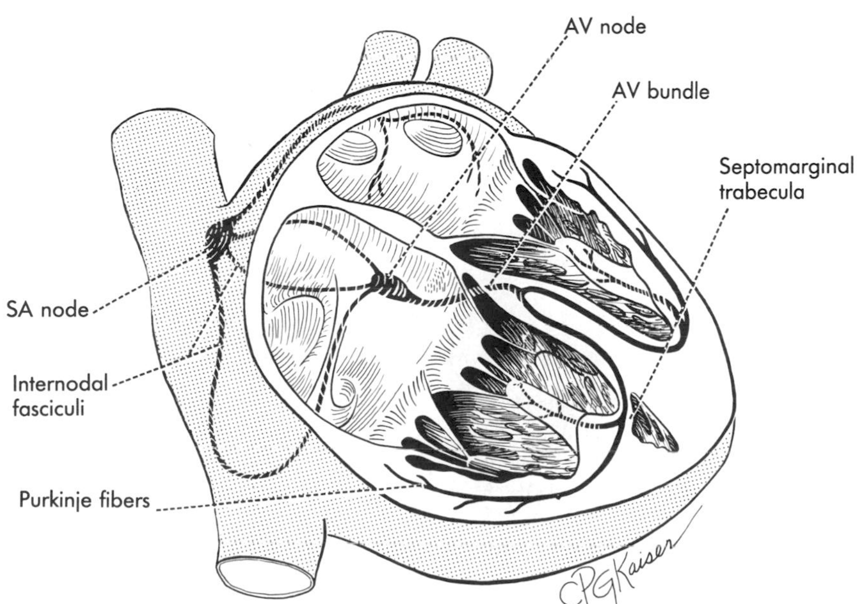

FIGURE *21-18.*
The conducting system of the heart.

The right crus of the atrioventricular bundle crosses from the septum to the ventricular wall along the *septomarginal trabecula*, whereas the left crus breaks up into branches and reaches the ventricular wall along several trabeculae carneae. These fasciculi spread out over the ventricular wall and the papillary muscles as the subendocardial **Purkinje fibers.** Because of this arrangement, the impulses dispatched from the atrioventricular node first activate ventricular muscle in the region of the apex, assuring a "milking" action of the ventricles toward the openings of the aorta and the pulmonary trunk.

The vicinity of the sinuatrial and atrioventricular nodes and of the atrioventricular bundle is richly innervated. Nerve fibers penetrate into the nodes and the bundle. Ganglion cells, however, are confined to the neighborhood of the atrial portion of the conducting system.

The blood supply of the conducting system is described in the previous section with the coronary arteries. Each node is closely associated with a small artery that is named after the node. Although the myocardium that surrounds the nodes, the atrioventricular bundle, and its crura is highly vascular, there are no capillaries in the nodes or the bundles.

Disease conditions that interfere with conduction along the atrioventricular system necessarily interfere with the normal rhythm of ventricular contraction. Interruption of transmission along the AV bundle produces *heart block*, which dissociates the contraction of the atria and the ventricles, so that the atria may beat at one speed and the ventricles at a slower one. As a consequence, the atria sometimes will attempt to force blood into an already filled or a contracting ventricle. Also, the ventricle may contract whether or not it is filled and, therefore, acts inefficiently. In some cases, only one branch of the atrioventricular bundle may be blocked (*bundle branch block*), which affects only one ventricle. In recent years, the condition has been alleviated by implanting in the ventricle an electrode connected to an electronic cardiac pacemaker that will deliver appropriate rhythmic shocks to the heart and produce proper ventricular contraction.

THE GREAT VESSELS

The great vessels include the ascending aorta, the pulmonary trunk, the two venae cavae, and the four pulmonary veins. All have been encountered in this chapter, and the purpose of the present section is to summarize their anatomy. Nothing needs to be added to the description of the inferior vena cava and pulmonary veins, each of which has a very short intrapericardial course.

The **pulmonary trunk** and the **ascending aorta** are each about 5 cm long and 3 cm in diameter. Although the pulmonary trunk conveys venous blood from the heart to the lungs, anatomically it is an artery (as are its branches, the pulmonary arteries), and the structure of its wall is similar to that of the aorta. Both vessels run a slightly twisted or spiral course within the pericardial sac. They entwine in such a manner that the pulmonary trunk obscures a substantial portion of the ascending aorta from view (see Fig. 21-4). The posterior wall of the pulmonary trunk is closely applied to the anterior wall of the aorta, as both walls develop from the spiral septum that divides the embryonic truncus arteriosus and bulbus cordis into these two vessels.

The pulmonary trunk begins at the pulmonary orifice of the right ventricle, and the aorta, at the aortic orifice of the left ventricle. Each orifice is surrounded by a fibrous ring (see Fig. 21-13) and can be closed by the pulmonary and aortic semilunar valves (described earlier) that separate the lumen of each vessel from that of the respective ventricle (see Fig. 21-11). The pulmonary orifice is anterior, and from it, the pulmonary trunk passes upward, backward, and to the left. The aortic orifice is posterior, and from it the aorta ascends toward the right and slightly forward. The pulmonary trunk terminates by dividing into the right and left pulmonary arteries opposite the left border of the sternum, behind the second costal cartilage. The ascending aorta reaches a similar position on the right side of the sternal angle and turns backward to become the arch of the aorta. Immediately above the cusps of the aortic and pulmonary valves, there are three dilations on the aorta and on the pulmonary trunk. These are the **aortic** and **pulmonary sinuses.** The coronary arteries arise from the left and right aortic sinuses (see Fig. 21-15). The dilated base of the aorta, on which the aortic sinuses bulge, is sometimes called the *bulb of the aorta*. As the ascending aorta becomes continuous with the arch of the aorta, it dilates again slightly to the right. This unnamed dilation is not present along the right margin of the cardiac outline in a posteroanterior x-ray film because to its right lies the superior vena cava. The pulmonary trunk, on the other hand, is visible along the left margin of the cardiac outline as it lies in the concavity of the arch of the aorta (see Fig. 21-7).

As described earlier (see The Serous Pericardium and Pericardial Cavity), the pulmonary trunk and the ascending aorta are enclosed by a common sleeve of serous pericardium. The relation of these vessels to intrapericardial structures is discussed in connection with the transverse sinus of the pericardium. The transverse sinus is posterior to the two great arteries.

Only the lower half of the **superior vena cava** is within the pericardial sac, which it enters behind the sternal angle. The vessel is formed in the superior mediastinum, and it is described in the next chapter. Its position and relations within the pericardial sac are dealt with earlier in this chapter.

THE HEART IN THE LIVING BODY

For assessing cardiac function, it is necessary to relate the general position of the heart and its specific anatomic features to landmarks on the precordium. The **precordium** is that part of the chest wall that roughly overlies the heart and the great vessels. This section deals with the position of the heart in the chest, the cardiac outline, and the location of the valves and auscultatory areas. The heart sounds are related to events in the cardiac cycle.

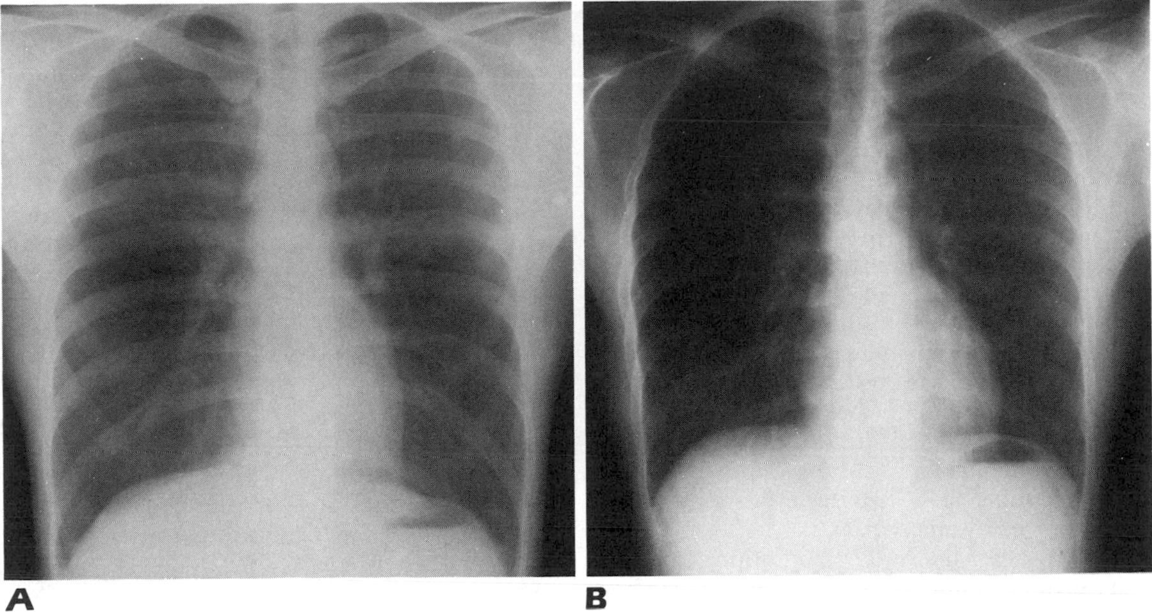

FIGURE *21-19.*
Radiograph of the chest of a young man, showing changes in the shape and position of the heart during (A) deep inspiration and (B) expiration.

Position. The heart rests with its inferior surface on the central portion of the diaphragm, and its inferior border is roughly on a level with the xiphisternal junction. The normal heart is somewhat larger than a person's clenched fist. One-third of it lies to the right of the median plane and extends slightly beyond the edge of the sternum; two-thirds lie to the left of the median plane. The exact position of the heart depends on many factors, and the surface projection described in the following is largely an approximation that holds true for the *average* heart in an *average individual.*

In the recumbent position the diaphragm is higher than it is in the standing position, and so is the heart. Because of its own weight, the heart shifts significantly toward the side the person is lying on, and it also approximates the chest wall on leaning forward. These are points to remember in palpation and auscultation of the heart. Figure 21-19 shows the changes in the same heart that are due to sustained, deep inspiration and expiration. The position of the heart is different in a narrow, slender person than in a person with a broad, stocky build (Fig. 21-20). Abdominal distention (e.g., pregnancy), unequal pressure

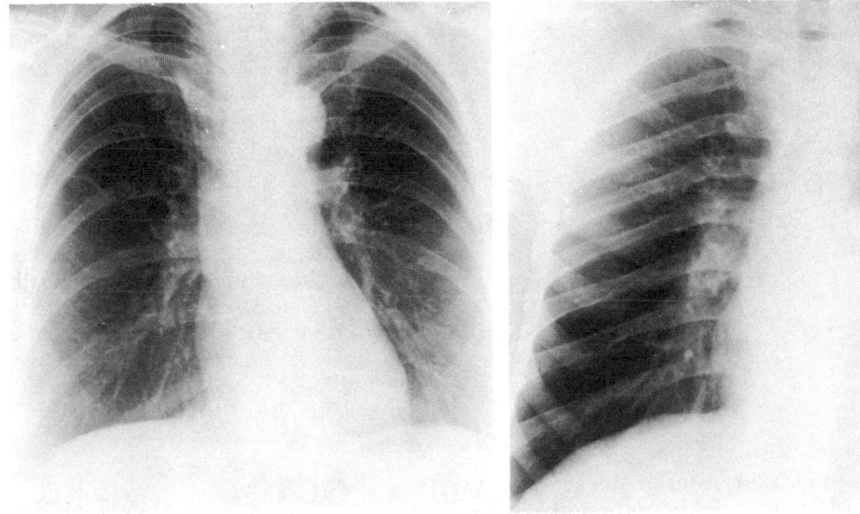

FIGURE *21-20.*
Contrasting types of hearts in persons of different body build: (left) the slender, more vertical type of heart; (right) a wider, more transverse type. There are numerous intergrades between these two extremes. (Courtesy of Dr. D. G. Pugh.)

or tension in the two pleural cavities, or shifts of the mediastinum caused by, for instance, spinal curvatures, all have an influence on the position of the heart regardless of whether or not the heart itself is normal.

Surface Projection. There is only one point of the heart that can be directly identified on the precordium: the apex. A **cardiac impulse** may be visible at the apex, and palpation over it will confirm the presence of the **apex beat.** In many normal individuals, the cardiac impulse is not visible, and the apex beat is felt with difficulty or not at all. In quiet breathing and in the supine position, the apex is located in the left fifth intercostal space just medial to the midclavicular line. The outflow tracts of the ventricles are behind the sternum just below the sternal angle. The region of the precordium that overlies the outflow tracts is known to clinicians as the **base of the heart.** It must be borne in mind that the term in this sense is different from that used by anatomists.

Figure 21-21 shows the surface projection of the cardiac borders, chambers, and valves. The right and left borders may be confirmed by percussion of the precordium, although the overlapping lungs make it difficult to map out cardiac dullness. The coronary sulcus runs diagonally from the left upper to the right lower corner of the quadrangular cardiac outline. It marks the position of the fibrous skeleton of the heart, which is seen almost edge on, but slightly from below. In it are located all the valves, which also appear edge on.

Heart Sounds and Auscultatory Areas. There is no unanimous agreement about precisely what physical events in the heart contribute to the generation of audible vibrations. There is no doubt, however, that the heart sounds are closely associated with the closure of valves. Opening of the valves in the normal heart is inaudible. Heart sounds can be heard over the entire precordium, but there are specific auscultation areas where sounds made by individual valves can be perceived to best advantage. For all but one valve, these areas do not coincide with the surface projection of the valves, probably because vibrations made by a valve are carried along with the blood to a point of optimal intensity.

Sounds generated by the **mitral valve** are best heard over the apex, and those of the **tricuspid valve** over the anterior wall of the right ventricle, which happens to superimpose on the projection of the valve itself. Sounds of the **aortic valve** radiate along the ascending aorta to the second costal cartilage at the sternal border on the right where the aorta is closest to the chest wall. This is the aortic auscultatory area. The **pulmonary,** or pulmonic, area is along the left sternal border in the second space, where the pulmonary trunk divides.

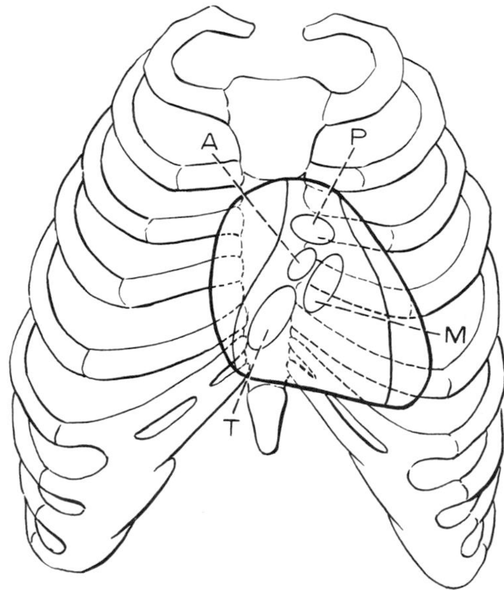

FIGURE *21-21.*
Approximate projection of the heart onto the anterior thoracic wall. The large middle portion of the anterior surface of the heart is formed by the right ventricle; the right and left borders are formed by the right atrium and left ventricle, respectively. The letters *P, A, M,* and *T* identify the positions of the pulmonary, aortic, mitral, and tricuspid valves, respectively.

A comprehensive discussion of the **cardiac cycle** is not the objective of this section, but correlation of the heart sounds with ventricular events serves a useful purpose in the present context.

There are two heart sounds, the first and the second, that follow each other in quick succession, and they are separated from the next doublet by a longer interval. During this interval, the ventricles are relaxed (**diastole**), whereas between the two heart sounds, the ventricles are contracting (**systole**). In diastole, the atrioventricular valves are open and the aortic and pulmonary valves are closed. Blood is pouring into the atria and flows freely into the ventricles through the open mitral and tricuspid valves. Then the ventricles begin to contract, and the rise in pressure closes the atrioventricular valves: the first heart sound is produced, signaling the beginning of ventricular systole. Simultaneously, contraction of the ventricular muscle makes the apex rise, resulting in the visible and palpable heart beat. Concurrent with the rising ventricular pressure, the aortic and pulmonary valves open silently and blood is ejected into the aorta and pulmonary trunk.

When the ventricles cease contracting, blood under pressure in the great vessels closes the aortic and pulmonary valves, an event that generates the second heart sound. The second heart sound signals the end of systole and the commencement of diastole. The ventricles relax, the atrioventricular valves open silently, and the cycle is repeated. Thus, the first heart sound is associated with atrioventricular valve closure and the second heart sound is associated with semilunar valve closure. Systole is between the first and second heart sounds and diastole between the second and first heart sounds.

EMBRYOLOGY

Normal Development

The heart first takes form by the fusion of two endothelial tubes that are formed in splanchnic mesoderm. The splanchnic mesoderm surrounding these tubes differentiates into the myocardium, and the outer layer of the mesodermal cells (the celomic epithelium) becomes the epicardium (see Fig. 19-12*B* and *C*). The endocardium of the fully formed heart corresponds to the primitive endothelial cardiac tubes; from this endothelium develop also the cardiac valves and most of the septa. The five divisions of the primitive heart tube (*truncus arteriosus, bulbus cordis, ventricle, atrium, sinus venosus*) were identified in the introductory section to this chapter (see Fig. 21-1). The purpose of the present section is to summarize the changes that lead to the establishment of the external form of the heart, the partitioning of its cavity into four chambers, and the development of the great vessels. External and internal changes progress concomitantly, although here they are discussed under separate headings.

Establishment of External Form

Four major events transform the simple endothelial cardiac tube into an organ that resembles the fully developed heart: 1) flexion of the heart tube between the bulbus and the ventricle; 2) fusion of the bulbus and the ventricle, 3) dorsal migration of the atrium in relation to the ventricle, which draws out the sinus venosus from the septum transversum into the pericardial cavity; 4) enlargement of the right horn of the sinus venosus and its merging with the right side of the atrium. Only the last of these events needs discussion; the first three have been mentioned in the introduction to this chapter.

The left horn of the sinus venosus atrophies, whereas its right horn enlarges, owing to the development of two major anastomoses that divert venous blood from the left side of the embryo to the right side of the heart (Fig. 21-22). One anastomosis is located caudal to the heart within the liver, the other, rostral to the heart in the mediastinum. The *caudal* anastomosis is the **ductus venosus,** which shunts blood from the left umbilical and vitelline veins to the proximal segment of the right vitelline vein. The terminal portion of the inferior vena cava develops from this terminal segment of the right vitelline vein (see Fig. 21-22*B* and *C*). The segments of the umbilical and vitelline veins that are excluded from the blood flow soon atrophy. The ductus venosus remains functional as long as placental blood has to reach the heart; after birth it is replaced by a fibrous cord, the *ligamentum venosum*, that is devoid of a lumen. The rostral anastomosis is between the left and right precardinal veins. The **precardinal anastomosis** persists as the left brachiocephalic vein, whereas the more caudal portion of the left precardinal vein atrophies, as does the left common cardinal vein. In the fully developed heart, the latter is represented by the oblique vein of the left atrium. On the right side, the precardinal vein, caudal to the anastomosis, and the common cardinal vein together make up the superior vena cava. As a consequence of these two venous shunts, the *right horn of the sinus venosus* enlarges whereas its *left horn shrinks* and becomes the *coronary sinus* (see Fig. 21-22). The enlarged right horn, the

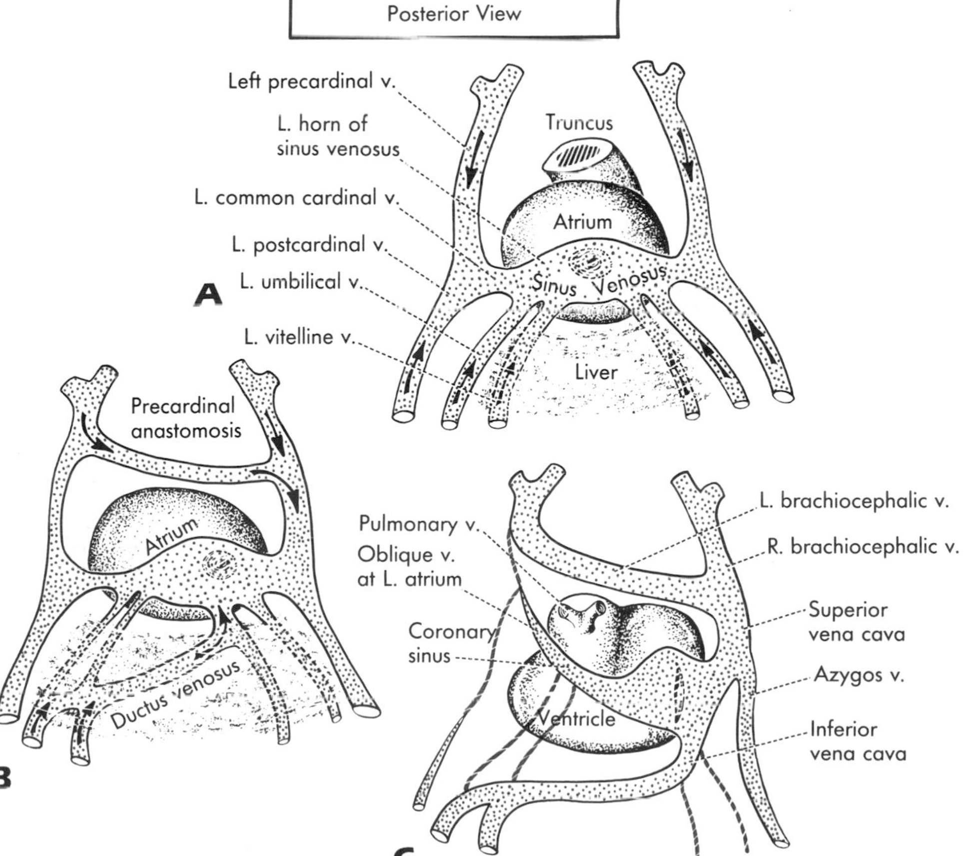

FIGURE *21-22.* **Schematic representation of developmental events that modify the sinus venosus. The primitive heart tube (shown in Fig. 21-1*A* and *B*) is seen here from a caudal or posterior view: (A) The most primitive arrangement is shown, with the sinus venosus receiving three pairs of veins and emptying into the common atrium. (B) Caudal and rostral anastomoses have developed between the tributaries of the sinus venosus at this stage, which leads to (C) the atrophy of certain venous channels and to the enlargement and persistence of others.**

tributaries of which can now be called the superior and inferior venae cavae and the coronary sinus, becomes incorporated into the right side of the atrium sinus venarum as this chamber is being partitioned. By the sixth week of embryonic development, the heart closely resembles that of its fully developed form.

Establishment of Internal Form

The merging of the bulbus cordis with the primitive ventricle and the sinus venosus with the right atrium modifies and enlarges the chambers of the primitive heart. The left atrium also is augmented by the incorporation of the developing pulmonary veins into its posterior wall. The division of the interior of the heart into its four definitive chambers is the result of four major events: 1) expansion and division of the atrioventricular canal; 2) partitioning of the common atrium; 3) partitioning of the common ventricle; 4) division of the truncus arteriosus and the adjoining portion of the bulbus cordis, and their shift toward the left.

The **atrioventricular canal** is the passage between the primitive atrium and the primitive ventricle, the forerunner of the anatomic left ventricle (see Fig. 21-1*D*). The atrioventricular canal soon expands to the right so that it opens also into the future right ventricle. The right ventricle is derived chiefly from the bulbus cordis, which is placed, by the looping of the heart, on the right side of the primitive ventricle. Following fusion of the bulbus and the primitive ventricle, the expansion of the atrioventricular canal to the right establishes connection between the primitive atrium and the common chamber of the future left and right ventricles. This expanded atrioventricular canal is marked on the exterior of the heart by the coronary sulcus. The canal soon becomes partitioned into two orifices by swellings that are produced by the proliferation of the endocardium in the dorsal and ventral walls of the canal (Fig. 21-23). These **endocardial tubercles** or **cushions** grow toward each other and, when they meet, divide the single atrioventricular canal into right and left atrioventricular orifices, which will now connect the right and left halves of the primitive atrium with the future right and left ventricles, respectively. The tricuspid and mitral valves develop in these orifices.

The **partitioning of the atrium** is accomplished by two overlapping septa, the septum primum and the septum secundum (see Fig. 21-23). The development of these septa, both produced by endothelial proliferation, is associated with three foramina: the foramen primum, the foramen secundum, and the foramen ovale. The **septum primum** descends as a curtain from the roof of the atrium toward the bridge formed by the fused endocardial cushions, and the gap between its inferior edge and the cushions is the **foramen primum.** When the septum contacts the endocardial cushions, the foramen primum is obliterated and a second opening, the **foramen secundum,** is formed by the breakdown of an area in the septum primum close to the atrial roof.

On its right, the foramen secundum becomes

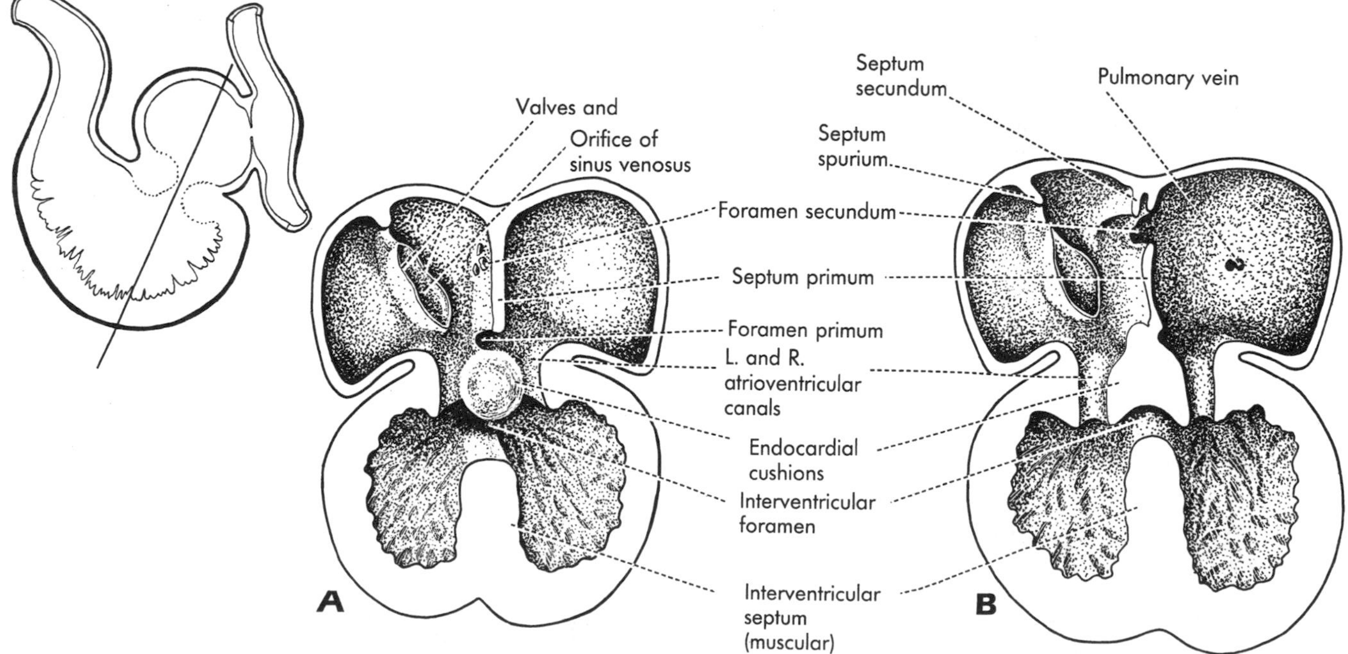

FIGURE *21-23.*
Two stages in the division of the common atrium into right and left chambers shown schematically; (Inset) the plane of section through the primitive heart tube permitting this view of the interior, which corresponds to Figure 21-1*D*. In (A) only the septum primum has formed; In (B) the septum secundum has commenced its growth on the atrial roof between the septum primum and the septum spurium. The septum spurium and the right valve of the sinus venosus give rise to the crista terminalis. At the stage shown in panel B, as yet only a single (common) pulmonary vein opens into the left atrium.

covered over by the **septum secundum,** but remains patent. Like the septum primum, the septum secundum grows from the roof of the atrium toward the endocardial cushions, but most of its crescent-shaped edge (known as the *limbus fossae ovalis*) fails to reach the cushions and leaves a defect that is the **foramen ovale.** Like the foramen secundum, the foramen ovale remains patent, but is overlapped on the left by the septum primum. The septum primum acts as a flap valve (and is sometimes called the *valvule of the foramen ovale*) that permits the flow of blood from the right atrium through the foramen ovale and foramen secundum into the left atrium. After birth, the two septa become pressed against each other by the rising pressure in the left atrium, and the foramina ovale and secundum become functionally closed. The two septa may not fuse, however, for a considerable period, and a cardiac catheter may be passed between the apposed septa from the right to the left atrium. The foramen ovale remains probe patent up to the age of 5 years in 50% of persons and up to 20 years of age in more than 25%.

The **interventricular septum** is derived from three elements: the muscular septum, the endocardial cushions, and the bulbar ridges. The *pars muscularis* of the interventricular septum commences its growth in the convex region of the cardiac loop opposite the flange of the bulboventricular septum (see Fig. 21-1) even before that septum becomes absorbed. The muscular septum grows upward toward the endocardial cushions, and its crescentic upper edge progressively reduces the *interventricular foramen* (see Fig. 21-23). This foramen is the communication between the right and left ventricles, which are derived from the greater part of the bulbus cordis and the primitive ventricle, respectively. The superior portion of the interventricular septum that fills in the interventricular foramen is derived from the endocardial cushions. An area in this portion of the septum remains transparent and membranous (*pars membranacea*). The anterior cusp of the mitral valve and the septal cusp of the tricuspid valve are also derived from the same endocardial tissue as the pars membranacea, and so is the lower portion of the interatrial septum. This explains the existence of the membranous atrioventricular septum.

The part of the interventricular septum that divides the outflow tracts of the right and left ventricles below the level of the semilunar valves is situated anterosuperiorly and is formed by the bulbar ridges. The **bulbar ridges** are two longitudinal swellings that meet in the midline and divide the lumen of the distal portion of the bulbus into the *conus arteriosus* or infundibulum of the right ventricle and the *aortic vestibule* of the left ventricle. Inferiorly, these bulbar ridges fuse with the components of the interventricular septum that are derived from the endocardial cushions and the muscular septum. The *crista supraventricularis* in the right ventricle marks the lower limit of the bulbar ridges.

Above the level of the semilunar valves, the **division of the truncus arteriosus** into the pulmonary trunk and ascending aorta is accomplished by the formation of the **spiral** (or *aorticopulmonary*) **septum.** This septum is formed by two longitudinal ridges in the truncus, which are continuous with the bulbar ridges. The spiraling of the truncal ridges is such that when the aorticopulmonary septum is completed, the pulmonary trunk connects with the right ventricle and the aorta connects with the left ventricle.

After the completion of the septa, the heart rotates in such a manner that the conus arteriosus and the pulmonary trunk come to lie more in front than to the right of the aorta and the aortic vestibule. In the fully developed heart, the aortic valve is posterior and to the right of the pulmonary valve. Distally, the pulmonary trunk is in communication with the sixth pair of aortic arches (the future pulmonary artery) and the aorta is in communication with the fourth pair of aortic arches (the future arch of the aorta). These changes are completed by the eighth week of human development, and only after birth does the heart adapt to maintaining separate pulmonary and systemic circulatory circuits.

Fetal Circulation

The circulation in the fetus differs in several important respects from that in the adult. The major changes that adapt the circulation to the exchange of blood gases in the lungs, rather than in the placenta, take place at the time of birth and during a relatively short transitional period that extends over the first few days of neonatal life. In the adult heart, the vascular circuits fed by the right and left ventricles are maintained independently of one an other, except for the minor anastomoses that exist between bronchial and pulmonary blood vessels, whereas in the fetus, there are large intracardiac and extracardiac shunts between the two circuits. In the adult, all of the right ventricle's output is spent in the perfusion of the lungs; in the fetus, the lungs offer a high resistance to blood flow so that more than 75% of the blood pumped by the right ventricle bypasses the lungs and flows from the pulmonary trunk through the **ductus arteriosus** directly into the aorta. The ductus arteriosus is a large connecting channel between the pulmonary trunk and the aorta and is a derivative of the sixth aortic arch. In the fetus, only approximately 50% of the combined ventricular output circulates through the lower part of the body, and the other 50% passes into a pair of **umbilical arteries** given off from the terminal branches of the descending aorta. These arteries leave the body of the fetus and perfuse the placenta. Blood traversing the placenta meets very little resistance and after it has been purified of metabolites and enriched with oxygen and nutrients, it is returned to the fetus along a single **umbilical vein.** Approximately half of this blood trickles through the substance of the liver before it enters the inferior vena cava; the other half bypasses the vascular liver parenchyma and reaches the inferior vena cava more directly through a large venous channel embedded in the liver, named the **ductus venosus** (see Fig. 21-22).

The entrance of the inferior vena cava into the right atrium is in line with the **foramen ovale.** About two-thirds of the stream of blood entering the right atrium from the inferior vena cava is directed, by the valve of the inferior vena cava, into the left atrium through the foramina ovale and secundum. The remaining one-third of the inferior vena caval blood passes into the right ventricle, together with the venous blood that is returned to the right atrium from the superior vena cava. The right ventricle pumps this blood into the pulmonary trunk and most of it enters the aorta through the ductus arteriosus, whereas only a small fraction passes through the lungs before it is returned to the left atrium. This venous blood, together with the inferior vena caval blood that entered the left atrium through the foramina ovale and secundum, passes into the left ventricle, which pumps it to the aorta. Because of the existence of the right-to-left shunt between the two atria (through the foramina ovale and secundum) and between the pulmonary trunk and aorta (through the ductus arteriosus), the two ventricles in the fetus work in parallel, pumping their combined output into the aorta, except for the small fraction that reaches the lungs from the pulmonary arteries.

Two important events change the dynamics of the circulation at the time of birth: (1) the first breath of air is taken; and (2) the newborn is separated from the placenta. The factors responsible for initiating the first breath remain conjectural, but with the entry of air into the lungs and the expansion of the lungs, pulmonary vascular resistance is suddenly reduced, which greatly increases pulmonary blood flow and causes a fall of pressure in the pulmonary trunk, right ventricle, and right atrium. On the left, or systemic, side, the abrupt exclusion of the low-resistance vascular bed of the placenta from the circulation results in an increase of overall systemic vascular resistance, causing the pressure to rise in the aorta, left ventricle, and left atrium. This increase in left atrial pressure, and the fall in right atrial pressure, presses the thin septum primum against the more rigid septum secundum and functionally closes the foramen ovale.

The combined effect of the decrease in pulmonary vascular resistance and the increase in systemic vascular resistance reverses the flow through the ductus arteriosus. During the first few hours of neonatal life, blood is shunted from the aorta into the pulmonary trunk, which greatly increases blood flow through the lungs and, consequently, augments the amount of blood returned to the left atrium. Functional closure of the ductus begins at birth by muscular contraction; the major impetus for this is oxygen. Anatomic closure may not be complete for several months, and in addition to the contraction, it is achieved by thickening of the intima and thrombosis. The duct eventually becomes converted into a fibrous cord, the **ligamentum arteriosum.**

Changes that continue to take place during the neonatal period include the obliteration of the ductus venosus, the umbilical vein, and the umbilical arteries; an increase in the muscle mass of the left ventricle compared with that of the right; and, consistent with the pressure changes in the pulmonary and systemic circulations, an increase in smooth muscle in the systemic vascular bed compared with a relative decrease in the amount of smooth muscle associated with pulmonary blood vessels.

ANATOMIC ABNORMALITIES OF THE HEART AND GREAT VESSELS

Anatomic abnormalities of the heart and great vessels may be *congenital* or *acquired.* The majority of congenital cardiac abnormalities are the result of interference with normal cardiac development during the first 7 weeks of intrauterine life. Acquired anatomic abnormalities are caused by diseases that exert their effect on the fully developed heart after birth. In the present context, anatomic defects of the heart and great arteries and veins will be considered chiefly to illustrate crucial points of development and functional anatomy. This is particularly instructive as far as congenital abnormalities are concerned.

Congenital Abnormalities

The Heart. Any of the developmental events discussed under the headings Establishment of External Form and Establishment of Internal Form may be arrested or interfered with. Discussion is limited here to a brief mention of abnormal looping of the heart and to defective development of the atrioventricular canal, the interatrial and interventricular septa, and the cardiac valves.

During **looping of the heart,** the bulbus may twist to the left side of the primitive ventricle, rather than to the right, as it normally does; that is, instead of normal *dextro*, or *d*, looping, *levo*, or *l*, looping takes place. The result of *l* looping is that the anatomic right ventricle will lie to the left of the anatomic left ventricle. Because the atria remain unaffected by the abnormal looping, the right atrium will empty into the anatomic left ventricle, now situated on the right side of the heart. After birth, venous blood would be pumped into the aorta. This malformation, however, is usually associated with transposition of the great arteries, which assures that the hemodynamics in such a grossly abnormal heart remain essentially normal as a result of the transposition: the pulmonary trunk comes off the anatomic left ventricle (located on the right), which receives blood from the normal right atrium. In such cases of *congenitally corrected transposition*, the heart is usually located in the left side of the chest, but sometimes it may be in the right side. These cases of *isolated dextrocardia* or *dextroversion* must be distinguished from *mirror image dextrocardia*, which is found in *situs inversus*. In this condition, the left-to-right orientation of all viscera is reversed. Although there is *l* looping, which reverses the normal orientation of the ventricles, the atria are also reversed; the hemodynamics in mirror image dextrocardia are normal.

Several cardiac abnormalities result from defective development of the **atrioventricular canal.** The canal initially connects the primitive atrium to the future left ventricle. If the atrioventricular canal fails to expand to connect the atrium to the future right ventricle, or bulbus, both atria will open into the left ventricle. A *double inlet left ventricle* results because the atrioventricular canal usually divides into mitral and tricuspid orifices. In such hearts, the right ventricle never develops normally: it may persist as a vestigial outflow channel or it may disappear altogether. This abnormality is also known, therefore, as *single ventricle.*

Interference with the development of the **endocardial cushions** may prevent their fusion completely or partially. If the endocardial cushions do not approximate each other, a large hole remains in the center of the heart, bordered by the defective interatrial and interventricular septa and the dorsal and ventral endocardial cushions. Such a defect is called a *complete persistent atrioventricular canal*. If the endocardial cushions approximate each other but do not fuse completely, the gaps left between the partially fused cushions remain as deficiencies in the corresponding valve leaflets: there may be a cleft in the septal cusp of the tricuspid and in the anterior cusp of the mitral valves.

When the endocardial cushions fail to approximate, the septum primum is usually also defective. Such a *septum primum defect* is one of several types of **atrial septal defects** (ASDs). Other types of ASD include the *secundum defect* and the *sinus venosus defect*. Incomplete development of the septum secundum generates an abnormally large foramen ovale, and such a rudimentary septum fails to cover the foramen secundum. The resultant uncovered hole is called an **ASD of the secundum type.** Alternatively, excessive breakdown of the upper part of the septum primum may generate an abnormally large foramen secundum, which will not be covered by a relatively normal septum secundum. Fenestration of the septum primum, as an extension of the foramen secundum, may create multiple holes in the valve of the foramen ovale that will permit communication between the two atria throughout life. Incomplete absorption of the sinus venosus into the atrium gives rise to **a sinus venosus defect.** In such a case, the superior vena caval orifice faces into the interatrial defect, which is situated close to the roof of the atria.

Ventricular septal defects (VSDs) likewise have several types. The defect may involve the muscular septum, the membranous septum, or the partition between the outflow tracts of the two ventricles. Muscular defects are placed low, may be single or multiple, and are usually located in the pits between trabeculae of the right ventricular myocardium. Defects in the membranous septum may give rise to communication between the left and right ventricles beneath the septal leaflet of the tricuspid valve or between the left ventricle and the right atrium above the same leaflet. These membranous defects are always below and posterior to the crista supraventricularis; the atrioventricular bundle passes along the lower margin of the defect. Defective development of the two bulbar ridges that partition the distal portion of the bulbus cordis leads to defects that are situated above the crista and permit communication between the infundibulum and aortic vestibule.

Valvular abnormalities may involve the atrioventricular and semilunar valves. Atresia of the tricuspid and mitral valves probably results from closure of the atrioventricular canals by fusion of the endocardial cushions. In the semilunar valves, complete fusion along the lunules produces atresia; partial fusion results in narrowing of the opening, which is known as *stenosis*.

A complex type of congenital cardiac abnormality is the **tetralogy of Fallot,** first described by Stensen in 1673 and later by Fallot in 1888. The primary abnormality is a narrowing of the right ventricular outflow tract caused by an unequal division of the bulbus cordis (Fig. 21-24*A* and *B*). This results in the displacement of the crista supraventricularis toward the anterolateral wall of the right ventricle. The displacement narrows the outflow tract of the right ventricle, and the gap it leaves posteriorly creates a VSD. Normally, fusion of the bulbar ridges takes place at the time when the undivided outflow tract still comes off the bulbus cordis (future right ventricle); only later does the aorta line up with the primitive (left) ventricle. In the tetralogy, movement of the aorta toward the left is arrested so that the aorta continues to come off partially from the right ventricle; in other words, the aorta overrides the interventricular septum (see Fig. 21-24*C*). Therefore, the right ventricle has to pump blood directly into the high-pressure systemic circulation through the aorta, as well as into its own abnormally narrow outflow tract. These two factors lead to right ventricular hypertrophy. Thus, the four features of the tetralogy consist of 1) infundibular narrowing (stenosis), 2) VSD, 3) overriding aorta, and 4) right ventricular hypertrophy.

The Great Arteries and Veins. Brief mention is made of selected abnormalities related to the anatomy discussed in this chapter: common truncus arteriosus, transposition of the great arteries, persistent left superior vena cava, and anomalous pulmonary veins.

When the truncus arteriosus is not partitioned by the spiral septum, the single arterial trunk leaves the outflow tract of both ventricles and supplies the coronary, pulmonary, and systemic circulations. This abnormality is called a *persistent truncus arteriosus*. In complete *transposition of the great arteries*, the aorta emerges from the right ventricle and usually lies anterior to, or side by side with, the pulmonary trunk. The pulmonary trunk is given off by the left ventricle. Postnatal survival depends on the persistence of a shunt between the right and left sides of the heart (ASD, VSD, or patent ductus arteriosus). The embryologic basis for the abnormality is not known. One hypothesis postulates that a mismatch occurs in the junction between the spiral ridges in the truncus and the more proximal ridges in the bulbus.

A *left superior vena cava* results from the persistence of the left common cardinal vein. Such a vessel runs down in front of the arch of the aorta and the left pulmonary artery to join a much enlarged coronary sinus. A right superior vena cava nearly always coexists with a left superior vena cava. In such cases of *double superior vena cava*, there is usually a connection in the superior mediastinum between the two vessels. A persistent left superior vena cava causes no clinical problems. Its recognition is important, however, if open heart surgery is to be undertaken.

Anomalous drainage of pulmonary veins also represents the persistence of embryonic venous channels and may occur in a variety of patterns. The venous plexus of the lungs develops as an extension of the veins that surround the foregut. The dominant veins that drain from the lung toward the foregut normally link up with the *common pulmonary vein*, which forms as an outgrowth of the primitive atrium. The common pulmonary vein is eventually absorbed into the wall of the left atrium, so that in the fully formed heart, its tributaries, the superior and inferior pulmonary veins, enter the left atrium. If the pulmonary venous plexus does not link up with the common pulmonary vein, or if this vein does not develop, blood will be returned from the lungs along the existing embryonic channels. Thus, some or all of the blood from the lungs may

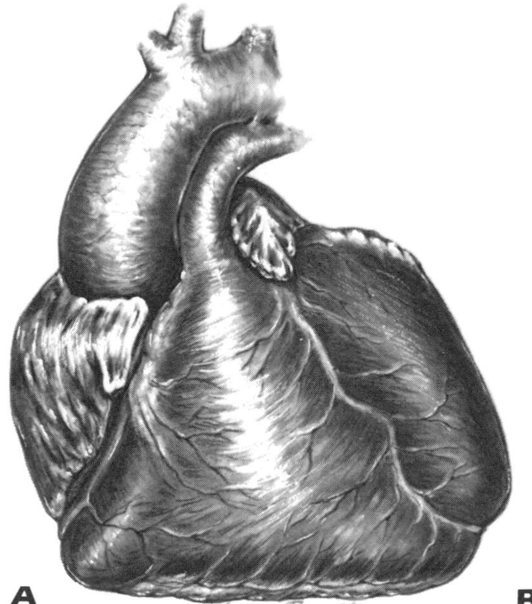

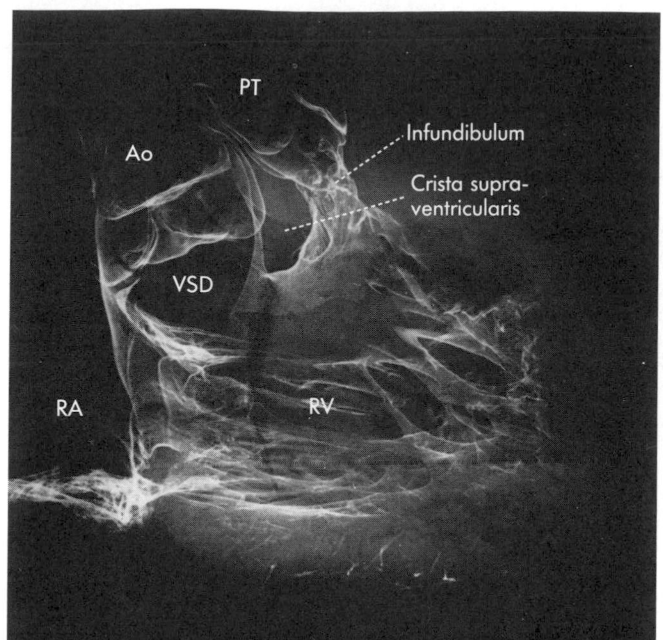

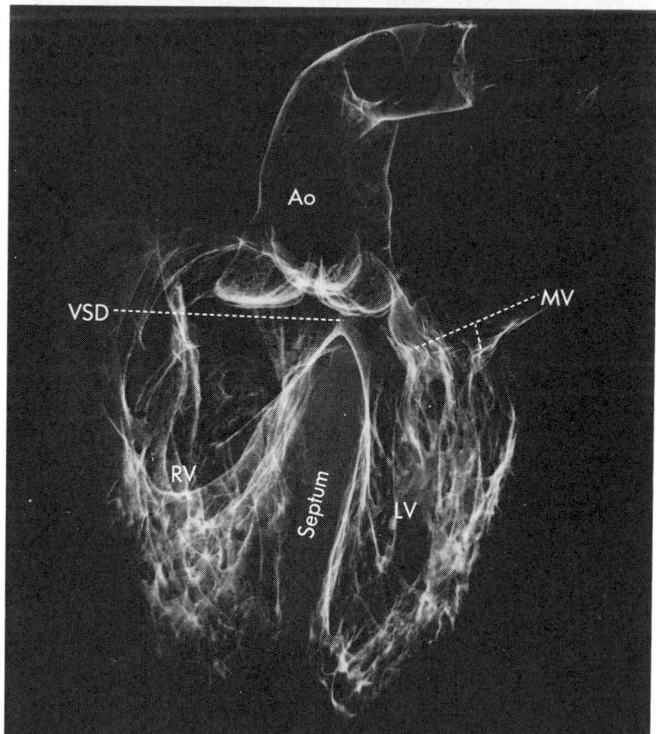

FIGURE *21-24.*
Tetralogy of Fallot: (A) the exterior of the heart with tetralogy; (B and C) radiographs taken of the heart by the method described in the legend of Figure 21-10. *Ao*, aorta; *PT*, pulmonary trunk; *RV*, right ventricle; *LV*, left ventricle; *MV*, anterior leaf of the mitral valve; *RA*, right atrium; *VSD*, ventricular septal defect. Notice the narrow outflow tract of the right ventricle (infundibulum) in panels A and B; the aortic and pulmonary valves at the base of the *Ao* and *PT*; the VSD in panels B and C; and the overriding of the ventricular septum by the aorta in panel C. (Prepared and kindly provided by Dr. Lore Tenckhoff.)

drain into the right or left superior vena cava or into the coronary sinus. A venous channel may persist on the anterior surface of the esophagus, which can receive anomalous pulmonary veins. Such a channel drains into the portal system (left gastric vein), the ductus venosus, or the inferior vena cava. In *total anomalous pulmonary venous return*, all the blood from the lungs is conveyed by abnormal channels to veins that empty into the right side of the heart; this leads to symptoms early in life and may constitute a surgical emergency in the neonate. More commonly, the anomalous venous drainage is only partial and may remain asymptomatic into adulthood, provided the volume of blood draining from the lungs to the right atrium is not large.

Clinical Classification of Congenital Cardiac Abnormalities. Broadly speaking, congenital cardiac malformations are classified clinically according to the presence or absence of cyanosis. *Cyanosis* is a bluish, discoloration of the skin and mucous membranes caused by an increase in the amount of deoxygenated hemoglobin in the blood. In **cyanotic congenital heart disease,** cyanosis results from the mixing of venous and arterial blood, a decrease in the volume of blood that reaches the lungs, or transposition of the great arteries. Double inlet left ventricle (single ventricle), complete persistent atrioventricular canal, and persistent truncus arteriosus are examples of mixing abnormalities. Obstruction of blood flow to the lungs is found in the tetralogy of Fallot, pulmonary atresia, and tricuspid atresia. In transposition of the great arteries, cyanosis is profound, as all the venous blood is pumped out directly into the transposed aorta. Survival depends on the shunting of some venous blood into the pulmonary artery through the ductus arteriosus, an ASD, or a VSD. An ASD is created within the first days of life, when transposition is diagnosed, by tearing the interatrial septum (balloon atrial septotomy).

Acyanotic congenital cardiac abnormalities comprise obstructive lesions and left-to-right shunts. Stenosis of the aortic and pulmonary valves makes up the most important obstructive lesions. Left-to-right shunts occur through a persistent patent ductus arteriosus or through atrial and ventricular septal defects.

Obstructive lesions lead to hypertrophy of the chamber situated proximal to the stenosed valve. Shunts produce volume overload, which results, primarily, in dilation and some hypertrophy of the overloaded chambers. ASDs cause right ventricular dilation; VSDs and patent ductus lead to left ventricular dilation.

Tremendous strides have been made in the surgical treatment of congenital heart disease. Many congenital heart defects are now amenable to corrective or palliative surgery. One of the most significant advances has been in the surgery, palliative and corrective, of the critically ill neonate and infant with congenital heart disease. In the past, this age group had the highest mortality.

Acquired Cardiac Abnormalities

Although not all functional disturbances of the heart are associated with anatomic abnormalities, many diseases can produce gross anatomic lesions in a heart that was normal to begin with (e.g., infections, rheumatic fever, hypertension, chronic pulmonary disease, myocardial infarction). Enlargement, dilation, or hypertrophy of the cardiac chambers may occur, but from an anatomic standpoint, valvular deformities are of the greatest interest.

Valvular abnormalities are of two kinds: stenosis or incompetence (also known as insufficiency). In *stenosis,* narrowing is caused by fusion of the leaflets, or cusps, of the valve along the commissures, or lunules, as a consequence of scar formation during the resolution of an inflammatory process that involves the valves and the associated tissues. The valve may become scarred and distorted in such a manner that the cusps cannot occlude the orifice completely and allow regurgitation of blood into the chambers separated by the defective valve. Such a valve is *incompetent.* Thus, one may speak, for example, of mitral stenosis or mitral incompetence and of aortic stenosis or aortic incompetence. Scarring and retraction of the cusps and their chordae tendineae may render a valve both stenosed and incompetent (e.g., mitral stenosis and incompetence).

The rigidity, thickening, and irregularity of deformed valves will alter the normal character of the heart sounds. Abnormal eddies will also be created as the blood passes the deformed valve. These added sounds generated by the abnormal eddies are known as *cardiac murmurs,* and they may be heard through systole, through diastole, or during both phases of the cardiac cycle. The diagnosis of a valvular abnormality is arrived at by the synthesis of several physical signs, including changes in the character of the heart sounds and the nature and timing of cardiac murmurs in relation to the cardiac cycle. Vibrations created by some valvular abnormalities may be so strong that they can be perceived not only through the stethoscope but also by a palpating hand placed on the precordium. The physical sign of such a palpable murmur is known as a *thrill.* In addition to physical signs, the shape and size of the heart on x-ray films and the electrocardiogram are routinely used in establishing the diagnosis.

Many acquired valvular abnormalities can be corrected surgically. If the cusps of a stenosed valve are not unduly deformed, the fused commissures may be divided (commissurotomy). Most cases of valvular incompetence, however, can be corrected only by replacing the defective valve with an artificial prosthetic valve.

RECOMMENDED READINGS

Anderson RH, Wilcox BR. Understanding cardiac anatomy: the prerequisite for optimal cardiac surgery. Ann Thorac Surg 1995;59:1366.

Anderson RH, Ho SY, Becker AE. The surgical anatomy of the conduction tissues. Thorax 1989;38:408.

Baptista CAC, Didio LJA, Teofilovski-Parapid G. Variation in the length and termination of the ramus circumflexus of the human left coronary artery. Anat Anz 1990;171:247.

Bezerra AJC, DiDio LJA, Prates JC. Variations of the area and shape of the left atrioventricular valve and its cusps and leaflets. Surg Radiol Anat 1994;16:277.

Conley D, Rosse C. The digital anatomist: interactive atlas of thoracic viscera (CD-ROM). Seattle: University of Washington School of Medicine, 1996.

Davies J, Anderson RH, Becker AE. The conduction system of the heart. London: Butterworth, 1983.

Davis CL. Development of the human heart from its first appearance to the stage found in embryos of twenty paired somites. Contrib Embryol 1927;19:245.

Demaria R, Godlewski G, De Guilhermier P, Tang J, Seguin J, Chaptal PA. Static morphometric bases for CT identification and evaluation of the outflow chamber of the left ventricle: preliminary study in formalin-fixed heart. Surg Radiol Anat 1993;15:145.

Dodge Jr JT, Brown BG, Bolson EL, Dodge HT. Diameter of the lumen of normal coronary arteries in man. Circulation 1993;13:111.

DuPlessis LA, Marchand P. The anatomy of the mitral valve and its associated structures. Thorax 1964;19:221.

Edwards JE, Dry TJ, Parker RL, et al. An atlas of congenital anomalies of the heart and great vessels. Springfield IL: Charles C Thomas, 1954.

Edwards WD, Tjik AJ, Seward JB. Standardized nomenclature and anatomic basis for regional tomographic analysis of the heart. Mayo Clin Proc 1981;56:479.

Ellison JP, Williams TH. Sympathetic nerve pathways to the human heart and their variations. Am J Anat 1969;124:149.

Felle P, Bannigan JG. Anatomy of the valve of the coronary sinus (thebesian valve). Clin Anat 1994;7:10.

Grande NR, Taveira De Silva AC, Pereira AS, Águas AP. Anatomical basis for the separation of four cardiac zones in the walls of human heart ventricles. Surg Radiol Anat 1994;16:355.

Hirsch EF, ed. The innervation of the vertebrate heart. Springfield IL: Charles C Thomas, 1970.

Hollinshead WH. Anatomy for surgeons: vol 2, the thorax, abdomen, and pelvis. 2nd ed. New York: Harper & Row, 1971.

James TN. Cardiac conduction system: fetal and postnatal development. Am J Cardiol 1970;25:213.

James TN. Anatomy of the human sinus node. Anat Rec 1961;141:109.

Kramer TC. The partitioning of the truncus and conus and the formation of the membranous portion of the interventricular septum in the human heart. Am J Anat 1942;71:343.

Mall FP. On the muscular architecture of the ventricles of the human heart. Am J Anat 1911;11:211.

McAlpine WA. Heart and coronary arteries: an anatomical atlas for clinical diagnosis, radiological investigation, and surgical treatment. New York: Springer, 1975.

Meredith J, Titus JL. The anatomic atrial connections between sinus and AV node. Circulation, 1968;37:566.

Nerantzis CE, Papachristos JCH, Gribizi JE, Voudris VA, Infantis GP, Koroxenidis GT. Functional dominance of the right coronary artery: incidence in the human heart. Clin Anat 1996;9:10.

Reig J, Jornet A, Petit M. Anatomical variations of the coronary perfusion as a basis of myocardial vulnerability to coronary artery occlusion. Clin Anat 1994;7:315.

Restivo A, Smith A, Wilkinson JL, Anderson RH. Normal variations in the relationship of the tricuspid valve to the membranous septum in the human heart. Anat Rec 1990;226:258.

Schlant RC, Alexander RW, eds. The heart, 8th ed. New York: McGraw-Hill, 1994.

Smith RB. The occurrence and location of intrinsic cardiac ganglia and nerve plexuses in the human neonate. Anat Rec 1971;169:33.

Von Lüdinghausen M, Ohmachi N, Besch S, Mettenleiter A. Atrial veins of the human heart. Clin Anat 1995;8:169.

Walmsley R. The orientation of the heart and the appearance of its chambers in the adult cadaver. Br Heart J 1958;20:441.

Walmsley R, Sinclair DW. Anatomy of membranous ventricular septum in the human heart. Clin Anat 1994;7:305.

Willius FA, Keys TE, eds. Classics of cardiology: a collection of classic works on the heart and circulation with comprehensive biographical accounts of the authors. New York: H Schuman, 1961.

Hollinshead's Textbook of Anatomy, by Cornelius Rosse and Penelope Gaddum-Rosse.
Lippincott-Raven Publishers, Philadelphia, © 1997.

CHAPTER 22

The Mediastinum

The mediastinum is a broad, median partition, or septum, that intervenes between the two pleural sacs and extends from the sternum to the vertebral bodies. As pointed out in Chapter 19, this mass of tissue incorporates the heart, the pericardial sac, and—practically speaking—all the contents of the thoracic cavity except the lungs and the pleura. The mediastinum is a conduit for the esophagus and trachea and, closely packed around them, the blood vessels, lymph vessels, and nerves as they enter or leave the thorax on their way to or from the neck, the upper limbs, or the abdomen. Only the pericardial sac, with its contents, and the thymus are confined to the mediastinum.

For descriptive purposes, the mediastinum is arbitrarily subdivided by a transverse plane that passes through the sternal angle and the lower border of the fourth thoracic vertebra (Fig. 22-1). The **superior mediastinum** is above this plane and is limited superiorly by the superior thoracic aperture; the **inferior mediastinum** is below the plane, and the diaphragm limits it inferiorly. The inferior mediastinum is further compartmentalized based on its relations to the pericardial sac: the sac and its contents compose the **middle mediastinum;** between the sac and the sternum is the **anterior mediastinum;** between the vertebral bodies and the pericardial sac is the **posterior mediastinum.**

This chapter is concerned chiefly with the superior and posterior mediastina, as there is little besides adipose tissue in the anterior mediastinum, and the middle mediastinum is described in Chapter 21.

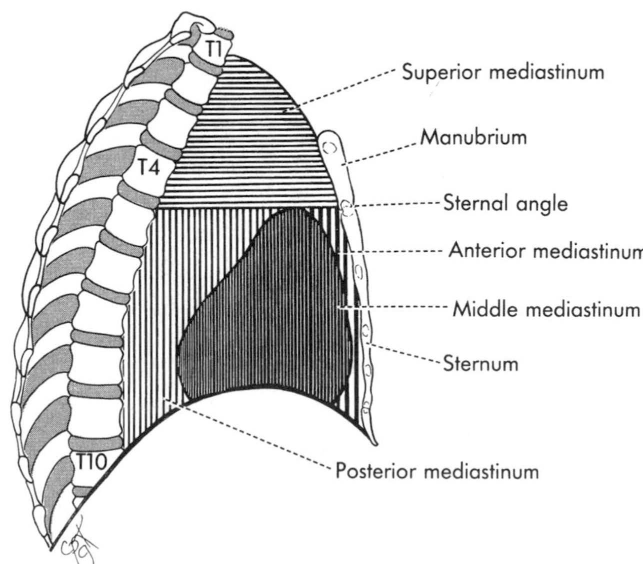

FIGURE *22-1.*
Subdivisions of the mediastinum: The superior mediastinum is shaded with *horizontal lines,* and the compartments of the inferior mediastinum are *shaded with vertical lines* in various patterns.

SUPERIOR MEDIASTINUM

The superior mediastinum is situated chiefly behind the manubrium sterni. Its posterior boundary, made up of the first four thoracic vertebrae, is considerably longer than its anterior one because the plane of the superior thoracic aperture slopes upward from the jugular notch. Above, the superior mediastinum is continuous with the neck; below, it is continuous with both the anterior and posterior mediastina. Its central portion is directly above the pericardial sac, and laterally, it is limited by parietal (mediastinal) pleura.

The main structures crowded into this small, wedge-shaped space are the trachea and esophagus, the arch of the aorta with its three large branches (brachiocephalic, left common carotid, and left subclavian arteries), the right and left brachiocephalic veins that form the superior vena cava, two phrenic nerves and two vagi, the recurrent laryngeal branch of the left vagus, the cardiac plexus and cardiac nerves, the thymus, the terminal portion of the thoracic duct, and a number of lymph nodes and lymph vessels. The key to understanding the relations of these numerous structures to one another is the asymmetry of the major arteries and veins on the right and left sides of the esophagus and trachea. The trachea, with the esophagus behind it, occupies a central position in the superior mediastinum. On the left, the superior mediastinum is dominated by arteries, whereas on the right, veins predominate (Fig. 22-2).

This asymmetry results from two major rearrangements of the primitive, symmetric pattern of embryonic vasculature:

1. On the right side, the segment of the fourth aortic arch that is incorporated into the right subclavian artery becomes displaced from the mediastinum, whereas on the left, the fourth aortic arch is retained in the mediastinum as a segment of the arch of the aorta (see Fig. 22-8).
2. On the left, the common cardinal vein (left superior vena cava) atrophies, whereas it persists on the right as the definitive superior vena cava. The anastomosis that develops between the left and right precardinal veins is represented by the more or less transverse left brachiocephalic vein that lies anterior to all major structures in the superior mediastinum except the thymus (see Fig. 21-22).

The vagus and phrenic nerves enter the superior mediastinum from the neck and continue toward the diaphragm. The vagi approach each other as they pass inferiorly to form the esophageal plexus behind the roots of the lungs in the posterior mediastinum. The right and left phrenic nerves, on the other hand, maintain a lateral position in the superior mediastinum and continue their course inferiorly on the lateral surfaces of the bulging

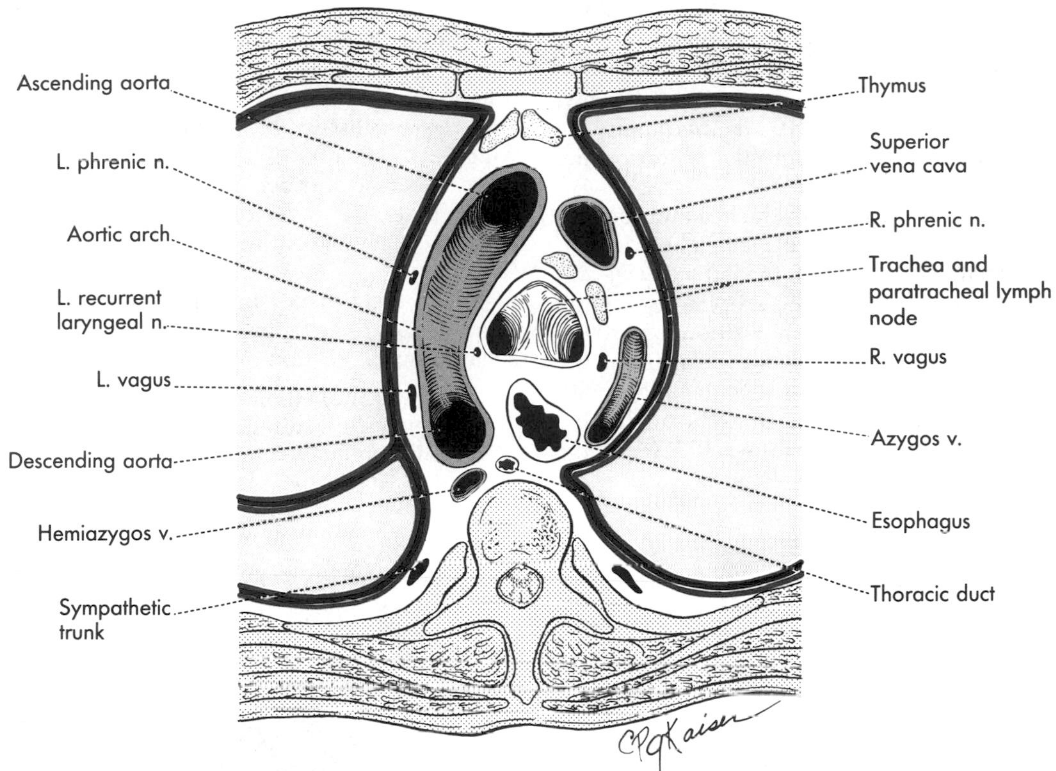

FIGURE 22-2.
A transverse section across the superior mediastinum, level with the body of the fourth thoracic vertebra: The section is being viewed from *above*. The pleura is indicated with solid *red lines*, and the pleural cavity is *solid black*.

pericardial sac as they head for the respective domes of the diaphragm.

The Thymus

The most superficial structure in the superior mediastinum is the thymus (see Figs. 19-14 and 21-2). It is a *primary* or *central lymphoid organ*, its most important function being the production of lymphocytes that are discharged into the bloodstream and are seeded to the rest of the lymphatic system. The thymus consists of two small, pyramidal *lobes*, each made up of many *lobules*. The two lobes are held together by connective tissue and can be distinguished from the surrounding fat by their pinkish gray color and the glandular appearance that is imparted by the lobular structure of the organ.

Each thymic lobe develops from the third pharyngeal pouch on its corresponding side. Following their separation from the pharynx, the epithelial primordia of the lobes descend into the thorax. Lymphocyte production is established during fetal development after the lobes become populated by immigrant lymphoid stem cells. Epithelial elements derived from ectoderm and endoderm, however, persist into postnatal life and may be responsible for the production of humoral factors that play some role in the differentiation of lymphocytes. The thymus continues to grow up to the age of 5 to 6 years, and progressively involutes thereafter, weighing hardly more than 10 g in the adult. It is largely replaced by fat and connective tissue, which maintain the form of the organ.

The thymus is directly behind the manubrium and may extend into the base of the neck and into the anterior mediastinum. The posterior surface of the organ is molded on the arch of the aorta, the left brachiocephalic vein, the trachea, and, more inferiorly, the pericardium. The two pleural sacs overlap the thymic lobes on each side (see Fig. 19-14). The blood supply is from branches of the internal thoracic or inferior thyroid arteries. A large thymic vein drains the gland into the left brachiocephalic vein, and smaller ones drain into the internal thoracic veins. Thymic lymphatics end in several mediastinal nodes. Small branches from cervical sympathetic ganglia and from the vagus enter the thymic lobes, and the connective tissue capsule is supplied by the phrenic nerves.

The Trachea and Esophagus

With the neck slightly flexed, the trachea is palpable in the jugular notch as it enters the superior mediastinum from the neck. Behind it is the esophagus lying on the anterior surface of the vertebral bodies. These two tubular structures fill the superior thoracic aperture in the median plane between the apices of the lungs. Bearing witness to their common embryologic origin, they remain in intimate contact with each other as they descend through the superior mediastinum. The trachea bifurcates into the right and left principal bronchi at, or slightly below, the lower boundary of the superior mediastinum, whereas the esophagus continues into the posterior mediastinum.

Above the root of the lung, both trachea and esophagus are crossed by the azygos vein on the right side (Fig. 22-3) and by the arch of the aorta on the left side (Fig. 22-4). The arch of the aorta indents the esophagus slightly and shifts the trachea from its median position toward the right. In its course through the superior mediastinum, the esophagus contacts the upper lobe of both lungs (with only the pleural sacs intervening), whereas the trachea becomes separated from the lung on the left side by the branches of the arch of the aorta (see Figs. 22-2 and 22-4).

The trachea and esophagus are mobile in the mediastinum and may be shifted from their more or less median position not only by endoscopic instruments (bronchoscope, esophagoscope, gastroscope) but also by neoplasms, abscesses, diverticula, curvatures of the spine, or pressure inequality in the two pleural cavities. The trachea is elastic and becomes elongated with each inspiration. Thus, the level of its bifurcation varies over the height of several centimeters, depending on body posture and respiratory movements.

The cervical portion of the trachea is dealt with in Chapter 30; the esophagus is described more fully in this chapter in the section on the posterior mediastinum.

Normal and Anomalous Development. The trachea is formed as a ventral diverticulum of the foregut. The lumen of the foregut, located dorsal to the diverticulum, develops into the esophagus, whereas

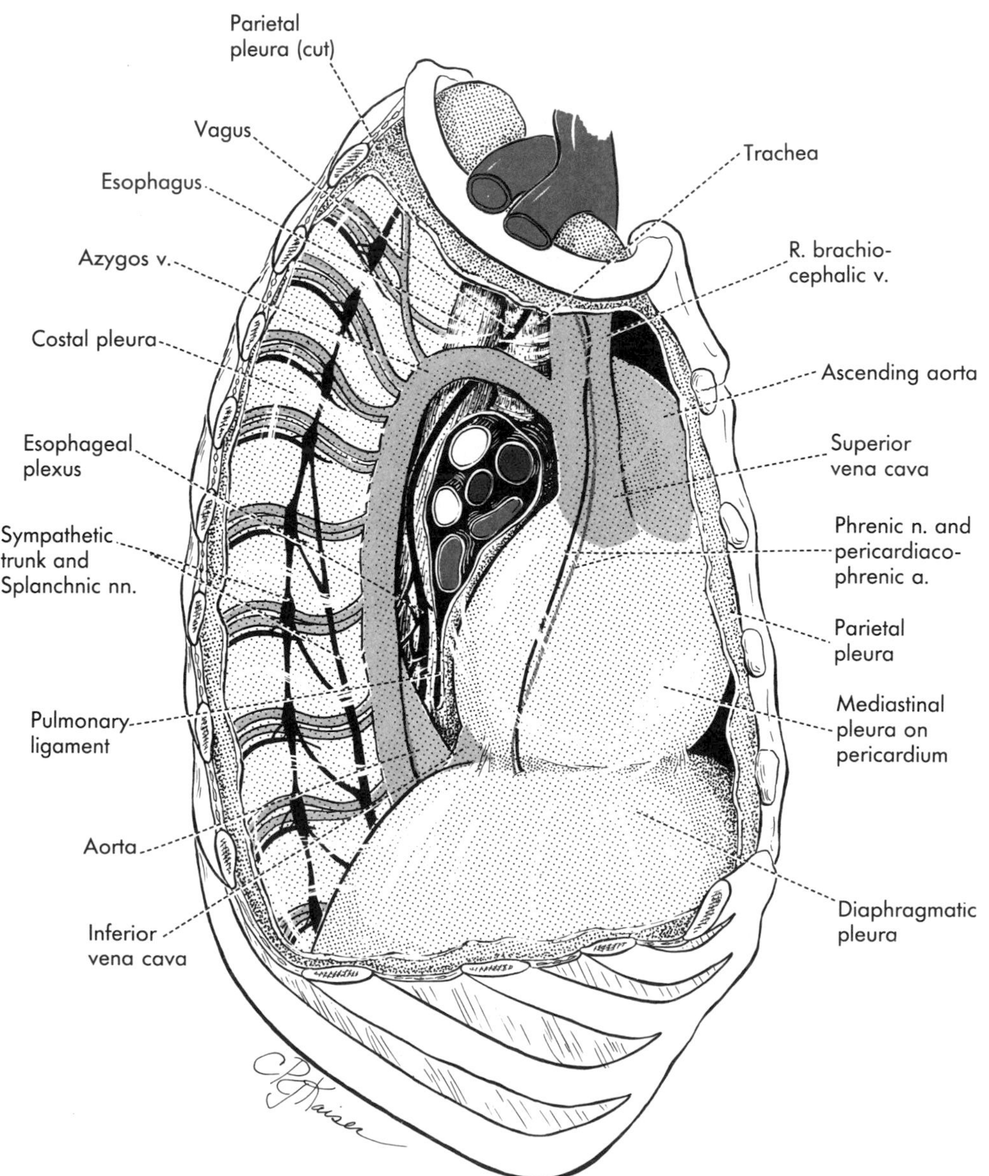

FIGURE 22-3.
The mediastinum seen from the right pleural cavity. The chest wall, a large portion of the costal pleura, and the right lung have been removed. The structures in the mediastinum are seen through the mediastinal pleura.

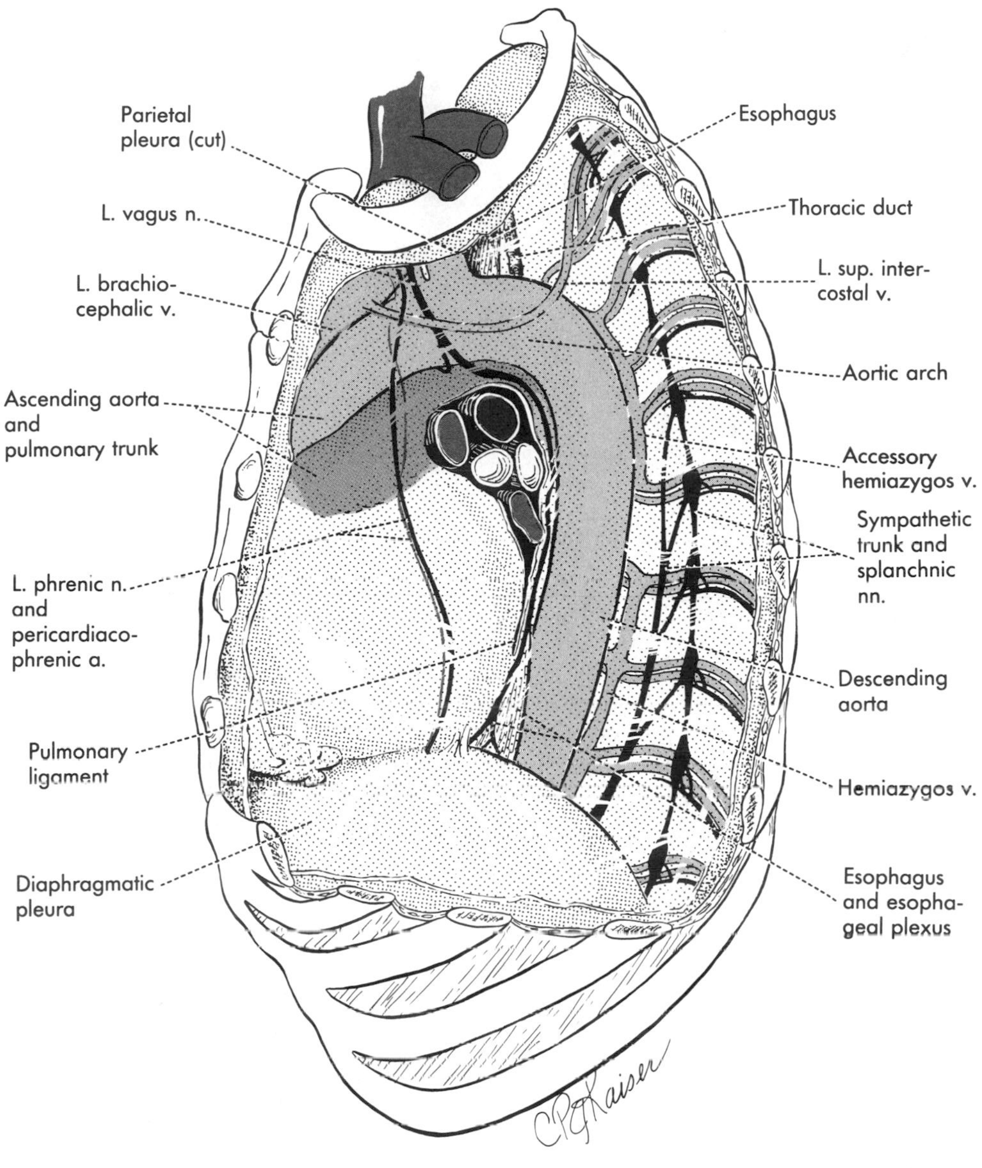

FIGURE 22-4.
The mediastinum seen from the left pleural cavity. The chest wall, a large portion of the costal pleura, and the left lung have been removed. The structures in the mediastinum are seen through the mediastinal pleura.

the diverticulum itself becomes pinched off and elongates (Fig. 22-5). Communication between the trachea and the esophagus is normally possible only through the pharynx and larynx. However, some type of maldevelopment is present in 1 of every 2000 to 3000 births. The esophagus or the trachea may become obliterated along a variable distance (**esophageal** or **tracheal atresia**), or there may be an abnormal communication between the trachea and the atretic or otherwise normal esophagus (**tracheoesophageal fistula;** Fig. 22-6). Such fistulae are usually the result of incomplete separation of the trachea and esophagus along the tracheoesophageal sulcus. Tracheal atresia is incompatible with postnatal life. However, it is important to recognize all tracheoesophageal abnormalities as soon after birth as possible. The more common types of these abnormalities are shown in Figure 22-6. To survive, the newborn must be able to swallow nourishment and saliva and prevent food from entering its lungs.

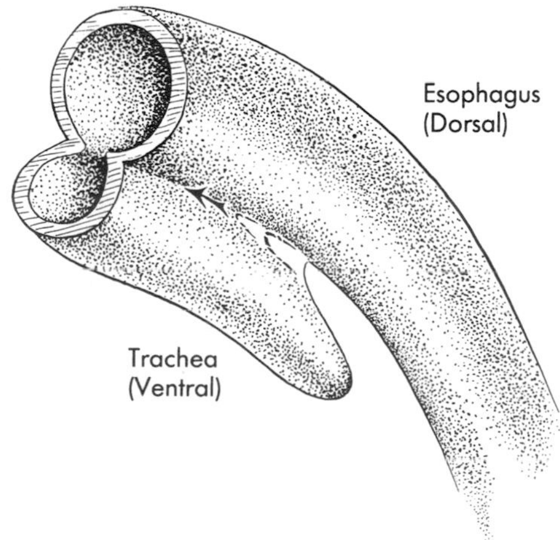

FIGURE 22-5.
Separation of the laryngotracheal diverticulum from the foregut.

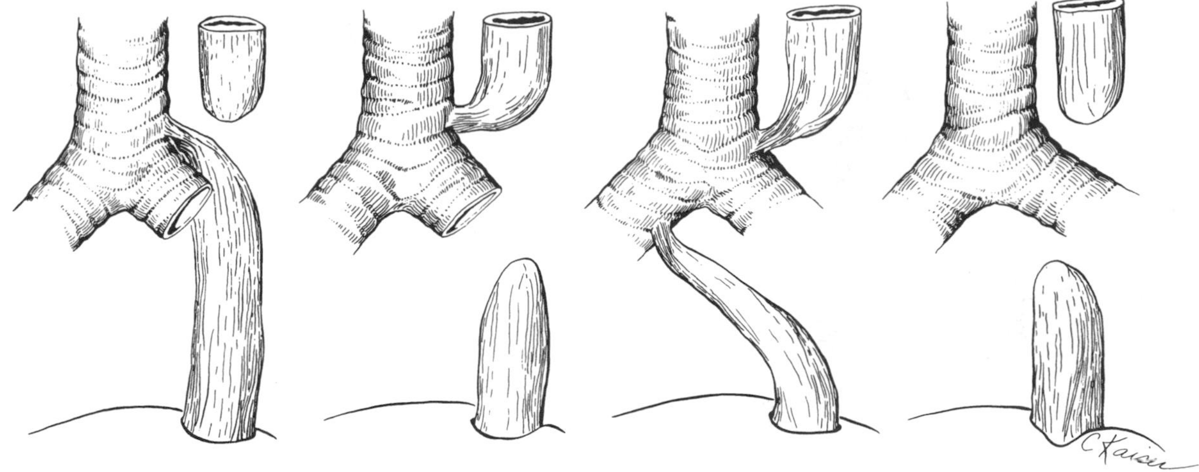

FIGURE 22-6.
The more common types of esophageal atresia and tracheoesophageal fistulae.

The Arch of the Aorta and Its Branches

As soon as the ascending aorta emerges from the pericardial sac, it begins to arch backward, and the segment that runs in a nearly sagittal plane in the superior mediastinum is known as the **arch of the aorta.** On reaching the fourth thoracic vertebra, the aorta becomes vertical, and in the posterior mediastinum, it is called the **descending thoracic aorta.** The arch of the aorta is convex upward and also to the left. It accommodates the right pulmonary artery and the left bronchus in its inferior concavity; the trachea and esophagus fit into the slight concavity that faces to the right. The profile of the left curve of the aorta creates the so-called *aortic knuckle*, identifiable on a posteroanterior chest x-ray film as the upward continuation of the cardiac silhouette (see Fig. 21-7). Through the pleura, the arch indents the medial surface at the left lung just above its hilum (see Fig. 20-3*B*). The **ligamentum arteriosum** connects the inferior surface of the arch of the aorta to the left pulmonary artery just as the artery is given off by the pulmonary trunk. The summit of the arch reaches more than halfway up behind the manubrium and from it arise in a row three major vessels: the brachiocephalic trunk, the left common carotid artery, and the left subclavian artery (Fig. 22-7).

The **brachiocephalic trunk,** the largest and most anterior of the branches, springs from the arch in the midline. Lying on the trachea, it ascends to its right side, and as the artery reaches the superior thoracic aperture, it divides into the **right subclavian** and **right common carotid arteries.**

The **left common carotid** and **left subclavian arteries**

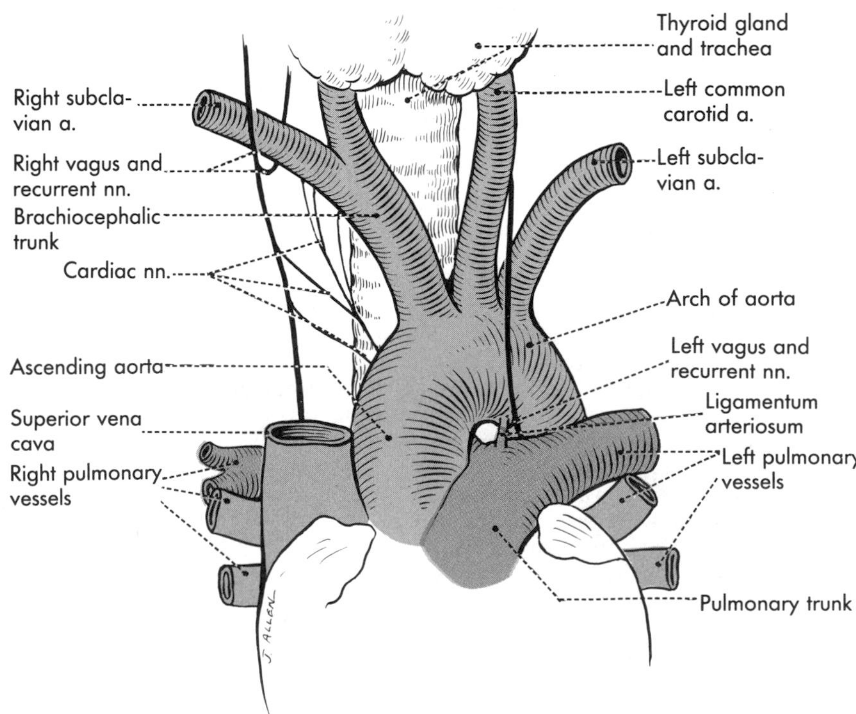

FIGURE 22-7.
The arch of the aorta and its branches with the vagus nerves and their branches.

arise independently from the arch of the aorta in close succession beyond the brachiocephalic trunk. The carotid and the subclavian ascend more or less vertically along the left side of the trachea. Near their origin all three arteries are crossed anteriorly by the left brachiocephalic vein. Between the vein and the superior thoracic aperture, their lateral surface is covered by parietal pleura (see Fig. 22-4).

The three major arteries do not give off any branches in the thorax. However, one of the branches of the subclavian artery, given off at the root of the neck, reenters the superior mediastinum and continues down through the anterior mediastinum. The vessel is the **internal thoracic artery** (see Figs. 19-11 and 30-23). A small inconstant branch, the **thyroidea ima artery,** may arise from the arch of the aorta, the right common carotid, or the subclavian arteries and ascends to the thyroid gland in the neck.

Normal and Anomalous Development

In the human embryo, six pairs of aortic arches arise from the distal dilation of the truncus arteriosus, which is known as the aortic sac. Each pair of aortic arches skirts around the foregut and connects to the dorsal

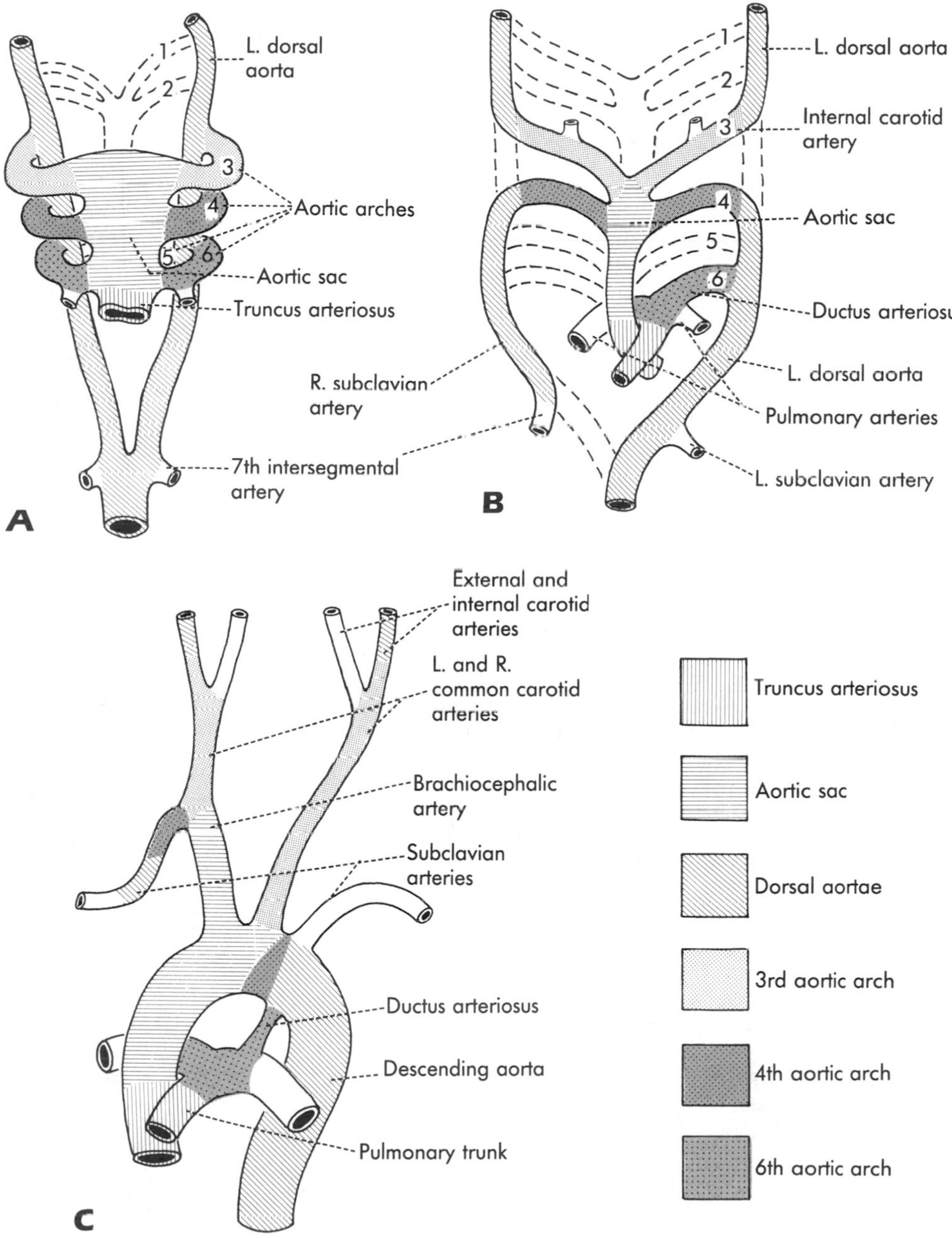

FIGURE *22-8.*
Transformation of the aortic arch system in the human embryo: (A) aortic arches *3, 4,* and *6* are seen connecting the aortic sac with the bilateral dorsal aortae; arches *1, 2,* and *5* have disappeared; (B) the channels that disappear are still indicated; (C) the derivatives of the arches at completion of development. (Adapted from Moore KL. The developing human: clinically oriented embryology. 3rd ed. Philadelphia: WB Saunders, 1982.)

aorta of the corresponding side (Fig. 22-8A see Fig. 21-1A). In fishes, these arteries run in the branchial arches and serve the gills. In the human, normally only the arch of the aorta retains an arcuate character, and this vessel incorporates the embryonic fourth aortic arch of the left side. Other components of the aortic arch system disappear altogether or become radically modified (see Fig. 22-8B and C).

Deviation from the usual set of developmental changes results in such congenital anomalies as a **double aortic arch** or a **right aortic arch** (Fig. 22-9). Both conditions predispose to compression of the esophagus and sometimes the trachea as well. Compression is due to the persistence of the vascular ring around the foregut derivatives in the case of a double arch, or to the continuity of the right aortic arch with a normal descending aorta that develops on the left side. An anomalous **retroesophageal right subclavian artery** that arises from the descending aorta rather than from the brachiocephalic artery (see Fig. 22-9), may also compress the esophagus.

The process that obliterates certain segments of the aortic arch system (e.g., ductus arteriosus) may involve a portion of the aorta, causing profound narrowing.

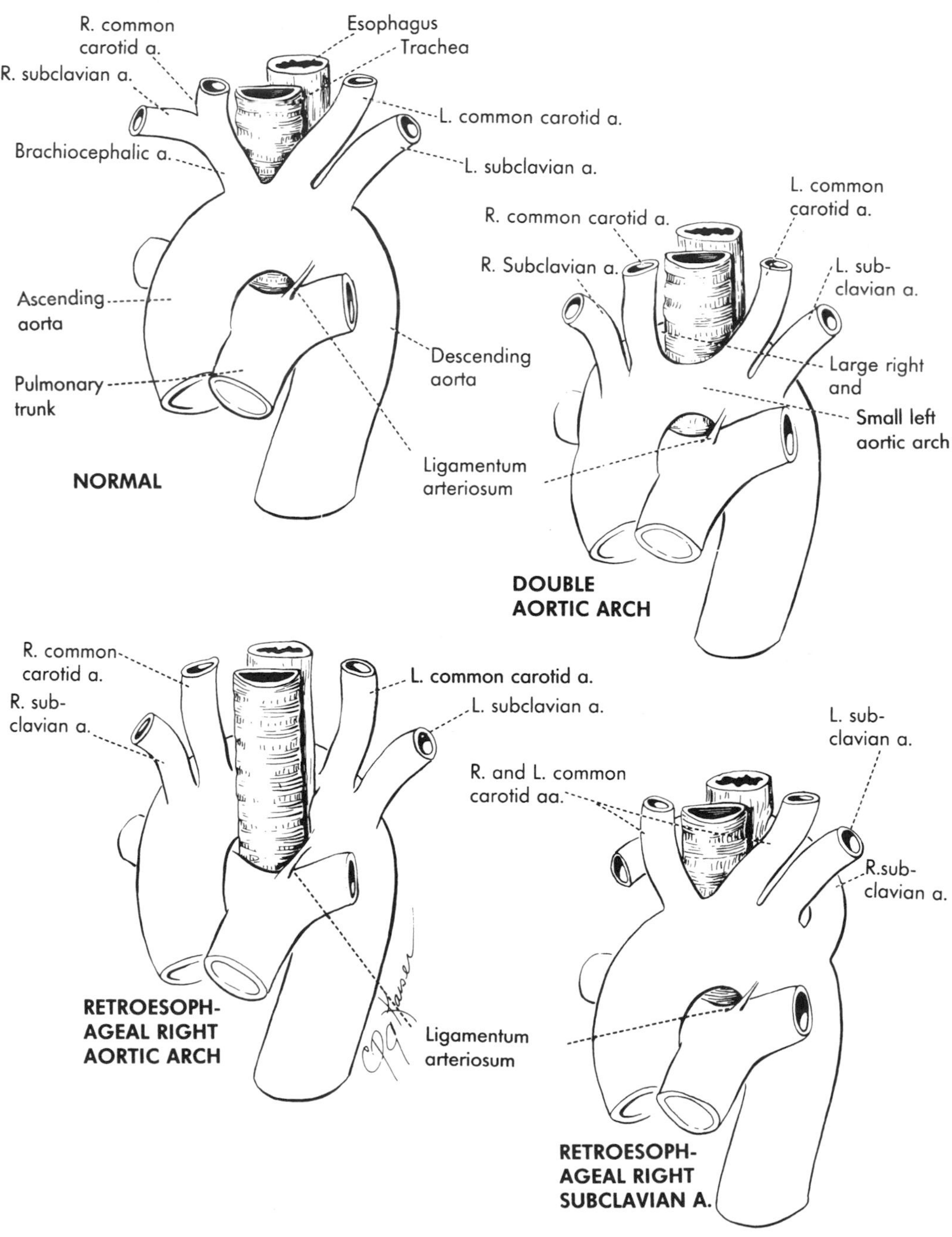

FIGURE 22-9.
Some abnormalities of the aortic arches compared with the *normal* arrangement.

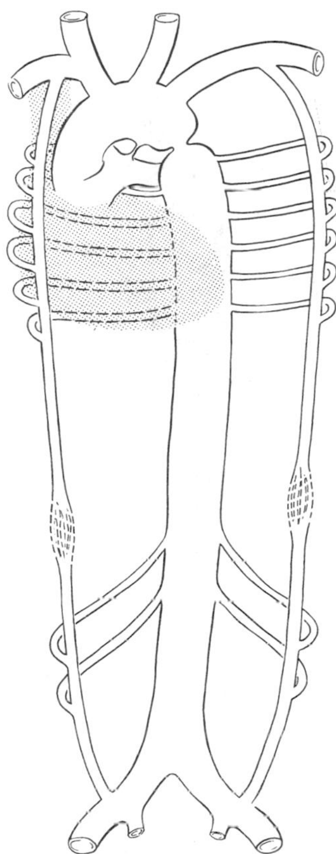

FIGURE *22-10.*
Schematic representation of coarctation of the aorta with the anastomotic channels that become enlarged.

The anomaly usually occurs in the vicinity of the ligamentum arteriosum and is known as **coarctation of the aorta.** The segment of the aortic arch between the left subclavian artery and the ductus arteriosus, known in the fetus as the *isthmus*, carries little blood before birth, and its narrowing may predispose to coarctation. Coarctation, however is more common just distal to the ligamentum arteriosum (Fig. 22-10). Blood supply to the body distal to the coarctation is assured by an extensive collateral circulation that develops between branches of the arch of the aorta and the descending aorta.

Of less clinical importance are the **variations in the branching pattern** of the arteries given off by the arch of the aorta. The left common carotid artery may share a common trunk with the brachiocephalic, or it may arise by a common trunk with the left subclavian. The left vertebral artery, normally a branch of the subclavian, may arise directly from the arch of the aorta.

The Brachiocephalic Veins and the Superior Vena Cava

The brachiocephalic veins are formed by the confluence of the subclavian and internal jugular veins on each side of the root of the neck just above the superior thoracic aperture. At their commencement, the veins lie in front of the main arteries and the cupula of the pleura. After entering the superior mediastinum, the brachiocephalic veins become overlapped by the pleura as they descend behind the manubrium sterni. The right brachiocephalic vein is vertical and is close to the right border of the manubrium. The left vein is much longer and its course is oblique behind the manubrium as it runs in an almost transverse direction toward the right (Fig. 22-11). Behind the sternal end of the right first rib, the left vein unites with the right brachiocephalic vein, and their confluence forms the superior vena cava. The tributaries of the brachiocephalic veins include the vertebral and the inferior thyroid veins from the neck and the internal thoracic, left superior intercostal, and thymic veins from the thorax.

The **superior vena cava** continues the vertical course of the right brachiocephalic vein, and just before it enters the pericardial sac, it receives the **azygos vein.** The azygos vein arches forward over the root of the right lung and enters the vena cava from the back. All the venous blood from the upper half of the body (except that from the heart itself) is delivered to the right atrium by the superior vena cava.

The lower half of the superior vena cava is in the pericardial sac (see Figs. 21-4 and 21-5). In the superior mediastinum, the vena cava is in contact on its left with the commencement of the arch of the aorta and behind, with the trachea. On the right, through the pleura, the superior vena cava contacts the upper lobe of the right lung, but it lies sufficiently forward to allow the trachea to contact the lung as well (see Fig. 22-3). In the front view, the left brachiocephalic vein, lying in the same coronal plane as the vena cava, obscures the summit of the arch of the aorta and the roots of its three branches. Just below it, one of the tributaries of the left brachiocephalic vein, the *left superior intercostal vein*, crosses the arch of the aorta and the left vagus nerve and itself is crossed by the phrenic nerve (see Fig. 22-11). Between the pleural sacs, the thymus prevents the brachiocephalic veins and the superior vena cava from coming in contact with the manubrium.

Nerves

The main nerves that enter the mediastinum through the superior thoracic aperture are the vagi, the phrenic nerves, and the sympathetic trunks. Branches from the vagi and the sympathetic trunks in the neck region (cervical cardiac branches) accompany the main nerves as they enter the aperture. The left recurrent laryngeal nerve, in contrast, ascends through the aperture from the mediastinum into the neck. The cardiac nerves and the cardiac and pulmonary plexuses are discussed in Chapters 20 and 21; the sympathetic trunks are described later in this chapter.

The *vagi*, the tenth pair of cranial nerves, furnish the parasympathetic innervation to all thoracic, and most abdominal viscera (see Fig. 7-8). The *phrenic nerves*, on the other hand, are anterior remi of spinal nerves derived mainly from the fourth and, to some extent, the third and fifth cervical segments of the spinal cord. They are the motor nerves of the diaphragm.

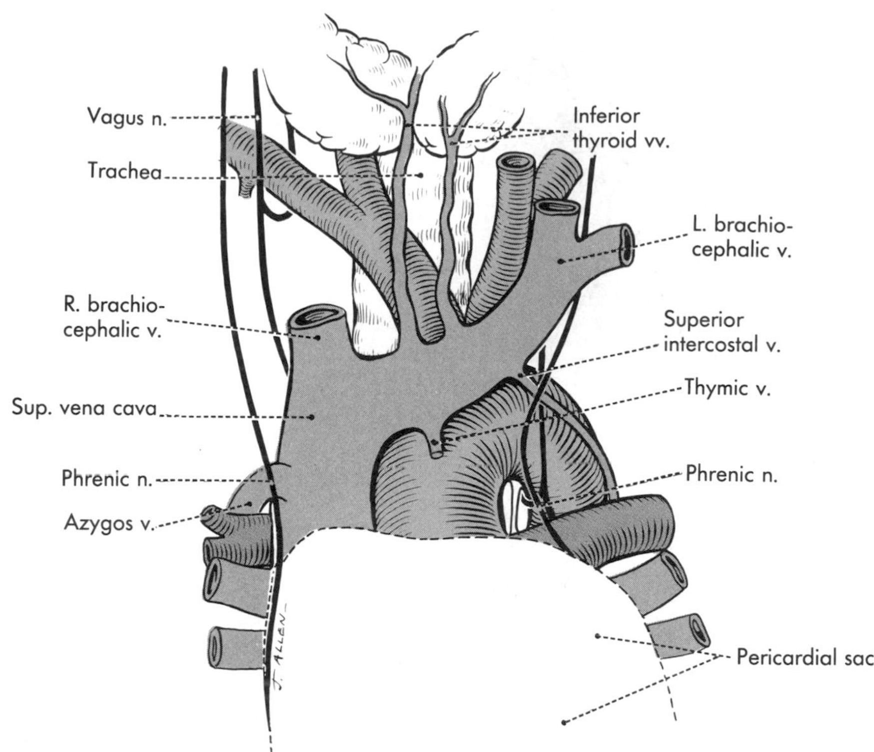

FIGURE *22-11.*
The brachiocephalic veins and the superior vena cava in the superior mediastinum.

The Vagi

At the root of the neck both right and left vagus nerves are between the internal jugular vein and the common carotid artery. Before they enter the mediastinum, they cross the first part of the subclavian artery as that vessel turns laterally. In their descent through the superior mediastinum, the vagi aim for the esophagus, on the surface of which the right and left nerves commingle and form the esophageal plexus. The structures contacted by the vagi differ on the two sides because of the asymmetry in the mediastinum. Starting behind the right brachiocephalic vein, the **right vagus** inclines posteriorly and crosses the trachea obliquely. It is easily identifiable in this position through the pleura (see Fig. 22-3). Just before reaching the esophagus behind the root of the right lung, the vagus is crossed by the azygos vein. The **left vagus** does not come in contact with the trachea; rather, it descends on the surface of the left subclavian artery lying behind the left brachiocephalic vein. It becomes identifiable through the pleura as it emerges from beneath this vein and crosses the arch of the aorta (see Fig. 22-4). Reaching the inferior concavity of the arch, the left vagus inclines backward and medially, passing behind the root of the left lung on its way to the esophagus.

In addition to their cervical cardiac branches, both vagi contribute **thoracic cardiac branches** to the cardiac plexus (see Figs. 21-17 and 22-7). These branches run downward and medially in the mediastinum, as do the cardiac branches that were given off in the neck. A **recurrent laryngeal branch** arises from each vagus, and these two nerves ascend to supply the larynx. The *left recurrent laryngeal nerve* arises from the left vagus at the lower border of the arch of the aorta (see Fig. 22-11), runs medially, skirting the concavity of the arch at its junction with the ligamentum arteriosum, and then ascends on the medial side of the arch in the groove between the trachea and the esophagus. The *right recurrent laryngeal nerve* does not enter the mediastinum because it arises from the right vagus in the base of the neck. Before it commences its ascent, it hooks around the right subclavian artery (an embryonic homologue of a segment of the arch of the aorta [see Fig. 22-8]) just above the plane of the superior thoracic aperture (see Fig. 22-11).

The Phrenic Nerves

In addition to carrying the motor innervation to the diaphragm (C-3 through C-5), the phrenic nerves convey somatic afferents (pain sensation) from the fibrous and parietal serous pericardium, from the mediastinal and diaphragmatic portions of the parietal pleura, and from parietal peritoneum on the inferior surface of the diaphragm, as well as proprioceptive impulses from the diaphragm itself. The phrenic nerves descend to the root of the neck (see Chap. 30) and enter the superior thoracic aperture just after they have crossed the subclavian vessels, passing between the artery and the vein. On each side, the phrenic nerve is lateral to the vagus and posterolateral to the commencement of the brachiocephalic vein (see Fig. 22-11). The right and left phrenic nerves contact different structures as they pass through the superior mediastinum lying subjacent to the mediastinal pleura. The **right phrenic nerve** remains in contact with veins, winding its way forward on the right brachiocephalic vein and the superior vena cava (see Fig. 22-3). The **left phrenic**

nerve parts company with the left brachiocephalic vein and inclines forward as it descends on the arch of the aorta (see Figs. 22-4 and 22-11). On the aorta, it crosses the left vagus and the left superior intercostal vein and is superficial to both. As the phrenic nerves enter the middle mediastinum, both nerves cross anterior to the root of the lung and descend along the greatest convexity of the bulging pericardial sac (see Figs. 22-3 and 22-4). They are accompanied by pericardiacophrenic vessels. The right phrenic nerve passes through the diaphragm with the inferior vena cava, and the left nerve pierces the diaphragm independently, in the vicinity of the apex of the heart.

POSTERIOR MEDIASTINUM

The posterior mediastinum is situated chiefly behind the pericardial sac. Posteriorly, it is limited by the vertebral column, and on each side, by the pleural sacs. Superiorly, it is continuous with the posterior part of the superior mediastinum; the division between the two compartments has no anatomic basis, only a descriptive one. Several of the structures, which for convenience are described in this section, do, in fact, pass through the superior mediastinum. Inferiorly, the posterior mediastinum is limited by the diaphragm, which transmits several mediastinal structures as they enter or leave the abdominal cavity. The contents of the posterior mediastinum include the esophagus with the esophageal plexus formed by the vagi; the descending thoracic aorta and its branches; the veins of the azygos system; the thoracic duct, the largest lymphatic channel in the body; several lymph nodes; and the thoracic portions of the sympathetic trunks with their branches.

The Esophagus

The esophagus is a muscular tube that connects the pharynx to the stomach. It is flattened by the collapse of its walls and its oval lumen is opened to diameters measuring approximately 2 × 3 cm by the passage of swallowed or regurgitated material. Sphincter mechanisms close off the esophagus from the pharynx and from the cardiac orifice of the stomach, which are approximately 25 to 35 cm apart. The esophagus is most firmly anchored at its junction with the pharynx and in the esophageal hiatus of the diaphragm. Apart from some slips of muscle that may connect it to the pleura or the left bronchus, it is relatively free along its more or less vertical descent as it follows the curvatures of the vertebral column, remaining apposed to the vertebral bodies until it approaches the diaphragm. To reach the esophageal hiatus, which is located in the muscular part of the diaphragm level with the tenth thoracic vertebra and to the left of the midline (see Fig. 25-3), the esophagus inclines forward and to the left, crossing from the right side of the aorta to the front of this vessel. In the hiatus, an extension of endoabdominal fascia, the so-called *phrenoesophageal ligament*, attaches circumferentially to the esophagus. It secures the esophagus to the diaphragm, defines the region of the lower esophageal sphincter, and provides a seal between the abdominal and thoracic cavities.

There are four places of narrowing along the esophagus where foreign bodies are prone to lodge and where swallowed corrosives produce the greatest injury. These are also the places most commonly traumatized by the passage of instruments and are the most frequently affected by carcinoma. The first narrowing is at the beginning of the esophagus in the neck, where it is surrounded by the upper esophageal sphincter; the second is the region of contact with the arch of the aorta; the third is where the esophagus is crossed by the left bronchus; and the fourth is in the esophageal hiatus of the diaphragm. Some of these narrow portions can be recognized on radiologic examination of a "barium swallow" (Fig. 22-12).

Structure and Sphincters. The *mucosa* that lines the esophagus is composed of nonkeratinized, stratified squamous epithelium supported by a *lamina propria* (connective tissue) and muscularis mucosae (smooth muscle). In the *submucosa* are embedded small mucous glands, the ducts of which empty into the esophageal lumen. The inner layer of the *muscle coat* proper forms a closely wound spiral of horizontal or circular orientation, whereas in the outer layer, the muscle fasciculi are more oblique, spiraling at a steeper pitch. From the pharynx to approximately the level of the arch of the aorta, the muscle is mostly striated (bronchial muscle); below this level, it is gradually

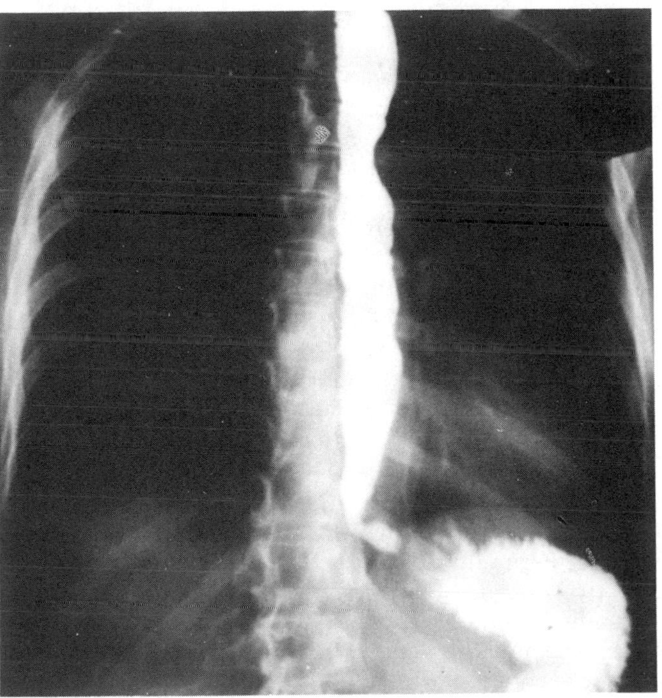

FIGURE *22-12.*
Anteroposterior view of the esophagus while a barium meal was being swallowed. The sharp indentation (at the level of the upper part of vertebra T-5) is caused by the arch of the aorta or the left bronchus. The esophagus appears particularly narrowed a little above the level of the stomach, because barium was passing into that organ.

replaced by smooth muscle. The *adventitia* that surrounds the muscle coat contains many elastic fibers. Unlike other parts of the gut, there is no *serosa* (serous membrane) around the esophagus, which accounts for the difficulties in suturing the esophagus and assuring a leakproof anastomosis.

The **upper esophageal sphincter,** so-called by clinicians, is part of the inferior constrictor of the *pharynx* and is analogous with the *cricopharyngeus* (see Fig. 34-3). The **lower esophageal sphincter**, called the *cardiac sphincter* by anatomises, cannot be demonstrated anatomically or histologically; however, there is decisive physiologic evidence for the existence of a sphincter mechanism around the lower portion of the esophagus. Many factors have been proposed to account for the resistance encountered here by swallowed material or by instruments that negotiate this region: circular esophageal muscle fibers, specialized diaphragmatic muscle (see Figs. 25-1 and 25-6), the phrenoesophageal ligament, and intra-abdominal pressure (see Chap 25). The most important function of this "physiologic sphincter" is to prevent regurgitation of gastric contents into the esophagus. Esophageal mucosa is eroded by the gastric juice, leading to inflammation and ulceration (*reflux esophagitis*).

The **relations of the esophagus** are important because abnormalities of some of its neighboring structures may be diagnosed by the displacement or distortion of esophageal contour on x-ray films. Such conditions include aneurysms of the aorta, distention of the left atrium, enlarged lymph nodes associated with the trachea and bronchi, and osteophytes (bone spurs) on the vertebrae. The relations of the cervical part of the esophagus are discussed in Chapter 29, and those of the upper portion of the thoracic part have been dealt with in the section on the superior mediastinum. For most of the length of the esophagus in the posterior mediastinum, the descending thoracic aorta is to its left. On its right side, it is covered by mediastinal pleura (see Fig. 22-3). Below the tracheal bifurcation, the following structures lie anterior to the esophagus: the right pulmonary artery, the left principal bronchus, the oblique sinus of the pericardium (see Fig. 21-2), and through it, the left atrium. The esophageal plexus formed by the vagi surrounds it (Fig. 22-13).

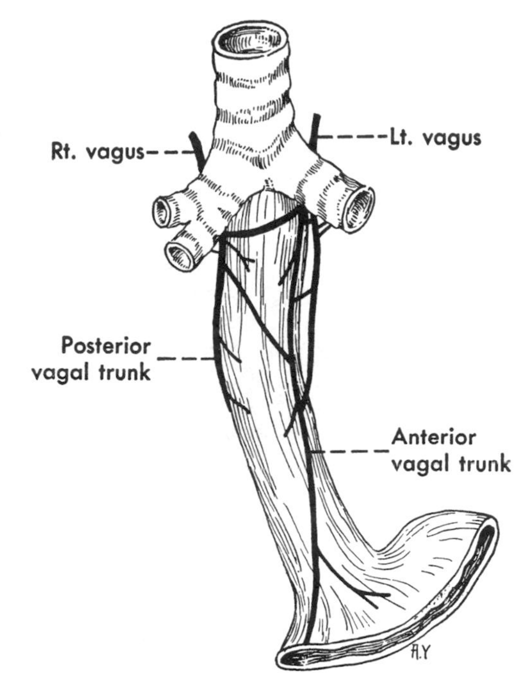

FIGURE *22-13.*
The esophageal plexus: In this example, only a few coarse branches were exchanged between the two vagi.

Blood Supply

The cervical part of the esophagus is supplied by branches of the inferior thyroid artery; the thoracic part is supplied by two or more *esophageal arteries* given off by the descending thoracic aorta and by twigs from the bronchial arteries; the abdominal portion is supplied by esophageal branches of the *left gastric artery*, which ascend along the esophagus and also supply a segment above the diaphragm. There are anastomoses between these territories of blood supply, but the anastomosis may be poor between the aortic and left gastric branches.

The **venous drainage** follows the arteries into the inferior thyroid, azygos, hemiazygos, and left gastric veins. It is important to remember that the latter vein belongs to the portal system, and in portal hypertension (for instance, due to cirrhosis or scarring of the liver) the veins of the submucosa of the lower part of the esophagus become greatly engorged and distended. Tearing or rupture of these **esophageal varices** can result in a fatal hemorrhage.

Lymph from the esophagus drains into deep cervical nodes, posterior mediastinal nodes, and left gastric nodes.

Innervation

The esophagus is supplied by branches of the vagi and the sympathetic trunks. Vagal branches to branchial striated muscle (branchial efferents) are comprised of the fibers of the *cranial accessory* (*11th cranial*) *nerve*, whereas the branches to smooth muscle are preganglionic, visceral efferents of the *10th cranial nerve*, the vagus. Cervical and thoracic sympathetic ganglia contribute visceral branches to the esophagus, and some branches from the splanchnic nerves ascend from the abdomen. Their effect on the esophageal muscle is unknown. The neurons that synapse with the parasympathetic fibers of the vagus are contained in the *myenteric* and *submucosal plexuses* located in the wall of the esophagus, and these plexuses give considerable autonomy to esophageal contraction, even when incoming vagal and sympathetic fibers are severed. A peristaltic wave of contraction is initiated in the esophagus by the voluntary act of swallowing. Unlike other portions of the alimentary canal, the esophagus does not engage in spontaneous peristaltic contractions.

Passage of food along the esophagus is aided by gravity; however, esophageal contractions definitely help to transmit the bolus of food into the stomach. This is clearly demonstrated by the effective swallowing of solids or liquids while standing on one's head. Swallowing requires coordination of segmental contractions and relaxation along the esophagus and of the sphincters.

Achalasia of the esophagus is a disorder in which the myenteric plexus and other vagal elements degenerate or are destroyed. The esophagus becomes grossly distended with food and fluid because the lower esophageal sphincter fails to relax. When the upper sphincter relaxes during sleep, the putrid contents of the esophagus may overflow into the pharynx and into the lung, causing aspiration pneumonia. In other cases, incoordination between the esophageal contraction and sphincter relaxation gives rise to so-called *diffuse spasm*, which builds up esophageal pressure and generates pain.

Esophageal pain is mediated along visceral afferents in the vagus and in the sympathetic nerves. The latter have their cell bodies in posterior root ganglia T-1 through T-10 and terminate in the corresponding segments of the spinal cord. Esophageal pain is felt substernally and may radiate to the back. Sometimes it can be confused with angina pectoris.

The Esophageal Plexus

The two *vagus nerves*, after they have passed behind the corresponding principal bronchi and given off their branches to the lungs, converge on the esophagus and run along it into the abdomen. As they reach the esophagus, each vagus tends to divide into several trunks, and there is an interchange of branches between the nerves of the two sides to form the *esophageal plexus*, which is of varying complexity from person to person (see Fig. 22-13). A little above the diaphragm, the plexus usually gives rise to two nerve trunks. The one on the left, in which fibers of the left vagus predominate, turns forward to run on the anterior surface of the esophagus; that on the right, containing mostly right vagal fibers, turns posteriorly to run on the posterior surface of the esophagus. This change in position is consistent with the embryonic rotation of the stomach. The two newly formed nerves are called the **anterior** and **posterior vagal trunks,** and they enter the abdomen on the esophagus.

Either vagal trunk may be split into two or more parts as it passes through the diaphragm. The trunks are not necessarily placed exactly anteriorly and posteriorly as their names imply. The variations in the vagal trunks are important to the surgeon who cuts these nerves on the lower portion of the esophagus (*vagotomy*) to reduce gastric secretion in the treatment of peptic ulcer.

The Descending Thoracic Aorta

The descending thoracic aorta is the continuation of the arch of the aorta, and it begins where the latter comes in contact with the vertebral column. In its descent through the posterior mediastinum, the aorta is related to the 5th to 12th thoracic vertebrae, first lying on the left side of the vertebral bodies and then gradually approaching the midline (see Figs. 22-2 and 22-4). At the lower border of the 12th thoracic vertebra, the aorta passes through the aortic hiatus of the diaphragm, but even in this hiatus it retains its intimate relation to the vertebrae. The portion of the descending aorta inferior to the hiatus is called the *abdominal aorta.*

Rarely, the aorta descends on the right side of the vertebral column rather than on the left. This anomaly is less frequent than a right aortic arch. Most right aortic arches continue into the descending aorta that is on the left side. When this occurs, the aortic arch passes posterior to the esophagus to link up with the descending aorta (see Fig. 22-9).

Branches

In its descent through the thorax, the aorta gives off several branches to supply the body wall (parietal branches) and some of the thoracic viscera (visceral branches). The paired *parietal branches* arise from the aorta's posterolateral surface: they comprise nine pairs of **posterior intercostal arteries** and one pair of **subcostal arteries.** The posterior intercostal arteries supply the lower nine intercostal spaces, and the subcostal arteries run along the inferior margins of the 12th ribs. The upper two of the 11 intercostal spaces receive posterior intercostal arteries that originate, as a rule, by a common stem (*supreme intercostal artery*) from the costocervical branch of the subclavian artery, and not from the aorta. The course, termination, and branches of these vessels are described in Chapter 19.

Several small *visceral branches* are given off from the anterior surface of the descending thoracic aorta. These include two or more **bronchial** and **esophageal arteries** and pericardial and mediastinal branches. Sometimes the bronchial and esophageal arteries arise from the posterior intercostal arteries, rather than from the aorta itself. A pair of **superior phrenic arteries** supply the posterior portion of the diaphragm.

The Azygos Venous System

The primary purpose of the azygos venous system is to drain blood from the body wall. In addition, the system receives venous blood from some of the thoracic viscera. It also provides an alternative route for venous return from the lower parts of the body should the main venous channel be obstructed.

Blood in the azygos system normally drains upward into the superior vena cava. Because of the complex development of these veins, there is much variation in their anatomy. The azygos system has largely replaced the postcardinal veins of the embryo (see Chap. 25), and portions of these primitive veins persist only at the commencement of the azygos system (ascending lumbar veins) and at its termination (the superior portion of the azygos vein).

The system is called *azygos* (unpaired, or lacking a mate) because the vessels of the two sides are asymmetric, although a common pattern of organization can be readily discerned (Fig. 22-14). The azygos system consists of

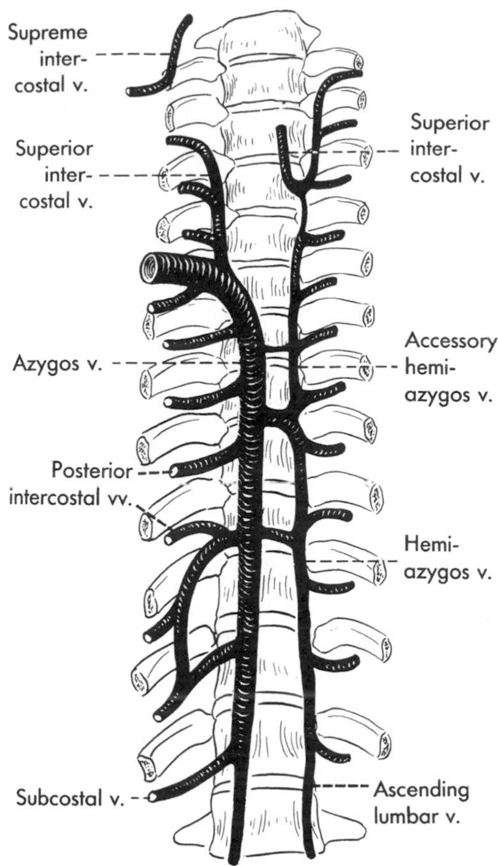

FIGURE *22-14.*
The azygos system of veins. In this example, there are connections among all parts of the hemiazygos system and several connections to the azygos vein.

two longitudinal venous channels, one on each side of the vertebral column. These channels receive the intersegmental veins of the body wall and are interconnected with each other across the vertebrae at irregular intervals. The longitudinal channel on the right is a continuous vessel called the **azygos vein**. On the left, the channel usually consists of two veins: the **hemiazygos vein** inferiorly and the **accessory hemiazygos vein** superiorly. These two veins on the left are interconnected with one another, and each empties independently into the azygos vein through one or more transverse connecting veins.

The azygos and hemiazygos veins are each formed by the union of two veins: the ascending lumbar vein and the subcostal vein. Inferiorly, the *ascending lumbar vein* is connected on the right to the inferior vena cava and on the left to the left renal vein (the segments of the latter are equivalent in their developmental origin). Each ascending lumbar vein receives some of the lumbar veins and passes through the diaphragm, or its aortic hiatus, to unite with the subcostal vein of the corresponding side. The azygos vein ascends in the posterior mediastinum to the level of the fourth thoracic vertebra, where it arches forward over the root of the right lung to terminate in the superior vena cava (see Fig. 22-3). The hemiazygos terminates in the azygos vein at about the level of the eighth thoracic vertebra.

As the azygos vein ascends on the right side, it receives the right **posterior intercostal veins** of all the spaces it passes (5th to 11th). There are four spaces above the level of its termination; the vein in the first space (*supreme intercostal vein*) turns upward to drain into the right brachiocephalic vein, whereas the next two drain into the *right superior intercostal vein*, and thence into the azygos. The fourth intercostal vein may join the right superior intercostal vein or it may, similar to its counterparts below, drain directly into the azygos. On the left side, the hemiazygos and accessory hemiazygos veins usually receive the left posterior intercostal veins of all but the first three spaces. The vein in the first space may drain directly into the left brachiocephalic vein as does its counterpart on the right, or it may join with the second and third intercostal veins to form the *left superior intercostal vein*, itself a tributary of the left brachiocephalic vein. There is a connection between the left superior intercostal vein and the accessory hemiazygos vein below it, thus completing a longitudinal anastomotic channel on the left side. Owing to transverse connections between this venous channel and the azygos vein, the azygos can collect venous blood from virtually all of the posterolateral parts of the thoracic and abdominal walls.

Through the anastomoses of the posterior and anterior intercostal veins, the azygos system is linked to the internal thoracic veins (see Chap. 19), and through the ascending lumbar veins, to the inferior vena cava. The azygos system is also in communication with the vertebral venous plexuses (see Fig. 13-18). The azygos system, devoid of venous valves, constitutes an important channel for collateral venous circulation when the inferior or superior venae cavae are obstructed.

Tributaries of the system from thoracic viscera include the bronchial, esophageal, pericardial, and some mediastinal veins.

Variations in the pattern of the azygos system are of no consequence. The most important, although exceedingly rare, anomaly of the azygos system is for it to receive all the blood from the inferior vena cava except that from the liver, so that the azygos vein drains practically everything below the level of the diaphragm except the digestive tract.

The Thoracic Duct and Mediastinal Lymph Nodes

Lymph draining from the greater part of the body is returned to the venous system by the thoracic duct. The duct is the upward continuation of the *cisterna chyli*, which is a saclike receptacle for lymph from the digestive tract and other abdominal and pelvic organs, from the abdominal wall and perineum, and from both lower limbs. As soon as the thoracic duct leaves the cisterna, it enters the thorax behind the aorta through the aortic hiatus of the diaphragm. In the posterior mediastinum, the duct ascends on the front of the vertebral bodies, running between the aorta and the azygos vein (Fig. 22-15; see Fig. 22-2). In the midthoracic region, it inclines toward the left and leaves the thorax behind the left subclavian artery. In

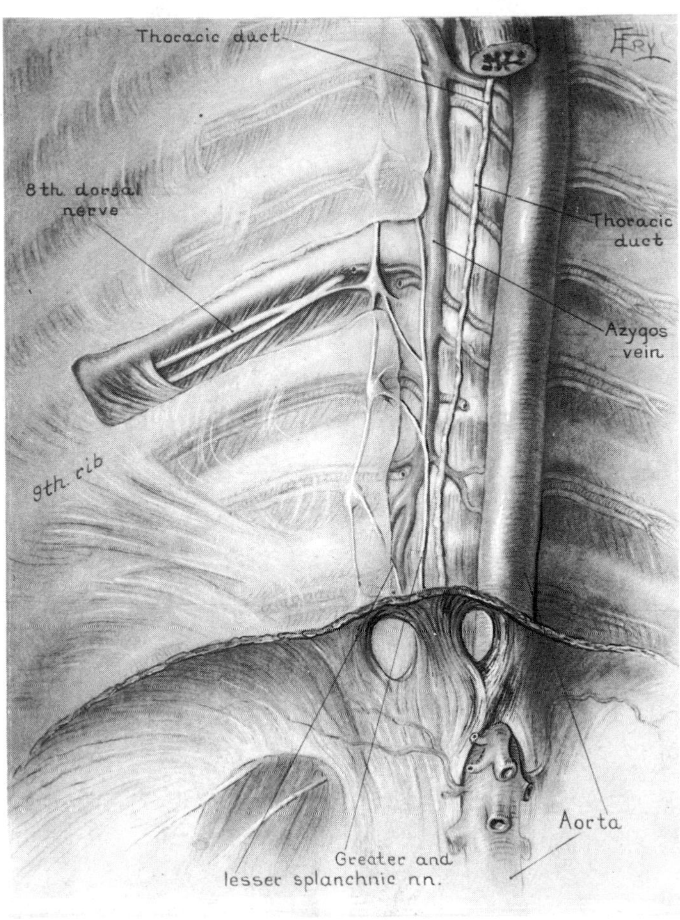

FIGURE *22-15.*
Structures on the posterior thoracic wall: Some of the lower right intercostal arteries have been partially removed. (Labat G. Regional anesthesia: its technique and clinical application. Philadelphia: WB Saunders, 1922.)

the base of the neck, the duct ends at the confluence of the left subclavian and left internal jugular veins (see Fig. 20-9). In most of its course, the thoracic duct lies behind the esophagus and is anterior to the right intercostal arteries and to the transverse, terminal portions of the hemiazygos and accessory hemiazygos veins as these vessels cross the vertebrae. On the right, it may come in contact with the retroesophageal recess of the pleura.

The duct receives tributary vessels from several groups of lymph nodes located in the mediastinum, although most of the nodes drain first into the *bronchomediastinal lymph trunks*. The **groups of lymph nodes** in the mediastinum include the *parasternal* and *intercostal nodes* (see Fig. 20-9), the large groups of *tracheobronchial lymph nodes*, the *posterior mediastinal nodes*, and the *diaphragmatic groups of lymph nodes*. The posterior diaphragmatic, the intercostal, and the posterior mediastinal lymph nodes of the left side send their efferent vessels directly into the thoracic duct. The latter nodes, situated behind the pericardial sac and esophagus, drain adjacent structures and the diaphragmatic surface of the liver. The efferents of the parasternal and tracheobronchial nodes form the right and left bronchomediastinal lymph trunks; the left one of these may join the thoracic duct in the base of the neck or may empty independently into the confluence of the left subclavian and internal jugular veins. Before its termination, the thoracic duct usually receives the left internal jugular and subclavian lymph trunks. The corresponding lymph trunks on the right side form the short **right lymphatic duct,** which has practically no intrathoracic course.

The lymph in the thoracic duct is usually white owing to the presence of *chyle*. The duct is like a small vein, but is less easily seen because of its white or colorless contents. Its somewhat varicose or beaded appearance is due to the presence of valves. One set of these at the termination of the duct prevents the backflow of venous blood, which does, however, occur at the time of death. The terminal portion of the duct in the cadaver may, therefore, be confused with a vein.

Variations of the duct are common, for the lower part of the duct represents the original right member of a pair of ducts, whereas the upper part represents the original left member. Sometimes two fairly large ducts parallel each other for a distance.

Because most of the immunocompetent lymphocytes that recirculate between the blood and lymphatic tissues pass along the thoracic duct, drainage of lymph through a *thoracic duct fistula* can eliminate these cells from the body. Thoracic duct drainage may form part of the immunosuppressive regimen in recipients of organ transplants. The thoracic duct may be injured inadvertently during operations in the posterior mediastinum, and sometimes it is ruptured by violence. When such an injury is associated with a tear or cut in the pleura, lymph will pour into the pleural cavity at a rate as high as 60 to 190 mL/hr. The condition is known as *chylothorax*, and the accumulation of lymph (chyle) may cause collapse of the lung. Unless the defect heals, the duct may have to be ligated. The ligation usually has no noticeable consequences because numerous collateral vessels divert the lymph flow, and several communications exist between the lymphatic and venous system, although these communications have not been defined anatomically. On the other hand, when widespread malignant infiltration causes extensive blockage of the duct and other lymphatics, lymph (or chyle) may accumulate in the pleural cavity and in the peritoneal cavity (*chyle ascites*).

The Sympathetic Trunks

The thoracic portion of the sympathetic nervous system is of particular importance because its paired trunks receive practically all of the preganglionic fibers that leave the spinal cord (see Chap. 7). Some of these fibers synapse in the thoracic sympathetic ganglia, and the postganglionic fibers either join the thoracic spinal nerves or proceed to innervate thoracic viscera. Other preganglionic fibers either ascend in the trunks to the cervical region or descend to the lumbar and sacral portions of the trunks. Preganglionic fibers also leave the thoracic sympathetic trunks as thoracic splanchnic nerves destined for the innervation of abdominal and pelvic viscera. In addition to these preganglionic and postganglionic fibers, the trunks contain visceral afferents that find their way to the thoracic portion of the trunks, not only from thoracic organs but also from viscera of the head, neck, abdomen, and pelvis.

The right and left sympathetic trunks are essentially symmetric. Each trunk consists of 11 to 12 ganglia linked to one another by interganglionic portions of the trunks (Fig. 22-16). Similar interganglionic branches connect the first and last thoracic ganglia to the cervical and lumbar portions of the trunks, respectively. The trunks lie behind the costal pleura (see Figs. 22-3 and 22-4) and, for the most part, rest on the front of the necks of the ribs. Their lower ends incline forward onto the sides of the vertebrae, such that by the time they penetrate the diaphragm, they are situated more anteriorly than laterally. Strictly speaking, therefore, only the inferior portions of the trunks are in the posterior mediastinum.

The **thoracic sympathetic ganglia** are numbered according to the intercostal nerve with which they connect. However, in 75% to 80% of persons, the uppermost or first thoracic ganglion is fused with the inferior cervical ganglion and forms the *cervicothoracic*, or *stellate, ganglion* (see Fig. 22-16); the last thoracic ganglion usually connects with both the 11th and the 12th thoracic nerve. Thus, there are, as a rule, 11 rather than 12 thoracic ganglia in each trunk. Each ganglion lies a little below the level of the corresponding intercostal nerve, to which it is connected by two of its branches. One of these branches consists predominantly of myelinated, preganglionic fibers and is called the *white ramus communicans*; the other consists predominantly of unmyelinated postganglionic fibers and is the *gray ramus communicans* (see also Chap. 7). Each of these rami may be split into two or more fascicles, or the gray and white rami may fuse into one.

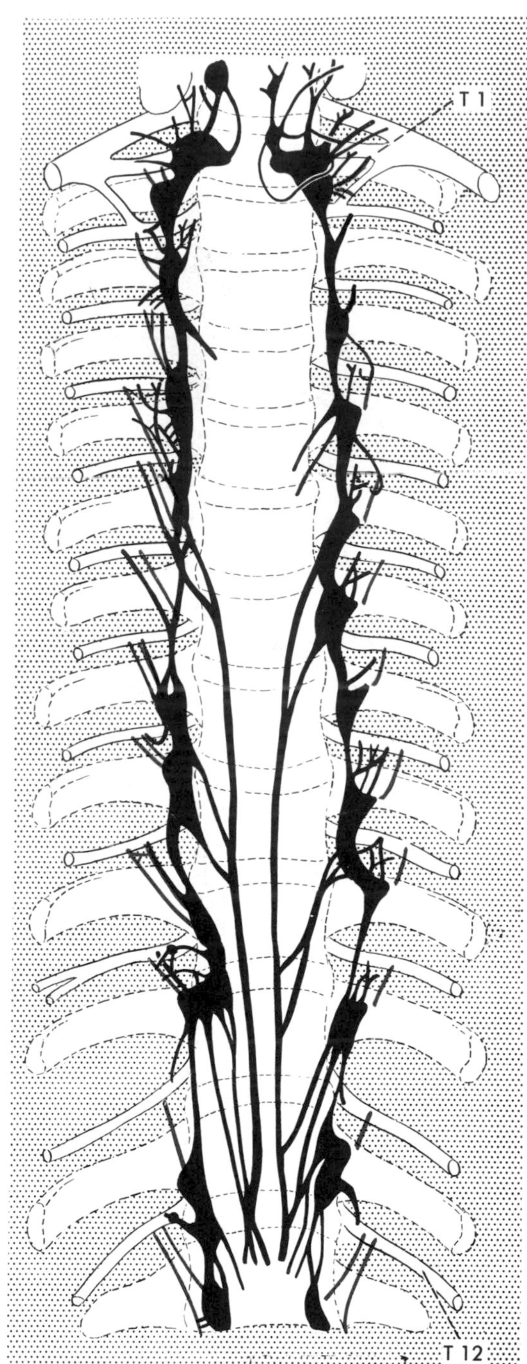

FIGURE *22-16.*
The thoracic sympathetic trunks, the splanchnic nerves, and the rami communicantes. The large ganglion is the cervicothoracic (stellate); the first lumbar ganglion appears at the lower end. The white rami communicantes are shown in *red*, and the gray are shown in *black*; that they were actually white and gray rami was determined by histologic investigation. (Redrawn from Pick J. Sheehan D. J Anat 1946;80:12.)

In addition to the rami communicantes and the interganglionic branches, each ganglion has one or more **medial branches** that serve the viscera. The medial branches destined for thoracic viscera are small and are postganglionic (postsynaptic); those for abdominal and pelvic viscera leave the ganglia as preganglionic (presynaptic) fibers and are gathered into two or three large nerves. These are the thoracic splanchnic nerves.

There are usually three **thoracic splanchnic nerves** called the greater, lesser, and lowest splanchnic nerves (Fig. 22-17). There is much variation in their origin; among 100 cadavers, for instance, 58 different patterns were found. The significant points to bear in mind are that these nerves are composed predominantly of preganglionic fibers that will relay in collateral ganglia of the abdomen (celiac, superior, and inferior mesenteric ganglia) and also contain afferent fibers (pain sensation) from abdominal and pelvic viscera.

The *greater splanchnic nerve* usually arises from the fifth (or sixth) to the ninth thoracic ganglia; the *lesser splanchnic nerve*, from the ninth and tenth; and the *lowest splanchnic nerve*, from the lowest thoracic ganglion. The lowest splanchnic nerve may also be represented merely by a branch of the lesser splanchnic. Nerves of considerable size are formed by the medial branches of the appropriate sets of ganglia; the greater splanchnic nerve is larger than the continuation of the sympathetic trunk into the abdomen (see Fig. 22-17). All three splanchnic nerves descend toward the diaphragm in front of the vertebral column, lying medial to the sympathetic trunks. They pierce the muscular part of the diaphragm and enter the celiac ganglion or one of the associated ganglia or plexuses. The lowest splanchnic nerve, or the corresponding branch of the lesser splanchnic, usually ends in the renal plexus.

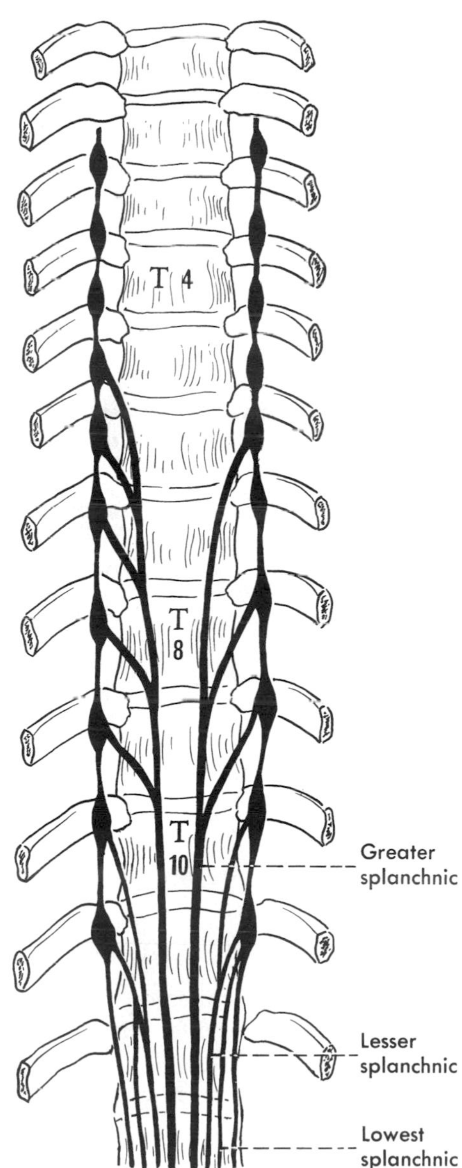

FIGURE 22-17.
Origin of the splanchnic nerves from the sympathetic trunks; they vary and are not necessarily symmetric on the two sides.

Visceral afferent fibers are found in many of the pathways described in the foregoing section. They travel in the medial branches of the sympathetic ganglia to reach the sympathetic trunks; from here each visceral afferent enters a white ramus communicans, joins the intercostal nerve to which the ramus is attached, and continues its way toward the corresponding spinal ganglion admixed with somatic afferent fibers in the intercostal nerve. (Not all visceral afferents travel this route using sympathetic pathways; others are found in parasympathetic pathways, notably the vagus nerves.)

RECOMMENDED READINGS

Congdon ED. Transformation of the aortic arch system during the development of the human embryo. Contrib Embryol 1922;14:47.

Conley DM, Kastella KG, Sundsten JW, Rauschning W, Rosse C. Computer-generated three-dimensional reconstruction of the mediastinum correlated with sectional and radiological anatomy. Clin Anat 1992;5:185.

Conley D, Rosse C. The digital anatomist: interactive atlas of thoracic viscera (CD-ROM). Seattle: University of Washington School of Medicine, 1996.

Edwards DAW. The esophagus. Gut 1971;12:985.

Glazer GM, Gross BH, Quint LE, Francis IR, Bookstein FL, Orringer MB. Normal mediastinal lymph nodes: number and size according to American Thoracic Society mapping. Am J Roentgenol 1985;144:261.

Heitzman ER. The mediastinum: radiologic correlations with anatomy and pathology. 2nd ed. New York: Springer-Verlag, 1988.

Hollinshead WH. Anatomy for surgeons: vol 2, the thorax, abdomen, and pelvis. 2nd ed. New York: Harper & Row, 1971.

Mahoney EB, Manning JA. Congenital abnormalities of the aortic arch. Surgery 1964;55:1.

Moore KL, Persaud TVN. The developing human: clinically oriented embryology. 5th ed. Philadelphia: WB Saunders, 1993.

Pillet JC, Papon X, Fournier H-D, Sakka M, Pillet J. Reconstruction of the aortic arches of a 28-day human embryo (stage 13) using the Born technique. Surg Radiol Anat 1995;17:129.

Proto AV. Mediastinal anatomy: emphasis on conventional images with anatomic and computed tomographic correlations. J Thorac Imaging 1987;2:1.

Riquiet M, Saab M, Le Pimpec Barthes F, Hidden G. Lymphatic drainage of the esophagus in the adult. Surg Radiol Anat 1993;15:209.

Sutliff KS, Hutchins GM. Septation of the respiratory and digestive tracts in human embryos: crucial role of the tracheoesophageal sulcus. Anat Rec 1994;238:237.

PART VI

ABDOMEN

Hollinshead's Textbook of Anatomy, by Cornelius Rosse and Penelope Gaddum-Rosse.
Lippincott-Raven Publishers, Philadelphia, © 1997.

CHAPTER 23

The Abdomen in General

The abdomen is the region of the trunk between the thorax and the pelvis. On the surface of the trunk, the abdomen is demarcated superiorly by the xiphisternal joint and the costal margins; inferiorly by the symphysis pubis, the inguinal folds, and the iliac crests; and posteriorly by the lumbar paravertebral musculature of the back. Within the trunk, the abdomen is much more extensive: the **abdominal cavity** bulges up into the rib cage and is separated from the thoracic cavity by the diaphragm, which has a highly concave abdominal surface (see Fig. 19-1); inferiorly, the abdominal cavity continues, without interruption, into the pelvis, being limited below by the pelvic floor, or pelvic diaphragm, which separates it from the perineum. The abdominal cavity is the inferior (caudal) compartment of the body cavity, or celom, and contains the major parts of the digestive and urinary systems, the internal organs of reproduction, and the peritoneum, which is the largest serous sac of the body intimately associated with the viscera.

It is customary, speaking both anatomically and clinically, to consider the abdominal cavity in two parts: the upper, larger portion is the **abdomen proper,** and the smaller part below is the **pelvic cavity.** The arbitrary plane that demarcates these two parts of the cavity coincides with the superior aperture or brim of the pelvis. The plane of the superior pelvic aperture slants forward from the sacral promontory to the upper border of the pubic symphysis. The pelvic cavity and its contents are considered separately in Chapter 27; this chapter, and the following two, deal primarily with the abdomen proper. It is important to remember, however, that through the superior pelvic aperture there is continuity of space, both within and outside the peritoneal sac, and several structures are transmitted through the aperture between the abdominal and pelvic portions of the cavity. Moreover, organs considered to be primarily abdominal (loops of small bowel, the appendix) may normally descend into the pelvis, and primarily pelvic viscera (distended bladder, pregnant uterus) normally rise up into the abdomen.

THE ABDOMINAL WALL

Above and anteriorly, the abdomen proper is surrounded by contractile and distensible walls, whereas the posterior wall is stable and bulky by comparison. The musculotendinous diaphragm forms the mobile, dome-shaped roof; and three concentric layers of sheetlike muscles, with their aponeuroses, enclose the abdomen anterolaterally. The bodies of the lumbar vertebrae and the alae of the iliac bones account for the stability of the abdominal wall posteriorly, and the three pairs of muscles associated with these bones (quadratus lumborum, psoas major, and iliacus) increase the bulk of the posterior abdominal wall (Fig. 23-1).

It is usual to consider the diaphragm and the posterior wall separately (see Chap. 25). Unless specifically qualified, the term *abdominal wall* is used by clinicians and anatomists alike to refer to the anterolateral abdominal wall only. In this sense, on the surface of the trunk, the extent of the abdominal wall corresponds to the extent of the abdomen defined in the first paragraph of this chapter. Over this region, the abdominal wall is made up of skin, superficial fascia, three layers of muscle (outer, inner, and innermost layers), and endoabdominal fascia (see Fig. 23-1). Except for the lack of ribs, the arrangement of these tissues resembles the structure of the thoracic wall (see Chap. 19).

The derivation and development of body wall muscles and fascias are considered in the introduction to the thoracic wall (see Chap. 19). The ventrolateral extensions of T-6 to T-12 myotomes into the somatopleure of the abdominal wall fuse with each other and give rise to all the muscles. Because of the absence of ribs, the only reminder of the segmental origin of the abdominal wall musculature is their segmental pattern of nerve and blood supply.

Fascial and muscular layers of the abdominal wall send extensions into the perineum. Most of these extensions provide fascial tunics for the ductus deferens in the male and the round ligament of the uterus in the female, as these structures pass through the abdominal wall. The passage through the abdominal wall, traversed by the ductus deferens or the round ligament, is known as the *inguinal canal.* Because of its clinical importance, the inguinal canal and the applied anatomy of inguinal and femoral hernia are considered separately in Chapter 26.

Muscles and Fascias

The outer, inner, and innermost muscle layers of the abdominal wall are formed by the external oblique, internal oblique, and transversus abdominis, respectively. These three pairs of broad, flat muscles, and their aponeuroses, form the major part of the anterolateral abdominal wall. On each side of the midline, a straplike muscle, the rectus abdominis, spans the abdominal wall between the rib cage and the symphysis pubis. The aponeuroses of the three flat muscles meet in a midline raphe, where the intertwining of their tendon fibers forms the *linea alba,* a white line of varying breadths. Before the aponeuroses meet in this raphe, they form a sheath around the rectus as they pass anteriorly or posteriorly to that muscle (see Fig. 23-1).

Each muscle is covered on its deep and superficial surface by *deep fascia.* This thin connective tissue membrane is firmly attached to the muscles and their aponeuroses. There is a small amount of loose connective, or areolar, tissue between the deep fascia of the adjacent muscle layers. The **neurovascular plane** is defined by such areo-

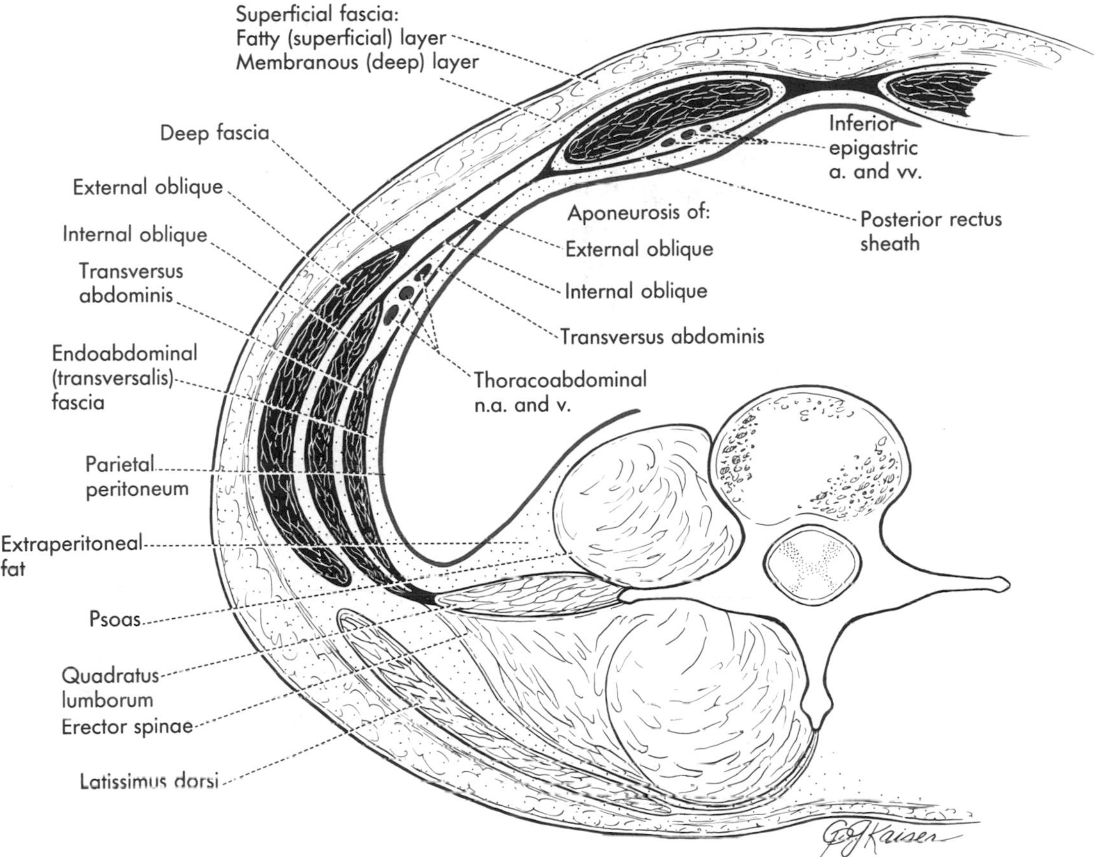

FIGURE 23-1.
A schematic transverse section of the abdomen to show the layers of the abdominal wall. The muscles of the anterolateral abdominal wall are shown in *black*; muscles associated with the vertebral column are *white*. Compare with Figure 19-2.

lar tissue between the internal oblique and the transversus abdominis. The segmental nerves and blood vessels of the body wall run in this plane and, from here, distribute their cutaneous and muscular branches that pierce the adjacent layers.

Superficial fascia separates the exterior of the muscular wall from the skin. On the interior, a layer of extraperitoneal, or *endoabdominal, fascia* attaches the parietal peritoneum to the transversus abdominis and merges with similar areolar tissue over the neighboring boundaries of the abdominal cavity.

Superficial Fascia

The subcutaneous tissue of the abdominal wall is a favorite repository for fat and may be several inches thick. Delicate fibrous strands, which surround the lobules of fat, are firmly anchored in the dermis, but adhere only loosely to the deep fascia of the external oblique. Consequently, the superficial fascia, and the skin with it, may be pinched up and moved around with ease, much more so than over the thigh, for instance. A cleavage plane can be readily defined by blunt dissection between the deep and the superficial fascia.

When the superficial fascia contains a moderate amount of fat, the deep surface appears membranous owing to a condensation of its overlapping, deeper fibrous strands into a definite lamella. Such a **membranous layer** can be demonstrated in most persons, and it may be dense enough to hold sutures. It can also be identified as a distinct layer by computed tomography. Thus, over the lower part of the abdomen, two layers can be defined in the superficial fascia: a *superficial fatty layer* and a *deep membranous layer*. The latter is similar in structure to the deep fascia, but it is quite distinct from it anatomically.

The attachments of the membranous superficial fascia are of some importance. In the midline, the fascia is attached to the linea alba, and in the region above the pubis, it forms a midline septum that is reinforced by contributions from the deep fascia. This septum extends onto the dorsum of the penis and is known as the suspensory, or *fundiform, ligament* of the penis. To each side of the midline, the superficial fascia descends into the perineum: in the male, the fat disappears over the penis, but the membranous layer invests the penis (*superficial penile fascia*) (Fig. 23-2*A*) and surrounds the scrotum (dartos fascia) (see Fig. 23-2*B*); in the female, both fatty and membranous layers continue into the labia majora. In both sexes, the membranous layer becomes, in effect, the *superficial fascia of the perineum*, and both superficial penile and dartos fas-

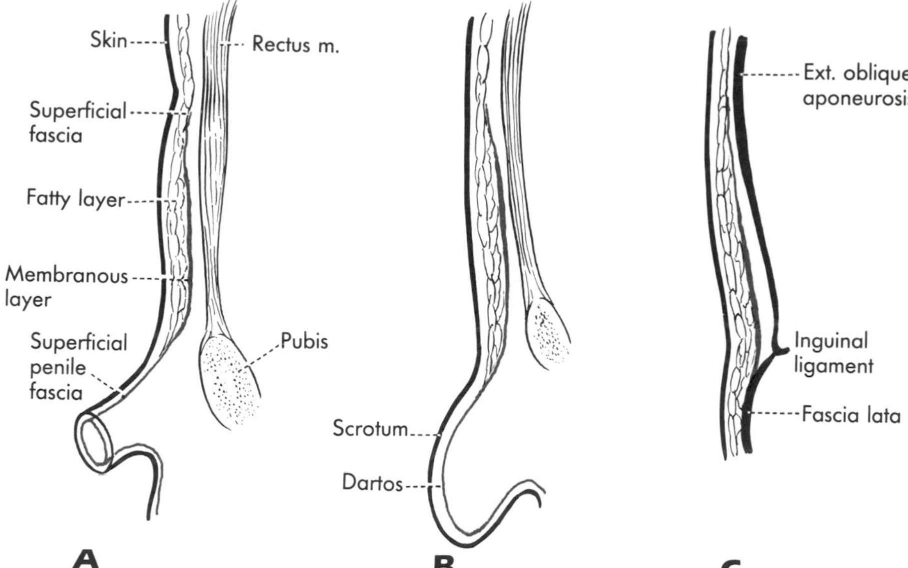

FIGURE 23-2.
Diagram showing the disposition of the superficial fascia of the lower part of the abdominal wall. The membranous layer is shown in *blue*. (A) a longitudinal section of the anterior abdominal wall just to one side of the midline; (B) a section a little more laterally; (C) a section far enough laterally to continue into the thigh.

cias can be considered as components of the superficial fascia of the perineum (see Chap. 28).

Further laterally, the superficial fascia continues into the thigh: the fat blends with the superficial fascia of the thigh, and the membranous layer becomes adherent to the fascia lata a finger breadth below the inguinal ligament (see Fig. 23-2C). Thus, in a dissection, a finger placed between the membranous superficial fascia and the deep fascia of the external oblique cannot be pushed into the thigh, but it can pass with relative ease into the penis, the wall of the scrotal sac, or the labia majora.

The superficial fascia is traversed by cutaneous nerves and blood vessels as well as by lymphatics. These nerves and vessels are considered in a separate section of this chapter.

The Oblique and Transversus Muscles

The **external oblique** (*m. obliquus externus abdominis*) is the most superficial and the largest of the flat muscles of the abdominal wall (Fig. 23-3). Rather more than the anterior half of the muscle consists of a strong tendinous membrane, the external oblique *aponeurosis*. The fleshy part of the muscle is attached superiorly to the exterior of the rib cage and inferiorly to the outer lip of the iliac crest. The muscle has two free margins: a posterior margin that is fleshy and more or less vertical; and an inferior margin that is entirely tendinous and runs obliquely between the anterior superior iliac spine and the pubic tubercle. This free inferior margin of the external oblique aponeurosis is thickened and is known as the *inguinal ligament*.

The fleshy slips of the external oblique attach to each of the last seven or eight ribs, but fuse almost immediately to form a broad muscle with no trace of segmentation. At their costal attachments, the costal slips interdigitate with the serratus anterior and the lower slips interdigitate with the latissimus dorsi. The muscle fibers slope downward and forward from their costal attachments, the posterior fibers being the most vertical. The slips attached to the last three to four ribs remain fleshy and attach below to the anterior half of the iliac crest. The remaining slips continue as the aponeurosis. Tendon fibers in the upper portion of the aponeurosis decussate in the linea alba, whereas those in the lower portion attach to the symphysis pubis and the pubic crest. More laterally, the aponeurosis terminates by forming the inguinal ligament and by attaching to the iliac crest for a short distance beyond the anterior superior iliac spine.

The decussation in the linea alba is rather complex: some of the tendon fibers in the external oblique aponeurosis can be traced directly into the aponeurosis of more than one of the flat muscles on the opposite side. Thus, the upper portion of each external oblique may be considered as a digastric muscle: one belly is the external oblique of one side, and the other, the internal oblique or transversus of the opposite side. Acting in unison with other flat muscles, the external obliques compress the abdomen. In this action, the costal attachment of the external oblique remains fixed and is appropriately designated as the muscle's site of origin. However, in producing movements of the trunk, the external oblique approximates the rib cage to the stable pelvis; therefore, the costal attachment should be designated as the muscle's site of insertion.

The **internal oblique** (*m. obliquus internus abdominis*) lies immediately deep to the external oblique (Fig. 23-4). The muscle arises from the upper surface of the anterior two-thirds of the iliac crest and, in continuity with this bony attachment, from the thoracolumbar fascia behind, and from the lateral third of the inguinal ligament (more precisely, from the line of fusion between the inguinal ligament and the iliopsoas fascia) in front. From this long, linear origin, fleshy fibers fan out and run mostly upward and medially, approximately at right angles to the fibers of the external oblique. The muscle does not have a free posterior border between the iliac crest and the ribs; rather, it is here that its posterior fibers arise from the thoracolumbar fascia, thereby obtaining indirect attachment to the vertebral column. These fibers, as well as the most

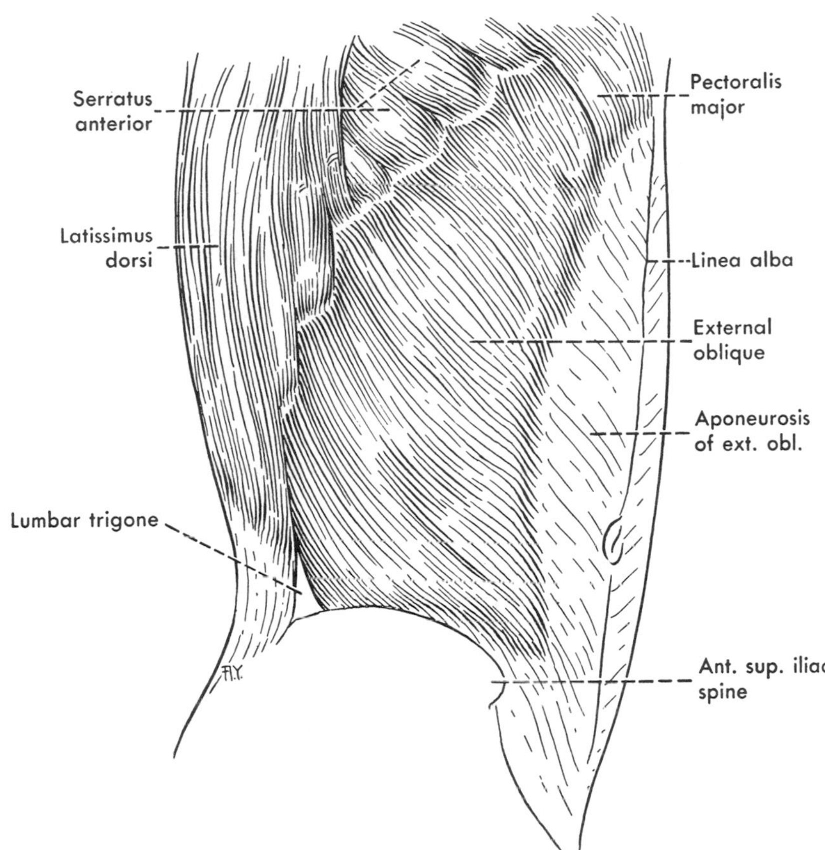

FIGURE 23-3.
The external oblique muscle.

posterior ones from the iliac crest, insert into the inferior border of the last three or four ribs. The rest of the fibers form an *aponeurosis*.

The aponeurosis and the most anterior fleshy fibers of the internal oblique have a free inferior border that passes downward and medially, running above and parallel with the inguinal ligament (see Fig. 26-28). This free border contributes to the formation of the **conjoint tendon** (*falx inguinalis*), so called because at some distance below the umbilicus, the aponeurosis of the internal oblique and the transversus abdominis fuse with each other. This fused aponeurosis passes anteriorly to the rectus, and its segment lateral to the rectus, the conjoint tendon, becomes anchored to the pecten of the pubis. The rest of the fused aponeurosis decussates with the aponeuroses of the other muscles in the raphe of the linea alba.

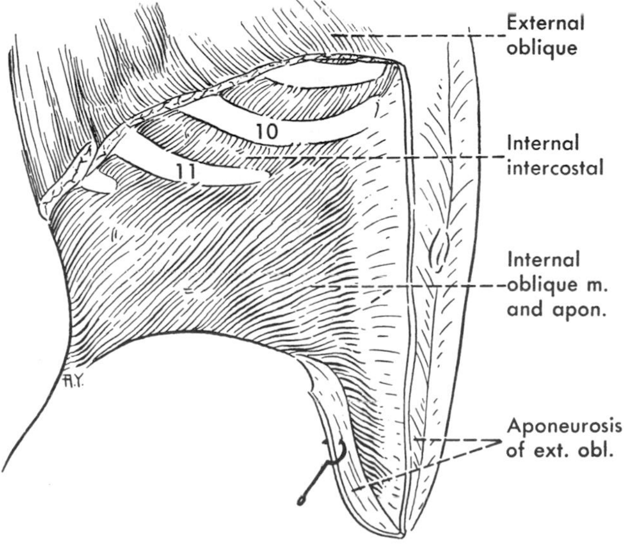

FIGURE 23-4.
The internal oblique muscle.

The more superior portion of the internal oblique aponeurosis splits into an anterior and posterior layer along the lateral edge of the rectus (see Fig. 23-8). The posterior layer remains fused to the transversus aponeurosis and passes with it behind the rectus; the anterior layer passes anteriorly to the rectus with the aponeurosis of the external oblique. These fused aponeurotic layers constitute the *rectus sheath* and meet their fellows of the opposite side in the linea alba. In the epigastrium, the internal oblique aponeurosis is attached to the inferior border of the costal margin.

The **transversus abdominis,** the innermost flat muscle of the abdominal wall, arises, like the internal oblique, from the iliopsoas fascia (adjacent to the lateral third of the inguinal ligament), from the iliac crest (the inner lip rather than the upper surface), and, between the iliac crest and the 12th rib, from the thoracolumbar fascia (Fig. 23-5). In addition, on the internal aspect of the lower six costal cartilages, slips of origin of the transversus interdigitate with those of the diaphragm. For the most part, the muscle fibers extend transversely and end in an *aponeurosis*. As it reaches the rectus, the aponeurosis fuses with the internal oblique aponeurosis to help form the *rectus sheath* (see Fig. 23-8). Below the level of the anterior superior il-

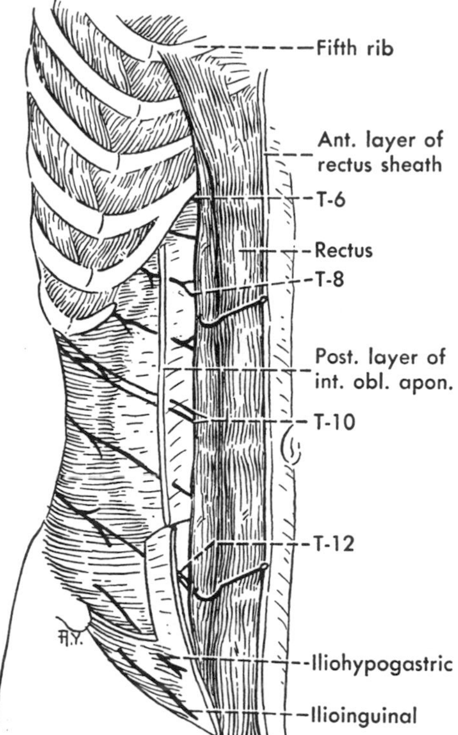

FIGURE *23-5.*
The transversus abdominis muscle and nerves of the anterior abdominal wall: The rectus sheath has been opened and the rectus muscle retracted medially to show the nerves penetrating the sheath and disappearing behind the muscle; the iliohypogastric and ilioinguinal nerves are shown as they come through the internal oblique.

iac spine, the muscle fibers tend to be directed downward and medially, paralleling the fibers of the internal oblique in this region. The lower fibers of the transversus, which arise from the iliopsoas fascia and the anterior superior iliac spine, form the portion of the aponeurosis that, after fusing with the internal oblique aponeurosis, makes up the **conjoint tendon** (*falx inguinalis*). Similar to the internal oblique, the transversus abdominis also has a free musculoaponeurotic border that arches over the spermatic cord or the round ligament of the uterus as these structures enter the inguinal canal.

The Rectus Abdominis and Its Sheath

The **rectus abdominis** arises from the pubic crest by a short tendon. A straplike muscle belly replaces the tendon and becomes progressively broader as it ascends to the rib cage, where it inserts into the fifth, sixth, and seventh costal cartilages and into the xiphoid process (Fig. 23-6). Not all the fibers of the muscle span this distance, however; *tendinous intersections*—usually three, sometimes four—divide the muscle transversely into segments. The intersections are, as a rule, not quite complete, especially posteriorly. They become prominent when the recti are contracted, and a median furrow over the linea alba appears between the two muscles (Fig. 23-7). The convex lateral border of each rectus is indicated by another shallow groove, the *linea semilunaris*. In a spare or muscular person, these three grooves are visible even when the recti are relaxed.

Overlapping the anterior surface of the rectus just above the pubis is the triangular **pyramidalis muscle** (see Fig. 23-6). This little muscle arises from the body of the pubis and inserts into the linea alba. It is a tensor of the

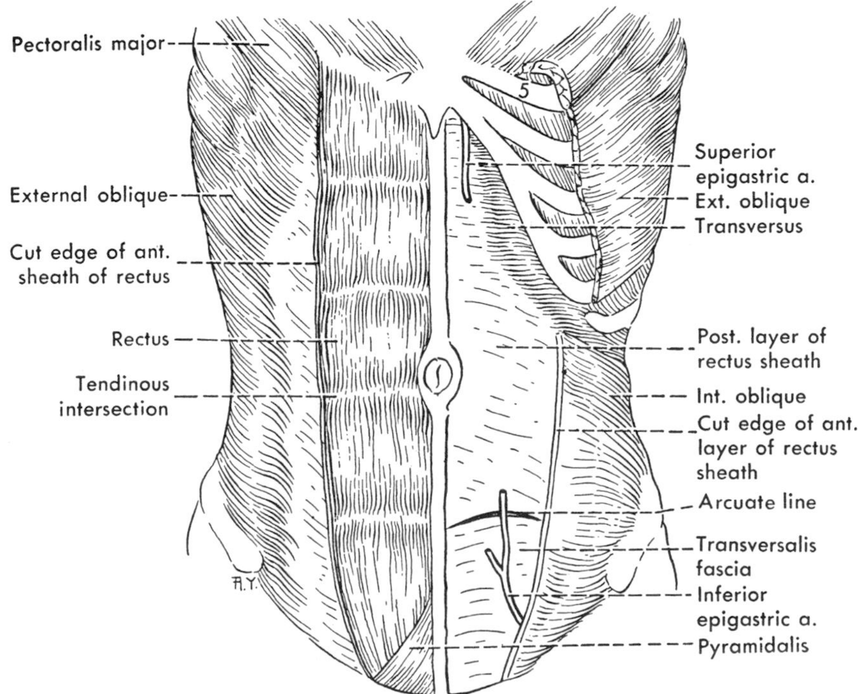

FIGURE *23-6.*
Rectus abdominis and pyramidalis muscles and the posterior layer of the sheath of the rectus.

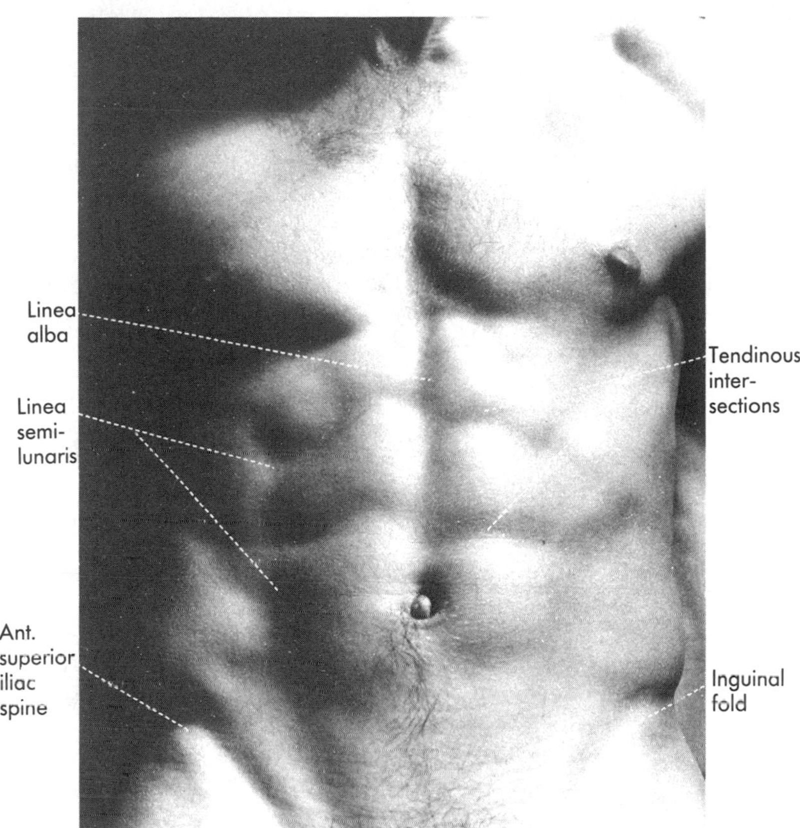

FIGURE 23-7.
The rectus abdominis contracted.

linea alba and is of no importance. The muscle may be missing on one or both sides.

The **rectus sheath** (*vagina m. recti abdominis*), formed by the aponeuroses of the three flat muscles of the abdominal wall, encloses the rectus (Fig. 23-8). The sheath has an anterior and a posterior lamina, and the two fuse with each other medially along the linea alba and laterally along the linea semilunaris. However, only the middle segment of the rectus is completely enclosed in this sheath; the posterior lamina is lacking behind both superior and inferior portions of the muscle.

The explanation for this arrangement is as follows: Along the lateral edge of the rectus, the internal oblique aponeurosis splits into an anterior and a posterior layer, and these pass, respectively, in front of and behind the middle portion of the rectus. The transversus aponeurosis becomes fused to the posterior layer, and the external oblique aponeurosis joins, in front, the anterior layer (see Fig. 23-8). The internal oblique aponeurosis does not extend up into the infrasternal angle, and the superior extent of the transversus is the costal margin. Therefore, in the infrasternal angle (epigastrium), the posterior lamina of the rectus sheath consists of some muscular and aponeurotic fibers of the transversus abdominis (see Figs. 23-5 and 23-8), whereas above the costal margin, the rectus lies directly on the costal cartilages.

Some distance below the umbilicus, the aponeurosis of the internal oblique changes its course and, rather than splitting into layers, passes unsplit in front of the rectus. Because the aponeurosis of the transversus remains fused

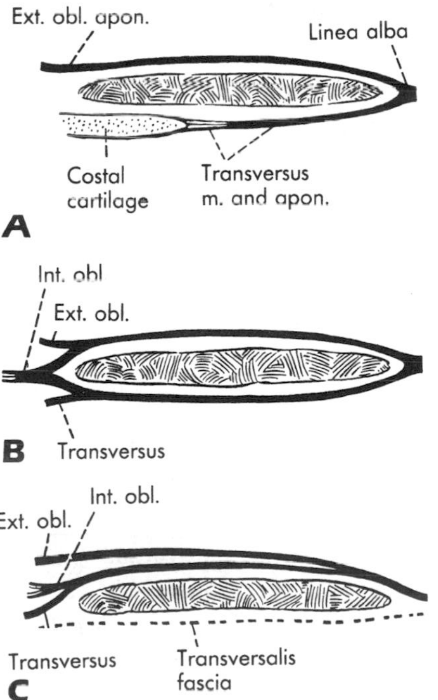

FIGURE 23-8.
Diagrams of the usually described method of formation of the rectus sheath: (A) a transverse section through the infrasternal angle (epigastrium); (B) one below the ribs, but above the arcuate line; and (C) one below the arcuate line.

with that of the internal oblique, it also passes to the front, creating a defect in the posterior lamina of the rectus sheath. Thus, over the inferior part of the rectus, all three aponeuroses are in the anterior lamina of the sheath, leaving the rectus in direct contact, posteriorly, with endoabdominal (transversalis) fascia (see Fig. 23-8C).

If the change in the course of the tendon fibers of the internal oblique and transversus aponeuroses is abrupt, the posterior lamina of the rectus sheath ends with a sharp crescentic border somewhere between the umbilicus and the pubis. This border, concave downward, is the **arcuate line** (Fig. 23-9).

The anterior wall of the rectus sheath is intimately attached to the tendinous intersections in the rectus; elsewhere, delicate connective tissue separates the muscles from the anterior and posterior walls of the sheath. Enclosed within the sheath are also the pyramidalis muscle, anterior to the rectus, and the superior and inferior epigastric vessels, posterior to it. The nerves that supply the rectus pierce the sheath along the linea semilunaris just before they sink into the lateral edge of the muscle (see Fig. 23-5).

The manner in which the sheath of the rectus is formed varies more than the usual descriptions indicate. Indeed, in one survey, the most common pattern was that in which the internal oblique aponeurosis passed entirely into the anterior lamina of the sheath, whereas the transversus split to contribute to both laminae. The integrity of the rectus sheath is of considerable importance from a functional point of view. Therefore, further reference to the more detailed arrangement of the tendon fibers in the rectus sheath is included in the discussion of the actions of the anterior abdominal wall muscles.

Innervation and Action of Abdominal Wall Muscles

The muscles of the abdominal wall are supplied segmentally by the anterior rami of T-6 to T-12 and L-1 spinal nerves. The course of these nerves in the abdominal wall is described in the next section. The rectus, external oblique, and transversus muscles with extensive fleshy attachment to the ribs receive muscular branches from the upper six of these nerves; rarely, L-1 may also supply the rectus. The main belly of the internal oblique is innervated by T-10 to T-12 and the ilioinguinal branch of L-1. The iliohypogastric branch of L-1 is chiefly cutaneous and is motor only to the inconsequential pyramidalis muscle.

The muscles of the anterior abdominal wall perform three functions: 1) support the abdominal viscera, 2) compress the abdomen, and 3) move the trunk.

Support. In the supine position, the muscles are completely relaxed. During sitting and standing, it is the flat muscles and their aponeuroses that support the abdominal contents; the recti are largely passive. In the standing position, continuous electrical activity can be recorded in the lower parts of the internal oblique (and probably also in the transversus), which constantly guards the inguinal region. The importance of this function will become apparent in the discussion of inguinal hernia (see Chap. 26).

The tendon fibers of the three pairs of aponeuroses are interwoven in the rectus sheath and the linea alba in such a manner that they permit the expansion of the abdomen while they support the viscera. Rather precise dissections of the aponeuroses have revealed that not only the internal oblique aponeurosis but also the

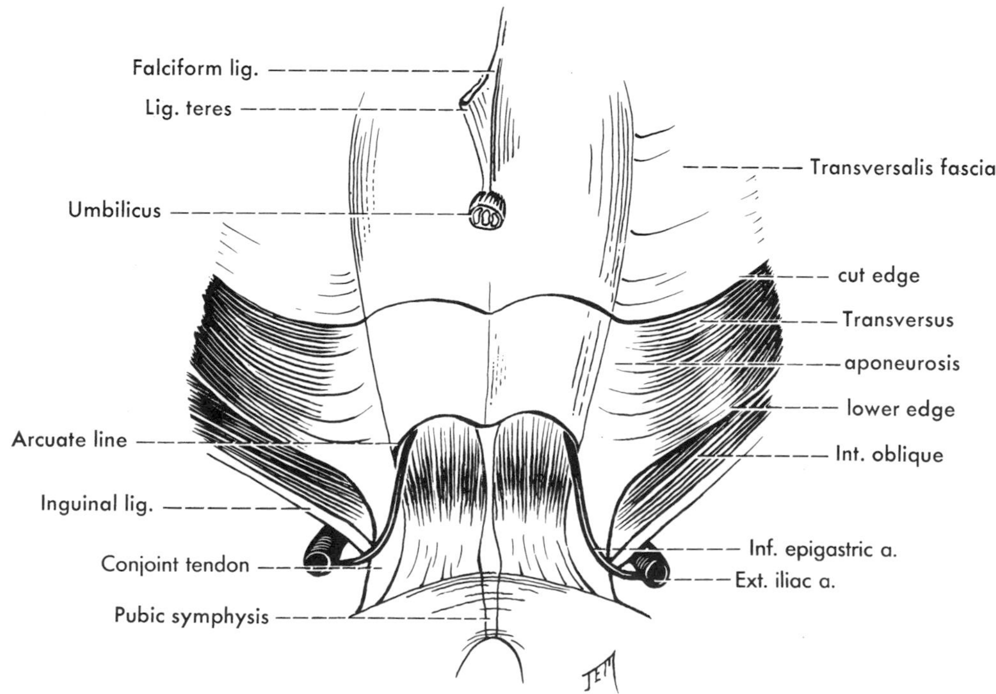

FIGURE 23-9.
The inner surface of the anterior abdominal wall, with the transversalis fascia removed below to show the arcuate line.

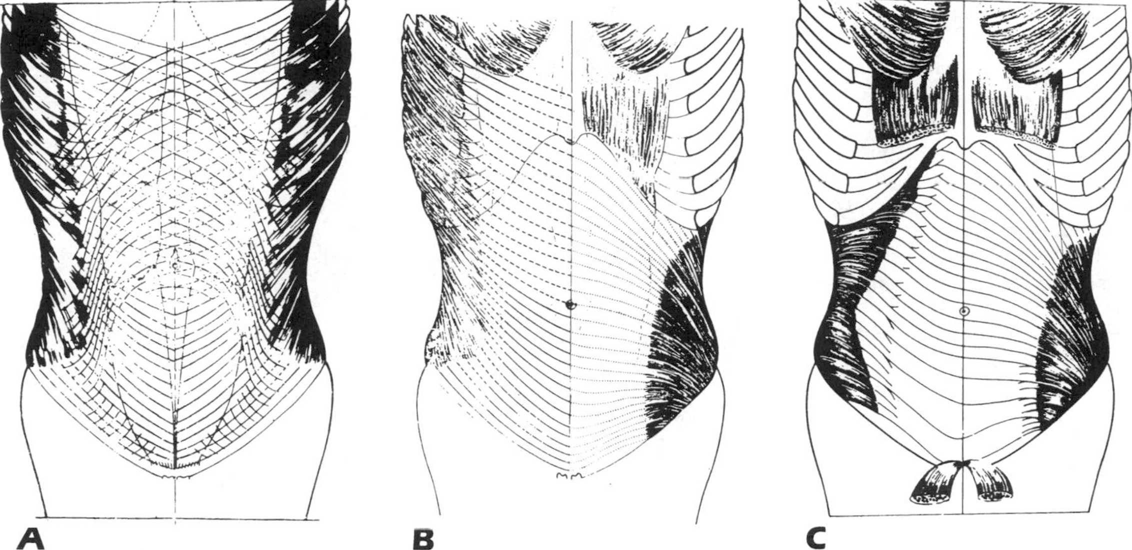

FIGURE *23-10.*
Continuities in tendon fibers across the linea alba between the aponeuroses of the flat muscles in the abdominal wall, creating digastric arrangements: (A) The superficial lamina of the external oblique aponeurosis is indicated in *continuous lines*, and the deep lamina is indicated in *interrupted lines*. Fibers in the superficial lamina on the *left side* are continuous with fibers of the deep lamina on the *right*. (B) Another set of fibers in the deep lamina of the right external oblique aponeurosis is continuous with those in the anterior lamina of the left internal oblique aponeurosis. (C) Fibers in the anterior lamina of the right transversus aponeurosis become continuous with those in the posterior lamina of the left internal oblique aponeurosis. (Askar OM. Ann R Coll Surg Eng 1977, 59:313.)

aponeuroses of both the external oblique and the transversus split into two strata. The three sheets of tendon fibers cross each other in different directions and become continuous across the linea alba, with fibers on the opposite side that are in a stratum either superficial or deep to that of their own.

For instance, the most superficial tendon fibers of the left external oblique aponeurosis are derived from some of the deep fibers of the right external oblique, which have come to the surface at the linea alba and have continued their course laterally and downward, crossing the deep stratum of the external oblique aponeurosis at right angles (Fig. 23-10). Other deep fibers of the right external oblique aponeurosis become continuous with the anterior lamina of the left internal oblique aponeurosis after they decussate in the linea alba (see Fig. 23-10*B*). Similarly, there are two strata to the transversus aponeurosis. Some fibers of the anterior stratum of the right transversus aponeurosis become continuous with the posterior lamina of the left internal oblique aponeurosis (see Fig. 23-10*C*). Other fibers in the anterior stratum of the right transversus aponeurosis become continuous with the posterior stratum of the left transversus aponeurosis (not illustrated). Thus, the rectus sheath, where it is completely formed, has three sets of fibers in both its anterior and posterior walls, and these fibers create a "plywoodlike" arrangement in each wall (Fig. 23-11).

This arrangement strengthens the abdominal wall considerably, owing to the perpendicular crossing of tendon fibers and the switching of tendon fibers from one stratum into another, which is chiefly responsible for holding the layers of the abdominal wall together without limiting their independent mobility. This is true also in the lower part of the abdomen, where all aponeurotic layers, with the possible exception of the posterior stratum of the transversus abdominis, pass in front of the rectus. Furthermore, the digastric arrangement created by these mechanisms ensures the unified action of the different muscle layers on the two sides.

Expansion of the abdomen is made possible, without increasing tension in the aponeuroses, by decreasing the angle of splitting in the strata, by decreasing the angles of decussation in the rectus sheath or linea alba, and by separating the parallel fiber bundles within the strata. Raising of the costal margin, which accompanies distention of the upper part of the abdomen, does, in fact, produce such an effect, because fibers in four of the six strata run parallel with the costal margin on each side.

Compression of the Abdomen. The obliques and the transversus, acting together bilaterally, function as a muscular girdle that exerts pressure on the abdominal contents. The digastric arrangement, established through the continuity of the tendon fibers between the aponeuroses of the two sides, ensures a uniform, bilaterally coordinated action of the muscle layers. The rectus participates little, if at all, in this function. Contraction of the flat muscles generates the increased pressure required for the

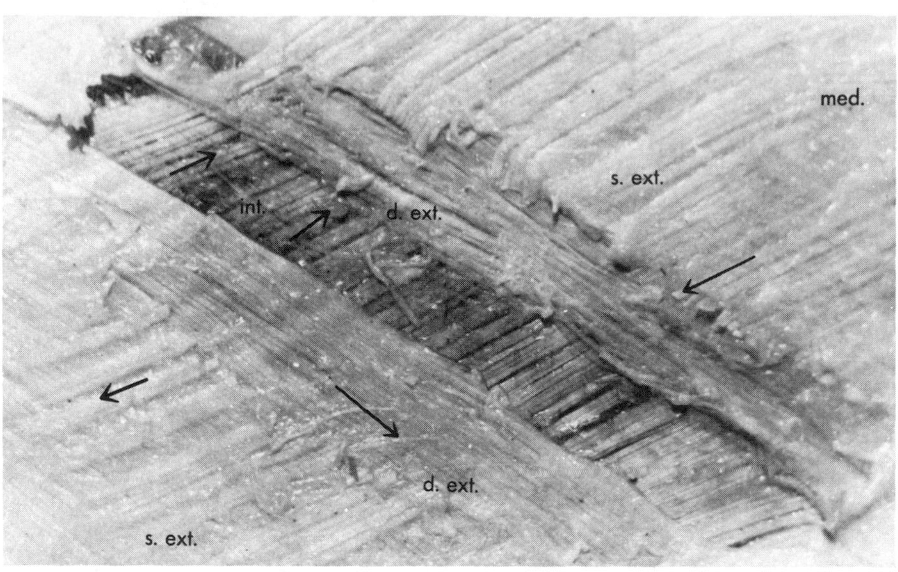

FIGURE *23-11.*
Plywoodlike arrangement of tendon fibers in the anterior sheath of the right rectus of a man aged 35 years. The superficial lamina (*s. ext.*), derived from the left external oblique aponeurosis, crosses at right angles the intermediate lamina (*d. ext.*), derived from the deep fibers on the right external oblique aponeurosis. The deepest lamina in the anterior sheath (*int.*) is derived from the anterior lamina of the right internal oblique, and the fiber direction coincides with that in the superficial lamina. (Rizk NN. J Anat 1980, 131:373.)

forceful expulsion of air from the lungs (coughing, sneezing, singing) or of gastric contents by vomiting. The same muscles raise abdominal pressure during bearing down (necessary to empty the rectum and the bladder and to deliver the fetus from the birth canal). The obliques and the transversus are not active during quiet respiration; they are, however, the most important and only indispensable muscles of maximal voluntary expiration. They not only push the relaxed diaphragm up into the chest but also depress and compress the lower part of the rib cage.

Trunk Movements. The abdominal muscles can approximate the rib cage to the pelvis and, thereby, indirectly move the vertebral column. The type of movement each muscle is capable of producing can be deduced from its bony attachments and the direction of its fibers. However, abdominal muscles are recruited to produce trunk movements only when resistance or the force of gravity must be overcome. Thus, the recti flex the trunk when a person rises from the supine to the sitting position (they contract even when only the head is raised), but they are inactive when a person bends forward from the erect position. The external and internal obliques, acting bilaterally, can assist flexion and are being exercised, along with the rectus, during sit-ups. The right external oblique, working together with the left internal oblique, can twist the trunk to the left. Without having to overcome resistance however, most of this movement is produced by the paravertebral muscles. Therefore, as a rule, trunk twisting exercises do not involve the abdominal wall muscles. The posterior vertical fibers of the external and internal obliques can produce lateral bending of the trunk. Their contraction will be more powerful, however, when they are called on to raise the trunk while a person is lying on his side. The transversus contributes little to trunk movement; its chief action is in raising abdominal pressure.

An important corollary function of the abdominal wall muscles is the stabilizing effect they exert on the vertebral column by raising abdominal pressure. Strengthening the abdominal wall musculature is part of all exercise programs that aim to improve standing and sitting posture and to alleviate certain types of backache.

Endoabdominal Fascia

In analogy with the endothoracic fascia, the loose areolar tissue that lines the entire abdominal cavity and attaches the parietal peritoneum to the abdominal walls may be designated as the *endoabdominal fascia* (see Fig. 23-1). Inferiorly, the endoabdominal fascia is continuous with the endopelvic fascia; superiorly, it lines the inferior surface of the diaphragm. This extraperitoneal connective tissue may become laden with fat, especially posteriorly, where it surrounds the kidneys. It is often referred to by radiologists as a *preperitoneal fat*. Fibrous strands of the endoabdominal fascia blend with the epimysium of the abdominal wall muscles, increasing the thickness of their deep fascia (see Fig. 23-1). These membranelike fascial layers over the inner surface of the transversus abdominis and its aponeurosis, and over the psoas and iliacus muscles, are of sufficient anatomic and clinical importance to designate them by specific names: *transversalis fascia, psoas fascia, iliacus fascia*.

In the lower part of the abdomen, the **transversalis fascia** completes the posterior rectus sheath below the arcuate line when the entire transversus aponeurosis passes to the anterior surface of the rectus (see Fig. 23-8). More laterally, the transversalis fascia attaches to the inferior upturned edge of the inguinal ligament (see Fig. 26-5), contributes to the formation of the *femoral sheath* that surrounds the femoral vessels as they enter or leave the thigh (see Fig. 26-17) and, by forming the *internal spermatic fascia*, provides one of the coverings of the spermatic cord or the round ligament of the uterus (see Fig. 26-7). The psoas and iliacus fascias are discussed in Chapter 25.

In the midline, the *transversalis fascia* ends by attaching to the upper border of the pubis, and the peritoneum, with some associated connective tissue, swings backward to cover the upper surface of the bladder (see Fig. 27-24). As a result, there is left between the lower part of the transversalis fascia and the pubis on the one hand, and between the peritoneum and the anterior wall of the bladder on the other, a potential *retropubic space* that is filled with a padding of extraperitoneal connective tissue, usually laden with fat.

The presence of loose endoabdominal fascia makes it possible for certain abdominal organs (e.g., kidneys) and structures (e.g., sympathetic trunks) to be approached surgically through abdominal incisions without entering the peritoneal cavity. For instance, resection of a segment of the lumbar sympathetic trunks (*lumbar sympathectomy*) may be performed by making an incision in each flank through the skin and the abdominal wall muscles. The sympathetic trunks lying on each side of the vertebral column can then be reached by blunt dissection in the extraperitoneal connective tissue without entering the peritoneum. Similarly, a surgeon can expose the bladder or the prostate, both lying in the pelvis, through an abdominal incision made above the pubic symphysis and then proceed inferiorly in the endoabdominal fascia of the retropubic space (e.g., retropubic prostatectomy). There will be no need to cut the peritoneum. Such a dissection is possible because endoabdominal and endopelvic extraperitoneal fascias are continuous with one another.

Nerves and Vessels

The innervation of the abdominal wall musculature, from the anterior rami of T-6 to L-1 spinal nerves, has already been discussed in a preceding section. The same nerves are sensory to the abdominal skin, all layers of fascia and muscle, and the parietal peritoneum associated with the abdominal walls. The arterial blood supply is from the lower posterior intercostal arteries and the lumbar arteries (both are branches of the aorta), and from a longitudinal, ventral anastomosis that comprises the superior and inferior epigastric arteries. These arteries are accompanied by corresponding veins. Lymph from the abdominal wall, above the umbilicus, drains to the axillary lymph nodes; below the umbilicus, it drains to the inguinal lymph nodes.

Nerves

The T-6 to T-11 anterior rami in the abdominal wall are the continuation of the *intercostal nerves*. T-12 is the *subcostal nerve*, and the two branches of L-1, the most distal nerve to supply the abdominal wall, are the *iliohypogastric* and *ilioinguinal nerves* (see Fig. 23-5). Maintaining their downward slope after they leave the intercostal space, the lower intercostal nerves enter the neurovascular plane of the abdominal wall by crossing the deep surface of the costal margin. Their collective name **thoracoabdominal nerves** aptly describes the distribution of these nerves to both thoracic and abdominal walls. These nerves and their accompanying vessels proceed between the internal oblique and transversus abdominis toward the linea semilunaris. They pierce the rectus sheath and penetrate the posterior surface of the rectus, which they supply. These nerves terminate as anterior cutaneous branches after piercing the rectus and emerging through the anterior lamina of its sheath. Nerve fibers may be interchanged between neighboring thoracoabdominal nerves, and sometimes a coarse plexus is formed before the nerves enter the rectus sheath, or the nerves may remain discrete and segmental.

The **subcostal, iliohypogastric,** and **ilioinguinal nerves** run in series and parallel with the thoracoabdominal nerves (see Fig. 23-5). However, unlike the intercostal nerves, they enter the neurovascular plane of the abdominal wall from within the abdominal cavity. Having crossed over the surface of the posterior abdominal wall muscles, they pierce the transversus abdominis at some point: the subcostal at the tendinous origin of the transversus from the thoracolumbar fascia, and the iliohypogastric and ilioinguinal above the iliac crest before they reach the anterior superior iliac spine. In the neurovascular plane, the iliohypogastric nerve divides into lateral and anterior cutaneous branches. Only the anterior branch supplies the abdominal wall; the lateral branch is distributed to the skin of the buttocks. The ilioinguinal nerve and the anterior branch of the iliohypogastric nerve soon pierce the internal oblique: the ilioinguinal nerve accompanies the spermatic cord in the inguinal canal, and the anterior branch of the iliohypogastric proceeds toward the medial area of the groin.

Branches. Muscular branches are given off by all these nerves directly from the main nerve, from a *collateral branch*, or from the cutaneous branches as these pierce the respective muscles. The innervation of the abdominal wall musculature is segmental, and the distribution of the individual nerves to the various muscles has already been discussed in a preceding section. The intercostal, subcostal, and iliohypogastric nerves give off, in addition to their terminal anterior cutaneous branches, a lateral cutaneous branch.

The **lateral cutaneous branch** of the last six intercostal nerves emerges below the corresponding rib, roughly along the midaxillary line (see Fig. 15-3). Each lateral cutaneous branch divides into a posterior and anterior branch. The posterior branches supply the skin over the thorax and the back as far posteriorly as the territory of the cutaneous branches given off by the thoracic posterior rami; the anterior branches run forward and downward supplying abdominal wall skin as far as the rectus. Skin over the recti and along the midline is supplied by the corresponding **anterior cutaneous branches** of the same nerves.

Knowledge of the segmental distribution of the cutaneous nerves over the abdomen has clinical uses. The key dermatomes to remember are T-10 in the region of the umbilicus and T-12 above the pubis (see Fig. 13-25). Skin between the costal margins (epigastrium) is supplied by T-6, T-7, and T-8. Parts of L-1 dermatome over the inguinal region (and buttocks) are served by the iliohypogastric nerve; other parts of L-1 dermatome over the upper part of the scrotum and root of the penis or the mons pubis and the adjoining part of the labium majus are served by the ilioinguinal nerve. There is considerable overlap between neighboring dermatomes of the trunk, and no anesthesia can be demonstrated clinically in a dermatome if its spinal nerve is the only one interrupted or blocked.

In the abdominal wall, as in the trunk in general, there is a superimposition of corresponding dermatomes and myotomes. Moreover, the innervation of the parietal peritoneum also conforms to this segmental arrangement. These anatomic facts explain the abdominal reflexes and the reflex contraction of the abdominal musculature when the peritoneum is irritated.

An **abdominal reflex** is the sudden, momentary contraction of the underlying musculature when the skin of certain dermatomes is unexpectedly scratched or touched with a pointed object. Strokes are made with the object diagonally across dermatomes T-7, T-8, and T-9, and then T-10, T-11, and T-12, first on one side of the abdomen and then on the other. When the reflex is present, the umbilicus will be drawn toward the side of the contraction. The reflex verifies the integrity of somatic afferents and efferents in the corresponding spinal nerves and the appropriate cord segments and gives information about the intactness of suprasegmental input from the brain to the motor neurons in the segments tested. Certain types of brain damage (e.g., some strokes) abolish these reflexes, even though the nerves and the spinal cord are uninjured.

Reflex contraction of the abdominal musculature protects the viscera. Blows to the abdomen rarely rupture the viscera, because the force is usually met by the reflex contraction of the muscles.

Guarding is the sustained involuntary contraction of segments of the abdominal musculature provoked by localized peritoneal inflammation. This may occur over an inflamed gallbladder or appendix. Somatic pain afferents excited in segments of the parietal peritoneum invoke reflex spasms of the muscles in the same segments to guard the underlying viscus from pressure. In cases of generalized peritonitis, the entire abdomen acquires boardlike rigidity because the entire peritoneum is inflamed.

Pain may be referred to the abdominal wall from certain abdominal viscera that send their visceral pain afferents into spinal cord segments that also receive somatic pain afferents from the abdominal wall. For instance, in the initial stages of appendicitis, before inflammation spreads to the parietal peritoneum, pain is felt over dermatome T-10 around the umbilicus, because pain afferents from the appendix relay in spinal cord segment T-10. Other examples of **referred pain** are discussed in the next chapter.

Arteries and Veins

The arteries of the abdominal wall are derived from two sources: 1) the thoracic and abdominal aorta and 2) the superior and inferior epigastric arteries. The aorta contributes the **posterior intercostal arteries** of the last five or six intercostal spaces, and the **subcostal** and the **lumbar arteries,** which are given off in series with the intercostals; the epigastric vessels have only small, unnamed branches. The aortic branches pass forward in the neurovascular plane, which they enter along with the nerves described in the previous section. They correspond to the branches of the nerves and terminate anteriorly by anastomosing with tiny branches of the epigastric arteries.

The **superior epigastric artery,** one of the terminal branches of the internal thoracic, enters first the rectus sheath and then the rectus, where it breaks up into branches (see Fig. 19-11). The **inferior epigastric artery,** a branch of the external iliac, ascends in the extraperitoneal fascia on the deep aspect of the abdominal wall, pierces the transversalis fascia behind the rectus, passes anteriorly to the arcuate line, and roughly at the level of the umbilicus, enters the posterior surface of the rectus. Branches of the two epigastric arteries anastomose with each other within the rectus; other branches anastomose with the intercostal, subcostal, and lumbar arteries; yet others pass to the skin along with the anterior cutaneous nerves.

Minor branches of the *musculophrenic artery* (see Fig. 19-11) augment the blood supply of the abdominal wall superiorly and anastomose with the superior epigastric. Inferiorly, small branches of the external iliac and femoral arteries help to supply deep and superficial tissues of the abdominal wall, respectively. The *deep circumflex iliac artery,* given off by the external iliac, and the *superficial circumflex iliac artery* (from the femoral) run toward and along the iliac crest. The *superficial epigastric artery* (from the femoral) ascends in the superficial fascia toward the umbilicus.

The superior and inferior epigastric arteries establish an anastomosis between the subclavian and external iliac arteries. This anastomosis enlarges and becomes an important channel for arterial blood to the lower part of the body when the aorta is obstructed. Blood will then flow posteriorly in the intercostal and lumbar vessels and inferiorly in the inferior epigastric artery. An example of aortic obstruction is coarctation (see Fig. 22-10). In such cases, all anastomotic connections of abdominal wall vessels assume considerable importance.

All arteries in the abdominal wall are accompanied by corresponding veins. Blood drains to the *superior vena cava* from the **intercostal** and **subcostal veins** through the azygos and hemiazygos veins and from the **superior epigastric veins** through the internal thoracic and brachiocephalic veins. The *inferior vena cava* receives blood from the **lumbar veins** directly or through the ascending lumbar vein; from the inferior epigastric and deep circumflex iliac veins, which are tributaries of the external iliac vein; and from the **superficial epigastric** and **superficial circumflex iliac veins,** tributaries of the femoral vein. In the superficial fascia of the lateral part of the abdominal wall, there are, in addition, longitudinal venous channels, the **thoracoepigastric veins,** that do not accompany arteries. These veins drain into the femoral vein and anastomose superiorly with tributaries of the axillary vein. All venous anastomoses correspond to those described for the respective arteries.

Anastomoses in the abdominal wall between tributaries of the superior and inferior venae cavae provide a potential alternative route for returning blood to the heart when one of the venae cavae becomes obstructed. The veins that drain the region of the umbilicus anastomose, furthermore, with **paraumbilical veins,** located on the deep aspect of the abdominal wall. These veins drain into the portal vein. Through the enlargement of these anastomoses, portal venous blood can find its way into systemic veins when there is an increased pressure in the portal venous system (*portal hypertension*; see Chap. 24). In such cases, the enlarged veins radiating away from the umbilicus, and visible on the surface of the abdomen, are a physical sign indicative of portal hypertension. The distended veins are known as the *caput medusae.*

Lymphatics

Lymphatics of the superficial fascia and skin above the umbilicus drain to the **axillary nodes;** those from below the umbilicus drain to the **superficial inguinal lymph nodes.** Lymphatics from the abdominal wall muscles, the extraperitoneal connective tissue, and parietal peritoneum drain along the arteries to nodes associated with the parent vessels (lateral aortic, parasternal, external iliac, and inguinal lymph nodes).

THE PERITONEUM AND THE PERITONEAL CAVITY

The peritoneum is a serous membrane that, like the pleura and the serous pericardium, forms a serous sac between its parietal and visceral laminae. The peritoneal sac encloses the peritoneal cavity. The **parietal peritoneum** lines the walls of the caudal compartment of the body cavity, constituted by the abdomen proper and the pelvis; the **visceral peritoneum** is applied closely to the surface of abdominal and pelvic viscera, and its reduplications form several peritoneal folds that are called *mesenteries, omenta,* or *ligaments.* Where the mesenteries or ligaments reflect onto the walls of the abdominopelvic cavity, visceral peritoneum becomes continuous with parietal peritoneum. The arrangement conforms, in principle, to that of the pleura or the pericardium. Anatomically, however, the peritoneum is much more complex, owing to the secondary peritoneal attachments that the primitive gut tube acquires after it has completed its elongation and rotation during development.

The major abdominal and pelvic viscera around which the peritoneal sac is wrapped are discussed in general terms in Chapters 9 and 10 and are dealt with in some detail again in subsequent chapters. For the purpose of orientation, Figures 23-12 and 23-13 present schematic anterior and posterior views of major abdominal organs.

The anatomy of the peritoneal cavity becomes intelligible only when the formation of the intraembryonic celom and the embryology of the gut are understood. The purpose of this section is a general anatomic survey of the peritoneal cavity along with some general developmental considerations. Further explanation of the peritoneal relations of abdominal and pelvic viscera may be found in subsequent chapters that deal with the particular anatomy of the respective organs.

Developmental Considerations

The Peritoneal Cavity and Mesenteries. Folding of the trilaminar embryonic disk defines the foregut (*proenteron*), midgut (*mesenteron*), and hindgut (*metenteron*) (see Chap. 9). The caudal portions of the bilateral celomic ducts, the pleuroperitoneal canals, become related to the primitive gut (see Fig. 9-3). As a consequence of the folding, the pleuroperitoneal canals, which initially rest on the upper surface of the yolk sac, become wrapped around the gut and expand (see Fig. 9-3*C*). This expansion approximates the two ducts to each other along the dorsal aspect of the gut; they will be separated only by splanchnic mesoderm through which vessels and nerves reach the gut. This median sagittal septum of mesoderm that, so to speak, suspends the gut along its entire length is the **common dorsal mesentery** (see Figs. 9-3*F* and 9-4). Around the midgut and the hindgut, the left and right pleuroperitoneal canals approximate each other also ventrally. As their walls contact each other on the ventral aspect of the gut, they form the ventral mesentery. This mesentery, however, conveys no vessels or nerves and rapidly disappears, so that a single cavity, U-shaped in cross-sectional profile, surrounds the midgut and the hindgut (see Fig. 9-4).

Ventral fusion of the two pleuroperitoneal canals around the foregut is prevented by the presence of the septum transversum, which has grown considerably in bulk because the liver cords, sprouting from the foregut, have invaded it. The septum fills the space between the ventrolateral body wall and the foregut which, with the two pleuroperitoneal canals alongside it, rests on the dorsal surface of the septum (Fig. 23-14).

Cavitation in the septum transversum and the expansion of the pleuroperitoneal canals into the septum define the surfaces of the liver and the *ventral mesentery of the foregut.* This mesentery will consist of two parts: 1) the *lesser omentum* between the stomach and the liver and 2) the *falciform ligament* between the liver and the ventral abdominal wall (see Fig. 23-14*C*). Unlike the ventral mesentery of the midgut and hindgut, the ventral mesentery of the foregut conveys blood vessels and nerves that pass to the liver; both portions of this mesentery are retained as permanent structures. The falciform ligament supports the umbilical vein on its way from the umbilicus to the liver; the lesser omentum contains the derivatives of the vitelline vessels (the hepatic artery and portal vein) and the gastric and hepatic nerve plexuses, as well as the bile duct, the stalk that retains a permanent connection between the liver and the foregut (see Fig. 23-14*D*).

A part of the septum transversum persists as the **diaphragm,** which, centrally, separates the peritoneal cavity from the pericardial cavity; more laterally, the diaphragm is interposed between the expanded pleural

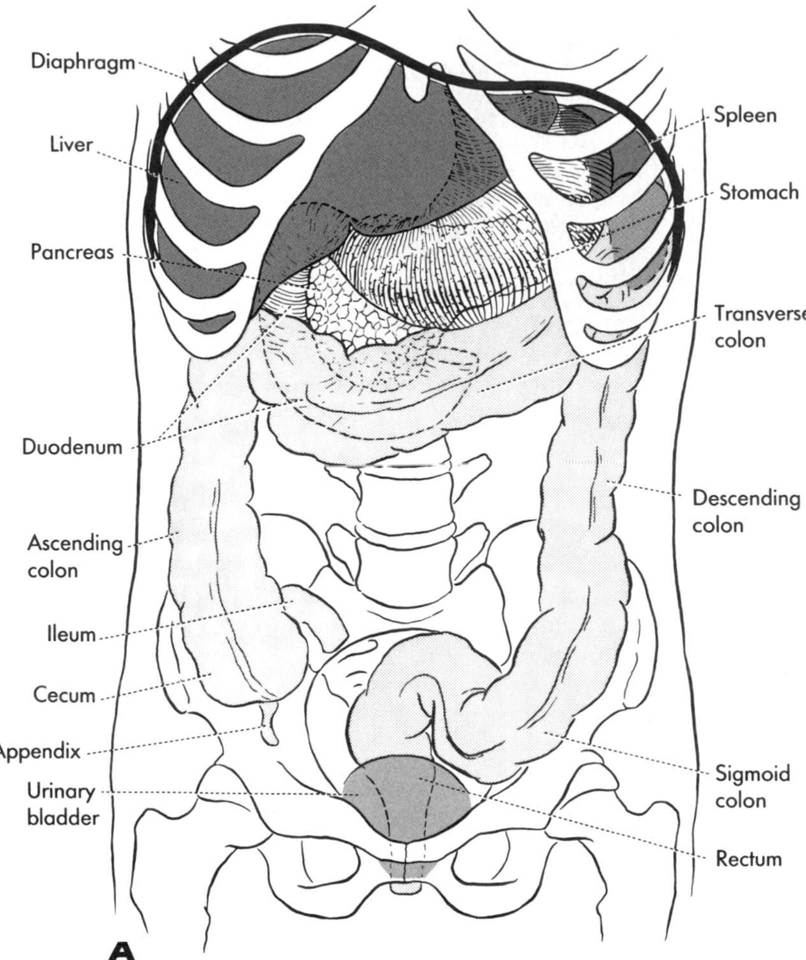

FIGURE *23-12.*
Anterior view of the chief abdominal viscera shown (A) schematically and (B) on a plain film. Panel A illustrates the overlap of the viscera in the supracolic compartmet. In Panel B, the gas contained in the various viscera helps identify them. The outline of other viscera is discernable, owing to the differential radiopacity of the fat that surrounds them. The jejunum and ileum are omitted from panel A.

cavities and the peritoneum. Dorsally, the diaphragm is completed by the development of the bilateral *pleuroperitoneal membranes*, which close off the pleuroperitoneal canals from the thorax, and by the dorsal mesentery of the esophagus (see Chap. 25).

It should be evident from this brief account of development that, unlike the lung and the heart, the gut does not invaginate a single serous sac to become suspended in the serous cavity by its mesentery, as is often implied by simplified explanations of the peritoneal cavity. Rather, the bilateral pleuroperitoneal canals become wrapped around the primitive gut and fuse with each other along much of its ventral aspect. By expanding, the canals create the dorsal mesentery along the entire length of the gut, and by growing into the septum transversum, the canals define the ventral mesentery along the foregut.

Differentiation of the Gut and Its Mesenteries. At the completion of the folding process, the gut consists of a roughly T-shaped tube: the vertical limb is the vitellointestinal duct connecting to the midgut; foregut and hindgut are along the horizontal bar of the T (see Fig. 9-3*B*). From the **foregut** will differentiate the esophagus (most of it located in the neck and the thorax), the *stomach*, and the *proximal half of the duodenum*. In addition, two buds appear on the caudal portion of the foregut: a *ventral diverticulum* grows into the septum transversum and give rise to the *liver*, *gallbladder*, and a portion of the *pancreas*; a *dorsal diverticulum* grows into the dorsal mesentery and gives rise to the remaining and major part of the pancreas (see Fig. 24-21*A*). From the **midgut** are derived the *second half of the duodenum*; the *jejunum*, *ileum*, *cecum* and *appendix*; *ascending colon*, and most of the *transverse colon*; from the **hindgut** are derived the terminal portion of the *transverse colon*, the *descending* and *sigmoid colon*, and the *rectum*.

The midgut and hindgut elongate greatly and form a large redundant loop suspended by the dorsal mesentery (see Fig. 23-14*D*). This loop and its mesentery become twisted and rotated (see Fig. 23-24). Later, portions of the gut and their mesentery become tethered to parietal peritoneum on the dorsal wall of the cavity. These secondary peritoneal attachments are achieved by visceral peritoneum fusing with parietal peritoneum. The fusion results in the disappearance of those portions of the dorsal mesentery that suspend the duodenum and the ascending and descending colons; consequently, these structures come to lie directly on the posterior abdominal wall. The fused layers of the peritoneum disappear behind them and these portions

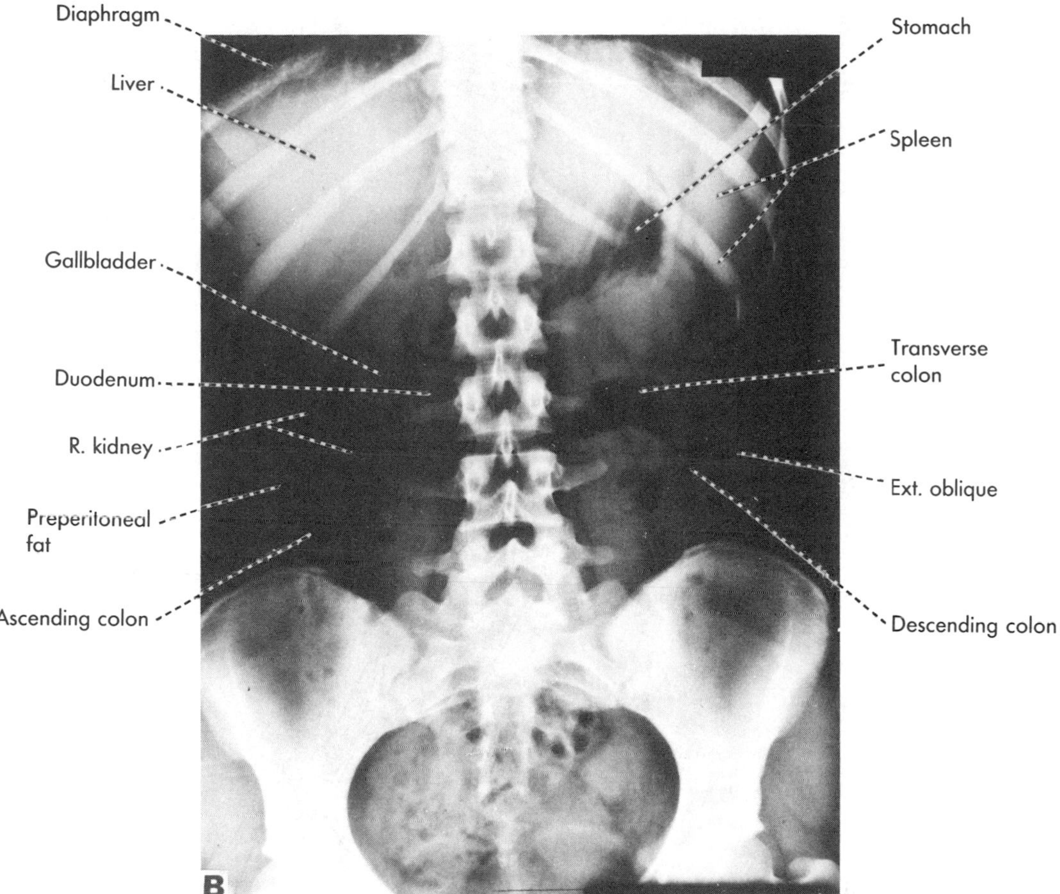

FIGURE 23-12. *(Continued)*

of the gut are directly in contact with the fascia of the abdominal wall. The pancreas also becomes immobilized in this fashion across the posterior abdominal wall. The jejunum and ileum retain their mesentery, which is known as the **mesentery proper**, and so do the transverse and the sigmoid colon, which are known as the **transverse mesocolon** and the **sigmoid mesocolon,** respectively. The rectum has not had a mesentery of any size to speak of, and peritoneum is draped over only the anterior and lateral surfaces of its cranial portion.

Owing to the displacements caused by the rotation of the gut (see Fig. 23-24), the secondary attachments of the persistent portions of the dorsal mesentery to the posterior abdominal wall become displaced from the dorsal midline. The dorsal mesentery of the stomach (*dorsal mesogastrium*) is modified by the development of the spleen, a collection of lymphoid tissue within the mesentery (see Fig. 23-14*D*). In addition, the dorsal mesogastrium expands greatly into a large apronlike fold known as the **greater omentum.** Furthermore, the stomach rotates so that its original right surface faces posteriorly and its left surface anteriorly, which not only exaggerates the bulging of the greater omentum toward the left but causes the orientation of the lesser omentum to change from a sagittal to a coronal plane.

The survey of the peritoneal cavity in the fully developed state relies, to some extent, on these elementary developmental considerations to relate the complex arrangement to a rather simple underlying basic plan. The developmental events of the rotation and mesenterial fusion will be summarized after the gross anatomy of the peritoneal cavity has been surveyed.

Survey of the Peritoneal Cavity and the Abdominopelvic Viscera

When the peritoneal sac is opened by an anterior incision of the parietal peritoneum, the first impression gained is that of a cavity filled by viscera: superiorly, the liver and the stomach, and more inferiorly, a fatty peritoneal fold, the greater omentum, and coils of intestine (Figs. 23-15 and 23-16). In truth, the peritoneal cavity contains only a small amount of serous fluid, which moistens the interior of the sac; all viscera are outside the peritoneum. Notwithstanding, certain viscera are frequently spoken of as lying in the peritoneal cavity or as being *peritoneal*, because they project into the cavity invested almost completely by visceral peritoneum; they

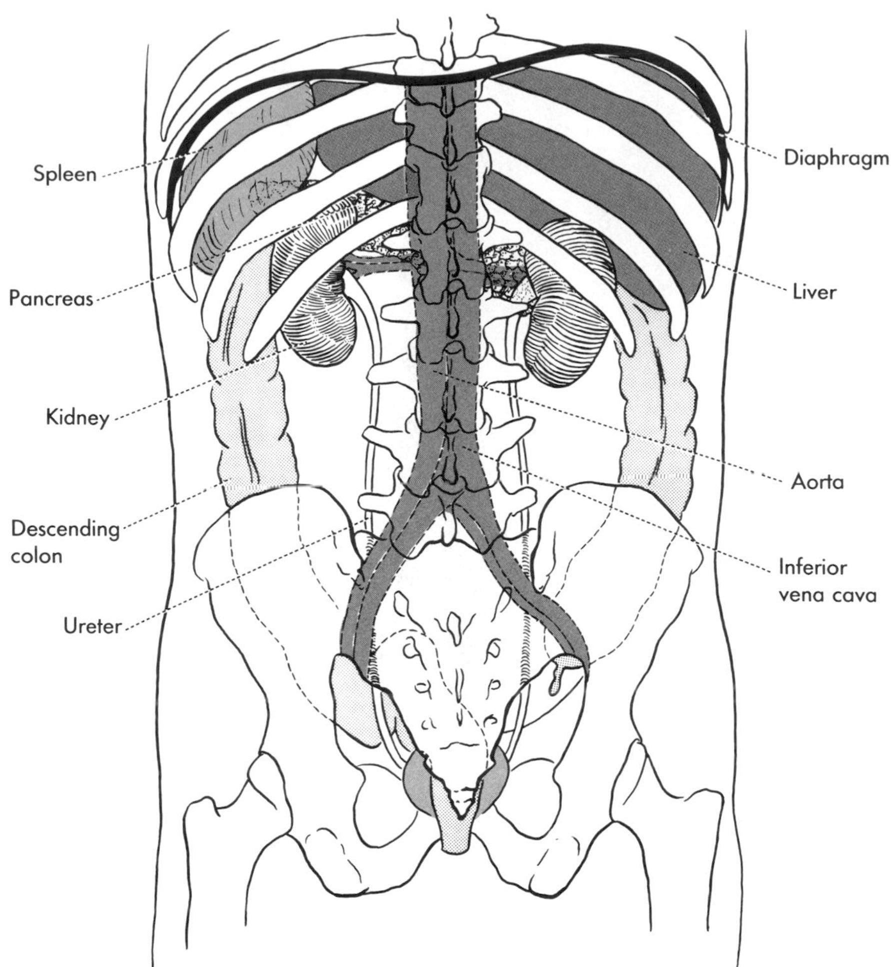

FIGURE *23-13.*
Diagram of the chief abdominal viscera from behind: The stomach and transverse colon are omitted.

can be reached only through the peritoneal cavity. Such organs are, for instance, the stomach, the jejunum, and the ileum. Visceral peritoneum is so closely bound to these viscera that it is considered an integral part of their wall: their *serosa.* On peritoneal organs that lack a lumen (liver, spleen), visceral peritoneum is closely bound to the organ's capsule. Other abdominal organs are spoken of as *retroperitoneal;* only their anterior surface is covered partly or completely by peritoneum. Such organs are not derived from the gut and include the kidneys and ureters, the suprarenal glands, the aorta and inferior vena cava, and the sympathetic trunks, as well as chains of lymph nodes lying along these structures. Those portions of the gut that lose their mesentery during development are sometimes described as *secondarily retroperitoneal.* Such organs are the pancreas and parts of the duodenum.

Diagrams and drawings cannot convey adequately the three-dimensional relations of the peritoneal cavity and the mesenteries. The following description will achieve its objective only if its reading is accompanied by the exploration of a cadaver, preferably one not hardened by fixatives. The study of an embalmed body, more readily accessible, can serve the purpose adequately if reference is made to the accompanying figures for appreciating relations that are difficult to explore in a hardened body.

Division of the Peritoneal Cavity

The peritoneal cavity consists of the greater sac and the lesser sac. The **greater sac** (*cavum peritonei*) is the main part of the cavity that extends from the diaphragm into the pelvis. This is the sac opened by incisions of the abdominal wall, and into this sac protrude all the peritoneal organs. The **lesser sac,** also known as the *omental bursa,* is a diverticulum of the greater sac, which forms a potential space mainly behind the stomach and the lesser omentum. It is confined largely to the left side of the upper abdomen and communicates on the right with the greater sac through a passage known as the *epiploic foramen.*

Exploration of the greater sac is aided by dividing it into a *supracolic* and an *infracolic compartment,* located, respectively, above and below the transverse colon and its mesentery, and into a third part, the *pelvic portion* of the peritoneal cavity, which is inferior to the pelvic brim. This division of the greater sac can be demonstrated by elevating the greater omentum, which hangs down from the greater curvature of the stomach and is fused to the anterior surface of the transverse colon and its mesocolon (see

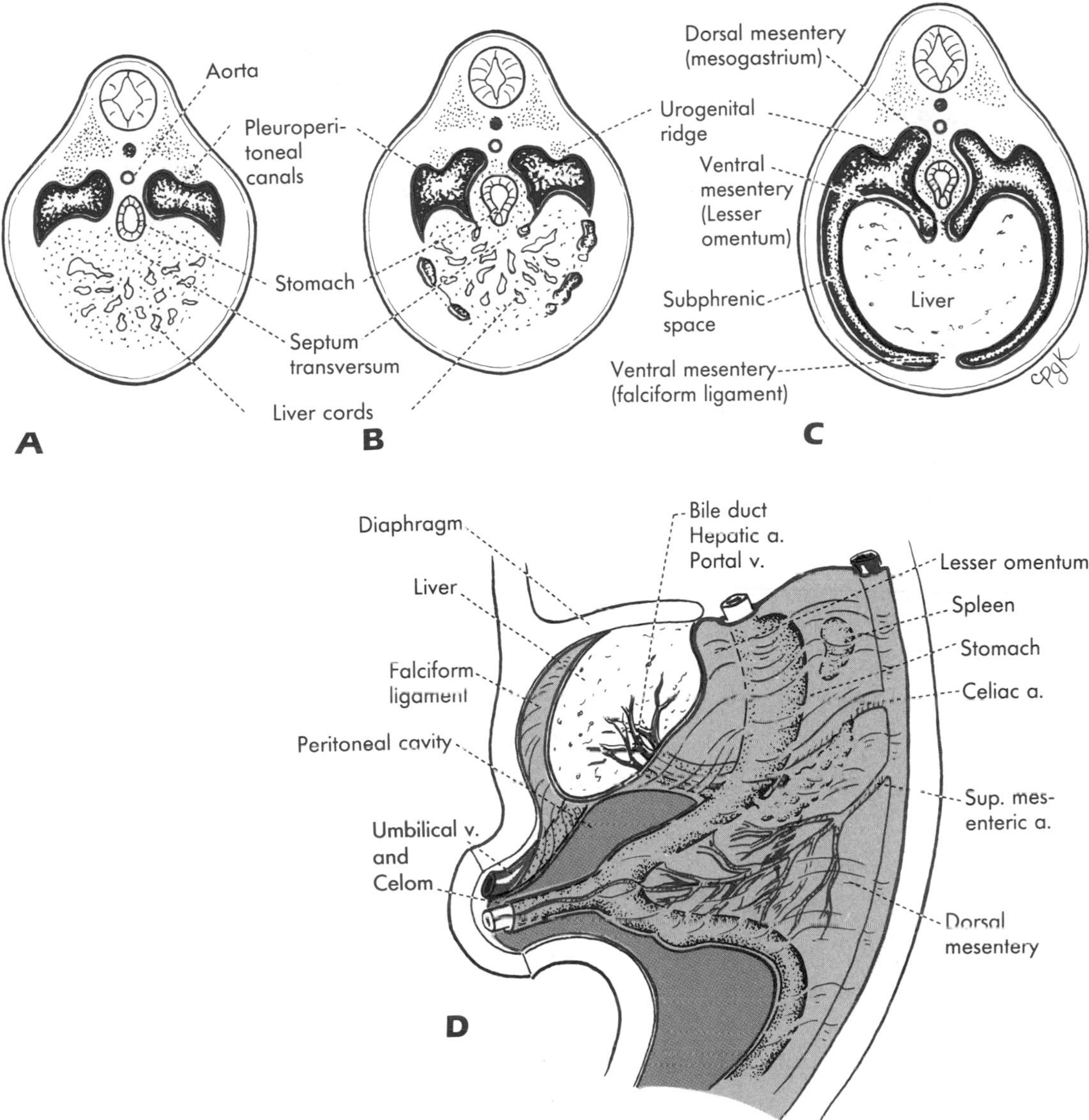

FIGURE 23-14.
Development of the ventral mesentery of the foregut from the septum transversum: (A) the pleuroperitoneal canals form the dorsal border of the septum transversum; (B) expansion of the canals into the septum; (C) formation of the lesser omentum and falciform ligament; (D) the ventral and dorsal mesenteries are viewed from the left side of the peritoneal cavity.

Fig. 23-16). The **supracolic compartment** of the greater sac is largely under cover of the costal margin and the diaphragm. In a fixed cadaver, much of it has to be examined by palpation unless the costal margin and the diaphragm are slit. The supracolic compartment contains the liver and stomach, the falciform ligament and the lesser omentum, and the greater omentum and the spleen, as well as the lesser sac. The **infracolic compartment** is filled with coils of jejunum and ileum and surrounded by the ascending, transverse, and descending colons; it leads into the pelvis inferiorly. The *pelvic portion* of the peritoneal cavity is revealed by lifting the coils of small intestine and sigmoid colon. Although its contents are the subject of a subsequent chapter, peritoneal relations in the pelvis will be studied in continuity with those of the abdomen proper.

The Supracolic Compartment of the Greater Sac

The Liver and Subphrenic Recesses. The peritoneal cavity between the liver and the diaphragm is divided anteriorly into right and left halves by the falciform ligament (see Fig. 23-15).

The **falciform ligament** is a double layer of peritoneum, the ventral portion of the ventral mesentery of the foregut (see Fig. 23-14). Right and left laminae of the ligament are continuous with one another around the inferior border of the ligament, which is falciform (sickle-

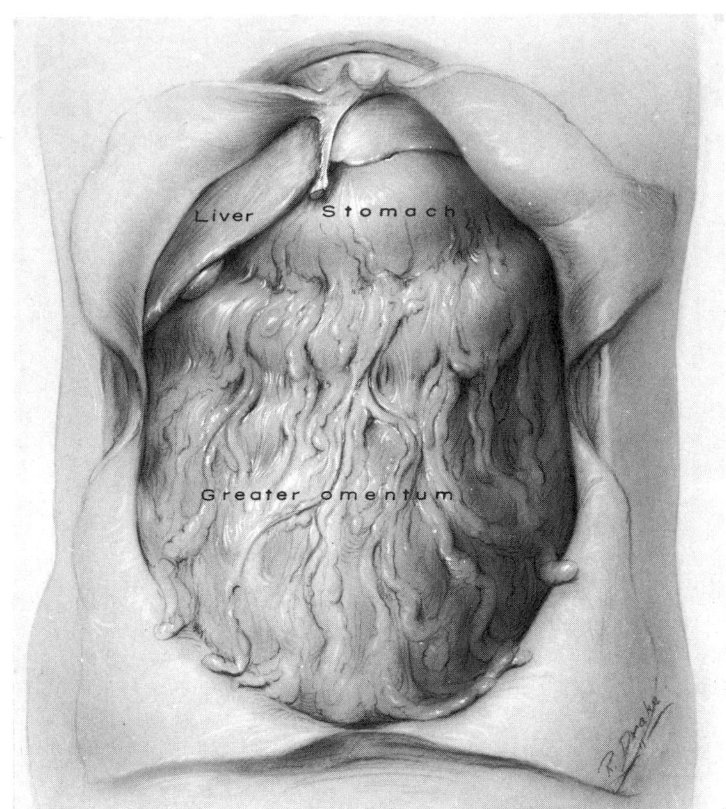

FIGURE *23-15.*
The abdominal organs in situ. The falciform ligament, on the liver, has been largely cut away from the abdominal wall to allow the wall to be reflected. The small intestine is completely hidden by the greater omentum, as is the large intestine, but the transverse colon shows as the bulge behind the upper part of the omentum.

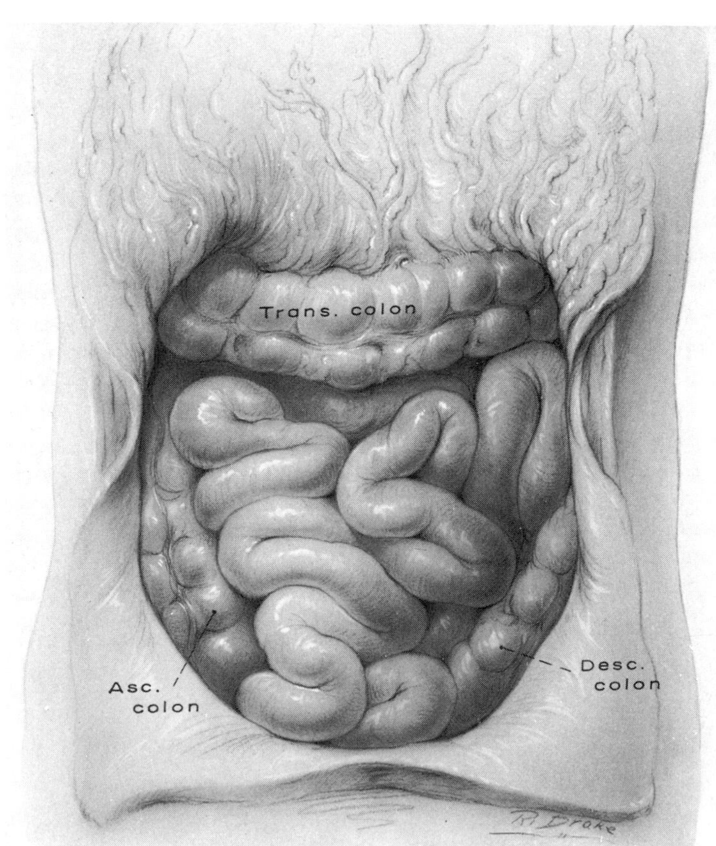

FIGURE *23-16.*
The digestive tract as seen after the greater omentum has been reflected upward. *Ascending, transverse,* and *descending* parts of the colon are identified; coils of small intestine fill most of the abdominal cavity.

shaped) and contains the obliterated umbilical vein, turned into a fibrous cord known as the *ligamentum teres hepatis* (round ligament of the liver). This ligament, enclosed in the free edge of the falciform ligament, spans the distance between the umbilicus and the notch on the sharp inferior border of the liver. Along the midline, right and left laminae of the falciform ligament reflect onto the deep surface of the abdominal wall and the diaphragm and become continuous with parietal peritoneum. Along their hepatic attachment, the same laminae of the falciform ligament continue as visceral peritoneum over the right and left lobes of the liver, respectively. Since this hepatic attachment is not directly opposite the line of attachment to the abdominal wall, rather to the right of the median plane, the falciform ligament itself lies in an oblique plane: its left leaf rests on the left lobe of the liver; its right leaf is in contact with parietal peritoneum of the abdominal wall and diaphragm.

On the right and left sides of the falciform ligament, the narrow peritoneal spaces confined between the liver and the diaphragm are known as the **right and left subphrenic recesses.**

These recesses may harbor infected exudate for some time after the primary abdominal pathology (cholecystitis, perforated peptic ulcer) has been treated. The resultant *subphrenic abscesses* are often difficult to detect clinically.

The subphrenic recesses are limited superiorly, just beyond the summit of the liver, by the **right and left coronary ligaments.** These are the narrow peritoneal reflections that suspend the liver from the diaphragm. Their name fancifully implies that, like a crown, albeit a much distorted one, the two ligaments encircle an area on the liver that is bare of peritoneum and is directly in contact with the diaphragm (see Figs. 24-27 and 24-28).

The part of each coronary ligament accessible in the subphrenic recess is the anterior layer (also known as the superior layer), which is continuous medially with the right and left laminae of the falciform ligament. Laterally, the left coronary ligament doubles back on itself and forms the *left triangular ligament* before it continues again medially as the posterior layer of the left coronary ligament (also known as the inferior layer; see Fig. 24-28). The *right triangular ligament* is similarly formed, but the posterior layer of this coronary ligament diverges widely from the anterior layer, enclosing a large bare area of the right lobe of the liver and the inferior vena cava; the bare area of the left lobe is virtually nonexistent. The meeting of the posterior layers of the right and left coronary ligaments forms the lesser omentum.

The Stomach and Lesser Omentum. The lesser omentum and the stomach are partly covered by the left lobe of the liver. Elevation of the inferior border of the liver reveals the anterior surface of the **stomach** demarcated by the *lesser curvature,* concave toward the right, and the *greater curvature,* convex toward the left (Fig. 23-17). Above, under the left lobe of the liver, the abdominal portion of the *esophagus* enters the stomach at the *cardia;* below, under the right lobe of the liver, just to the right of the midline, the *pylorus* of the stomach leads into the first part of the *duodenum.*

The **lesser omentum** connects the inferior surface of the liver to the esophagus, the lesser curvature of the stomach, and the first part of the duodenum. Like the falciform ligament, the lesser omentum is a double layer of peritoneum, consisting of anterior and posterior (rather than left and right) laminae. It is the portion of the ventral mesentery between the liver and the foregut (see Fig. 23-14). The part of the lesser omentum between the liver and the stomach is known as the *hepatogastric ligament;* this is continuous with the *hepatoduodenal ligament,* the portion of the omentum between the liver and the duodenum (see Fig. 23-17). The hepatoduodenal ligament terminates in a more or less vertical free border on the right. Around this border, anterior and posterior laminae of the lesser omentum are continuous with one another. The left border of the lesser omentum is not free: between the liver and the esophagus, anterior and posterior laminae reflect onto the inferior surface of the diaphragm.

Enclosed in the *free border of the hepatoduodenal ligament* are the bile duct, hepatic artery, and portal vein, the triad or pedicle that connects the liver to the foregut and its vasculature. On the inferior surface of the liver in line with this pedicle is the *gallbladder* (see Fig. 23-17).

The lesser omentum and the stomach lie more or less in a coronal plane: their anterior surfaces face into the greater sac; their posterior surfaces face into the lesser sac. The **lesser sac,** otherwise known as the **omental bursa,** is a large irregular peritoneal *cul-de-sac,* the main portion of which is behind the stomach and the lesser omentum. The **epiploic foramen,** located behind the free edge of the lesser omentum, provides the slitlike communicating passage between the greater sac and the lesser sac. Posteriorly, the foramen is bounded by the inferior vena cava; above, by the liver; and below, by the first part of the duodenum and pancreas, all covered in peritoneum.

The Hepatorenal Recess. The part of the greater sac into which the epiploic foramen opens is called the *hepatorenal recess* or pouch, one of the subhepatic peritoneal spaces. This recess is between the inferior surface of the right lobe of the liver and the anterior surface of the right kidney (Fig. 23-18). Superiorly, this space is limited by the posterior layer of the right coronary ligament (*hepatorenal ligament*) and inferiorly, by the right flexure of the colon. Laterally, the space leads into the right paracolic sulcus (*vide infra*).

The Greater Omentum. The greater omentum is a large apronlike peritoneal fold attached to the greater curvature of the stomach and the adjacent part of the duodenum (see Fig. 23-15). Owing to the complex developmental changes, which will be explained later, it is difficult to appreciate that the greater omentum is the dorsal mesentery of the stomach (*dorsal mesogastrium*), composed of two peritoneal laminae folded upon themselves that connect the stomach to the posterior abdominal wall. The anterior, or outer, and the posterior, or inner, peritoneal lam-

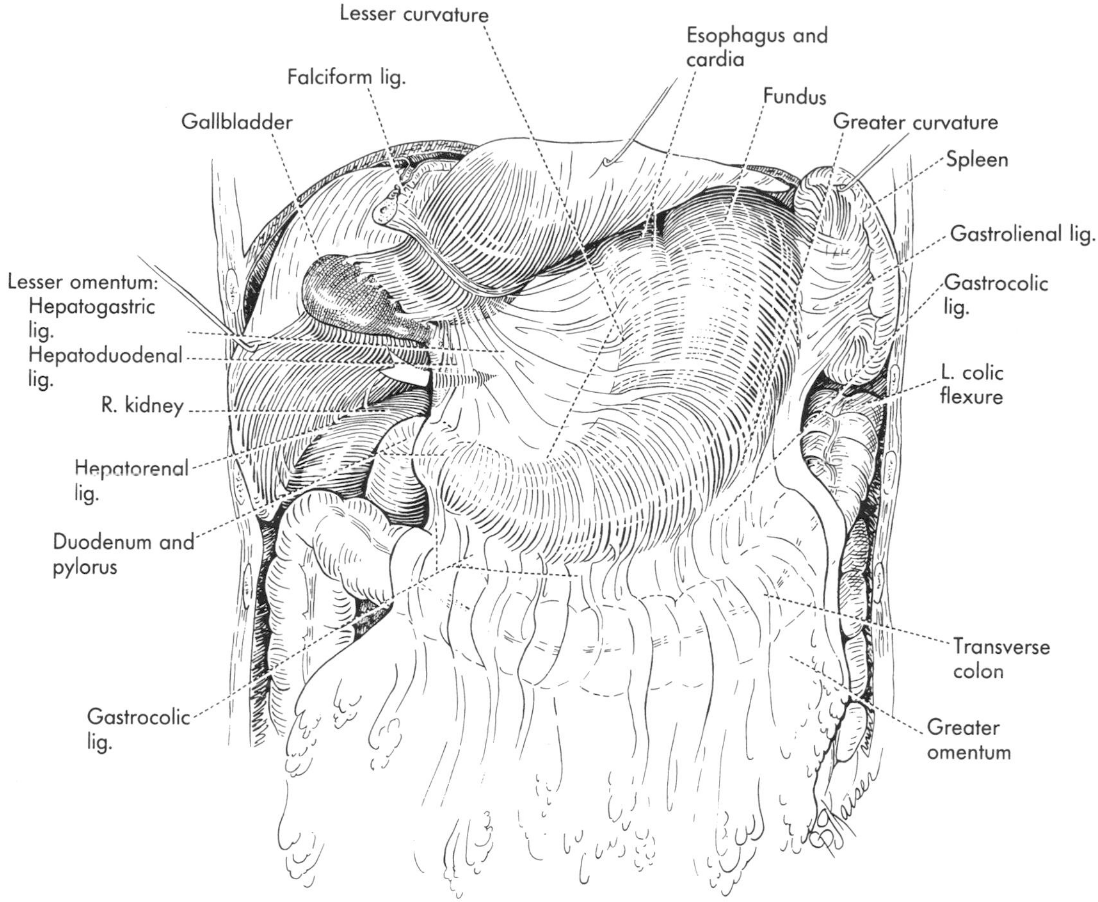

FIGURE 23-17.
The supracolic compartment showing the stomach, lesser omentum, and greater omentum: The inferior border of the liver has been elevated to reveal its inferior surface, and the anterior border of the spleen has been lifted away from the fundus of the stomach to reveal the upper part of the greater omentum. The *arrow* is in the epiploic foramen.

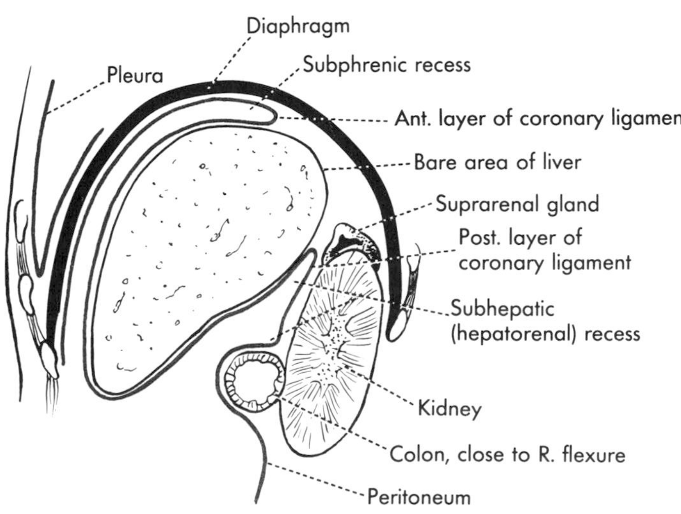

FIGURE 23-18.
Diagram of the subphrenic and subhepatic recesses.

inae of the greater omentum are derived from the corresponding laminae of the lesser omentum after they have embraced the stomach. The anatomy of these laminae is best understood by considering the component parts of the greater omentum separately: these are the gastrocolic ligament and the gastrolienal and lienorenal ligaments. That these so-called ligaments are confluent and constitute the greater omentum would be more easily appreciated if they were designated as omenta rather than ligaments.

The **gastrocolic ligament** (omentum) is the portion of the greater omentum attached to the first part of the duodenum and the adjacent two-thirds of the greater curvature (see Fig. 23-17). Its anterior and posterior peritoneal laminae are rather redundant; both double back on themselves along the inferior edge of the greater omentum before being draped over the transverse colon and its mesentery (Fig. 23-19; see Fig. 23-16); hence, the name of the ligament. This name, however, is deceptive, because the laminae do not terminate on the colon; they continue

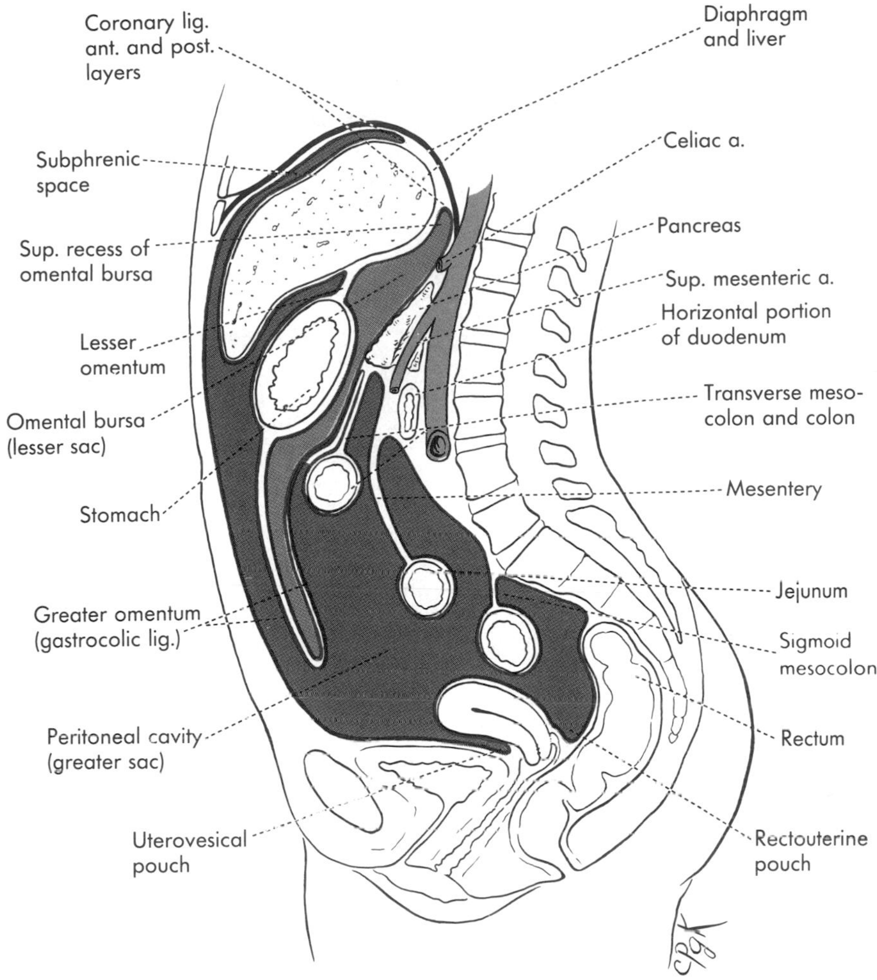

FIGURE *23-19.*
Schematic sagittal section of the abdominal cavity to show the peritoneal continuity: The cut surface of the peritoneum facing into the greater sac is shown in *solid red line*; that facing into the omental bursa is shown in *solid blue line*. The cavity of the greater sac is *red*, that of the omental bursa, *blue*. To illustrate the disposition of the peritonium, the cavity of the lesser sac is shown to extend as far down as the inferior margin of the greater omentum. The sigmoid mesocolon has been included in the section to emphasize the peritoneal reflections from the posterior abdominal wall; actually, the base of the sigmoid mesocolon is attached well to the left of the midline (*see* Fig. 23-20).

to the posterior abdominal wall (see Fig. 23-19). Along the inferior edge of the greater omentum, the *anterior (outer) lamina* (red in Fig. 23-19) will become the most posterior layer of the greater omentum. It ascends to the posterior abdominal wall and immediately reflects forward to become the superior lamina of the transverse mesocolon. These two adjacent laminae are usually fused to one another along a "bloodless" plane and, hence, may be stripped apart. The *posterior (inner) lamina* (blue in Fig. 23-19) of the gastrocolic ligament, derived from the posterior surface of the stomach, follows the anterior lamina and lines the inferior recess of the lesser sac. The latter extends into the greater omentum for a variable distance, but rarely beyond the level of the transverse colon; below this point, the omentum usually consists of four fused peritoneal laminae. Thus the cavity of the lesser sac becomes obliterated and extends for a much shorter distance inferior to the stomach than is illustrated in Figure 23-19.

As the posterior lamina reaches the posterior abdominal wall, it becomes continuous with parietal peritoneum covering the posterior wall of the lesser sac.

The posterior attachments of the gastrocolic portion of the omentum and the posterior attachment of most of the transverse mesocolon coincide. These two mesenteries are attached to the posterior abdominal wall along a horizontal line that lies for the most part along the pancreas (Fig. 23-20).

On the right, the greater omentum has a free border created by the fusion of the anterior and posterior laminae of the gastrocolic ligament. The same is true on the left below the transverse colon (see Fig. 23-17). Above the colon, the gastrocolic portion of the omentum continues superiorly as the **gastrolienal** (gastrosplenic) and **lienorenal** (splenorenal) **ligaments** or omenta. This superior part of the greater omentum connects the upper third of the greater curvature and the fundus of the stomach to the posterior abdominal wall. The parietal line of attachment is largely over the left kidney. This part of the dorsal mesogastrium is divided by the spleen into the gastrolienal and lienorenal ligaments (Fig. 23-21).

The *anterior or outer lamina of the gastrolienal ligament* (red in Fig. 23-21) passes from the stomach to the anterior lip of the hilum of the spleen, surrounds that organ, and, from the posterior lip of the splenic hilum, continues posteriorly as the outer lamina of the lienorenal ligament. The *posterior or inner lamina of the gastrolienal ligament* (blue in Fig. 23-21) is derived from the posterior aspect of the

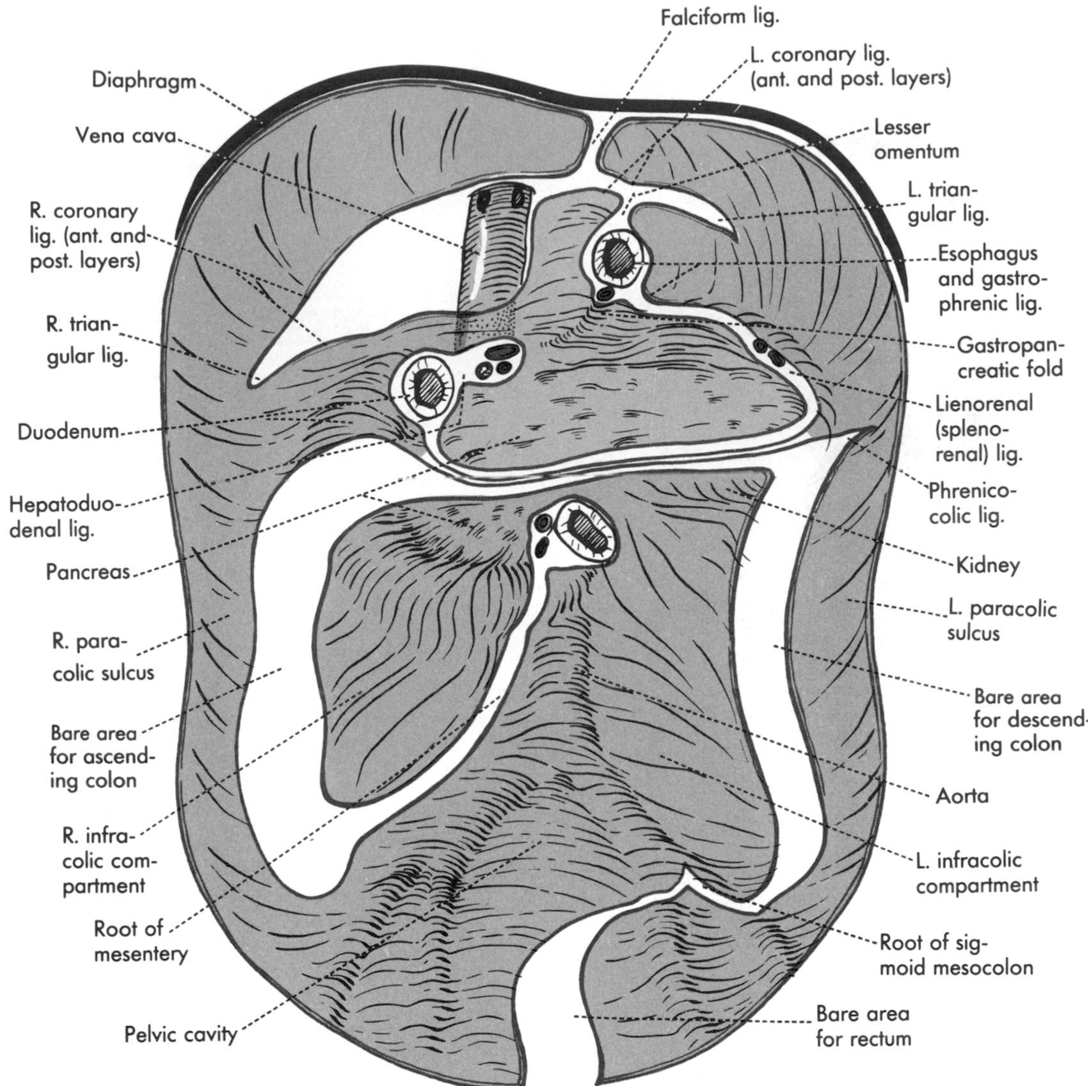

FIGURE *23-20.*
Peritoneal attachments to the posterior abdominal wall and the diaphragm. The duodenum and pancreas have been left in situ, but all the other parts of the digestive system have been removed. The peritoneum lining the greater sac is *pink*, that lining the omental bursa is *blue*.

stomach, doubles back on itself at the splenic hilum, and passes posteriorly as the inner lamina of the lienorenal ligament. Lining the splenic recess of the lesser sac, this lamina only touches the hilum of the spleen; it does not cover any surface of that organ.

The small part of the greater omentum located above the spleen is called the **gastrophrenic ligament** (or omentum), because it connects the fundus of the stomach, and also the esophagus, to the diaphragm superior to the left kidney.

> If the left hand were placed in the lesser sac and the right hand on the anterior surface of the stomach, the two hands could touch between the stomach and the spleen, with only the gastrolienal ligament intervening; between the spleen and the left kidney, with only the lienorenal ligament intervening (see Fig. 23-21); and below the greater curvature of the stomach, with only the gastrocolic ligament intervening (see Fig. 23-19). If the right hand were placed in the infracolic compartment, it would be separated from the left hand, still in the lesser sac, by the transverse mesocolon fused to the two laminae of the gastrocolic ligament (see Fig. 23-19).
>
> When the peritoneal cavity is opened, the *greater omentum* is seldom found spread evenly in front of the intestine as anatomic illustrations suggest. The omentum is moved around, presumably by peristaltic activity of the stomach and bowel, and it may be packed into any part of the peritoneal cavity. The greater omentum can thus seal off the spread of infection. Should, for instance, the gallbladder, appendix, or other viscera become inflamed, the omentum wraps itself around the inflamed organ and may be retained there permanently by the adhesions resulting from the inflammatory process.

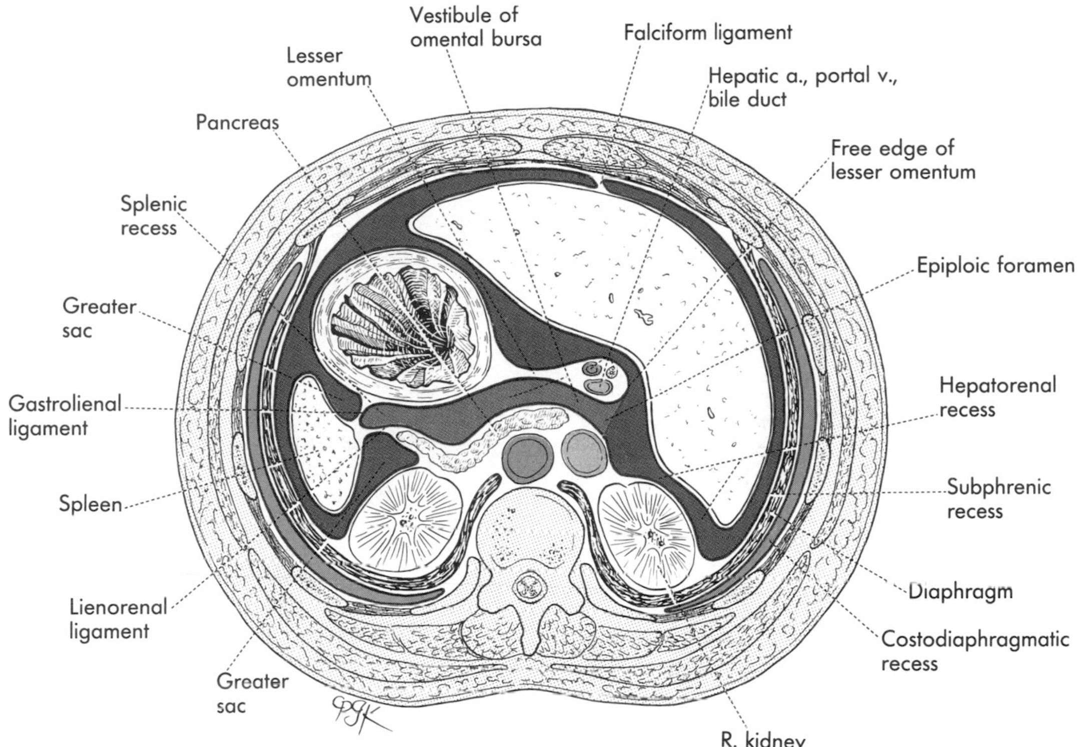

FIGURE *23-21.*
A schematic representation of a transverse section across T-12 vertebra seen from *above* to correspond with the orientation of the reader's own body. The peritoneal continuities are shown around the stomach and its mesenteries: the lining of the omental bursa is *blue*, and that of the greater sac is *pink*.

The Lesser Sac (Omental Bursa)

The description of the greater and the lesser omentum has touched on much of the anatomy of the lesser sac. To comprehend the lesser sac more fully, it is necessary to consider its divisions and its posterior wall in particular (see Fig. 23-20).

The epiploic foramen leads into the **vestibule** of the lesser sac, and from the vestibule diverge the three recesses of the sac: a superior, inferior, and splenic recess (see Fig. 23-21).

The upward continuation of the vestibule behind the liver is the **superior recess.** In the anterior wall of the superior recess is the highly convex caudate lobe of the liver, which projects into this narrow, slitlike space (see Fig. 23-27*A*). The recess is roofed over by the diaphragm, which also forms the posterior wall (see Fig. 23-19). The peritoneal lining over the diaphragm in the recess is continuous in front and on the right with the posterior layer of the right coronary ligament, and it is this ligament that limits the recess above and to the right of the caudate lobe. The posterior layer of the right coronary ligament in the vestibule and superior recess is the continuation of the hepatorenal ligament across the inferior vena cava and, beyond the epiploic foramen, upward along the left side of the vena cava (see Fig. 23-20). As the vena cava passes through the diaphragm, the line of peritoneal reflection turns to the left, along the upper margin of the caudate lobe. On the left side of this lobe, the posterior layer of the right coronary ligament terminates by becoming the posterior lamina of the lesser omentum. (In other words, the lamina joins the anterior lamina of the lesser omentum, continuous with the posterior layer of the left coronary ligament.) Thus, on the left, the superior recess is closed off from the greater sac by the hepatogastric portion of the lesser omentum: the omentum runs from the deep groove of the left side of the caudate lobe to the esophagus and the lesser curvature of the stomach. As mentioned earlier, superiorly, the recess is sealed by the reflection of the posterior lamina of the lesser omentum onto the diaphragm.

Two peritoneal ridges mark the boundary between the vestibule and its inferior and splenic recesses. These ridges are the *gastropancreatic folds*, raised up from the posterior wall of the lesser sac by the branches of the celiac trunk (see Fig. 23-20). The **inferior recess** is below the right gastropancreatic fold (containing the common hepatic artery) and extends behind the stomach into the greater omentum. In its posterior wall lies the pancreas and below that the posterior lamina of the greater omentum, fused with the anterior lamina to the transverse mesocolon. The **splenic recess** is to the left of the left gastropancreatic fold (containing the left gastric artery) and extends behind the stomach and in between the gastrolienal and lienorenal ligaments. In its posterior wall lie, retroperitoneally, the left suprarenal gland, the upper pole of the left kidney, and the diaphragm. The splenic artery running along the upper border of the pancreas demarcates the splenic and inferior recesses from one another. The splenic vessels and the tail of the pancreas pass forward to the hilum of the spleen, being enclosed in the lienorenal ligament (see Fig. 23-21). A small portion of the abdominal aorta, from which the short celiac trunk springs, is in the posterior wall of the lesser sac where the two gastropancreatic folds converge with each other.

The lesser sac is normally empty except for the serous fluid that moistens its walls. An ulcer on the posterior wall of the stomach may perforate into the lesser sac, as may a pancreatic cyst or abscess. The gastric contents and exudate may become sealed off in the lesser sac, which may then become distended, giving rise to a *pseudocyst*. Infected material may also track its way from the lesser sac, through the epiploic foramen, into the hepatorenal space and then along the paracolic sulcus into the pelvis. Exudate or pus may also form in the hepatorenal space as a complication of gallbladder disease.

The epiploic foramen is usually too small for exploring the lesser sac through it. To do this adequately in the dissecting laboratory or at surgery, an opening has to be made in the lesser omentum or in one of the ligaments of the greater omentum. The lesser sac may also be entered from the infracolic compartment through the transverse mesocolon and the two laminae of the greater omentum fused to it.

Development of the Spaces and Mesenteries in the Supracolic Compartment

To explain satisfactorily the anatomy of the supracolic compartment at a time when development is complete, it is necessary to expand somewhat on the introductory remarks made in Chapter 9 and earlier in this chapter.

Dorsal Mesogastrium. To begin with, the foregut lies largely dorsal to the septum transversum, and its dorsal mesentery, the dorsal mesogastrium, is a relatively thick structure that separates the right and left pleuroperitoneal canals from one another (see Fig. 23-14*A* through *C*). The attachment of the dorsal mesogastrium to the foregut identifies the greater curvature of the stomach and the future medial border of the duodenum, both of which at this stage face posteriorly. The lesser curvature of the stomach abuts against the septum transversum.

In addition to the vitelline arteries, which will be known as branches of the celiac trunk, the dorsal mesogastrium contains the spleen, the pancreas, and the vitelline veins, which in their final configuration pass as a single vessel (the portal vein) from the dorsal mesogastrium into the septum transversum (see Fig. 23-14*D*).

Septum Transversum. The ventral mesentery of the foregut at this stage is the septum transversum, a wedge-shaped block of mesoderm ventral to the foregut and the pleuroperitoneal canals. The cranial surface of the septum is defined by the pericardial cavity, and the caudal surface is defined by a portion of the intraembryonic celom that extends into the umbilical cord around the vitellointestinal duct and around the loop formed by the midgut. The following structures pass forward toward the central point of the septum transversum buried just beneath the surface of the septum that faces toward the body stalk. 1) from the body stalk, the umbilical vein runs posteriorly to enter the liver; 2) from the caudal end of the foregut, the bile duct runs forward, forming the pedicle of the liver, which is expanding in the septum transversum; 3) the hepatic artery; and 4) the portal vein accompanies the bile duct, both having entered the septum transversum from the dorsal mesogastrium as they pass along the right side of the foregut (duodenum) (see Fig. 23-14*D*).

The peripheral cell layers of the septum transversum contribute to the formation of the *diaphragm*, especially cranially, forming its central tendon (the floor of the pericardial cavity; see Figs. 21-2 and 25-4); the more central cells become incorporated into the liver as its connective tissue elements and the walls of its vessels. The *subphrenic recesses* of the peritoneal cavity develop in the cleavage plane between the peripheral cells of the septum and the liver, becoming confluent posteriorly with the pleuroperitoneal canals and caudally with the umbilical part of the celom that extends into the umbilical cord (see Fig. 23-14*C*).

The expansions of the celomic ducts into the septum transversum define the peritoneal surfaces of the liver but stop short of surrounding it completely in three places: 1) anteriorly, where the falciform ligament remains as a mesentery supporting the umbilical vein along its inferior edge; 2) posteriorly, where the lesser omentum remains, supporting along its inferior edge the bile duct, hepatic artery, and portal vein; 3) posterosuperiorly, where the coronary ligaments surround the bare area of the liver, retaining it in contact with the portion of the diaphragm that is derived from the septum transversum.

These events transform the septum transversum into the ventral mesentery that consists of the falciform ligament and the lesser omentum, with the liver between the two.

The definitive anatomy of the ventral mesentery is established by reorientation of its component parts: 1) the free edge of the falciform ligament becomes vertical and sickle-shaped owing to the elongation of the ventral body wall between the liver and the umbilicus; 2) the free edge of the lesser omentum becomes vertical, owing to the descent of the stomach and duodenum; 3) the lesser omentum changes from a sagittal to a coronal plane owing to the rotation of the stomach and duodenum (vide infra).

It is to be emphasized that the **epiploic foramen** is created by the reorientation of the free edge of the lesser omentum into a plane that is parallel with, rather than perpendicular to, the posterior abdominal wall. The epiploic foramen is the slitlike space trapped behind the now vertical free edge, rather than a hole created in some existing structure.

Omental Bursa. The *rotation of the stomach* and duodenum, in a manner that turns their original right surface posteriorly, is probably promoted by the destabilization of the dorsal mesogastrium (Fig. 23-22). The rather bulky **dorsal mesogastrium** is invaded by the cavity of the right pleuroperitoneal canal. This cavity created in the mesogastrium thins out the dorsal mesentery and is known as the omental bursa. The location of the spleen in the far left wall of the omental bursa may contribute to the buckling of the dorsal mesogastrium upon itself, causing the spleen to bulge into the left pleuroperitoneal canal and aiding the stomach in pointing its greater curvature toward the left (see Fig. 23-22). The buckling, which hinges on the spleen, divides the dorsal mesogastrium into an anterior portion between the greater curvature of the stomach and the spleen (*gastrolienal ligament*) and a posterior portion between the dorsal midline attachment of the mesentery and the spleen (*lienorenal ligament*). The latter comes to lie parallel with the surface of the left kidney and contains the pancreas and the splenic vessels.

This folded dorsal mesogastrium can now be called the **greater omentum,** and it becomes even more expanded to the extent that it hangs from the greater curvature of the stomach far down into the more caudal part of the peritoneal cavity. The definitive anatomy of the greater omentum is established by secondary adhesions to adjacent structures: posteriorly, it becomes tethered to the surface of the left kidney and fuses its original left lamina with the parietal peritoneum on the mesonephros (antecedent of the kidney), immobilizing the pancreas on the posterior abdominal wall (see Fig. 23-22); after the midgut and hindgut obtain their definitive position in the peritoneal cavity, the greater omentum adheres to the superior surface of the transverse colon and its mesocolon.

The **cavity of the omental bursa** grows with the greater omentum, and its *splenic recess* follows the spleen toward the left; its *inferior recess* is contained in the redundant fold of the greater omentum, and part of it may become obliterated. The *vestibule* of the lesser sac is the portion of the peritoneal cavity that becomes trapped behind the lesser omentum when the stomach and the lesser omentum complete their 90° turn. The *superior recess* of the lesser sac is the cranial extension of the vestibule and is the infradiaphragmatic portion of the *pneumatoenteric recess*, for the explanation of which the literature should be consulted.

The Infracolic Compartment of the Greater Sac

The upper limit of the infracolic compartment is the transverse colon and its mesentery (see Fig. 23-16). Inferiorly, the compartment communicates with the pelvis. The attachment of the transverse mesocolon to the retroperitoneal pancreas has been discussed. To the right of the pancreas, this attachment line crosses the vertical segment of the duodenum, and the mesocolon terminates at the hepatic flexure of the colon; on the left, beyond the pancreas, the attachment line terminates at the left, or splenic, flexure of the colon (see Fig. 23-20). These colonic flexures lie on the anterior surface of the kidneys and mark the junction of the transverse colon with the ascending colon on the right and the descending colon on the left. These vertical segments of the large bowel form the lateral boundaries of the infracolic compartment.

Both the ascending and the descending colon have lost their mesenteries during the development of the colon. Their posterior surfaces, bare of peritoneum, lie directly on the posterior abdominal wall. The visceral peritoneum on their anterior and lateral surfaces is continuous laterally with parietal peritoneum in the **paracolic sulci.** The right paracolic sulcus, or gutter, communicates above with the hepatorenal space; the left paracolic sulcus, or gutter, is limited above by a small peritoneal fold, the *phrenicocolic ligament*, pinched up between the left flexure and the diaphragm. Below, the two paracolic gutters lead into the *iliac fossae* and then into the pelvis. Medially,

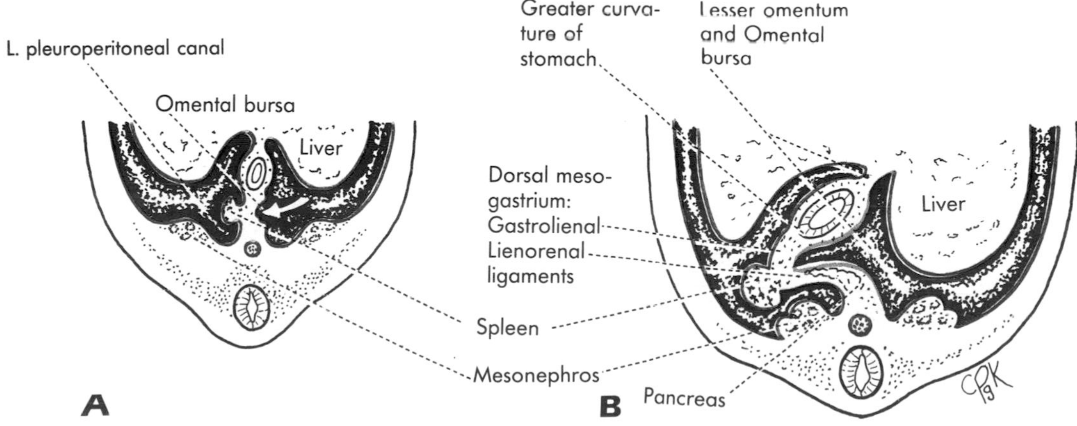

FIGURE 23-22.
Development of the omental bursa and the dorsal mesogastrium: (A) commencement of cavitation in the dorsal mesogastrium (compare with Fig. 23-14C), (B) the stomach has rotated; fusion of the lienorenal ligament to parietal peritoneum over the kidney will establish the definitive anatomy.

peritoneum from the anterior and medial surfaces of the ascending and descending colon is continuous with parietal peritoneum on the posterior wall of the infracolic compartment.

On the posterior abdominal wall, the *duodenum* descends behind the transverse mesocolon, crossing the boundary between the supracolic and infracolic compartments (Fig. 23-23). Only the first part of the duodenum, seen in the supracolic compartment, has mesenteries; the rest lies with the pancreas across the posterior abdominal wall. In front of the third lumbar vertebra, the duodenum passes horizontally from the right to the left side of the infracolic compartment. Turning upward and then abruptly forward, it becomes the *jejunum*, the union of the two creating the acute *duodenojejunal flexure*. Distally, the jejunum continues as the *ileum*. The numerous coils of the jejunum fill the upper part of the infracolic compartment; below, the coils of the ileum usually also fill the pelvis. The ileum opens into the medial side of the large intestine in the right iliac fossa. The large intestine above this *ileocecal junction* is the ascending colon; below, it is the saclike *cecum*, from which the *vermiform appendix* takes origin.

The jejunum and ileum are suspended from the posterior abdominal wall by a large continuous peritoneal fold, the **mesenetry.** The mesentery is fan-shaped and fluted: its intestinal border is about 40 times longer than its root, which is attached diagonally across the posterior wall of the infracolic compartment from the duodenojejunal flexure to the ileocecal junction (see Fig. 23-23). Between its two peritoneal laminae, the mesentery contains the blood vessels, lymphatics, lymph nodes, and nerve plexuses that serve the jejunum and ileum. These structures are embedded in a considerable amount of fat.

Along the root of the mesentery, its right peritoneal lamina becomes continuous with peritoneum covering the pancreas and duodenum in the upper part of the infracolic compartment; below, the same lamina is continuous with parietal peritoneum, covering the ureter and the lower pole of the right kidney, as well as the muscles of the posterior abdominal wall (see Fig. 23-23). The left lamina of the mesentery also reflects over the duodenum above; below, it becomes continuous with the parietal peritoneum of an extensive quadrangular area that leads down into the pelvis. In this area, retroperitoneal structures include the lower pole of the left kidney, the left ureter, the inferior vena cava, the aorta, and both left and right common iliac vessels.

In the left iliac fossa, the infracolic compartment is limited inferiorly by the *sigmoid colon* and its mesentery, the **sigmoid mesocolon.** The sigmoid colon is the distal continuation of the descending colon. Passing into the pelvis, the sigmoid colon loses its mesentery and becomes the rectum. The sigmoid mesocolon is attached to the posterior abdominal wall along the line of an inverted V. The left limb of the V is in the iliac fossa; the right limb descends into the pelvis (see Fig. 23-23).

Developmental Events in the Infracolic Compartment: Rotation of the Gut

The midgut and hindgut increase in length quite early in development and, although they remain suspended by the common dorsal mesentery, they soon form a loop, the apex of which is connected to the yolk sac through the umbilical cord by the vitellointestinal duct (Fig. 23-24; see Fig. 23-14*D*). This loop will become highly convoluted as the intestine continues to grow. The intraembryonic celom fails to keep pace with this growth, and therefore, the loop herniates into the umbilical portion of the celom.

The midgut and its mesentery become twisted and turned in a particular manner during this process. When the abdominal cavity is sufficiently expanded, this physiologic hernia is reduced, and the intestine

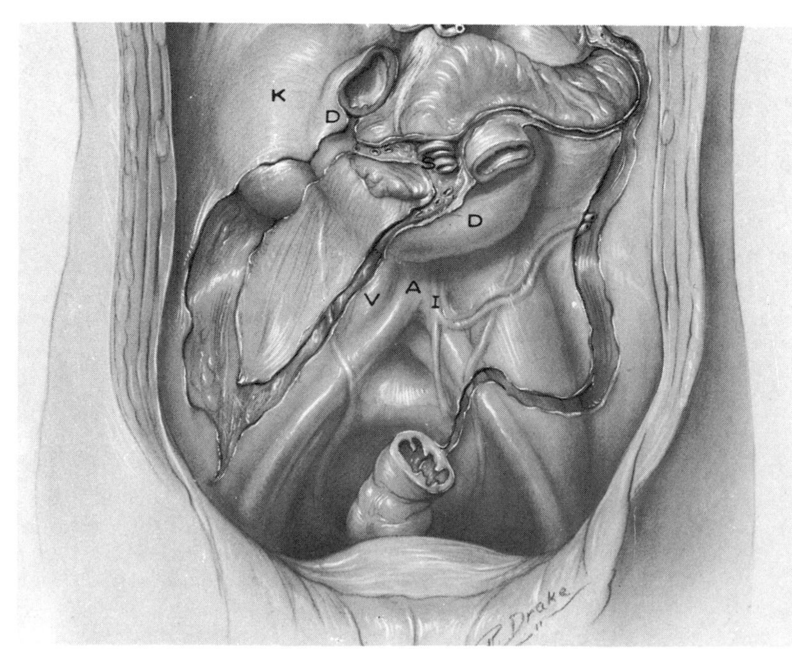

FIGURE 23-23.
The peritoneal attachments and retroperitoneal structures in the infracolic compartment: *A*, aorta; *D*, duodenum; *I*, inferior mesenteric vein; *K*, kidney; *V*, inferior vena cava (correlate with Fig. 23-20).

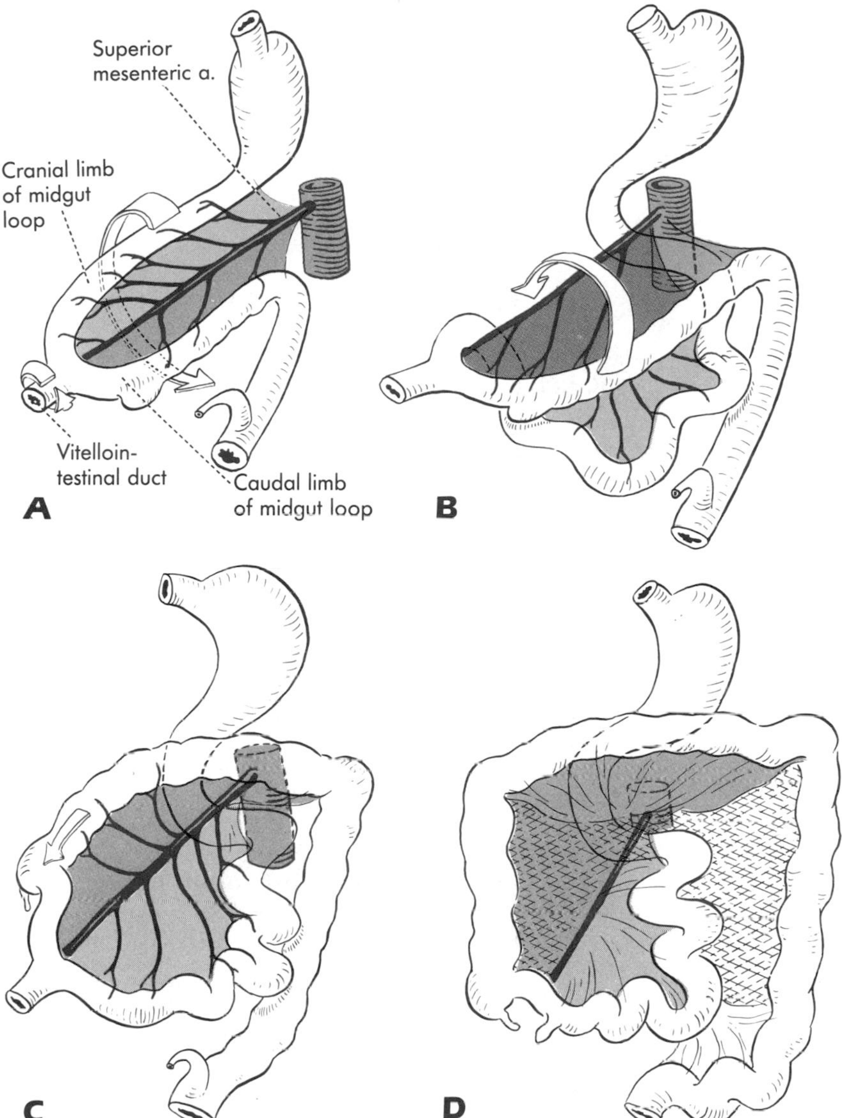

FIGURE 23-24.
Schematic representation of the rotation the midgut. Events that occur simultaneously are arbitrarily divided into discrete steps to accord with descriptions in the text. (A) The primitive midgut loop is viewed from the *left side* (compare with Fig. 23-14*D*). The umbilical celom is not illustrated. (B) The cranial limb of the loop has descended into the left side of the peritoneal cavity; the duodenum is placed behind the superior mesenteric artery. (C) The caudal limb has ascended and is moving downward in the right side of the peritoneal cavity. (D) The definitive arrangement has been attained and mesenterial fusion is complete.

returns from the umbilical cord into the abdominal cavity. The rearrangement of the intestine that results from the rotation of the midgut becomes stabilized through the fusion of extensive portions of the mesentery with parietal peritoneum on the posterior wall of the infracolic compartment.

The key to understanding the infracolic compartment is the fate of the midgut loop, which is best discussed in its simplest form (see Fig. 23-24). The cranial limb of the loop is made up of the duodenum and jejunum; the future ileum is in the region of the apex of the loop and from it arises the vitellointestinal duct; on the caudal limb of the loop, the cecum is identified by a saccular dilation, and the rest of the caudal limb continues as the colon into the hindgut.

The vitelline arteries and veins, from which the superior and inferior mesenteric vessels develop, are contained in the dorsal mesentery. The superior mesenteric artery runs to the apex of the loop (and beyond it to the yolk sac), distributing numerous branches to the cranial limb of the loop and only three branches to the caudal limb (see Figs. 23-14 and 23-24*C*).

For our purpose, the specific sequence of events in the rotation of the gut is immaterial; the following points are important:

1. The superior mesenteric artery and the vitellointestinal duct in line with it can be considered the axis of the rotation, which takes place counterclockwise and amounts to roughly 270°.
2. The cranial limb of the loop moves downward on the right side of the celom, and once its excursion exceeds 180°, the limb must pass *behind* (or caudal to) the superior mesenteric artery, ending in the left side of the celom (see Fig. 23-24*A* and *B*). This is the component of the rotation that carries the future horizontal portion of the duodenum *behind* the superior mesenteric artery and lays it across the vertebral column, placing the duodenojejunal junction and all of the cranial limb of the loop into the left side of the infracolic compartment. The

duodenum becomes fixed in this position quite early in the process of rotation.

3. The caudal limb of the loop ascends in the left side of the celom, and once its excursion exceeds 180°, the limb must cross *anterior* to the proximal end of the cranial limb and then continue its movement by descent in the right side of the celom (see Fig. 23-24*B* and *C*). This is the component of the rotation that lays the future transverse colon across the descending portion of the duodenum and carries the cecum into the right side of the peritoneal cavity.

It is important to remember that during this process the mesentery does not behave as a passive sheet of tissue, but as one capable of adjusting to the movement of the intestine by growth as well as by twisting and folding. Viewed from the front at the completion of the rotation, the mesentery presents an arrangement resembling a funnel: the rim of the funnel is made up of the caudal loop (in essence, the large intestine); the coils of the cranial loop (most of the small intestine) are suspended on their mesentery within the funnel; the cavity of the funnel tapers toward the origin of the superior mesenteric artery or the duodenojejunal flexure (see Fig. 23-24*C* and *D*).

The definitive arrangement is arrived at by fusion of the mesentery of the ascending and descending colons to the posterior parietal peritoneum in the infracolic compartment and the fusion of the mesentery of the jejunum and ileum to the same parietal peritoneum across a diagonal line that slopes from the duodenojejunal flexure to the ileocecal junction now located in the right iliac fossa (see Fig. 23-24*D*). Such extensive fusion of the dorsal mesentery and portions of the intestine to the posterior abdominal wall is a feature peculiar to the human and some of the anthropoid apes.

Abnormal Rotation. Abnormalities of rotation are of three major types: failure of mesenterial fusion, reversed rotation, and entrapment of portions of the gut in mesenterial folds.

The most common abnormality is failure of the mesentery of the ascending colon to fuse to the posterior wall. This is usually limited to the distal part of the ascending colon, but in its most severe form will leave the entire small and large intestine, up to the left colic flexure, suspended on a free mesentery. In such a case, the root of the mesentery is limited to the vicinity of the duodenojejunal flexure, and this predisposes to the twisting of the unfixed intestine and its mesentery upon itself. The twisting, called *volvulus*, obstructs the lumen of both the intestine and the blood vessels in the mesentery, constituting a major emergency.

The descending colon and its mesentery may also fail to fuse. Usually, this leaves the descending colon suspended on a short mesentery attached to the posterior abdominal wall well to the left of the midline.

The cranial limb of the midgut loop may fail to move in the appropriate direction and may cross in front of, rather than behind, the superior mesenteric artery. Such reversed rotation places the duodenum anterior, rather than posterior, to the large intestine, and if mesenterial fusion fixes the gut in this position, obstruction may result. Other types of abnormalities in rotation may produce abnormal peritoneal bands, which may be responsible for transitory or acute obstruction of either the small or the large intestine.

The rotating gut may be caught in a pocket of the mesentery, which it will distend. The most striking example of this is *paraduodenal hernias*. The small intestine becomes trapped behind the mesentery of the ascending or descending colon, and when the mesentery fuses with the posterior wall, the small intestine will be encased in a peritoneal bag on the right or left side of the duodenum.

The Pelvic Portion of the Peritoneal Cavity

The major pelvic organs covered by peritoneum include the rectum, urinary bladder, and, in the female, uterus and its adnexae as well. The rectum is largely accommodated in the curvature of the sacrum; the bladder, when empty, is confined to the pelvis, sheltered behind the body of the two pubes and the symphysis between them. The uterus protrudes upward and forward in the space between the rectum and the bladder, and the uterine tubes extend from it laterally. Peritoneal relations that are different in the pelves of the two sexes are examined in detail in Chapter 27. The purpose here is to understand peritoneal continuities between the abdomen proper and the pelvis.

Continuing down from the infracolic compartment, peritoneum covers the anterior and lateral surfaces of the rectum in its upper portion; bare of peritoneum are the lower third of the rectum, embedded in extraperitoneal fascia, and its entire posterior surface in contact with the sacrum.

In the male, the peritoneum sweeps forward from the rectum to the bladder, creating a peritoneal recess between the two organs that is the *rectovesical pouch* (Fig. 23-25*A*). Just before the peritoneum comes in contact with the bladder, it is draped over the upper part of the seminal vesicles. From the superior surface of the bladder, the peritoneum ascends toward the umbilicus on the deep aspect of the anterior abdominal wall. Laterally, the peritoneum of the rectum and the bladder become continuous with parietal peritoneum of the pelvic wall, which then merges across the pelvic brim with parietal peritoneum in the iliac fossae. Visible and palpable through the parietal peritoneum on each side are the ureter and ductus deferens: the ureter runs anteromedially from the pelvic wall to the bladder, and the ductus deferens runs posteromedially from the inguinal fossa in front toward the seminal vesicles in the back.

In the female, the peritoneum sweeps forward from the rectum onto the uterus; the peritoneal space between them is the *rectouterine pouch* (see Figs. 23-19 and 23-25*B*). Just before the peritoneum comes in contact with the uterus, it covers the posterior fornix of the vagina. The peritoneum invests completely the posterior and anterior surfaces of the uterus before reflecting onto the superior surface of the bladder. The *vesicouterine pouch* is between the two organs.

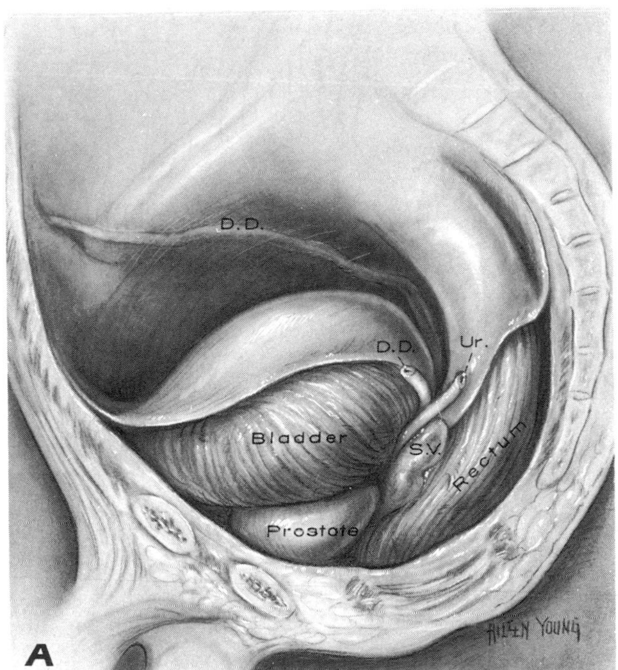

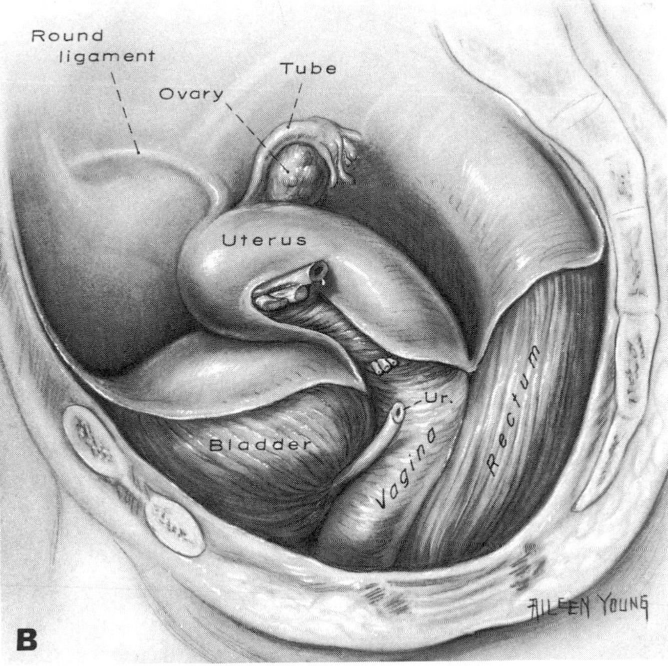

FIGURE 23-25.
The pelvic viscera with their peritoneal covering in (A) the male and (B) female pelvis. Over the rectum and bladder, the *cut edges* indicate the reflection of the peritoneum to the lateral pelvic wall. Over the uterus, the *cut edges* of the peritoneum indicate the attachment of the broad ligament to the uterus: *D.D.* identifies the right and left ductus deferentes; *Ur*, the left ureter; and *S.V.*, the left seminal vesicle. In panel B, at the base of the broad ligament, above the ureter, are the stumps of the uterine vessels as they enter the uterus. Between the cut edges of the leaves of the uppermost part of the broad ligament are stumps of the left uterine tube, of the ovarian ligament just below this, and of the round ligament just anterior to the ovarian ligament.

Lateral to the uterus, a transverse fold of peritoneum is raised up from the floor of the pelvic cavity. The name of this fold is the **broad ligament,** which, similar to a mesentery, encloses the uterine tube in its superior border. Anterior and posterior laminae of the broad ligament merge with the peritoneum on respective surfaces of the uterus; reaching the lateral wall of the pelvis, the laminae reflect to become parietal peritoneum. Through the anterior lamina is visible and palpable the *round ligament of the uterus*, spanning the distance between the inguinal fossa and the uterus; through the posterior lamina, the *ligament of the ovary* can be traced from the ovary to the uterus. A reduplication of the posterior lamina suspends the ovary from the posterolateral aspect of the broad ligament. The lateral fimbriated end of the uterine tube fuses with the posterior lamina of the broad ligament in such a manner that the *ostium* of the tube surrounded by the fimbriae opens into the peritoneal cavity. Through the vagina, the uterine cavity, and the lumen of the tubes, communication is thus established between the exterior and the peritoneal cavity. In the male, the peritoneal cavity is completely closed. In the female, the ova that are shed into the peritoneal cavity can enter through the ostium into the uterine tubes, where they may be fertilized by spermatozoa deposited in the vagina.

Many spermatozoa that are ejaculated in the vagina find their way into the uterine tube and, escaping through the ostium, may accumulate in the rectouterine pouch. These spermatozoa may be aspirated from the pouch by a needle inserted into the posterior fornix of the vagina. Their presence in the aspirate rules out bilateral blockage of the uterine tubes as a cause of infertility. Infection in the female genital tract may spread along the same route as the spermatozoa and may cause peritoneal inflammation and later extensive adhesions in the pelvis.

Deep Aspect of the Anterior Abdominal Wall

In the peritoneal tissue of the anterior abdominal wall, three ligaments extend from the region of the bladder to the umbilicus and in so doing produce more or less prominent peritoneal folds (Fig. 23-26). The **median umbilical ligament** is the remains of the *urachus*, an extension of the embryonic bladder to the umbilicus; it is attached to the apex of the bladder and produces the *median fold*. The **medial umbilical ligaments,** on each side of the median fold, are the fibrous remains of the *umbilical arteries* of the fetus, which passed just lateral to the bladder and raised up the *medial umbilical folds*. The **lateral umbil-**

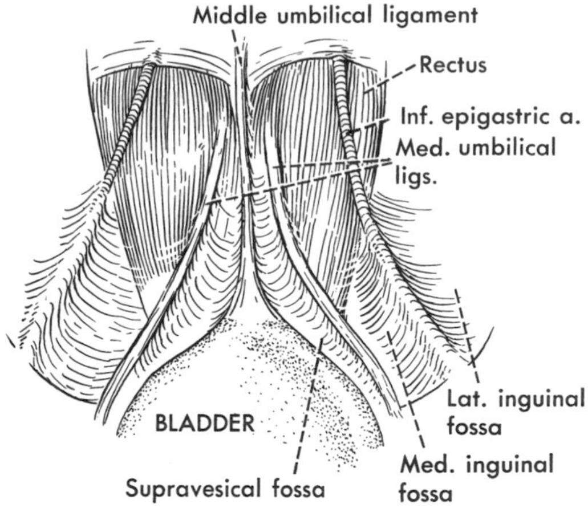

FIGURE 23-26.
View of the posterior surface of the lower part of the anterior abdominal wall, showing the structures that produce the folds and fossae related to the bladder and inguinal region.

ical folds, which may not be at all prominent, are produced by the *inferior epigastric arteries*.

On each side of the median umbilical fold, just above the bladder, is a *supravesical fossa*; a *medial inguinal fossa* lies between the medial and lateral folds, and a *lateral inguinal fossa* lies lateral to each lateral fold. The medial inguinal fossa represents the *inguinal triangle*, the peritoneal area through which direct inguinal hernias occur; indirect inguinal hernias occur in the lateral inguinal fossa (see Chap. 26).

At the inguinal triangles, the anterior and posterior abdominal walls meet each other. Parietal peritoneum of the iliac fossae passes from the anterior surface of the iliacus and psoas muscles onto the deep aspect of the anterior abdominal wall. Parietal peritoneum of the medial umbilical folds and the supravesical fossae is the forward continuation of the pelvic peritoneum.

Vertical and Horizontal Continuities of the Peritoneum

Tracing peritoneal continuities in sagittal and transverse sections of the abdomen contributes greatly to understanding abdominal anatomy. Figure 23-19 illustrates that starting at the umbilicus, it is possible, in a sagittal section, to trace with a pencil the peritoneum of the greater sac into the upper abdomen, down into the pelvis, and back to the umbilicus without lifting the pencil. The same is possible in the lesser sac, starting with the hepatic attachment of the lesser omentum, for instance. A transverse section across the epiploic foramen permits tracing of the peritoneum from the left leaf of the falciform ligament into the lesser sac and back again to the starting point (see Fig. 23-21). Higher and lower sections aid in defining communication of various peritoneal spaces or the lack of such communication (Fig. 23-27).

THE ABDOMINAL REGIONS AND LOCATION OF ABDOMINAL VISCERA

Abdominal viscera are located in reference to the surface of the body with the help of landmarks, planes that intersect the surface of the body along lines, and regions determined by some of the planes. Although in the course of a physical examination, lines are seldom drawn on the surface of the body, the student engaged in studying anatomy and acquiring the skills of physical examination benefits much from drawing these lines as an aid to learning the positions of various viscera. Such knowledge forms the basis for the examination of the abdomen. Symptoms and signs of abdominal disease are located and recorded with reference to abdominal regions mapped out on the abdominal wall.

Landmarks. The anatomic landmarks on the anterior abdominal wall have been described earlier in this chapter and include the xiphisternal joint, the costal margins, the umbilicus, the iliac crests and their tubercles, the anterior superior iliac spines, the inguinal folds, and the symphysis pubis (Fig. 23-28*A*).

Planes and Lines. There are sagittal and horizontal planes used for locating viscera (see Fig. 23-28*B*). Of the **sagittal planes,** the *median plane* coincides with the linea alba and passes through the umbilicus. The *midclavicular lines* drawn vertically from the midpoint of each clavicle define bilateral sagittal planes (often called *lateral planes*) that intersect the costal margin close to the tip of the ninth costal cartilage and the inguinal fold halfway between the anterior superior iliac spine and the symphysis pubis.

The **horizontal planes** are the transpyloric, subcostal, supracristal, and intertubercular planes. All are useful in defining vertebral levels. The *transpyloric plane* is halfway between the jugular notch and the upper border of the symphysis pubis. It is more readily found, with sufficient accuracy, along the ulnar border of the subject's hand when the thumb is laid across the xiphisternal joint. The transpyloric plane intersects the costal margins and the midclavicular lines at the tip of the ninth costal cartilage and crosses the lower border of L-1 vertebra. It is so called because it usually passes through the pylorus of the stomach. The *subcostal plane* connects the lowest points of the two costal margins and lies across the upper border of L-3 vertebra. The *supracristal plane* joins the highest points of the two iliac crests; in it lies the spinous process of L-4 vertebra and, in young and lean individuals, the umbilicus. The *intertubercular plane* connects the tubercles of the right and left iliac crests and passes through L-5 vertebra. The plane connecting the two anterior superior iliac spines is unnamed; it passes below the level of the sacral promontory and is not longer used in mapping abdominal regions.

Quadrants and Regions. The most commonly used regions are the four **quadrants** of the abdomen (see Fig.

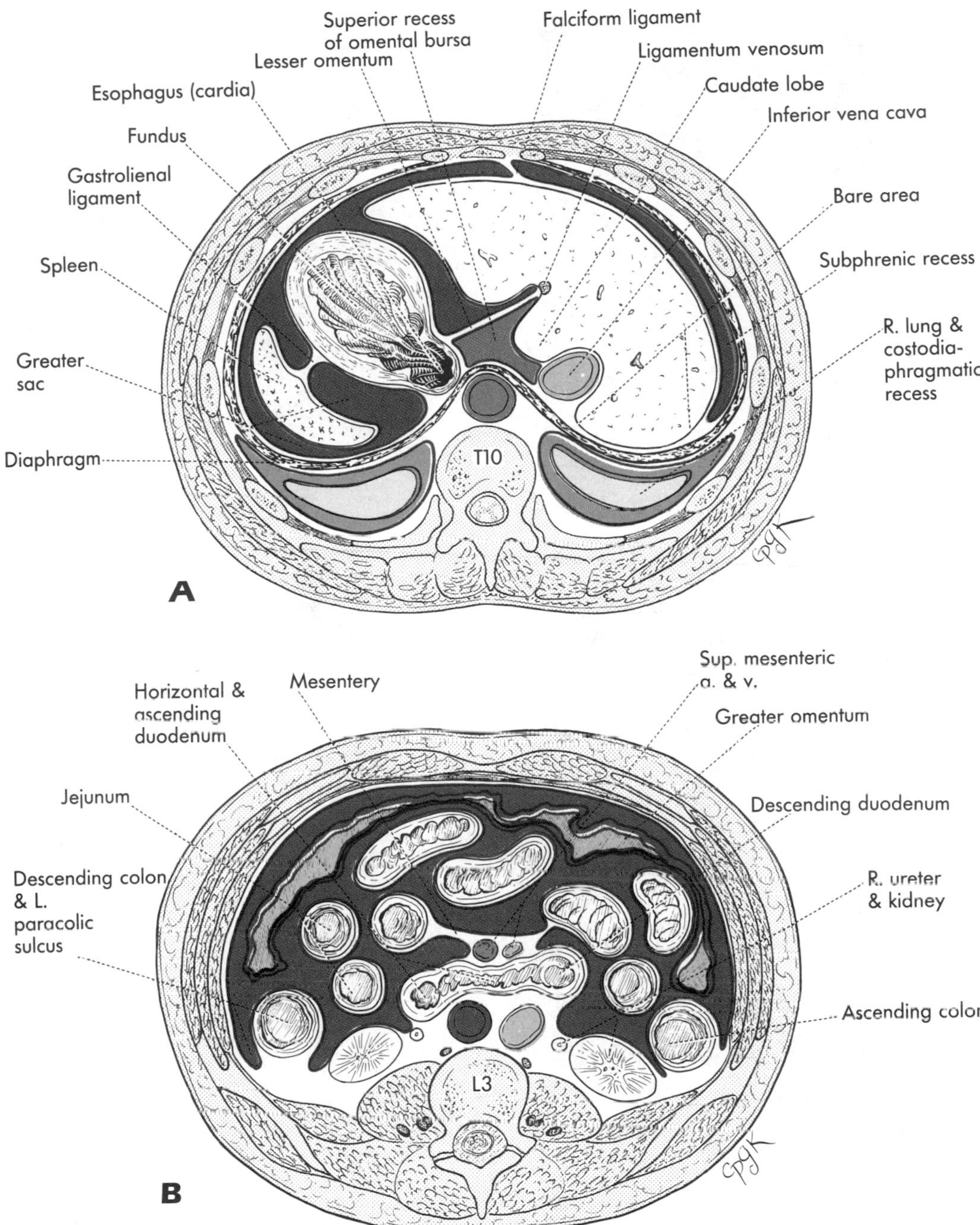

FIGURE 23-27.
Schematic transverse sections at the level of (A) T-10 and (B) L-3. The orientation and color scheme correspond to those of Figure 23-21.

23-28*C*). The median plane and the horizontal plane across the umbilicus (usually the supracristal plane) divide the abdomen into right and left *upper quadrants* and right and left *lower quadrants*.

An alternative method divides the abdomen into nine **regions** by two sagittal and two horizontal planes (see Fig. 23-28*D*). The sagittal planes are in the right and left midclavicular lines, and the horizontal planes are the transpyloric and intertubercular planes.

Superiorly, sheltered by the costal cartilages, are the right and left *hypochondriac regions* extending beneath the diaphragm; between them, bounded by the costal margins and the transpyloric plane, is the *epigastrium*. The middle zone of the abdomen is made up of the *umbilical region* in the center, with the right and left *lateral regions* in the flanks. Inferiorly, the *pubic region* is in the center with each *inguinal region*, limited below by the inguinal folds, on each side. Alternative names are still in use for the re-

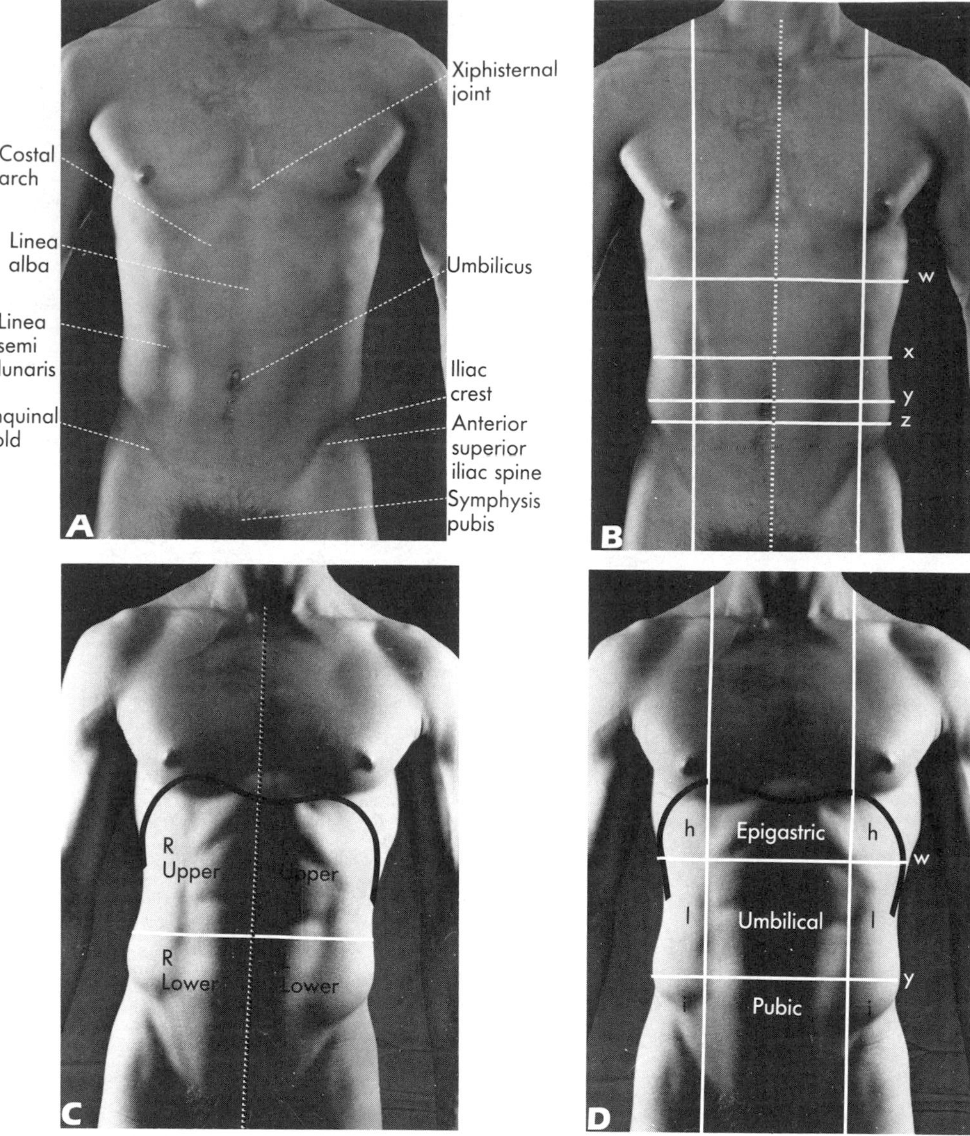

FIGURE 23-28.
Surface landmarks and regions on the anterior abdominal wall: (A) surface landmarks; (B) lines and planes: The median plane is indicated by a *fine, interrupted line*, and the midclavicular or lateral planes are indicated by *solid vertical lines* (*w*, transpyloric plane; *x*, subcostal plane; *y*, supracristal plane; *z*, intertubercular plane), (C) quadrants; (D) regions: *h*, hypochondrium; *l*, lumbar region; *i*, inguinal region.

gions in this lower zone: the pubic region is also known as the *hypogastrium* and the inguinal regions as the *iliac fossae*.

Named parts of the abdomen not usually recognized as clearly delimited regions are the flank (latus), loin (lumbus), and groin (inguen). In general, the *flank* is the anterolateral part of the abdominal wall, including the lateral region between the thoracic cage and the bony pelvis; the *loin* is the posterolateral part in the same area, including the paraspinal musculature; and the *groin* is the meeting point of the abdomen and the thigh along the inguinal fold.

Contents of the Abdominal Regions

Of the abdominal organs, only the liver, the duodenum, and the pancreas are relatively fixed. The location of most other abdominal viscera is rather variable. Nevertheless, some idea of the usual location of the major abdominal organs is valuable to both the anatomist and the clinician.

The *right hypochondrium* is filled by the liver (see Fig. 23-12). For this reason, the region is dull to percussion. The *left hypochondrium* contains the fundus of the stomach, which is usually full of air (see Fig. 23-12). Consequently, the percussion tone in the left hypochondrium is usually resonant. The spleen is located quite far posteriorly in the left hypochondrium, and it may be mapped out there by percussion as a dull area (see Fig. 23-13). The *epigastrium* is crossed obliquely by the liver and contains a portion of the stomach, as well as part of the pancreas (see Fig. 23-12). The right and left *lateral regions* contain the ascending and descending colon, respectively (see Fig. 23-12). With some experience the lower poles of the kidneys may be identified here by bimanual palpation (see Fig. 23-13). The *umbilical region* is filled with coils of small intestine and usually contains also the transverse colon and the greater omentum. In the *right inguinal region* are the cecum and the root of the appendix, and in the *left inguinal region* is the sigmoid colon. Into the *pubic region* rises the full bladder and the pregnant uterus. When these organs are empty, the pubic region, or hypogastrium, contains small bowel. It is through this region that the uterus and ovaries may be felt by bimanual palpation.

In addition to giving an indication of the vertebral levels, some of the horizontal planes are useful guides to the following organs: not only the pylorus, but also the fundus of the gallbladder lies in the transpyloric plane. The hilum of the right kidney is usually just inferior, and the hilum of the left kidney is just superior, to the transpyloric plane. This plane also identifies the inferior tip of the spinal cord. In the subcostal plane lies the horizontal part of the duodenum, and the supracristal plane is a good guide to the bifurcation of the abdominal aorta.

Situs Inversus

In perhaps one of 5,000 to 20,000 persons, the disposition of the abdominal viscera is the mirror image of that just recounted: the stomach runs from right to left, the liver is largely on the left side, the cecum and appendix are on the left, and so forth. This is known as *situs inversus viscerum*. Either the thoracic or the abdominal organs alone may exhibit situs inversus, but commonly both do together. In the absence of knowledge of the presence of the condition, faulty diagnosis and even operative approaches on the wrong side may occur, for in situs inversus, the pain from a diseased appendix or gallbladder may be localized by the patient either on the left side, where the organ is, or on the right side, where it should be.

RECOMMENDED READINGS

Anson BJ, Lyman RY, Lander HH. The abdominal viscera in situ: a study of 125 consecutive cadavers. Anat Rec 1936;67:17.

Baron MA. Structure of the intestinal peritoneum in man. Am J Anat 1941;69:439.

Basmajian JV, DeLuca CJ. Anterior abdominal wall and perineum. In: Muscles alive: their functions revealed by electromyography. 5th ed. Baltimore: Williams & Wilkins, 1985.

Batson OV. Anatomic variations in the abdomen. Surg Clin North Am 1955;35:1527.

Bodin JP, Gabelle P, Bouchet Y, Caix M, Descottes B. The greater omentum: surgical anatomy. Anat Clin 1981;3:149.

Brizon J, Castaing J, Hourtoulle FG. Le peritoine. Paris: Libraire Maloine SA, 1956.

Chudnoff J, Shapiro H. Two cases of complete situs inversus. Anat Rec 1939;74:189.

Demoulin C, Yucel K, Vock P, et al. Two- and three-dimensional phase contrast MR angiography of the abdomen. J Comput Assist Tomogr 1990;14:779.

Firor HV, Harris VJ. Rotational abnormalities of the gut: re-emphasis of a neglected facet, isolated incomplete rotation of the duodenum. Am J Roentgenol 1974;120:315.

Flint MM, Gudgell J. Electromyographic study of abdominal muscular activity during exercise. Res Q, 1965;36:29.

Hollinshead WH. Anatomy for surgeons: vol 2, the thorax, abdomen, and pelvis. 2nd ed. New York: Harper & Row, 1971.

Huntington GS. The anatomy of the human peritoneum and abdominal cavity considered from the standpoint of development and comparative anatomy. Philadelphia: Lea Brothers, 1903.

Jackson CM. On the developmental topography of the thoracic and abdominal viscera. Anat Rec 1909;3:361.

Johnson D, Dixon AK, Abrahams PH. The abdominal subcutaneous tissue: computed tomographic, magnetic resonance, and anatomical observations. Clin Anat 1996;9:19.

Juskiewenski S, Guitard J, Vaysse PH, Fourtanier G, Moscovici J. Anomalies of rotation and fixation of the primitive midgut. Anat Clin 1981;3:107.

Krupski WC, Sumchai A, Effeney DJ, Ehrenfeld WK. The importance of abdominal wall collateral blood vessels: planning incisions and obtaining arteriography. Arch Surg 1984;119:854.

MacConaill MA, Basmajian JV. Thoraco-abdominal wall. In: Muscles and movements: a basis for human kinesiology. Baltimore: Williams & Wilkins, 1969.

McVay CB, Anson BF. Aponeurotic and fascial continuities in the abdomen, pelvis and thigh. Anat Rec 1940;76:213.

Milloy FJ, Anson BJ. The rectus abdominis muscle and the epigastric arteries. Surg Obstet Gynecol 1960;110:293.

Moody RO. The position of the abdominal viscera in healthy, young British and American adults. J Anat 1927;61:223.

Naylor CD, McCormack DG, Sullivan SN. The midclavicular line: a wandering landmark. Can Med Assoc J 1987;136:48.

Quinn TH, Annibali R, Dalley AF II, Fitzgibbons RJ Jr. Dissection of the anterior abdominal wall and the deep inguinal region from a laparoscopic perspective. Clin Anat 1995;8:245.

Rizk NN. A new description of the anterior abdominal wall in man and mammals. J Anat 1980;131:373.

Taylor GI, Watterson PA, Zelt RG. The vascular anatomy of the anterior abdominal wall: the basis for flap design. Perspect Plast Surg 1991;2:1.

Tobin CE, Benjamin JA. Anatomic and clinical re-evaluation of Camper's, Scarpa's and Colles' fasciae. Surg Gynecol Obstet 1949;88:545.

Waters RL, Morris JM. Effect of spinal supports on the electrical activity of muscles of the trunk. J Bone Joint Surg Am 1970;52:51.

Hollinshead's Textbook of Anatomy, by Cornelius Rosse and
Penelope Gaddum-Rosse.
Lippincott-Raven Publishers, Philadelphia, © 1997.

CHAPTER 24

The Gut and its Derivatives

This chapter deals with the stomach and intestine, the spleen, the liver, the gallbladder, and the pancreas. Before discussing the anatomy of the individual viscera, it will be useful to gain an overall appreciation of the developmental relations between portions of the digestive tract and to understand the system of their blood supply, lymph drainage, and innervation. This can be done quite profitably as an introduction to the anatomy of these organs in view of the survey of abdominal contents presented in the preceding chapter.

Developmental Considerations

It is explained in Chapter 23 which parts of the alimentary canal are derived from the foregut, midgut, and hindgut. The general patterns of blood and nerve supply of the gut and its derivatives are best described by relating them to these three subdivisions of the primitive gut.

Blood is supplied to the primitive gut by a number of vitelline arteries and is drained by the vitelline veins. The **vitelline arteries** are ventral branches of the aorta. Three of the vitelline arteries persist, one for each of the main segments of the gut: the foregut is supplied by the *celiac artery* (celiac trunk), the midgut by the *superior mesenteric artery*, and the hindgut by the *inferior mesenteric artery*. **Vitelline veins** from respective segments of the gut follow the arteries in the peripheral part of their course; proximally, they all terminate in the *portal vein*, derived from a central anastomosis of the vitelline veins. The portal vein delivers the venous blood collected from all segments of the gut to the liver. After percolating through the hepatic sinusoids, the *hepatic veins* drain blood from the liver into the inferior vena cava. The vascular perfusion of the liver is augmented by the *hepatic artery*, a branch of the celiac trunk, and, in the fetus, also by placental blood brought to the liver by the *umbilical vein*. Most of the blood from the placenta is conducted through the liver toward the inferior vena cava by the *ductus venosus*. The ductus venosus, similar to the umbilical vein, is transformed into a fibrous cord known as the *ligamentum venosum*, which is embedded in the inferior surface of the liver.

Abdominal viscera derived from **intermediate mesoderm,** rather than from the gut (kidneys, gonads, suprarenal glands), are supplied by paired lateral visceral branches of the aorta; their venous blood is returned to the cardinal veins of the embryo and the anastomoses that develop in association with these veins. From these venous channels is formed the *inferior vena cava.*

The inferior vena cava with all its tributaries, the abdominal aorta with its branches that supply the body wall, and the viscera derived from intermediate mesoderm, all are outside the peritoneal sac. The blood vessels of the gut derived from the vitelline arteries and veins, on the other hand, are enclosed between the two laminae of the dorsal mesentery of the gut; those destined for the liver pass from the dorsal mesentery into the lesser omentum. Because of the eventual fusion of extensive portions of the dorsal mesentery to the parietal peritoneum, many of the veins and arteries that serve the gut become fixed to the posterior wall of the lesser sac and the infracolic compartment; by the completion of development these vessels appear to be retroperitoneal.

General Pattern of Blood Supply

The **abdominal aorta** descends retroperitoneally, lying on the lumbar vertebrae. In front of the fourth lumbar vertebra, it bifurcates into right and left common iliac arteries. The abdominal aorta gives off three sets of branches: paired segmental lateral branches to the body wall; paired visceral branches to organs derived from intermediate mesoderm; and three unpaired ventral branches: the celiac, superior mesenteric, and inferior mesenteric arteries. This chapter deals with only the latter groups of vessels derived from the vitelline arteries that supply the gut and its derivatives.

The **celiac trunk** is the artery of the foregut. It originates from the aorta in front of T-12 vertebra, immediately below the margin of the aortic hiatus of the diaphragm. The celiac trunk is very short, and it breaks up into three branches: the *common hepatic, left gastric,* and *splenic arteries,* all of which run retroperitoneally in the posterior wall of the lesser sac. The hepatic branch of the common hepatic enters the hepatoduodenal ligament to reach the liver.

The **superior mesenteric artery** is the artery of the midgut. It arises from the aorta only a little below the celiac, in front of L-1 vertebra. At its origin, it is behind the pancreas, and on its way to enter the root of the mesentery, it passes through the pancreas and crosses in front of the horizontal portion of the duodenum. Its branches to the jejunum and ileum are in the mesentery, those to the ascending colon behind the peritoneum of the infracolic compartment, and those to the transverse colon in the transverse mesocolon.

The **inferior mesenteric artery** is the artery of the hindgut. It originates from the aorta in front of L-3 vertebra just behind the horizontal portion of the duodenum. At first, all its branches are retroperitoneal; those to the descending colon remain so. Branches to the transverse colon and to the sigmoid colon enter the respective mesocolons; the terminal branch supplies the rectum.

There are extensive **anastomoses** between the arteries of the gut along the stomach and the intestine. These anastomoses are of two types: those within each arterial system (e.g., most branches of the celiac trunk freely anastomose with each other), and those within neighboring systems. (Branches of the celiac anastomose with those of the superior mesenteric, and branches of the superior mesenteric anastomose with those of the inferior mesenteric.)

The **superior and inferior mesenteric veins** are formed by tributaries that correspond with the branches of the respective arteries. There is no celiac vein; veins corresponding to the branches of the celiac artery enter the portal vein. The **portal vein** is formed behind the pancreas by the union of the superior mesenteric and splenic veins, and it ascends to the liver in the hepatoduodenal portion of the lesser omentum. The inferior mesenteric vein usually terminates in the splenic vein; hence, the portal vein drains all the blood from the entire intestine, the stomach, the spleen, and the pancreas. After percolating through the liver, the hepatic veins drain this blood into the inferior vena cava just before the vena cava ascends through the diaphragm.

The **inferior vena cava** drains the lower limbs, the contents of the perineum and pelvis, and the extraperitoneal abdominal organs, as well as the abdominal wall. As mentioned, the gut and its derivatives send their blood indirectly into the inferior vena cava through the liver and the hepatic veins. The inferior vena cava is formed by the union of the common iliac veins just above the sacral promontory, and it ascends along the right side of the aorta, lying in the posterior wall of the infracolic compartment, behind the pancreas and the epiploic foramen; more superiorly, it is embedded in the bare area of the liver.

There are extensive **anastomoses** between the tributaries of the portal system. Of considerable clinical importance are the potential *portasystemic anastomoses* that exist in defined locations between tributaries of the portal vein and the inferior and superior venae cavae.

General Pattern of Lymphatic Drainage

Lymph vessels draining the gut and its derivatives accompany the blood vessels and are interrupted by a series of lymph nodes. The peripheral nodes are close to the viscera and within the mesenteries; the central nodes are in front of the aorta, around the origin of the main arteries (*preaortic lymph nodes*). Lymph from these nodes is drained by two to three large *intestinal lymph trunks* to the *cisterna chyli*, a saclike receptacle of lymph lying in front of the body of L-1 vertebra. The cisterna also receives bilateral *lumbar lymph trunks*, which convey lymph to it from the lower limbs, perineum, pelvis, and abdominal wall, as well as kidneys and gonads. These lumbar lymph trunks are interrupted by a series of lymph nodes located along the vertebrae (*paraaortic or lumbar lymph nodes*).

General Pattern of Nerve Supply

Visceral efferent and visceral afferent nerves reach and leave abdominal organs through **autonomic nerve plexuses** associated with blood vessels. These plexuses are usually named according to the artery they accompany. The *parasympathetic innervation* of the foregut and midgut is furnished by the vagi; that of the hindgut by the pelvic splanchnic nerves derived from S-2 to S-4 segments of the spinal cord. *Sympathetic innervation* of all abdominal and pelvic viscera is provided by the lower thoracic and upper lumbar segments of the spinal cord. Both sympathetic and parasympathetic nerves contain visceral efferents and visceral afferents.

Synaptic relay of parasympathetic efferents occurs in small *intramural* or *enteric ganglia* of the organs they serve; synaptic relay of sympathetic efferents occurs in *collateral ganglia* located on the aorta, chiefly at the origin of the three main vessels (celiac and superior and inferior mesenteric, as well as smaller *aortic* ganglia).

Parasympathetic activity stimulates glandular secretions and peristalsis and causes dilation of the sphincters. *Sympathetic activity* constricts the sphincters and the blood vessels. Parasympathetic **visceral afferents** are primarily concerned with general visceral sensations (hunger, nausea) and afferent impulses contributing to visceral reflexes. The pseudounipolar cell bodies of parasympathetic afferents from the foregut and midgut are in the vagal ganglia at the base of the skull; those from the hindgut, in spinal ganglia of S-2 to S-4 spinal nerves. Visceral afferents in the sympathetic system are primarily concerned with pain that is induced by tension in the viscera and mesenteries. The pseudounipolar cell bodies are located in the spinal ganglia of the lower thoracic and upper lumbar posterior roots.

The **basic plan** of the autonomic plexuses in the abdomen is best appreciated by considering the sympathetic input into them. After entering the abdomen through the diaphragm, the *thoracic splanchnic nerves* (see Figs. 22-16 and 22-17) commingle with each other in front of the aorta, giving rise to the *aortic plexus*. This plexus is augmented by *lumbar splanchnic nerves*, medial branches of the lumbar sympathetic chain ganglia, which feed preganglionic fibers into the plexus. The *celiac, superior, and inferior mesenteric plexuses* are offshoots of the aortic plexus. Before entering the celiac or superior or inferior mesenteric plexuses, preganglionic sympathetic nerve fibers relay in the celiac or superior or inferior mesenteric ganglia. The aortic plexus, below the origin of the inferior mesenteric artery, continues down into the pelvis and is known as the *superior hypogastric plexus*.

Parasympathetic fibers of vagal and pelvic splanchnic origin commingle with the sympathetic fibers in the aortic plexus and its offshoots. The vagi enter the abdomen with the esophagus, and their branches join the aortic plexus in the celiac region; the pelvic splanchnics ascend into the abdomen along branches of the inferior mesenteric artery.

Visceral afferents of both parasympathetic and sympathetic systems run along with the efferent fibers of each system. The sympathetic afferents ascend through the splanchnic nerves, the sympathetic chains, and the white rami communicantes into the spinal nerves. Parasympathetic afferents from the foregut and midgut ascend with the vagus; those from the hindgut descend to pelvic splanchnic nerves located in the pelvis.

THE ESOPHAGUS, STOMACH, AND SPLEEN

The Abdominal Portion of the Esophagus

Of its total length of 25 cm, only the terminal 1.5 cm of the esophagus is in the abdomen. Entering the abdomen through the esophageal hiatus of the diaphragm, to the left of the midline opposite T-10 vertebra, the esophagus curves to the left and joins the cardia of the stomach (Fig. 24-1). In the abdomen, the esophagus is compressed: its right margin is continuous with the lesser curvature of the stomach; its left margin creates a sharp angle with the fundus of the stomach, which is the *cardiac incisure*.

Relations

The esophagus, together with the most superior part of the lesser omentum attached to its right margin, forms the left boundary of the superior recess of the lesser sac (see Fig. 23-27*A*). The anterior lamina of the lesser omentum continues over the anterior surface of the esophagus, which faces into the most superior part of the greater sac, one of the subphrenic spaces. Limited anteriorly by the posterior lamina of the left coronary ligament, this is only a potential space (see Fig. 23-20). The esophagus is in contact with the posterior surface of the liver and may create a shallow indentation on it behind the left coronary ligament.

The posterior surface of the esophagus rests directly on the diaphragm. Peritoneum reflecting onto the diaphragm from the right and left margins of the esophagus forms the upper part of the *gastrophrenic ligament*. Behind the esophagus, the two laminae of this ligament do not become apposed to each other; in between them the left gastric vessels pass forward from the posterior wall of the lesser sac (leaving the left gastropancreatic fold) and make contact with the esophagus and the lesser curvature of the stomach. The anterior and posterior vagal trunks, derived from the esophageal plexus, lie on respective surfaces of the esophagus (see Fig. 22-13). Their position, as well as the number of the trunks, may vary.

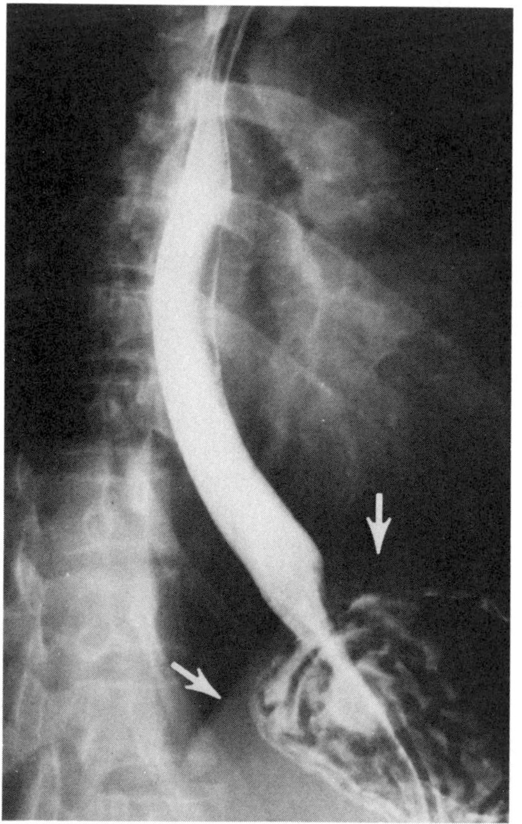

A

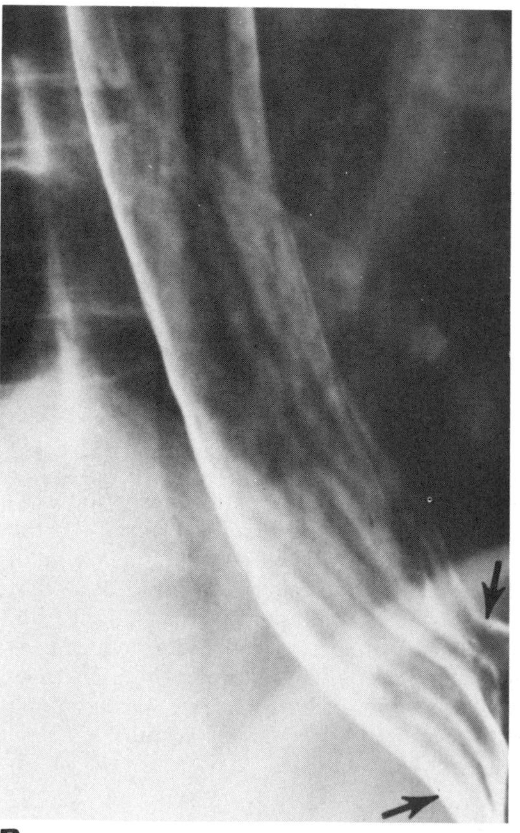

B

FIGURE *24-1.*
Radiographs of the esophagus and cardia seen in oblique views: (A) the swallowed barium outlines most of the thoracic part of the esophagus, demarcated from the abdominal part by the left dome of the diaphragm (*white arrows*). Barium is entering the stomach through the cardia. (B) A close-up view of the lower part of the esophagus terminating at the cardia (*black arrows*). When the viscera contain air, the barium adhering to their lining outlines the mucosal folds.

Stomach (Ventriculus, Gaster)

The stomach is a saclike dilatation of the alimentary canal, closed off from the esophagus by the *cardiac sphincter* and from the duodenum by the *pyloric sphincter*. By its peristaltic activity, the stomach churns and homogenizes the swallowed foods, liquids, and saliva, adding to them its own secretions before propelling the resultant, partially digested *chyme* in aliquots into the duodenum.

The stomach lies largely under cover of the ribs and costal cartilages that form the left costal margin. It is fixed only at two points: the cardia above and the pylorus below. Between these two points, its position and shape may vary considerably, depending on the habitus (body build) of the individual, the fullness and muscle tone of the stomach itself, and the status of the surrounding viscera (Fig. 24-2).

The cardia is located behind the seventh costal cartilage, 2.5 cm to the left of the midline; the pylorus is 2.5 cm to the right of the midline in the transpyloric plane. The pylorus lies on the body of L-1 vertebra, but the cardia is some distance anterior to T-11.

The stomach has several **named parts,** which are not, however, demarcated by clear lines or anatomic features. Its two openings, the *cardiac and pyloric ostia*, connect it to the esophagus and the duodenum; the regions of the stomach adjacent to these openings are known as the *cardia* and the *pylorus*, respectively. Between the cardia and the pylorus, the stomach is made up of the fundus, the body, the pyloric antrum, and the pyloric canal (Fig. 24-3). The upper left margin of the cardia is indicated by the *cardiac incisure*, the sharp angle between the left border of the esophagus and the stomach. The line drawn horizontally across the stomach, starting at the cardiac incisure, separates the *fundus* above from the *body* below. The body is also continuous above with the cardia and below with the *pyloric antrum*, which leads into the more or less tubular *pyloric canal*. The pylorus is marked on the surface of the stomach by a shallow groove in which the small prepyloric vein may be identified during surgery.

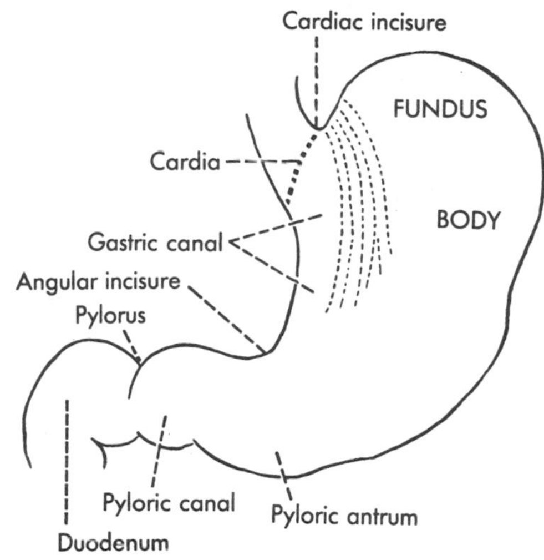

FIGURE 24-3.
Parts of the stomach: The *broken lines* indicate the innermost or oblique layer of muscle that bounds the gastric canal.

The empty stomach, especially in the fixed cadaver, presents well-defined anterior and posterior surfaces that are separated from one another by the greater and lesser curvatures. In the collapsed stomach, the curvatures form

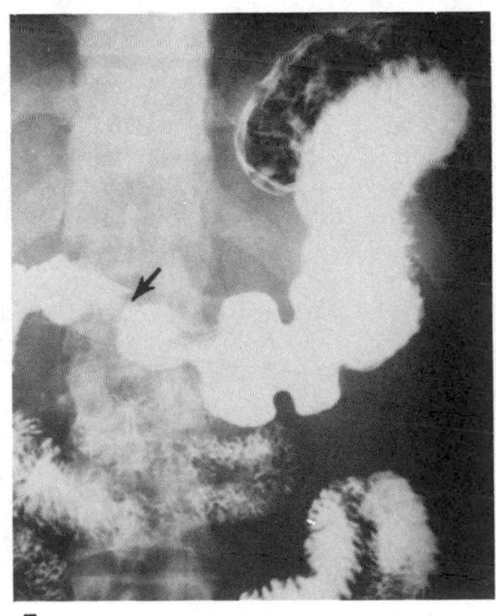

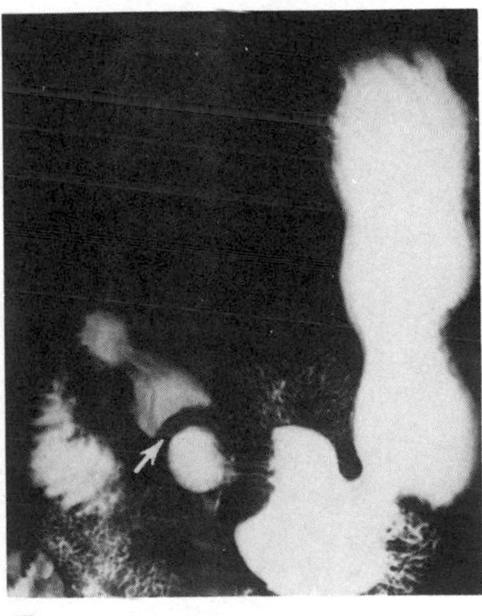

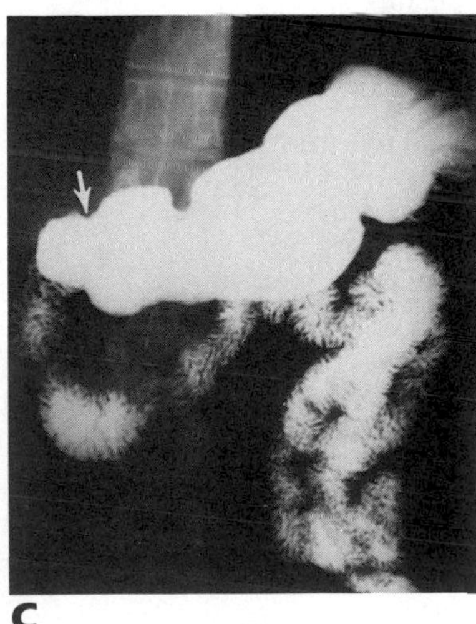

FIGURE 24-2.
Variation in the shape and position of the stomach as revealed by radiographs following a barium meal. In all three cases illustrated, the cardia is concealed by the gastric fundus, which is filled with air; the body, pyloric antrum, pyloric canal, and duodenum are filled with barium. Peristaltic contraction distorts both greater and lesser curvatures. The pylorus is indicated by an *arrow*: or (A) typical configuration of the stomach; (B) a vertical and elongated (J-shaped) stomach; (C) a short and horizontal stomach.

definite borders. Distention of the stomach obliterates these borders, but the curvatures remain identifiable even in the full stomach and are chiefly responsible for the characteristic shape of the organ. The *lesser curvature* is continuous with the right margin of the esophagus. It is concave to the right and faces upward. An *angular incisure* indicates the junction between the body and the pyloric antrum. To the lesser curvature is attached the hepatogastric portion of the lesser omentum; the left and right gastric arteries and veins run in the omentum closely skirting the curvature. The *greater curvature* commences at the cardiac incisure and is convex to the left as well as downward. The various named ligaments of the greater omentum are attached to it in continuity (see Fig. 23-17). The right and left gastroepiploic vessels skirt the greater curvature between the two laminae of the gastrocolic ligament.

Relations

In addition to the omenta, the stomach has many important relations. The *anterior surface*, covered with peritoneum, faces into the greater sac and is overlapped by the left lobe of the liver; the spleen overlaps the fundus. Between the liver and the spleen, the left dome of the diaphragm separates the stomach from the left lung and the heart (Fig. 24-4). Below the costal margin, the stomach is in contact with the anterior abdominal wall unless the greater omentum and the transverse colon have been displaced upward and lie in front of the stomach. The *posterior surface*, covered in peritoneum, faces into the lesser sac (see Figs. 23-21 and 23-27). The so-called *stomach bed*, on which the stomach rests, is made up of retroperitoneal structures in the posterior wall of the lesser sac (pancreas, with the splenic artery along its superior border; diaphragm; left kidney and suprarenal gland); as well as the transverse mesocolon with the laminae of the greater omentum fused to it and, outside the lesser sac, the spleen (Fig. 24-5).

Musculature and Interior

The form of the stomach is largely due to its musculature, which is rather thicker than in other parts of the alimen-

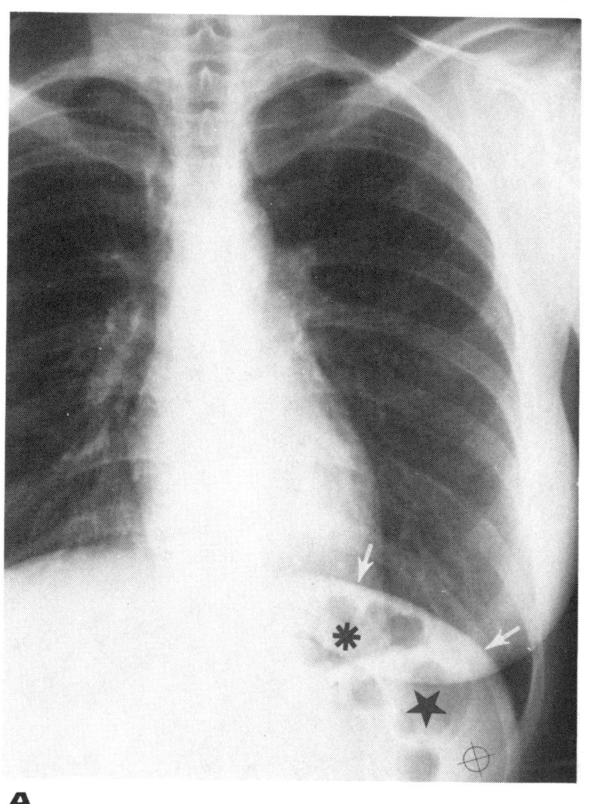

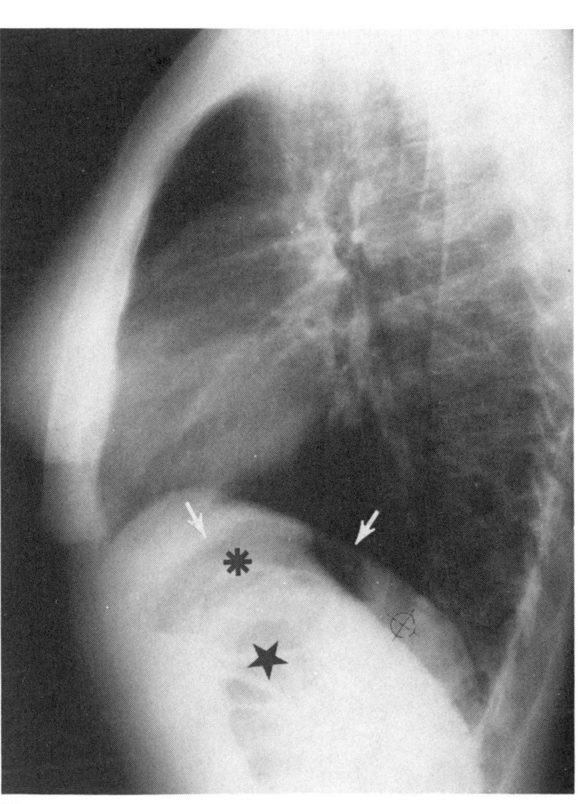

FIGURE *24-4.*
Plain films of the left side of the chest and upper abdomen to show the relation of the stomach to thoracic and some abdominal viscera: (A) anteroposterior (frontal) view; (B) left lateral view. The left dome of the diaphragm is indicated by *arrows*. The gas in the fundus of the stomach (*) is overlapped slightly by the shadow of gas in the left colic flexure (★); the opacity posterolateral to the gastric fundus is the spleen (+). Through the diaphragm, the fundus is related to the left lung, seen as a radiolucent area. The breast shadow is clearly seen in front of the left dome of the diaphragm.

tary canal. The outer, *longitudinal layer* of muscle is best developed along the curvatures and is continuous with the longitudinal muscle of the esophagus and duodenum. The inner, *circular layer* is uniform over the stomach, but forms a thickened muscular ring at the pylorus; this is the *pyloric sphincter*. During gastric contractions, the sphincter is usually also contracted; its intermittent relaxation permits gradual emptying of the stomach.

There is no anatomically identifiable muscular ring or sphincter at the cardia, yet a sphincter mechanism does exist at the *esophagogastric junction*, where intraluminal pressure is higher than in either the esophagus or the stomach. Swallowed, radiopaque material can be seen to be held up momentarily before entering the stomach until relaxation of the cardiac sphincter permits its passage. Similarly, splashing sounds made by swallowed water as it is transmitted by the cardia are delayed some seconds after swallowing. These sounds can be heard by a stethoscope placed over the surface projection of the cardia. Delay or absence of the sound is a sign of obstruction at the cardia. Several mechanisms have been postulated for the functional cardiac sphincter and for the prevention of regurgitation of gastric contents into the esophagus (see Chap. 22).

Prolonged spasm of both cardiac and pyloric sphincters may occur. In the case of cardiospasm, food is held up in the thoracic part of the esophagus, which may become greatly dilated. The condition, known as *achalasia*, is thought to be due to a paucity of parasympathetic ganglion cells in the wall of the esophagus and the cardia. Spasm of the pyloric sphincter causes gastric retention and distention. *Congenital pyloric stenosis*, due to hypertrophy of the pyloric sphincter, is seen in the newborn. Division of the pyloric sphincter provides the cure. In later life, *pylorospasm* may be caused by irritation from an adjacent ulcer or by division of the vagi performed to reduce gastric secretion of acid in the treatment of peptic ulcer. The condition may require division of the sphincter (pyloroplasty), as in the treatment of congenital stenosis, or the creation of an anastomosis between the jejunum and the stomach (gastrojejunostomy) to bypass the stenosis.

Unlike other parts of the alimentary tract, the stomach possesses, internal to the circular muscle coat, an incomplete layer of *oblique muscle* fibers (see Fig. 24-3). From the cardiac incisure, the oblique muscle fans out into both anterior and posterior walls and descends parallel with the lesser curvature. These oblique bundles define the *gastric canal* adjacent to the lesser curvature. Swallowed fluids first enter the gastric canal, explaining why ingested corrosive materials particularly affect the lesser curvature.

The **mucosa** of the stomach is rather thick and velvety. When the stomach is empty, it is thrown into characteristic ridges or *rugae*. These rugae are most prominent

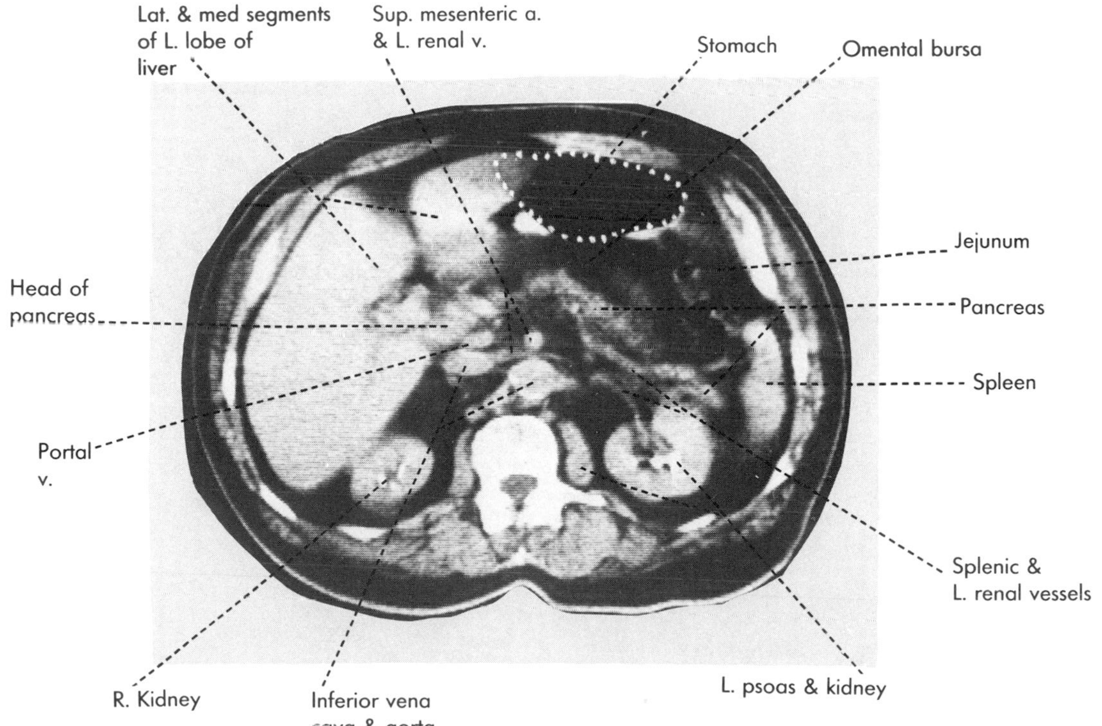

FIGURE 24-5.
Posterior relations of the stomach shown in a computed tomogram (CT scan). The section passes through the lower part of the body of the stomach and its antrum (*outlined*); loops of jejunum are tucked between the lateral aspect of the stomach and the spleen (compare with Fig. 24-4). The section is seen from *below* and, therefore, the left-to-right orientation is reversed to that in Figures 23-21 and 23-27; nevertheless, comparison with this CT scan should be instructive.

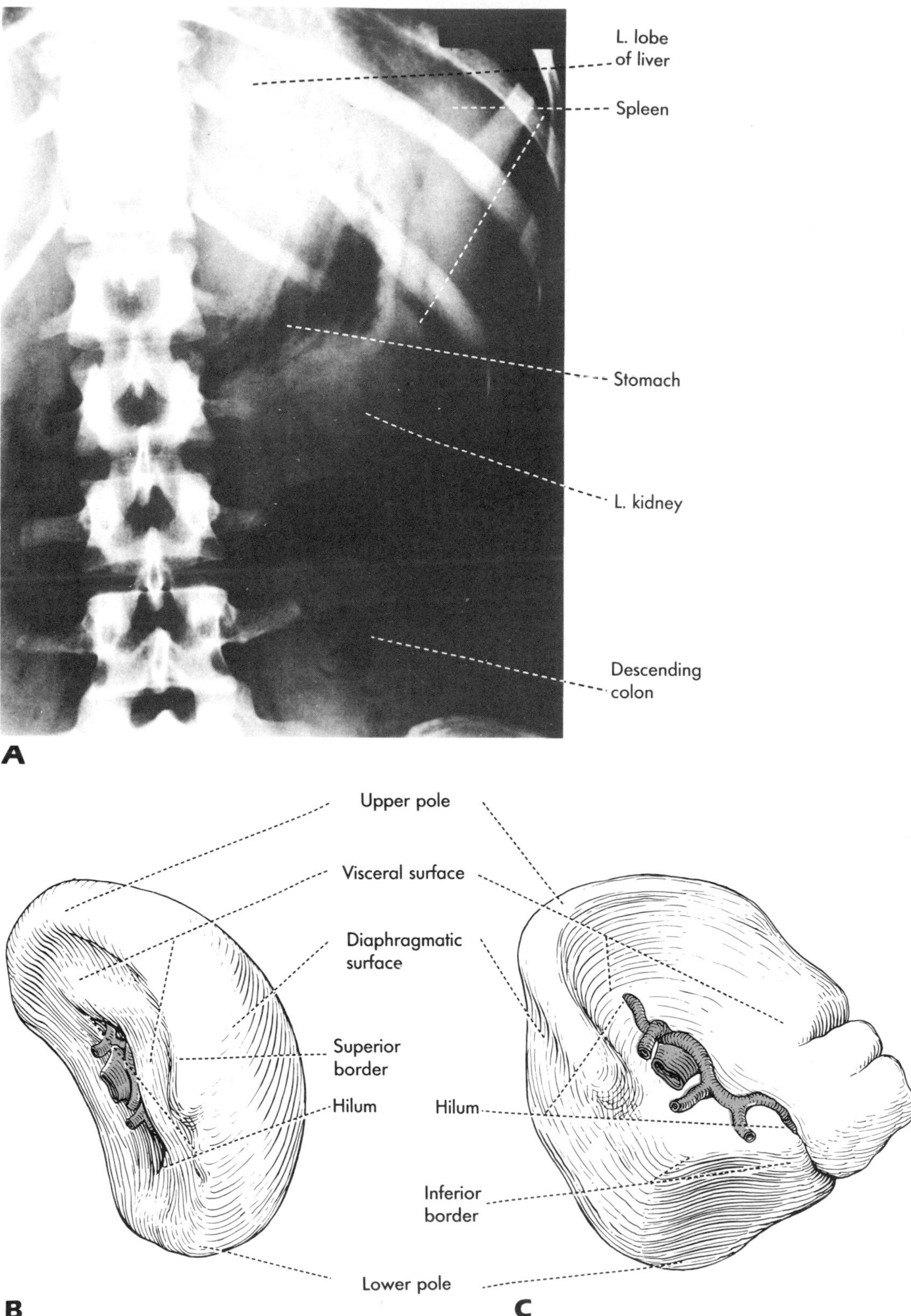

FIGURE *24-6.*
The spleen: (A) the position of the spleen is shown in a plain anteroposterior x-ray film of the left upper abdomen. Note its relation to the stomach and the ribs. (B) The spleen in more or less the position it occupies in the body; (C) the spleen with its visceral surface turned forward.

in the body and fundus of the stomach (see Fig. 24-1); the mucosa of the pyloric antrum and the canal presents a smoother pattern. Gastric ulcers and neoplasms distort the mucosal pattern and can be detected radiologically.

The Spleen

Although strictly speaking the spleen is not a derivative of the gut, it is best discussed along with the stomach because it is enclosed in the dorsal mesogastrium, it is anatomically closely related to the stomach, it derives its blood and nerve supply from arteries and nerves of the foregut, and its venous blood is drained into the portal vein.

The spleen is an irregular, roughly wedge-shaped, lymphoid organ. Functionally, it is a member of the immune system and is primarily called on to eliminate senescent and damaged cells from the circulation, filter antigens and other particulate matter from the blood, and contribute to the immune response against such agents. Its removal, however, does not seriously impair the immune response.

The spleen is located in the greater sac of the peritoneum between the diaphragm and the stomach, sheltered entirely by the ribs (Fig. 24-6). The normal spleen cannot be palpated; however, it may be mapped out by percussion. The spleen is roughly as large as a clenched fist, but it varies considerably in size. It has a rather smooth, convex diaphragmatic surface that faces posterolaterally and a more irregular concave visceral surface that presents the hilum; a superior border, which may be notched, and a more rounded inferior border; and blunt upper and lower poles. The longitudinal axis of the spleen lies along the tenth rib: the upper pole is 3 to 4 cm from the spinous process of the tenth thoracic vertebra, and the lower pole, which is more rounded, reaches normally as far forward as the midaxillary line.

The spleen develops in the dorsal mesogastrium, so that, save for its hilum, it is completely invested with peritoneum, which is fused to its fibrous capsule. The peritoneum is derived from the left lamina of the mesogastrium; the right lamina, lining the splenic recess of the lesser sac, comes in contact with the spleen only at the hilum (see Fig. 23-21). The *hilum* is a longitudinal fissure on the visceral surface. It admits the branches of the splenic vessels, which are conveyed to the spleen in the lienorenal ligament. This ligament, attached to the posterior lip of the hilum, also usually contains the tail of the pancreas, the only organ that may make direct contact with the spleen. The gastrolienal ligament, attached to the anterior lip of the hilum, conveys branches of the splenic vessels to the stomach. These two ligaments attached to the hilum make up the *splenic pedicle.*

Through the greater sac, the spleen is in contact with the stomach, the left kidney, and the splenic flexure of the colon, all of which create impressions on the visceral surface. The lower pole is in contact with the phrenicocolic ligament, which is thought to support the spleen.

The posterolateral surface of the spleen is related through the diaphragm to the base of the left lung, the costodiaphragmatic recess of the left pleura, and the ninth, tenth, and eleventh ribs (see Fig. 24-6). Without necessarily tearing the diaphragm, fractures or violent displacements of these ribs may rupture the spleen, which is highly vascular and rather friable.

> Owing to a variety of causes, the spleen may increase in size by as much as tenfold. When it more than doubles its size, it becomes palpable at the left costal margin, and further enlargement will extend it diagonally across the abdomen beyond the midline. Sometimes, there may be *accessory spleens,* usually located in the splenic pedicle. *Splenectomy* is performed when the spleen is ruptured or accidentally nicked at operation and its bleeding cannot be stopped. Splenectomy is also performed in the treatment of certain blood dyscrasias. In these cases, accessory spleens must also be removed.

Vessels and Nerves

Blood Supply

Because they are derived from or associated with the foregut, the abdominal esophagus, the stomach, and the spleen are supplied by branches of the celiac trunk. This artery also provides blood to the liver, gallbladder, pancreas, and a part of the duodenum, which are also derived from the foregut and are discussed later.

Celiac Trunk. As soon as the aorta enters the abdomen, it gives off the short celiac trunk, which juts forward from the anterior surface of the aorta and breaks up almost immediately into its three branches (Fig. 24-7). The two larger branches, the *common hepatic* and *splenic arteries,* diverge from one another along the upper border of the pancreas; the *left gastric artery* ascends toward the cardia. All these vessels are behind the posterior peritoneal wall of the lesser sac: the common hepatic in the right and the left gastric in the left gastropancreatic fold and the splenic along the upper margin of the pancreas.

The **common hepatic artery** reaches the inferior boundary of the epiploic foramen formed by the duodenum and the pancreas and passes forward into the hepatoduodenal portion of the lesser omentum. Here, it divides into a *hepatic artery proper* (which ascends in the hepatoduodenal ligament) and the *gastroduodenal artery* (which descends behind the first part of the duodenum). Two arteries arise on the right for the supply of the stomach: the *right gastric,* a branch of the hepatic artery proper, and the *right gastroepiploic,* a branch of the gastroduodenal.

On the left, the **splenic artery** reaches the hilum of the spleen along the pancreas and in the lienorenal ligament and gives off two sets of branches to the stomach: the *short gastric arteries* to the fundus and the *left gastroepiploic artery* to the body. Both sets reach the stomach in the gastrolienal ligament.

The **left gastric artery,** the smallest branch of the celiac trunk, on reaching the cardia, leaves the left gas-

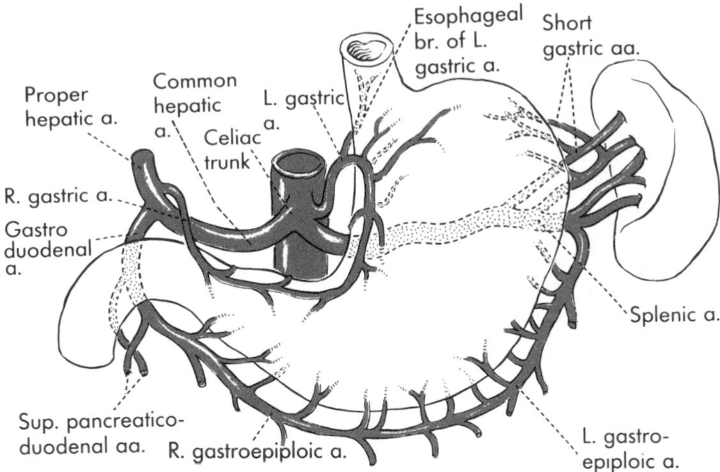

FIGURE 24-7.
Arteries of the stomach.

tropancreatic fold by turning forward onto the lesser curvature of the stomach. The artery runs toward the pylorus in the lesser omentum to meet the right gastric artery.

The **abdominal esophagus** is supplied by esophageal branches of the left gastric, given off in the gastrophrenic ligament before the left gastric enters the lesser omentum. The **stomach** receives its blood supply from two arterial arcades, one on each of its curvatures (see Fig. 24.7). Each arcade is created by the anastomosis of two arteries: the right and left gastric arteries anastomose along the lesser curvature; the right and left gastroepiploic arteries anastomose along the greater curvature. Each arcade gives off numerous gastric branches to both anterior and posterior surfaces of the stomach and also epiploic branches to the lesser and greater omenta (epiploa). Anastomoses between the gastric branches link the two arcades to one another. These arteries anastomose with the short gastric arteries in the region of the fundus.

As many as 15 different branching patterns have been described for the celiac trunk. Angiography is effective in detecting these variations. In 1% of cases, the celiac trunk is completely missing and its branches arise from a common stem with the superior mesenteric (celiacomesenteric). Some branches may arise directly from the aorta.

Veins. All arteries are accompanied by veins of similar names. Those draining the esophagus and stomach terminate either directly in the portal vein or in the splenic vein. There is no celiac vein. The **portal vein** receives both *left* and *right gastric veins*; the *splenic vein* receives the *short gastric veins* and may receive both left and right *gastroepiploic veins*. The right gastroepiploic vein, however, usually drains into the superior mesenteric vein.

All the veins anastomose as freely as the arteries. The noteworthy anastomosis is in the wall of the abdominal part of the esophagus. Here, branches of the left gastric vein, part of the portal venous system, anastomose with esophageal tributaries of the accessory hemiazygos vein, part of the systemic veins. In cases of raised portal venous pressure (portal hypertension), veins subjacent to the esophageal and gastric mucosa become engorged and varicose (*esophageal and gastric varices*) and may bleed copiously.

Lymphatics

Lymphatics in the submucosa of the esophagus and stomach form a dense anastomosing plexus. The clinical importance of the gastric lymph nodes that receive lymph from this plexus is the propensity of gastric carcinoma to spread along lymphatics. The groups of lymph nodes that first receive lymph from the stomach are named according to their location: *right* and *left gastric*, *right* and *left gastroepiploic*, *pyloric*, and *pancreaticolienal nodes*.

Four areas of the stomach have been defined with primary drainage to one or two of these groups of nodes (Fig. 24-8). The largest area of the stomach along its lesser curvature, including the cardia, fundus, and esophagus, drains to the *left gastric nodes* along the left gastric vessels.

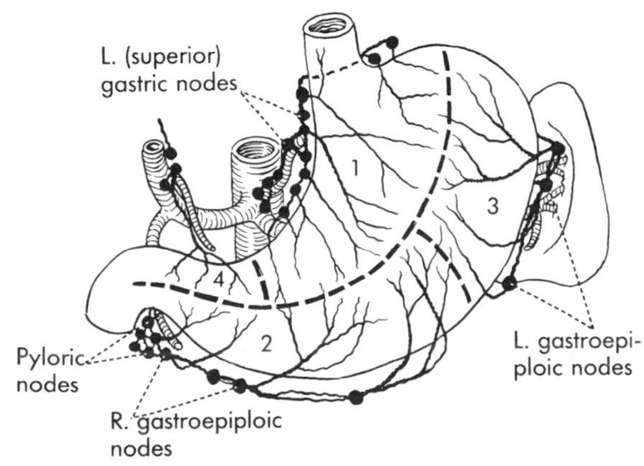

FIGURE 24-8.
The general lymphatic drainage of the stomach: The four zones described in the text are *numbered*, and the major groups of lymph nodes receiving this drainage are shown.

The second area, where carcinoma is the most frequent, includes the pyloric antrum and canal along the greater curvature and is drained by the *right gastroepiploic* and *pyloric nodes,* both located on the right part of the greater curvature. The third area of drainage is along the left part of the greater curvature to the *left gastroepiploic* and *pancreaticolienal nodes*; the latter are along the splenic artery. The fourth area, the pyloric antrum along the lesser curvature, is drained by the *right gastric nodes.* The efferent lymph from all these nodes passes through the *celiac nodes* before it enters the cisterna chyli through an intestinal lymph trunk.

The **spleen** is one of the few organs that is not pervaded by lymphatics: Tissue fluid formed in the spleen evidently freely enters the venous sinusoids. Splenic lymphatics are largely confined to the capsule and the visceral peritoneum of the organ. They drain along the splenic vessels into the pancreaticolienal nodes. It is a peculiarity of the spleen that, in comparison with the liver, cancerous metastases rarely establish themselves in it.

Nerve Supply

Innervation of the abdominal esophagus and the stomach is provided directly by the vagi and through the subsidiary plexuses of the celiac plexus that accompany the arteries. The latter consist chiefly of sympathetic efferents and afferents.

The *anterior vagal trunk,* derived largely, but not entirely, from the left vagus nerve, enters the abdomen usually as a single trunk on the anterior surface of the esophagus (Fig. 24-9); sometimes, however, this trunk is double or triple. The anterior vagal trunk gives off three branches in the vicinity of the lesser curvature: the *hepatic branch* runs through the upper part of the lesser omentum and joins the plexus on the hepatic artery and portal vein; the *celiac branch* follows the left gastric artery to the celiac plexus; and the *gastric branch,* the largest of the three, follows the lesser curvature and distributes anterior gastric branches to the stomach as far as the pylorus. Innervation of the pyloric part of the stomach is reinforced by vagal

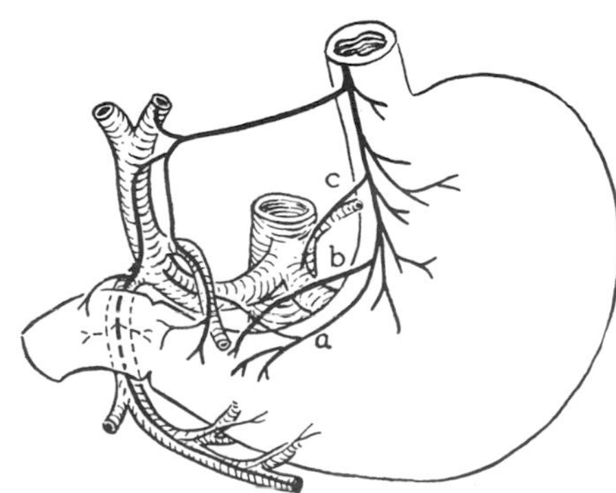

FIGURE *24-9.*
Distribution of the anterior vagal trunk: *a* is its principal branch along the lesser curvature of the stomach; *b* is a branch that runs through the lesser omentum to reach the pyloric end of the stomach; and *c* is a branch running higher in the lesser omentum to join the hepatic plexus.

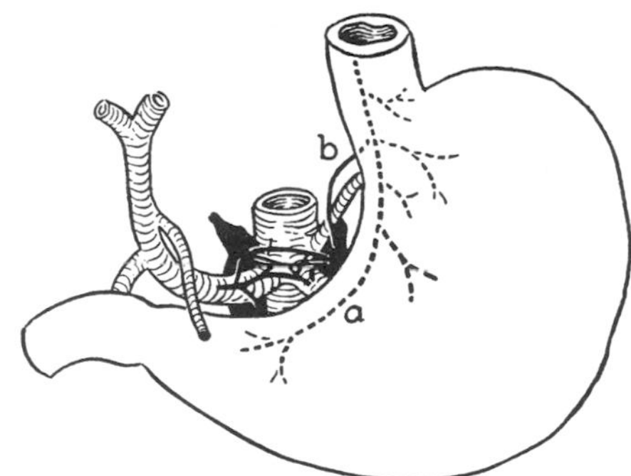

FIGURE *24-10.*
Diagram of the posterior vagal trunk: *a* is its chief branch along the lesser curvature; *b* is its branch to the celiac plexus.

fibers that run in the lesser omentum and along the hepatic artery.

The *posterior vagal trunk,* derived largely, but not entirely, from the right vagus nerve, enters the abdomen on the posterior surface of the esophagus and also runs along the lesser curvature (Fig. 24-10). It usually has a celiac and sometimes a hepatic branch; the continuation of the main trunk, the posterior gastric nerve, distributes its branches to the posterior surface of the stomach.

> The vagus nerves largely control the secretion of acid by the parietal cells of the stomach. Because excess acid secretion is associated with the formation of peptic ulcers (found in both the stomach and the duodenum), section of the vagus trunks as they enter the abdomen is carried out to reduce the production of acid. *Vagotomy* is usually done in conjunction with resection of the ulcerated area, including the pyloric part and a portion of the body, where most of the acid-producing cells are located. More recently, a "selective vagotomy" is sometimes performed in which only the gastric branch of the vagus is cut, thus sparing the remainder of the abdominal distribution of the vagi and avoiding some of the sequelae, such as dilation of the gallbladder, that follow total vagotomy.

Both **sympathetic efferent and afferent nerves** to the stomach are derived from T-6 to T-9 spinal cord segments. These nerve fibers are transmitted by the *greater thoracic splanchnic nerve*; preganglionic fibers relay in the celiac ganglia, and the nerves reach the stomach, esophagus, and spleen along the branches of the celiac artery. The innervation of the spleen seems to be purely sympathetic; sympathetic stimulation produces contraction of the spleen, which forces many of its red cells into the circulation.

THE DUODENUM AND PANCREAS

The Duodenum

The duodenum is the first, the shortest, and the widest part of the small intestine. It is particularly important because, in addition to contributing its own secretions (*suc-*

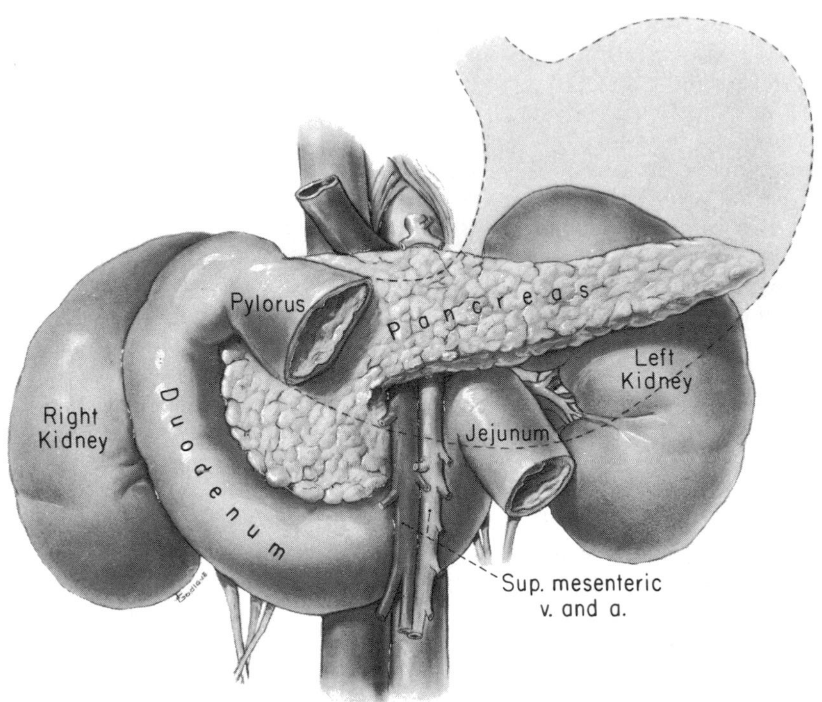

FIGURE *24-11.*
Duodenum and pancreas: Except for part of the pylorus, the stomach is indicated only in outline. The uncinate process is obscured by the superior mesenteric vessels.

cus entericus) to the chyme discharged into it by the stomach, it receives bile and pancreatic juice through the common bile duct and pancreatic duct. Ancient anatomists found the length of the duodenum to be 12 finger breadths, hence its name, which means twelve. From the pylorus to the duodenojejunal flexure, the duodenum measures about 25 cm. Together with the pancreas, which is intimately associated with it, it is the most deeply lying portion of the alimentary tract and the least accessible to physical examination. Both organs have been thrown against the posterior abdominal wall by rotation of the gut and have become fixed there by fusion of their peritoneal covering and mesentery with parietal peritoneum (Fig. 24-11). Therefore, only the anterior surface of the duodenum and pancreas is covered in peritoneum; posteriorly, they are devoid of peritoneum.

For descriptive purposes, the duodenum is divided into four parts: the *superior*, *descending*, *horizontal*, and *ascending* portions, which are also referred to by number. A superior and inferior *duodenal flexure* separates the second, or descending, part from the first part above and the horizontal part below, respectively. Owing to the variation of the angle in the flexures, the overall shape of the duodenum varies, but it always resembles an almost complete circle that encloses the head of the pancreas (Fig. 24-12).

At its commencement, the *first* or **superior part** of the duodenum forms the *duodenal ampulla*, or cap, into which protrudes the pylorus (Fig. 24-13). The rest slopes upward and posteriorly along the right side of L-1 vertebral body. Approximately the medial half of the first part of the duodenum forms the inferior margin of the epiploic foramen, and attached to its upper margin is the free edge of the lesser omentum; to its lower margin is attached the greater omentum. These peritoneal attachments lend the first part of the duodenum a considerable degree of mobility not possessed by more distal portions. The liver overlaps the first part anteriorly, and the gallbladder is in contact with it. Posterior to it is the pancreas, the portal vein, the common bile duct, and the gastroduodenal artery, all of which cross it vertically, being partially embedded in the pancreas.

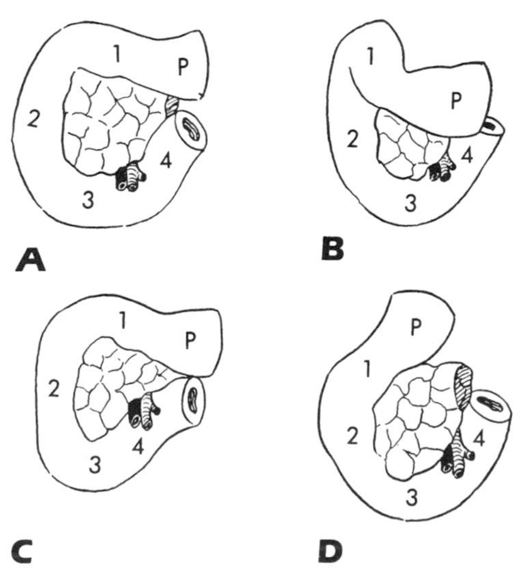

FIGURE *24-12.*
Some variations in the shape of the duodenum; these depend in part on variations in the position of the pylorus *(P)* and of the movable superior part (*1*) of the duodenum; *2* is the descending part; *3* and *4* are the horizontal and ascending parts. These four parts are clearly distinguishable in (A), less so in (B and C) and not at all in (D).

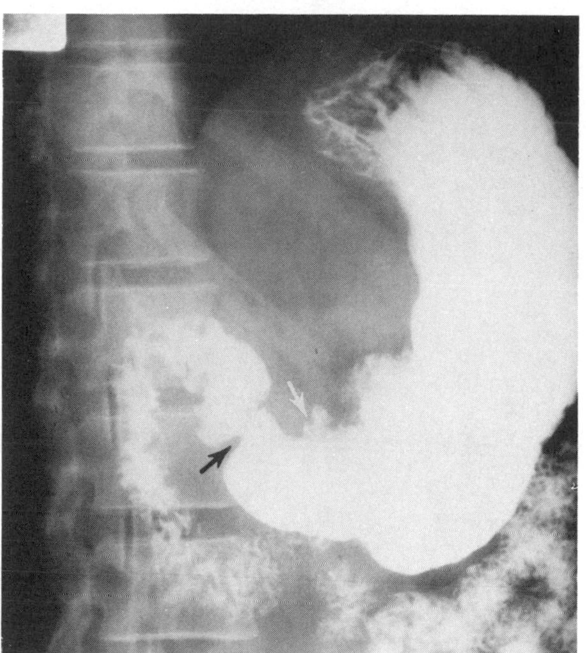

FIGURE 24-13.
The duodenum shown in an oblique view following a barium meal. The vertebrae are seen from the right side; the stomach overlaps anteriorly, the duodenojejunal junction, which is located at a level above the lesser curvature. Note the direction of the four parts of the duodenum in relation to the vertebrae and also the transverse mucosal folds. ***Black arrow,*** **pylorus;** ***white arrow,*** **duodenojejunal flexure.**

The **second part** of the duodenum descends vertically along the right side of the bodies of L-1, L-2, and L-3 vertebrae and lies with its posterior surface on the hilum of the right kidney and its vessels. The anterior surface is covered with peritoneum except along the attachment line of the transverse mesocolon, which crosses the descending portion of the duodenum at its midpoint (Fig. 24-14). The descending duodenum is overlapped above the transverse mesocolon by the liver and below it by the transverse colon and coils of jejunum. The head of the pancreas is in direct contact with the medial surface of the descending duodenum. The common bile duct embedded in the pancreas descends parallel with the posteromedial surface of the duodenum; it is joined by the main pancreatic duct before the two pierce the duodenal wall and open into its lumen at the tip of the *major duodenal papilla* (see Fig. 24-35). A *minor duodenal papilla,* located more superiorly, may mark the opening of the accessory pancreatic duct into the duodenum. These papillae are usually concealed by the circular folds of the mucosa present throughout the small intestine.

The third or **horizontal part** of the duodenum crosses to the left in front of L-3 vertebra and in so doing passes over the inferior vena cava and aorta. In front of the aorta, it becomes continuous with the short **ascending** or **fourth part,** which returns to L-2 vertebra on the left side of the aorta, where the sharp duodenojejunal flexure marks its junction with the jejunum. The anterior surface of both the third and fourth parts is covered by peritoneum, except where the root of the mesentery crosses them (see Fig. 24-14). The superior mesenteric artery enters and the vein

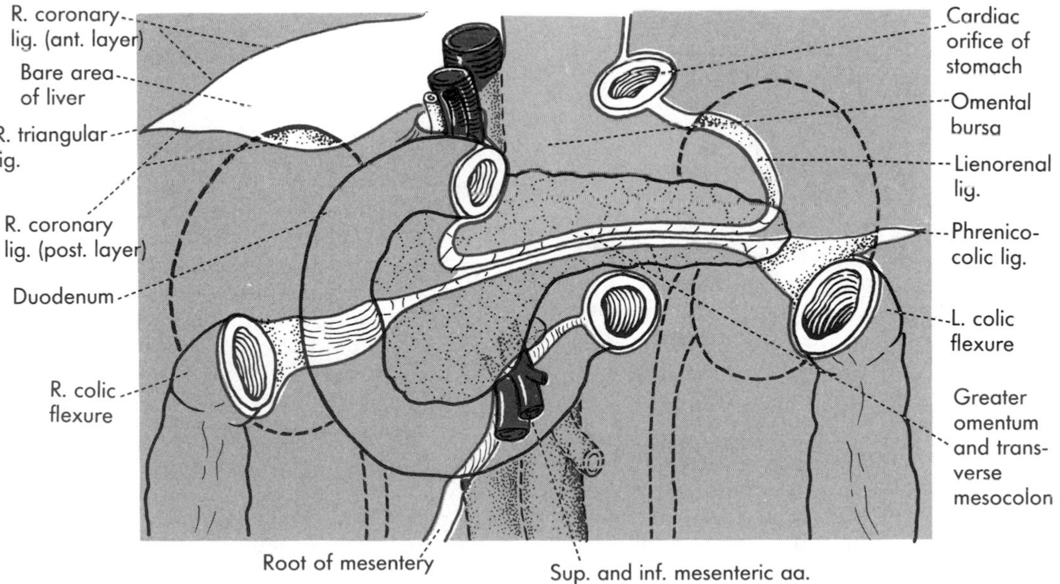

FIGURE 24-14.
Some relations of the duodenum and pancreas, anterior view. Most of the vessels related to the duodenum and pancreas are not shown. The common bile duct, the hepatic artery, and the portal vein are in the hepatoduodenal ligament (cut) above the first part of the duodenum; the superior mesenteric vessels emerge between the pancreas and the duodenum and enter the root of the mesentery.

leaves the root of the mesentery over the third part of the duodenum. Both vessels cross the horizontal segment of the duodenum anteriorly.

Superior Mesenteric Artery Syndrome. The rather unusual relation of the superior mesenteric vessels to the horizontal part of the duodenum comes about because of the rotation of the gut (see Chap. 23). The superior mesenteric vessels form the axis around which the midgut rotates. The most proximal portion of the midgut, represented by the distal half of the duodenum, is carried behind this axis from the right side of the abdomen to the left side. This is the event that lays the horizontal portion of the duodenum across the inferior vena cava and aorta and places it posterior to the superior mesenteric vessels. These vessels may compress the duodenum, leading to distention of the proximal duodenum and the stomach (*superior mesenteric artery syndrome*). The condition is manifest by abdominal pain, nausea, and vomiting, and it is not easy to diagnose.

Suspensory Muscle of the Duodenum. The posterior surface of the duodenum and pancreas is attached to the posterior abdominal wall by loose connective tissue. This tissue plane may be opened up and the two organs mobilized by incising the peritoneum along the groove between the right kidney and the descending duodenum. This approach provides access to the pancreas and the portion of the bile duct embedded in it. The duodenum is secured to the posterior abdominal wall by a fibromuscular ligament known as the *suspensory muscle of the duodenum*, described in 1853 by Treitz. This ligament is variable and has two parts: one derived from the diaphragm, which contains striated muscle; the other from the duodenal wall, which contains smooth muscle. The two parts blend with each other in the region of the celiac artery. It is thought that the presence of the suspensory muscle, which is most constant and best developed in the region of the fourth part of the duodenum, accounts for the acute angle of the duodenojejunal flexure.

Paraduodenal Recesses. Some peritoneal folds may be raised up on the left side of the duodenojejunal flexure (paraduodenal folds), and the pockets, or **paraduodenal recesses,** thus created present a potential danger for the entrapment of a loop of bowel (Fig. 24-15). Such *internal hernias* are quite rare, but when they have to be reduced, the surgeon must be mindful of the inferior mesenteric vein and the left colic artery, which are related to these folds.

Development and Anomalies. The developmental events that establish the topographic relations of the duodenum are dealt with in Chapter 23. Most positional abnormalities of the duodenum are related to malrotation of the gut. Excluding congenital pyloric obstruction and imperforate anus, the duodenum is the most common site of congenital obstruction of the digestive tract. The explanation is the complex developmental history of the duodenal lumen. Subsequent to the formation of the primitive endodermal gut tube, the lumen of the duodenum becomes occluded by epithelial proliferation. Recanalization of the duodenum is achieved by cavitation and resorption of the epithelial core, which progresses parallel with the differentiation of the surrounding splanchnic mesoderm into the muscular and connective tissue components of the duodenal wall. If a given segment remains solidly epithelial beyond a critical period, it will be replaced later by mesoderm and its derivative tissues, creating a stenosis or complete obstruction known as **atresia.** The most common site of obstruction is at the level of the major duodenal papilla. If complete, or severe, the obstruction requires surgical correction in the neonate.

Duodenal diverticula are diagnosed much later in life, and they may or may not be congenital. They are thought to be caused by herniation of the duodenal lining through gaps in the muscle coat where blood vessels or ducts pierce the wall. Most diverticula occur along the concavity of the second and third parts of the duodenum. The majority are found close to the entrance of the common bile duct and chief pancreatic duct into the duodenal wall.

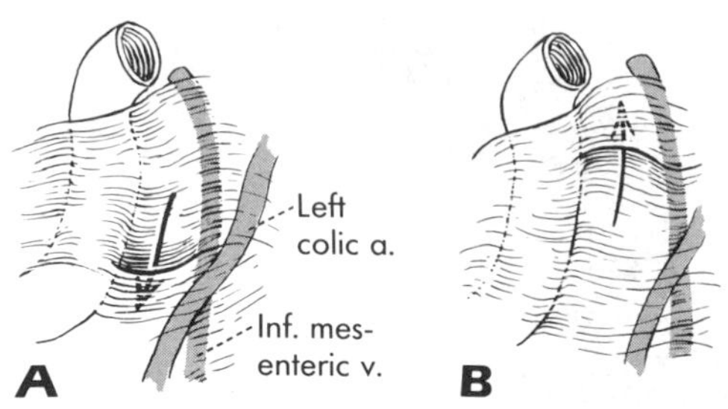

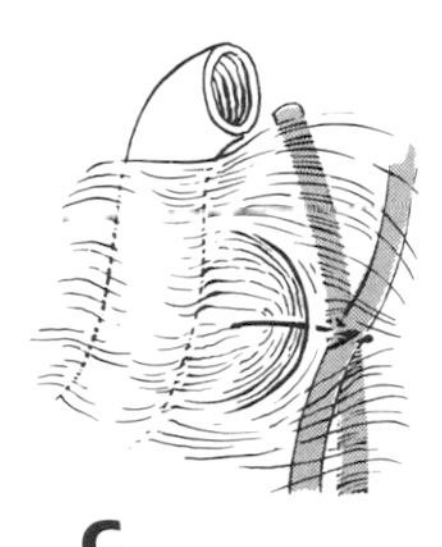

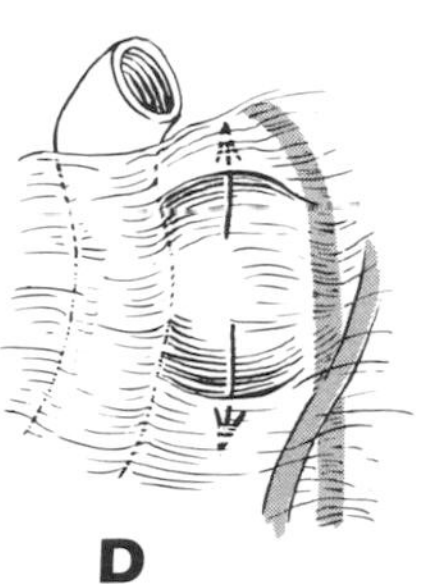

FIGURE *24-15.*
Some of the folds and recesses that may be associated with the duodenum: (A) shows an inferior duodenal fold and recess; (B) a superior fold and recess; (C) a paraduodenal recess; and (D) combined superior and inferior folds and recesses. (These also may be associated with a paraduodenal fold and recess.)

The Pancreas

The pancreas is a large, flat, finely lobulated gland associated with the duodenum (see Fig. 24-11). It produces both exocrine and endocrine secretions. The former, discharged into the duodenum, contain some of the most important enzymes for digestion; the latter, discharged into the venous system, are essential for the regulation of carbohydrate metabolism.

The pancreas is located in the upper part of the abdomen, hidden by many organs. It is not accessible by

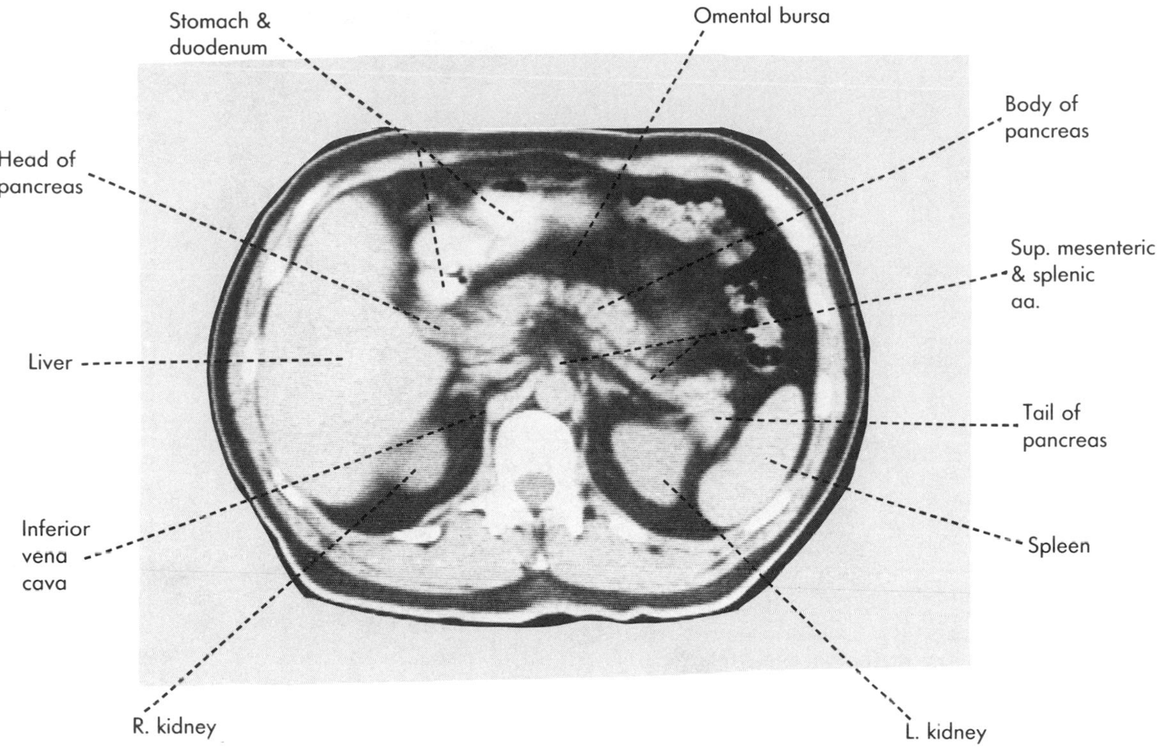

FIGURE *24-16.*
The relations of the pancreas shown on a CT scan section of the abdomen (compare with Fig. 24-5).

physical examination. It lies retroperitoneally, molded on the posterior abdominal wall, mostly behind the lesser sac. The pancreas extends from the right side of L-1, L-2, and L-3 vertebrae, over the median eminence created by the bodies of these vertebrae, with the inferior vena cava and aorta in front of them, to the left as far as the hilum of the spleen. In so doing, the pancreas projects a sinuous profile in a transverse section (Fig. 24-16) that is not evident from the anterior view (see Fig. 24-11).

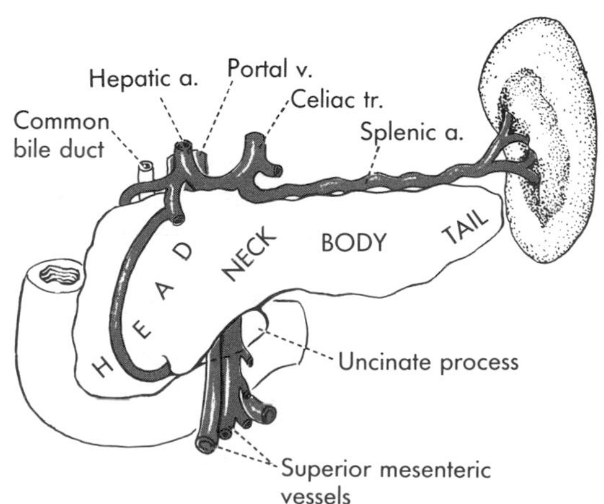

FIGURE *24-17.*
The parts of the pancreas, and some of its vascular relations, anterior view.

The pancreas consists of a head, neck, body, and tail (Fig. 24-17). The broad, flat **head** fits snugly into the curve of the duodenum. Toward the left, the upper part of the head is continuous with the neck; from the lower part of the head toward the left projects the uncinate process. The **neck** is constricted by the superior mesenteric vessels, which lie in the *pancreatic incisure,* a deep groove on the posterior surface of the neck. The **uncinate process** is inferior to the neck of the pancreas and lies largely behind the superior mesenteric vessels. These vessels are trapped, so to speak, between the neck above and anteriorly and the uncinate process below and posteriorly (Fig. 24-18). The **body** lies above the duodenojejunal flexure and on the left kidney, over which it tapers into the **tail** (see Fig. 24-11), which often extends into the lienorenal ligament.

Relations

Both anterior and posterior surfaces of the pancreas are related to many organs. The base of the transverse mesocolon attaches across the head and along the lower margin of the neck and body (see Fig. 24-14). Consequently, most of the anterior surface faces into the omental bursa and, through the bursa, is related to the stomach. Above the lesser curvature, the lesser omentum, and through it the liver, may also be in contact with the pancreas (see Fig. 24-11). The first part of the duodenum is either above or on the anterior surface of the head (see Fig. 24-12). The

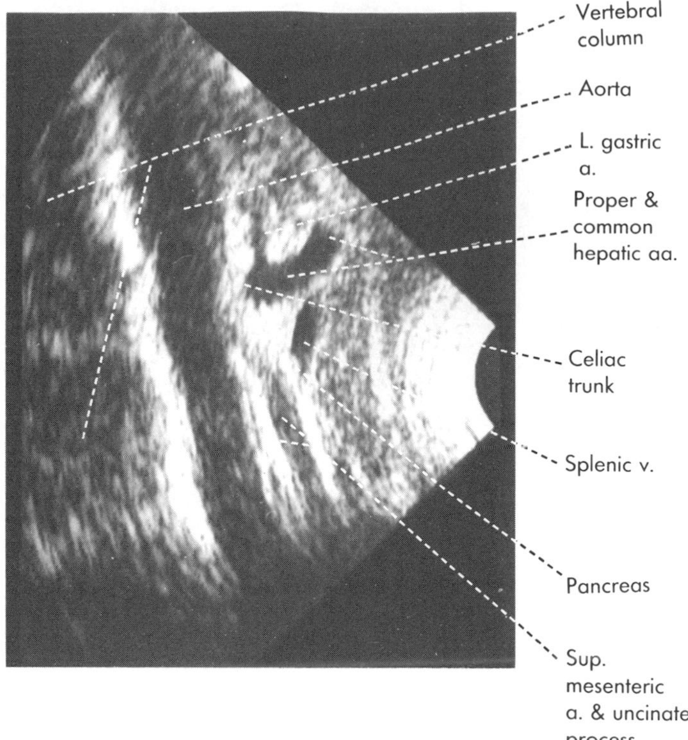

FIGURE 24-18.
Ultrasound imaging of some of the vascular relations of the pancreas. The cone of ultrasound emanates from the generator placed on the anterior abdominal wall on the right of the figure.

lower part of the head and the narrow inferior surface of the neck and body face into the infracolic compartment (see Fig. 24-14) and are in contact with loops of bowel.

The posterior surface of the head lies on the hilum of the right kidney and its vessels, the portal vein and the inferior vena cava. Close to the duodenum, the upper part of the posterior surface of the head is grooved or tunneled by the common bile duct (Fig. 24-19). The neck and uncinate process lie in front of the aorta; the body crosses the left kidney just above its hilum and also overlaps the left suprarenal gland and the right crus of the diaphragm.

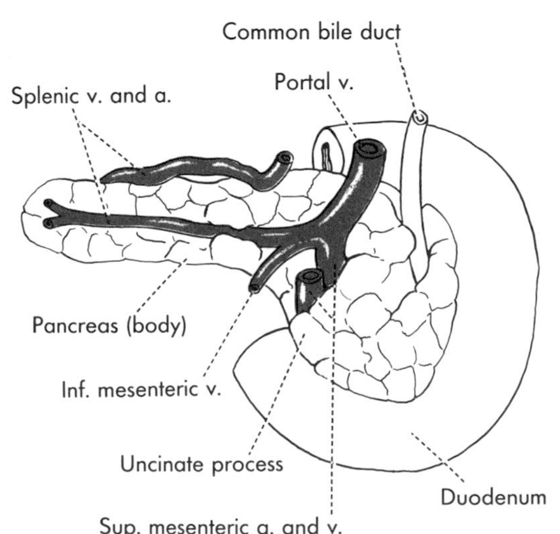

FIGURE 24-19.
Posterior view of the pancreas.

In addition to the superior mesenteric vessels, the celiac trunk and two of its branches are also intimately associated with the pancreas (see Fig. 24-17). The celiac trunk originates at the upper margin of the pancreas and may often be buried in pancreatic tissue; the common hepatic artery runs to the right along the upper margin of the neck and the head; the splenic artery runs to the left along the upper margin of the body and crosses to the front of the tail. The splenic vein is behind the pancreas and is joined there by the inferior mesenteric vein. The confluence of the splenic and superior mesenteric veins forms the portal vein on the posterior surface of the pancreas (see Fig. 24-19). The tip of the tail frequently makes contact with the spleen at its hilum and must not be damaged during splenectomy.

The Pancreatic Ducts

The exocrine secretions of the pancreas are collected by two ducts, the chief and accessory pancreatic ducts; both drain into the second part of the duodenum (Fig. 24-20). The **chief pancreatic duct** runs the length of the pancreas, collecting radicles from the entire tail and body and from the posteroinferior part of the head, including the uncinate process. At the concave border of the duodenum, the chief duct joins the common bile duct and with it enters the duodenum (see Figs. 24-32 and 24-35). The **accessory pancreatic duct** drains the anterosuperior part of the head and empties independently into the second part of the duodenum. Its opening is 2 cm above and somewhat anterior to the joint opening of the chief pancreatic and common bile duct at the major duodenal papilla.

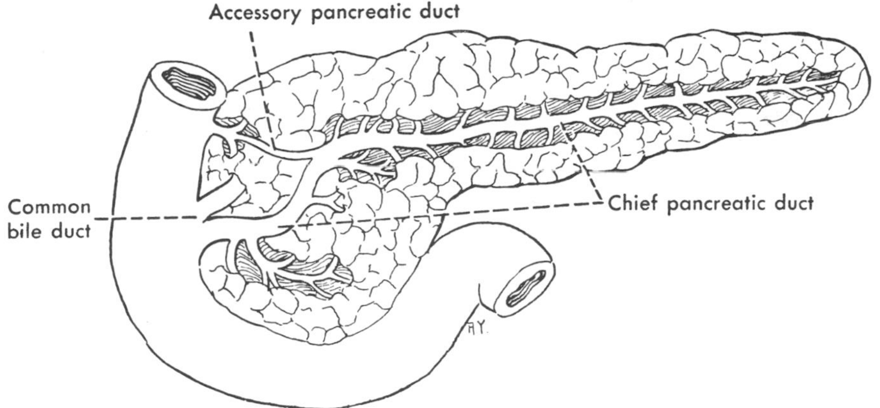

FIGURE *24-20.*
The common arrangement of the pancreatic ducts.

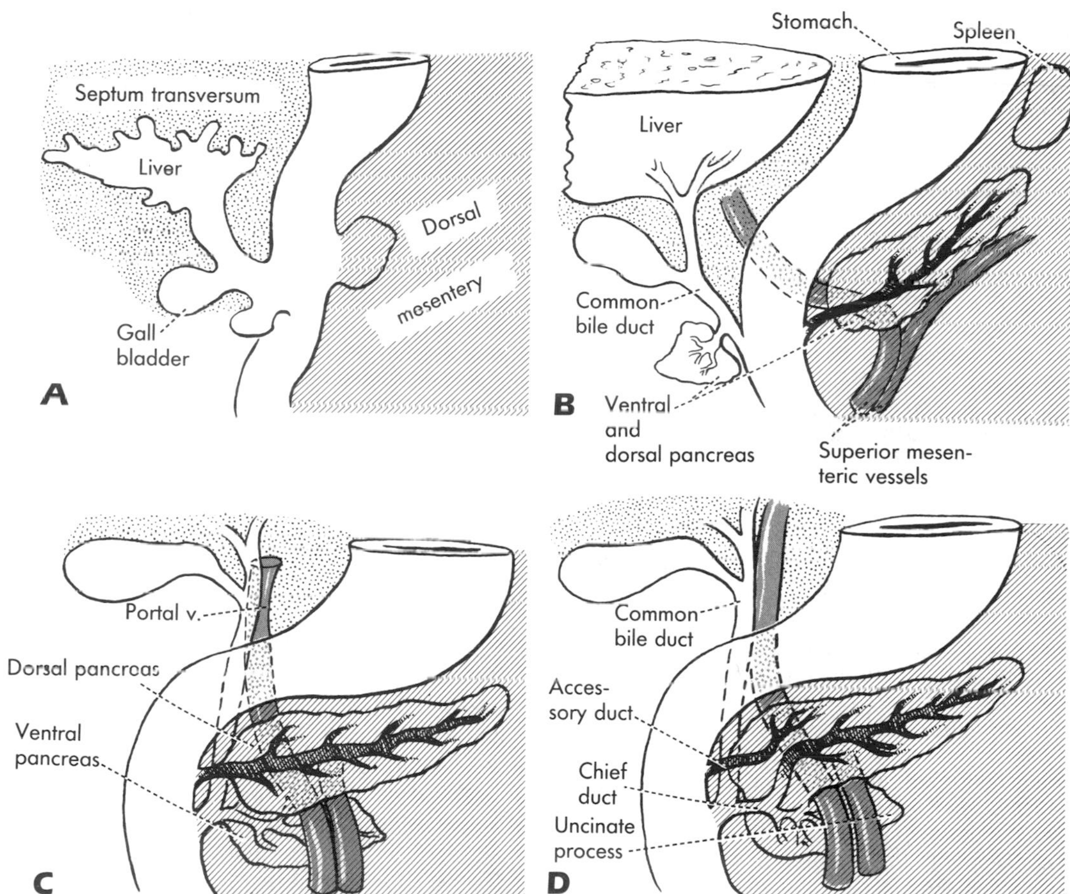

FIGURE *24-21.*
Development of the pancreas: (A) The ventral diverticulum of the duodenum has differentiated into the liver, gallbladder, and ventral pancreas (*unlabeled*); the dorsal diverticulum enclosed in the dorsal mesentery forms the dorsal pancreas. (B) The ducts for bile and pancreatic secretions have been defined. The position of the portal vein and the superior mesenteric vessels is indicated. (C) Differential growth involving the left half of the circumference of the duodenum displaces the ventral pancreas and the common bile duct posteriorly and to the left, trapping the superior mesenteric vessels between the dorsal and ventral pancreas. (D) The two pancreatic primordia fuse; the ducts of the dorsal and ventral pancreas (shown in *black* and *white*, respectively) anastomose, and the chief duct will empty its contents into the duodenum through the duct of the ventral pancreas. The proximal portion of the dorsal pancreatic duct becomes the accessory pancreatic duct.

Development

The pancreas develops from the union of a dorsal and a ventral primordium (Fig. 24-21*A*). The **dorsal primordium** gives rise to the upper part of the head, the neck, body, and tail; from the ventral primordium develops the lower part of the head, including the uncinate process.

The dorsal pancreas arises as a bud from the dorsal side of the duodenum and grows into the dorsal mesentery toward the spleen (see Fig. 24-21*B*). The ventral pancreas arises from the base of the liver diverticulum, which also gives rise to the gallbladder.

The two primordia become approximated to each other by differential growth limited to the left circumference of the duodenum, which transports both the common bile duct and the ventral pancreas to the posterior aspect of the duodenum. As a consequence of this migration, the ventral pancreas is swung against the right side of the dorsal mesentery and overlaps the lower border of the dorsal pancreas contained in the mesentery (see Fig. 24-21*C*). Between the two pancreatic primordia, within the mesentery, are the vitelline arteries and veins of the midgut, from which the superior mesenteric vessels develop. The topographic relation of these vessels to the neck and uncinate process of the pancreas thus becomes intelligible (see Fig. 24-18).

Development is completed by rotation of the gut, which swings the duodenum to the right, and by the subsequent fusion of the right leaf of its mesentery to the posterior parietal peritoneum. Anastomosis between the dorsal and ventral pancreatic ducts rechannels the main stream of pancreatic secretions to the ventral pancreatic duct: although most of the chief pancreatic duct is derived from the duct of the dorsal pancreas, the ventral pancreatic duct forms the terminal portion of the chief duct; the terminal portion of the dorsal duct gives rise to the accessory pancreatic duct (see Fig. 24-21*D*).

A common variation in the accessory pancreatic duct is whether or not it has a patent connection with the chief pancreatic duct and, therefore, can serve as an accessory drainage to the pancreas if the chief pancreatic duct is occluded close to or within the wall of the duodenum. The combined results of several studies indicate that, in about 40% of adults, the accessory pancreatic duct has no patent connection to the chief duct; in about 7%, the accessory duct is as large as, or larger than, the chief duct and, therefore, appears as the direct continuation of this duct in the body of the pancreas. Occasionally, the accessory duct does not connect with the duodenum but drains only into the chief duct (Fig. 24-22).

Accessory or **aberrant pancreatic tissue** may develop in association with the duodenum and less frequently with the stomach, the jejunum, and the ileal diverticulum. A band of pancreatic tissue may encircle and constrict the second part of the duodenum. The cause of this congenital anomaly, known as *annular pancreas*, remains unknown, although several theories of its embryogenesis have been proposed.

The endocrine cells of the pancreas, which form the *pancreatic islets*, are believed to differentiate and sequestrate from the acinar cells of the organ quite early in development. Failure of some of the acini of the exocrine pancreas to connect during development with the duct system may give rise to *congenital pancreatic cysts*.

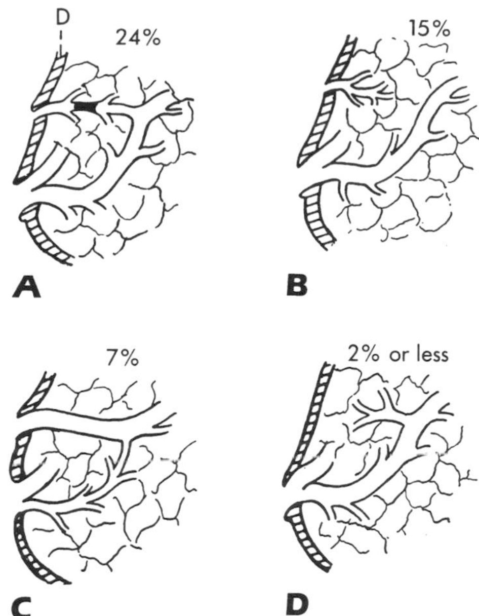

FIGURE *24-22.*
Variations in the duct system of the pancreas: The duodenal wall is *shaded* and the duodenal lumen is on the *left* of each figure: (A) occlusion of the accessory duct; (B) discontinuity between the two ducts; (C) so-called inversion of the ducts, in which the accessory duct is larger; and (D) absence of the duodenal end of the accessory duct. The percentages indicate the approximate incidence of each of these conditions.

Vessels and Nerves

Blood Supply

The duodenum and pancreas are supplied by branches of the celiac trunk and the superior mesenteric artery. The first part of the duodenum has a poor blood supply furnished by small branches of the gastroduodenal artery; the second, third, and fourth parts of the duodenum and the head of the pancreas are served by two parallel arterial arcades located in the concavity of the duodenum on the surface of or embedded in the head of the pancreas. The arcades are fed from above by branches of the gastroduodenal artery and from below by the superior mesenteric artery. The neck, body, and tail of the pancreas are supplied by the splenic artery.

The **first part of the duodenum** is supplied by the *supraduodenal* and *retroduodenal arteries*, branches of the gastroduodenal (Fig. 24-23). These vessels may be given off by the gastroduodenal artery directly or by one or other of its named branches.

The **arterial arcades,** on the head of the pancreas, are made up of four freely anastomosing *pancreaticoduodenal arteries;* anterior and posterior vessels above, given off by the gastroduodenal artery, and anterior and posterior

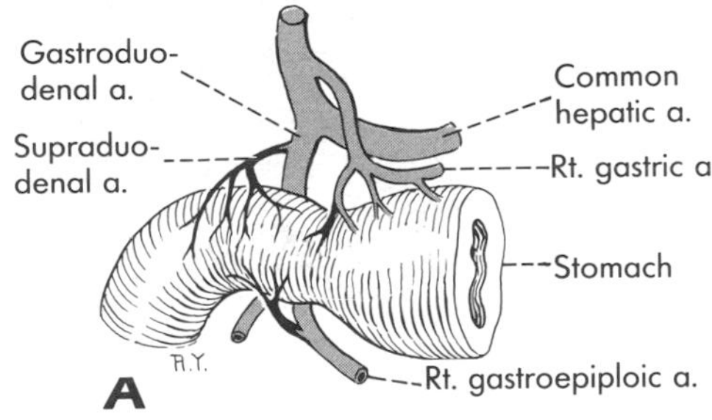

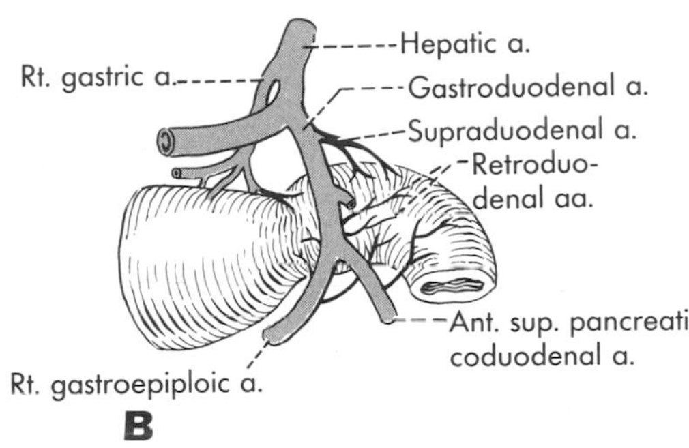

FIGURE 24-23.
(A) Anterior and (B) posterior views of the blood supply to the first part of the duodenum.

vessels below, given off by the superior mesenteric (Fig. 24-21). Either the anterior or the posterior arcades may be incomplete, but for such small channels, they are remarkably constant.

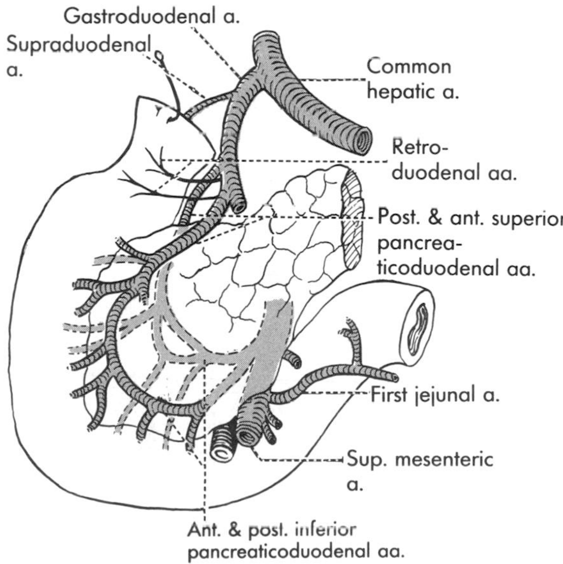

FIGURE 24-24.
The pancreaticoduodenal arcades and the blood supply to the duodenum and the head of the pancreas. The first part of the duodenum has been elevated and turned to the left, revealing its posterior surface.

The *anterior superior pancreaticoduodenal artery* arises as one of the terminal branches of the gastroduodenal artery after this artery has descended behind the first part of the duodenum. The other terminal branch, the right gastroepiploic, has already been traced to the greater curvature of the stomach. The *posterior superior pancreaticoduodenal artery* is given off by the gastroduodenal before it divides into its terminal branches. The posterior superior pancreaticoduodenal artery runs inferiorly along the left side of the common bile duct.

The two *inferior pancreaticoduodenal arteries* arise by a common stem (the first branch given off by the superior mesenteric artery), which divides into an anterior and a posterior vessel. These ascend on or in the head of the pancreas to anastomose with the respective arteries derived from the gastroduodenal. Both anterior and posterior arcades give off branches into the head of the pancreas and a series of straight vessels to the second, third, and fourth parts of the duodenum. The blood supply of the fourth part and that of the duodenojejunal flexure is augmented by duodenal branches of the *superior mesenteric artery* and the first *jejunal artery*.

The rest of the pancreas beyond the head is supplied by a series of **pancreatic branches** given off by the splenic artery (Fig. 24-25). The most proximal of these vessels anastomose with the arteries that supply the head. The named vessels are large and constant: the *dorsal pancreatic artery* is usually given off by the splenic close to its origin from the celiac trunk, or it may arise from the trunk itself or from the common hepatic artery; the *great pancreatic artery* (*a. pancreatica magna*) enters the middle of the body of the pancreas; the *caudal pancreatic artery*, or arteries to the tail, is from a branch of the splenic or from the left gastroepiploic artery. Numerous other splenic branches to the pancreas anastomose freely with other pancreatic vessels. One of these anastomotic arteries is sometimes designated as the *inferior pancreatic*.

The **venous drainage** of the duodenum and pancreas follows, in general, the arterial supply. There are anterior and posterior venous arcades that parallel the arterial arcades and several small twigs from the first part of the duodenum that empty into pancreaticoduodenal veins or the right gastroepiploic or the portal vein. One of these veins, the *prepyloric vein*, was discussed earlier, as a landmark for the pylorus.

The venous drainage of the body and tail of the pancreas is by a variable number of veins that empty into the splenic vein as this lies embedded in the posterior surface of the pancreas.

Lymphatics

The lymphatics of the duodenum and pancreas tend to follow the blood vessels. Those from the duodenum and the head of the pancreas drain, in part, into celiac and superior mesenteric lymph nodes. Some lymphatics also terminate in lumbar lymph nodes. Anterior lymphatics drain also into the pyloric nodes already mentioned in connection with the lymphatic drainage of the stomach.

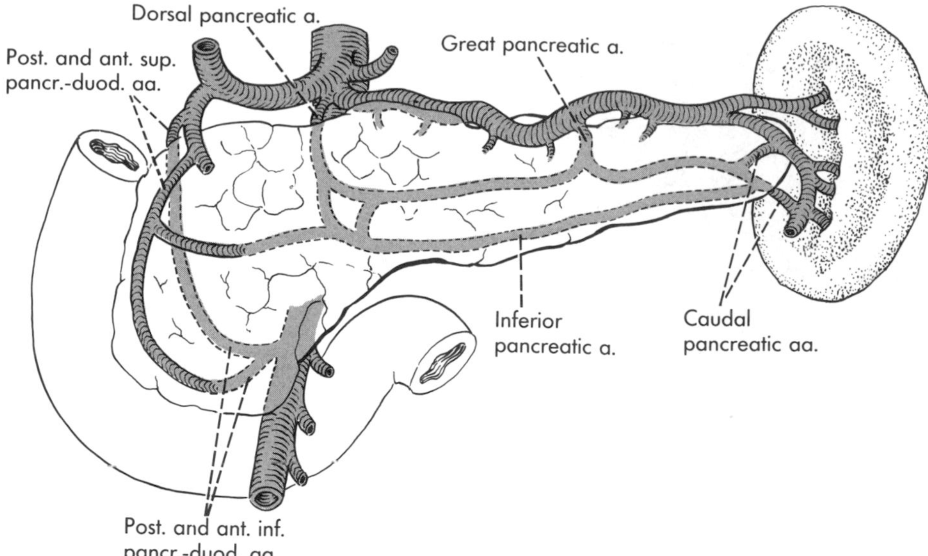

FIGURE *24-25.*
The chief arteries of the pancreas and their anastomoses.

From the body and tail of the pancreas, there is drainage into the pancreaticolienal nodes along the splenic vessels, which send their efferents to the celiac nodes. Carcinoma of the head of the pancreas or the duodenum may, therefore, involve three major groups of lymph nodes: celiac, superior mesenteric, and upper lumbar.

Nerve Supply

The nerves to the duodenum and pancreas are derived from the **celiac** and **superior mesenteric plexuses,** which are continuous with each other. The nerves to the duodenum follow the vessels, and those to the pancreas (*pancreatic plexus*) arise directly from the two major plexuses and enter the posterior surface of the pancreas.

It has been claimed that the sympathetic fibers to the pancreas end exclusively on the blood vessels, but that the parasympathetic vagal fibers end in connection with both the acinar cells and the cells of the islets. The physiology of the vagal innervation of the pancreas is not well understood, for although vagal fibers are presumably concerned with some phase of the formation or release of the pancreatic enzymes, the pancreas is largely controlled by a duodenal hormone, secretin. Vagotomy produces no clear effect on the composition or the amount of pancreatic secretions.

The pain fibers from the pancreas run in the thoracic splanchnic nerves and are conveyed to spinal cord segments T-6 to T-10. Pancreatic pain is manifest as a constant severe pain in the upper two-thirds of the abdomen. Pancreatic pain may also be referred to the back over T-10 to L-2 vertebrae. The explanation of this may be related to the somatic innervation by the spinal cord segments of the structures upon which the pancreas lies or to the excitation of the somatic receptor neurons in the spinal cord by relay of the visceral pain afferents.

THE LIVER, GALLBLADDER, AND BILIARY DUCTS

The Liver

The liver (*hepar*) is the largest and most vascular organ in the body. In addition to being the chief site of intermediary metabolism, the liver secretes bile and a number of hormones, synthesizes serum proteins and lipids, and processes not only the products of digestion, but also most endogenous and exogenous substances, including toxins and drugs, that enter the circulation. It participates in the elimination of senescent cells and particulate matter from the bloodstream and during much of fetal life produces hematopoietic cells of all types.

Position

The liver lies largely under cover of the costal cartilages, occupying much of the upper abdomen, especially on the right. It extends from the right hypochondrium, which it fills almost completely, across the epigastrium into the left hypochondrium as far as the left lateral line (Fig. 24-26).

> The upper extent of the liver under the right dome of the diaphragm is readily demonstrated by the transition of a resonant percussion tone into a dull one. This occurs just below the nipple in the fourth intercostal space when the subject is supine and about one intercostal space lower in the standing or sitting position. In the midline, the upper limit of the liver is behind the xiphisternal joint and along the left lateral line, one or two intercostal spaces lower than on the right side. The liver is difficult to percuss on the left owing to the gas in the gastric fundus, which the liver overlaps.

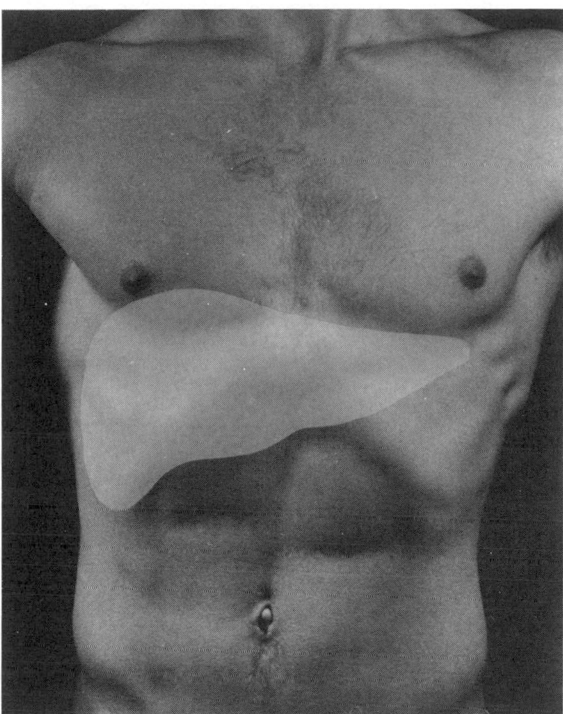

FIGURE 24-26.
The surface markings of the liver.

The lower limit of the liver is sheltered by the right costal margin as far medially as the tip of the ninth costal cartilage, then it crosses the epigastrium obliquely, less than a hand's breadth below the xiphisternal joint; beyond the left costal margin, the lower border of the liver tapers upward into the tongue-shaped left lobe.

The liver follows the excursions of the diaphragm: ascent and descent of its lower edge during respiratory movements may be detected by an experienced examining hand provided the abdominal musculature is relaxed. In the newborn and the young infant, the lower border of the liver extends below the costal margin.

Size, Shape, and Surfaces

The liver weighs 1 to 2 kg, contributing close to 1/40 of the total body weight. In the newborn and infant, its relative size is considerably greater.

The liver is an irregular, wedge-shaped organ (Fig. 24-27) on which only two surfaces and one margin can be defined distinctly: a diaphragmatic and a visceral surface and an inferior margin.

The **diaphragmatic surface** includes smooth *peritoneal areas* that face upward, anteriorly and to the right (see Fig. 24-27) and an irregular *bare area* devoid of peritoneum facing posteriorly (Fig. 24-28).

The most notable features on the diaphragmatic surface are the inferior vena cava and the peritoneal ligaments that connect the liver to the diaphragm. The *inferior vena cava* is embedded in the liver in a deep *sulcus* located in the left portion of the bare area (see Fig. 24-28). This sulcus is usually roofed over by fibrous tissue, called the *ligament of the inferior vena cava,* which may contain hepatic tissue converting the sulcus into a tunnel. The *peritoneal ligaments* are the falciform ligament and the left and right coronary and triangular ligaments, which are described in Chapter 23 (see Figs. 24-27 and 24-28).

The relatively flat **visceral surface**, also covered by peritoneum, is divided into several areas by deep fissures and impressions adjacent viscera have made on it (Fig. 24-29). This surface faces downward as well as posteriorly and is separated in front from the diaphragmatic surface by the sharp *inferior margin* and in the back by the posterior lamina of the coronary ligament (see Fig. 24-28).

The most notable features of the visceral surface are the gallbladder, the fissure for the ligamentum teres hepatis (round ligament), the fissure for the ligamentum venosum, and the porta hepatis (see Fig. 24-29). The *gallbladder* lies in an elongated *fossa* that runs from the inferior margin of the liver in front toward the inferior vena cava in the bare area and leads into the porta hepatis. The gallbladder is retained in the fossa partly by the continuity of the hepatic peritoneum across the inferior surface of it. The *ligamentum teres* continues from the free edge of the falciform ligament toward the porta hepatis, buried in its fissure, which is more or less parallel with the gallbladder. Beyond the porta hepatis, in line with the fissure for the ligamentum teres, is a second fissure in which is buried the *ligamentum venosum.*

The **porta hepatis** is a transverse fissure located between the neck of the gallbladder and the junction of the fissures for the ligamenta teres and venosum. Through the porta hepatis, the hepatic artery and portal vein enter

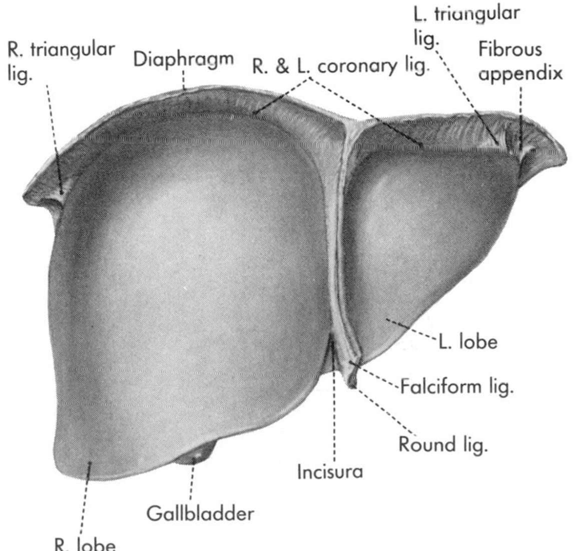

FIGURE 24-27.
Anterior view of the liver and its peritoneal ligaments. (Popper H, Schaffner F. Liver: structure and function. New York: McGraw-Hill, 1957.)

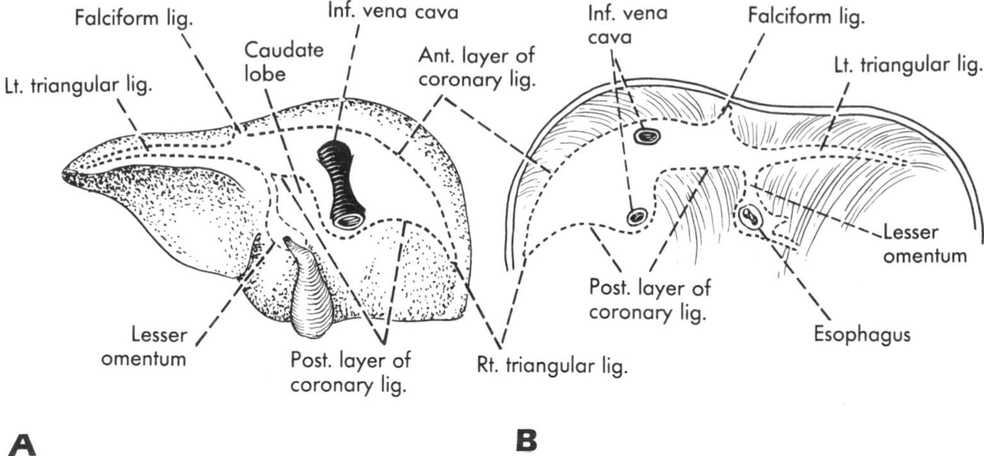

FIGURE 24-28.
Posterior view of the liver and its peritoneal attachments illustrated schematically: (A) the posterior diaphragmatic and visceral surfaces, with *lines of reflection* of peritoneum and ligaments indicated; (B) shows attachments to the diaphragm.

the liver, and the hepatic ducts leave it. Just below the porta, the hepatic ducts are joined by the cystic duct from the gallbladder. Right and left leaves of the lesser omentum, attached in the fissure for the ligamentum venosum, prolong their hepatic attachment to the anterior and posterior lips of the porta hepatis, respectively. At the right limit of the porta, the two leaves become continuous with one another as they form the uppermost portion of the free edge of the lesser omentum (hepatoduodenal ligament), embracing in it the structures that enter and leave the porta hepatis. These structures in the hepatoduodenal ligament are often referred to as the *hepatic pedicle*.

Lobes and Segments

On the diaphragmatic surface, the attachment of the falciform ligament of the liver demarcates the right lobe from the left (see Fig. 24-27). The right lobe, which forms the base of the wedge-shaped liver, is approximately six times the size of the tongue-shaped left lobe. On the visceral surface, the two fissures, the porta hepatis, and the gallbladder define four lobes: the **right lobe** to the right of the gallbladder; the **left lobe** to the left of the fissures of the ligamenta teres and venosum; the **quadrate lobe** between the gallbladder and the fissure for the ligamentum teres in front of the porta hepatis; and, behind the porta, the **caudate lobe** between the fissure for the ligamentum venosum and the inferior vena cava (see Fig. 24-29).

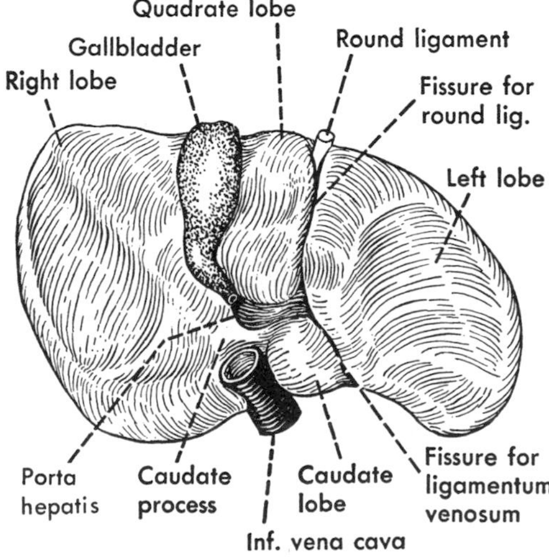

FIGURE 24-29.
The visceral surface of the liver continuous with the posterior diaphragmatic surface.

These lobes, demarcated by surface features, are useful landmarks, but they do not correspond to the structural units or hepatic segments that are established by the intrahepatic branching of the bile ducts, to which the branches of the hepatic artery and the portal vein conform. Although not as well defined as the bronchopulmonary segments, the hepatic segments can be demonstrated by injection techniques and corrosion casts of the bile ducts and hepatic blood vessels.

There are **four hepatic segments**—*anterior, posterior, lateral,* and *medial*—and each segment is divided into an *upper* and a *lower area* (Fig. 24-30). The *anterior and posterior segments* are on the right; they are drained by the right hepatic duct and served by the right branches of the hepatic artery and portal vein and, therefore, constitute the "true" right lobe. The *medial and lateral segments* constitute the "true" left lobe. These two true lobes are of equal size and weight, and the junction between them falls in a nearly sagittal plane, passing through the fossa of the gallbladder and the sulcus for the inferior vena cava. This plane is some distance to the right of the falciform ligament.

There is no identifiable demarcation between the anterior and posterior segments of the right lobe; the fissures of the ligamenta teres and venosum mark the junction between the lateral and medial segments of the left lobe. The caudate and quadrate lobes are incorporated into the upper and lower areas of the medial segment, respectively.

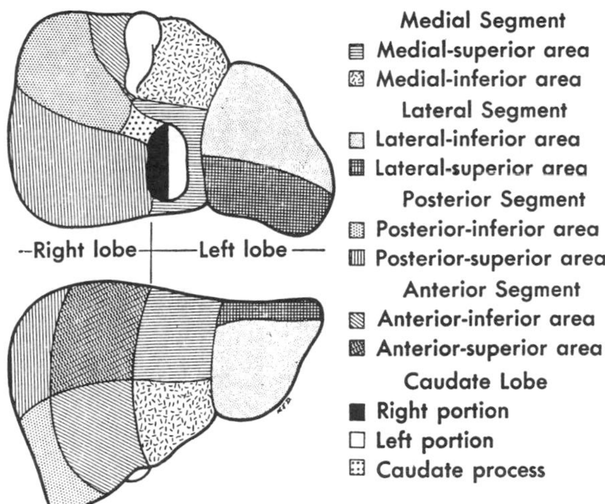

FIGURE *24-30.*
Divisions of the liver, based on the biliary drainage of the organ. The upper figure is an inferior view of the liver, and the lower figure is an anterior view. (Healey JE Jr, Schroy PC, Sorenson RJ. J Int Coll Surg 1953;20:133.)

The caudate lobe, in fact, could be considered as a special segment; it is supplied by an independent branch of the right and left hepatic arteries and the right and left radicles of the portal vein and is drained into both right and left hepatic ducts.

The anatomy of hepatic segmentation is still of controversial usefulness in partial resection of the liver: a true lobe, rather than a segment, must be resected in most instances of partial hepatectomy.

Relations

The peritoneal areas on the **diaphragmatic surface** of the liver are related to the diaphragm through the *subphrenic spaces* described in Chapter 23. Through the diaphragm, the costodiaphragmatic recesses and the base of the right and, to a lesser extent, the left lung are related to the liver. The central tendon of the diaphragm separates the liver from the pericardial cavity and the heart, which makes a shallow impression on the upper surface of the liver.

> The clinical importance of these relations can be emphasized by some examples: A liver biopsy is obtained by thrusting a small trocar and cannula into the right lobe of the liver. After withdrawal of the trocar, a small core of liver parenchyma is aspirated. The trocar and cannula are usually inserted into the seventh or eighth intercostal space in the midaxillary line. Before reaching the hepatic peritoneum, the instrument has to traverse the tissues of the intercostal space, the costal pleura, the costodiaphragmatic recess, the diaphragmatic pleura, the diaphragm, the diaphragmatic peritoneum, and the subphrenic recess. Another example is the discharge of a hepatic abscess: it may burst, not only into a subphrenic space, but through the diaphragm into the pleural cavity or even into a basal bronchus when the inflammatory process fixes the base of the lung to the diaphragm.

Most of the **bare area** of the liver is in direct contact with the diaphragm and, in addition, with the inferior vena cava and, just to its right, with the right suprarenal gland and a small area of the right kidney (Fig. 24-31). The potential anastomoses of venous capillaries between the liver and the diaphragm that exist in the bare area will open up and become functional under certain pathologic conditions.

To the left of the inferior vena cava, the liver is indented by the vertebral column and the aorta; both are separated from it by the diaphragm.

The **visceral surface** makes contact with many viscera, all, except for the gallbladder, through the peritoneal cavity (see Fig. 24-31). To the right of the gallbladder, the duodenum, the right kidney, and, farther anteriorly, the right flexure of the colon and the transverse colon make impressions on the *right lobe.* Between the kidney and the liver is the hepatorenal recess, which communicates with

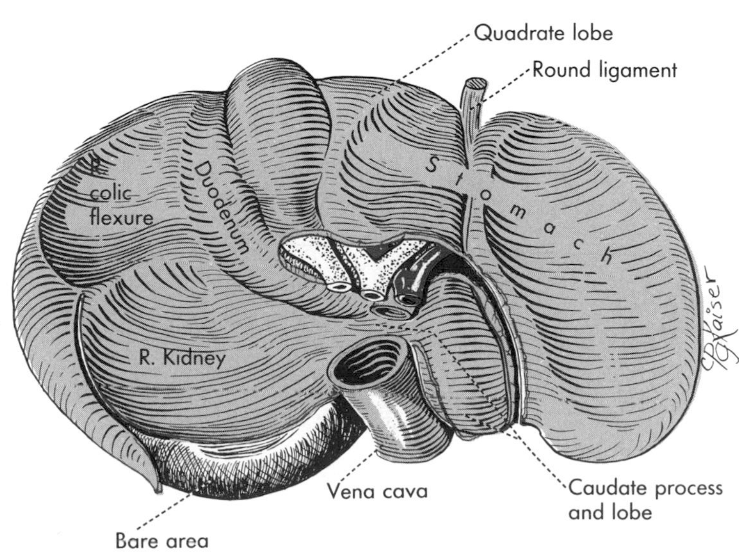

FIGURE *24-31.*
Relations of the visceral surface of the liver.

the omental bursa (see Fig. 23-18). To the left of the gallbladder, the *quadrate lobe* is in contact with the lesser omentum and the pyloric part of the stomach. Behind and above the porta hepatis, the *caudate lobe* faces into the slit-like superior recess of the lesser sac (see Fig. 23-27). The narrow *caudate process* between the porta hepatis and the inferior vena cava forms the roof of the epiploic foramen. The inferior surface of the *left lobe* is in contact with the fundus and body of the stomach. Along the blunt posterior border of the liver, the esophagus makes an impression just to the left of the lesser omentum.

Development

The liver develops from the interaction of endodermal cells derived from the rostral lip of the archenteron (the region of the junction between the yolk sac and the primitive gut) and prochordal splanchnic mesoderm which, after completion of the head fold, becomes the septum transversum. The mesodermal cells induce the endoderm to proliferate and form the hepatic diverticulum, which grows into the septum transversum; the endodermal cells induce the mesoderm to form the hepatic sinusoids.

The septum transversum contains the vitelline veins and the umbilical veins before the hepatic diverticulum invades it. These vessels subdivide to form the sinusoids, and the sinusoids invade the hepatic diverticulum, breaking it up into cords of hepatocytes, which later become rearranged to create the radially disposed sheets of liver cells in the hepatic lobules. Some cells lose connection with the hepatic diverticulum and develop independently.

Bile canaliculi and ductules are formed in the substance of the liver, and these tubes establish connections with the extrahepatic bile ducts as a secondary event at a later stage. This process of intrahepatic bile duct formation is responsible for establishing the hepatic segments. Failure of union between some of these bile ducts with the biliary tree may be the cause of cyst formation in the liver.

It has been proposed that some hepatocytes arise from the mesothelium of the celomic lining and become commingled with the endoderm-derived hepatocytes, being indistinguishable from them in every respect. The mesoderm of the septum transversum contributes to the liver all its connective tissue, peritoneal coverings, blood vessels, and, except for the epithelial lining, walls of all bile ducts.

The rapidly growing liver distends the septum transversum and acquires peritoneal surfaces, except for the bare area, where the original relation with the septum transversum is retained. Extrahepatic portions of the septum transversum form a part of the diaphragm and the ventral mesentery. After the ninth week, the growth rate of the left lobe of the liver regresses, and some of its hepatocytes degenerate. Such degeneration affects mainly the left lobe and may be so complete as to leave a *fibrous appendage* at the left extremity of the lobe (see Fig. 24-27).

There are numerous **variations** in the segmental division of the liver, as well as in the branchings of its ducts and vessels. Few abnormalities of lobulation exist. *Riedel's lobe* is an extension of normal hepatic tissue from the inferior margin of the liver, usually from the right lobe. Its significance is that it may be mistaken for an abnormal abdominal mass. Rarely, there may be an anomalous extension of hepatic tissue through the diaphragm into the chest.

The Gallbladder and the Biliary Ducts

Bile is produced by hepatocytes and collected in the tiny canaliculi bordered by the hepatocytes themselves. These *bile canaliculi* drain at the periphery of the hepatic lobules into thin-walled *bile ductules* that run toward the porta hepatis along the branches of the portal vein and hepatic artery. They coalesce into larger and larger ducts, eventually forming the *segmental bile ducts* and the ducts of the true right and left lobes (see Fig. 24-36). The *right and left hepatic ducts* emerge from the liver in the fissure of the porta hepatis and unite to form the *common hepatic duct*. This duct is joined by the cystic duct, the duct of the gallbladder, and the two form the common bile duct. As already recounted, the common bile duct is joined in turn by the chief pancreatic duct before the two open together into the duodenum (Fig. 24-32).

The Common Hepatic Duct

The usual length of the common hepatic duct varies from 2.5 to 5 cm, for the right and left hepatic ducts may join deep in the porta hepatis or may descend into the lesser omentum before joining. On the other hand, there may be no common hepatic duct at all, for the cystic duct may join the right hepatic duct before the latter joins the left hepatic duct. Normally, the cystic duct joins the right side of the common hepatic duct at an acute angle in front of the portal vein. In the porta hepatis and the lesser omentum, the common hepatic duct lies on the right side of the hepatic artery in front of the portal vein.

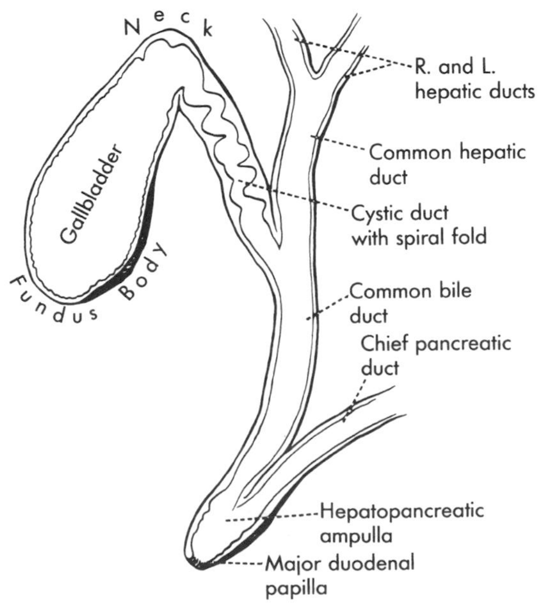

FIGURE 24-32.
The extrahepatic biliary ducts and the gallbladder.

In about one-fifth of all bodies, a hepatic duct that normally joins the duct system within the substance of the liver emerges independently to join one of the extrahepatic ducts, most often the common bile duct. Such a duct is called an *aberrant* or *accessory bile duct*.

The Gallbladder and the Cystic Duct

The gallbladder (*vesica fellea; fel* meaning bile or gall) is an elongated pear-shaped sac in which bile is stored and concentrated. Bile enters and leaves the gallbladder through the cystic duct. The gallbladder lies on the visceral surface of the liver (see Fig. 24-31); its position and peritoneal covering on this hepatic surface have already been discussed. The nonperitoneal upper surface of the gallbladder is attached by connective tissue to a shallow fossa on the liver located between the right lobe and the quadrate lobe. Sometimes the gallbladder is invested almost completely by peritoneum and may be suspended from the liver from a mesentery (floating gallbladder).

The gallbladder is rarely congenitally absent; it may be intrahepatic or may not have its normal position on the visceral surface of the liver. Rarely, the fundus of the gallbladder is bifid, or there may be two gallbladders.

The gallbladder consists of the fundus, body, and neck (see Fig. 24-32). The **fundus** is the expanded blind anterior end of the organ projecting beyond the inferior margin of the liver. It is covered completely in peritoneum and is in contact with the anterior abdominal wall just below the tip of the ninth costal cartilage. The **body** tapers toward the neck, which lies in the porta hepatis. The junction of the body and neck is sometimes straight, more often angular. The **neck** may show a pouchlike dilation toward the right (Hartmann's pouch); it has been shown to be a pathologic feature. The neck turns sharply downward as it becomes continuous with the cystic duct.

The **cystic duct** is up to 5 cm long and runs backward and downward from the neck of the gallbladder. The junction with the common hepatic duct usually takes place immediately below the porta hepatis; however, the two ducts may parallel each other for some distance and, on occasion, may not join until they have almost reached the duodenum.

The mucous membrane of the cystic duct is raised up into a *spiral fold* that consists of five to ten irregular turns (Fig. 24-33; see Fig. 24-32); it is continuous with a similar fold in the neck of the gallbladder. The spiral fold (sometimes called a valve) is believed to serve the purpose of keeping the duct open so that bile can pass through it both in and out of the gallbladder. When the common bile duct is closed at its inferior end, bile secreted by the liver fills the duct and passes along the cystic duct into the gallbladder. When the common bile duct is open, bile flows into it from the common hepatic and cystic ducts. The flow of bile is augmented by the contraction of the gallbladder, which is coordinated with the relaxation of the sphincter of the common bile duct through the action of cholecystokinin, a hormone released by the duodenal mucosa.

Relations. The relations of the gallbladder and biliary ducts have clinical relevance for the diagnosis of gallbladder disease and for its surgical treatment.

The inferior surface of the gallbladder, close to its neck, is in contact with the first part of the duodenum; fur-

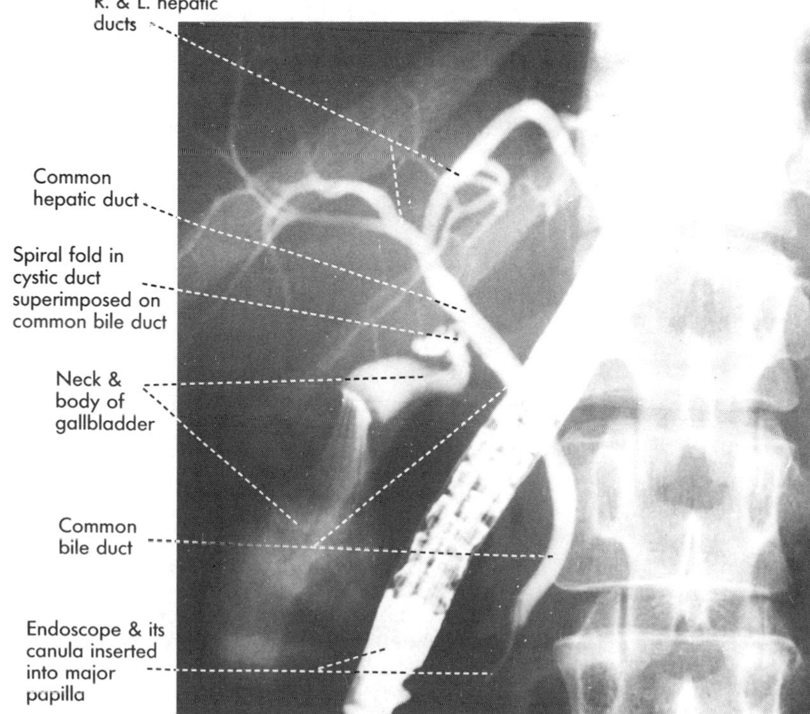

FIGURE *24-33.* **The gallbladder, extrahepatic ducts, and some intrahepatic biliary ducts revealed by endoscopic retrograde cholecystography. For explanation of the procedure, see text.**

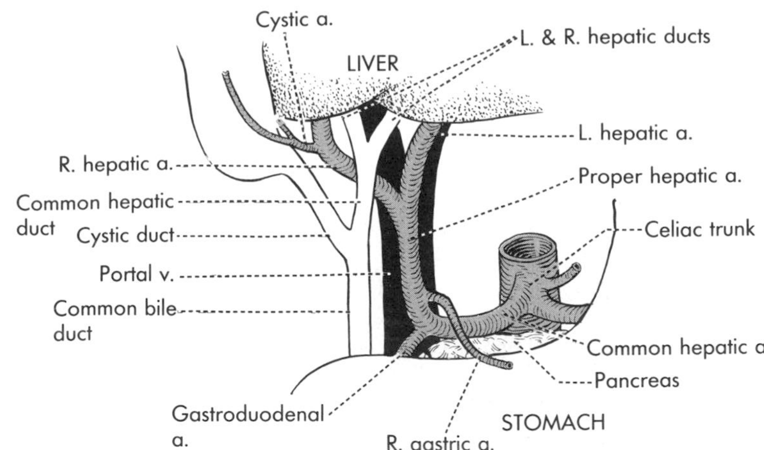

FIGURE *24-34.*
Normal arrangement of the biliary duct system, the hepatic artery, and the portal vein as they run in the free edge of the lesser omentum (hepatoduodenal ligament).

ther anteriorly, the body rests on the descending part of the duodenum and on the tranverse colon. In the cadaver, green stain is usually present on the organs with which the gallbladder is in contact. Inflammation of the gallbladder (*cholecystitis*) may cause it to adhere to its neighboring organs and also to the greater omentum. Inflamed and suppurating tissue may break down, creating a fistula between the gallbladder and the duodenum or the transverse colon.

The region of union of the **cystic** and **common hepatic ducts** is of particular interest in the common operative procedure of *cholescystectomy* (removal of the gallbladder). The cystic duct and common hepatic duct define two sides of a triangle, the base of which is formed by the liver (Fig. 24-34). This *cystohepatic triangle* (of Calot) contains the right hepatic artery, the cystic artery, and most aberrant or accessory bile ducts that may be present. There is, however, considerable variation in the position of structures in this region, and successful cholecystectomy demands a meticulous dissection and careful identification of all ducts and vessels. Damage to the common hepatic or common bile duct usually results in stricture from scar formation, and this may also impede biliary flow to the extent that it will threaten the life of the individual.

The Common Bile Duct

The common bile duct (*ductus choledochus*) drains bile from both the liver and the gallbladder. The duct descends almost vertically from just below the porta hepatis in the right free border of the lesser omentum. It parallels the hepatic artery and portal vein, lying to the right of both structures and in front of the portal vein (see Fig. 24-34). Artery, vein, and duct can be grasped together between finger and thumb with the forefinger inserted into the epiploic foramen. Leaving the lesser omentum, the bile duct descends behind the first part of the duodenum along the gastroduodenal artery and comes to lie on, or embedded, in, the posterior surface of the head of the pancreas (see Fig. 24-19). Here it lies anterior to the inferior vena cava and a variable distance to the left of the posteromedial wall of the descending duodenum. In the head of the pancreas, the duct turns right and is joined by the chief pancreatic duct, and the two enter the posterior aspect of the duodenal wall obliquely at the midpoint of the descending part (see Fig. 24-20).

Embedded in the duodenal wall, the two ducts empty into the **hepatopancreatic ampulla** (of Vater), a short dilated chamber protruding from the wall into the duodenal lumen as the *major duodenal papilla* (Fig. 24-35). The ampulla, as well as the intramural parts of the bile duct and pancreatic ducts, is surrounded by smooth-muscle **sphincters.** The sphincter around the ampulla has long been known as the *sphincter of Oddi.* All three sphincters are apparently independent of the muscle coat of the duodenum. The longitudinal and circular muscles of the duodenum swing around the ducts, creating potential weaknesses in the duodenal wall, predisposing to duodenal diverticula. These sphincters remain closed until gastric contents enter the duodenum, stimulating its mucosa to release cholecystokinin. This hormone, in addition to causing contraction of the gallbladder, relaxes the sphincters, permitting bile and pancreatic secretions to enter the duodenum.

Clinical and Radiologic Examination

The position of the fundus of the gallbladder can be located at the tip of the right ninth costal cartilage by the intersection of the right costal margin and the transpyloric plane or by extrapolating the line that joins the left anterior superior iliac spine to the umbilicus as far as the costal margin. During the movements of respiration, the gallbladder moves up and down with the inferior edge of the liver. Although the position of the gallbladder is known to vary with body type of the individual, the landmarks discussed here are clinically useful.

In the normal subject, the gallbladder cannot be felt by palpation. When the gallbladder is inflamed or distended, the patient will experience pain and will catch his or her breath as the gallbladder descends with

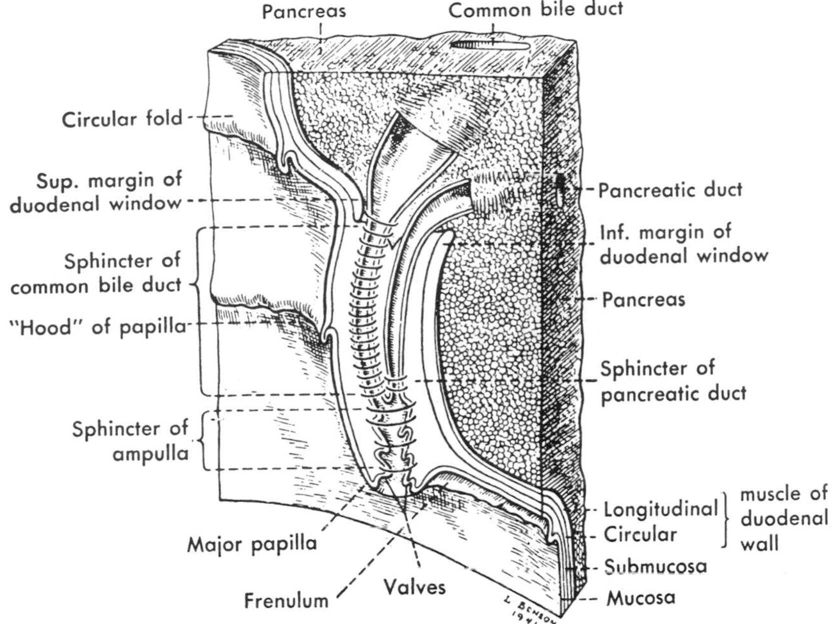

FIGURE *24-35.* **Diagrammatic representation of the sphincter of the hepatopancreatic ampulla. Note that much of it, represented by the encircling lines, actually is around the common bile duct, rather than the ampulla, and that there is also a small sphincter of the pancreatic duct. (Boyden EA. Surgery 1941;10:567.)**

an inspiration and meets the pressure of the palpating hand placed just below the right costal margin.

The gallbladder may be visualized radiographically following the ingestion of iodinated lipid-soluble substances, which, consequent to absorption, are secreted in the bile. Concentration of the substance in the gallbladder renders the organ radiopaque (*oral cholecystography*). The emptying of such a radiopaque gallbladder can be demonstrated by feeding the patient substances that effectively stimulate the release of cholecystokinin (e.g., egg yolk and cream). The rate and extent of emptying can be monitored on serial x-ray films.

Some iodinated compounds are excreted rapidly in the bile following their intravenous administration (*intravenous cholangiography*) and, therefore, are suitable for radiologic examination of the major bile ducts Concentration of the bile in the gallbladder is not required.

A small catheter containing fiber optics for endoscopy can be swallowed by the patient and advanced into the duodenum. Under direct vision through the endoscope, the catheter may be inserted into the hepatopancreatic ampulla, and the bile duct or the pancreatic duct or both may be injected with x-ray-opaque contrast medium (*endoscopic retrograde cholangiography* [Figs. 24-36; see Fig. 24-33]). The retrograde injection outlines the extrahepatic and intrahepatic bile ducts for radiologic examination. *Percutaneous transhepatic cholangiography* is performed by inserting a flexible metal needle through the skin into the liver and injecting contrast medium into a bile duct.

Biliary Obstruction and Gallstones. An obstruction to flow of bile into the duodenum causes distention of the bile ducts and the gallbladder, leading eventually to absorption of the yellow bile pigments into the circulation; this becomes manifest as a type of *jaundice*. Obstruction of bile flow may occur anywhere along the biliary tree and may be caused by spasm of the sphincters, gallstones, or external pressure on the ducts by an adjacent neoplasm. Biliary stasis predisposes to infection and to the formation of gallstones.

Not all the factors leading to the formation of gallstones are understood, but one of them seems to be sluggish flow of bile with the resultant absorption of water from it and precipitation of some of the contents in the form of stones. Gallstones can be formed within the hepatic duct, within the radicles in the liver, or in the gallbladder. Many gallstones are radiolucent and cannot be seen on x-ray film. They may be revealed as filling defects on cholangiograms or on cholecystograms.

Stones that pass into the cystic duct may obstruct this duct, or if they enter the common bile duct, they may be arrested anywhere along its length, causing obstruction and spasms. The common bile duct is narrowest at the point of its entry into the duodenal wall; stones may get held up here or at the ostium of the hepatopancreatic ampulla. There may be excruciating pain as a result of stretching of the duct or spasm of its wall and the sphincters. The intensity of the pain would warrant the use of morphine; however, this drug is known to induce spasm of the ampullary sphincter and, therefore, cannot be used to relieve the pain of biliary colic.

It remains controversial as to what extent backflow of bile into the pancreatic ducts contributes to *pancreatitis* when the ampulla is occluded. Spasm of the ampullary sphincter has been held responsible for certain cases of pain originating in the biliary system and for some cases of pancreatitis. The sphincter has, in fact, been sectioned to relieve these conditions.

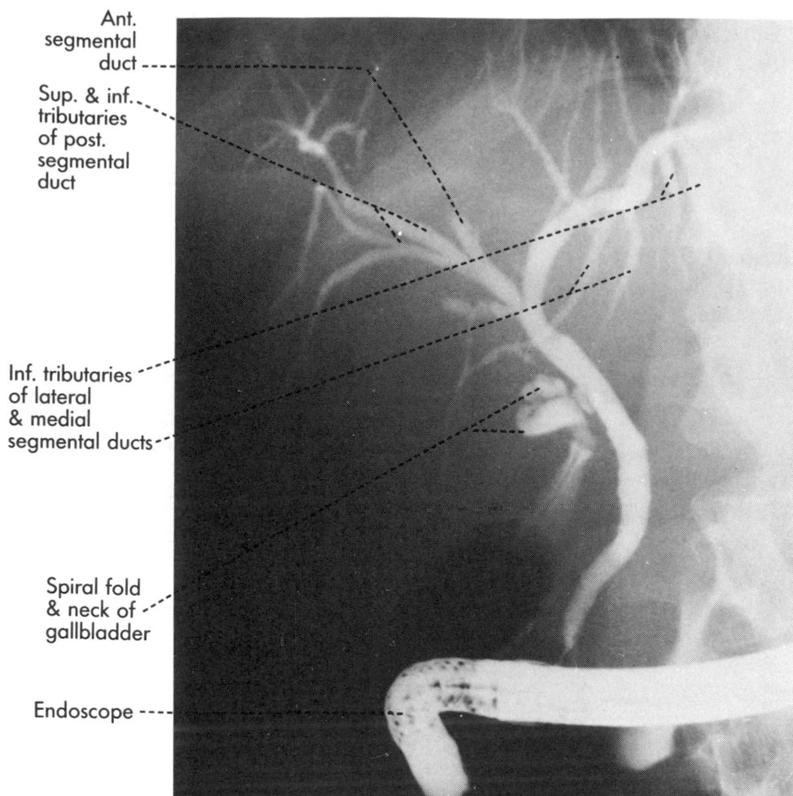

FIGURE *24-36.*
Some of the segmental bile ducts revealed by endoscopic retrograde cholangiography (see also Fig. 24-33).

Vessels and Nerves

Blood Supply

The **liver** is perfused with blood from two sources: the hepatic artery proper and the portal vein. In a recumbent normal adult, nearly one-third of the cardiac output passes through the liver. Roughly 80% of this is delivered through the portal vein; the 20% delivered through the hepatic artery furnishes up to 80% of the oxygen requirements of the liver. After the arterial and portal blood percolates through the sinusoids of the hepatic lobules, it is collected at their center by radicles of the hepatic veins, which convey it to the inferior vena cava.

The **gallbladder** and some of the extrahepatic biliary ducts receive their arterial supply from branches of the hepatic artery proper and, lower down, from the gastroduodenal arteries; their venous blood is returned for the most part to the liver or the portal vein.

In contrast to the arteries of the stomach, duodenum, pancreas, and the rest of the digestive tract, the hepatic artery does not form any anastomoses, and its branches are end arteries. Furthermore, the segmental arteries within the liver can also be considered end arteries, as the only anastomoses between the territories of distribution are through tiny vessels of the subcapsular region. The few arterial twigs that enter the liver over its bare area from the phrenic vessels in the diaphragm have no functional importance.

The Hepatic Artery Proper. On reaching the inferior margin of the epiploic foramen, the *common hepatic artery,* one of the three branches of the celiac trunk, divides into two vessels: the gastroduodenal artery descends behind the first part of the duodenum; the hepatic artery proper ascends in the hepatoduodenal ligament toward the porta hepatis (see Fig. 24-34).

In the lesser omentum, the *proper hepatic artery* lies to the left of the common bile duct and in front of the portal vein. As it nears the liver, it divides into right and left hepatic arteries. This division typically takes place to the left of the common hepatic duct. The left hepatic artery retains this relation to the hepatic duct as they disappear into the porta hepatis. The right hepatic artery runs upward and turns to the right, crossing behind the common bile duct in approximately 85% of persons (see Fig. 24-34); in 15% of persons, it crosses in front of the duct.

If the bifurcation of the proper hepatic artery is low, the right hepatic artery may lie in front of the common bile duct or may cross in front of both the common bile duct and the cystic duct. In any event, the right hepatic artery will be found in the *cystohepatic triangle* (see Fig. 24-34). In this triangle, lying close to the cystic duct and the neck of the gallbladder, the right hepatic artery gives off the cystic artery.

As the **cystic artery** reaches the gallbladder, it divides into two branches, one of which runs on the serous surface of the gallbladder, the other on its hepatic surface between the gallbladder and hepatic substance.

The **blood supply to the extrahepatic biliary ducts** is somewhat variable, but the major supply typically comes from the *posterior superior pancreaticoduodenal artery,* a branch of the gastroduodenal, and is supplemented above by branches from the right or left hepatic arteries or cystic artery.

The **venous drainage of the gallbladder** is partly through veins that pass directly into the substance of the liver, joining branches of the portal vein, and partly through veins that cross the neck to enter the liver or join the ascending veins of the common bile duct that follow the hepatic ducts into the liver. Only rarely does a cystic vein enter the portal vein directly. The major venous drainage of the common bile duct is upward, but veins from its lower end may communicate with veins of the duodenum and pancreas and also with the portal vein.

Variations

Variations in the arterial supply of the liver and gallbladder are extremely common, particularly if the relations of the arteries to the duct system are taken into consideration as well.

In approximately a third of all bodies, an artery of abnormal origin (not derived from the proper hepatic) can be found entering the liver. Such arteries are called **aberrant hepatic arteries.** These arteries usually replace a segmental branch of the hepatic artery that would normally be given off in the substance of the liver.

Aberrant arteries may go to either side or both sides of the liver. Those that go only into the left side are more commonly derived from the left gastric artery. An aberrant right hepatic artery usually arises from the superior mesenteric artery or the aorta. There may be two aberrant arteries of different origin. In about 4% of bodies, the entire common or proper hepatic artery is aberrant, arising from the superior mesenteric, the aorta, or the left gastric artery.

Aberrant arteries of superior mesenteric and aortic origin may run behind, instead of in front of, the portal vein. Aberrant arteries always present a hazard in biliary surgery because of the varied relations that they may present. This is also true of arteries of normal origin that pursue unusual courses.

The **cystic artery** also may show a number of variations, both in its manner of origin and course.

It should be obvious by now that when variations, both in the duct system and in the hepatic artery and its branches, are considered, what can be thought of as an absolutely normal set of ducts, arteries, and interrelations is actually not common—one estimate has been that this occurs in only about one-third of bodies.

The Portal Vein. The portal vein is formed behind the pancreas by the union of the splenic and superior mesenteric veins (Fig. 24-37). It drains, indirectly, the inferior mesenteric vein, which enters the terminal part of the splenic vein, and receives the veins from the duodenum and stomach. The portal vein thus collects blood from the entire digestive tract except the liver, to which it carries its blood. On entering the liver, the portal vein breaks up into branches that end in the hepatic sinusoids, where portal blood is brought into intimate contact with the hepatocytes.

After its formation, the portal vein emerges above the upper border of the pancreas and enters the lesser omentum, usually being crossed anteriorly before it does so by the hepatic artery; it then lies behind and to the left of the common bile duct and behind the proper hepatic artery (see Fig. 24-34). Between its level of formation and its disappearance into the liver, the portal vein typically receives tributaries from the stomach and from the upper part of the pancreas and duodenum. The *left gastric vein* usually joins it low, and the *right gastric vein* often runs up some distance in the lesser omentum to reach it. It also receives the pancreaticoduodenal vein, other veins from the pancreas, and the *paraumbilical veins* running along the ligamentum teres in the falciform ligament. Rarely, the portal vein receives the cystic vein before ending in the porta hepatis and dividing into right and left branches. The left branch of the portal vein is joined by the *round ligament of the liver*, and the same branch gives off the *ligamentum venosum*, which connects it to the left hepatic vein (Fig. 24-38).

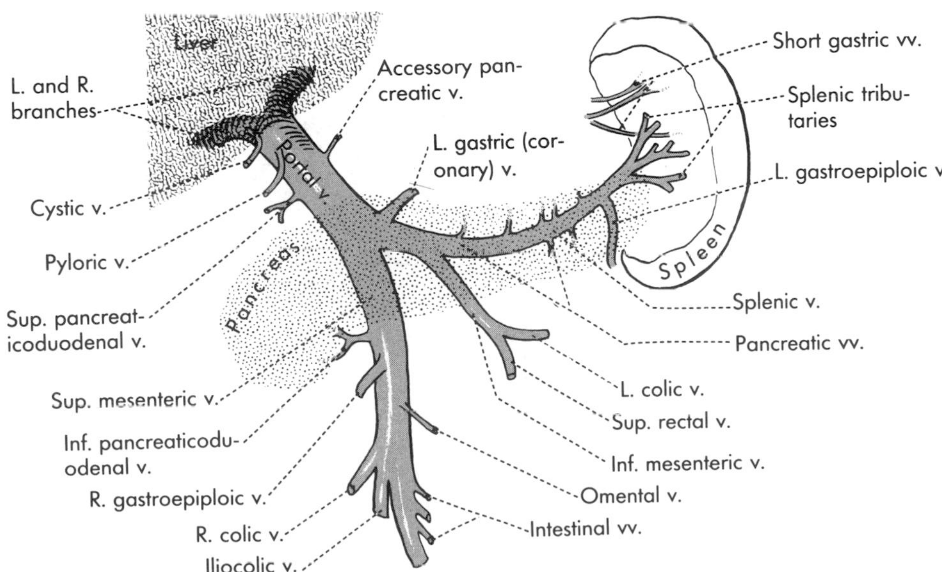

FIGURE 24-37. **Formation of the portal vein and the most frequent sites of terminations of its tributaries in it. (Modified from Douglass BE, Baggenstoss AH, Hollinshead WH. Surg Gynecol Obstet 1950;91:562).**

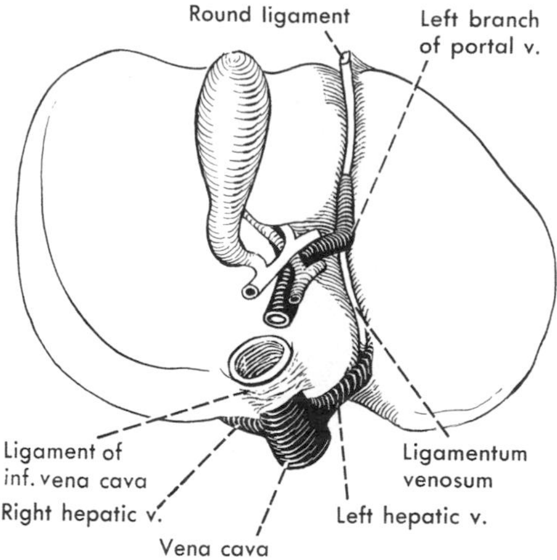

FIGURE *24-38.*
Relations of the round ligament (ligamentum teres) and the ligamentum venosum. The left hepatic artery and duct have been cut away, and the fissures for the ligaments have been spread to show their contents.

The **ligamenta teres hepatis and venosum** represent two segments of the major venous channel through which the placental blood reaches the fetal heart. The *round ligament of the liver* represents the obliterated left umbilical vein (the right umbilical vein having disappeared early in development), and the *ligamentum venosum* represents the ductus venosus. The *umbilical vein* runs from the umbilicus in the free border of the falciform ligament to the porta hepatis, creating a furrow on the visceral surface of the liver. Only a portion of the nutrient and oxygen-rich placental blood delivered by the umbilical vein is spent in the liver, mixing in the hepatic sinuses with blood from both the hepatic artery and the vitelline veins, which give rise to the portal vein. Much of the placental blood is diverted from the liver parenchyma by the **ductus venosus.** This large venous channel is embedded in the liver and shunts blood from the umbilical vein to the proximal end of the vitelline vein, from which the hepatic veins and the proximal segment of the inferior vena cava develop.

After birth, both the umbilical vein and the ductus venosus become nonfunctional, occluded, and fibrosed, but a lumen can be opened up in the umbilical vein for a considerable time, permitting the withdrawal or transfusion of blood during the neonatal period. In the hepatic end of the round ligament, a lumen may persist into adulthood, and the "ligament" can be used to inject substances into the portal vein or to withdraw blood from it.

The left branch of the portal vein makes a sharp angle with the umbilical vein, whereas the right branch lies more directly in line with it. In the fetus, this arrangement places the left lobe at a circulatory disadvantage, causing the growth rate of the left lobe to lag behind that of the right. As a consequence, hepatocytes may disappear from the tip of the tongue-shaped left lobe, leaving behind the fibrous capsule and the hepatic peritoneum as the *fibrous appendix of the liver* at the left extremity of the left lobe (see Fig. 24-27).

Hepatic Veins. The blood in the sinusoids of the liver derived from the arterial and portal venous circulation is collected into radicles of the hepatic veins. These veins, however, do not accompany their portal triads made up of branches of the bile duct, hepatic artery, and portal vein; rather, they run between them. The major stems of the hepatic veins lie between subsegments and segments, rather than in the segments; they are intersegmental. The largest hepatic veins are three: the *left hepatic vein*, between the medial and lateral segments of the true left lobe; the *middle hepatic*, between the true right and left lobes; and the *right hepatic*, between the anterior and posterior segments of the right lobe (Fig. 24-39). These three veins may enter the inferior vena cava independently, but the left and middle veins usually join, so that only two major hepatic veins enter the vena cava. They enter while the vena cava is in its sulcus on the bare area of the liver and immediately before it pierces the diaphragm to end in the heart.

Cirrhosis of the Liver and Portal Hypertension. The liver consists of polyhedral *lobules*, each of roughly 1 mm diameter and made up of anastomosing sheets or laminae of hepatocytes radiating away from a central canal containing a radicle of the hepatic vein. At the periphery of the lobules, in the corners of the polyhedron, run the *portal triads*, consisting of a bile duct and branches of the hepatic artery and the portal vein. The radially arranged venous sinusoids occupy the lacunae between the sheets of liver cells within a lobule and connect the portal vein of the triad to the central vein of the lobule. The sinusoids also receive minute branches given off by the hepatic arteries of the triads. The permeable sinusoidal wall, consisting of endothelial cells and some macrophages (Kupffer cells), separates the blood from the lacunar surfaces of hepatocytes. The portal triads are embedded in perilobular connective tissue, which pervades the liver and is continuous with the capsule of the organ lying subjacent to the hepatic peritoneum.

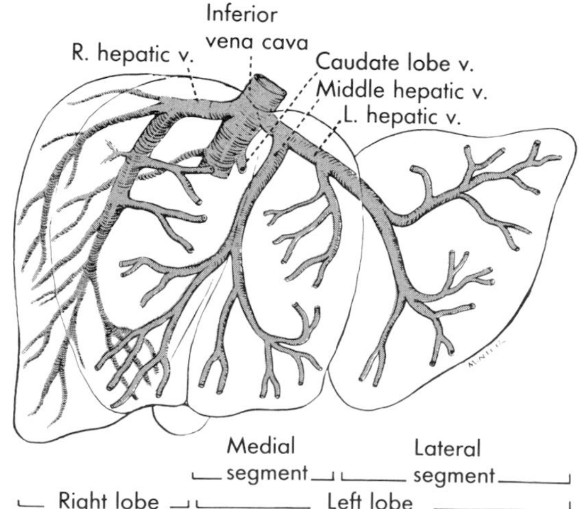

FIGURE *24-39.*
The hepatic veins. (Healey JE Jr. J Int Coll Surg 1954;22:542.)

Following injury and death of the hepatocytes (caused by infection, toxins, alcohol, poisons), their regeneration is usually prevented by excessive scar-tissue formation produced by proliferation of the perilobular connective tissue. The resultant hepatic fibrosis exhibits a variety of patterns and is known as *cirrhosis*. Resistance to blood flow through the fibrosed or cirrhotic liver is increased, causing a build up of pressure in the radicles of the portal vein in the triads. Since no valves exist in the portal vein and its tributaries, the increased venous pressure will affect the entire portal venous system, causing engorgement and distention of all its tributaries, as well as of the spleen. This condition is known as *portal hypertension*.

Some relief of high venous pressure is obtained by opening up anastomoses between veins that drain into the portal system and those that drain into tributaries of the two venae cavae. There are three specific locations where such **portasystemic anastomoses** produce grossly dilated venous varicosities: *esophageal varices* at the lower end of the esophagus, the *caput medusae* around the umbilicus, and *hemorrhoids* or *piles* in the anal canal and lower end of the rectum. In the wall of the esophagus, the tributaries of the left gastric vein anastomose with those of the azygos system; around the umbilicus, the paraumbilical veins connect to tributaries of the epigastric veins, which drain into both superior and inferior venae cavae; in the wall of the anal canal and rectum, superior rectal veins, tributaries of the inferior mesenteric vein, anastomose with the middle and inferior rectal veins, both of which drain eventually into the inferior vena cava.

It is well to note that most hemorrhoids have causes other than portal hypertension. Caput medusae may occur also when the superior or inferior vena cava is obstructed. The sole cause of esophageal varices is portal hypertension.

In addition to the three specific sites of portasystemic anastomoses, anastomoses develop between the portal and systemic venous systems wherever nonperitoneal areas of the intestine, liver, and pancreas are in contact with the body wall. These include the posterior surface of the pancreas, the duodenum, and the ascending and descending colon, as well as the bare area of the liver.

The common method of reducing portal pressure is to divert blood from the portal to the caval system by an operative anastomosis. This usually is done by creating a fistula between the portal vein and the inferior vena cava as they lie close together below the liver (*portacaval anastomosis*) or by anastomosing the splenic vein to the left renal vein (*splenorenal anastomosis*) after removal of the spleen. The effectiveness of the latter procedure is a consequence of the absence of valves in the portal system whereby blood can run retrogradely through the splenic vein into the renal vein more easily than it can run through the engorged esophageal veins.

Lymphatics

A network of superficial lymphatics exists in the capsule of the liver underneath its peritoneum; lymphatics accompanying the portal triads constitute the deep lymphatics. Most of the **superficial lymphatics** from the posterior aspect of both the diaphragmatic and visceral surfaces of the liver converge toward the bare area and pass with the inferior vena cava through the diaphragm to terminate in the *posterior mediastinal lymph nodes*. These lymph nodes drain into the thoracic duct. The posterior part of the left lobe drains to the *left gastric nodes*. Superficial lymphatics from the lower part of the anterior aspect of the diaphragmatic surface run around the inferior edge of the liver, join with those of the anterior portion of the visceral surface, and drain into *hepatic nodes* located at the porta hepatis and, lower down, along the hepatic artery. These hepatic nodes also receive lymph from the gallbladder and the extrahepatic biliary ducts. They drain their lymph to the celiac nodes and through an intestinal lymph trunk into the cisterna chyli. Many superficial lymphatics from the upper part of the diaphragmatic surface of the liver run through the falciform ligament, turn upward along the superior epigastric vessels, and terminate in *parasternal lymph nodes*.

Deep lymphatics of the liver form ascending and descending lymph trunks. The ascending trunk follows the hepatic veins and the inferior vena cava to the posterior mediastinal lymph nodes; the descending trunk passes through the porta hepatis to the hepatic lymph nodes.

Nerve Supply

The nerves to the liver, gallbladder, and extrahepatic ducts run in the **hepatic plexus,** which, for the most part, originates from the celiac plexus and follows the hepatic arteries and the portal vein to the liver. Close to the liver, the plexus is usually joined by one or more hepatic branches from the anterior vagal trunk and sometimes from the posterior vagal trunk. These vagal fibers reach the hepatic plexus through the lesser omentum. A part of the plexus surrounds the hepatic arteries and gives off twigs to the duct system and to the gallbladder. Both sympathetic and vagal fibers are said to end on the gallbladder and the extrahepatic and intrahepatic ducts; blood vessels receive sympathetic fibers only.

Sympathetic stimulation causes constriction of the branches of both the hepatic artery and the portal vein. The nerves in the liver apparently do not affect the rate of bile formation. In humans, sympathectomy does not appear to affect the gallbladder, but vagotomy leads to its enlargement and seems to slow its emptying. Vagotomy has been suspected to increase the incidence of gallstones.

Among the fibers of the hepatic plexus are *visceral afferents* concerned with visceral pain. These fibers belong to the sympathetic components of the autonomic nervous system and reach the sympathetic trunks by passing through the celiac plexus and the splanchnic nerves. They enter the spinal cord through posterior roots of the sixth to ninth thoracic nerves. Pain from the gallbladder tends to be referred to the right side of the thoracic wall in the region of the sixth to ninth ribs and extends back toward the inferior angle of the scapula. Most of the pain fibers seem to be in the right splanchnic nerves, but some may also reach the cord through the left splanchnic nerves.

Pain from the spasm of the sphincters and the muscle of the wall of the biliary ducts can be excruciating. Distention of the hepatic capsule and hepatic peritoneum by swelling and inflammation of the liver, as in hepatitis, is also painful, felt in the epigastrium and sometimes referred to the shoulder.

THE SMALL AND LARGE INTESTINE

The Jejunum and Ileum

The small intestine (*intestinum tenue*) is made up of the rather short and thick duodenum, discussed earlier in this chapter, and of the much longer and more mobile jejunum and ileum. The jejunum and ileum are specialized for the absorption of digested foodstuffs, vitamins, and electrolytes, and this specialization is reflected in the large surface of their mucosa. Their combined length, when excised from an unembalmed body, varies from 5 to 10 m, with an average length of approximately 7 m. By definition, the upper two-fifths of the intestine between the duodenojejunal junction and the cecum is designated as the jejunum and the distal three-fifths is designated as the ileum.

In the abdominal cavity, this long tube is disposed in a series of coils and loops that fill almost completely the infracolic compartment and the pelvic portion of the peritoneal cavity (Fig. 24-40). Visceral peritoneum completely invests the jejunum and ileum except along a narrow strip where it becomes continuous with the two peritoneal laminae of the *mesentery*, which suspends the coils of the small bowel from the posterior abdominal wall.

The jejunum begins at the **duodenojejunal flexure** on the left side of L-2 vertebra; its first loops lie in the upper part of the left infracolic compartment. Although some of its coils may extend into the pelvis, it generally occupies the umbilical region (see Fig. 24-40).

There are histologic differences between the upper end of the jejunum and the lower end of the ileum, but the transition between them is gradual. Loops of ileum are found mainly in the hypogastrium and the pelvic cavity, from which the terminal portion of the ileum ascends to open into the posteromedial side of the junction between the cecum and the ascending colon, located in the right iliac fossa.

The jejunum is slightly wider than the ileum and has a thicker wall because of its thick mucosa. The mucosa is thrown into *circular folds* in the jejunum, whereas circular folds in the ileum are small and sparse. Distinctive *lymphoid follicles* (Peyer's patches), formed in the submucosa of the ileum, are visible through the epithelium and may be several centimeters long; such large follicles are absent in the jejunum.

The lumen of the jejunum and ileum is filled with liquid and gas. In the recumbent position, the gas rises to the surface, and for this reason, percussion of the abdomen in the umbilical region yields a resonant sound. Peristaltic activity in the small intestine is responsible for generating most of the *bowel sounds*,

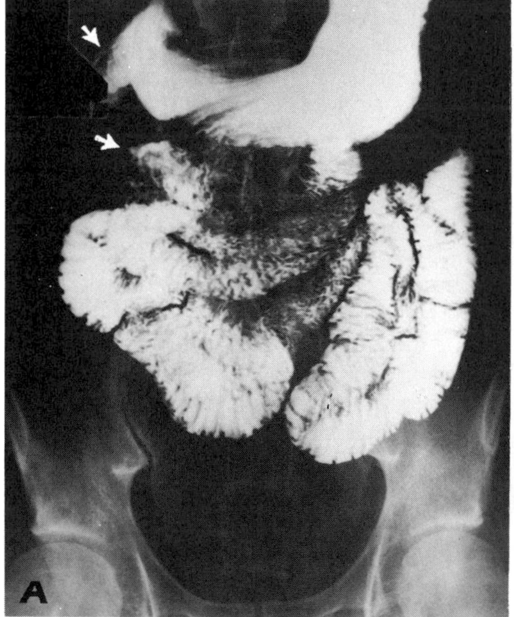

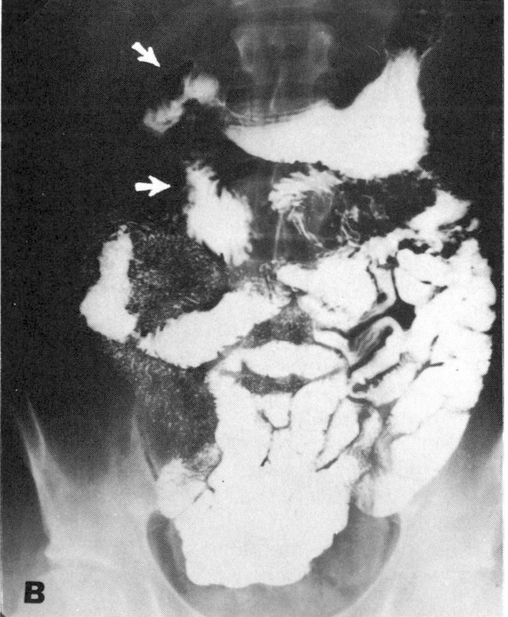

FIGURE *24-40.*
Radiographs of the digestive tract after a barium meal: *(A)* The stomach, parts of the duodenum (*arrows*), and the jejunum are well visualized; *(B)* taken 1 hour and 45 minutes later, some material still remains in the stomach, duodenum, and jejunum, but most of it is now in the ileum. The *upper arrow* in each figure points to the "duodenal cap," partly hidden in the first figure by the pyloric end of the stomach; the *lower arrow* points to the lower part of the descending limb of the duodenum. (Courtesy of Dr. D. G. Pugh.)

which are often audible to the unaided ear. In the normal abdomen, bowel sounds can always be detected with a stethoscope. In the cadaver, the jejunum is usually empty and collapsed (*jejunum* meaning empty; *ileum* meaning coiled).

The absorptive surface of the mucosa is increased not only by the circular folds but also by the characteristic *villi*, which give the fresh mucosal surface a lush, pink, velvetlike appearance. Because most of the absorption takes place in the jejunum and ileum, removal of large segments of the jejunum and ileum leads to grave nutritional problems.

The mobility of the jejunum and ileum is enhanced by the **mesentery,** described in Chapter 23. Its attachment to the posterior abdominal wall, known as the *root* or *base of the mesentery*, is about 15 cm long.

During development, the midline attachment of the mesentery has shifted to become oblique. Starting at the duodenojejunal junction, the root of the mesentery descends into the right iliac fossa; in so doing, it crosses the horizontal part of the duodenum, the aorta, the inferior vena cava, the right ureter, and the right psoas muscle, terminating at the junction of the ileum with the large intestine. The height of the mesentery from root to intestinal border varies between 12 and 25 cm, being the broadest in the central portion. Although the root of the mesentery is essentially straight, the intestinal border is very much folded as it follows the coils of the jejunum and ileum.

The Ileal Diverticulum. The most common anomaly of the small intestine is the ileal diverticulum or *Meckel's diverticulum*, a protrusion from the antimesenteric border of the ileum (Fig. 24-41). It represents a persistence of part of the vitelline duct that joined the midgut loop to the yolk sac. The diverticulum has been found in 1% to 2.5% of persons in whom it was sought. It usually is located 10 to 15 cm from the ileocecal junction, and it may be 2 to 5 cm long. Occasionally, it is attached to the umbilicus by a fibrous cord, and, very rarely, a patency in the cord persists, in which case the diverticulum opens to the exterior at the umbilicus. The ileal diverticulum is particularly prone to pathologic change; therefore, if it is discovered during an abdominal operation, it is usually removed.

The Large Intestine

General Anatomy

The large intestine (*intestinum crassum*) begins at the ileocecal junction and ends at the anus. It is approximately 1.5 m long and consists of the cecum and appendix, the ascending, transverse, descending, and sigmoid colons, the rectum, and the anal canal. The function of the large intestine is to convert the liquid contents of the ileum into semisolid feces by the time the sigmoid colon is reached. This is accomplished by the absorption of fluid and electrolytes.

The ascending and descending colons are located in the flanks on the right and left side of the abdominal cavity, respectively. With the transverse colon above and the sigmoid colon below, they surround a quadrangular space in the peritoneal cavity (Fig. 24-42) that is filled with the coils of small intestine. The transverse and sigmoid colons possess considerable mobility, as each is suspended on a mesentery; the ascending and descending colons, as well as the rectum, are fixed to the posterior abdominal or pelvic wall. The cecum and appendix are completely peritoneal as they hang free from the inferior end of the ascending colon.

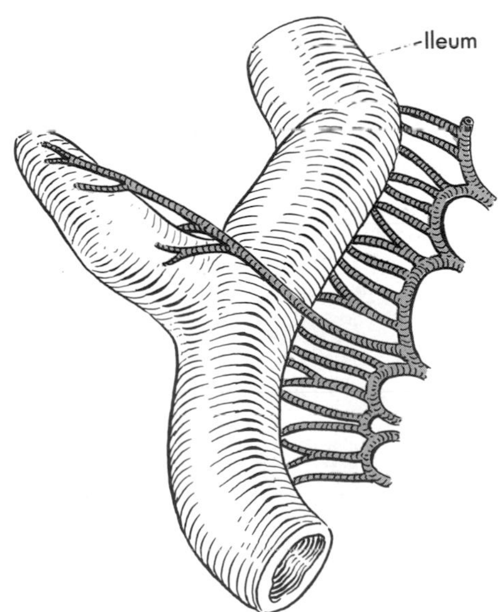

FIGURE *24-41.*
Ileal or Meckel's diverticulum. It has an independent blood supply from an arcade of the intestinal arteries.

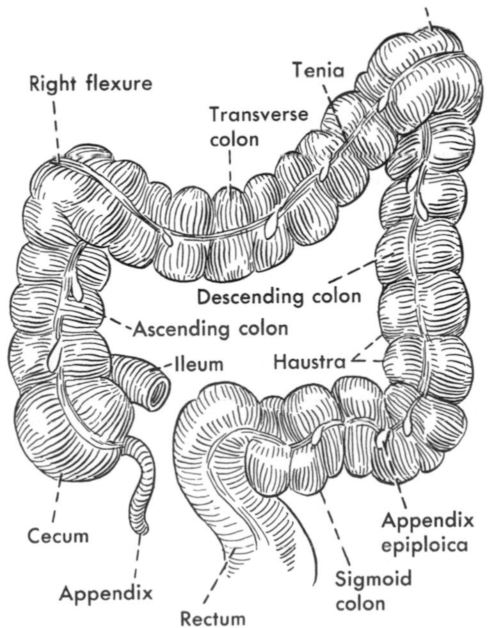

FIGURE *24-42.*
The large intestine.

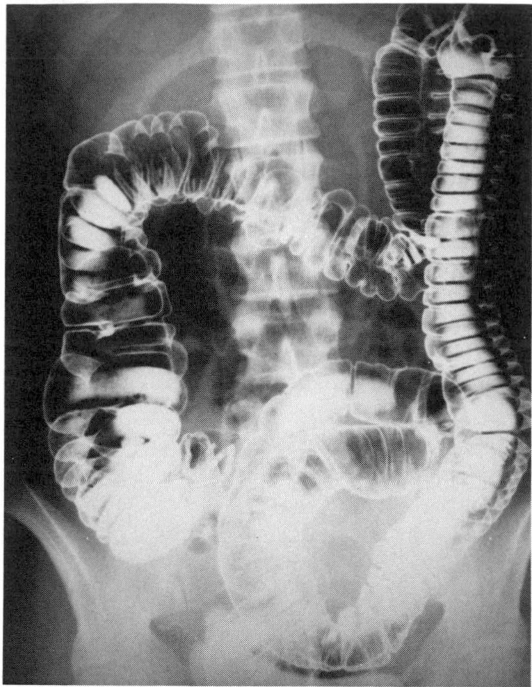

FIGURE *24-43.*
A radiograph of the large intestine using "double contrast." Following a barium enema, air was introduced into the bowel. Note the haustra, the different levels of the right and left colic flexures, the narrow appendix related to the terminal ileum (seen end on), and the sigmoid colon, which forms a loop larger than usual.

This chapter is concerned with the large intestine as far distally as the sigmoid colon; the rectum is dealt with along with other pelvic organs (see Chap. 27).

There are several features that distinguish the large intestine from the small. In general, the large intestine has a larger caliber, although it may contract to a diameter smaller than that of the small intestine. The longitudinal muscle of the cecum and colon, rather than forming a continuous coat on the exterior of the circular muscle, as in most parts of the digestive tube, is gathered into three narrow ribbonlike bands called the *teniae* (taeniae) *coli.* One tenia is at the antimesenteric border or on the anterior surface of the colon and cecum, and the other two are equidistance, each one-third around the circumference of the bowel. Because the teniae are shorter than the gut tube itself, or because some fibers of the teniae stray from the main band and invaginate the gut wall, the cecum and colon present a series of sacculations called *haustra coli* (Fig. 24-43, also see Fig. 24-42). These haustrations involve the circular muscle, the submucosa, and the mucosa. Another typical feature of the cecum and colon are the *appendices epiploicae,* pendant-shaped bodies of fat enclosed by peritoneum, hanging from the teniae.

The Cecum

The cecum (*intestinum caecum;* blind intestine) is the saccular commencement of the large intestine located in the right iliac fossa (Fig. 24-44*A*). At its base, the cecum is continuous superiorly with the ascending colon; their junction is marked on the interior by the *ileocecal valve.* The frenula of the valve encircle approximately the posteromedial third of the cecocolic junction and guard the opening of the ileum (see Fig. 24-44*B*). The *vermiform* (wormlike) *appendix* is attached to the posteromedial surface of the cecum, some 2 cm inferior to the ileocecal opening, and its narrow lumen communicates with the spacious cecum.

Development. The cecum and appendix commence their development as the cone-shaped, blind end of the large intestine, the apex of which is the tip of the appendix. Growth of the appendix becomes retarded, while that of the cecum proceeds, creating an abrupt demarcation between the two. Moreover, in the majority of cases, the right anterior haustrum of the cecum expands more than the remaining two haustra, which displaces the base of the appendix from the inferior tip of the cecum to the posteromedial wall and converts the anterior haustrum into the spacious blind inferior end of the cecum. The three teniae of the cecum, however, retain their fetal position and meet each other at the root of the appendix.

In 78% to 90% of cases, development proceeds as described; in the remaining cases, it may be arrested at some stage, explaining the variations in the shape of the cecum and the location of the base of the appendix.

Peritoneal Folds and Recesses. The cecum has no mesentery; it projects from the antimesenteric side of the gut and is therefore, covered on all sides with serosa. However, fusion of the ascending colon to the posterior abdominal wall may extend and involve the cecum for a variable distance, reducing its mobility.

The cecum is connected to the parietal peritoneum of the iliac fossa, usually by two **cecal folds** of peritoneum that limit, on each side, a peritoneal space behind the cecum called the **retrocecal recess.** When the fusion of the ascending colon to the posterior wall is halted, the retrocecal recess will continue as a *retrocolic recess* behind the ascending colon. Additional cecal folds may divide these recesses into compartments.

There are two other peritoneal recesses associated with the medial side of the cecum that are formed by two small peritoneal folds. The **superior ileocecal recess** is behind a peritoneal fold raised up by the anterior cecal artery as it approaches the medial side of the cecum, passing anterior to the termination of the ileum (see Fig. 24-44*A*); therefore, this fold is called the *vascular fold of the cecum.* The **inferior ileocecal recess** is behind the *ileocecal fold,* which is a bloodless fold of the cecum that joins the antimesenteric border of the terminal ileum to the cecum and the base of the appendix (see Fig. 24-44*A*).

Relations. The cecum is located just above the lateral third of the inguinal ligament. Its anterior surface is in contact with the parietal peritoneum of the anterior abdominal wall; posteriorly, the retrocecal recess separates it from the iliacus and the psoas muscle. It is accessible to palpation in the right iliac fossa; its liquid contents do not

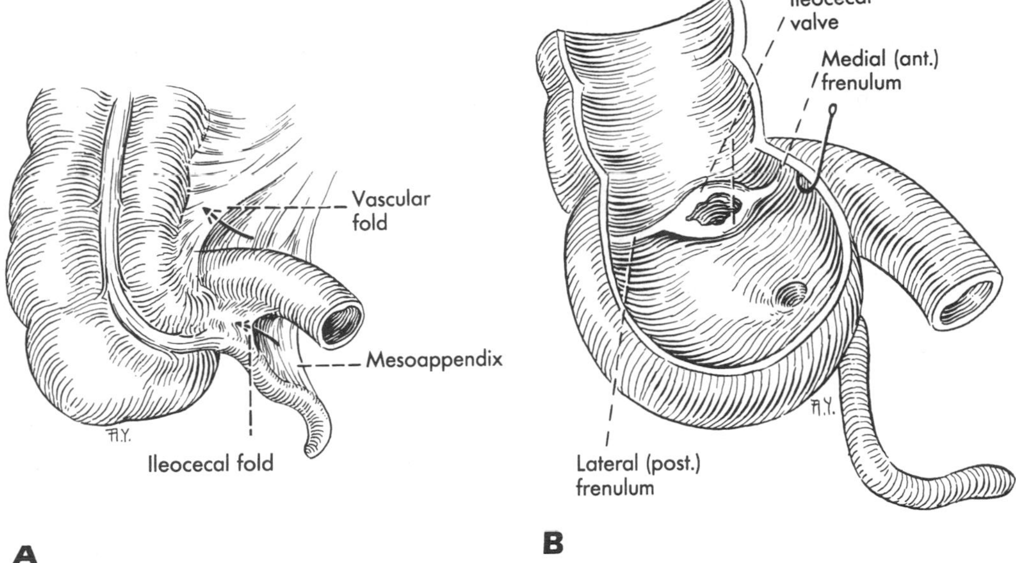

FIGURE *24-44.*
(A) Peritoneal folds associated with the terminal portion of the ileum and with the cecum: The *arrows* indicate the superior and inferior ileocecal recesses. (B) The cecum opened by removal of parts of its anterior wall.

offer resistance to the palpating fingers, which can readily reach the underlying firm iliacus. Consequently, the right iliac fossa feels empty to palpation.

The Ileocecal Ostium. On the interior of the cecum, the ileocecal ostium is surrounded by lips or flaps that protrude into the lumen of the cecocolic junction and contain some circular muscle derived partly from ileal and partly from cecal musculature: this is the *ileocecal valve.* Upper and lower lips unite and continue circumferentially at the frenula of the ileocecal valve. This valve is not particularly efficient, for x-ray films often reveal backflow through it into the ileum when the colon and cecum are filled with contrast material.

The Appendix

The length of the appendix is quite variable; it may be as much as 20 cm, although usually it is half as long. In addition to being fixed by its base to the posteromedial surface of the cecum, the appendix is attached by its own mesentery, the *mesoappendix*, to the inferior border of the terminal portion of the ileum (see Fig. 24-44*A*). The *appendicular artery* and *vein* enter the mesoappendix from behind the terminal ileum and run in the mesentery to the tip of the appendix. Usually, the appendicular artery is an end artery and its thrombosis, caused by appendicitis, results in gangrene of the appendix.

The appendix may lie in several positions. Most often it is hidden in the retrocecal recess. It may hang down into the pelvis or curve along the inferior margin of the cecum, or it may lie on the anterior surface of the terminal ileum or be tucked behind it. The physical signs that permit diagnosis of appendicitis are greatly influenced by the position of the appendix.

Appendicitis. The appendix is a specialized part of the digestive tract; its function is not completely understood. It has thick walls because its submucosa is filled with numerous lymphoid follicles. Its narrow lumen becomes readily occluded, and water may be absorbed from its contents to the extent that a *fecolith* (calcified bolus of feces) may form, which is often visible on x-ray films. Occlusion and stasis predispose to infection and inflammation, presenting the clinical picture of appendicitis. Until surgical treatment of appendicitis was introduced at the end of the last century, most cases were fatal.

Inflammation of the appendix induces visceral pain owing to distention of the organ and its covering serosa. This pain is perceived in the central abdomen and is poorly localized. When the inflammation spreads to parietal peritoneum, the pain shifts to the right iliac fossa. The precise location of the pain and the nature of tenderness are greatly influenced by the location of the appendix. A subcecal or preileal appendix will produce inflammation of the parietal peritoneum on the anterior abdominal wall with the attendant localized spasm in the anterior abdominal wall muscles and hypersensitivity of the overlying skin. This makes diagnosis relatively straightforward. The physical sign of *rebound tenderness*, that is, eliciting pain by slowly and progressively pressing on the abdominal wall in the iliac fossa and then suddenly letting it go, is explained by the sudden stretch experienced by the parietal peritoneum when the palpating hand lets go and the abdominal muscles jump back into position.

A pelvic appendix may cause signs and symptoms suggestive of pelvic disease (inflammation of the uterine tubes or ovary) and may be palpated rectally. Least definite are the physical signs of an inflamed retrocecal or retroileal appendix, because the appendix is inaccessible to palpation in these locations. Inflamed parietal peritoneum in the iliac fossa may cause spasm of the iliopsoas or may irritate the right ureter.

The tip of the appendix may be in variable positions, but its base is relatively constant at the junction of the middle and lateral thirds of a line that joins the right anterior superior iliac spine to the umbilicus (McBurney's point). In cases of *situs inversus*, the appendix, together with the cecum, is located on the left, rather than on the right, side.

The Colon

The **ascending colon** begins at the upper border of the ileocecal junction and continues up the posterior body wall until just below the liver. In front of the right kidney, it makes a sharp bend to the left (see Figs. 24-42 and 24-43). This bend creates the *right colic flexure* (sometimes called the hepatic flexure), beyond which the large intestine is called the transverse colon. Traced from the root of the mesentery of the small intestine, the peritoneum of the right infracolic compartment passes over the anterior surface of the ascending colon and swings back a little before continuing on the posterior abdominal wall. This creates the right *paracolic sulcus*, or gutter, lateral to the ascending colon.

The **paracolic sulcus** tends to conduct infectious material originating in the region of the appendix to the hepatorenal recess or, in the reverse direction, from a subphrenic or subhepatic abscess into the pelvis. It is also along the paracolic sulcus that the surgeon incises peritoneum when it is necessary to mobilize the ascending colon and its blood vessels. The blood vessels and lymphatics lie in the retroperitoneal connective tissue between the root of the mesentery of the small intestine and the left border of the colon, but this is tissue that once composed the mesentery of the ascending colon. By mobilizing the large intestine on its lateral avascular border and loosening it gently toward the midline, the connective tissue, containing the blood vessels and lymphatics, can be split from endoabdominal fascia and lifted as if it were still part of the mesentery.

The **transverse colon** begins at the right colic flexure and runs across in front of the coils of the small intestine to the left side, where it ends in the *left colic flexure* (also called the splenic flexure). The left colic flexure is situated higher and further posteriorly than the right colic flexure. An empty transverse colon may run obliquely upward from right to left, but a full one, especially when the person is standing, usually loops down a variable distance in front of the small intestine (see Fig. 24-43). The *transverse mesocolon* has already been described with its relations to the omental bursa and the infracolic compartment (see Figs. 23-19 and 23-20). Its attachments to the posterior abdominal wall have also been recounted (see Fig. 24-14). The blood vessels and lymphatics of the transverse colon course through the transverse mesocolon. The first part of the transverse colon lies against the liver and gallbladder. Sometimes the lesser omentum extends farther to the right than usual to form the *hepatocolic ligament*, which connects the liver and gallbladder to the right colic flexure.

The **descending colon** begins at the left colic flexure, where the large intestine loses its mesentery in front of the left kidney. It passes down on the left side with a *paracolic sulcus*, like that of the ascending colon, related to it laterally. At or below the crest of the ilium, the colon acquires a mesentery once again and its name changes to sigmoid colon.

There is great variation in the length of the **sigmoid colon** (so called because it frequently takes the form of a Greek letter sigma). A loop of it may be so long that it is susceptible to *volvulus*, twisting on itself to produce obstruction. The attachment of the *sigmoid mesocolon* to the posterior body wall varies. It may run obliquely downward and medially across the pelvic brim; more often, the attachment resembles an inverted V that encloses between its limbs an *intersigmoid recess* of the peritoneum at the pelvic brim. The external and common iliac vessels are in the floor of the recess, and if the recess is deep, the ureter frequently passes across the vessels here on its way from the abdomen to pelvis. The sigmoid colon becomes the rectum when it loses its mesentery; this usually takes place in front of the third sacral vertebra.

Diverticulitis. Diverticulitis is a common affliction of the colon, particularly on the left side. It is thought that pockets of colic mucosa herniate through the gaps created in the muscle coat of the colon by the entry of blood vessels along the mesenteric border or what was the mesenteric border. Fecal material may become impacted in these diverticula, which subsequently become inflamed; this is *diverticulitis*. Diverticulitis may present a clinical picture similar to that of appendicitis and may be confused with a left-sided appendix.

Vessels and Nerves

Blood Supply

The jejunum, ileum, cecum, ascending colon, and most of the transverse colon belong to the midgut; their arterial supply is furnished by the *superior mesenteric artery*. The hindgut, consisting of the left portion of the transverse colon, the descending and sigmoid colon, and the rectum, is supplied by the *inferior mesenteric artery*. The territories of drainage of the *superior and inferior mesenteric veins* conform to this basic plan of arterial distribution, and tributaries of the veins receive names that correspond with those of the arterial branches.

The Superior Mesenteric Artery. The origin and initial course of the superior mesenteric artery (Fig. 24-45) behind and through the pancreas have already been encountered (see Figs. 24-11 and 24-14), but some recapitulation may not be redundant here. It is the second *ventral branch* of the aorta, given off slightly below the celiac trunk, opposite the lower border of L-1 vertebra. The

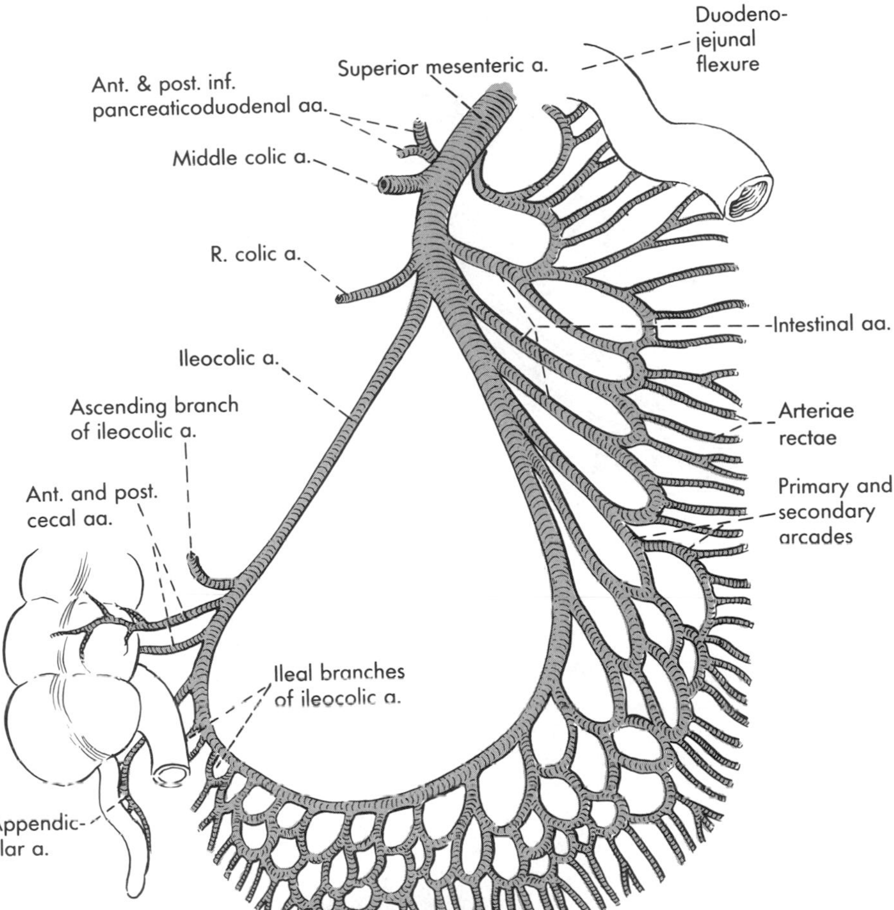

FIGURE 24-45.
The blood supply to the jejunum and ileum: the ileocolic artery lies at the base of the mesentery of the intestine; the stem of the superior mesenteric artery swings into the mesentery.

artery descends in a groove on the posterior surface of the neck of the pancreas. Immediately below its origin, it crosses the left renal vein, which lies between it and the aorta. Below the inferior margin of the neck of the pancreas, it crosses anteriorly to the uncinate process and the horizontal portion of the duodenum; these also separate it from the aorta (see Fig. 24-18). As it passes over the duodenum, it enters the root of the mesentery (see Fig. 24-14). Within the mesentery, the main arterial stem describes an arc that spans the distance between the horizontal duodenum and the ileocecal junction, where the superior mesenteric artery terminates by anastomosing with one of its own branches, the ileocolic artery (see Fig. 24-45).

The superior mesenteric artery gives off three sets of **branches:** 1) several small arteries before it enters the root of the mesentery; 2) three large arteries for the supply of the large bowel from the right side of the proximal part of its course; and 3) an uninterrupted series of arteries for the jejunum and ileum from the left side of the arc it describes in the mesentery (see Fig. 24-45).

The first group of small arteries include the **inferior pancreaticoduodenal stem,** which divides into anterior and posterior vessels (see Fig. 24-25), and the first few of the jejunal arteries. Of the arteries to the large intestine, the **middle colic artery** is the first to arise from the right side of the superior mesenteric. This branch is usually given off at the inferior margin of the neck of the pancreas before the superior mesenteric artery enters the mesentery. The middle colic artery passes into the transverse mesocolon. On approaching the colon, it divides into *right and left branches* (Fig. 24-46). They contribute to the *marginal artery* by anastomosing with the adjoining vessels along the inner border of the colon (Fig. 24-47). The second branch given off from the right side is the **right colic artery**. It crosses the right half of the infracolic compartment retroperitoneally and, nearing the ascending colon, divides into an *ascending and descending branch,* which also contribute to the formation of the marginal artery (see Figs. 24-46 and 24-47). The third artery given off from the right side of the superior mesenteric is the **ileocolic artery.** It runs a more or less straight course toward the ileocecal junction along the root of the mesentery or retroperitoneally, along the right side of the root of the mesentery. Near the ileocecal junction, it gives off several branches (see Figs. 24-45 and 24-46): the *ascending colic artery,* which passes up along the ascending colon and contributes to the formation of the marginal artery; anterior and posterior *cecal arteries* (the anterior one contained in the vascular fold of the cecum, the posterior one passing retroperitoneally); the *appendicular artery,* which de-

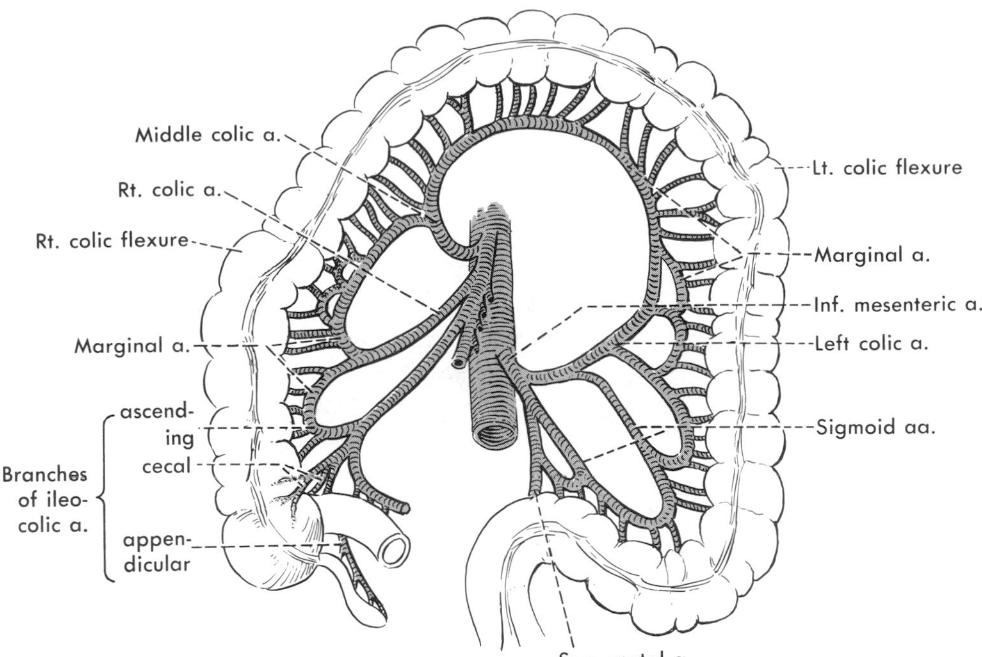

FIGURE 24-46.
The blood supply of the colon.

scends behind the ileum and enters the mesoappendix; and the *ileal branch,* which anastomoses with the terminal portion of the superior mesenteric artery.

The **jejunal and ileal arteries,** given off in the mesentery from the convex left side of the superior mesenteric artery, may number up to 20. Each of these parallel vessels terminates in two branches that anastomose with the branch of their neighbors, forming a row of *arterial arcades.* The secondary branches that spring from these arcades reduplicate this pattern, adding tiers of arcades as the height of the mesentery increases (see Fig. 24-45). From the last tier of arcades, straight vessels (*arteriae rectae*) approach the jejunum and ileum and enter their wall without anastomosing again along the mesenteric border of the gut.

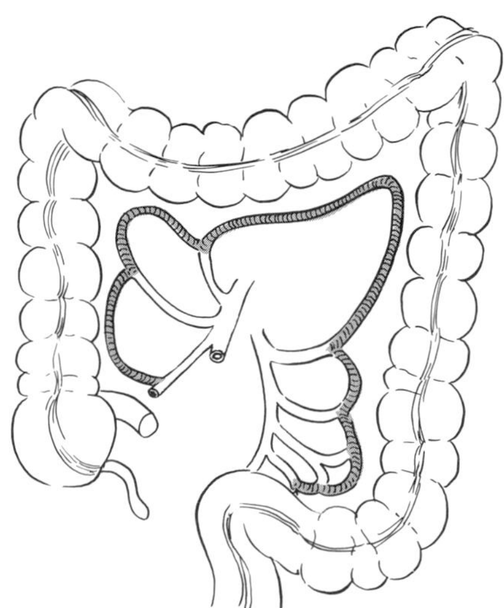

FIGURE 24-47.
The marginal artery (*colored*).

In summary, the superior mesenteric artery supplies the distal half of the duodenum, part of the head of the pancreas, and the entire jejunum, ileum, cecum, appendix, and ascending colon, and also most of the transverse colon. The branches to the small intestine form anastomosing arcades in the mesentery; the branches to the colon anastomose to form the marginal artery.

Intestinal Strangulation and Gangrene. After reaching the small intestine, the arteriae rectae pass deep to the peritoneum of one side or the other; sometimes an artery may branch and supply both sides simultaneously. These arteries anastomose at the antimesenteric border with those from the other side of the gut. Thus, although normal twisting of the mesentery does not disturb the circulation of the small intestine because of the collateral circulation afforded by the arcades, occlusion of a series of arcades or straight vessels seriously interferes with circulation and may lead to surgical emergency because of strangulation of the bowel.

When a loop of small intestine is caught in a peritoneal recess or in a hole in one of the mesenteries, not only may its lumen become obstructed but its blood vessels will also become compressed. Such compression first closes off the veins. The artery continues to pump blood into the trapped coil of bowel with no possibility for return flow through the veins. This causes edema and swelling, gradually obstructing the arteries. Thus, intestinal obstruction in such cases of so-called **internal hernias** will be complicated by *strangulation* of the bowel, and this, in turn, leads to *gangrene.* The same sequence of events may ensue when a part of the small or large intestine enters the inguinal or femoral canal in the form of a hernia (see Chap. 26).

The Inferior Mesenteric Artery. The third ventral branch of the aorta arises about 4 cm above the aortic bifurcation behind or immediately below the horizontal part of the duodenum at the level of the third lumbar vertebra. The inferior mesenteric artery descends in front and then along the left side of the aorta, lying beneath the peritoneal floor of the left infracolic compartment (see Fig. 24 46). Reaching the left common iliac vessels, the artery enters the sigmoid mesocolon and continues into the pelvis as the *superior rectal artery*.

The **branches** of the inferior mesenteric artery are the left colic artery, two to four sigmoid arteries, and its terminal branch, the superior rectal artery. The **left colic artery** runs retroperitoneally toward the left and divides into *ascending* and *descending branches* that contribute to the marginal artery along the descending colon, the left colic flexure, and the transverse colon. Often before the left colic divides, it gives off a sigmoid artery that anastomoses with the **sigmoid arteries** proper given off directly by the inferior mesenteric. Sigmoid branches are also usually contributed by the superior rectal artery.

The Marginal Artery. Although not recognized by *Nomina Anatomica* as being worthy of a name of its own, a continuous arterial channel can be identified and dissected in many bodies that skirts the inner margin of the large intestine from the cecocolic junction to the rectosigmoid junction: surgeons call it the *marginal artery* (see Fig. 24-47). This anastomotic channel consists of the ascending branch of the ileocolic artery; the descending and ascending branches of the right colic; the right and left branches of the middle colic; the ascending, descending, and sigmoid branches of the left colic; the sigmoid branches of the inferior mesenteric; and the superior rectal. When well developed, the marginal artery can serve as a good source of collateral circulation to a part of the colon for which the chief arterial stem has been obstructed or ligated.

The collateral circulation to the left side of the colon is frequently made use of when, for instance, some of the sigmoid colon or rectum must be removed. In certain of these operations, the inferior mesenteric artery is ligated close to its origin, and in these instances, an adequate collateral circulation downward from the middle colic and upward from the middle rectal arteries usually can be obtained.

Although anastomoses in the rectum have traditionally been considered as inadequate, and the anastomoses at the left colic flexure sometimes so, injection experiments have shown that both the middle colic and middle rectal arteries may be filled through the marginal artery by injection into the other vessel. The weakest part of the marginal artery is often between the ileocolic and right colic arteries, where there may be no anastomosis at all.

The marginal artery may be close to the wall of the bowel or some distance away from it; in the latter circumstance, there may be more than one arcade formed by the anastomosing branches. From the arcades straight arteries (*arteriae rectae*) are given off that pass to the colon, some penetrating the wall of the colon at the mesenteric tenia, others running anteriorly and posteriorly around its surfaces to enter the other teniae.

There is some variation in the distribution of all the vessels to the colon. Perhaps the most variable is the distribution of the middle colic artery. This typically supplies the major part of the transverse colon, but not the colic flexures, which are supplied by the right and left colic arteries, respectively. Sometimes, however, the middle colic supplies one or both flexures. Ligation of the middle colic artery predisposes more often to ischemia of a part of the colon than does ligation of any other colic artery. Occasionally, a colic vessel or one of its branches may be entirely absent.

Veins. All the major veins of the digestive tract in the abdomen (except the hepatic veins) are part of the portal system.

The **superior mesenteric vein** receives the drainage from a part of the head of the pancreas and duodenum, from the entire length of the jejunum and ileum, from the cecum and appendix, and from the ascending and most of the transverse colon; it thus parallels the artery. The veins of the jejunum and ileum follow essentially the same pattern as the arteries and unite to form the *superior mesenteric vein*. There are typically *ileocolic* and *right colic veins* joining the superior mesenteric vein. There may be more than one *middle colic vein*, and it may join the superior mesenteric or unite with pancreatic veins or veins from the stomach to enter the portal vein instead of the superior mesenteric.

At the upper part of the root of the mesentery, the superior mesenteric vein lies in front and slightly to the right of the superior mesenteric artery and passes in front of the duodenum to end by uniting behind the pancreas with the splenic vein, thereby forming the portal vein.

The superior rectal, sigmoid, and left colic veins unite to form the **inferior mesenteric vein,** which drains the descending colon, sigmoid colon, and much of the rectum, plus the left part of the transverse colon. It ends at a higher level than the artery originates, passing upward on the left of the aorta and the duodenojejunal flexure (see Fig. 24-15) to disappear behind the pancreas, where it joins the splenic vein. Sometimes, instead, it curves medially at the lower border of the pancreas to join the superior mesenteric vein or the angle between the splenic and superior mesenteric veins.

Since all venous drainage of the digestive tract, including that of the stomach and upper duodenum, reaches the liver, venous spread of gastrointestinal neoplasms almost always results in metastases to the liver.

Lymphatics

As in other parts of the digestive tract, lymphatics of the small and large intestine follow the blood vessels and lymph is filtered through several sets of lymph nodes. Lymph nodes are situated both close to the digestive tract and more centrally. Drainage is, in general, through a converging series of lymphatics and nodes, of which the chief and terminal ones are the *superior mesenteric* and *inferior mesenteric lymph nodes*, lying in front of the aorta. Lymph leaving the digestive tract does not necessarily run through each node along its pathway, for only a few lymphatics end in any one node; others bypass it and go to neighboring or more proximal nodes. In general, however, by the time lymph from the digestive tract has reached the superior or inferior mesenteric nodes, it has passed through several sets of regional lymph nodes.

It is for this reason that resection of a part of the gut containing a cancerous growth must be coupled with extensive excision of the mesenteries and all the draining lymph nodes.

Lymphatics of the small intestine perform a special function, the absorption of fat. Because of the emulsified fat in the lymph, the lymphatics of the mesentery are milky white and, therefore, are called *lacteals*. Their lymph is the *chyle*. Lacteals can be readily demonstrated in experimental animals by laparotomy following a fatty meal.

The lymphatics from most of the small intestine and the ascending and transverse colons drain into *superior mesenteric lymph nodes* (Fig. 24-48). The main nodes of this group are large, lying around the origin of the artery. They communicate with the adjacent celiac and upper lumbar nodes. Efferent lymphatics of the celiac and superior mesenteric lymph nodes together form an *intestinal lymph trunk* that terminates in the cisterna chyli (see Fig. 25-14).

Subsidiary nodes of the superior mesenteric group are the well over 100 *mesenteric nodes* situated in the mesentery of the small intestine along the arcades and branches of the superior mesenteric artery; *ileocolic nodes* along that artery, receiving the drainage of the cecum and appendix; and *right and middle colic nodes*, along the vessels of the same name. Because the superior mesenteric artery helps supply the pancreas and duodenum, a part of the drainage of these organs is also into the superior mesenteric nodes.

The lymphatics accompanying the inferior mesenteric vessels (Fig. 24-49) drain the major part of the rectum, the sigmoid and the descending colon, the left colic flexure, and the left end of the transverse colon. The lymph passes through one or more *left colic nodes* associated with the branches of the inferior mesenteric vessels, and the lymphatics converge on the large **inferior mesenteric lymph nodes** associated with the stem of the inferior mesenteric artery. Lymphatics that leave the inferior mesenteric nodes enter **lumbar nodes** situated along the aorta and the inferior vena cava.

The lymphatics from the left colic flexure and approximately the left third of the transverse colon drain

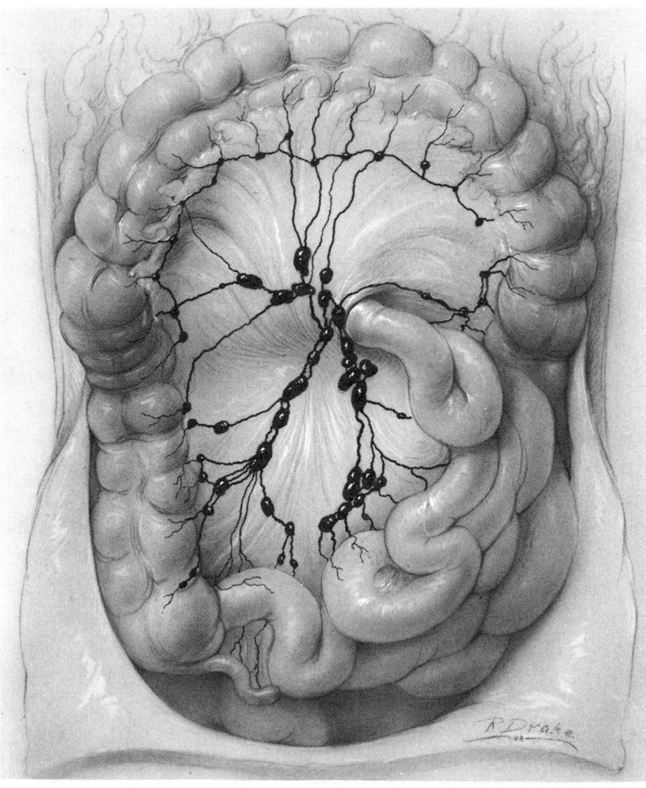

FIGURE *24-48.*
Lymphatics and nodes associated with the superior mesenteric artery and its branches and draining the ascending and transverse parts of the colon and most of the small intestine. Nodes along the marginal artery, the middle and right colics, the ileocolic, and the stem of the superior mesenteric artery in the mesentery are all recognizable. (Desjardins AU. Arch Surg 1939;38:714.)

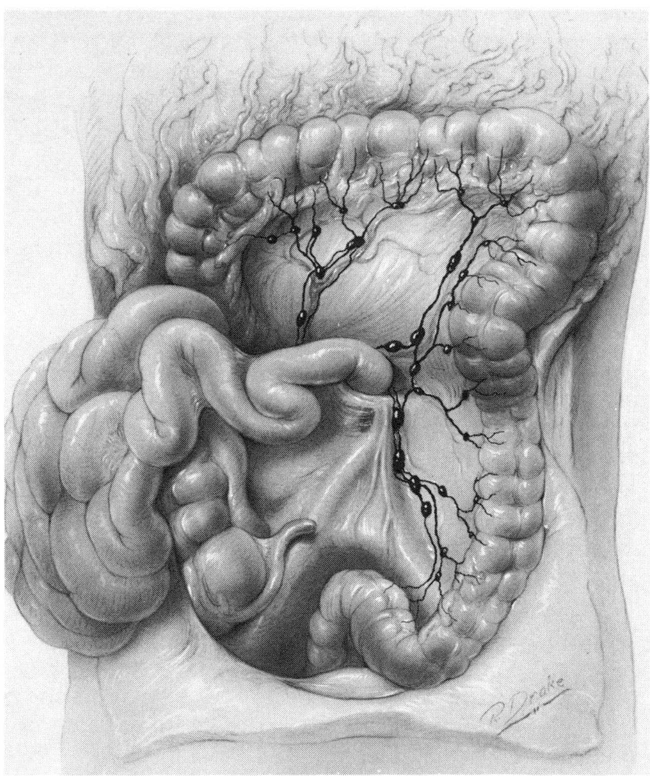

FIGURE *24-49.*
Lymphatics and lymph nodes associated with the inferior mesenteric and middle colic arteries and draining the transverse, descending, and sigmoid parts of the colon (the rectal drainage see Fig. 27-20, is not shown here). Note that lymphatics from the region of the left colic flexure diverge close to the duodenojejunal junction, so that lymph can pass either above this junction to superior mesenteric nodes or continue downward to inferior mesenteric nodes. (Desjardins AU. Arch Surg 1939;38:714.)

downward along the ascending branch of the left colic artery. Only some of them join the inferior mesenteric nodes; others diverge from them at the duodenojejunal flexure and follow the terminal course of the inferior mesenteric vein superiorly and terminate in the superior mesenteric nodes. Thus, the left colic flexure and the left third of the transverse colon have dual lymphatic drainage: along branches of the middle colic artery to the superior mesenteric node, and along branches of the left colic artery to both superior and inferior mesenteric nodes.

Efferent lymphatics of the celiac and superior mesenteric nodes together form the **intestinal lymph trunk** (sometimes more than one). That trunk delivers lymph into the cisterna chyli from the visceral surface of the liver, the spleen, stomach, pancreas, and duodenum, and from all the small intestine and the right side of the colon, including the major portion of the transverse colon. The *lumbar nodes* receive the drainage of the left side of the colon through the inferior mesenteric nodes and empty into the cisterna chyli. The lumbar nodes also receive the drainage from the kidneys, suprarenal glands, gonads, lower limbs, lower parts of the abdominal wall, perineum, and most of the pelvic viscera; thus, they are not primarily associated with the digestive tract and are discussed later.

Nerve Supply

Nerve fibers to and from the small and large intestine are conveyed in the *superior* and *inferior mesenteric plexuses*, which are offshoots of the *aortic plexus* along the arteries of corresponding name and along subsidiary plexuses that follow branches of the two mesenteric vessels. The superior mesenteric plexus is continuous above with the celiac plexus and below through the *intermesenteric segment* of the *aortic plexus* with the inferior mesenteric plexus. Below the origin of the inferior mesenteric artery, the aortic plexus continues inferiorly and, beyond the aortic bifurcation, becomes the *superior hypogastric plexus*, which descends into the pelvis.

All the plexuses contain sympathetic collateral ganglia in which sympathetic preganglionic efferent fibers synapse. The largest of these ganglia are the celiac, superior mesenteric, and inferior mesenteric ganglia, located at the root of the respective vessels. There are, however, numerous other smaller aortic ganglia, the majority of microscopic size.

The **superior mesenteric plexus** and its subsidiary plexuses are composed of *vagal* parasympathetic fibers of both *efferent* and *afferent* functional types and of visceral efferents and afferents that connect the plexus to the sympathetic chain, passing through the thoracic splanchnic nerves.

The **vagal fibers** reach and leave the celiac plexus through the celiac branches of the vagal trunks, given off as they lie on the abdominal esophagus (Fig. 24-50; see Figs. 24-9 and 24-10). Separate branches of the vagal trunks can be traced to the liver and stomach (see Fig. 24-9), but the vagal fibers for the rest of the foregut and midgut are intermingled with sympathetic fibers in the celiac and superior mesenteric plexuses. Vagal fibers running along the middle colic and marginal arteries reach possibly as far distally in the digestive tract as the left colic flexure. *Vagal efferents* pass through the aortic ganglia without a synapse; their postganglionic cell bodies are located in the *enteric ganglia*. Vagal efferents, in general, increase peristaltic activity and, at least in part, secretory activity; they inhibit the ileocecal sphincter. However, the vagi apparently have their chief effect on the stomach; the main results of vagotomy are decreases in the acid secretion and rate of emptying of the stomach, with no apparent change in the function of the small or large intestine.

The function of the *vagal visceral afferents* is largely unknown; they are believed to mediate the feelings of nausea and distention and are probably also involved in visceral reflexes (e.g., gastrocecal reflex that activates the discharge of ileal contents into the cecum when food enters the stomach).

The sympathetic components of the superior mesenteric plexus reach it through the *thoracic splanchnic nerves* which, having passed through the diaphragm, enter the celiac plexus and, through it, descend to the superior mesenteric plexus (see Fig. 24-50). Sympathetic *visceral efferents* synapse in the superior mesenteric and neighboring smaller aortic ganglia. The postsynaptic fibers reach the enteric plexus along the offshoots of the superior mesenteric plexuses that run with the branches of the superior mesenteric artery. Their function is to inhibit the smooth muscle of the digestive tract and possibly its secretory activity. Their most marked effect, however, is on blood vessels, which they constrict.

Thoracolumbar sympathectomy produces dilation of abdominal blood vessels, and the vasodilation in the extensive abdominal vascular bed contributes to lowering the blood pressure. Sympathectomy does not, however, produce any marked or constant change in the activity of the digestive tract.

Visceral afferents in the sympathetic nerves are chiefly concerned with the mediation of pain. They ascend through the plexuses, the ganglia, and the splanchnic nerves; pass through the sympathetic trunks and their ganglia; and, through their white rami communicantes, join the spinal nerve and its posterior root. Their cell bodies are located in the spinal ganglia. The spinal segments that receive afferent input from abdominal viscera are, in general, the same as those that contain the visceral efferent neurons for the appropriate organs (Fig. 24-51).

The **inferior mesenteric plexus** receives sympathetic fibers from the superior mesenteric plexus through the intermesenteric plexus (see Fig. 24-50). The connections and distribution of both efferent and afferent nerves belonging to the sympathetic system conform to the same principles and pattern as those just described for the superior mesenteric plexus. The sympathetic input into the inferior mesenteric plexus is reinforced, however, by the *lumbar splanchnic nerves*, visceral branches of the upper lumbar ganglia, which are in series with the thoracic splanchnic nerves.

The *parasympathetic components* of the inferior mesen-

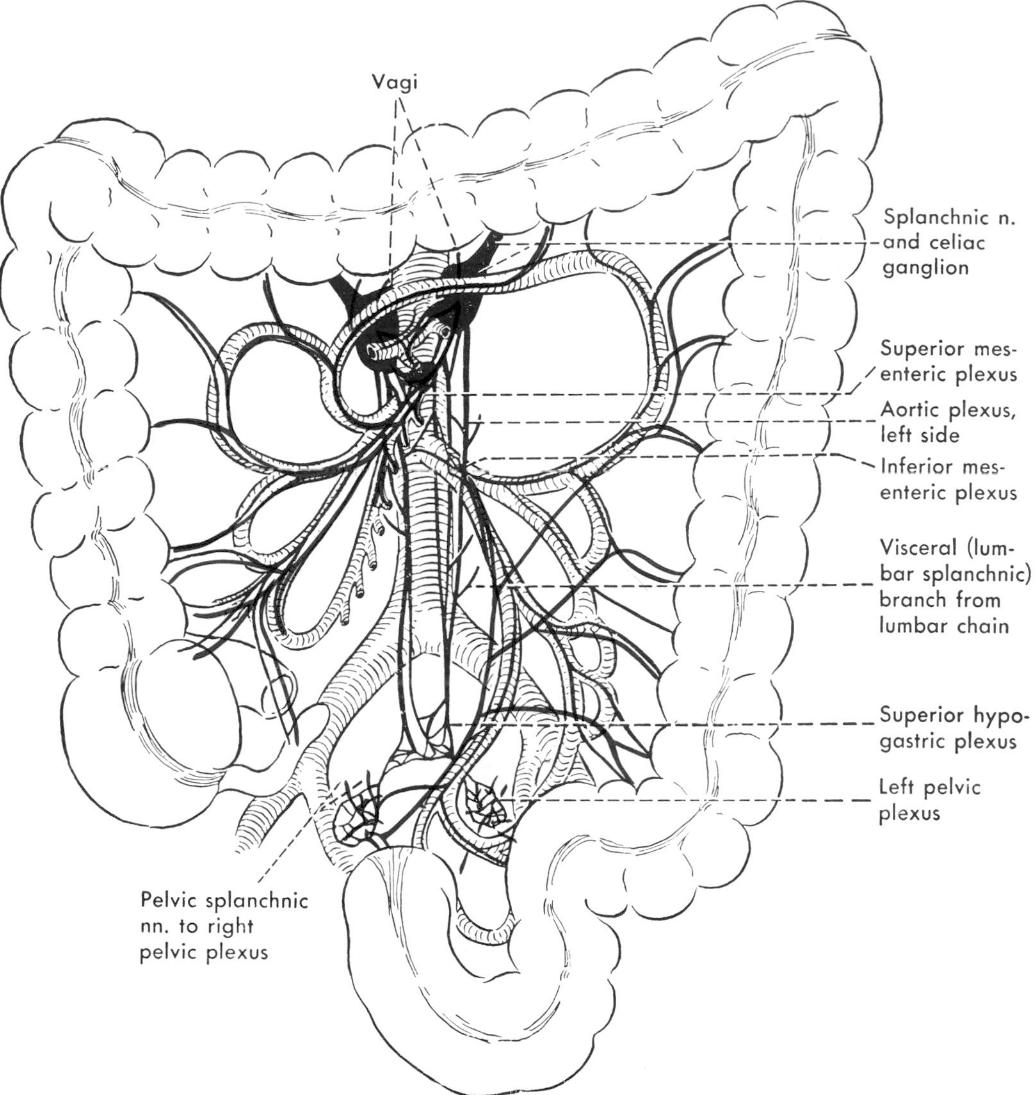

FIGURE *24-50.*
Nerves of the large intestine: Sympathetic efferents and the visceral afferents that accompany them are represented by *black lines*; vagal parasympathetic fibers and sacral parasympathetic fibers are represented by *red lines*. In this diagram, the vagi are shown distributed as far as the transverse colon; parasympathetic fibers of sacral origin are shown supplying the descending colon.

teric plexus are not derived from the vagi, but rather, from pelvic splanchnic nerves. *Visceral efferents* of the **pelvic splanchnic nerves** have their cell bodies in the intermediolateral cell column of S-2 to S-4 spinal cord segments. Their axons enter the pelvis and ascend through the pelvic plexus into the mesentery of the sigmoid colon, where they commingle along the marginal artery with the sympathetic fibers derived from the inferior mesenteric plexus. Similar to the vagal fibers in the foregut and midgut, they synapse in enteric ganglia in the wall of the hindgut (descending and sigmoid colon and the rectum). It is uncertain whether any *visceral afferents* of the descending and sigmoid colons pass along the pelvic splanchnic nerves, but pain afferents definitely follow the sympathetic pathway in the inferior mesenteric plexus. Exactly where the vagal parasympathetic and sacral parasympathetic fibers meet is unknown, but it is believed to be no farther distally than the left colic flexure. Although pelvic splanchnic nerves certainly reach the sigmoid and the descending colon, it seems that parasympathetic fibers are absent from the plexus around the stem of the inferior mesenteric artery and also from the aortic plexus between the artery and the aortic bifurcation.

Visceral Pain. Most accounts indicate that afferent fibers accompany the vagus from abdominal organs; however, the presence of sacral parasympathetic afferents from the descending and sigmoid colon is controversial. On the other hand, it has been clearly shown that all pain from abdominal viscera is conducted by fibers that run with the sympathetic

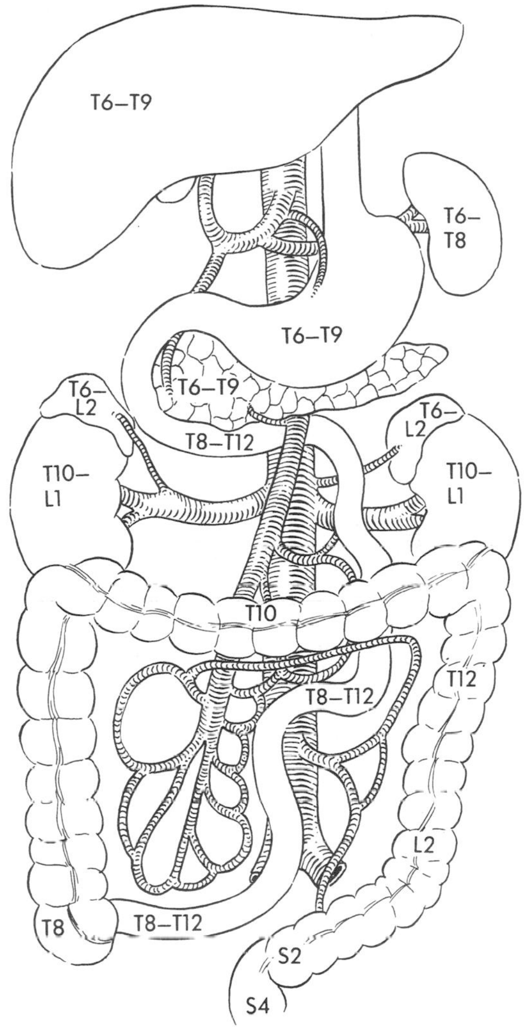

FIGURE *24-51.*
The approximate segmental distribution of sympathetic efferent and visceral afferent fibers to the abdominal viscera.

system and enter the spinal cord through posterior roots of the same nerves that give rise to the preganglionic sympathetic fibers to the viscera (see Fig. 24-51). Although pain arising in the abdominal viscera can be alleviated by sectioning the splanchnic nerves or removing the thoracolumbar parts of the sympathetic trunks, the pain will not be eliminated if disease also involves parietal peritoneum, which is innervated through somatic nerves of the body wall. A sympathectomy may be carried out for the relief of pain, for instance, in severe pancreatitis or, in some cases, a painful and inoperable carcinoma. The sympathectomy will be effective in the relief of pain only as long as the disease is confined to the organs. Once invasion of somatic structures occurs, the pain will return and be of a different character.

It should be remembered that afferent pathways from the viscera that run in the sympathetic system pass through the posterior roots of the spinal nerves, where they join somatic afferents from the body wall. Moreover, within the spinal cord, visceral afferents may end on the same group of interneurons as somatic afferents that have entered the cord in the same posterior root. Thus, some pain fibers from the viscera and from the body wall may share the same neurons in the posterior horn of the spinal cord. This sharing of a common interneuronal pool is believed to be the chief explanation for "**referred pain**." Referred pain is pain that actually originates in a viscus but is perceived as if located in a somatic structure such as the skin or the underlying musculature. This somatic pain is rather well localized and quite distinct from visceral pain, which is deep seated and poorly localized. Because of the shared interneuron pool, the sufferer cannot distinguish whether the pain stimulus reaches the spinal cord along somatic or visceral pain afferents. He will allocate the pain to the somatic region, because this has good cortical representation.

RECOMMENDED READINGS

Anuras S, Cooke AR, Christensen J. An inhibitory innervation at the gastroduodenal junction. J Clin Invest 1974;54:529.

Benson EA, Page RE. A practical reappraisal of the anatomy of the extrahepatic bile ducts and arteries. Br J Surg 1976;63:853.

Bertelli E, Di Gregorio F, Bertelli L, Mosca S. The arterial blood supply of the pancreas: a review. I. The superior pancreaticoduodenal and the anterior superior pancreaticoduodenal arteries. An anatomical and radiological study. Surg Radiol Anat 1995;17:97.

Boyden EA. The anatomy of the choledochoduodenal junction in man. Surg Gynecol Obstet 1957;104:61.

Cortés JA, Gómez Pellico L. Arterial segmentation in the spleen. Surg Radiol Anat 1988;10:323.

DiDio LJA, Anderson MC. The sphincters of the digestive system: anatomical, functional and surgical considerations. Baltimore: Williams & Wilkins, 1968.

Dott NM. Anomalies of intestinal rotation: their embryology and surgical aspects; with report of five cases. Br J Surg 1923;11:251.

Douglass BE, Bagenstoos AH, Hollinshead WH. The anatomy of the portal vein and its tributaries. Surg Gynecol Obstet 1950;91:562.

Flament JB, Delattre JF, Hidden G. The mechanisms responsible for stabilising the liver. Anat Clin 1982;4:125.

Fuller GN, Hargreaves MR, King DM. Scratch test in clinical examination of the liver. Lancet 1988;2:181.

Gillot C, Hureau J, Aaron C, Martin R, Thaler G, Michels N. The superior mesenteric vein. J Int Coll Surg 1964;41:339.

Gómez Pellico L, Labrador Vallverdu J, Fernández Camacho FJ. Venous segmentation of the spleen. Surg Radiol Anat 1994;16:157.

Hayes MA, Goldenberg IS, Bishop CC. The developmental basis for bile duct anomalies. Surg Gynecol Obstet 1958;107:447.

Healey JE, Schroy PC. Anatomy of the biliary ducts within the human liver (analysis of the prevailing pattern of branchings and the major variations of the biliary ducts). Arch Surg 1953;66:599.

Henderson JR. Why are the islets of Langerhans? Lancet 1969;2:469.

Henderson JR, Daniel PM, Fraser PA. The pancreas as a single organ: the influence of the endocrine upon exocrine part of the gland. Gut 1981;22:158.

Hollinshead WH. Anatomy for surgeons: vol 2, the thorax, abdomen, and pelvis. 2nd ed. New York: Harper & Row, 1971.

Homes RO, Lowitt WV. Studies of the portal venous system. Gastroenterology 1951;17:209.

Lewis FT. The form of the stomach in human embryos with notes upon the nomenclature of the stomach. Am J Anat 1912;13:477.

Michels NA. The blood supply and anatomy of the upper abdominal organs. Philadelphia: JB Lippincott, 1995.

Michels NA. The variational anatomy of the spleen and splenic artery. Am J Anat 1942;70:21.

Millat B, Chevrel JP. The pylorus: an anatomical and physiological study. Anat Clin 1981;3:161.

Mizumoto R, Suzuki H. Surgical anatomy of the hepatic hilum with special reference to the caudate lobe. World J Surg 1988;12:2.

Mourad N, Zhang J, Rath AM, Chevrel JP. The venous drainage of the pancreas. Surg Radiol Anat 1994;16:37.

Nylander G, Tjernberg B. The lymphatics of the greater omentum. Lymphology 1969;2:3.

O'Connor CE, Reed WP. In vivo location of the human vermiform appendix. Clin Anat 1994;7:139.

Ray BS, Neill CL. Abdominal visceral sensation in man. Ann Surg 1947;126:709.

Roberts WH, Engen PC, Mitchell DA. When the marginal artery is not marginal. Anat Anz 1984;155:269.

Rosenberg JC, Didio LJA. In vivo appearance and function of the termination of the ileum as observed directly through a cecostomy. Am J Gastroenterol 1969;52:411.

Sapira JD, Williamson DL. How big is the normal liver? Arch Intern Med 1979;139:971.

Severn CB. A morphological study of the development of the human liver. 11. Establishment of liver parenchyma, extrahepatic ducts and associated venous channels. Am J Anat 1972;133:85.

Slack JMW. Developmental biology of the pancreas. Development 1995;121:1569.

Sow ML, Dia A, Ouedraogo T. Anatomic basis for conservative surgery of the spleen. Surg Radiol Anat 1991;13:81.

Soyer P, Bluemke DA, Bliss DF, Woodhouse CE, Fishman EK. Surgical segmental anatomy of the liver: demonstration with spiral CT during arterial portography and multiplanar reconstruction. Am J Roentgenol 1995;163:99.

Sylvester PA, Stewart R, Ellis H. Tortuosity of the human splenic artery. Clin Anat 1995;8:214.

Trutmann M, Sasse D. The lymphatics of the liver. Anat Embryol 1994;190:201.

Underhill BML. Intestinal length in man. Br Med J 1955;2:1243.

VanDamme JP, Bonte J. The blood supply of the stomach. Acta Anat 1988;131:88.

Wakely C. The position of the vermiform appendix as ascertained by an analysis of 10,000 cases. J Anat 1933;67:277.

Weinberg J, Greaney EM. Identification of regional lymph nodes by means of a vital staining dye during surgery of gastric cancer. Surg Gynecol Obstet 1950;90:561.

Zhang J, Rath AM, Boyer JC, Dumas JL, Menu Y, Chevrel JP. Radioanatomic study of the gastrocolic venous trunk. Surg Radiol Anat 1994;16:413.

Hollinshead's Textbook of Anatomy, by Cornelius Rosse and Penelope Gaddum-Rosse.
Lippincott-Raven Publishers, Philadelphia, © 1997.

CHAPTER 25

The Posterior Abdominal Wall and Associated Organs

As noted in Chapter 23, the posterior abdominal wall is constructed on a different plan than the distensible anterolateral walls of the abdomen (see Fig. 23-1). The posterior abdominal wall is bulky and stable because of the lumbar vertebral column and the iliac bones, to which are attached the quadratus lumborum, psoas, and iliacus muscles (Fig. 25-1). These muscles, rather than supporting the abdominal viscera and controlling abdominal pressure as the muscles of the anterior abdominal wall do, act on the vertebral column and the hip joint.

The posterior part of the abdominal wall is formed, in the midline, by the lumbar portion of the *vertebral column*; laterally, on each side of this, by the *psoas major* and *quadratus lumborum muscles*; and in the iliac region, by the *iliacus muscle*, which covers the internal surface of the wing of the ilium. Lateral to the quadratus lumborum is the *transversus abdominis*. The *diaphragm* may be considered along with the posterior abdominal wall, because it not only forms the roof of the abdominal cavity, but it completes the posterior wall superiorly.

Embedded in the psoas major is the *lumbar plexus*, formed by anterior rami of the lumbar spinal nerves. From the plexus issue major nerves for the supply of the lower limb and the inguinal region. These nerves descend on the abdominal surface of the muscles of the posterior wall.

On the anterior surface of the lumbar vertebral bodies lie the *abdominal aorta*, with its associated *autonomic nerve plexuses*, and the *inferior vena cava* (see Fig. 25-1). On the lateral aspects of the same vertebrae are the *sympathetic trunks* and chains of *lymph nodes* and *lymphatics*. The organs that are developmentally associated with the posterior abdominal wall are derived from *intermediate mesoderm* and the overlying celomic epithelium. They are the *kidneys*, the *suprarenal glands*, and the *gonads*. In the female, the gonads have descended, with their ducts, into the pelvis; in the male, they have descended into the perineum. They will be considered in the appropriate chapters. The kidneys, ureters, and suprarenal glands remain on the posterior abdominal wall outside the peritoneal sac and will be dealt with in the last section of this chapter.

THE MUSCLES AND FASCIAS

The Quadratus Lumborum

A roughly quadrilateral muscle, the quadratus lumborum fills the medial half of the gap between the last rib, the iliac crest, and the tips of the lumbar transverse pro-

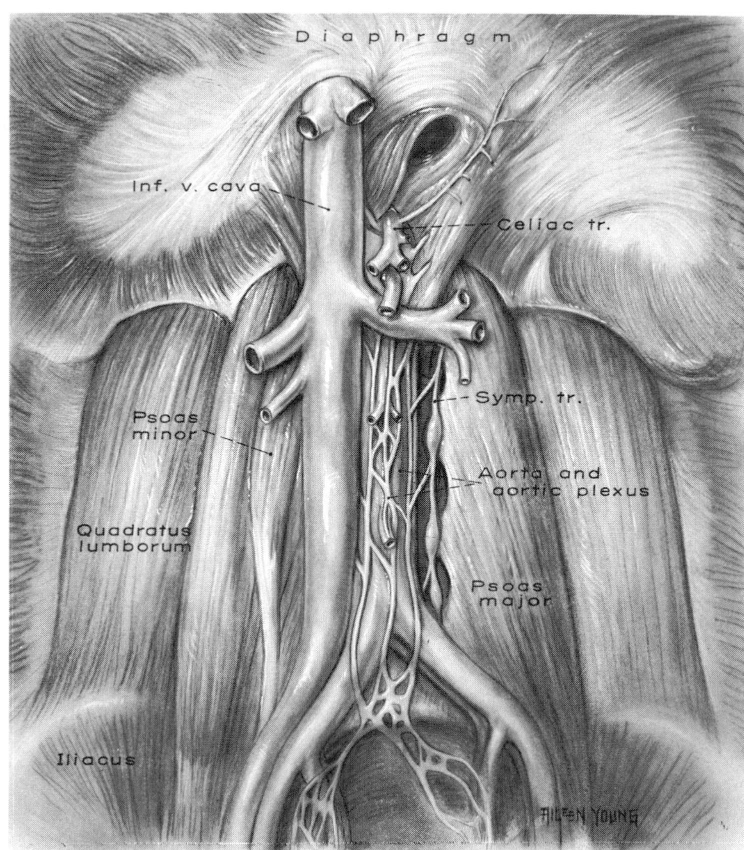

FIGURE *25-1.*
The great vessels and the autonomic nerves on the posterior abdominal wall. Around the celiac and superior mesenteric stems as they arise from the aorta are ganglia of the celiac plexus, and below these, the aortic plexus lies on the front of the aorta and then, crossing the aortic bifurcation, proceeds into the pelvis. The left lumbar sympathetic trunk is visible alongside the aorta; the right one is hidden by the inferior vena cava.

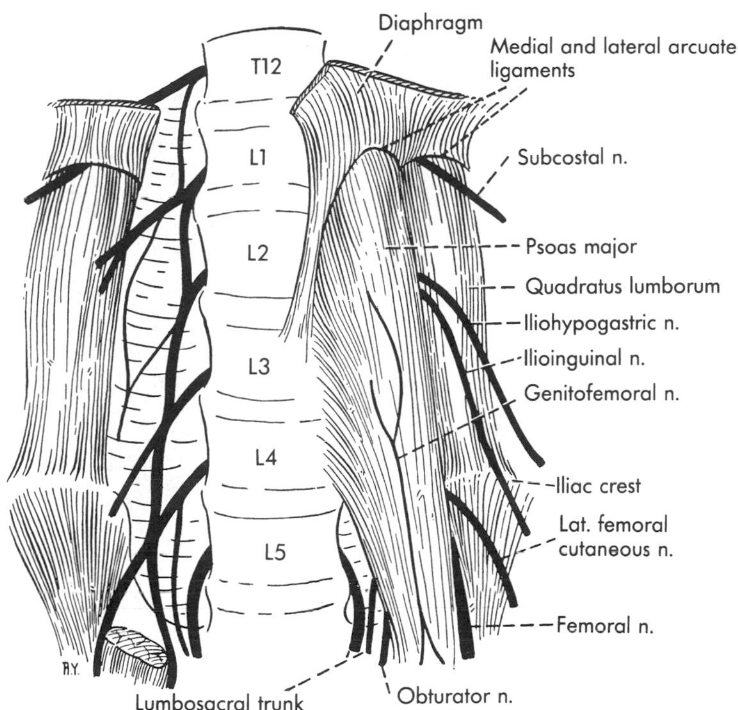

FIGURE 25-2.
The lumbar plexus: The right psoas muscle and the associated part of the diaphragm have been removed.

cesses (see Fig. 25-1). It is attached to all of these bones and to the iliolumbar ligament.

The **actions** of the quadratus lumborum include depression and stabilization of the 12th rib and lateral bending of the trunk. In forced expiration, when the diaphragm is relaxed, the quadratus lumborum depresses the 12th rib, providing the base for intercostal muscle action that can then depress the other ribs. Fixation of the 12th rib provides the stable base for diaphragmatic contraction, a chief factor in inspiration. In lateral bending of the trunk, the quadratus lumborum approximates the rib cage to the iliac crest on its own side. Acting together, the muscles of the two sides may extend the lumbar spine, increasing its lordosis.

The quadratus lumborum is supplied by the anterior rami of T-12 and L-1 to L-4.

Relations

The most medial portion of the quadratus lumborum is overlapped anteriorly by the psoas major (see Fig. 25-1). Along its lateral edge, the transversus abdominis and internal oblique arise from the anterior layer of the thoracolumbar fascia, lying behind the muscle (see Fig. 12-31). Close to the 12th rib, the quadratus lumborum is crossed anteriorly by the *lateral arcuate ligament* (see Fig. 25-3). The *subcostal nerve* enters the abdomen by passing behind the ligament and then crosses the quadratus lumborum. It descends on the anterior surface of the muscle, more or less parallel with branches of the lumbar plexus that emerge along the lateral border of the psoas (Fig. 25-2). The *subcostal artery* and the anterior branches of the *lumbar arteries*, however, pass posterior to the muscle. In addition to the nerves, the anterior relations of the quadratus lumborum on each side are the kidneys and the colon.

The Psoas and Iliacus

The psoas and iliacus are two separate muscles in the abdomen, but they exert their flexor action on the hip through a common tendon inserted into the lesser trochanter. In this context, they are described in Chapter 17 (see Figs. 17-22 and 18-12).

The **psoas major** is shaped like an elongated cone; its apex, represented by the tendon of insertion, points into the thigh. The psoas covers the anterolateral surface of the lumbar vertebral bodies, largely filling the space between the transverse processes and the vertebral bodies (see Figs. 25-23 and Fig. 23-1). The muscle arises by several sets of slips: from the anterior margin of the lower edge of all lumbar transverse processes; from the anterolateral circumference of the intervertebral disks between vertebrae T-12 to L-5 and the adjacent margins of the vertebral bodies; and from five small, tendinous arches that span the slight concavity of each vertebral body between its upper and lower margin (see Fig. 17-22).

The lumbar plexus is enclosed within the muscle between the fibers that arise from the transverse processes and those attached to the disks and vertebral bodies. The lumbar arteries and veins and the rami communicantes of lumbar sympathetic ganglia skirt the vertebral bodies running underneath the five tendinous arches of the psoas origin.

From this wide vertebral attachment, the psoas tapers downward, crosses in front of the ala of the sacrum and the sacroiliac joint, and then runs along the pelvic brim where the iliacus is immediately lateral to it.

The fan-shaped iliacus arises from most of the inner surface of the wing of the ilum (iliac fossa) and inserts many of its fibers into the tendon of the psoas as the two muscles leave the abdomen between the inguinal ligament and the superior ramus of the pubis (see Fig. 17-22).

A slender muscle bundle, the **psoas minor,** is present on the anterior surface of the psoas major in less than half of the bodies. It arises with the highest fibers of the psoas major and its long, narrow tendon inserts at or near the iliopubic eminence.

Actions

In addition to flexing the thigh on a stabilized trunk, the iliopsoas is an important flexor of the trunk at the hip. In the erect position, the force for this movement is provided by gravity. However, when the trunk is flexed against gravity, as during sit-ups, most of the required force is generated by the iliopsoas, especially when the movement is performed with the knees straight on the ground. The psoas major is not an effective flexor of the lumbar spine itself, in view of its rather posterior attachment to the vertebrae in relation to the lumbar curvature. The contribution of the psoas to vertebral movements and of the iliopsoas to rotation at the hip remains controversial.

The psoas is innervated by anterior rami L-1 to L-3, and the iliacus by branches of the femoral nerve (L-2 and L-3).

Relations

The psoas is crossed superiorly by the *medial arcuate ligament,* and on its anterior surface lie the kidneys (see Fig. 25-1). Lower down, the muscles are crossed anteriorly by the ureters, the testicular or ovarian vessels, and the vessels of the ascending and descending colon. The right psoas is crossed also by the root of the mesentery of the small intestine and the left psoas by the root of the sigmoid mesocolon. The lumbar portions of the two sympathetic trunks lie on the front of the psoas major and on the vertebral column just at the origin of the muscle. The lower and medial part of the psoas is covered by the common iliac and external iliac vessels as these run to and along the pelvic brim.

The *lumbar plexus* takes form within the substance of the psoas major. The plexus can be displayed only by tearing the muscle, for it does not divide the muscle into planes. Its branches emerge through the psoas anteriorly, along its lateral border, or along the medial border (see Fig. 25-2). The *genitofemoral nerve,* a branch of the lumbar plexus, runs downward on the front of the psoas major and may be mistaken for the tendon of the psoas minor. The genitofemoral nerve divides on the lower part of the iliopsoas into a genital and a femoral branch; the former leaves the abdomen through the deep inguinal ring, and the latter by passing along the external iliac artery. The branches that emerge through the lateral border of the psoas are, in order from above downward, the iliohypogastric and ilioinguinal nerves, the lateral femoral cutaneous nerve, and the femoral nerve.

The *femoral nerve* emerges from the muscle close to the iliac crest, runs down in the groove between the psoas and iliacus muscles, and enters the thigh with these muscles. The *lateral femoral cutaneous nerve,* emerging slightly higher, passes across the lower part of the quadratus lumborum and across the iliac crest to run on the surface of the iliacus muscle. It makes its exit from the abdomen behind the lateral part of the inguinal ligament, or it may pierce through the ligament. The *iliohypogastric* and *ilioinguinal nerves* emerge separately or together through the upper part of the muscle and run laterally and downward across the quadratus lumborum before turning forward on the internal surface of the transversus abdominis. They enter the transversus only slightly above the iliac crest, some 2 to 3 cm posterior to the anterior superior iliac spine.

On the wing of the sacrum, concealed by the common iliac vessels, three important structures lie on the medial side of the psoas: 1) the *lumbosacral trunk,* made up of fibers from L-4 and L-5 anterior rami, which connect the lumbar plexus to the sacral plexus; 2) the *obturator nerve,* a branch of the lumbar plexus, which leaves the pelvis through the obturator foramen to supply the adductor compartment of the thigh; and 3) the *iliolumbar artery,* a branch of the internal iliac, which ascends from the pelvis and gives off a branch that, along the lateral side of the psoas, fans out into the iliacus.

The iliacus muscle is covered with peritoneum, except where the cecum and ascending colon or the descending colon lies against its upper part.

Fascias of the Posterior Abdominal Muscles

Although the fascia on the abdominal surface of the quadratus lumborum, psoas, and iliacus can be considered analogous with the transversalis fascia, there are sufficient specializations to merit mention. The membranous fascia on the surface of these muscles is distinct from the extraperitoneal fat that may be quite voluminous in this region and will be considered with the kidneys.

The tranversalis fascia, which clothes the inner surface of the transversus muscle, is continued onto the lower surface of the diaphragm as the *diaphragmatic fascia;* it also continues over the anterior surfaces of the quadratus lumborum and psoas major muscles as the fascia of these muscles. After attachment to the iliac crest, the transversalis fascia clothes the iliacus muscle as the iliacus fascia.

The fascia of the quadratus lumborum and psoas major muscles is thickened above where the diaphragm crosses the muscles. The thickenings, called the *lateral* and *medial arcuate ligaments* (lumbocostal aches), give rise to fibers of the diaphragm and are considered a part of this muscle. Through the ligaments, the diaphragm is tightly attached to the muscles, thus sealing any potential aperture behind the diaphragm in this location.

Branches of the lumbar plexus are beneath the psoas and quadratus lumborum fascia, but the common and external iliac vessels lie on the surface of the psoas fascia. The psoas fascia descends into the thigh with the muscle and its tendon. An abscess of one of the lumbar vertebral bodies may discharge its contents into the psoas fascia and track down into the groin, where the resultant swelling (*psoas abscess*) may be confused with a hernia. Behind the external iliac vessels, the iliacus fascia contributes to the formation of the posterior wall of the femoral sheath (see Fig. 26-17), through which a femoral hernia protrudes into the groin.

The Diaphragm

The diaphragm is a curved, musculotendinous sheet intervening between the thoracic and abdominal cavities. Those structures that pass between the thorax and the abdomen necessarily penetrate the diaphragm or pass behind it.

Parts

The fibers of the diaphragm are arranged radially around a **central tendon** and are divisible into sternal, costal, and lumbar portions (Fig. 25-3).

The small **sternal portion** of the diaphragm arises from the posterior surface of the xiphoid process and runs upward and backward to insert into the central tendon. The extensive **costal portion** of the muscle arises from the inner surface of the seventh, eighth, and ninth costal cartilages and the distal ends of the last three ribs. Between the origin from the 12th rib and the origin from the vertebral column, the muscular fibers arise from the arcuate ligaments.

The *lateral arcuate ligament* extends across the quadratus lumborum from the 12th rib to the transverse process of the first lumbar vertebra. The *medial arcuate ligament* extends from this transverse process across the psoas major to the side of the body of L-1 or L-2 vertebra to blend here with the corresponding crus of the lumbar part of the diaphragm. That part arising from the arcuate ligaments, therefore, represents the region of transition between the costal and lumbar part of the diaphragm.

Sometimes the diaphragm is thin and nonmuscular above the lateral arcuate ligament, apparently as a result of degeneration of the muscle that should be here. This weak place is the *lumbocostal trigone* and is more commonly present on the left side than on the right. It is of clinical importance because the kidney lies directly in front of it, and in operations on the kidney, inadvertent breakthrough of the thin lumbocostal triangle into the pleural cavity may occur because the pleura of the costodiaphragmatic recess is immediately posterior.

The **lumbar part** of the diaphragm arises by two **crura,** tendinous in their lower parts where they are firmly attached to the front of the vertebral column and becoming muscular as they curve forward into the diaphragm. The crura are separated by a gap, the *aortic hiatus*. The *right crus* of the diaphragm is usually wider and about one vertebral segment longer than the *left crus* and is attached to the front of the upper three or four lumbar vertebrae. At the level of the 12th thoracic vertebra, the two crura are united over the front of the aortic hiatus by a tendinous arch, the *median arcuate ligament*. Beyond this, the muscular fibers derived from the right crus spread out so that they regularly pass on both sides of the esophageal hiatus. In contrast, the left crus typically sends few or no fibers to the right of the esophageal hiatus, its fibers curving primarily to the left of this.

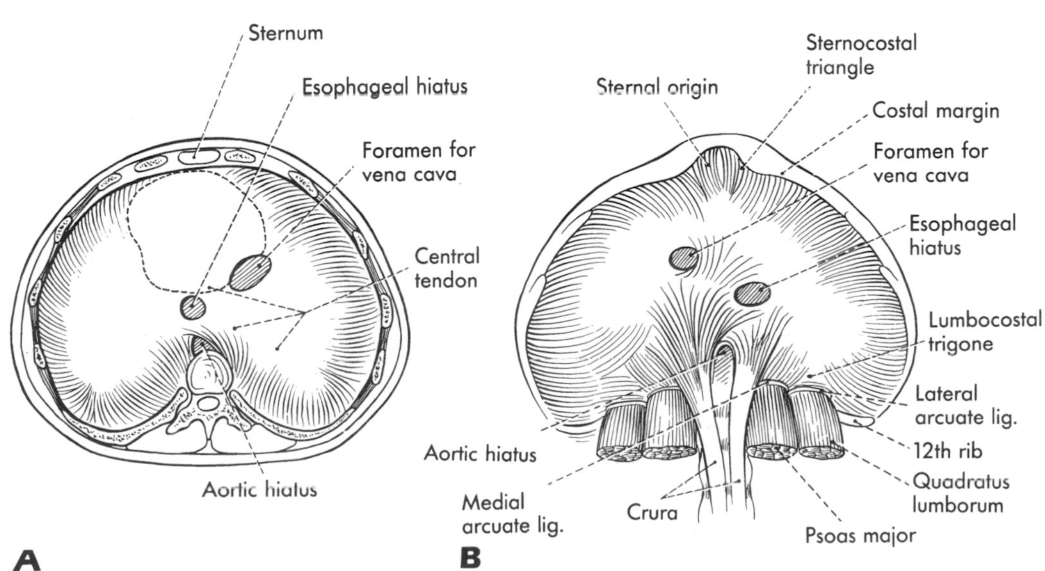

FIGURE 25-3.
(A) Superior and (B) inferior views of the diaphragm.

Apertures

Structures that pass between the thoracic and abdominal cavities do so through three large, named apertures and through several unnamed, smaller openings or gaps. The three major apertures are the aortic and esophageal hiatuses and the foramen for the inferior vena cava.

The **aortic hiatus** is located behind, rather than within, the diaphragm. It is enclosed by the 12th thoracic vertebra, the two crura, and the median arcuate ligament. Through the hiatus, the *aorta* descends, changing its name as it does so from the descending thoracic aorta to the descending abdominal aorta. The *thoracic duct* ascends through the hiatus as does, sometimes, the *azygos vein*. Because these structures are located behind the diaphragm, they are not compressed by its contraction.

The **esophageal hiatus** lies slightly to the left of the midline and is enclosed by the insertion of the medial fibers of the right crus into the central tendon. Because it is situated farther forward on the curve of the diaphragm than is the aortic hiatus, it also lies higher, approximately at the level of the tenth thoracic vertebra in the relaxed diaphragm. Through the hiatus pass, with the *esophagus*, the *vagal trunks*, and the *esophageal branches of the left gastric vessels*.

Communication between the thoracic and abdominal cavities through the hiatus is sealed off by the *phrenoesophageal ligament*. This ligament is a lamina of transversalis (diaphragmatic) fascia that surrounds the esophagus as it lies in the hiatus and attaches to its muscular wall some distance above the gastroesophageal junction, penetrating as far as the submucosa of the esophagus. Enlargement of the hiatus involves stretching the diaphragmatic muscle and the phrenoesophageal ligament. Protrusion of abdominal contents into the thorax through such an enlarged opening is known as a *hiatus hernia*.

It is controversial whether or not diaphragmatic contraction, especially that of the fibers of the right crus, provide a sphincter action around the esophageal hiatus. Factors implicated in the sphincter mechanisms at the cardia are discussed in Chapter 24.

The **foramen for the inferior vena cava** lies still farther forward and correspondingly higher than the esophageal hiatus at the height of the right dome of the diaphragm. In the cadaver, the foramen lies at the level of the eighth thoracic vertebra. It is within the tendinous part of the diaphragm, and the inferior vena cava is firmly attached to the margins of the foramen as it passes through the diaphragm. Thus, contraction of the muscular parts of the diaphragm stretches the caval opening, aiding venous flow from the abdomen toward the right atrium. Branches of the right phrenic nerve pass through the opening along with the inferior vena cava.

Of the **smaller structures** passing between the thorax and abdomen, the superior epigastric vessels are anterior, and all others pass behind the posterior part of the diaphragm. The *sternocostal triangle* is a small gap between the sternal and costal fibers of the diaphragm (see Fig. 25-3). Through it, on each side of the xiphisternum, pass the *superior epigastric vessels* (the continuation of internal thoracic vessels to the anterior abdominal wall). These vessels are accompanied by some lymphatics.

The path of the posterior structures is not constant; they simply pierce through the muscular fibers or pass behind the arcuate ligaments without producing a real hiatus in the diaphragm. The *sympathetic trunks* descend behind the medial end of the medial arcuate ligaments; the *subcostal nerves* descend behind the lateral arcuate ligaments. In addition, three *splanchnic nerves* pierce each crus; the abdominal beginnings of the *azygos and hemiazygos veins* pass behind the crura. The *phrenic nerves* pierce the central tendon of the diaphragm or the muscle fibers close to the tendon, the left phrenic at the apex of the pericardial sac and the right near the foramen of the inferior vena cava.

Relations

The upper surface of the diaphragm is largely covered by pleura and pericardium and, through these, is in contact with the base of the *lungs* and with the *heart*. The lower surface is, in part, covered by adherent peritoneum, continuous with the peritoneum of the falciform, coronary, and triangular ligaments of the liver and, between the liver and esophagus, the lesser omentum. Through this peritoneum, the diaphragm is in contact with the *liver* on the right side and with the *stomach* and *spleen* on the left. The peritoneal spaces between the diaphragm and these organs are the *subphrenic spaces*. The lower posterior part of the diaphragm, facing mostly forward, is widely separated from the peritoneum by the *kidneys*, with their adipose capsules and surrounding fat, and those retroperitoneal structures that lie in front of the kidneys. Except for intervening fat, the *suprarenal glands* and the upper poles of the kidneys rest directly on the diaphragm.

Blood Supply

The chief blood supply to the diaphragm reaches its abdominal surface from the *inferior phrenic arteries*. These paired arteries, as a rule, arise from the aorta just as it enters the abdomen. A branch of each pierces the diaphragm to help supply the pericardial sac and becomes continuous with the *pericardiacophrenic arteries* (branches of the internal thoracics). Other vessels to the diaphragm are the small *superior phrenic arteries* from the thoracic aorta, and branches from the *musculophrenic*, the terminal branch of the internal thoracic that runs along the costal attachment of the diaphragm.

Of the veins, the most important are the inferior phrenic veins. The right inferior phrenic vein ends in the upper part of the inferior vena cava; the left may do so, but it usually descends and ends in the left suprarenal vein or the left renal vein.

Innervation and Action

The **motor innervation** of the diaphragm appears to be entirely from the two phrenic nerves (C-3 to C-5), which descend through the thorax between the pericardium and pleura and enter the diaphragm. The **sensory innervation** is from two sources. A large central area of the diaphragm is supplied with sensory fibers from the phrenic nerves, but its peripheral part is supplied by twigs of the intercostal nerves that run into it where it is attached to the ribs. In consequence of this sensory innervation, pain from the central part of the diaphragm is referred to the base of the neck and to the shoulder, the cutaneous area innervated by the third to fifth cervical nerves; pain from the periphery of the diaphragm is referred to the costal area or the anterior abdominal wall.

The diaphragm is the most important **muscle of respiration.** Its contribution to respiratory movements is described in Chapter 19. Together with the anterior abdominal muscles, the diaphragm is also important in raising abdominal pressure necessary for the evacuation of abdominal contents: defecation, micturition, and parturition.

Development. The diaphragm develops from tissue derived from four sources: the septum transversum, the dorsal mesentery of the esophagus or mesoesophagus, the pleuroperitoneal membranes, and the somatic mesoderm of the body wall (Fig. 25-4).

The **septum transversum,** which has been discussed before in several contexts, forms the central tendon and most of the muscular part of the diaphragm anterior to it. The **mesoesophagus** contributes the median portion of the diaphragm behind the central tendon, including the crura and the parts that surround the esophageal hiatus. The **pleuroperitoneal membranes** grow from the walls of the pleuroperitoneal canals toward the posterolateral edge of the septum transversum and the mesoesophagus and, thereby, close off the communication between the pleural and peritoneal parts of the celomic ducts. The tissue they contribute to the diaphragm is in the posterolateral portion of the central tendon. The most peripheral muscular parts of the diaphragm, forming the medial walls of the costodiaphragmatic recesses, are derived from **body wall.** The expansion of the pleural sacs in a caudal direction splits off an inner lamina of somatic mesoderm, with which the septum transversum is continuous, and pushes it medially, creating the costodiaphragmatic recesses. This process is similar to the one that forms the fibrous pericardium from the same lamina of somatic mesoderm (see Fig. 19-12).

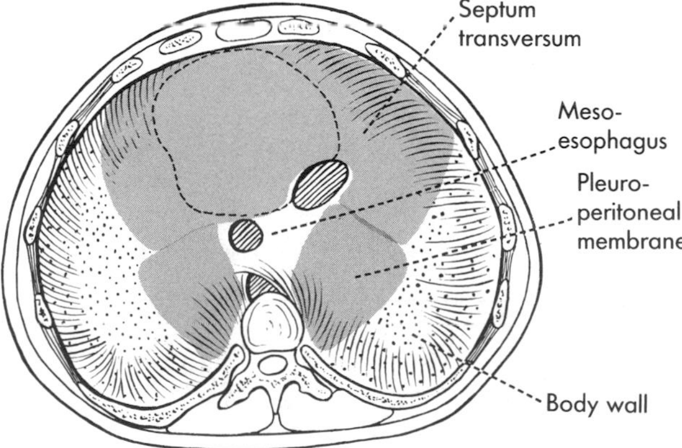

FIGURE 25-4.
Development of the diaphragm. Parts derived from the septum transversum are shown in *pink*; those from the mesoesophagus are *uncolored*. Parts derived from the pleuroperitoneal membranes are *blue*; those from the body wall are *stippled*.

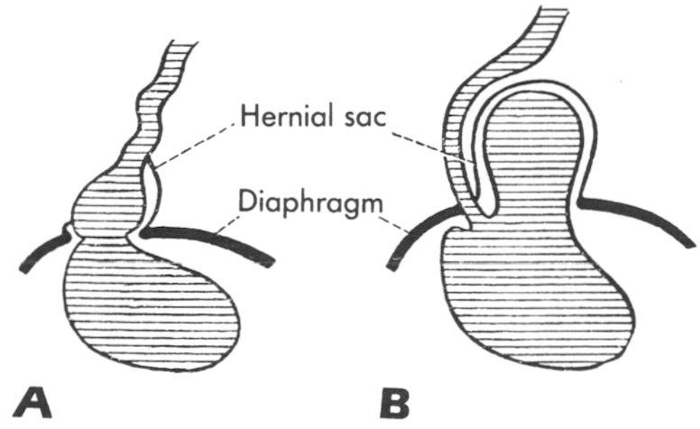

FIGURE 25-5.
Schema of the two chief types of hernia through the esophageal hiatus, viewed from the right side: (A) the sliding type, shown here with some redundancy of the esophagus; *(B)* the paraesophageal type. Note the difference both in the location of and in the angle formed by the esophagogastric junction.

Congenital and Acquired Diaphragmatic Hernias. Probably because of the presence of the liver, the right pleuroperitoneal canal closes early. The left one persists longer, and if it has not closed by the time the intestine is returned to the peritoneal cavity from the umbilical celom, abdominal contents will herniate up into the thorax. The most common type of *congenital diaphragmatic hernia* is one in which the stomach or loops of small or large intestine have passed through the left pleuroperitoneal canal to lie in the left pleural cavity. Both cardiac and pyloric ends of the stomach remain below the diaphragm, but the organ is pushed "upside down" into the pleural cavity.

Much more rarely, a similar herniation occurs after the diaphragm has been completed, but before the thin pleuroperitoneal membrane has been strengthened by muscle. In these cases, the herniated intestines lie in a sac consisting of peritoneum internally and pleura externally that projects up into the thoracic cavity (*eventration of the diaphragm*).

The two other locations in which diaphragmatic hernias ordinarily occur are the esophageal hiatus and the sternocostal triangle. Hernia in either location may be congenital; however, esophageal hiatal hernia, the more common, is far more frequently acquired. In the common type of **hiatal hernia,** the cardia and fundus of the stomach slide upward through an enlarged esophageal hiatus, somewhat as if the esophagus had pulled them up. In such *sliding hernias*, the cardiac notch is obliterated, and the upper end of the stomach seems to be simply a widening of the esophagus (Fig. 25-5A). In the other type of hiatal hernia, called *paraesophageal hernia*, the gastroesophageal opening remains in the abdomen, but the fundus and perhaps a part of the body of the stomach balloon up through the hiatus into the thorax (see Fig. 25-5B).

THE VESSELS OF THE POSTERIOR WALL

The Abdominal Aorta

The aorta enters the abdomen through the aortic hiatus and passes downward on the front of the vertebral column to end by bifurcating in front of the lower part of the fourth lumbar vertebra (Figs. 25-6 and 25-7; see Fig. 25-1). On the surface of the body, the abdominal aorta can be represented as a midline structure extending from about 3 cm above the transpyloric plane to the supracristal plane (usually the umbilicus). Its pulsations may be palpated and in lean individuals can also be seen.

Relations

A complex *plexus of autonomic nerves* is closely applied to the anterior surface of the aorta from the aortic hiatus to the bifurcation. Several large structures cross the anterior surface of the aorta: just below the origin of the celiac trunk, the *pancreas;* just below the origin of the superior mesenteric artery, the *left renal vein;* and slightly lower, the horizontal portion of the *duodenum*. The terminal segment of the aorta and its bifurcation are covered by *parietal peritoneum* of the left infracolic compartment. The *inferior vena cava* is on the right of the abdominal aorta throughout its course; only the right crus of the diaphragm intervenes partially between the two parallel vessels. Below the pancreas, on the left of the aorta, the fourth part of the duodenum ascends to the duodenojejunal flexure, and lower down, the *inferior mesenteric artery* remains in contact with the left side of the aorta for some distance.

Branches

The abdominal aorta gives off four types of branches: unpaired ventral visceral branches to the gut and its derivatives, paired visceral branches to organs derived from intermediate mesoderm, dorsal branches to the body wall, and terminal branches.

There are three **ventral visceral branches:** the celiac trunk and the superior and inferior mesenteric arteries, all of which are described in detail in Chapter 24.

Paired Visceral Branches. The paired visceral branches are the inferior phrenic and middle suprarenal

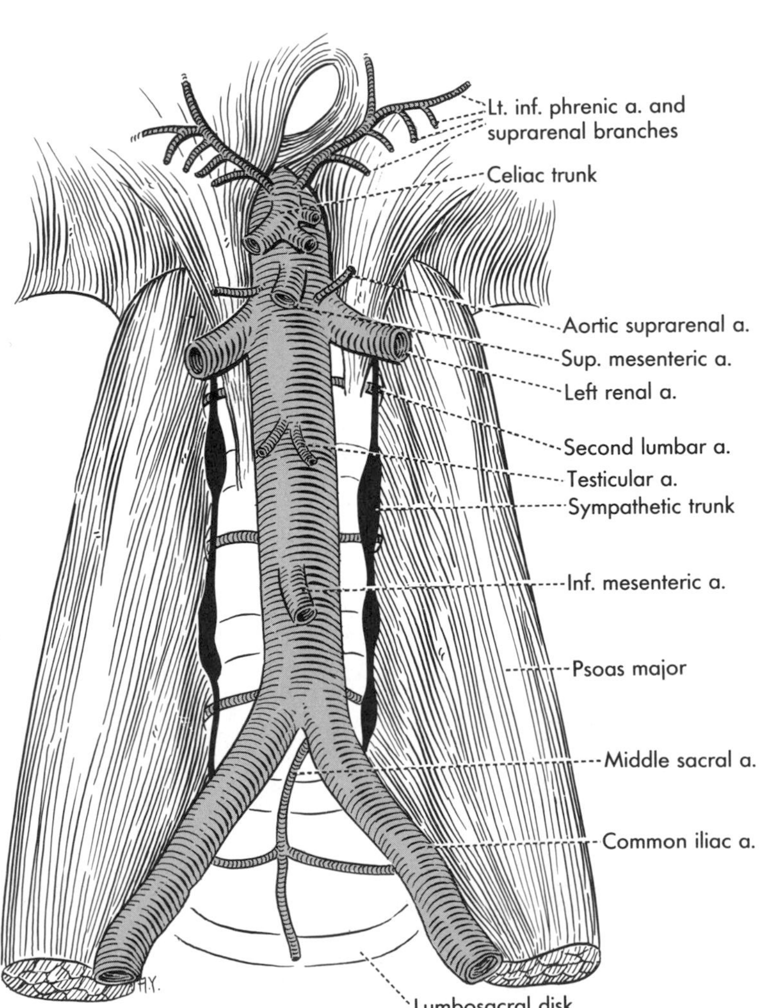

FIGURE 25-6.
The abdominal part of the aorta and its branches: The inferior vena cava is omitted from the drawing.

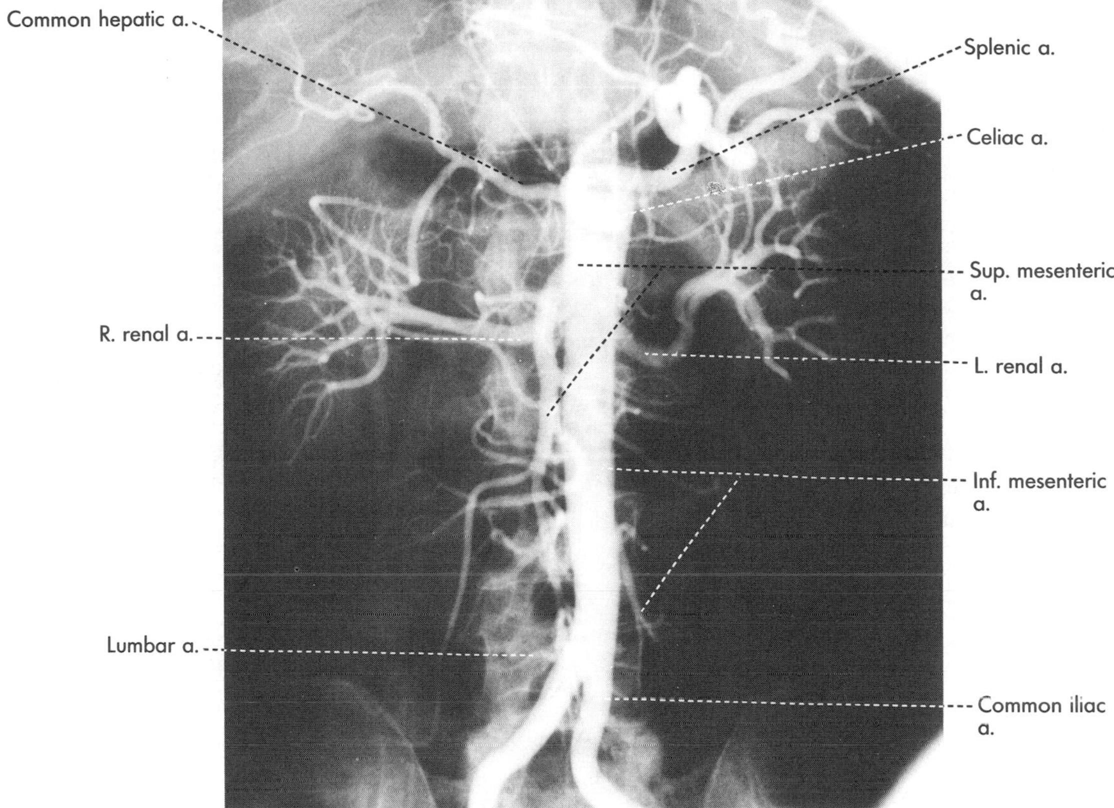

FIGURE 25-7.
An abdominal arteriogram: Contrast medium was injected into the aorta just above the origin of the celiac artery through a catheter. The catheter, barely visible along the left margin of the aorta, was inserted into the right femoral artery and advanced superiorly in the lumen of the external and common iliac arteries into the aorta (compare with Fig. 24-7*B*).

arteries, both of which supply the suprarenal glands, and the renal and gonadal (testicular or ovarian) arteries.

The **inferior phrenic arteries** may arise separately or by a common stem from the aorta in the aortic hiatus. Sometimes they are given off by the celiac trunk. They run upward and laterally, passing medial to the suprarenal glands, and furnish these glands with a major part of their blood supply before they disappear into the diaphragm (see Figs. 25-6 and Fig. 25-26).

The small and variable **middle suprarenal arteries,** given off from the lateral aspect of the aorta just above the origin of the renal artery, help supply the suprarenal glands and anastomose with branches of the inferior phrenic and with the *inferior suprarenal arteries,* branches of the renal arteries.

The **renal arteries** are given off at right angles from the lateral aspect of the aorta at the level of L-1 vertebra, only a little below the origin of the superior mesenteric. The right artery passes behind the inferior vena cava; the left is behind the left renal vein.

The origin and much of the abdominal course of the **testicular** and **ovarian arteries** are similar. The paired vessels usually arise from the front of the aorta, below the origin of the renal arteries, either at the same or at different levels, or even by a common stem. The left artery may loop upward to pass behind and above the renal vein before turning down. Otherwise, both vessels run downward and laterally on the anterior surface of the psoas muscle (see Fig. 25-19). Throughout most of its course, each artery is accompanied by the corresponding vein. The arteries usually give off a branch to the adipose capsule of the kidney and, as they pass in front of the ureter, contribute to its blood supply.

After crossing the ureters, the vessels pursue a different course in the two sexes. *In the male,* the vessels cross the iliac fossa in a continuation of their downward and forward course and then enter the deep inguinal ring. They become incorporated into the spermatic cord and reach the testis with it. *In the female,* they approach the pelvic brim and turn downward and medially as they enter the pelvis.

The high origin of the vessels indicates the embryonic position of the gonads, which have migrated caudally in the female as well as in the male.

Dorsal Branches. There usually four pairs of lumbar arteries given off from the dorsal aspect of the aorta and a single median sacral artery.

The first two pairs of **lumbar arteries** run behind or through the crura of the diaphragm. All four pairs are

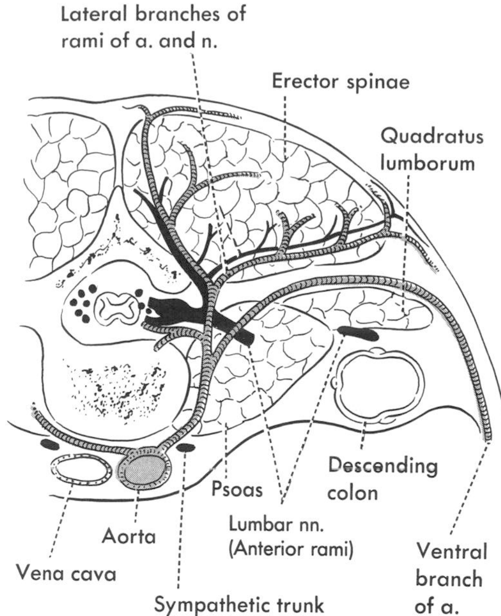

FIGURE 25-8.
Diagram of a lumbar artery.

closely applied to the front of the vertebral bodies. As they pass laterally, they lie behind the lumbar lymphatic chains and the lumbar sympathetic trunks on both sides; on the right, they lie behind the inferior vena cava. They disappear between the psoas major muscle and the vertebral bodies through the tendinous arches from which the psoas arises (see Fig. 25-6).

Like the posterior intercostal arteries, each lumbar artery gives off a *dorsal branch* that turns backward to supply the musculature of the back and, in turn, gives off a *spinal branch* to the vertebral column and the nerve roots. The rest of the artery continues behind the psoas and quadratus lumborum muscles into the anterolateral abdominal wall (Fig. 25-8).

The true continuation of the aorta is the **median sacral artery,** a small vessel that arises from the posterior surface of the aorta just above the level of its bifurcation (see Fig. 25-6). This vessel emerges between the common iliac arteries, closely applied to the front of the vertebral column and covered anteriorly by peritoneum and the continuation of the aortic plexus in the retroperitoneal tissues. Before it reaches the pelvis, the median sacral artery may give off a fifth, or lowest, pair of small lumbar arteries. Sometimes, the fourth lumbar arteries may arise from the median sacral artery as well, or the median sacral may arise from one of the lumbar arteries instead of from the aorta.

Terminal Branches. The large terminal branches of the aorta are the right and left **common iliac arteries.** These diverge and run downward and laterally with the corresponding common iliac veins (see Fig. 25-19). The arteries follow the medial border of the psoas major muscle to the pelvic brim, where each common iliac artery divides into an internal and an external iliac artery. The *internal iliac artery* enters the pelvis. Its course and branches are described in Chapter 27. The *external iliac artery* continues to follow the iliopsoas and leaves the abdomen between the inguinal ligament and the superior ramus of the pubis.

Usually, there are no branches of the common iliac arteries other than their terminal branches. The branches of the external iliac are described in Chapter 26.

The Inferior Vena Cava and Its Tributaries

The inferior vena cava is formed by the junction of the two common iliac veins on the right anterior surface of the fifth lumbar vertebra and conveys venous blood to the right atrium from all parts of the body below the diaphragm. It ascends in front of the lumbar vertebrae on the right of and parallel with the abdominal aorta (Fig. 25-9). Passing behind the right lobe of the liver, it inclines forward with the curvature of the diaphragm to pierce its central tendon, where it is on level with, but some distance anterior to, the eighth thoracic vertebra. In the thorax, the inferior vena cava has a short intrapericardial course before it opens into the lower posterior corner of the right atrium.

On the surface of the body, the position of the inferior vena cava may be indicated by a band extending from a point in the intertubercular plane 2 to 3 cm to the right of

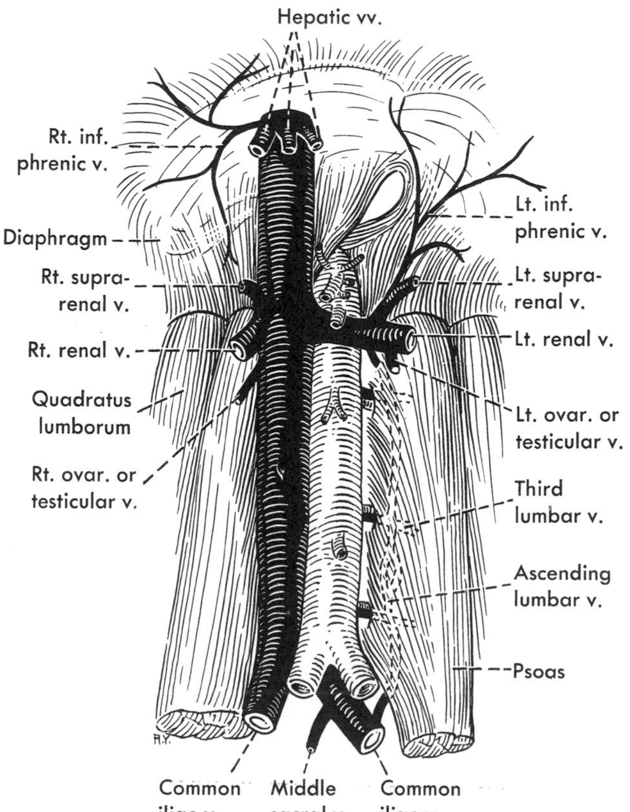

FIGURE 25-9.
The inferior vena cava and its tributaries.

the midline to the sternal end of the right sixth costal cartilage.

Relations

The inferior vena cava begins behind the *right common iliac artery,* above which it is covered by parietal peritoneum of the infracolic compartment and is crossed by the *root of the mesentery.* Retroperitoneally, the right *ureter* may overlap it, and the right *testicular* or *ovarian artery* passes over it. The anterior surface of the vena cava is crossed by both the horizontal and superior parts of the *duodenum,* and in between the two, the head of the *pancreas,* the *common bile duct,* and the **portal vein** lie in direct contact with it. Above the duodenum, the inferior vena cava is again covered by peritoneum as it forms the posterior boundary of the *epiploic foramen.* Beyond the posterior layer of the right coronary ligament, the vena cava lies in a deep groove, or tunnel, of the *liver,* which forms the boundary between the right and caudate lobes.

The more important structures upon which the inferior vena cava lies include some of the *lumbar arteries;* the *right renal, suprarenal,* and *inferior phrenic arteries;* and the *right sympathetic trunk.* On its right, the inferior vena cava is in contact with the right suprarenal gland, the right kidney and ureter, and the descending part of the duodenum; on the left, below the aortic hiatus, lies the abdominal aorta.

Tributaries

Through the *common iliac veins,* the inferior vena cava collects all the blood from the pelvis, the perineum, and the lower limbs. The pelvis and perineum are drained by the *internal iliac vein,* and the lower limbs by the *external iliac vein;* the two unite to form the *common iliac vein* on each side. Blood from the digestive tract, having been collected by the portal system and passed through the liver, enters the vena cava through two or three *hepatic veins* that open into the vena cava just below the diaphragm (see Fig. 24-39). Between the hepatic veins and common iliac veins, the inferior vena cava receives the *right inferior phrenic, right suprarenal,* and *right testicular* or *ovarian veins,* both *renal veins,* and a variable number of the four pairs of *lumbar veins.* The left inferior phrenic, the left suprarenal, and the left testicular or ovarian veins drain into the left renal vein, a developmental homologue of a segment of the inferior vena cava. Only the lumbar veins need to be described here, as all other tributaries of the inferior vena cava are dealt with in the sections on the organs they drain.

The **lumbar veins** follow the distribution of the corresponding arteries, as do, in general, the other tributaries of the vena cava. The lumbar veins enter the inferior vena cava in an irregular pattern; the second left lumbar vein frequently enters the left renal vein. In the abdominal wall, the tributaries of the lumbar veins communicate with those of the epigastric veins. In front of the transverse processes, the lumbar veins of each side are connected to one another, just before they enter the inferior vena cava, by a vertical anastomotic venous channel, the *ascending lumbar vein.* These veins are the abdominal counterparts of the azygos and hemiazygos veins of the posterior mediastinum (see Fig. 22-14). Inferiorly, the ascending lumbar vein connects the lumbar veins with the common or internal iliac veins and the iliolumbar vein. Superiorly, the ascending lumbar veins pass through the crura of the diaphragm or through the aortic hiatus and, uniting with the subcostal veins, form the azygos vein on the right and the hemiazygos vein on the left. Through a small vein, the right ascending lumbar vein connects with the inferior vena cava and the left ascending lumbar vein connects with the left renal vein.

The ascending lumbar vein, therefore, is a potential source of collateral circulation from the lower part of the body when the inferior vena cava is occluded. Because the lumbar veins communicate with the internal vertebral venous plexuses as well, the plexuses around the spinal cord form an important part of this collateral drainage. Other channels that may be involved are the epigastric veins, the superficial veins of the abdomen, and the gonadal veins. Sudden obstruction of the vena cava above the renal level, however, interferes too much with renal function to be tolerated.

Development. The inferior vena cava is a composite of several generations of longitudinal venous channels and anastomoses that interlink these channels. These vessels appear at different stages and disappear partially or completely in the course of development. The tributaries of the vena cava are persistent segments of some of these embryonic veins. A description of these veins is not our purpose here, and mention of them is made only to indicate that the explanation of the anatomy of the inferior vena cava and its tributaries may be found in the manner in which these veins unite to form a single vessel. Errors or arrests in this process provide the clues for the congenital anomalies associated with the inferior vena cava.

The embryonic veins are concerned with draining the body wall, the lower limb buds, and the mesonephric ridges. Some of the veins are located behind the mesonephric ridges, others within them. The so-called *postrenal segment* of the inferior vena cava, lying caudal to the renal vessels, develops from veins that are most dorsally placed, whereas the so-called *prerenal segment,* cranial to the renal veins, develops from more ventrally lying veins. This explains the forward inclination of the vena cava in its course above the level of the renal veins and also why the right inferior phrenic, suprarenal, and renal arteries pass behind the vena cava, whereas the right testicular or ovarian artery passes in front of it.

The first set of bilateral veins is the **postcardinal veins**, which disappear except at the cranial end, where they form the azygos vein and the left superior intercostal vein, and at the caudal end, where anastomosis between the two postcardinal veins persists as the left common iliac vein (white area in Fig. 25-10*A*). The postcardinal veins are replaced by the **supracardinal veins;** the right one of the pair forms the postrenal segment of the inferior vena cava (see blue in Fig. 25-10*B* and *C*). The third set, called the **subcardinal veins,** is formed more ventrally within the mesonephros, which it drains through its tributaries. The right subcardinal vein becomes incorporated into the prerenal segment of the inferior vena cava below the liver (see red in Fig. 25-10).

The subcardinal veins establish connections with both the supracardinal veins (*the subsupracardinal anastomosis*; (black in Fig. 25-10) and, ventral to the aorta, with each other (*subcardinal anastomosis*). The left renal vein is derived from the subcardinal anastomosis, explaining its position anterior to the aorta. The continuity between postrenal and prerenal segments of the inferior vena cava is established by a portion derived from the subsupracardinal anastomosis. The tributaries of the inferior vena cava are all derived from the subcardinal system.

The most cranial portion of the prerenal segment of the vena cava is formed by the right vitelline vein, which also gives rise to the hepatic veins, and by a special vessel that grows from the hepatic veins to link up with the subcardinal portion of the inferior vena cava; the latter vein constitutes the hepatic segment of the fully formed vessel (see purple in Fig. 25-10).

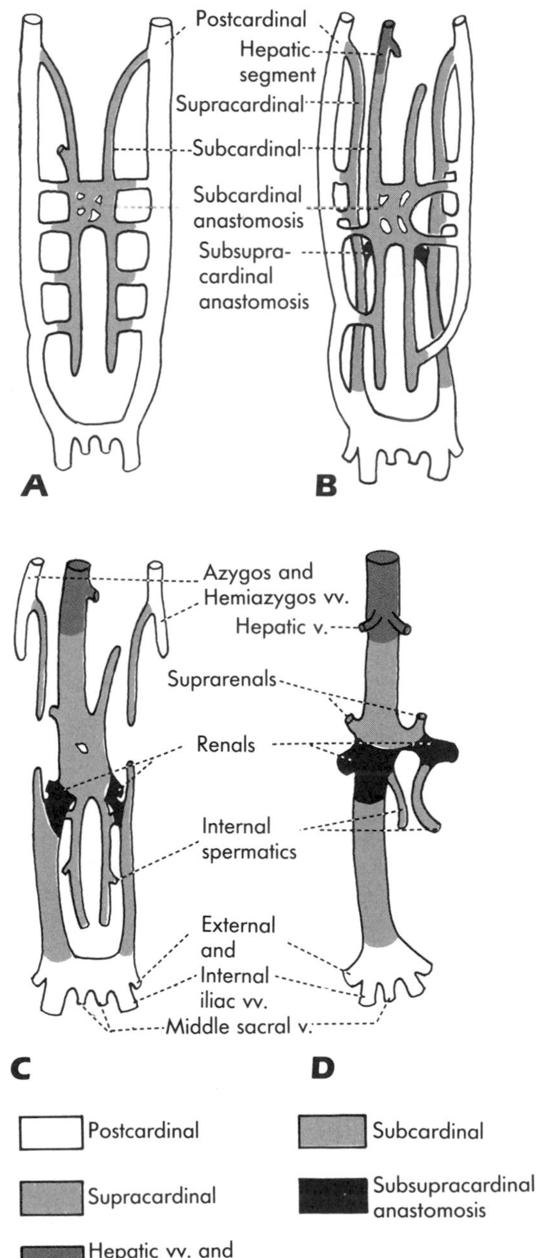

FIGURE *25-10.*
Development of the inferior vena cava and its tributaries: (A) the postcardinals are the chief drainage of the caudal part of the body; (B) the supracardinals have developed and are taking over this drainage; (C) the lower portions of the supracardinals are draining into the subcardinal system; and (D) the definitive condition is shown.

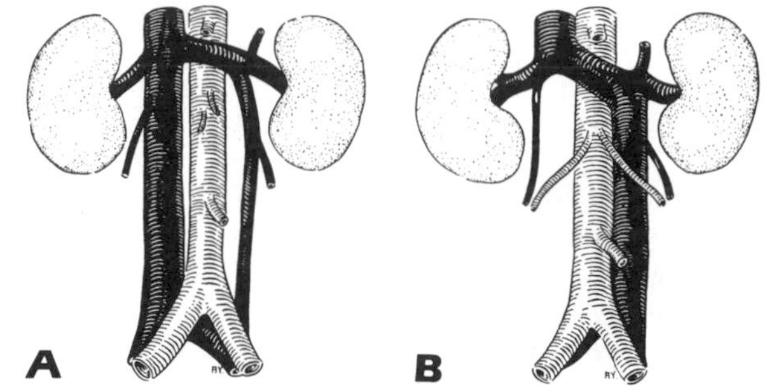

FIGURE *25-11.*
(A) Double inferior vena cava and (B) left inferior vena cava: Note that above the renal level, however, the inferior vena cava is single and on the right side in both cases.

Anomalies. Most anomalies of the inferior vena cava involve the postrenal segment. The usual ones are *double vena cava* and *left inferior vena cava*, caused by persistence on the left side of veins that normally disappear (Fig. 25-11). If the left vena cava is the smaller of a pair, it may seem to join the left renal vein. If it is larger or the only one, it crosses to the right side in front of the aorta at the renal level and receives the left renal, suprarenal, and gonadal veins. If the right subcardinal rather than the right supracardinal, vein persists to form the postrenal segment of the vena cava, the whole vessel is displaced ventrally, causing the ureter to pass behind it (retrocaval ureter).

Very rarely, also, the lower end of the inferior vena cava is so formed that it lies anterior, rather than posterior, to the right common iliac artery.

The hepatic portion of the prerenal segment may fail to develop, in which case the bilateral supracardinal veins that form the azygos and hemiazygos systems are the channels through which blood can return from below the diaphragm to the heart.

THE LYMPHATICS

Lymph from all parts of the body below the diaphragm is directed toward lymph vessels and chains of lymph nodes that ascend around the great vessels of the posterior abdominal wall. The lymphatics from the lower limb, the perineum and buttocks, and the lower part of the anterior abdominal wall converge on the *inguinal lymph nodes* which, in turn, drain upward to a series of *external* and *common iliac nodes* lying along and around the vessels of the same name. Being located along the pelvic brim, these nodes also receive the drainage from the *internal iliac nodes* which, in turn, drain most of the urinary and genital organs in the pelvis and a part of the rectum, the chief drainage of which is along the inferior mesenteric artery. Right and left sets of common iliac nodes meet and exchange lymphatics at the level of the aortic bifurcation.

Above the aortic bifurcation, lymphatics continue upward along the aorta and inferior vena cava (Figs. 25-12 and 25-13). These chains of nodes are known as the **lumbar nodes** (also called *aortic* or *caval nodes*). Although they interchange lymphatics across the midline, these nodes are best thought of as a left chain and a right chain lying along the aorta and the inferior vena cava, respectively. The lumbar nodes receive lymphatics not only from the common iliac nodes, but also directly from the body wall, kidneys, and suprarenals, as well as from the testes or ovaries.

At the level of origin of the inferior mesenteric artery, the lumbar nodes also receive the lymphatic drainage from the left side of the colon; at the level of origin of the superior mesenteric and celiac arteries, they exchange lymphatics with the superior mesenteric and celiac nodes. In this region, lumbar nodes are so mingled with these nodes that it is impossible to say exactly which is a lumbar node and which are nodes connected more directly with the digestive tract.

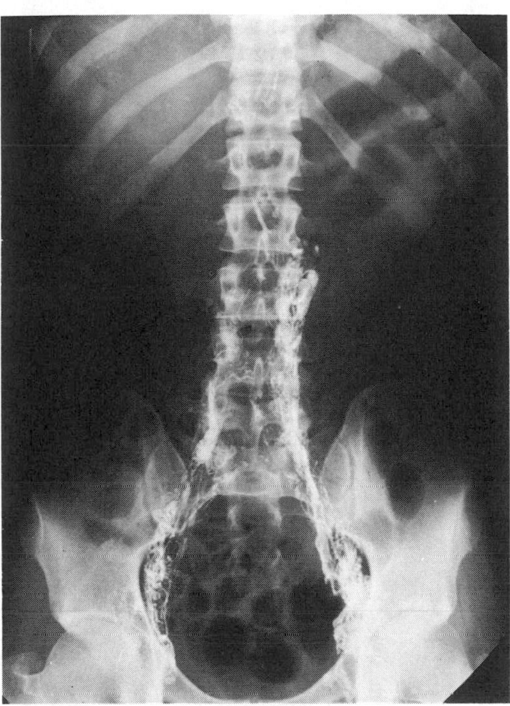

FIGURE 25-13.
Iliac and lower lumbar nodes injected through lymphatics of the feet. (Courtesy of Dr. W. E. Miller.)

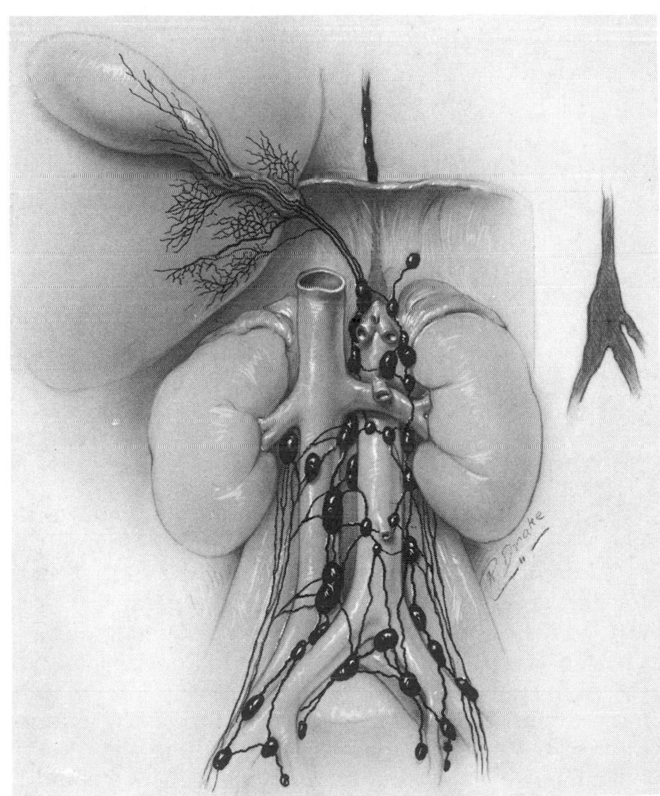

FIGURE 25-12.
Iliac and lumbar lymph nodes: Some of the nodes above the left renal vein are superior mesenteric and celiac nodes, and lymph vessels from the liver and gallbladder can be seen joining the latter. The lower part of the thoracic duct is indicated, and the small inset shows one type of cisterna chyli. (Desjardins AU. Arch Surg 1939,38:714).

The chief efferent vessels from the upper lumbar nodes on each side unite to form the lumbar lymphatic trunk, and the two **lumbar trunks** are joined by the intestinal trunk in the formation of the cisterna chyli. The **intestinal trunk** (there may be more than one) is a short stem formed by efferent lymphatics from the superior mesenteric and celiac nodes. It usually joins the left lumbar trunk before the two lumbar trunks unite.

The **cisterna chyli** is the lower expanded end of the thoracic duct. It lies in the upper part of the abdomen behind the right side of the aorta, in front of the upper right lumbar vessels, on the bodies of L-1 and L-2 vertebrae (Fig. 25-14). Its continuation, the thoracic duct, passes through the aortic hiatus and ascends through the thorax as previously described.

The cisterna chyli varies considerably in its mode of formation, its size, and its placement (see Fig. 25-14). There may be no visible enlargement, and the lymph trunks may unite in highly variable patterns. However, regardless of its method of formation, the important point is that the thoracic duct receives, at its lower end, practically all the lymphatic drainage from the body below the level of the diaphragm, including that from the digestive tract.

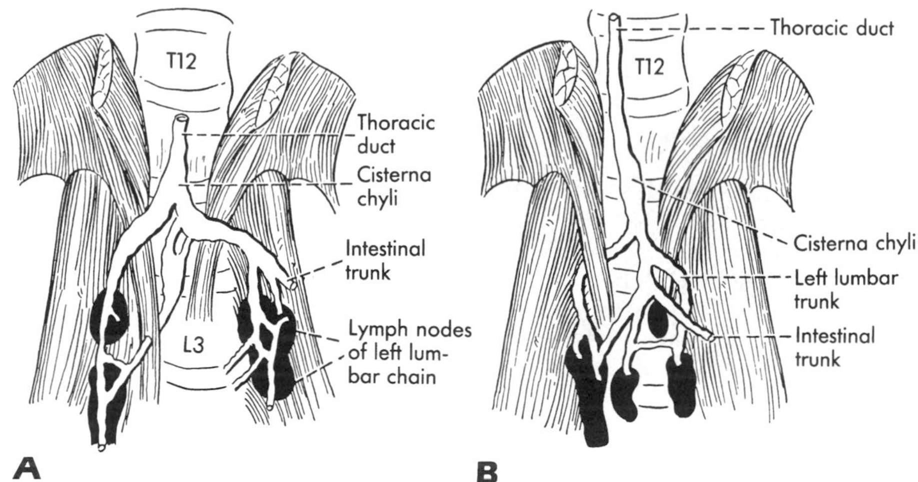

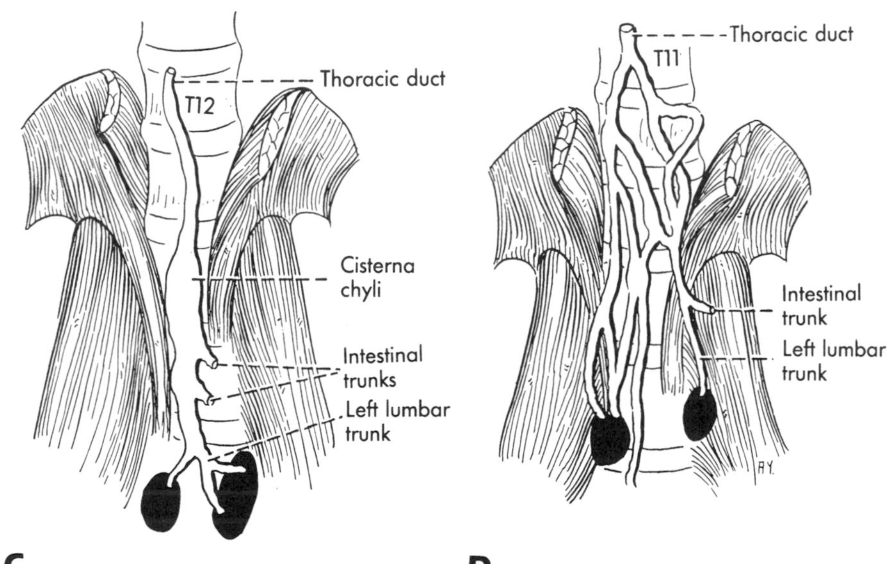

FIGURE *25-14.*
Some variations in the formation of the thoracic duct. (Adapted from Jossifow GM. Arch Anat Physiol Anat Abt 1906; p 68.)

THE NERVE PLEXUSES AND THE SYMPATHETIC TRUNKS

Two qualitatively distinct nerve plexuses are associated with the posterior abdominal wall: the lumbar plexus, composed of somatic nerves, and the aortic plexus, composed of autonomic nerves. The lumbar plexus is enclosed in the psoas major, and its branches have already been identified earlier in this chapter as they emerge from the psoas. The aortic plexus is disposed on the anterior surface of the abdominal aorta, and its subsidiary plexuses are described in the previous chapter in relation to the innervation of the gut and its derivatives. The two sympathetic trunks concerned with relaying sympathetic efferents to the lumbar plexus (i.e., to the lower limbs) and, to a lesser extent, to abdominal viscera lie lateral to the aorta and inferior vena cava on the sides of the lumbar vertebral bodies.

Lumbar Plexus

The lumbar plexus is the upper part of the lumbosacral plexus, the nerve plexus of the lower limbs. Although located on the posterior abdominal wall, the composition, formation, and main branches of the plexus are described in Chapters 14 and 17, because understanding of the plexus is essential for comprehending the innervation of the lower limbs (see Figs. 14-6 and 17-9). The lumbar part of the lumbosacral plexus is formed by anterior rami of L-2 to L-4 spinal nerves. The lumbar plexus is linked, however, by connections superiorly to L-1 and T-12 anterior rami, and inferiorly by the *lumbosacral trunk* (composed of anterior rami of L-4 and L-5) to the sacral plexus (Fig. 25-15). This section describes the relations of the lumbar plexus and the course of the branches that issue from it.

The anterior rami of T-12 to L-4 nerves enter the psoas major muscle as soon as they split off from their parent

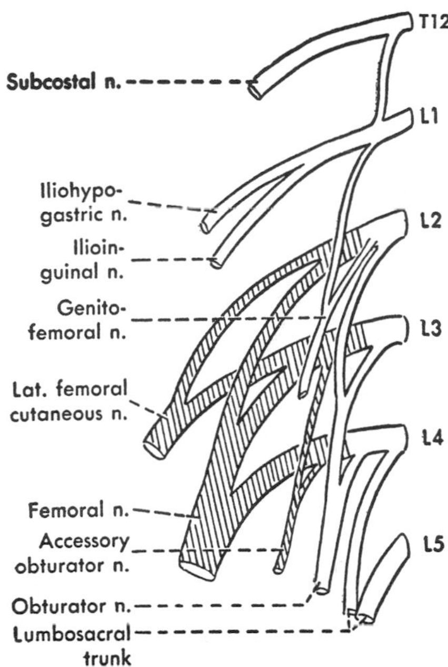

FIGURE 25-15.
A common form of the lumbar plexus: The anterior rami of the nerves, identified by the lettering, and the anterior divisions of the plexus, are *unshaded*; the posterior divisions and branches of the plexus are *shaded*. The accessory obturator nerve is sometimes considered as an anterior branch, and sometimes as a posterior one.

spinal nerves in the intervertebral foramina. As they proceed laterally they are enclosed between the posterior component of the psoas that is attached to the lumbar transverse processes and the anterior part of the muscle arising from the vertebral bodies and intervetebral disks. The splitting of L-2 to L-4 anterior rami into anterior and posterior divisions, and the subsequent union of these divisions to form the nerves that arise from the plexus, takes place within the substance of the psoas.

The nerves that arise from T-12 to L-4 anterior rami are illustrated in Figures 25-2 and 25-15. The *subcostal nerve* (T-12), the *iliohypogastric* (L-1) and *ilioinguinal nerves* (L-1), the *lateral femoral cutaneous nerve* (L-2 and L-3), and *femoral nerve* (L-2, L-3, and L-4), emerge from the psoas major along its lateral border, the *genitofemoral nerve* (L-1 and L-2) pierces the anterior surface of the muscle; the *obturator* (L-2, L-3, and L-4) and *accessory obturator* (L-3 and L-4) nerves appear along the medial border of the muscle (see Fig. 25-2). The *lumbosacral trunk* (L-4 and L-5) descends into the pelvis medial to the latter two nerves without entering the psoas major.

The distributions of the obturator, accessory obturator, femoral, and lateral femoral cutaneous nerves to the lower limb are described in chapters concerned with the lower limb. The iliohypogastric and ilioinguinal nerves are distributed mostly to the skin of the lowest part of the abdomen and upper part of the thigh and buttock. The iliohypogastric nerve may also innervate the pyramidalis muscle. The femoral branch of the genitofemoral goes to the skin of the thigh, and the genital branch goes to the cremaster muscle and to the skin of the scrotum and labia majus.

Variations. The chief variation of the lumbar plexus is in its lower boundary. The lumbar plexus is considered to be normal if it receives more than half the fibers of the fourth lumbar anterior ramus, all of those from the third and none from the fifth. If, in contrast, the plexus receives a minor contribution from the fourth lumbar root, or only some of the fibers from the third lumbar root, with or without those of the fourth the plexus is considered *prefixed* (that is, moved somewhat cranially). If, on the other hand, almost all or all of the fourth root joins the lumbar plexus, and some of the fifth root does likewise, the plexus is considered *postfixed* (that is, having a caudal border that is lower than usual). The cranial border of the plexus (the highest level from which it receives fibers) also may vary, and this variation is apparently independent of the level of the caudal border.

Variations in the composition of the lumbar plexus may affect the composition of the individual branches of the plexus. Although the reported variations are numerous, the basic pattern described is a useful guide to clinical evaluation of the plexus. For instance, the femoral nerve usually receives fibers from the second, third, and fourth lumbar nerves, and the noted variations from this are that it may receive fibers from L-1 or from L-5 or from both. Thus, the shift in the composition of the femoral nerve usually is not more than a segment, which, clinically, is not critical.

The Lumbar Sympathetic Trunks

The lumbar parts of the paired sympathetic trunks lie on the sides of the vertebral bodies at the origin of the psoas major muscle from these bodies (see Fig. 25-6). Each is a continuation of the thoracic part of the trunk on its own side. The interganglionic branch from the lowest thoracic to the uppermost lumbar ganglion is typically slender and usually runs behind the medial arcuate ligament to enter the abdomen. The upper part of the lumbar trunk lies somewhat behind the crus. Each trunk is continued over the sacral promontory as the sacral part of the sympathetic trunk. In the abdomen, the left trunk lies to the left of, but slightly behind, the aorta; the right trunk lies behind the inferior vena cava. However, they are located in front of the lumbar arteries and veins.

Although five *lumbar ganglia* would be expected, because there are five lumbar segments of the body, their number and placement on each side vary (Fig. 25-16). The definitive ganglia are the result of fusion and splitting of the primitive ganglia. Because of the simultaneous variations in number and connections of the ganglia, it is difficult to number them logically or to be sure that similarly numbered ganglia are similar in their connections.

Owing to the variability of the lumbar ganglia, there is considerable variation in their *rami communicantes.* As a rule, however, only the upper lumbar ganglia receive *white rami,* which bring to the sympathetic trunk preganglionic fibers, but they may receive several of these because of the fusion of the ganglia (Fig. 25-17). All ganglia give off *gray rami communicantes,* some of them more than

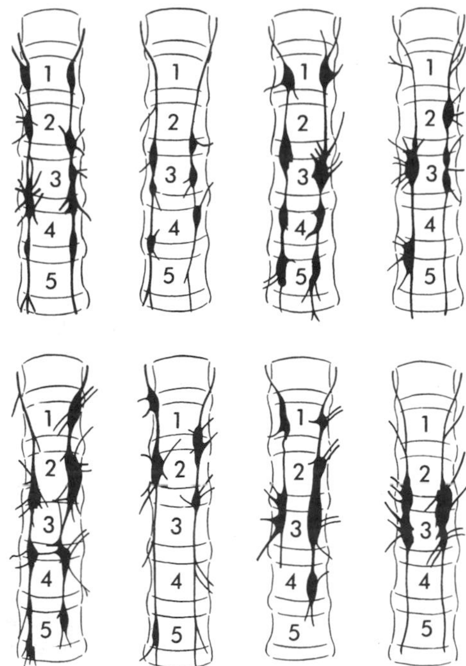

FIGURE 25-16.
Variations in the lumbar sympathetic trunks. The two sides of the same body are rarely symmetric for both number and placement of the lumbar ganglia. (Redrawn from Yeager GH, Cowley RA. Ann Surg 1948;127:953.)

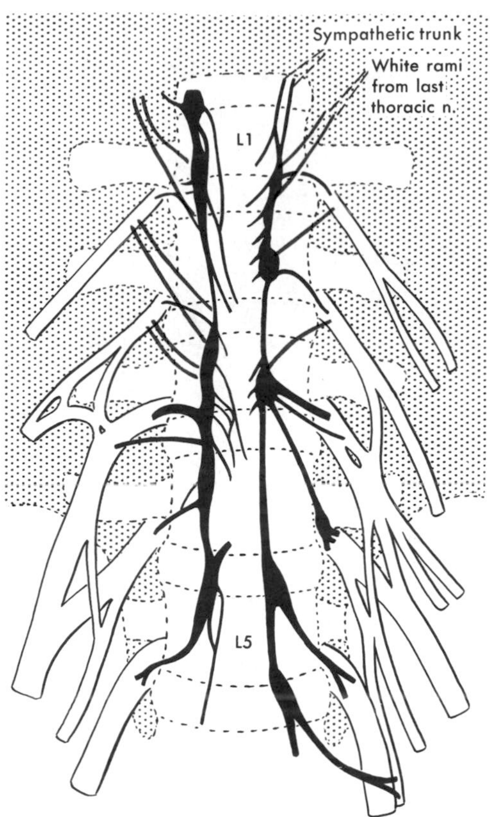

FIGURE 25-17.
The rami communicantes of the lumbar sympathetic trunk in a specimen in which the rami were both dissected and examined histologically. The white rami, as determined by histologic examinations, are shown in *red*; the gray rami, in *black*. (Redrawn from Pick J, Sheehan D. J Anat 1946;80:12.)

one, to the anterior rami of the lumbar nerves. Also, each lumbar nerve usually receives gray rami from more than one ganglion. Some of these postganglionic sympathetic efferents find their way into the posterior rami of these nerves as well, running medially to the point of division of the spinal nerve.

The upper lumbar ganglia give medial branches that are the *lumbar splanchnic nerves* (See Fig. 25-17). These nerves contain preganglionic visceral efferent fibers that relay in the aortic ganglia after the lumbar splanchnic nerves join the aortic plexus, which they help form. The lumbar splanchnic nerves also convey visceral afferents from the aortic plexus to the lumbar ganglia and, through them and their white rami communicantes, to the upper lumbar spinal nerves.

Sympathectomies

Segments of the sympathetic trunks have been removed (sympathectomy), mainly with two objectives: 1) improving the circulation in the lower limbs by reducing vasospasms caused by increased sympathetic activity; and 2) lowering the blood pressure by vasodilation in the large vascular bed of abdominal viscera. Because of the availability of a variety of suitable drugs, sympathectomies are now done less frequently.

For the sympathetic innervation of the lower limb, which receives all its postganglionic fibers through the lumbar and sacral nerves by way of the gray rami communicantes, the standard operation is to remove the upper segment of the lumbar trunk, which receives all the white rami communicantes. For hypertension caused by sympathetic overactivity, cutting the splanchnic nerves and removing the upper parts of the lumbar trunks, often together with the lower parts of the thoracic sympathetic trunks (thoracolumbar sympathectomy), has been the operation of choice. The effect of denervation on the abdominal and pelvic organs is generalized vasodilation. In the male, a complicating, undesirable effect is interference with ejaculation.

The Aortic Plexus

The functional components and the anatomic subdivisions of the aortic plexus are mentioned in Chapter 24 with relation to the innervation of the gut and its derivatives. The aortic plexus is a continuous network of nerves extending on the surface of the aorta from the aortic hiatus to the bifurcation and, below that, into the pelvis (Fig. 25-18). It has several parts named according to the major branches of the aorta.

The superior and most dense portion of the plexus is the **celiac plexus,** continuous below with the **superior mesenteric plexus.** The part of the aortic plexus intervening between the superior and inferior mesenteric arteries is called the **intermesenteric plexus.** Some of the fibers of

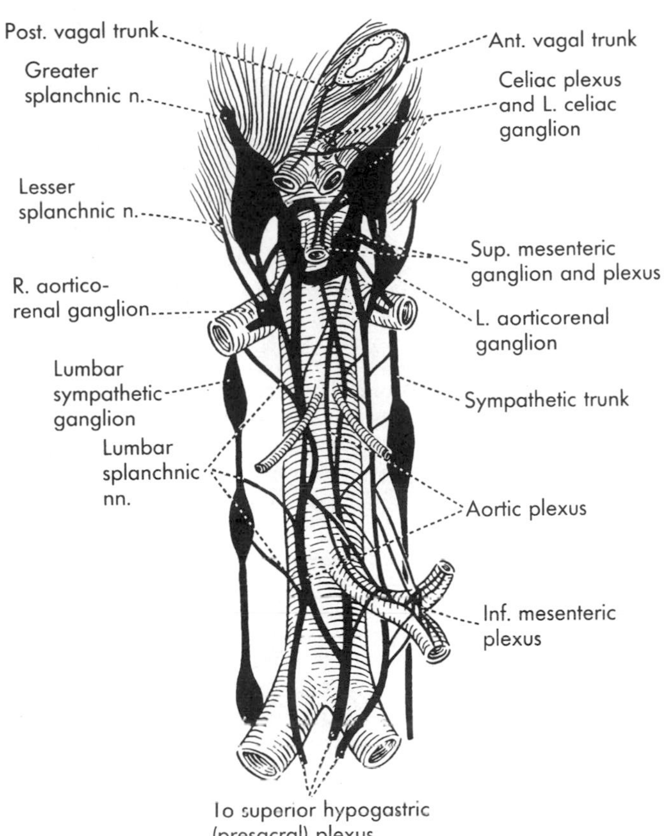

FIGURE *25-18.*
The autonomic nerve plexuses and ganglia associated with the aorta: The aortic plexus is below the level of the superior mesenteric artery.

the intermesenteric plexus continue along the inferior mesenteric artery as the **inferior mesenteric plexus;** others descend toward the sacral promontory and, beyond the bifurcation, are designated the **superior hypogastric plexus.**

The aortic plexus receives input from the following sources: 1) thoracic splanchnic nerves (greater, lesser, and lowest), composed of the visceral branches of the lower thoracic sympathetic ganglia; 2) lumbar splanchnic nerves, visceral branches of lumbar sympathetic ganglia; 3) celiac branches of the vagi. The plexus also contains visceral afferents from all abdominal and most pelvic viscera, which leave the plexus along the vagi and the thoracic and lumbar splanchnic nerves. The pelvic splanchnic nerves, which furnish parasympathetic fibers to the descending colon and the rest of the hindgut, do not enter the aortic plexus; they follow the sigmoid arteries on their ascent from the pelvis (see Fig. 24-50). Thus, the aortic plexus is composed chiefly of sympathetic fibers with some vagal fibers admixed in its superior parts.

The branches of the aortic plexus are the subsidiary plexuses that accompany the branches of the aorta (e.g., hepatic, and inferior mesenteric).

Throughout its length, from the uppermost part of the abdomen down into the pelvis, the aortic plexus contains numerous minute ganglia within which preganglionic sympathetic fibers synapse. It also contains a few large ganglia. The **celiac ganglia,** the largest ones, are paired structures lying in the lateral parts of the celiac plexus on the sides of the aorta and the crura of the diaphragm at about the level of the origin of the celiac trunk. They regularly receive the greater splanchnic nerves and may receive the lesser; through them, therefore, come most of the fibers that descend from the thorax. More or less continuous with the celiac ganglia are the **superior mesenteric ganglia,** which are sometimes identifiable as separate ganglia and sometimes not. These lie on each side of the origin of the superior mesenteric artery and may unite below the artery to form an unpaired ganglion. A smaller ganglion, the **aorticorenal ganglion,** frequently is identifiable a little lower, lying close to the origin of the renal artery. The **inferior mesenteric ganglion** often is so embedded in the inferior mesenteric plexus or so subdivided into smaller ganglia that it is difficult or impossible to find.

THE KIDNEYS, URETERS, AND SUPRARENAL GLANDS

The kidneys, ureters, and suprarenal glands are located in the retroperitoneal connective tissue of the posterior abdominal wall (Fig. 25-19). Their close anatomic association is a consequence of their developmental history. The three structures commence their development far away from each other. The close association of the kidneys with the ureters, their excretory ducts, is essential for function; the kidneys and suprarenal glands have nothing in common functionally, although both are essential to life. Following the separate anatomic descriptions of these three paired organs, their relations, blood supply, lymph drainage, innervation, and development will be considered together.

The Kidneys

The kidneys (*renes*) are two somewhat bean-shaped, reddish-brown organs the function of which is the maintenance of the body's fluid and electrolyte balance. They regulate the volume and composition of the urine, which they excrete and discharge through the ureters into the urinary bladder. The kidneys also secrete substances into the circulation that regulate blood pressure and certain processes of hematopoiesis.

Each kidney is about 11 cm long, 6 cm wide, and 3 cm thick.

Parts and Structure

Each kidney has a smooth anterior and posterior *surface,* separated by the lateral and medial *margins.* The two margins become confluent with each other around the rather blunt superior and inferior extremities or *poles* of the kidneys. Much of the medial margin is occupied by the *hilum,*

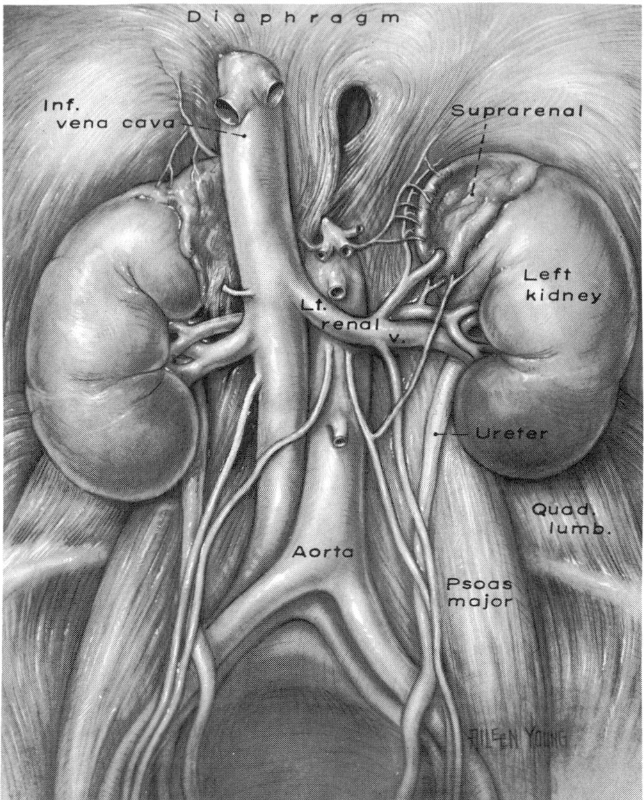

FIGURE *25-19.*
The kidneys and suprarenal glands.

through which the renal vessels, lymphatics, and nerves enter or leave the *renal sinus*, the space enclosed by the renal tissue. The sinus and hilum contain also, along with some fat, the *renal pelvis*, which is the expanded upper end of the ureter, shaped like a complex funnel and distinct from the renal *parenchyma*.

A section through the hilum in a plane parallel with the renal surfaces reveals the renal sinus with its contents and the structure of the renal parenchyma (Fig. 25-20). The parenchyma is enclosed by the *fibrous capsule*, which fits the kidney tightly but is not bound to it; once incised, it can be easily stripped from the kidney. The renal parenchyma consists of two parts: the outer *cortex*, which forms a continuous broad band of tissue subjacent to the capsule, and the inner *medulla*, which is discontinuous owing to the projections of the cortex toward the renal sinus. These projections are the *renal columns*, and the individual portions of the medulla between them are known as *renal pyramids*.

The renal cortex, which is rather pale, dense, and homogeneous on macroscopic examination, contains mainly the *renal corpuscles* (about 1 million in each kidney) and the convoluted portions of the *renal tubules*, whereas the renal pyramids, distinguishable from the cortex by their darker color and longitudinal striations, contain the descending and ascending limbs of the renal tubules and the *collecting tubules*. With the aid of a hand lens, it is possible to see the extension of the striations from the base of the pyramids into the cortex. These striations are the *medullary rays* and, similar to the medulla, contain collecting tubules.

The nipplelike apex of each pyramid points into the renal sinus and is known as the *renal papilla*. The renal papillae are perforated by the termination of collecting tubules and drain the urine into the *minor calices*, subdivisions of the renal pelvis. A minor calix may receive several papillae, as there are, in each kidney, 5 to 18 renal papillae and only up to 13 minor calices. Each pyramid, with the peripheral cortex between its base and the capsule, constitutes a *lobe* of the kidney; there are 5 to 18 lobes in each kidney.

Microscopic Structure. The renal parenchyma consists of a mass of *uriniferous tubules* and blood vessels. Each uriniferous tubule has two component parts, distinct both functionally and developmentally: 1) the *nephron*, composed of a *renal corpuscle* and a *renal tubule*; and 2) *collecting tubules*, in which several renal tubules terminate. Urine is produced by the nephron and is then conducted to the minor calices by the collecting tubules.

The renal corpuscle consists of the *glomerulus*, a tuft of capillaries that produces a filtrate of blood plasma discharged into the *glomerular capsule*, the expanded end of the renal tubule around the glomerulus. The rest of the renal tubule has several named segments that are concerned with the modification of the glomerular

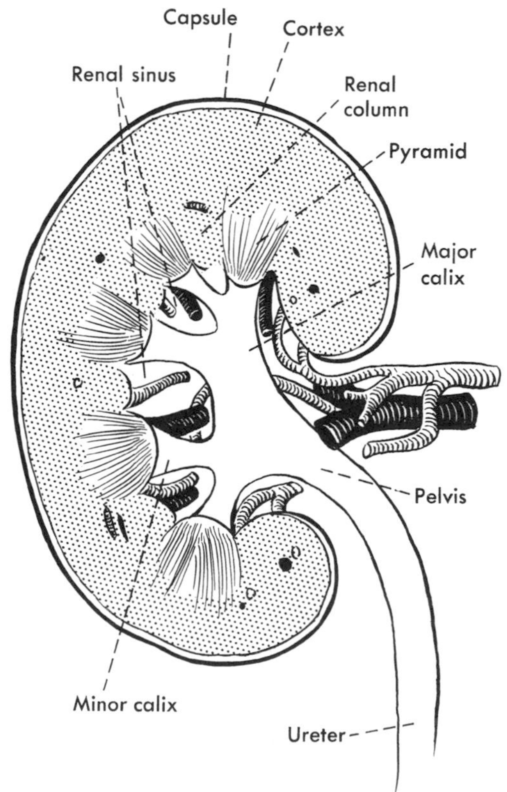

FIGURE *25-20.*
The kidney: The renal vessels anterior to the renal pelvis have been cut in removing the anterior half of the kidney; the fat in the renal sinus has also been removed.

filtrate, converting it into urine by the time the collecting tubule is reached.

Position

The kidneys lie in the paravertebral gutters, the depth of which is reduced by the psoas major. The vertebral levels of the kidney vary somewhat with body build and posture and also with the excursions of the diaphragm. However, when a person is in the supine position, the kidneys tend to extend from the 12th thoracic to the 3rd lumbar vertebra, with the right kidney usually a little lower than the left. The transpyloric plane passes through the upper part of the hilum of the right kidney and through the lower part of the hilum of the left. The upper poles of the kidneys are closer to one another than the lower poles; thus, both their long and transverse axes are oblique. The hila face anteriorly as well as medially, the lateral margin being more posterior.

The kidneys are difficult to palpate; the rib cage and the bulky paravertebral muscles make them inaccessible. When the abdominal wall is relaxed in a supine subject, the lower poles of the kidneys may be caught in the lumbar region of the abdomen between a hand placed just below the costal margin and the other posteriorly between the last rib and the iliac crest. Projected to the anterior abdominal wall, the renal hila are just medial to the point where the transpyloric plane intersects the costal margin and, on the back, 5 cm from the spinous process of L-1 vertebra. The upper poles are in the epigastrium, each 2.5 cm from the midline, approximately 5 cm above the hilum. The lower poles are 7.5 cm from the midline, slightly above the supracristal plane.

The Renal Pelvis and Ureter

In the sinus of the kidney, the renal pelvis divides into two or three **major calices** which, in turn, divide into **minor calices** (Fig. 25-21). Into the minor calices, urine is discharged through the pores of the *cribriform plate*, which caps the tip of each renal papilla.

The renal pelvis extends through the hilum and, as it tapers to a narrow tube outside the kidney, becomes the ureter. The ureteropelvic junction is rather indefinite and is located approximately opposite the lower pole of the kidney. From here the ureter descends more or less vertically in the extraperitoneal fascia of the posterior abdominal wall (Fig. 25-22). At the pelvic brim, where the ureters cross the common iliac vessels, they incline medially and continue their intrapelvic course to the urinary bladder (see Chap. 27).

Hydronephrosis. After its discharge from the renal tubule into the collecting ducts, the urine is not

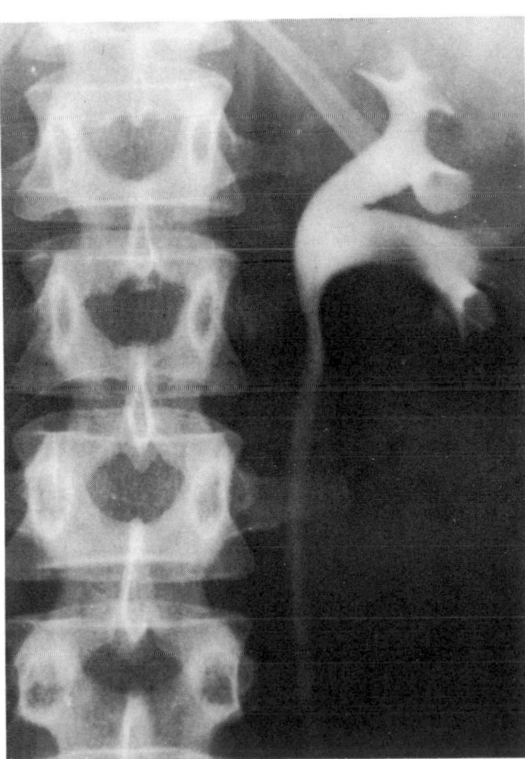

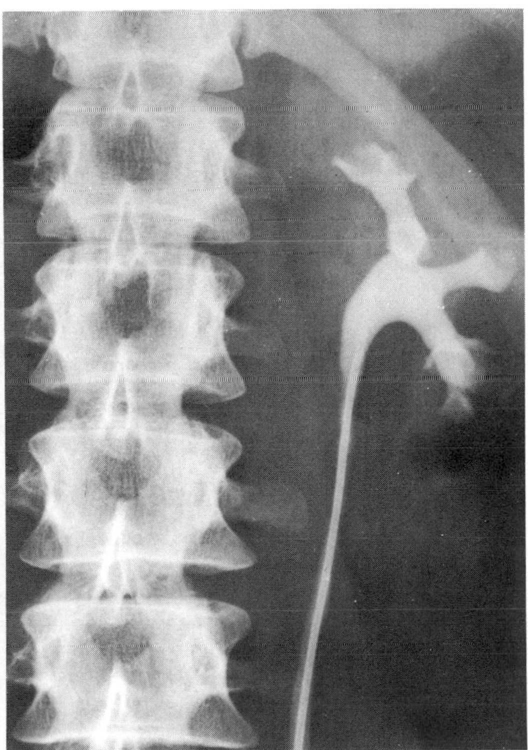

FIGURE *25-21.*
Retrograde pyelograms of the kidneys: Contrast medium is introduced into the renal pelvis through a catheter (visible in the film on the right) that was inserted into the ureter from the bladder. One of the kidneys has two and the other has three major calices. Only one of the minor calices shows, but their pattern is obviously different in the two kidneys. (Braasch WF, Emmett JL. Clinical urography. Philadelphia: WB Saunders 1951.)

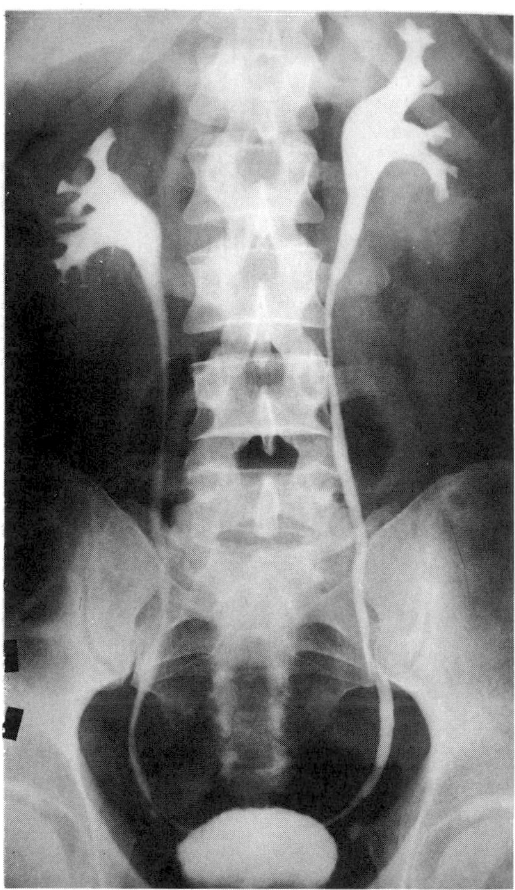

FIGURE 25-22.
An ascending or retrograde pyelogram showing the renal pelves and calices and the courses of the ureters: The urinary bladder also is visualized. (Braasch WF, Emmett JL. Clinical urography. Philadelphia: WB Saunders, 1951.)

changed until it is voided from the bladder. Its passage through the renal pelvis and ureters is aided by peristaltic activity. There is constant production of urine by the kidneys, and obstruction of its flow along the ureters causes pressure to build up proximal to the obstruction, producing distention of the renal pelvis and its calices. This condition is known as hydronephrosis and also involves the ureter above the obstruction. Persistent and severe hydronephrosis results in damage to, and eventually atrophy of, the kidney.

The obstruction may be caused by stenosis of the ureteropelvic junction, by compression of the ureter, or by a urinary calculus (stone) lodged anywhere along the ureter. Hydronephrosis may result also from abnormalities in ureteric peristalsis or from abnormalities at the junction of the ureter with the bladder.

Urinary Calculi. Urinary stasis in the renal pelvis predisposes to the formation of stones, especially if certain substances are excreted in abnormally high concentrations in the urine. There are several types of renal calculi. If they are small, they are passed down the ureter and are voided. Larger ones may cause spasm and obstruction of the ureter, announced by excruciating pain. Still larger ones may not leave the renal pelvis, where they may form a cast of one or more of the calices. As they increase in size, they may eventually fragment.

The Suprarenal Gland

The two suprarenal glands are roughly triangular, compact bodies, closely applied to the upper poles of the kidneys (see Fig. 25-19). They consist of an outer, pale cortex and an inner, almost black, medulla; the two regions are quite distinct, not only macroscopically and histologically, but also in development and function. The composition and function of both cortex and medulla are described in Chapter 11.

The right suprarenal gland is rather pyramidal in shape; the left one is semilunar, larger, and flatter. The largest dimension of the glands does not exceed 5 cm. Their base, molded on the upper pole of the kidneys, is concave, and each gland has an anterior surface, covered partly with peritoneum on the right and completely on the left, and a posterior surface that rests against the diaphragm. Each gland has a small hilum on its anterior surface; a single vein issues from it. Many arterial twigs enter the glands around their periphery.

Related Fascias and Organs

The retroperitoneal connective tissue that surrounds the kidneys, ureters, and suprarenal glands is organized in a particular manner to form the *renal fascia* and the *adipose capsule* of the kidney. Other organs and structures are related through this connective tissue to the kidneys, ureters, and suprarenal glands.

Adipose Capsule and Renal Fascia

The *perirenal fat,* in immediate contact with the kidney, ureter, and suprarenal glands, is considered to be the *adipose capsule.* This perirenal fat extends through the hilum, and in the renal sinus, the renal vessels, lymphatics, nerves, and calices of the renal pelvis are embedded in it. A membranous condensation of connective tissue surrounds this perirenal fat and separates it from the general adipose tissue of the posterior abdominal wall. The membranous component is the *renal fascia,* and the fat outside this fascia is known as the *pararenal fat* (Fig. 25-23).

It is the **renal fascia,** rather than the adipose capsule, that is of importance. The renal fascia surrounds each kidney as a separate sheath, and it must be incised in any operation on the kidney, whether from an anterior or a posterior approach. Descriptions of the fascia and its continuities vary, but it is usually described as a complete covering of both the kidney and suprarenal gland, sometimes sending a septum between them.

The renal fascia on the anterior surface of the kidney passes around the lateral border to become continuous with that on the posterior surface (see Fig. 25-23). Traced medially, the two layers are continuous in a similar way over the medial margin of the kidney, except around the renal vessels, where they have been described as being

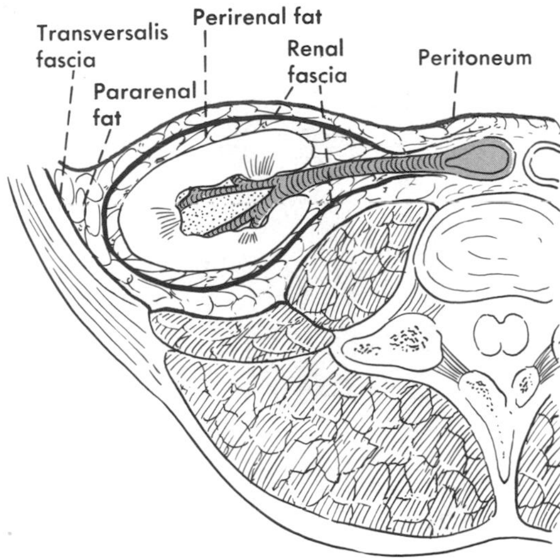

FIGURE 25-23.
Diagram of the renal fascia in a cross section through the posterior body wall.

traceable across the vertebral column, both in front of and behind the great vessels, to the corresponding layers around the other kidney. It is generally granted, however, that passage of material other than injected gas does not occur across the midline. Traced upward, the renal fascia passes over the suprarenal gland, and its anterior layer merges with that of the posterior layer above the gland. The layers have been described as meeting also below the kidney, except where the ureter leaves. Because the renal fascia is open below, around the ureter, infections around the kidney may descend into the pelvis, and infections in the pelvis ascend to the kidney. The fat within the fascia forms a potential space in which fluid or injected air can accumulate and be more or less retained by the fascia.

Gas is sometimes injected into the extraperitoneal tissue of the pelvis and is permitted to ascend into the adipose capsule to outline the kidney and suprarenal gland for roentgenographic examination, particularly when a tumor is suspected.

Radiology. The outline of the kidneys can often be made out on a plain x-ray film of the abdomen because of contrast in the density of the radiolucent pararenal and perirenal fat and the more radiopaque renal parenchyma (see Fig. 23-12*B*). *Excretory urography* is a procedure that makes use of the ability of the kidneys to concentrate and excrete rather rapidly certain substances injected intravenously. When such substances are tagged with radiopaque molecules (e.g., iodine), the kidneys become radiopaque soon after the injection, and their anatomy, as well as that of the renal pelvis, can be examined on x-ray films (Fig. 25-24). Such an x-ray film is called an *intravenous pyelogram* (IVP). The anatomy of the ureters and renal pelves can be studied with greater accuracy if they are filled with contrast medium directly through a catheter inserted through the bladder into the orifice of the ureter (see Figs. 25-21 and 25-22; *ascending or retrograde urography; retrograde pyelogram*).

Related Structures and Organs

The posterior relations of the kidneys, ureters, and suprarenal glands are quite similar on the two sides, whereas anteriorly, there are major differences.

Posterior Relations. Both suprarenal glands and roughly the upper third of both kidneys lie on the diaphragm. Through the costal parts and the lumbocostal trigones of the diaphragm, these organs are related to the

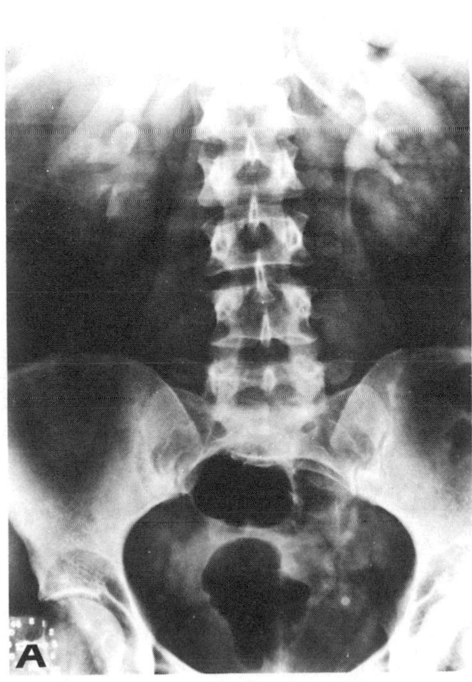

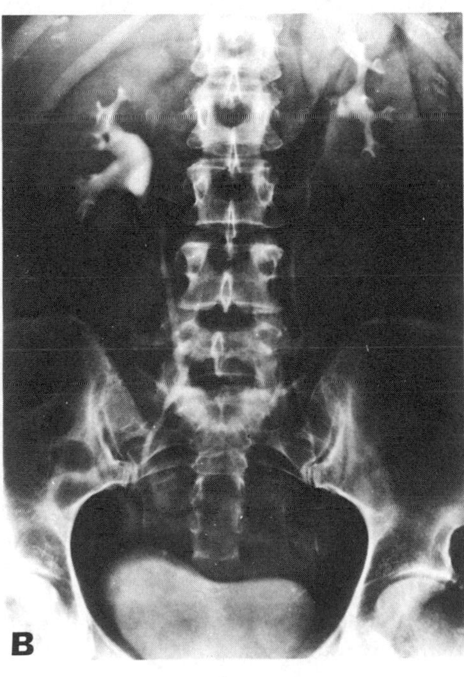

FIGURE 25-24.
Two intravenous pyelograms (IVPs) in two different subjects: In (A) exposed shortly after intravenous injection of the contrast medium, the renal parenchyma is radiopaque owing to the concentration of the contrast medium by the kidneys, which is also beginning to outline the calices and the renal pelvis. (B) Exposed much later, the contrast medium fills the renal pelves, the ureters, and the bladder.

pleura, quite intimately if there are few or no muscle fibers present in the trigones. The 11th and 12th ribs are behind the suprarenal glands and the left kidney. The costodiaphragmatic recess and the diaphragm intervene between the 11th rib and the renal fascia, whereas the 12th rib is in direct contact with the fascia of both kidneys. Fractures or displacements of this rib may cause injury to the kidney. The pleural sacs extend below the lower border of the last rib and are present behind the kidneys and the diaphragm in the triangular area bounded by the 12th rib, the medial arcuate line, and L-1 transverse process.

Both lateral and medial lumbocostal arches (arcuate lines) cross behind the kidneys. Below the medial arch, the medial margin of the kidney rests on the psoas major, as does the renal pelvis and, lower down, the ureter. The posterior branches of the renal artery enter the renal hilum, running posteriorly to the upper part of the renal pelvis. Each ureter is separated from the tips of the lumbar transverse processes by the psoas major muscle. As noted before, the ureter lies on the psoas as far down as the pelvic brim, where the ureters cross anterior to the common iliac vessels.

Below the lateral arcuate line, the renal fascia is in contact with the quadratus lumborum. Near their lateral margins, the kidneys lie on the transversus abdominis. The subcostal and iliohypogastric nerves cross these two muscles behind the kidney.

Anterior Relations on the Right. The upper half of the right suprarenal gland and, to its right, the upper pole of the right kidney lie behind the bare area of the liver. Medially, the suprarenal gland is overlapped by the inferior vena cava (Fig. 25-25; see Fig. 25-19). The kidney and the suprarenal gland are crossed by the posterior layer of the right coronary ligament (hepatorenal ligament), and below this ligament, both are covered by parietal peritoneum. Their anterior surface here faces into the hepatorenal recess (compare Figs. 25-25 and 23-18). Through this recess, the kidney and suprarenal gland are in contact with the inferior surface of the right lobe of the liver (see Fig. 24-31). The medial margin of the kidney, in the region of the hilum, is nonperitoneal; the descending part of the duodenum lies on it. Just above the inferior pole, the right colic flexure is in direct contact with the renal fascia (see Fig. 25-25). The lower pole itself, however, is covered by parietal peritoneum of the right infracolic compartment.

The right *renal pelvis* is crossed anteriorly by the anterior branches of the renal vessels, which, together with the pelvis, are behind the duodenum. Below the duodenum, the right ureter descends behind the peritoneum of the right infracolic compartment, where it is crossed by the testicular or ovarian vessels, the right colic and iliocolic vessels, and the root of the mesentery.

Anterior Relations on the Left. The left suprarenal gland and the upper pole of the left kidney face into the omental bursa and are covered by parietal peritoneum (see Fig. 25-25). Through the cavity of the bursa, the stomach is in contact with this area, limited toward the left by the attachment of the lienorenal ligament to the kidney.

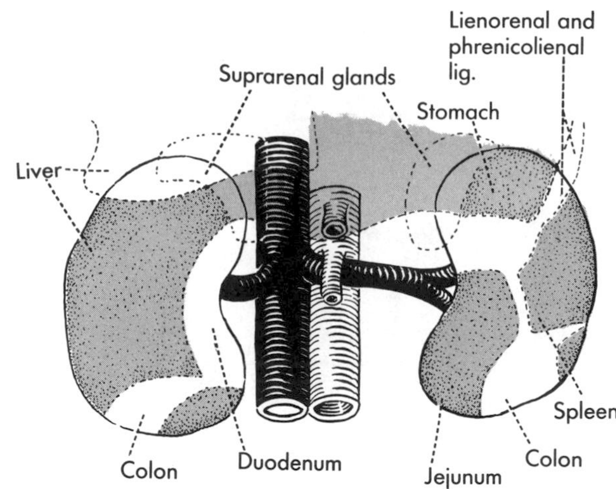

FIGURE 25-25.
Peritoneal relations of the kidneys: The *stippled areas* are those in which the kidneys are directly related to the peritoneum through the fat and connective tissue over them. Peritoneum of the greater sac is *pink;* that of the omental bursa is *blue.*

On the left side of the ligament, parietal peritoneum of the greater sac covers the kidney, and through the cavity of this sac, the spleen is in contact with the anterior surface and the lateral margin of the kidney. Below the gastric area, the tail of the pancreas rests directly on the renal fascia, and it overlaps much of the hilum and its vessels. The lower pole and the adjoining anteromedial surface are covered by parietal peritoneum of the left infracolic compartment; loops of jejunum are in contact with it. Lateral to the lower pole, the left colic flexure and descending colon are in direct contact with the renal fascia.

The *renal pelvis* is crossed anteriorly by branches of the renal vessels and the tail of the pancreas. The left ureter is retroperitoneal in the left infracolic compartment and is crossed by the left colic vessel and, just above the pelvic brim, by the root of the sigmoid mesocolon.

Vessels and Nerves

Arterial Supply and Venous Drainage

Suprarenal Glands. The arterial supply to the suprarenal gland is derived from three or four sources: the inferior phrenic arteries, the aorta, and the renal and, on occasion the gonadal arteries (Fig. 25-26).

As the *inferior phrenic arteries* pass just above and medial to the suprarenal glands, each artery usually gives off a series of branches into the gland of its own side before it supplies the diaphragm. These arteries constitute the **superior suprarenal arteries,** and they have long been named as though there were only a single artery. They enter the upper part of the gland over a considerable expanse of its anterior and posterior surface.

There usually is at least one artery to each gland given off by the aorta just above the origin of the renal arteries. This artery (or arteries) is called the **middle**

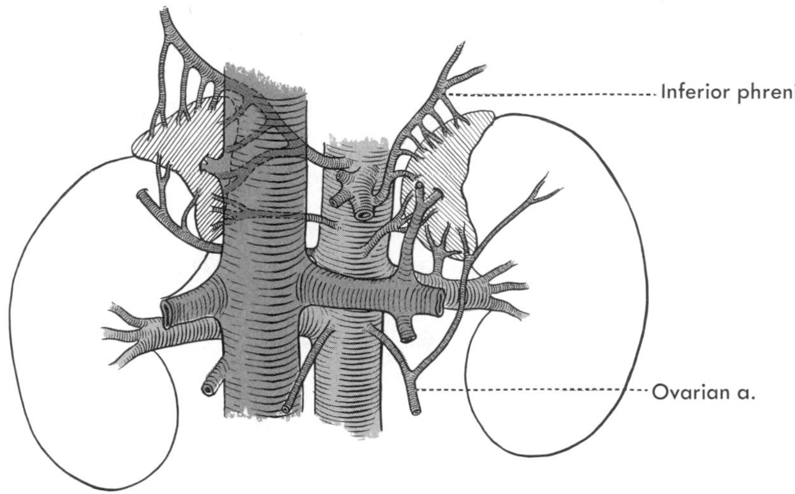

FIGURE 25-26.
Vessels of the suprarenal glands; note the single vein from each gland, and the multiple arteries. (Modified from Hollinshead WH. Surg Clin North Am 1952;32:1115.)

suprarenal artery. Also, one or more arteries reach the suprarenal gland from the adjacent renal artery and are called the **inferior suprarenal artery.** In addition to these three regular sources of blood supply, other vessels running close by may also supply branches to the suprarenal gland. Most constant of these are the arteries to the gonads.

Since any of the arteries approaching the gland may branch or rebranch, the number of vessels entering it may be quite numerous—as many as 50 individual stems have been counted. There is no regular position in which these branches enter the gland; they enter over much of the surface. In contrast with the arteries, the main drainage of the gland is into a single **suprarenal vein** that leaves the gland through its hilum, although there are also several tiny venous twigs that connect with veins in the adjacent connective tissue. On the left side, the suprarenal vein is usually joined by the inferior phrenic vein of that side, and separately or together, they empty into the left renal vein. On the right side, the suprarenal vein joins the inferior vena cava. Usually, the suprarenal vein is very short, emerging from the gland close to the vena cava.

Kidneys. The two renal arteries arise from the lateral aspects of the aorta, only a little below the origin of the superior mesenteric artery, most commonly at the level of the lower third of the first lumbar vertebra to the upper third of the second. The right artery tends to arise a little lower than the left one (Fig. 25-27) and passes behind the inferior vena cava. The renal veins lie in front of the renal arteries, largely hiding them (see Fig. 25-19). On their way to the renal hilum, the renal arteries give off their nonrenal branches and, just before reaching the hilum, divide into *segmental renal arteries,* which pass around the renal pelvis into the renal sinus.

The renal artery gives off its *suprarenal branch,* sends one or more *ureteric arteries* downward and one or more *capsular branches* into the adipose capsule of the kidney. Usually, fairly close to the renal pelvis, the renal artery divides into *anterior* and *posterior rami* that pass on respective sides of the renal pelvis and the major calices. Each of these arteries supplies a vascular segment of the kidney and each is known as a segmental artery (Fig. 25-28).

Vascular Segments. Within the renal sinus, anterior and posterior arterial rami rebranch. Although the pattern is quite variable, the distribution is constant enough to allow the division of the kidney into vascular segments that correspond to the prevailing vascular pattern.

There are three anterior rami of the renal artery; the **superior, anterior,** and **inferior segmental arteries;** they supply segments of the kidney named correspondingly (Fig. 25-28). There is usually a **posterior ramus** of the renal artery supplying the

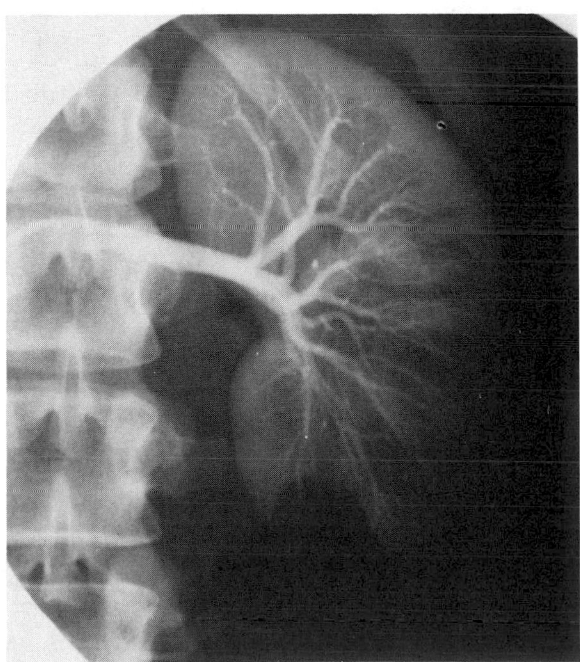

FIGURE 25-27.
A renal arteriogram: Contrast medium was injected into the left renal artery through a catheter, just visible in the aorta close to the origin of the artery.

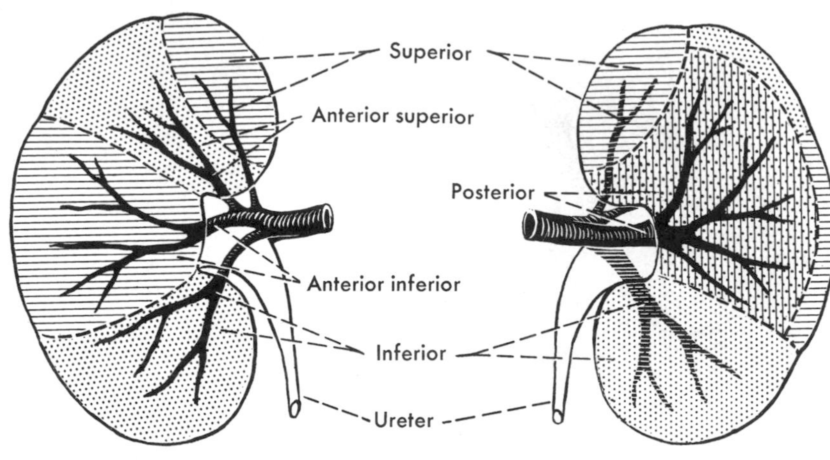

FIGURE *25-28.*
The segmental renal arteries and the renal segments.

posterior segment. Superior and inferior segments occupying the region of the upper and lower poles are represented on both anterior and posterior surfaces of the kidney; the anterior and posterior segments are limited to the corresponding surfaces. Vascular patterns that depart markedly from the one described here have also been reported.

As the branches of the renal artery run through the renal sinus, they give off twigs to the connective tissue of the sinus and to the renal pelvis and calices. Their major branches penetrate the renal parenchyma as **interlobar arteries.** These become the **arcuate arteries** after a sharp turn reorients them across the bases of the pyramids. In this position, they give rise to the **interlobular arteries** from which the smaller vessels of the kidney are derived.

The segmental arteries do not anastomose with each other; obstruction of a segmental artery leads to cessation of function and death of that segment of the kidney served by the artery.

In contrast with the arteries, the **veins** within the kidney anastomose with each other and have no segmental distribution. All tributaries of the renal vein usually pass in front of the renal pelvis, but sometimes one may pass behind it.

The **left renal vein** crosses in front of the aorta and behind the descending stem of the superior mesenteric artery to join the inferior vena cava. The short **right renal vein** joins the inferior vena cava at about the same level.

The right renal vein usually receives no tributaries other than those from the kidney; the left renal vein usually receives the *upper lumbar vein*, a communication from the *ascending lumbar vein*, the combined stem of the *left inferior phrenic* and *suprarenal veins*, and the vein from the left gonad (*ovarian or testicular*). The right ovarian or testicular vein typically enters the inferior vena cava below the entrance of the right renal vein, whereas the right suprarenal vein and the right inferior phrenic enter the vena cava separately above the renal vein.

Variations. The renal, inferior phrenic, suprarenal, and gonadal arteries are all members of a series of segmental mesonephric arteries that supplied the urogenital ridges. These ridges contain the suprarenal glands the developing kidneys, and the gonads. In approximately one-third of bodies, more than one artery persists to an otherwise normal kidney. Almost a third of such kidneys receive two or more of these so-called accessory renal arteries. Two or three renal arteries occur as often on one side as the other.

Whether these accessory renal arteries pass behind or in front of the inferior vena cava depends on their level of origin from the aorta. When they arise in the vicinity of normal renal arteries or above them, they will pass behind the prerenal segment of the inferior vena cava, along with the inferior phrenic or suprarenal branches of the aorta. Should they arise from the part of the aorta that parallels the postrenal segment of the inferior vena cava, they will pass in front of it and also in front of the renal pelvis or ureter. These inferior accessory arteries may compress the ureter or the renal pelvis, predisposing to hydronephrosis.

Although most of the branches of the renal artery and most of the tributaries of the renal vein pass through the hilum of the kidney, arterial branches that do not do so are fairly common. Such extrahilar arteries penetrate the parenchyma of the kidney on its external surface. They may arise from the renal artery or the aorta, or they may have an aberrant origin from a different vessel. Their unexpected presence is a hazard in operations on the kidney. They are particularly frequent to the upper pole.

None of the so-called accessory renal arteries, be they hilar or extrahilar, can be considered as truly accessory to the normal renal vasculature. They do not anastomose with the segmental arteries. Although these arteries are sometimes called by surgeons "aberrant," this term should be applied to them only when they do not arise from the renal artery or the aorta.

Multiple **renal veins** are almost as frequent as multiple arteries on the right side, but are rare on the left. However, the left renal vein may bifurcate and pass both in front of and behind the aorta, thus forming a *circumaortic venous ring*, or it may have no anterior connection at all and will pass behind, rather than in front of, the aorta.

Unlike the arteries, the venous tributaries anastomose within the kidney, and there are also minor anastomoses, through the fibrous capsule, with veins that are not tributaries of the renal vein. However, because of the inefficiency of these anastomoses, sudden occlusion of the right renal vein causes necrosis of the whole kidney. The left renal vein, on the other hand, has larger connections to the extrarenal veins that enter the caval system. It has been ligated and divided in a number of cases, with no evidence of impairment of renal function, owing, it is believed, to larger anastomoses on the left.

Ureter. In its course through the abdomen, the ureter receives twigs from adjacent vessels, but in no fixed pattern. The *renal artery* rather regularly supplies the upper end. Ureteric branches can often be found from the aorta, the testicular or ovarian, and the iliac arteries. After it has entered the pelvis, the ureter receives one or more branches from pelvic arteries. Typically, all the vessels reaching the ureter divide into ascending and descending branches that form a longitudinal anastomosis along it. This anastomosis may be poor in places because of the uneven spacing of the vessels.

The **veins** of the ureter conform to the pattern of arterial supply.

Lymphatics

The suprarenal glands, kidneys, and ureters drain their lymphatics into the lumbar nodes.

Innervation

Suprarenal Glands. As the greater splanchnic nerves pass the suprarenal glands on their way to the celiac plexus, they give off fibers directly to the glands, which mingle with fibers derived from the celiac plexus. The *suprarenal plexus* formed by these nerves consists of *preganglionic* sympathetic fibers that terminate on the cells of the suprarenal medulla. These cells are equivalent to the autonomic ganglia and release their neurotransmitter substances directly into the venous sinusoids of the medulla (see Chap. 11). The suprarenal cortex has no nerve supply.

Kidneys. Extensions of the celiac plexus form a *renal plexus* around the renal artery. This plexus is joined by the lowest splanchnic nerve or by the renal branch of the lesser splanchnic nerve. The plexus contains small *renal ganglia*, one of which, the *aorticorenal ganglion*, is of macroscopic size and is located close to each renal artery.

The sympathetic fibers in the renal plexus are concerned with the control of blood vessels to the kidney. A surgical section of them increases the blood flow through the kidney and thereby produces diuresis, but apparently has no other effect on renal function and no effect upon the pressure of urine in the renal calices. The renal plexus also contains visceral afferent fibers concerned with pain, which terminate in T-10 to L-1 spinal cord segments. Renal pain is usually referred to the back.

Ureters. The *ureteric plexus* is formed by delicate nerve filaments derived from various parts of the aortic plexus. The nerves contain sympathetic efferents and afferents. Stimulation of the renal plexus, which contributes to the ureteric plexus, increases peristaltic activity of the ureter, but surgical section of the plexus does not interfere with ureteric peristalsis. The visceral afferents concerned with pain relay in segments T-11 to L-2. Ureteric pain, mentioned in relation to urinary calculi, is referred to a wide area, including parts of the abdominal wall above the iliac crest, the suprapubic region, the genitals, and the medial aspects of the thigh and leg.

Development and Congenital Anomalies

Normal Development

The Urogenital Ridges. The kidneys, gonads, and suprarenal cortex develop from intermediate mesoderm. The longitudinal, bilateral mass of **intermediate mesoderm** becomes defined in the trilaminar embryo lateral to the somites. Once the intraembryonic celom is formed, the lateral surface of this bar of mesoderm comes to face into each celomic duct (see Figs. 9-2 and 9-3). Growth and differentiation of the intermediate mesoderm produce two longitudinal ridges that bulge into the celomic ducts on either side of the dorsal mesentery of the primitive gut (see Fig. 9-3). These so-called *urogenital ridges* extend from the lower cervical to the caudal regions of the embryo. The celomic or abdominal surface of the urogenital ridges is covered with the celomic mesothelium derived from cells of the intermediate mesoderm itself. This mesothelium is destined to become parietal peritoneum in this region and to contribute to the gonads and suprarenal gland. The attachment of the ridges to the dorsal wall of the celom is spoken of as the *urogenital mesentery*.

The anterolateral part of the urogenital ridges is occupied by *nephrogenic tissue*, from which develop three successive and overlapping generations of kidneys: *pronephros*, *mesonephros*, and *metanephros*. The anteromedial portion of the ridges is occupied by the primitive gonads, and behind them is the suprarenal gland (Fig. 25-29).

Gonads and Suprarenal Glands. Proliferation of the celomic mesothelium that overlies the gonadal and suprarenal surfaces of the urogenital ridges contributes to the formation of both the gonads (ovaries and testes) and the suprarenal cortex. In addition, each organ becomes invaded by immigrant cells: the gonads by the primitive germ cells from the yolk sac and the suprarenal glands by cells derived from the neural crest. The primitive germ cells are the ancestors of oogonia and spermatogonia; from the neural crest cells develops the suprarenal medulla. All autonomic ganglia, the function of which is similar to the suprarenal medulla, are also derived from neural crest cells.

Kidneys. The pronephros and mesonephros are segmental organs located in the lower cervical and thoracolumbar regions of the embryo. They receive a series of segmental branches from the aorta. Early in development, urine is discharged directly into the celom; later, it is discharged into bilateral longitudinal ducts called at first the pronephric ducts and later the mesonephric ducts, which empty into the cloaca. The metanephros, located in the sacral region of the embryo, becomes functional as its predecessors, the pronephros and mesonephros, decline and disappear.

Although the mesonephric duct persists in the male (see Fig. 27-15), urine produced by the metanephros will be conveyed to the cloaca by a new duct that sprouts from the caudal end of the mesonephric duct in the form of the **metanephric diverticulum,** known also as the *ureteric bud* (see Fig. 27-15). This diverticulum elongates and grows cranially to invade the metanephros, located at the caudal end of the urogenital ridges (see Fig. 25-29). Contact between the metanephric diverticulum and the metanephros induces differentiation of the renal corpuscles and renal tubule from metanephric tissue and differentiation of the collecting tubules from the cranial end of the diverticulum. This establishes the definitive kidney. More caudal parts of the metanephric diverticulum become the renal pelvis and the ureter.

Changes in Relations. Disappearance of the pronephros and mesonephros leaves the ovary or testis, the mesonephric duct, and an additional duct called the paramesonephric duct (see Chap. 27) suspended in the urogenital mesentery. This mesentery with its contents slides down the posterior abdominal wall into the pelvis (further discussed in Chap. 27), leaving behind the suprarenal glands in a retroperitoneal position.

The definitive kidneys, after they have been formed in the pelvis, ascend on the posterior abdominal wall, but the mechanisms of this migration are unknown. It is probable that differential growth of the various vertebral regions and the elongation of the ureteric bud are responsible for the relative and absolute cranial migration of the definitive kidneys. This takes place behind the peritoneum and brings the kidneys in contact with the suprarenal glands which, up to the time of birth, are larger than the kidneys themselves. As the kidney ascends, its connections to the segmental arteries that originally supply the mesonephros also change. The reduction of these mesonephric branches of the aorta normally results in a single artery for each kidney.

Congenital Abnormalities

Gross abnormalities of the kidneys or ureters occur in at least 3% to 4% of persons. There are a large variety of congenital abnormalities that can be broadly classed as 1) agenesis and hypoplasia, 2) duplications,

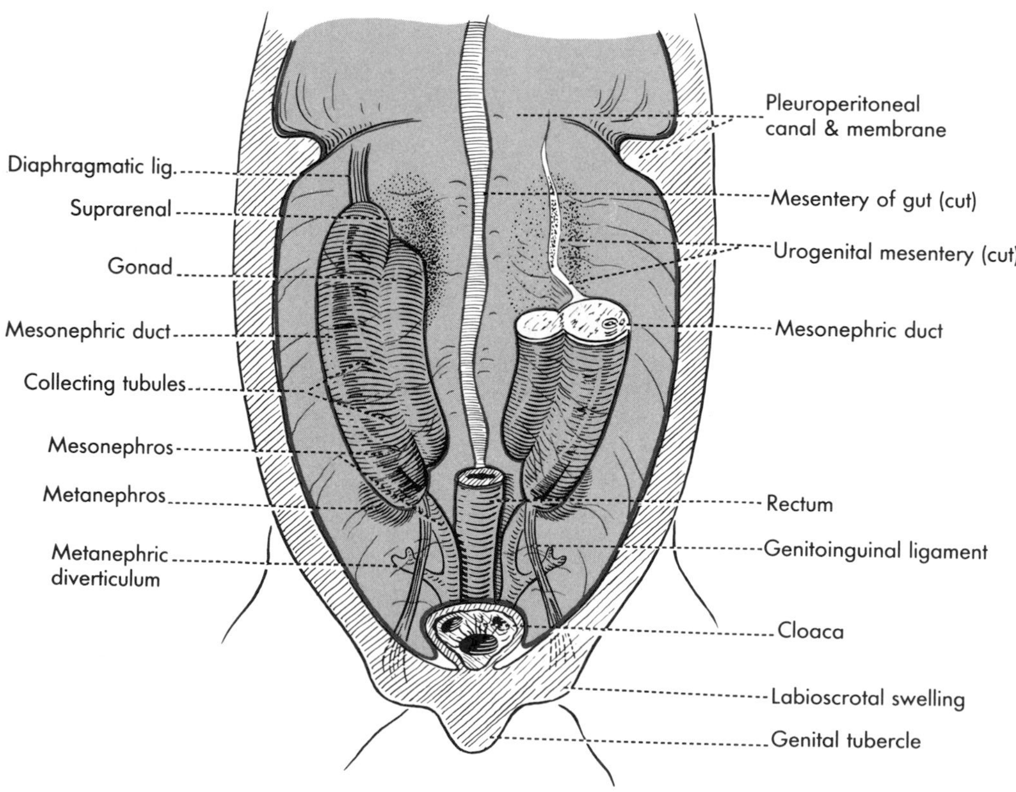

FIGURE 25-29.
The urogenital ridges, their mesentery and associated ligaments, illustrated diagrammatically: Except for the rectum, the gut has been excised with its mesentery. The mesothelial lining of the celom is *pink*. The paramesonephric ducts are omitted from this scheme, although they develop in both sexes. For the relation of the paramesonephric ducts to the mesonephros and the mesonephric duct, see Figure 27-16*A*.

3) malposition and malrotation, and 4) congenital cystic disease. By far the most common are abnormalities of position.

Fetuses in whom both kidneys fail to develop (**renal agenesis**) survive to term, but die within a few days after their separation from the placental circulation. One functioning kidney, however, is entirely compatible with life. A single kidney, resulting from unilateral renal agenesis, may be abnormally located, as may be one or both of an otherwise normal pair of kidneys.

Splitting of the ureteric bud during its growth leads to partial or complete **duplication** of the kidney, owing to reduplication of the induction process in the metanephros. The renal duplication is usually incomplete, and the kidney consists of two fused masses, one above the other, with separate renal pelves that empty into a bifid ureter or into two separate ureters. The extra ureter may open into the normal ureter (bifid ureter), in which case the ureteric bud probably split close to the metanephros. If the split was close to the mesonephric duct, the extra ureter may end independently in the bladder (into which the distal portion of the mesonephric duct, bearing the metanephric diverticulum, becomes absorbed), or it may end ectopically in the urethra. It is interesting that usually the upper part of a "double kidney" and the upper ureter are the abnormal structures. In such cases, usually the upper ureter terminates ectopically and the lower one has a normal course into the bladder.

Arrests or errors in the ascent of the kidney result in **ectopia.** In *simple renal ectopia*, one or both kidneys are placed lower than usual, owing to the arrest of a normal process. A large proportion of ectopic kidneys are in the pelvis, and they typically receive their blood supply from whatever artery lies close to them. Many such kidneys have multiple blood supplies.

It is a general rule that the lower the kidneys lie, the closer together they are. Thus, ectopic kidneys placed low in the abdomen tend to fuse together, usually at their lower poles, to form a somewhat horseshoe-shaped mass called *horseshoe kidneys* (Fig. 25-30).

In *crossed ectopia*, a kidney crosses to the opposite side during its ascent. Usually, when this occurs, the kidney that is crossed fuses with the kidney on the normal side, so that there is a single renal mass. However, that one ureter descends on one side and the other crosses the vertebral column to descend on the other distinguishes such a mass from that of a partial duplication of the kidney.

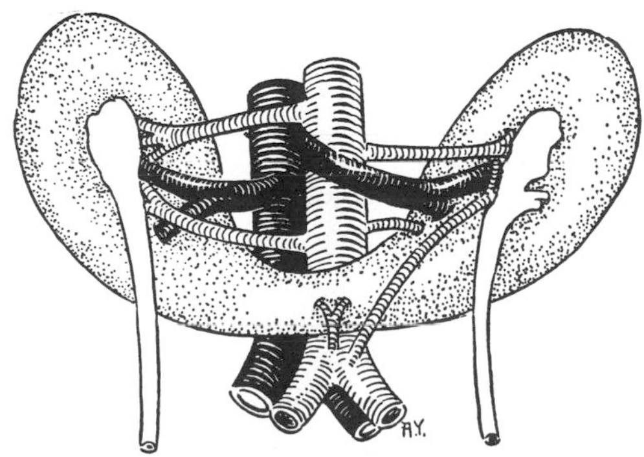

FIGURE *25-30.* **Horseshoe kidney.**

Among the most common abnormalities of position of the kidneys is **abnormal rotation.** The definitive kidneys begin their development with their hila facing forward. Subsequently, they turn 90° and point their hila medially. This rotation may fail to occur, go too far, or be in the reverse direction—thus, a renal pelvis may face posteriorly or laterally. Abnormal rotation is regularly associated with abnormally low kidneys, but may occur in normally placed ones.

A rare *abnormality of the right ureter* is for it to run behind the inferior vena cava. The anomaly, called **retrocaval** or *postcaval ureter*, is a consequence of abnormal formation of the postrenal segment of the inferior vena cava. Retrocaval ureter usually calls attention to itself eventually because of obstruction by the vena cava.

Several types of **renal cysts** have congenital origin. The most widely accepted explanation of *polycystic kidneys*, a condition in which the organs are riddled with multiple cysts, is the widespread failure of the renal tubules, derived from metanephric tissue, to join up with the collecting tubules derived from the ureteric bud. The cysts arise because the urine produced by the nephrons cannot be drained into the calices.

RECOMMENDED READINGS

Boyarsky L, Labay P, Glenn JF. More evidence for ureteral nerve function and its clinical implications. J Urol 1968;99:533.

Boyd W, Blincoe H, Hayner JC. Sequence of action of the diaphragm and quadratus lumborum during quiet breathing. Anat Rec 1965;151:579.

Carey JM, Hollinshead WH. Anatomic study of the esophageal hiatus. Surg Gynecol Obstet 1955;100:196.

Carriero A, Magarelli N, Tamburri L, Tonni AG, Iezzi A, Bonomo L. Magnetic resonance angiography of the left renal vein. Surg Radiol Anat 1994;16:205.

Castellino RA, Marglin MI. Imaging of abdominal and pelvic lymph nodes: lymphography or computed tomography? Invest Radiol 1982;17:433.

Chuang VP, Mena CE, Hoskins PA. Congenital anomalies of the inferior vena cava: review of embryogenesis and presentation of a simplified classification. Br J Radiol 1974;47:206.

Debatin J, Spritzer C, Grist T, et al. Imaging of the renal arteries: value of MR-angiography. Am J Roentgenol 1991;157:981.

Dorfman RE, Alpen MB, Gross BH, Sandler MA. Upper abdominal lymph nodes: criteria for normal size determined with CT. Radiology 1991;180:319.

Gauthier AP, Verbanck S, Estenne M, Segebarth C, Macklem PT, Paiva M. Three-dimensional reconstruction of the in vivo human diaphragm shape at different lung volumes. J Appl Physiol 1994;76:495.

Graves FT. Anatomy of the intrarenal arteries and its application to segmental resection of the kidney. Br J Surg 1954;42:132.

Hollinshead WH. Anatomy for surgeons: vol 2, the thorax, abdomen, and pelvis. 2nd ed. New York: Harper & Row, 1971.

Lau J, Lo R, Chan F, Wong K. The posterior "nutcracker": hematuria secondary to retroaortic left renal vein. Urology 1986;28:437.

Listerud MB, Harkins HN. Anatomy of the esophageal hiatus. Arch Surg 1958;776:835.

Magnusson A. Size of normal retroperitoneal lymph nodes. Acta Radiol 1983;24:315.

Mitchell GAG. The innervation of the kidney, ureter, testicle and epididymis. J Anat 1938;72:508.
O'Rahilly R, Meucke EC. The timing and sequence of events in the development of the human urinary system during the embryonic period proper. Z Anat Entwicklungsgesch 1972;138:99.
Pick J. The autonomic nervous system: morphological, comparative, clinical, and surgical aspects. Philadelphia: JB Lippincott, 1970.
Pollak R, Prusak BF, Mozes MF. Anatomic abnormalities of cadaver kidneys procured for purposes of transplantation. Am Surg 1986;52:233.
Potter EL. The normal and abnormal development of the kidney. Chicago: Year Book, 1974.
Reddy V, Sharma S, Cobanoglu A. What dictates the position of the diaphragm—the heart or the liver? J Thorac Cardiovasc Surg 1994;108:687.
Ross JA, Samuel E, Millar DR. Variations in the renal vascular pedicle: an anatomical and radiological study with particular reference to renal transplantation. Br J Urol 1961;33:478.
Satyapal KS, Rambiritch V, Pillai G. Additional renal veins: incidence and morphometry. Clin Anat 1995;8:51.
Satyapal KS, Kalideen JM. The left renal vein: a major collateral system. Clin Anat 1994;7:352.
Schulman CC. Innervation of the ureter: a histochemical and ultrastructural study. Anat Clin 1981;3:127.
Sénécail B, Colin D, Person H, Vallée B, Lefèvre C. The "anatomic" view of the suprarenals in medical imaging. Surg Radiol Anat 1994;16:211.
Smith GT. The renal vascular patterns in man. J Urol 1963;89:275.
Smith HW. The kidney. New York: Oxford University Press, 1969.
Tarney TJ. Diaphragmatic hernia. Ann Thorac Surg 1968;5:66.
Tobin CE. The renal fascia and its relation to the transversalis fascia. Anat Rec 1944;89:295.
Wells LJ. Development of the human diaphragm and pleural sacs. Contrib Embryol 1954;35:107.

Hollinshead's Textbook of Anatomy, by Cornelius Rosse and Penelope Gaddum-Rosse.
Lippincott-Raven Publishers, Philadelphia, © 1997.

CHAPTER 26

The Inguinal and Femoral Canals; The Scrotum; The Applied Anatomy of Hernia

On the surface of the body, the inguinal region is the meeting place of the anterior abdominal wall and the thigh; in the interior of the body, the anterior and posterior walls of the abdomen meet each other in the inguinal region. This area has particular clinical importance because it is here that abdominal contents most commonly protrude through the abdominal wall and present themselves as hernias.

The key to the anatomy of this region is the **inguinal ligament,** already encountered in Chapter 23. Structures that pass between the abdominal cavity and the scrotum or the labia majora do so *above* the inguinal ligament; the slitlike passage in the abdominal wall that transmits them is the **inguinal canal.** In the female, only a fibromuscular band, the *round ligament of the uterus*, passes through the inguinal canal to attach to the skin of the labia majora. In the male, on the other hand, the canal transmits the duct of the testis (*ductus deferens*) with its associated vessels and nerves; wrapped in fascial tunics, together they form the *spermatic cord*. Consequently, the inguinal canal is of greater significance in the male than in the female.

In both sexes, abdominal contents that should normally remain in the abdomen may descend through the inguinal canal to form an **inguinal hernia.** Inguinal hernias emerge as swellings from the inguinal canal and will eventually distend the scrotum or the labium majus.

Structures that pass between the abdominal cavity and the thigh do so *beneath* the inguinal ligament. These are the external iliac artery and vein, wrapped in a fascial tunic called the *femoral sheath*. The potential space within the femoral sheath is the **femoral canal.** This canal may become distended by abdominal contents that should normally remain in the abdomen, forming a **femoral hernia,** which descends beneath the inguinal ligament into the thigh; it cannot enter the scrotum or the labia majora.

To explain the anatomy of the inguinal and femoral canals, a requisite for understanding inguinal and femoral hernia, the inguinal ligament will be described first. This chapter also deals with the scrotum, because it is anatomically continuous with the inguinal canal, despite the fact that the scrotum is located in the perineum. The description of the labia majora, however, is deferred to Chapter 28, where it is included with other parts of the vulva.

THE INGUINAL LIGAMENT

The inguinal ligament is not a true ligament; rather, it is the inferior free border of the external oblique aponeurosis, thickened and reinforced by collagen fiber bundles that run from the anterior superior iliac spine to the pubic tubercle. (Fig. 26-1). When viewed from the front, the external oblique aponeurosis is rounded because its free border is turned posteriorly; anteriorly, there is a smooth transition between the fibers of the ligament and those of the aponeurosis proper. Thus, the inguinal ligament has an upper and a lower surface.

The inguinal ligament is not visible readily on either the superficial or the deep aspect of the anterior abdominal wall. It is concealed by the fascias attached to it. Anteriorly, the **fascia lata** is attached to the rounded lower border of the external oblique aponeurosis; posteriorly, the attachment of the **transversalis fascia** along the free edge of the ligament obscures that edge to some degree.

Because of the pull of the fascia lata on the inguinal ligament, the ligament is convex downward when the lower limbs are in line with the trunk; flexion of the hip relaxes and straightens the ligament.

Attachments. The inguinal ligament is best exposed for the study of its attachments by incising the external oblique aponeurosis just above and parallel with the inguinal ligament. Laterally, the inguinal ligament is attached to the *anterior superior iliac spine* and medially, to the *pubic tubercle* (Fig. 26-2). Before the ligament reaches the pubic tubercle, some fibers diverge from its posterior free edge and attach to the medial 2 to 3 cm of the *pecten* of the superior ramus of the pubis. This crescent-shaped expansion is called the **lacunar ligament,** and it fills in a triangular gap between the medial end of the inguinal ligament and the pecten pubis (see Fig. 26-2). At the apex of this triangle is the pubic tubercle; the base is formed by the sharp, free edge of the lacunar ligament, which faces laterally and forms the medial boundary of the *lacuna vasorum*, the space through which the external iliac vessels leave and enter the thigh (see Fig. 26-2). Some fibers of the lacunar ligament continue laterally along the pecten pubis and contribute to the formation of a strong fibrous band, the **pectineal ligament,** which is fused with the periosteum of the superior ramus of the pubis.

As the inguinal ligament ends on the pubic tubercle, it gives off a few fibers that reflect upward and run through the aponeurosis into the linea alba. These fibers constitute the **reflected part** of the inguinal ligament (Fig. 26-3). This ligament lies in the posterior wall of the *superficial inguinal ring*.

Relations. The space between the inguinal ligament and the superior ramus of the pubis is divided into two compartments by a fascial septum, the **iliopectineal arch,** continuous both with the inguinal ligament and with the iliopsoas fascia (see Fig. 26-2). The lateral compartment, the *lacuna musculorum*, contains the iliopsoas muscle with the femoral nerve lying on it; the medial compartment, the *lacuna vasorum*, transmits the external iliac vessels, as mentioned earlier. The medial half of the inguinal ligament has a free surface facing into the lacuna vasorum; its lateral half is bound to the iliopsoas fascia. The most inferior fibers of the internal oblique and transversus abdo-

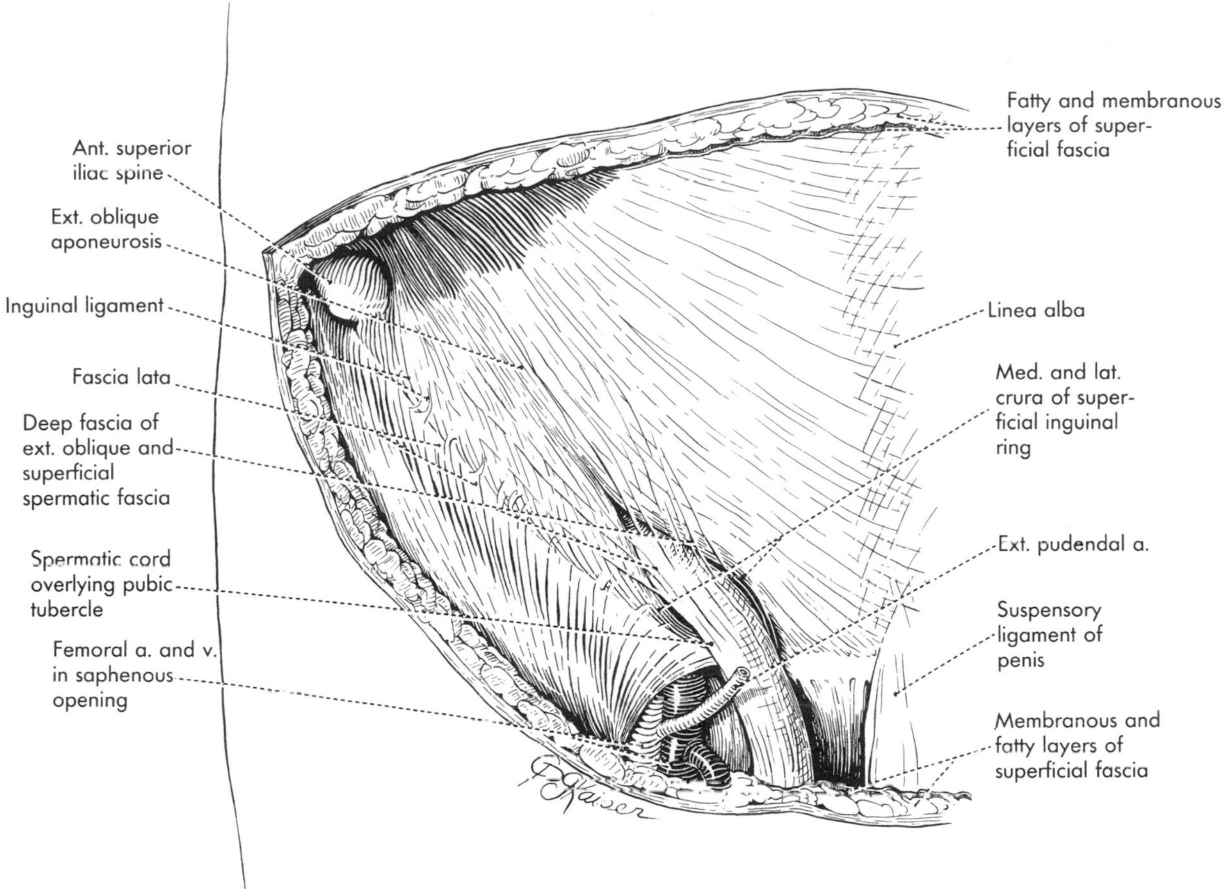

FIGURE 26-1.
A dissection of the inguinal region showing the anterior view of the inguinal ligament, the related fascias, the superficial inguinal ring, and the saphenous opening.

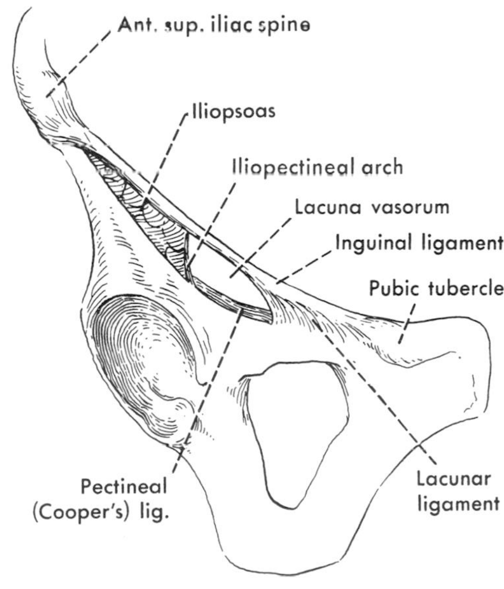

FIGURE 26-2.
Inguinal, lacunar, and pectineal ligaments and the muscular and vascular compartments behind the inguinal ligament, seen from below. The pelvis has been tilted backward from the anatomic position to one that it would assume during sitting.

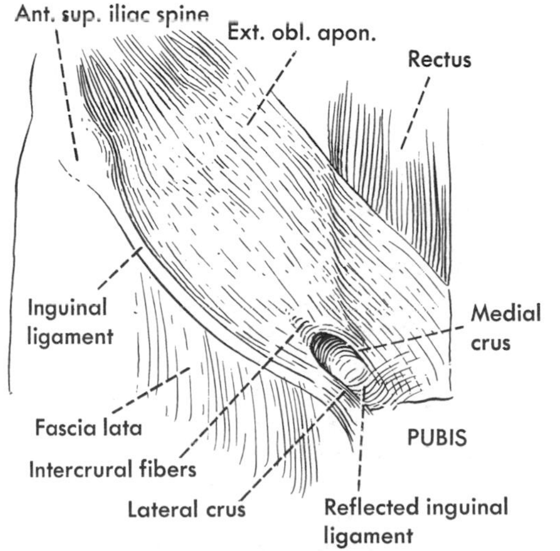

FIGURE 26-3.
The superficial inguinal ring.

minis arise from the line of fusion between the inguinal ligament and the iliopsoas fascia. The upper surface of the medial half of the ligament forms the floor of the inguinal canal. Just medial to the anterior superior iliac spine, the inguinal ligament is usually pierced by the *lateral femoral cutaneous nerve*. The nerve may be compressed by the ligament, giving rise to pain in the area of the nerve's distribution (see Fig. 18-7). The medial end of the ligament, attached to the pubic tubercle, forms the inferior boundary of the *superficial inguinal ring* and is designated as the lateral crus of the ring.

THE INGUINAL CANAL

The inguinal canal is an oblique passage through the anterior abdominal wall connecting the extraperitoneal space of the abdomen to the scrotum or the labia majora. The canal commences at the *deep inguinal ring* and terminates at the *superficial inguinal ring*. It is 4 to 5 cm long and slopes medially and downward.

Boundaries

The Deep Inguinal Ring

The deep inguinal ring appears as an oval defect in the transversalis fascia when the deep aspect of the fascia is exposed by reflecting the parietal peritoneum from it. In truth, the transversalis fascia, rather than being defective, is prolonged anteriorly from the margins of the deep ring into the inguinal canal. It forms a fascial sleeve that surrounds the ductus deferens or the round ligament of the uterus, both of which enter the deep ring from the abdomen with their accompanying vessels and nerves. This fascial sleeve is the **internal spermatic fascia,** and the structures enclosed in it constitute the **spermatic cord** in the male or the **round ligament** in the female. The deep ring is best defined, therefore, as the junction of the internal spermatic fascia with the transversalis fascia proper.

The deep ring is located at the *midinguinal point*, midway between the anterior superior iliac spine and the pubic symphysis, slightly more than 1 cm above the inguinal ligament. Immediately anterior to the deep inguinal ring is the lower border of the **transversus abdominis,** and the spermatic cord enters the inguinal canal by passing below the inferior margin of this muscle. The fibers constituting this part of the transversus arise farther laterally from the line of fusion between the inguinal ligament and the iliopsoas fascia. As the fibers arch medially, they cross in front of the ring, so that only part of the ring is below the inferior border of the muscle (Fig. 26-4). When the transversus contracts, as it always does when abdominal pressure is raised, its lower border moves downward, providing a firm covering for the deep inguinal ring. On its deep surface, the ring is covered by extraperitoneal fat and parietal peritoneum.

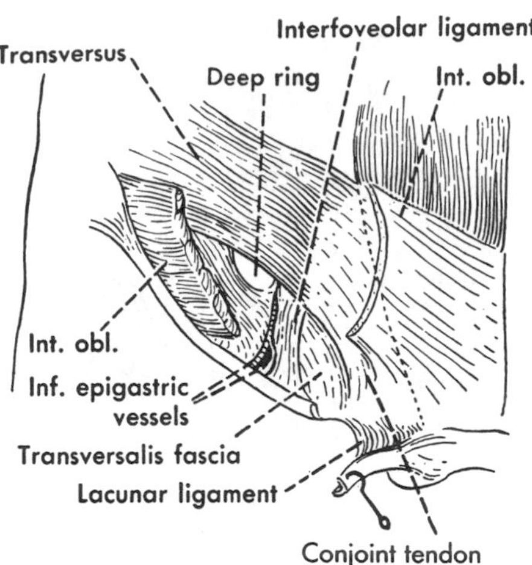

FIGURE *26-4.*
Anterior view of the deep inguinal ring: The inguinal region deep to the internal oblique; the internal spermatic fascia, derived from the transversalis fascia, has been cut away from this fascia at the deep inguinal ring. The sloping fibers bordering the deep ring inferiorly constitute the iliopubic tract.

The Superficial Inguinal Ring

The superficial inguinal ring is a somewhat triangular defect in the aponeurosis of the external oblique, formed by the separation of its fibers (see Fig. 26-1). The base of this triangular hiatus is the pubic crest, and its sides are the *crura* of the ring. The **lateral crus** lies really inferiorly and is the inguinal ligament attached to the pubic tubercle; the **medial crus** is superior and is formed by that part of the external oblique aponeurosis that attaches to the symphysis and the body of the pubis. Laterally, at the apex of the triangle, the two crura are bound together by the more or less obvious *intercrural fibers* of the aponeurosis. If these are well defined, they give the lateral margin of the superficial ring a rounded rather than an angular contour (see Fig. 26-3).

The superficial inguinal ring, like the deep inguinal ring, is not a true opening. A thin layer of connective tissue continues from the margins of the superficial ring toward the scrotum or the labium majus and invests the spermatic cord or the round ligament as these exit from the inguinal canal (see Fig. 26-1). This connective tissue sleeve is the **superficial spermatic fascia** and is derived from the deep fascia that covers both superficial and deep surfaces of the external oblique aponeurosis. Therefore, although the margins of the superficial ring are much better defined than those of the deep ring, they are not clearly visible until the superficial spermatic fascia is cut away from the edges of the crura.

Walls

The **floor** of the inguinal canal is formed by the medial half of the inguinal ligament and the lacunar ligament. The roof is open; the canal communicates superiorly with the tissue spaces that separate the external and internal obliques and the transversus.

The entire length of the **anterior wall** of the inguinal canal is formed by the external oblique aponeurosis. In front of the deep ring, the transversus abdominis reinforces the anterior wall of the canal and so does the internal oblique (see Fig. 26-4). This inferior part of the **internal oblique** arises just in front of the transversus on the lateral half of the inguinal ligament, and as its fibers run medially, they lie in front of the deep ring. Here, the internal oblique splits to allow the spermatic cord or the round ligament to pass through it. Beyond this hiatus in the muscle, the internal oblique becomes rather thin and aponeurotic, and as it continues medially, now in the posterior wall of the inguinal canal, its inferior free border rests on the posterior edge of the inguinal ligament. The internal oblique terminates by fusing with the aponeurosis of the transversus; the two form the conjoint tendon and contribute to the inferior part of the anterior rectus sheath (see Fig. 23-9).

The **posterior wall** of the inguinal canal is rather complex and important because it is here that weaknesses predispose to the formation of inguinal hernia. The posterior wall is made up of the transversalis fascia, the conjoint tendon, and the inferior fibers of the internal oblique just described.

The **transversalis fascia** fills the hiatus between the inferior border of the transversus and the inguinal ligament. The fascia is thickened along the ligament and forms a more or less distinct band that runs from the iliopsoas fascia to the pubis. When this band is recognizable, it is called the *iliopubic tract* (Fig. 26-5). At its lateral end, the tract forms the inferior boundary of the deep inguinal ring. The medial boundary of the deep ring is also reinforced by a thickening of the transversalis fascia; this is the *interfoveolar ligament*. When present, this ligament extends from the lower border of the transversus to the inguinal ligament, more or less in front of the inferior epigastric vessels (see Fig. 26-5). Medially, the interfoveolar ligament blends into the conjoint tendon.

The **conjoint tendon** (*falx inguinalis*) is the combined aponeurosis of the transversus and internal oblique inserted into the pectineal ligament along the superior ramus of the pubis (see Fig. 26-5). Most of the fused aponeurosis passes in front of the rectus as part of its sheath and inserts into the pubic crest; only the part lateral to the rec-

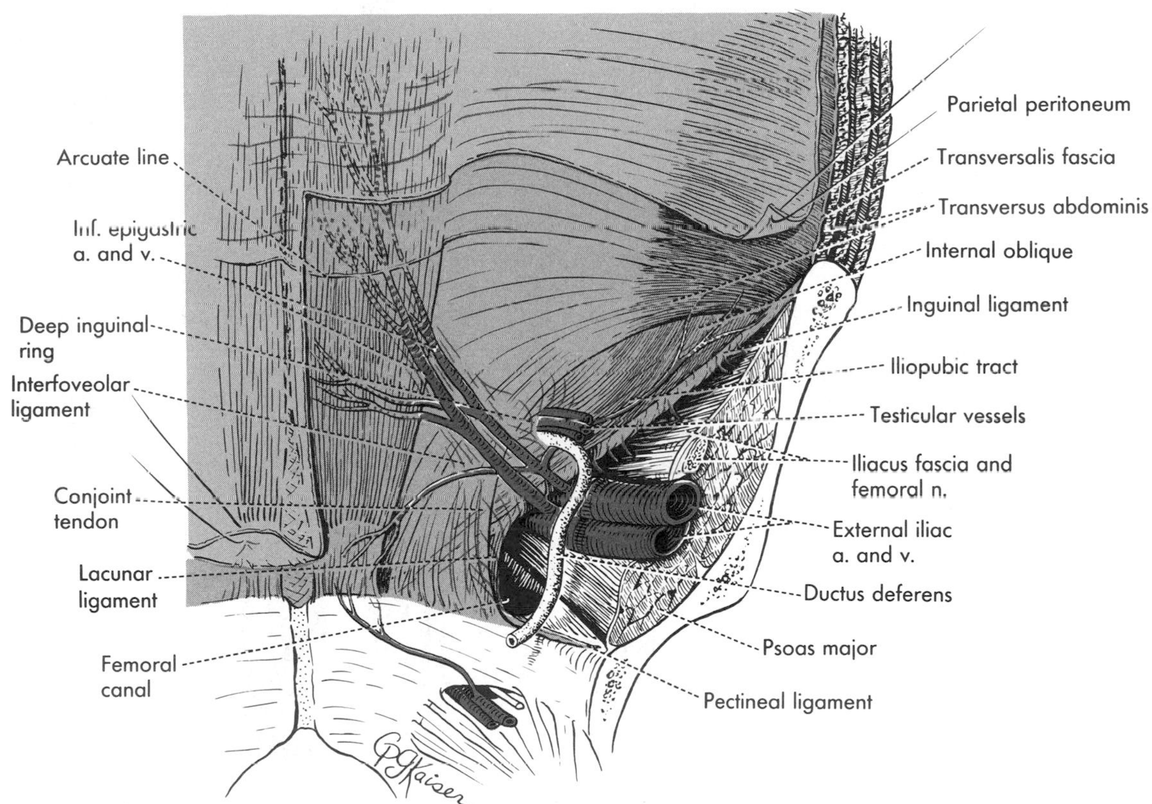

FIGURE 26-5.
The posterior aspect of the anterior abdominal wall. The peritoneum (*pink*) has been cut away to reveal the features of the transversalis fascia (*blue*) and the tendons and ligaments (*black*) that contribute to the posterior wall of the inguinal canal. The femoral canal and the structures that pass inferior to the inguinal ligament are also illustrated. The inguinal triangle is bordered by the rectus (*unlabeled*), the inferior epigastric artery, and the medial portion of the inguinal ligament.

tus is designated as the conjoint tendon. The conjoint tendon forms the posterior wall of the most medial portion of the inguinal canal, more or less directly behind the superficial inguinal ring. It varies how far laterally the conjoint tendon extends, as does how strong it is and how distinct it is from the interfoveolar ligament with which its lateral border merges.

The deep aspect of the posterior wall of the inguinal canal is covered by parietal peritoneum of the **lateral** and **medial inguinal fossae** described in Chapter 23 (see Fig. 23-26). The deep inguinal ring is located in the lateral inguinal fossa just lateral to the inferior epigastric vessels. The medial inguinal fossa overlies a triangular area bordered by the rectus, the inguinal ligament, and the inferior epigastric vessels: it is known as the *inguinal triangle* (see Fig. 26-5).

A summary of the posterior wall of the inguinal canal according to these landmarks is relevant to the applied anatomy of inguinal hernia. **In the inguinal triangle,** the medial portion of the posterior wall consists of the *conjoint tendon* (with transversalis fascia on its deep surface) and, in front of it, the inconsequential *reflected part of the inguinal ligament* (see Fig. 26-3). Lateral to the crescentic edge of the conjoint tendon, *transversalis fascia*, incorporating the interfoveolar ligament and the iliopubic tract, completes the posterior wall as far as the inferior epigastric vessels. Directly in front of this fascia, the *hiatus* in the internal oblique transmits the spermatic cord and a few attenuated fibers of the *internal oblique* and its aponeurosis, paralleling the inguinal ligament. **Lateral to the inferior epigastric vessels** is the deep inguinal ring, the lower margin of which is formed, as noted earlier, by the iliopubic tract.

Contents

The inguinal canal contains the spermatic cord or the round ligament and the ilioinguinal nerve. The structures that constitute the spermatic cord and the round ligament pass through both deep and superficial inguinal rings; the ilioinguinal nerve enters the canal laterally and leaves it through the superficial ring.

The **ilioinguinal nerve**, a branch of the lumbar plexus (see Fig. 25-15), enters the abdominal wall by piercing the deep surface of the transversus abdominis just above the anterior superior iliac spine and soon after that passes through the internal oblique. It supplies both muscles and descends into the inguinal canal between the internal and external obliques. In the canal, the nerve runs along the inferior aspect of the spermatic cord to the superficial inguinal ring, where it pierces the external spermatic fascia and distributes its branches to the skin of the upper part of the thigh, scrotum, and penis, or the labia majora and mons pubis.

The Spermatic Cord

The spermatic cord is the pedicle of the testis, and it also connects the scrotum to the abdomen. It is composed of the structures that pass through the deep inguinal ring and fascial coverings contributed to it by the layers of the abdominal wall.

In the male, the principal structures that pass through the deep inguinal ring include the ductus deferens, the testicular artery and veins, lymphatics, and autonomic nerve plexuses around the testicular artery and the ductus deferens. Less important structures that enter the deep ring are the genital branch of the genitofemoral nerve and small arteries that supply the ductus itself and the cremaster muscle.

The Ductus Deferens. The ductus deferens, also known as the *vas deferens,* conveys spermatozoa and secretions produced by the testis to the ejaculatory ducts. The deferent duct commences behind the lower pole of the testis as the continuation of the duct of the epididymis (Fig. 26-6) and terminates in the pelvis just above the prostate by forming the ejaculatory duct (see Fig. 27-29). The deferent duct ascends in the scrotum behind the testis and then in the spermatic cord, entering the inguinal canal through the superficial ring and leaving it through the deep ring. At the deep ring, the duct bends sharply medially and, embedded in pelvic fascia, pursues its intrapelvic course toward the prostate.

The deferent duct can be identified as a 2- to 3-mm–thick palpable cord when the neck of the scrotum is rolled between finger and thumb. The lumen of the duct is quite narrow, and its thickness is due to longitudinal and circular smooth muscle in its walls. The duct is usually filled with spermatozoa; contraction of its walls, induced by sympathetic activity, discharges the spermatozoa into the ejaculate.

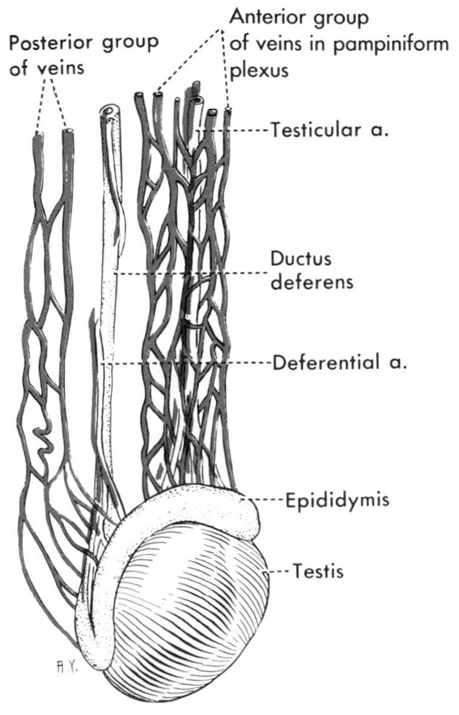

FIGURE **26-6.**
Blood supply of the testis.

The ductus (or vas) deferens may be exposed under local anesthetic by an incision in the skin in the neck of the scrotum before the vas enters the superficial inguinal ring. Bilateral division and closure of at least one end of the vas is called **vasectomy**. It renders an individual permanently sterile unless the duct is surgically reanastomosed.

The vasectomized individual will retain full sexual function and will continue to produce an ejaculate, but spermatozoa will be absent from it. Although vasectomy may seem an ideal method of contraception in the male, it has not been resolved to what degree absorption of the sperm (which continue to be produced at an apparently normal rate) contributes to certain manifestations of autoimmunity sometimes observed in vasectomized individuals.

The Testicular Artery. The testicular artery, a branch of the abdominal aorta, descends on the posterior abdominal wall to the deep inguinal ring, where it joins the ductus deferens (Fig. 26-7). Enclosed in the spermatic cord, the artery enters the scrotum where it lies anterior to the ductus and surrounded by the *pampiniform plexus*, formed by the veins that drain the testis (see Fig. 26-6). These veins emerge from the back of the testis and epididymis and give rise to some 10 to 12 veins, which, as they ascend, anastomose with each other, mainly around the testicular artery. This is the **pampiniform** (tendrillike) **plexus,** drained superiorly by three to four veins that pass through the inguinal canal and terminate on each side in two **testicular veins** at the deep inguinal ring. These veins ascend with the testicular artery to end in the inferior vena cava on the right and in the left renal vein on the left (see Chap. 25).

There is experimental evidence, obtained mainly in the dog and ram, that the cooler venous blood in the pampiniform plexus lowers the temperature of the blood in the testicular artery. This contributes to providing the temperature optimal for spermatogenesis, which has to be below that of the abdominal cavity.

The testicular vein and the pampiniform plexus are devoid of valves except for an occasional one at their termination in the inferior vena cava or the left renal vein. Engorgement and distention of these veins leads to varicosities in the pampiniform plexus that are palpable through the scrotum. The condition, known as **varicocele**, is much more common on the left than on the right, presumably related, in many cases, to the fact that the superior mesenteric artery crosses, and partially compresses, the left renal vein just before its termination. In the supine position, both the varicosities and the discomfort caused by the distention of the veins disappear because the venous pressure is relieved from the pampiniform plexus.

The two small arteries that enter the deep ring are the **artery of the ductus deferens,** a branch of the internal iliac, and the **cremasteric artery,** a branch of the inferior epigastric. The latter supplies only the tunics of the spermatic cord, but the artery of the ductus supplies the ductus and the epididymis and anastomoses with the testicular artery. These anastomoses, however, are not large enough to provide an adequate blood supply to the testis when the testicular artery becomes occluded. Such occlusion most often results from **torsion of the testis.** Twisting of the testis, with the spermatic cord as its pedicle, occludes the veins and the testicular artery, and unless this is relieved, the testis will die. Indeed, this has been the outcome in the majority of cases.

The Spermatic Fascias. The fascial coverings contributed to the spermatic cord by layers of the abdominal wall are the internal and external spermatic and the cremasteric fascias (see Fig. 26-7). As explained already with the description of the deep and superficial inguinal rings, the **internal spermatic fascia** is derived from the transversalis fascia and the **external spermatic fascia** is derived

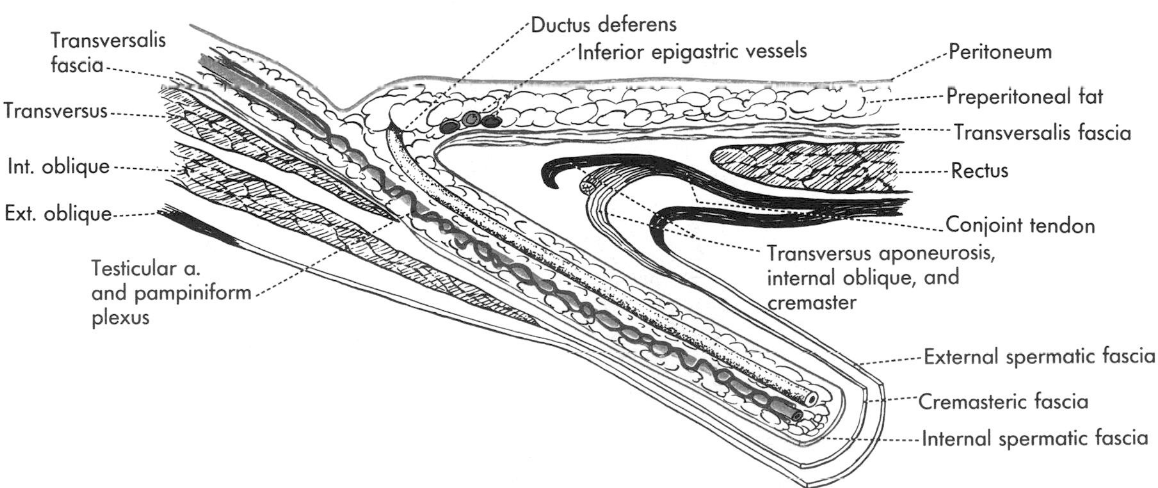

FIGURE *26-7.*
The continuity between the layers of the abdominal wall and the tunics of the spermatic cord in a hypothetical longitudinal section through the upper part of the spermatic cord. As in Figure 26-5, the peritoneum is *red* and the transversalis fascia and its continuation, the internal spermatic fascia, are *blue*.

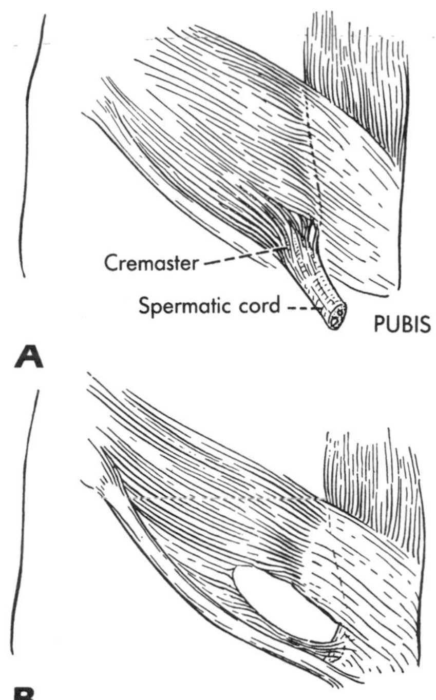

FIGURE 26-8.
(A) Course of the spermatic cord through the internal oblique muscle; (B) the cremaster muscle and the cord have been removed to show the defect in the internal oblique.

from the fascias of the external oblique. The **cremasteric fascia** is derived chiefly from the internal oblique (Fig. 26-8). In the inguinal canal, the fascia is wrapped around the internal spermatic fascia, forming the outer covering of the spermatic cord. However, inferior to the superficial ring, the cremasteric fascia is inside the external spermatic fascia. All these fascias become continuous with layers of the scrotal sac (Fig. 26-9).

The cremasteric fascia differs from the other fascial tunics of the spermatic cord in that it contains loops of muscle fasciculi constituting the **cremaster muscle.** As the lower fibers of the internal oblique part to let the spermatic cord pass through, not only the deep fascia, but also some of the muscle fibers of the internal oblique are carried along the cord in the form of loops that reach down into the scrotum (see Fig. 26-8). Although most of the loops of the cremaster are traceable to the internal oblique, some of the loops may be derived from the lower border of the transversus and others may have an independent origin on the inguinal ligament.

Contraction of the cremaster elevates the testis. Both testes are elevated just before ejaculation. The cremaster is innervated by the genital branch of the *genitofemoral nerve* (L-1), which enters the inguinal canal through the deep inguinal ring. Sudden stroking of the skin on the medial side of the thigh provokes unilateral reflex contraction of the cremaster, manifest by momentary elevation of the testis, particularly well seen when the scrotal sac is relaxed. This phenomenon is known as the **cremasteric reflex;** it tests the L-1 segment of the spinal cord.

The Round Ligament

The *ligamentum teres uteri* is a fibromuscular band that passes retroperitoneally from the uterus, located in the pelvis, to the deep inguinal ring. After traversing the inguinal canal, the ligament breaks up into fibrous strands that merge with the connective tissue of the labium majus.

In the inguinal canal, the round ligament acquires the same fascial tunics as the spermatic cord. However, apart from the ligament itself, these fascias contain no structure of significance and no genital duct or major vessel; they usually fuse with the round ligament almost as soon as they are formed. Therefore, the portion of the ligament surrounded by the fascial tunics is known by the same name as its intrapelvic portion devoid of fascial coverings.

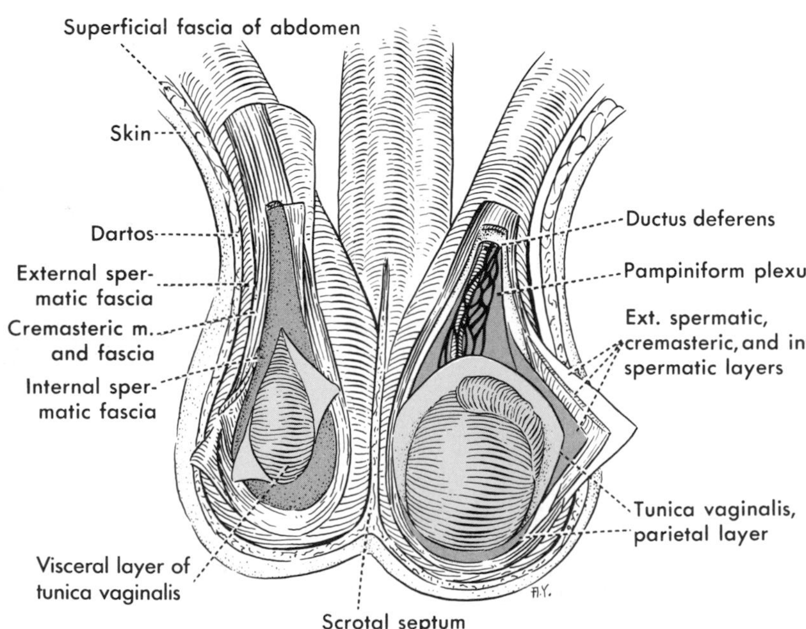

FIGURE 26-9.
The scrotum and the coverings of the spermatic cord and testis from the front. On the reader's right, the tunica vaginalis has been opened to show the testis and the epididymis, which here are covered by the visceral layer of the tunic. Parietal and visceral layers of the tunica vaginalis are *pink*, and the internal spermatic fascia is *blue*.

THE SCROTUM AND ITS CONTENTS

The Scrotum

The scrotum is a sac formed by the continuation of the skin and superficial fascia of the abdominal wall into the perineum. It hangs below the pubis and the root of the penis and, together with the penis, constitutes the **external genitalia** of the male. Its interior is divided into right and left halves, each containing a testis with its associated ducts, a serous sac called the *tunica vaginalis* applied to the surface of the testis, and the inferior portion of the spermatic cord, including its fascial tunics.

The appearance of the dark, sparsely hairy **scrotal skin** is influenced by the smooth muscle contained in the dermis and underlying fascia. The skin may be smooth and flaccid or wrinkled and drawn closely around the testis. A median *scrotal raphe* indicates the fusion of the bilateral labioscrotal swellings that formed the scrotum. The raphe extends onto the inferior surface of the penis and posteriorly in the perineum as far as the anus.

Beneath the skin, and closely bound to it, is the **dartos** (*tunica dartos*), the continuation of the membranous layer of the superficial fascia from the abdominal wall into the scrotum (see Fig. 23-2). This fascia in the scrotum is devoid of fat and contains a significant amount of smooth muscle, the *dartos muscle*. Deep to the scrotal raphe, the dartos extends inward as the *scrotal septum*, forming a partition between the right and left halves of the scrotum (Fig. 26-9). In addition to its connection with the abdominal superficial fascia, the dartos is continuous with the superficial penile fascia and, posteriorly, with the superficial fascia of the perineum.

Within each scrotal cavity, the **tunics of the spermatic cord** end as a trilaminar sac enclosing the tunica vaginalis and the testis (see Fig. 26-9). The *external spermatic, cremasteric*, and *internal spermatic fascias* are all present in the scrotum, although their fusion with each other may make it difficult to dissect them separately.

The **tunica vaginalis testis** is an extension of the peritoneal sac into the scrotum. Beyond the neonatal period, however, the tunica vaginalis normally does not communicate with the peritoneal cavity. The *processus vaginalis*, which connected the two in the fetus, becomes obliterated along the inguinal canal and the upper part of the scrotum and either disappears altogether or persists as a thin fibrous band. The tunica vaginalis has a *parietal layer*, fused by its nonserous external surface with the internal spermatic fascia, and a *visceral layer*, bound to the anterolateral surface of the testis and epididymis (see Fig. 26-9). The cavity of the tunica vaginalis contains a small amount of serous fluid that moistens the apposed, inner mesothelial surfaces of the visceral and parietal laminae of the tunica.

The cavity of the tunica vaginalis may become distended with serous fluid, forming what is known as a **hydrocele**. Unless the anteroposterior orientation of the testis is reversed (anteversion of the testis), such a swelling, quite translucent when a beam of light is shone through it, is always located anterior to the testis.

Hydrocele exists in many varieties. *Congenital hydrocele* is present at birth and is associated with the persistence of a communication between the peritoneal cavity and the tunica vaginalis through a patent *processus vaginalis*. Even when there is no communication, a hydrocele may suddenly appear in young children or at any age, caused by inflammation of the tunica vaginalis. When the hydrocele is chronic, the swelling may attain quite an enormous size and needs to be drained periodically.

The **blood supply, lymph drainage,** and **innervation of the scrotum** are quite distinct from that of the testis and the spermatic cord. The main scrotal vessels and nerves belong to the perineum and are discussed in Chapter 28.

The Testis and Its Ducts

The testis is the male gonad: its function is the production of spermatozoa and the secretion of testosterone (or dihydrotestosterone), a hormone responsible for the development and maintenance of the secondary sex characteristics of maleness. The spermatozoa leave the testis through the *ductuli efferentes*, which unite to form the *duct of the epididymis*. This highly coiled duct forms a compact body, the *epididymis*, and gives rise to the *ductus deferens*.

The Testis

Each testis is a firm, ellipsoid organ, measuring approximately $4 \times 3 \times 2.5$ cm. The longest diameter is between the rounded superior and inferior poles, and this axis is tilted slightly anteriorly and laterally. The testis, convex and smooth on all surfaces, is slightly flattened from side to side, presenting rounded anterior and posterior borders and more extensive lateral and medial surfaces. The epididymis is applied to the posterior border and protrudes from it laterally; it is in contact with the testis from its superior to its inferior pole (see Fig. 26-6).

The testis and the epididymis invaginate the **tunica vaginalis** from behind. Therefore, the visceral lamina of the tunica covers the testis and epididymis everywhere except along their posterior border and along the posterior part of the area of contact between the two. Anteriorly, a deep groove, the *sinus epididymidis*, intervenes between the testis and the epididymis and is lined by the tunica vaginalis. The tunica vaginalis also covers the anterior surface of the spermatic cord for a variable distance above the testis.

The appearance and structure of the tunica vaginalis is identical with that of the peritoneum. It has been conjectured that, similar to the ovary, the testis is devoid of visceral peritoneum because the celomic epithelium covering the surface of the embryonic gonads (*germinal epithelium*) becomes incorporated into both ovary and testis to form their cortex. Whether it is the remnant of the germinal epithelium or the celomic lining, mesothelium covers the surfaces of the testis that face into the cavity of the tunica vaginalis, and this mesothelium is continuous with that of the parietal lamina of the tunica vaginalis.

When the tunica vaginalis is particularly extensive, the "bare area" along its posterior border will be

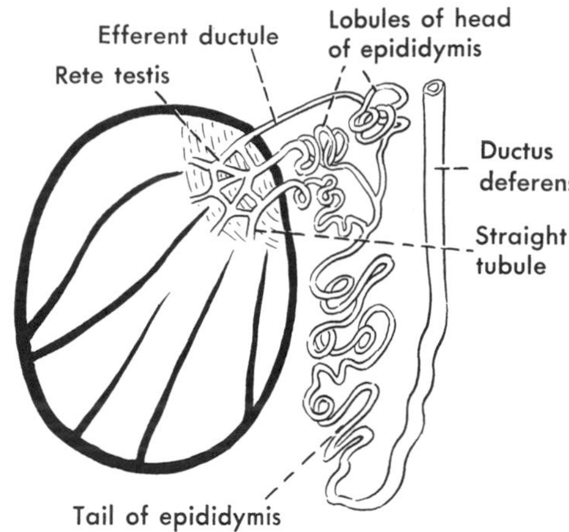

FIGURE 26-10.
Diagram of the duct system of the testis.

narrow, and the testis will appear as if suspended on a short mesentery. Such a mesentery may be designated the *mesorchium* (orchid is one of the Greek names for the testis). A well-defined mesorchium predisposes to torsion of the testis.

Mediastinum Testis. Vessels, nerves, and lymphatics enter and leave the testis and epididymis along their posterior border, which is devoid of the tunica vaginalis (see Fig. 26-6). The **seminiferous tubules** in the interior of the testis also converge toward the posterior border and discharge their contents into a duct system, the **rete testis** which, in turn, is connected to the epididymis by the **ductuli efferentes,** located near the superior pole of the testis (Fig. 26-10). The posterior segment of the testis, containing the rete, is known as the *mediastinum testis.*

Internal Structure. Subjacent to the tunica vaginalis, the testis is invested by a dense layer of fibrous tissue, the **tunica albuginea** which is thinner over the mediastinum. Small septa (*septula testis*) extend from the deep surface of the tunica albuginea into the testis and subdivide it into 200 to 300 roughly pyramid-shaped compartments or **lobules.** The apex of each lobule points toward the mediastinum, and within the lobule lie one to three **seminiferous tubules.** These tubules are 0.1 to 0.3 mm in diameter and may measure nearly 1 m in length. Most of the tubule packed into the lobule is highly convoluted (*tubuli seminiferi contorti*), but one or both ends of all tubules pointing toward the mediastinum become straight (*tubuli seminiferi recti*). In the mediastinum these straight seminiferous tubules terminate in a labyrinth of intercommunicating channels that form the **rete testis**. As the rete passes through the tunica alburginea, it links up with 10 to 20 efferent ductules.

The Epididymis

Didymos is the Greek equivalent of the Latin word *testis.* The epididymis is a comma-shaped, compact body formed by tortuous tubules bound together by areolar tissue. The epididymis consists of a head (*caput*) overlying the superior pole of the testis, a tapering body (*corpus*), and a tail (*cauda*). The body lies along the posterolateral aspect of the testis, and the tail reaches below the inferior pole of the testis.

The head of the epididymis is made up of 10 to 20 lobules, each consisting of an efferent ductule that becomes highly convoluted after leaving the testis. These ductules unite with each other in the epididymis to form the **duct of the epididymis** (see Fig. 26-10). The body and tail are made up of convolutions of this duct. Beyond the tail, the duct is called the **ductus deferens** and becomes more and more straight as it ascends behind the testis into the spermatic cord.

Although the epididymis itself measures barely more than 4 cm, the length of its duct exceeds 6 m. During their passage through the epididymis, the spermatozoa undergo maturation and acquire the capacity for motility. It is not yet known to what extent this maturational process is influenced by the secretions of the epididymal epithelium.

Vestigial Structures. There are vestigial structures associated with the epididymis and the upper pole of the testis. These are the *appendices of the testis and the epididymis*, the *aberrant ductules*, and the *paradidymis* (Fig. 26-11). All these vestiges are remnants of embryonic structures associated with the mesonephros and the developing gonads, discussed in the next section. Their clinical significance is that either appendix may undergo torsion, giving rise to intense pain. The condition must be distinguished clinically from torsion of the testis itself. The aberrant ductules or the paradidymis may give rise to cysts within the scrotum. Such cysts must be distinguished from hydrocele and from cysts of the processus vaginalis.

Blood Supply, Lymph Drainage, and Innervation

Blood Supply. The testicular artery and vein and the pampiniform plexus were discussed with the spermatic

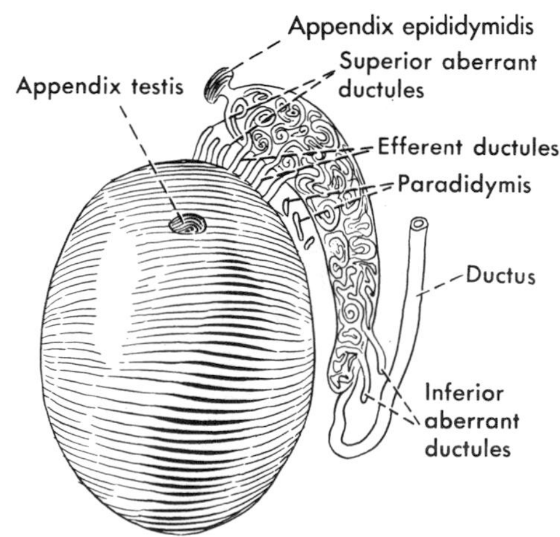

FIGURE 26-11.
Embryonic remains sometimes associated with the testis and its ducts: The appendix testis is a remnant of the paramesonephric duct, and the others are remains of the mesonephric system.

cord earlier in this chapter. The distribution of the intratesticular branches of these vessels follows a connective tissue lamina (*tunica vasculosa*) that is subjacent to the tunica albuginea and is continuous with the mediastinum testis. Extensions of this vascular lamina along the septula testis supply blood to the lobules. However, capillaries do not penetrate the seminiferous tubules. There is evidence that a barrier exists between the blood and the lumen of the duct systems in which spermatozoa are produced and transported.

Lymphatics. The lymphatics of the testis and epididymis drain upward as components of the spermatic cord. After they have passed through the inguinal canal, they run upward in the abdomen along the testicular vessels and join the upper lumbar nodes. In consequence of this drainage, metastatic carcinoma from the testis first involves the lymph nodes close to the renal level, rather than the inguinal nodes, which are nearer topographically.

Nerve Supply. Autonomic nerves accompany both the testicular vessels and the ductus deferens. The **testicular plexus** is derived from the aortic and renal plexuses, and the sympathetic efferent and afferent fibers connect chiefly to T-10 and T-11 segments of the spinal cord through the thoracic splanchnic nerves. The efferent fibers are evidently vasomotor; the visceral afferents are concerned with pain. The testis is quite sensitive to pressure, and the pain of it is localized in the testis as long as the cutaneous nerves of the scrotum are intact. Testicular pain may also be referred to the lower thoracic segments.

The **deferential plexus** becomes associated with the ductus during its intrapelvic course and is derived from branches of the superior and inferior hypogastric plexuses. The exact origins and pathways of the nerves are unknown. Sympathetic efferents in this plexus are responsible for contraction of the muscle wall of the epididymis and ductus deferens, and there is some evidence that parasympathetic fibers derived from the pelvic splanchnics relax the smooth muscle of these ducts. Pain afferents seem to end in the same cord segments as those in the testicular plexus. Epididymal pain cannot be distinguished from testicular pain.

Development and Descent of the Testis

The Testis and Its Ducts

The testis develops in the urogenital ridge lying along the medial side of the mesonephros (see Fig. 25-29). It is connected to the mesonephros by a peritoneal fold, the *mesorchium.*

The primitive testis consists of a *cortex*, formed chiefly by the proliferation of celomic mesothelium (*germinal epithelium*), and a *medulla*, adjacent to the mesonephros and derived from the mesenchyme of intermediate mesoderm. Both the cortex and medulla form cords of cells: from the former develop the seminiferous tubules, from the latter, the rete testis. The seminiferous tubules incorporate the primitive germ cells that migrate to the testis from the yolk sac, and these tubules inosculate with the rete.

Although the mesonephros atrophies and disappears, its collecting tubules and its chief duct persist. Some of the collecting tubules establish connections with the rete testis and become the ductuli efferentes. The mesonephric duct is thus put in communication with the seminiferous tubules. (Fig. 26-12). The definitive pathway for spermatozoa is established by the transformation of the urinary duct of the mesonephros into ducts that transport spermatozoa. From the mesonephric duct differentiates the duct of the epididymis, the ductus deferens, and the ejaculatory duct. Its blind cranial end persists as the appendix of the epididymis. Some mesonephric collecting tubules do not connect with the rete and become the *aberrant ductules* and the *paradidymis,* associated with the epididymis (see Fig. 26-11); those that do connect with the rete form not only the ductuli efferentes but the lobules of the caput epididymidis.

Descent of the Testis

The caudal pole of the urogenital ridges is connected to the skin of the labioscrotal swellings by the *genitoinguinal ligament* (see Fig. 25-26). Once the mesonephros disappears, this ligament spans the distance between the lower pole of the testis and the future scrotal skin; it is renamed in the male the **gubernaculum testis.**

Concomitant with the differentiation of the abdominal wall musculature, the fascial coverings of the spermatic cord develop around the gubernaculum in the region of the inguinal canal. At this stage, the future inguinal canal is essentially vertical.

Similar to the testis, the gubernaculum is retroperitoneal on the posterior abdominal wall and in the lateral inguinal fossa. From the lateral inguinal fossa a tubular extension of the peritoneal sac grows into the mesenchyme of the gubernaculum and forms the **processus vaginalis.** The processus vaginalis extends through the inguinal canal into the scrotum, forming, with the layers of the spermatic cord, what is called the *inguinal bursa* (Fig. 26-13). Some unknown factors initiate the descent of the testis after the inguinal bursa has been formed.

Presumably guided by the gubernaculum, the testis slides down from the posterior abdominal wall, through the inguinal canal, to pass retroperitoneally outside and behind the processus vaginalis, but within the sleeve of the internal spermatic fascia. The gubernaculum shortens as the testis progresses and pulls its ducts with it into the inguinal canal. After the testis has reached the scrotum, the processus vaginalis becomes obliterated and persists only in the scrotum as the tunica vaginalis. The gubernaculum cannot be identified as a discrete structure in the fully developed scrotum. Descent of the testis occurs during the eighth month of fetal life, but may be delayed for a year or so after birth.

In the female, the **round ligament of the uterus** is the equivalent of the caudal portion of the gubernaculum. Although the ovary does not descend into the inguinal canal, the inguinal bursa is formed the same way as in the male.

Abnormalities of Descent. Failure of the testis to descend properly results in **cryptorchidism** or **ectopia testis.** In the former, the testis remains in the abdominal cavity or lodges in the inguinal canal rather than emerging through the superficial inguinal ring; in

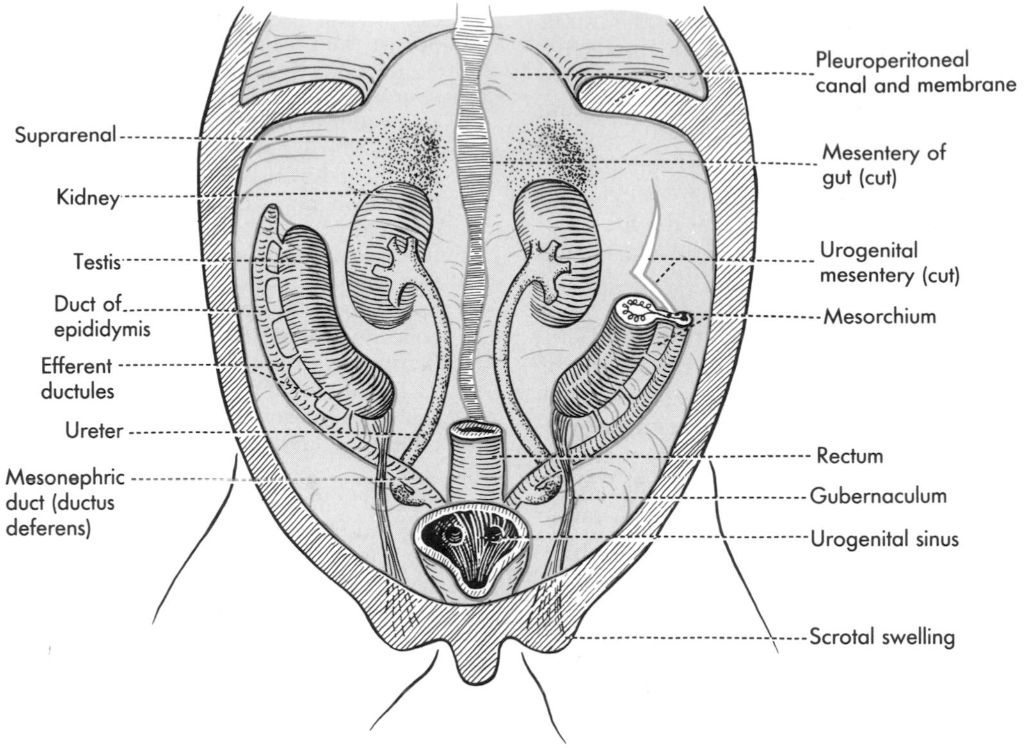

FIGURE *26-12.*
Development of the testis and its duct system shown diagrammatically: This represents a stage later than that in Figure 25-29. The mesothelial lining of the celom is *pink*. The definitive kidneys have ascended the posterior abdominal wall; the testis, with its ligaments and ducts, is still highly placed.

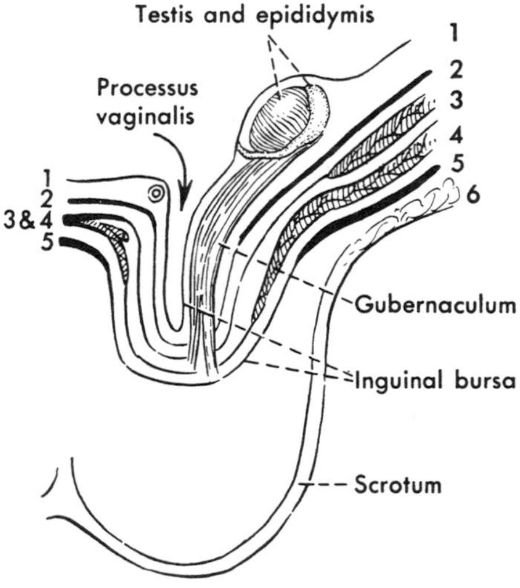

FIGURE *26-13.*
Diagram of the testis, inguinal bursa, and scrotum before descent of the testis: The numbered layers are *1*, peritoneum; *2*, transversalis fascia; *3*, transversus muscle and tendon; *4*, internal oblique muscle and tendon; *5*, aponeurosis of the external oblique; *6*, skin and subcutaneous tissue (superficial fascia). Note that the wall of the inguinal bursa consists of all the layers through the derivative (external spermatic fascia) of the external oblique; the considerable space existing at this stage between the bursa and the scrotum proper is occupied by loose connective tissue. The gubernaculum, along the course of which the testis descends, is shown here somewhat smaller than it really is; at the time of descent, it is as large in diameter as the combined testis and epididymis.

the latter, the testis may emerge through the ring but will lie between the superficial abdominal fascia and the abdominal muscles above the ring or will assume various anomalous positions (Fig. 26-14). Testes that do not descend into the scrotum usually are sterile. An undescended testis is kept at too high a temperature to permit spermatogenesis. It begins to show increasing evidence of damage after the age of 5 years; therefore, if neither testis is in the scrotum by that time and the descent cannot be induced by appropriate administration of hormones, at least one testis should be placed in the scrotum by surgical means.

INGUINAL HERNIA

Hernias In General

The protrusion of any structure through an opening or passage that it normally does not traverse is called a hernia or "rupture." The most well-known types of hernias are protrusions of abdominal contents through the anterolateral abdominal wall. There are many hernias, however, that are entirely internal and may not involve abdominal contents. For instance, the heart may herniate through a defect in the pericardium or a muscle through a defect in its deep fascia. Previous chapters have already mentioned several types of internal abdominal hernia: hiatus hernia, a protrusion of the stomach through the diaphragm, and paraduodenal and other internal intestinal hernias through holes in the mesentery or behind peritoneal folds.

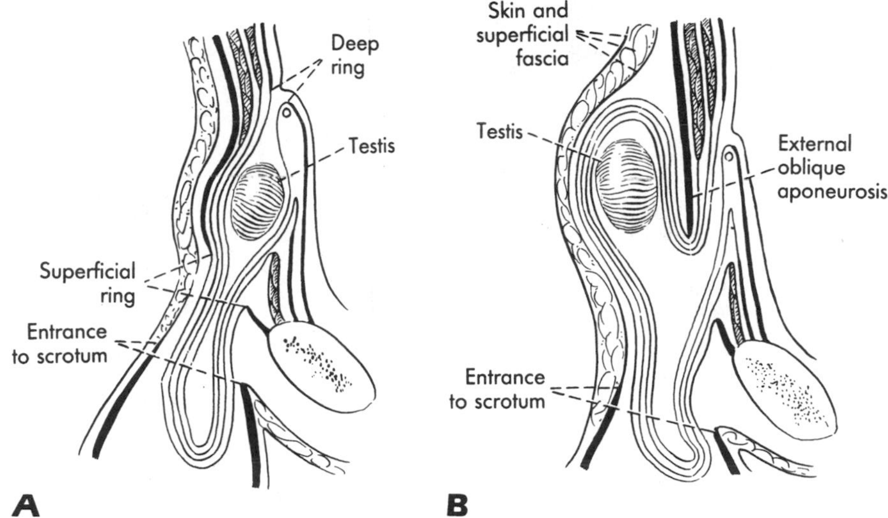

FIGURE *26-14.*
Two types of maldescent of the testis: (A) the testis has lodged in the inguinal canal; and (B) it has emerged through the superficial ring, but is lying deep to skin and superficial fascia of the inguinal region.

Hernias through the abdominal wall may occur through the inguinal and femoral canals, through or along the umbilicus, through tears in the linea alba or rectus sheath, or through the scar of an incision that has been made in the anterolateral abdominal wall, as well as in some other rather unusual places.

In the planning of abdominal incisions, consideration is given to factors that will prevent the formation of hernias through the weakness created by the scar tissue. For instance, the appendectomy incision takes advantage of the fact that the internal and external oblique muscles run at right angles to one another, and the incision separates rather than transects the fibers of each muscle. Paramedian incisions often are made through the anterior sheath of the rectus, and after retraction of the muscle laterally, the posterior rectus sheath is incised, so that when the muscle is replaced, it guards the scars created.

Direct and Indirect Inguinal Hernias

Abdominal contents may enter the inguinal canal directly through its posterior wall or indirectly through the deep inguinal ring. Consequently, two types of inguinal hernias are distinguished: *direct* and *indirect*. Both types emerge through the superficial inguinal ring and present themselves as swellings in the groin, and both types may eventually descend into the scrotum. The hernias that enter the inguinal canal directly through its posterior wall bulge more or less directly into the superficial inguinal ring, especially if the ring is rather large; this is another reason for designating them direct hernias.

Both direct and indirect inguinal hernias are usually contained in a peritoneal sac that surrounds a herniating loop of small or large intestine or a portion of the greater omentum. It is possible, however, for a nonperitoneal structure, most commonly the bladder, to form an inguinal hernia without any peritoneal covering around it.

By definition, an inguinal hernia, the neck of which is located lateral to the inferior epigastric vessels, is called *indirect*; one that commences medial to the inferior epigastric vessels is designated as *direct*. Indirect inguinal hernias may be *congenital* or *acquired*; essentially all direct inguinal hernias are acquired.

A **congenital indirect hernia** is the result of a *patent processus vaginalis* that connects the peritoneal cavity with the tunica vaginalis (Fig. 26-15). The hernia may not appear until adulthood. In **acquired indirect hernias,** the peritoneal sac of the hernia does not communicate with the tunica vaginalis. It is suspected, however, that the majority of acquired indirect inguinal hernias occur because a variable length of the proximal part of the processus vaginalis remains patent. Such hernias are within the spermatic cord, and in the inguinal canal, their peritoneal sac is surrounded by the internal spermatic and cremasteric fascias. Beyond the superficial ring, they are also covered by the external spermatic fascia.

The effective shutter mechanisms of the transversus and internal oblique over the deep inguinal ring prevent such hernias from occurring even when the proximal portion of the processus is patent (see Fig. 26-4). The precipitating factors of hernias remain speculative.

After an indirect inguinal hernia has been reduced, its reappearance may be prevented by firm pressure applied, even by one finger, over the deep inguinal ring. If the hernia reappears when the patient increases abdominal pressure, while the deep inguinal ring is controlled by the finger placed over it, the hernia is likely to be a direct one.

Because of its narrow neck and the obliquity of its passage through the inguinal canal, an indirect hernia is likely to obstruct and strangulate. Strangulation implies that the blood supply to the contents of the hernia has been cut off and gangrene is likely to set in. Either of these complications is a surgical emergency. Therefore, the surgical repair of indirect hernias is indicated once the diagnosis is established.

The neck of a **direct inguinal hernia** is wide. The hernial sac is formed by parietal peritoneum of the

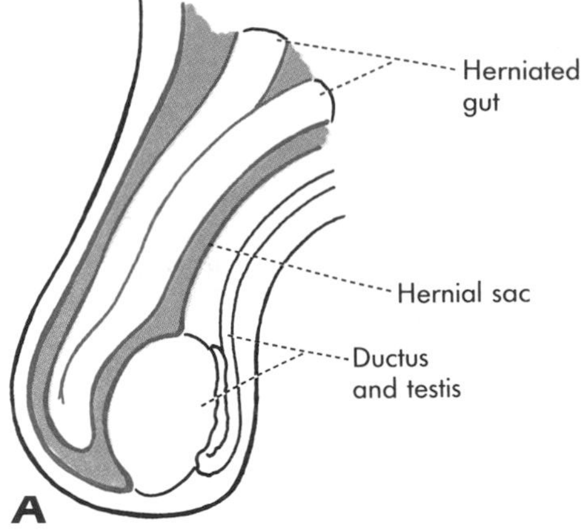

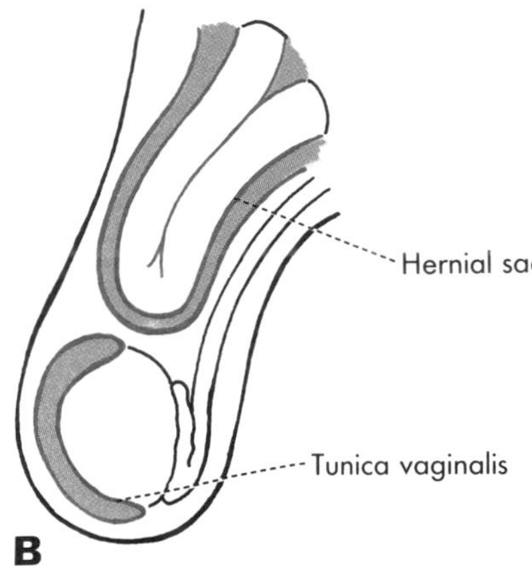

FIGURE *26-15.*
Two types of indirect inguinal hernia: (A) the type usually called congenital; (B) the type usually called acquired.

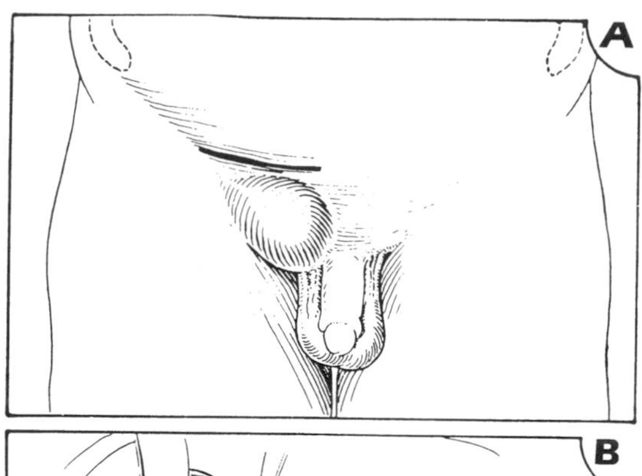

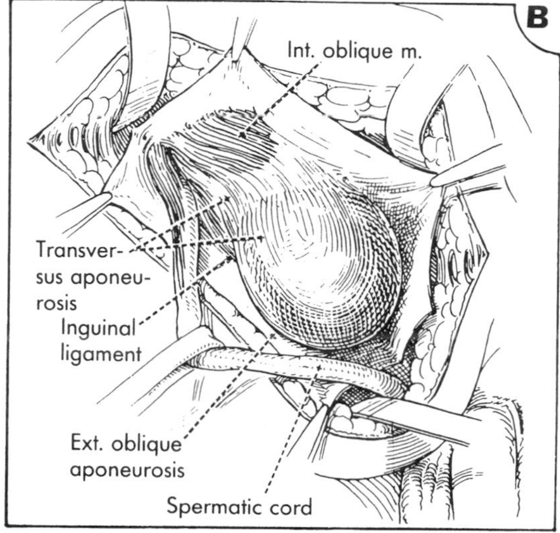

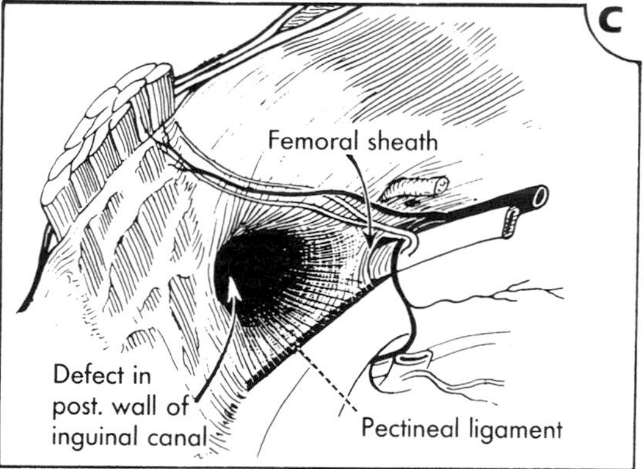

FIGURE *26-16.*
(A) The appearance of a direct inguinal hernia in an anterior view, with the line of incision marked on the skin; (B) with the external oblique and internal oblique aponeuroses divided, opening up the inguinal canal; (C) the deep or posterior aspect of the inguinal canal with the forward herniation of the transversalis fascia and the conjoint tendon into the inguinal canal. (Anson BJ, McVay CB. Surgical anatomy. 5th ed. vol 1. Philadelphia; WB Saunders, 1971.)

medial inguinal or supravesical fossae (see Fig. 23-26). Pushing transversalis fascia in front of it, the hernial sac may slip under the crescentic edge of the conjoint tendon and under the inferior fibers of the internal oblique, which lie parallel with the inguinal ligament, or it may stretch and push the conjoint tendon and the internal oblique in front of it. Until such a hernia emerges through the superficial inguinal ring, it will not be inside the spermatic cord (Fig. 26-16); beyond the superficial ring, it will lie between the superficial spermatic and cremasteric fascias. A direct inguinal hernia may also enter the inguinal canal through the hiatus of the internal oblique, through which the spermatic cord passes, especially if this hiatus is large (see Fig. 26-8). In such a case, the hernia will be within the cremasteric fascia. Because of their wide neck, direct inguinal hernias are more readily reduced than indirect inguinal hernias, and they are less likely to obstruct or strangulate.

Hernial Repair. Repair of any abdominal hernia includes reducing it, ligating the neck of the peritoneal hernial sac so that the peritoneum possesses a smooth surface rather than a funnel-shaped diverticulum that invites further herniation, closing the enlarged opening through which the hernia has escaped, and strengthening the region to mitigate a recurrence.

In the female, both the deep and superficial inguinal rings may be closed. In the male, however, they can be narrowed only to the extent that they allow passage of the spermatic cord. The specific technique used to strengthen the walls of the inguinal canal varies with the size of the hernia, its type, and the preference of the surgeon. In indirect hernia, the technique usually includes 1) narrowing the enlarged superficial and deep rings so that they accommodate the cord with little room to spare and 2) reinforcing the wall of the inguinal canal in one manner or another. The best-known techniques involve bringing down the borders of the internal oblique and transversus muscles and suturing them to the inguinal ligament or the pectineal ligament.

THE FEMORAL SHEATH AND FEMORAL HERNIA

In the upright anatomic position, the pelvis is so oriented that the inguinal ligament lies anterior and somewhat below the level of the superior ramus of the pubis. The psoas and iliacus muscles pass vertically behind the lateral part of the inguinal ligament into the thigh (see Fig. 17-22) and fill the *lacuna musculorum* (Fig. 26-17). Between the two muscles is the femoral nerve. The transversalis fascia on the deep surface of the transversus meets and becomes continuous with the iliopsoas fascia along the lateral part of the inguinal ligament.

Behind the medial part of the inguinal ligament in the lacuna vasorum, the external iliac artery descends vertically into the thigh to become the femoral artery; the external iliac vein, the continuation of the femoral vein, ascends on the medial side of the artery (see Figs. 18-16 and 26-17). The space behind the inguinal ligament, through which these vessels pass, is bounded medially by the free edge of the lacunar ligament and the conjoint tendon, posteriorly by the pectineal ligament and the superior ramus of the pubis, and laterally by the iliopectineal arch, which separates the artery from the psoas and the femoral nerve.

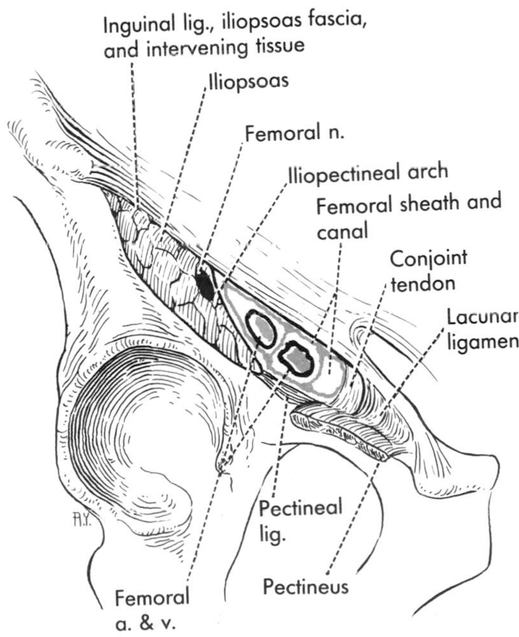

FIGURE *26-17.*
The space between the inguinal ligament and the coxal bone: The iliopectineal arch divides this into the laterally lying lacuna musculorum, occupied by the iliopsoas muscle and the femoral nerve, and the medially lying lacuna vasorum, occupied by the femoral vessels and the femoral canal enclosed in the femoral sheath, shown in *blue*.

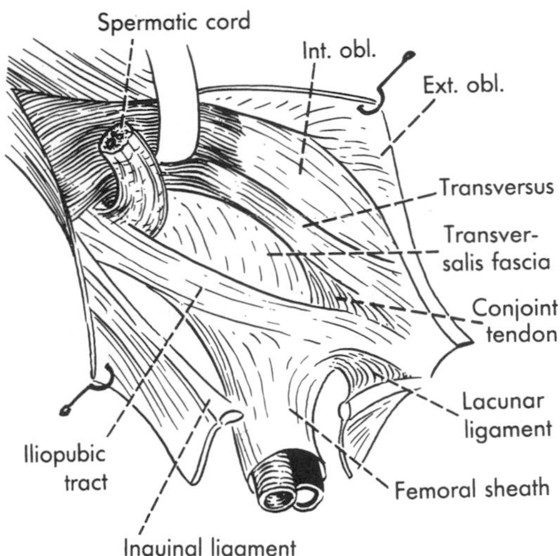

FIGURE *26-18.*
The transversalis fascia in the inguinofemoral region seen from the front, showing the continuity with the femoral sheath and the transverse thickening ("iliopubic tract") across the femoral ring. The internal oblique is elevated; the spermatic cord and the inguinal ligament are cut and displaced. (Redrawn from Clark JH, Hashimoto EI: Surg Gynecol Obstet 1946; 82:840.)

Just above the inguinal ligament, the transversalis fascia forms a reinforced band, the *iliopubic tract;* below the inguinal ligament, the iliopubic tract continues into the lacuna vasorum and forms a sheath around the femoral vessels (Fig. 26-18). This funnel-shaped diverticulum of the transversalis fascia, called the **femoral sheath,** extends around the femoral vessels into the femoral triangle as if the vessels had drawn it out into the thigh (see Fig. 18-16). It is described in Chapter 18.

Two septa divide the femoral sheath into three compartments: the lateral compartment contains the femoral artery; the intermediate compartment contains the femoral vein; and the medial compartment is essentially empty except for some areolar tissue, lymphatics, and a lymph node. The medial compartment of the femoral sheath is the **femoral canal,** a potential space into which the femoral vein can expand when the venous return through it increases during walking and running. The femoral canal is cone-shaped, with its base, the **femoral ring,** facing into the abdomen. The medial margin of the femoral ring is formed by the lacunar ligament and the conjoint tendon (Fig. 26-19); its anterior lip is formed by the iliopubic tract along the inguinal ligament; the pectineal ligament borders it posteriorly.

The ring, measuring just over 1 cm in diameter, is open above except for a filmy layer of extraperitoneal tissue that stretches across it and is known as the *femoral septum.* Only extraperitoneal connective tissue intervenes between the femoral ring and the parietal peritoneum. The ring represents an area of potential weakness through which femoral hernias descend into the femoral canal. The apex of the 1- to 1.5-cm–long canal points into the

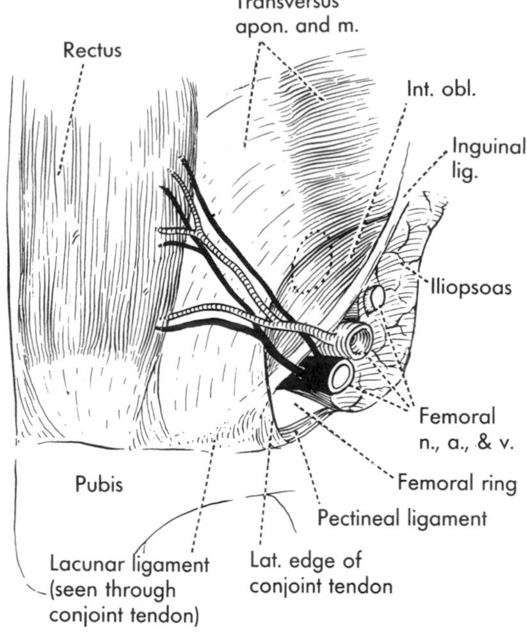

FIGURE *26-19.*
The inguinal region and the upper end of the femoral canal from the inner aspect of the anterior abdominal wall, after removal of the transversalis fascia. The location of the deep inguinal ring is indicated by the *broken oval.* Figure 26-5 shows the same view, but with the transversalis fascia intact.

femoral triangle and is formed by the fusion of the femoral sheath with the adventitia of the femoral vein behind the saphenous opening (see Fig. 18-16).

Femoral Hernia

Femoral hernias are always acquired; a pre-formed peritoneal sac is never present in the femoral canal. A hernia is likely to occur when the femoral ring is large, but the exact predisposing causes are variable and largely unknown. The peritoneal sac forced into the canal by the hernia is covered by extraperitoneal fat. The hernia dilates the femoral sheath and protrudes into the subcutaneous tissue of the upper part of the thigh, through the *saphenous hiatus*, stretching before it the *cribriform fascia* (see Chap. 18; Fig. 26-20).

The femoral hernia is always inferior to the inguinal ligament and can be further distinguished from an inguinal hernia by verifying that it does not emerge through the superficial inguinal ring. After a hernia has been reduced, a finger (usually the little finger) may be inserted into the superficial inguinal ring by invaginating the skin of the scrotum. When abdominal pressure is raised, an inguinal hernia can be felt pushing against the finger in the superficial ring; a femoral hernia will appear below the ring without contacting the finger.

Because of the sharp ligamentous lips of the femoral ring, a femoral hernia is particularly likely to obstruct and strangulate. Repair of the hernia follows the same principles as that of an inguinal hernia. The femoral ring may be closed completely by suturing the conjoint tendon or the inguinal ligament to the pectineal ligament.

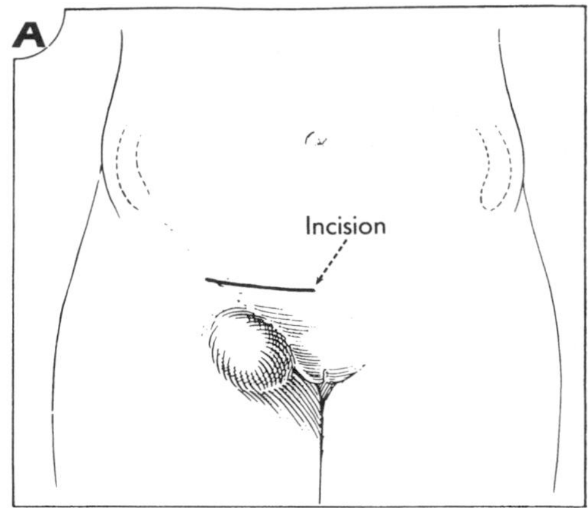

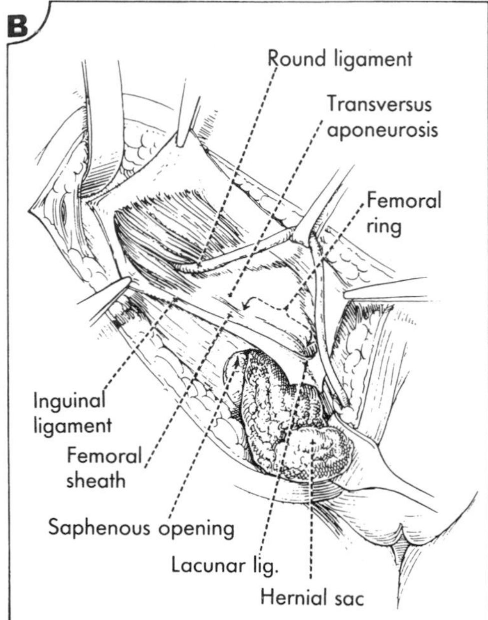

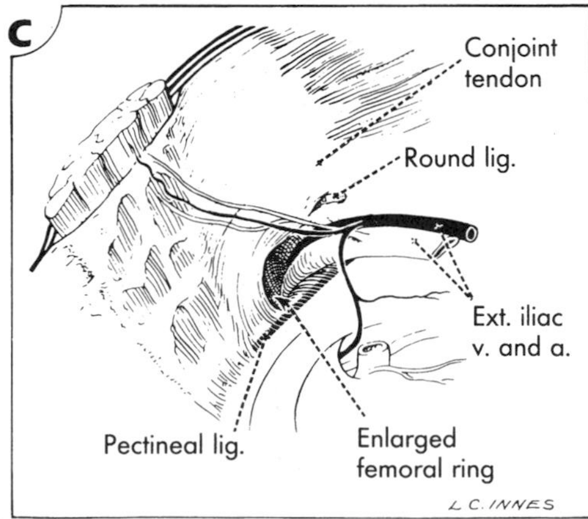

FIGURE *26-20.*
(A) The appearance of a femoral hernia in an anterior view with the line of incision marked on the skin. (B) The external oblique aponeurosis has been divided. The hernial sac pushes forward inferior to the inguinal ligament. (C) the posterior aspect of the inguinal region with the parts named and the hernial sac omitted from the enlarged femoral ring. (Anson BJ, McVay CB: Surgical anatomy. 5th ed. vol 1. Philadelphia; WB Saunders, 1971)

Vascular Relations

Just before it leaves the abdomen, the **external iliac artery** gives rise to two named branches, the inferior epigastric and the deep circumflex iliac.

The **inferior epigastric artery** arises from the front of the external iliac artery and turns forward and upward on the anterior abdominal wall between the peritoneum and the transversalis fascia (see Fig. 26-19). As it runs upward, it is directed also somewhat medially; it passes just on the medial side of the deep inguinal ring and in its course raises the lateral umbilical fold of peritoneum (see Fig. 23-26). It pierces the transversalis fascia below the arcuate line to reach the deep surface of the rectus abdominis and, shortly thereafter, enters the muscle to run upward in its substance. Close to its origin, the inferior epigastric artery gives off, in the male, the **cremasteric artery,** which follows the spermatic cord and supplies the tunics of the cord and testis, or in the female, a small **artery of the round ligament** that follows the round ligament of the uterus. The inferior epigastric also gives rise to a **pubic branch** that runs medially and downward, passing close to the femoral ring. It sends anastomotic twigs to the obturator artery and, behind the pubic symphysis, anastomoses with its fellow of the opposite side and with vessels on the adjacent surface of the bladder. The connection to the obturator artery may become the anomalous stem of this pubic branch. The obturator artery leaves the pelvis through the obturator foramen just below the superior ramus of the pubis.

The **deep circumflex iliac artery** arises from the lateral side of the external iliac and runs laterally and upward across the iliopsoas toward the anterior superior iliac spine. It pierces the transversus to run above the iliac crest, between the transversus and the internal oblique.

RECOMMENDED READINGS

Anson BJ, Morgan EH, McVay CB. Surgical anatomy of the inguinal region based upon a study of 500 body-halves. Surg Gynecol Obstet 1960;111:707.

Arregui ME, Nagan RF, eds. Inguinal hernia: advances or controversies? Oxford: Radcliffe Medical Press, 1994.

Blunt MJ. Posterior wall of the inguinal canal. Br J Surg 1951;39:230.

Doyle JF. The superficial inguinal arch: a reassessment of what has been called the inguinal ligament. J Anat 1971;108:297.

Gilroy AM, Marks S Jr, Lei Q, Page DW. Anatomic characteristics of the iliopubic tract: implications for repair of inguinal hernias. Clin Anat 1992;5:255.

Gunn SA, Gould TC. Vasculature of the testes and adnexa. In: Handbook of physiology. Sect 7, vol II. Washington DC: American Physiological Society, 1975.

Hadziselimovic F. Embryology of testicular descent and maldescent. In: Hadziselimovic F, ed. Cryptorchidism: management and implication. Berlin: Springer, 1983:11.

Heyns CF, Hutson JM. Historical review of theories on testicular descent. J Urol 1995;153:754.

Hodson N. The nerves of the testis, epididymis, and scrotum. In: Johnson AD, Gomes WR, Vandemark NL, eds. The testis, vol 1. New York: Academic Press, 1970.

Hollinshead WH. Anatomy for surgeons: vol 2, the thorax, abdomen, and pelvis. 2nd ed. New York: Harper & Row, 1971.

Holstein AF, Roosen-Runge EC. Atlas of human spermatogenesis. Berlin: Grosse, 1981.

Johnson FP. Dissections of human seminiferous tubules. Anat Rec 1934;59:187.

Johnson AD, Gomes WR, Vandemark NL, eds. The testis. New York: Academic Press, 1970.

Kohler FP. On the etiology of variocele. J Urol 1967;97:741.

McVay CB. The normal and pathologic anatomy of the transversus abdominis muscle in inguinal and femoral hernia. Surg Clin North Am 1971;51:1251.

Rowe PC, Gearhart JP. Retraction of the umbilicus during voiding as an initial sign of a urachal anomaly. Pediatrics 1993;91:53.

Scheye TH, Vanneuville G, Amara B, Francannet PH, Dechelotte P, Campagne D. Anatomic basis of pathology of the urachus. Surg Radiol Anat 1994;16:135.

Shafik A. The cremasteric muscle. In: Johnson AD, Gomes WR, eds. The testis, vol 4. New York: Academic Press, 1977.

Waites GMH. Temperature regulation and the testis. In: In: Johnson AD, Gomes WR, Vandemark NL, eds. The testis, vol 1. New York: Academic Press, 1970.

Yeager VL. Intermediate inguinal ring. Clin Anat 1992;5:289.

PART VII

THE PELVIS AND PERINEUM

Hollinshead's Textbook of Anatomy, by Cornelius Rosse and Penelope Gaddum-Rosse.
Lippincott-Raven Publishers, Philadelphia, © 1997.

CHAPTER 27

The Pelvis

The primary function of the **bony pelvis,** made up of the two *ossa coxae* and the *sacrum,* is the transmission of forces between the lower limbs and the axial skeleton. The anatomy of these bones is described in Chapters 12, 14, and 17. The osseoligamentous ring, formed by the bony pelvis, encloses the **pelvic cavity,** the inferior portion of the body cavity introduced in Chapter 23.

The word "pelvis" means "basin" and is used for referring to both the bony pelvis and the pelvic cavity. In this chapter, the term is used chiefly in the latter sense, because the purpose is to describe the pelvic cavity with its apertures, walls, and contents.

Insofar as the pelvis contains most of the internal genitalia of the female and some of those of the male, pelvic contents differ in the two sexes. In the female, the pelvic internal genitalia include the ovaries, the uterine tubes, and the uterus, with their associated peritoneal and fibromuscular ligaments, and the upper part of the vagina; the male pelvic internal genitalia are the deferent ducts, the seminal vesicles and ejaculatory ducts, and the prostate. Notwithstanding these sexual differences, and those evident in its skeleton, the basic anatomy of the pelvis is the same in the two sexes: this is true of the boundaries, fascias, vessels, and nerves of the pelvis, as well as of its nongenital viscera, the bladder and the rectum. Except for the ovaries and, to some extent, the rectum, pelvic viscera are supplied by branches of the internal iliac artery; the internal iliac vein drains them. Pelvic lymphatics generally follow the blood vessels but do not all empty into the internal iliac nodes. The pelvis contains the *sacral plexus,* the largest plexus of somatic nerves in the body, from which issue some of the major nerves of the lower limb. The autonomic plexus for the supply of pelvic viscera is the *inferior hypogastric,* or *pelvic, plexus;* its offshoots reach the viscera along the arteries.

The first section of this chapter discusses the boundaries of the pelvic cavity, including its apertures and the bony, ligamentous, and muscular elements in its walls. These features have a bearing on the anatomy of the birth canal, the passage through which the fetus is delivered. The sections dealing with pelvic viscera are preceded by developmental considerations that explain not only the embryologic but also the topographic relations between pelvic viscera.

BOUNDARIES OF THE PELVIC CAVITY

The boundaries of the pelvic cavity are formed by the pelvic skeleton and the pelvic musculature. The pelvis has a wide, more or less oval, *superior aperture,* or *inlet,* and a more narrow, somewhat rectangular, *inferior aperture,* or *outlet.* Through the superior aperture, the pelvic cavity communicates freely with the abdominal cavity proper; inferiorly, the pelvic cavity is limited by a muscular floor, the *pelvic diaphragm,* which is attached to the pelvic walls. The *inferior pelvic aperture* is below the pelvic diaphragm and, therefore, outside the pelvic cavity; it provides the osseoligamentous frame of the perineum. The walls of the pelvic cavity taper downward like those of a basin and are formed anteriorly by the body of the two pubes and the symphysis between them; posteriorly, they are formed by the sacrum, and anterolaterally, by the obturator internus muscle, covering most of the lower half of the internal surface of the coxal bone (see Fig. 17-3). Posterolaterally, between the greater sciatic notch of the coxal bone and the sacrum, the greater sciatic foramen provides exit for nerves and vessels from the pelvis to the gluteal region and the perineum. The foramen is largely filled by the piriformis muscle (see Fig. 17-19).

The Pelvic Skeleton

The size of the pelvic cavity is determined by the pelvic skeleton. The limits imposed by the bony pelvis are so important in obstetric considerations that the muscles and fascias contributing to the pelvic walls are not taken into account at all in assessments of the size of the pelvis. The pelvic apertures are bordered largely by bones and, as already noted, the anterior and posterior walls of the pelvic cavity are formed by bare bone.

The Pelvic Apertures

The **pelvic inlet** is bordered by the pelvic brim, formed on each side by the *pubic crest,* the *linea terminalis* (consisting of the pecten pubis and the arcuate line on the ilium (see Fig. 17-3), and the *ala of the sacrum* (Fig. 27-1). Posteriorly, the sacral promontory, perched on a level higher than the linea terminalis, juts forward into the pelvic inlet, rendering it somewhat heart-shaped rather than oval. The two sacroiliac joints and the symphysis pubis firmly unite these bones and permit essentially no change in the di-

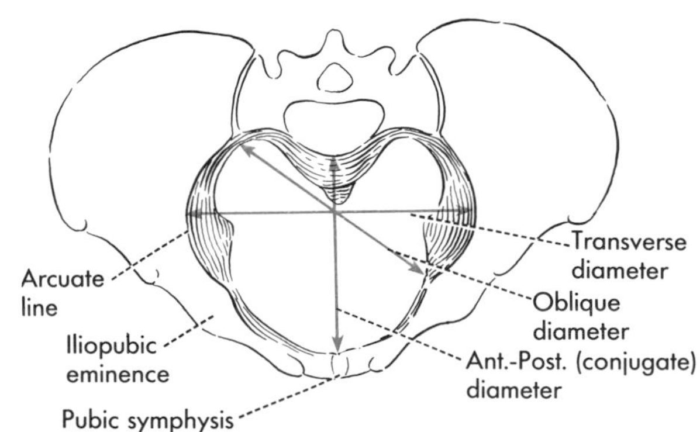

FIGURE *27-1.*
Commonly measured diameters of the pelvic inlet of the female.

mensions of the pelvic inlet, although during pregnancy, the ligaments of the joints may slacken, and there may be some play between the bones.

During much of its growth and development, the fetus enclosed in the enlarged uterus is located in the abdominal cavity above the pelvic brim. For delivery to take place, the fetal head has to be admitted into the pelvic cavity through the pelvic inlet. This "engagement" of the fetal head usually occurs sometime before the commencement of labor. Clearly, the shape and dimensions of the pelvic inlet have obstetric consequences, and these are assessed by physical and radiologic measurements of various pelvic diameters.

The commonly measured **diameters of the superior aperture** are the conjugate and transverse diameters (see Fig. 27-1). The *conjugate*, or anteroposterior, *diameter* is measured from the upper border of the symphysis pubis to the sacral promontory (*true conjugate diameter*; this can only be done radiologically), or from the lower border of the symphysis pubis to the promontory (*diagonal conjugate*; this can be obtained by vaginal examination, because the fingers of the examiner can reach the sacrum). The *transverse diameter* is the greatest distance obtainable between bilateral symmetric points on the linea terminalis. Apart from radiologic measurements, this can be inferred from the external dimensions of the pelvis or from the transverse diameter of the pelvic cavity measured between the ischial spines, palpable *per vaginam*. Various other diameters may be measured for obstetric diagnosis and prognosis in the pelvic inlet, outlet, and cavity; however, because the superior pelvic aperture is the most variable in shape, pelves are classified according to the ratio of the conjugate and transverse diameters in this aperture.

Four major **types of pelves** are recognized: anthropoid, android, gynecoid, and platypelloid pelves. In the first two, the conjugate diameter is longer than the transverse; in the latter two, the reverse is true. Anthropoid and android pelves predominate in males; most women have gynecoid or android pelves. Platypelloid pelvis is rare and shows a pronounced anteroposterior flattening; an anthropoid pelvis is flattened from side to side. Both types, as well as an android pelvis, may make engagement of the fetal head difficult.

The **inferior pelvic aperture** is formed anteriorly by the *pubic arch*, made up of the inferior margin of the pubic symphysis, and the conjoint rami of the pubis and ischium, terminating behind in the ischial tuberosity. Posteriorly, the aperture is bordered by the *sacrotuberous ligaments*, which connect the ischial tuberosities to the dorsal aspect of the sacrum and the coccyx. The coccyx juts forward into the inferior aperture (see Fig. 28-1).

After the fetal head progresses beyond the pelvic floor into the perineum, it is delivered through the inferior pelvic aperture, its occiput usually passing in the pubic arch. A narrow pubic arch, characteristic of anthropoid and android pelves, may displace the fetal head posteriorly to the extent that the soft tissues of the perineum will be torn.

Orientation of the Bony Pelvis

Correct orientation of the pelvis is necessary for appreciating the topographic relations of pelvic and perineal viscera and the mechanisms that support them. In the upright anatomic position, the pelvis is so oriented that the right and left anterior superior iliac spines and pubic tubercles are in the same coronal plane. Indeed, it is possible for a lean person facing a wall to bring all four bony points in contact with the wall. If a transverse plane is placed at right angles to the vertical plane across the superior border of the symphysis pubis, it will pass through the ischial spines and, in the female, also through the tip of the coccyx (Fig. 27-2). The plane of the pelvic inlet makes approximately a 60° angle with such a horizontal plane, whereas the plane of the pelvic outlet lies almost parallel with it. Consideration of these planes makes it clear that 1) the superior pelvic aperture faces more anteriorly than upward; 2) the anterior wall of the pelvic cavity is much shorter than its posterior wall; and 3) the axis of the pelvic cavity, which runs through the central point of the inlet and the outlet, is curved, almost paralleling the sacral curvature (see Fig. 27-2).

Skeletal Sex Differences

Adaptations of the female pelvis to childbearing are reflected in several features of the pelvic skeleton. Although the absolute measurements of any part of the pelvis may be greater in the male than in the female, the relative proportions of the female pelvis give it a more roomy cavity, wider apertures, and a lighter skeletal frame.

The pelvic cavity of the male tends to be more conical; that of the female is more cylindrical. The female *sacrum* is shorter and wider than the male, and its concavity is deeper. In the female, more than two-thirds of the base of the sacrum is made up by the alae, whereas in the male, the width of the first sacral vertebral body occupies more than one-third of the

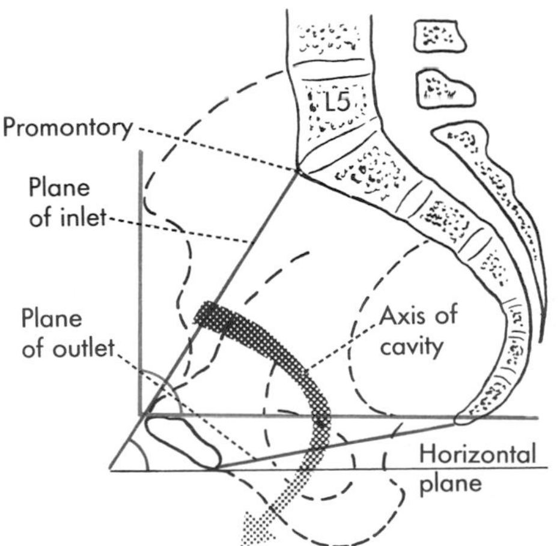

FIGURE 27-2.
Orientation of the pelvis: the *red vertical line* shows the alignment of the anterior superior iliac spine with the pubic tubercle; the *red horizontal line* shows the alignment of the pubic symphysis, ischial spine, and tip of the coccyx. The planes of the pelvic inlet and outlet are *blue*.

base at the expense of the alae. The anterolateral wall of the pelvis is relatively wider in the female, as expressed by several features: the pubic tubercles are farther apart; the distance between the symphysis and the anterior lip of the acetabulum is greater in the female than the diameter of the acetabulum, whereas in the male, these measurements are approximately equal. This gives a triangular shape to the obturator foramen in the female; in the male, the foramen is more or less round.

The greater sciatic notch and pubic arch are wider in the female than in the male. In the male, the pubic arch makes an acute angle considerably less than 90°. In the female, the arch is smooth and rounded; the line of the two inferior pubic rami, if extrapolated forward, would make an angle close to 90°. In the male, the ischiopubic rami are rather robust and everted to give attachment to the crura of the penis; in the female, the rami are rather delicate.

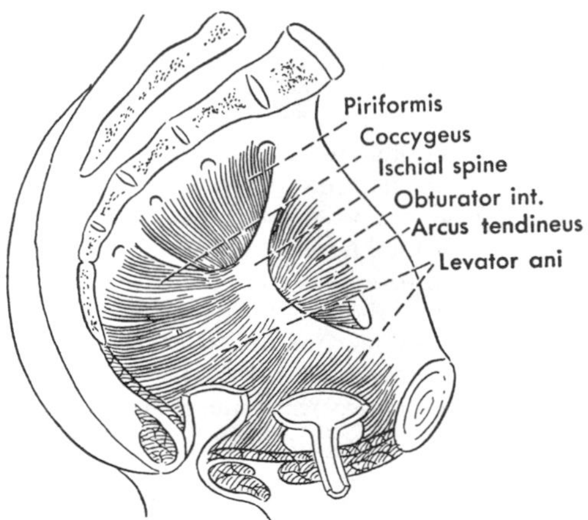

FIGURE 27-3.
Muscles of the pelvic wall and floor: Stumps of the hemisected rectum and the bladder and prostate have been left in place, and the sphincter ani externus and the urogenital diaphragm are shown, *unlabeled*, below the levator ani.

The Pelvic Musculature

Although the pelvic cavity is part of the body cavity derived from the intraembryonic celom, the muscles in its walls bear no resemblance to those of the thorax and abdomen proper. The *piriformis* and *obturator internus* are both muscles of the lower limb that lie on the interior of the pelvic skeleton and, consequently, line part of the pelvic cavity. The several named parts of the levator ani muscle and the coccygeus arise in continuity from the wall of the pelvic cavity and, fusing with their counterparts of the opposite side along the midline of the gutter-shaped pelvic floor, constitute the *pelvic diaphragm*. This diaphragm separates the pelvic cavity from the perineum. The levator ani and coccygeus have evolved from the musculature of the tail, supplying a diaphragm across the pelvic outlet, necessitated by an erect posture and wide bony pelvis.

The Piriformis and Obturator Internus

Both the piriformis and the obturator internus are lateral rotators of the thigh; both are found in the gluteal region (see Chap. 17).

The **piriformis** arises on the posterior wall of the pelvis from the area of bone in between and lateral to the pelvic foramina of the sacrum. Between the two muscles, the bodies of the second, third, and fourth sacral vertebrae are bare, covered only with periosteum, as are the first sacral vertebra and the ala of the sacrum above the origin of the piriformis. The muscle completes the posterior wall laterally and leaves the pelvis through the greater sciatic foramen, which it nearly fills (Fig. 27-3). The anterior rami of sacral spinal nerves emerging from the pelvic foramina of the sacrum unite on the pelvic surface of the piriformis to form the sacral plexus, and the major branches of the plexus leave the pelvis with the muscle.

The **obturator internus** covers a large area on the internal surface of the coxal bone below the pelvic brim. It arises from the medial surface of the obturator membrane, from the adjoining margins of the obturator foramen (except the superior pubic ramus, which is bare), and from the broad strip of bone above and behind the obturator foramen formed by the fused bodies of the ilium and the ischium (see Fig. 17-3). The fan-shaped muscle tapers to a narrow tendon lodged in the lesser sciatic notch, where it turns abruptly laterally and heads with the tendon of the piriformis toward the greater trochanter. Less than the upper half of the muscle faces into the pelvic cavity; the lower part forms the lateral wall of the perineum. The medial surface of the muscle is covered by the dense *obturator fascia*, and to this fascia is attached the major part of the pelvic diaphragm.

The Pelvic Diaphragm

The pelvic diaphragm consists of the *coccygeus muscle* posteriorly and the more extensive and complex *levator ani* anterolaterally (Fig. 27-4; see Fig. 27-3). The diaphragm is a thin sheet of muscle and its halves form the sloping floor of the pelvis, through which the pelvic effluents, the urethra, vagina, and anal canal, pass into the perineum. The diaphragm is sometimes compared to, and may be demonstrated as, a funnel slotted into the pelvic cavity. The rim of the funnel on each side fits snugly against the body of the pubis, the obturator internus, the ischial spine, and the sacrum. The stem of the funnel may represent the urethra, the vagina, or the anal canal. Unlike the funnel, however, the diaphragm is incomplete both posteriorly and anteriorly: posteriorly, the two coccygeus muscles leave the coccyx and sacrum bare between them; anteriorly, there is a U-shaped deficiency between the two levator ani muscles, through which the urethra, vagina, and anal canal pass. The anterior deficiency is known as the **urogenital hiatus.** It is closed completely, largely by the pelvic effluents accommodated in it and by fibers of the levator ani that attach to the urethra, vagina, and anal canal. The pelvic fascia that covers half of the pelvic diaphragm fuses with that of the opposite side and with the fascias that surround the pelvic effluents, sealing any communication between the pelvis and the perineum through the hiatus.

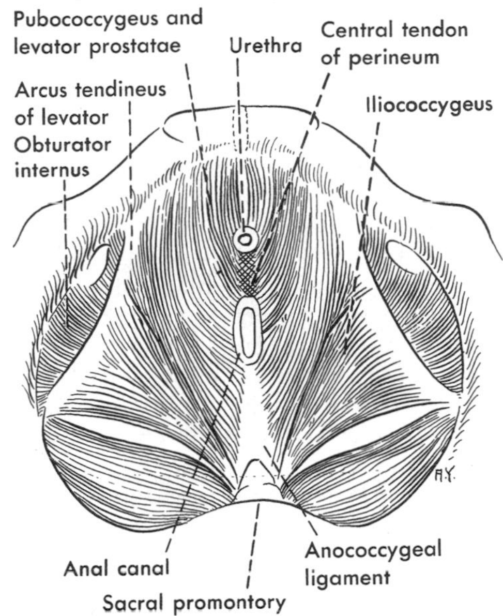

FIGURE 27-4.
The levator ani from above.

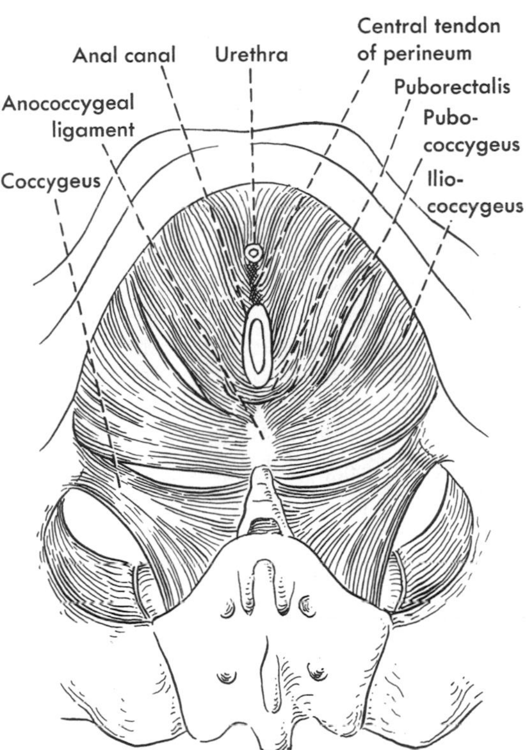

FIGURE 27-5.
The pelvic diaphragm of the male from below.

The Levator Ani. The muscle originates along a semicircular line that skirts the pelvic walls from the pelvic surface of the body of the pubis to the ischial spine. In between these bony points, the levator ani is attached to a bandlike reinforcement in the obturator fascia known as the *arcus tendineus* (or the *tendinous arch of the levator ani*). The fibers of the muscle sweep backward as well as downward, with varying degrees of obliquity, and insert into the walls of the urethra, vagina, and anal canal and, beyond the urogenital hiatus, into the *anococcygeal ligament*, or raphe, and the coccyx.

The named parts of the levator ani are the pubococcygeus (levator prostatae or pubovaginalis), the puborectalis, and the iliococcygeus. None of these parts is a distinct entity, but their fibers have different directions and relations.

The **pubococcygeus muscle** runs posteriorly from the body of the pubis and the anterior part of the tendinous arch to the anococcygeal ligament and the coccyx (Fig. 27-5; see Fig. 27-4). The medial fasciculi of the two muscles border the urogenital hiatus, and some of their fibers terminate by inserting into the structures that fill the hiatus between the pubic symphysis and the anococcygeal ligament. The most anterior of these fibers insert into the urethra, or sweep behind the prostate or the vagina, and end in the central tendon of the perineum, a fibromuscular body (*perineal body*) projecting from the perineum into the urogenital hiatus. In the male, this part of the muscle is called the **levator prostatae;** in the female, it is called the **pubovaginalis.** Some fibers of the pubovaginalis blend with the wall of the vagina and will be surrounded in the perineum by the sphincter vaginae; others, bypassing the vagina, can act as an additional sphincter around it.

The **puborectalis** is a relatively thick bundle in the levator ani, best defined on the perineal surface of the pubococcygeus (see Fig. 27-5). On each side, the muscle sweeps backward from the pubis and fuses with its fellow of the opposite side behind the junction of the rectum with the anal canal, forming a sling around the anorectal junction. Some fibers blend with the longitudinal muscle coat of the anal canal. The puborectalis is chiefly responsible for the angulation at the perineal flexure between the rectum and the anal canal. As it pulls the anorectal junction forward, the muscle has a sphincterlike action and contributes to anal continence.

The **iliococcygeus** arises from the posterior part of the arcus tendineus and the ischial spine. It inserts into the anococcygeal raphe and the coccyx, just below the insertion of the coccygeus.

The Coccygeus. In conformity with the parts of the levator ani, the coccygeus could be called the ischiococcygeus. The small triangular muscle arises from the ischial spine and expands to insert on the lateral borders of the lower two sacral and upper two coccygeal segments. On its external surface, it is blended with the *sacrospinous ligament*, which forms the inferior limit of the greater sciatic foramen.

Innervation and Actions

The **piriformis** and **obturator internus** are supplied chiefly by S-1 segment through small branches of the sacral plexus (see Chap. 17). The **levator ani** is innervated on its pelvic surface by twigs from the fourth (sometimes also the third) sacral anterior ramus. The anterior part of the muscle, particularly the puborectalis, usually receives a branch from the pudendal nerve after this nerve has left the pelvis and lies on the inferior surface of the muscle. The **coccygeus** is supplied by the fourth and fifth sacral anterior rami.

The levator ani has important functions in the regulation of abdominal and pelvic pressure and contracts whenever abdominal pressure is raised. The muscle is particularly involved with the voluntary control of micturition and the support of the uterus, both described later. The pelvic diaphragm supports all the pelvic viscera, and insertion of some of its fibers into the central tendon of the perineum is an important factor in this respect. Its contraction raises the entire pelvic floor. Prenatal exercises are aimed at conscious relaxation of the pelvic diaphragm, whereas the strengthening of the muscle has been advocated for preventing the prolapse of pelvic viscera.

PELVIC FASCIA, VESSELS, AND NERVES

The major pelvic organs protrude into the cavity of the pelvis from its floor, lined up between the anterior and the posterior wall along the midline; only the ovaries, uterine tubes, and deferent ducts are laterally placed. The pelvic peritoneum is draped over these organs, and, although it descends into the recesses between the viscera, it does not make contact with the pelvic floor. The voluminous, irregular space between the pelvic peritoneum and the pelvic floor and walls is filled with *pelvic fascia*. Although much of this fascia is loose areolar tissue, capable of accommodating to the changing dimensions of the distensible pelvic viscera, specialized condensations in this fascia form neurovascular sheaths, whereas others support and separate the pelvic organs (Fig. 27-6).

Blood vessels and nerves are arranged in the pelvis more or less in layers concentric with the posterolateral pelvic wall. They are embedded in fascial laminae that can be defined in the plane of these vessels and nerves. The most exterior lamina in contact with the muscular walls is that of the somatic nerves and contains the sacral plexus with its branches. Internal to this are the blood vessels, branches of the internal iliac artery and vein. On the medial surface of these vessels, embedded in the same fascia as the ureters, is the inferior hypogastric plexus of nerves, a continuation of the superior hypogastric plexus, which descends into the pelvis from the anterior surface of the abdominal aorta.

Visceral branches of the internal iliac vessels and the inferior hypogastric plexuses reach the pelvic organs by passing from the periphery of the cavity toward its center between the pelvic peritoneum and the pelvic floor. Condensations of pelvic fascia around these vessels and nerves form some of the neurovascular sheaths and the supporting ligaments of the pelvic organs.

Pelvic Fascia

The connective tissue continuum within the pelvis can be divided into *parietal* and *visceral pelvic fascias* and *subperitoneal pelvic connective tissue.*

Parietal pelvic fascia forms somewhat dense mem-

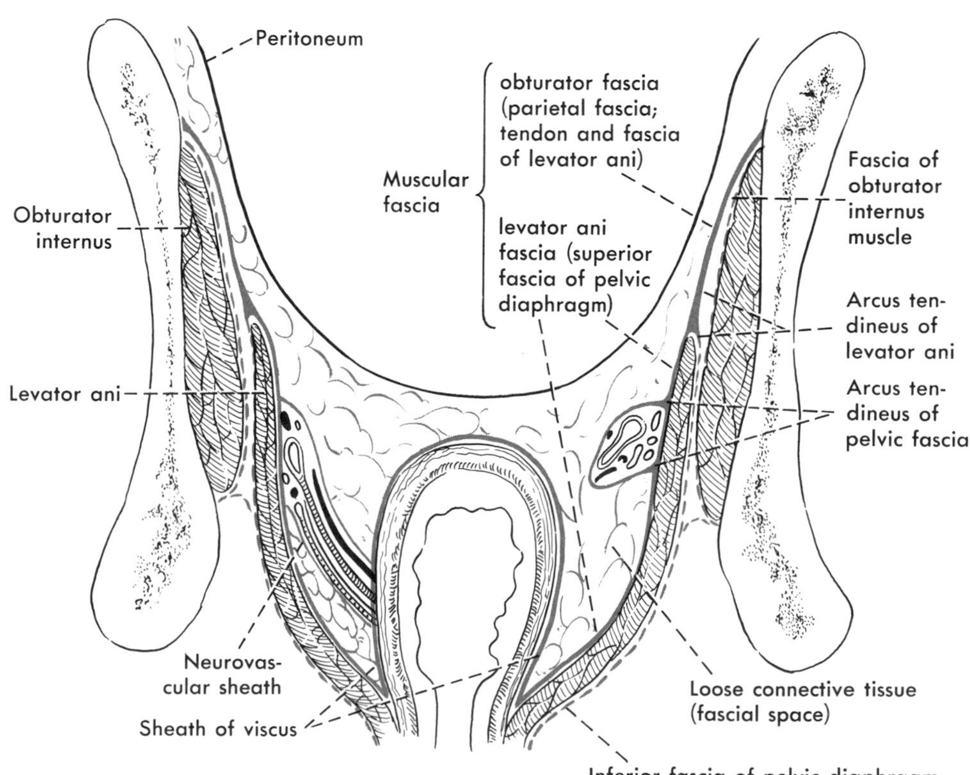

FIGURE 27-6.
Highly diagrammatic schema of the fascia of the pelvis in a coronal section: The closely related fascia on the obturator internus muscles and the outer surface of the levator ani is indicated by *broken lines*.

branes on the pelvic surface of the muscles and blends with the periosteum of the bony pelvic boundaries. Particularly well defined is the *obturator fascia* (see Fig. 27-6). Indeed, it is thought that this fascia between the linea terminalis and the arcus tendineus of the levator ani is a vestige of the levator ani itself that, in the course of evolution, lowered its origin from the pelvic brim to the tendinous arch. Much thinner layers of fascias exist over the piriformis and the pelvic diaphragm. The latter, called the *superior fascia of the pelvic diaphragm,* is continuous across the pelvic floor and blends with the obturator fascia laterally and with the visceral pelvic fascias at the urogenital hiatus.

The **visceral pelvic fascia** invests the bladder, prostate, vagina, uterus, and rectum in sheaths, or sleeves, of connective tissue in a manner that allows their distention. In the male, the heaviest of these fascias is the *prostatic fascia,* or sheath, which is nondistensible and surrounds not only the prostate but also the prostatic venous plexus.

The **subperitoneal pelvic connective tissue** is the continuation of extraperitoneal fascia from the abdomen into the pelvis. There has been much controversy as to whether condensations of this fascia, which ensheaths blood vessels and nerves, can be considered as ligaments and to what extent these putative ligaments support the pelvic contents. Although, with the exception of the puboprostatic ligaments, none are named in *Nomina Anatomica,* the following ligaments have been described (albeit by various names) and are considered in the applied anatomy of the pelvis by gynecologists and urologists: in the female, the uterosacral ligaments, the lateral cervical ligaments (or cardinal ligaments of the uterus), and the pubovesical ligaments (Fig. 27-7*A*); in the male, the fibrous tissue of the sacrogenital folds, the lateral ligaments of the bladder (or prostate), and the puboprostatic ligaments (Fig. 27-7*B*).

The puboprostatic and pubovesical ligaments, equivalent in the two sexes, are sometimes considered part of the superior fascia of the pelvic diaphragm; they do not contain any blood vessels. All ligaments blend medially with the visceral fascia of either the prostate, bladder, vagina, or cervix and laterally with the superior fascia of the pelvic diaphragm. The latter junction is often evident as the *arcus tendineus of the pelvic fascia,* distinct from that of the levator ani, located at a higher level (see Fig. 27-6). Many of these ligaments incorporate some smooth muscle. Their contents and relations are discussed with the respective vessels, nerves, and organs.

There are a number of **fascial septa** in the subperitoneal connective tissue of the pelvis, some of which at times are considered part of the visceral fascial sheaths. These septa include the *vesicovaginal septum* in front of the vagina and the uterine cervix and the *peritoneoperineal fascia,* called the *rectovesical septum* in the male and the *rectovaginal septum* in the female. It has been both asserted and denied that this septum represents the peritoneum of the rectovesical or rectouterine pouch, which during development receded from its original contact with the pelvic floor. More pronounced in the male, the rectovesical septum is attached above to the peritoneum of the rectovesical pouch and blends on each side with the parietal fascia on the lateral pelvic walls and below with the fascia of the pelvic floor (see Fig. 27-24). It may be a strong white membrane, or it may be quite thin. It divides, in essence, the subperitoneal connective tissue space of the pelvis into anterior and posterior compartments.

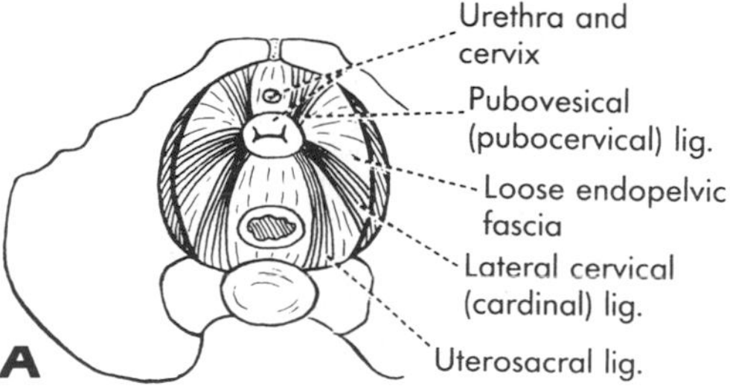

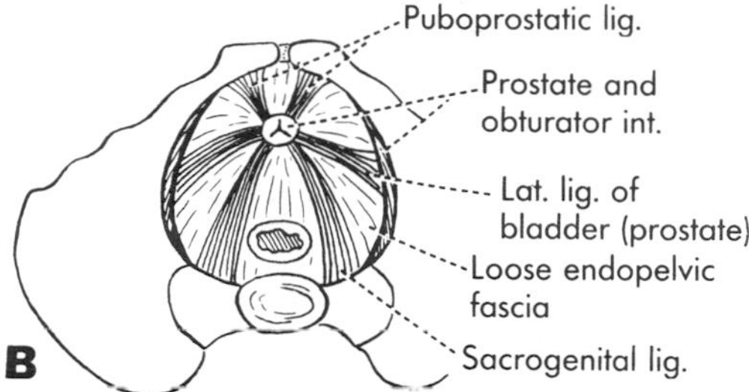

FIGURE 27-7.
Schematic representation of condensations of the subperitoneal pelvic connective tissue into so-called ligaments (A) in the female and (B) in the male, seen from a superior view after removal of the pelvic viscera.

Blood Vessels and Lymphatics

Although the internal iliac vessels supply and drain all pelvic structures, there are other vessels that significantly contribute to the circulation in the pelvis. These smaller vessels are the ovarian artery and vein, the superior rectal artery and vein, and, much less important, the median sacral artery and vein.

Internal Iliac Artery

The internal iliac artery is one of the terminal branches of the common iliac artery, arising at the pelvic brim in front of the sacroiliac joint. The other terminal branch, the external iliac artery, continues in the direction of the common iliac artery along the pelvic brim, whereas the internal iliac passes downward into the pelvis across the common or external iliac vein.

In front of the greater sciatic foramen, the artery breaks up into a number of branches that supply the pelvic viscera as well as the perineum and the proximal parts of the lower limbs (Fig. 27-8).

In the fetus, blood is returned to the placental circulation through the umbilical artery, the first branch of the

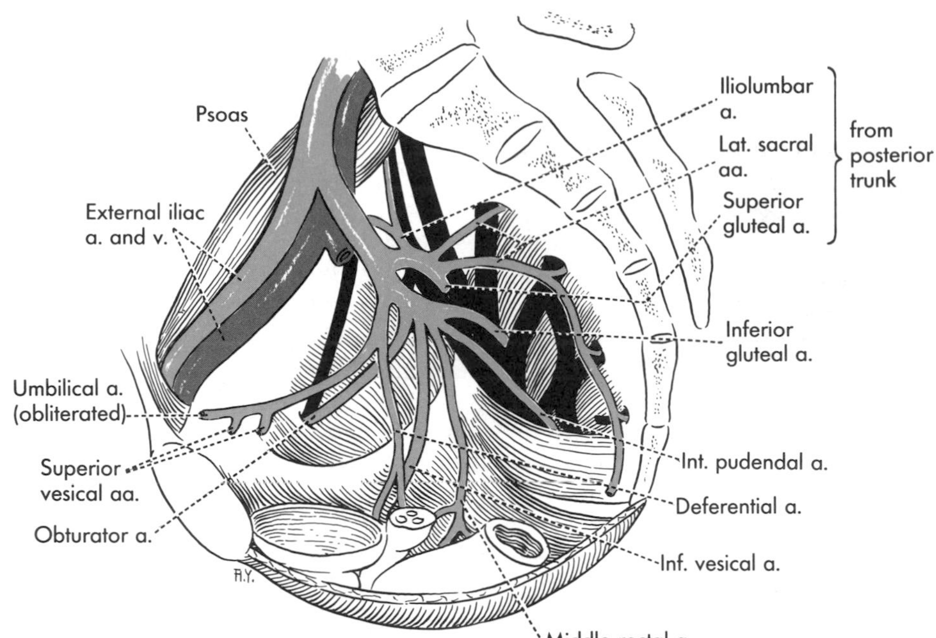

FIGURE 27-8.
Branches of the internal iliac artery in the male: The pattern seen here is common, but varies greatly among bodies. The obturator nerve and nerves of the sacral plexus are shown in *black*.

internal iliac. The umbilical artery, after passing forward just below the pelvic brim, ascends to the umbilicus. After birth, the extrapelvic portion of the umbilical artery becomes obliterated, and the intrapelvic portion decreases in relative size and supplies the bladder.

There is great variation in the precise branching pattern of the internal iliac artery. Nine major types of branching and 49 subtypes have been described. The structures and regions supplied by the branches of the artery, however, are quite constant (Fig. 27-9). Before the artery breaks up into its named branches, it usually divides into an **anterior** and a **posterior trunk**. It is common for all the pelvic visceral branches to arise from the anterior trunk, along with the artery of the perineum called the internal pudendal.

Branches. The **visceral branches** of the internal iliac artery include the following:

1. The *umbilical artery*, which gives off the *superior vesical arteries* to the upper part of the bladder and the *artery of the ductus deferens*, continues forward as the medial umbilical ligament. The artery of the ductus supplies, in addition to the deferent duct, the ureter, the seminal vesicles, and part of the bladder.
2. The *inferior vesical artery* is present in the male. It reaches the bladder and the prostate along the lateral ligament of the bladder and supplies both.
3. The *middle rectal artery* may arise from a common stem with the inferior vesical; it enters the rectum just above the pelvic floor and supplies chiefly its muscle coat. It anastomoses in the rectal wall with both superior and inferior rectal arteries.
4. The *uterine artery* descends on the pelvic wall and turns medially along the lateral cervical ligament. It passes above and in front of the ureter, just lat-

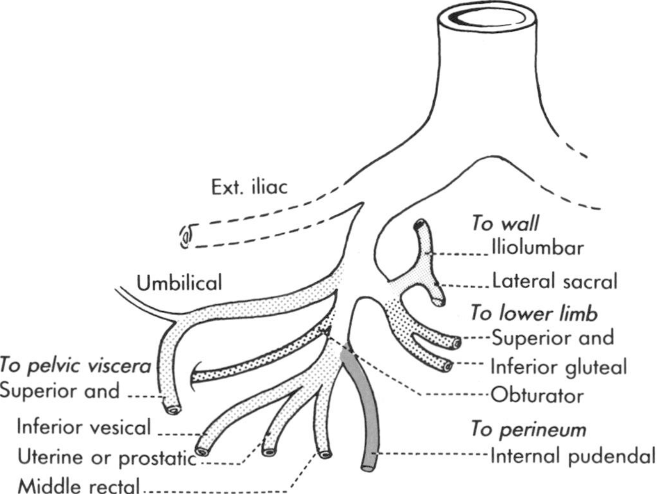

FIGURE 27-9.
Groups of branches of the internal iliac artery given off for the supply of the pelvic wall, the pelvic viscera, the perineum, and the lower limb, identified by *different colors* and *patterns of shading*.

eral to the cervix. In addition to supplying the uterus, it gives rise to the vaginal arteries and terminates in its tubal branch. It also helps supply the ovary. The artery replaces the inferior vesical artery of the male.

5. One or more *vaginal arteries* may arise from the internal iliac with the uterine artery or independently. They run to the side of the vagina in the pelvis and descend in its wall to the perineum. In the pelvis, they also supply the bladder and the rectum. Some anatomists consider the vaginal arteries as replacing the inferior vesical arteries of the male.

All five visceral branches arise from the anterior trunk of the internal iliac (see Figs. 27-8 and 27-9).

Branches to the pelvic wall are given off by the posterior trunk of the internal iliac artery. The *iliolumbar artery* leaves the pelvis by ascending along the lumbosacral trunk in front of the ala of the sacrum. It divides into an iliac branch, which supplies the iliacus, and a lumbar branch, which replaces the fifth lumbar arteries.

There are usually two *lateral sacral arteries*. The upper artery disappears into the first sacral foramen; the other descends close to the pelvic sacral foramina and sends a branch into the foramina. If there is only one artery, it gives a large branch into the first sacral foramen before descending. The lateral sacral arteries correspond essentially to the dorsal branches of the intercostal and lumbar arteries. They give rise to branches that supply the bone of the sacrum and the dural sheaths of the nerve roots. Some twigs emerge from the dorsal sacral foramina to supply the musculature and skin on the dorsal surface of the sacrum.

Branches to the lower limb include the obturator artery and the superior and inferior gluteal arteries. The *obturator artery* is a branch of the anterior trunk and runs parallel with the umbilical artery along the pelvic wall on the surface of the obturator internus muscle, to which it gives branches. The obturator nerve runs above the artery and the obturator vein runs below it. They all converge upon the obturator canal and disappear into the thigh. The obturator artery thereafter is distributed primarily to the obturator externus muscle and the hip joint. Fairly commonly (in about 25% to 30% of sides) the obturator artery arises from the inferior epigastric artery or the external iliac, rather than from the internal iliac. A large anastomotic vessel between the pubic branch of the inferior epigastric and the obturator artery may function as a second origin of the obturator artery. Such an anastomotic vessel or an anomalous obturator artery runs close to or across the femoral ring to reach the obturator canal. Because of its close relation to the neck of a femoral hernia, such an artery is in danger of being divided when a strangulated or obstructed femoral hernia is relieved.

Of the two *gluteal arteries*, the inferior is usually given off by the anterior trunk of the internal iliac and the superior gluteal artery is usually given off by the posterior trunk. Both arteries leave the pelvis through the greater sciatic foramen, the superior artery above and the inferior artery below the piriformis.

The **internal pudendal artery,** a large branch of the anterior trunk, leaves the pelvis between the piriformis and coccygeus and descends vertically on the exterior of the levator ani into the perineum (see Figs. 28-22 and 28-23).

The Internal Iliac Vein and Its Tributaries

The internal iliac vein lies, for the most part, between the lateral pelvic wall and the internal iliac artery. It joins the external iliac vein to form the common iliac vein. Its tributaries largely parallel the branches of the artery, except that there is no umbilical vein in the pelvis.

The tributaries of the internal iliac vein communicate freely with each other and also with veins lying outside their territory of drainage. Most important of these venous communications are those with the vertebral venous plexus and with the veins of the portal system. Veins passing through the pelvic foramina of the sacrum link the tributaries of the internal iliac vein to the vertebral venous plexus. Metastases from neoplasms of the pelvic viscera or infected emboli from the same organs may pass through these veins and lodge in the cancellous bone of the vertebrae or may even reach the cranial cavity.

In the wall of the rectum, the middle and inferior rectal veins, tributaries of the internal iliac vein, anastomose with the superior rectal vein, part of the portal venous system. As a result of portal hypertension, blood may be shunted from the superior rectal veins into the tributaries of the internal iliac vein. On the other hand, because there are no valves in the veins of the pelvis, venous blood may leave the pelvis along the route of least resistance. This includes the internal iliac veins, the vertebral venous plexus, or the anastomosis in the wall of the rectum.

Other Vessels

The **ovarian artery** and its two accompanying veins cross the pelvic brim some distance anterior to the internal iliac vessels. Their course, on the posterior abdominal wall, is traced in Chapter 25. Below the pelvic brim, the vessels run in the suspensory ligament of the ovary and in the broad ligament before reaching the ovary and anastomosing with tubal branches of the uterine vessels.

The **superior rectal vessels** cross the pelvic brim of the left side in the sigmoid mesocolon. They are described in Chapter 24, and their pelvic distribution is discussed with the rectum.

Although the **median sacral artery** was originally the terminal part of the aorta, it arises from that vessel's posterior aspect a little above the aortic bifurcation. It descends over the sacral promontory close against the bone and behind the superior hypogastric plexus. It runs downward for the length of the sacrum, embedded in connective tissue on the anterior surface of this bone, and gives off twigs into the bone and lateral twigs that anastomose with the lateral sacral vessels. Just beyond the tip of the coccyx, it ends and is connected with the median sacral veins by a series of arteriovenous anastomoses that form the *coccygeal body*. Two **median sacral veins** parallel the artery and unite before ending in the left common iliac vein as this crosses to the right to help form the inferior vena cava.

Lymphatics and Lymph Nodes

The lymph nodes in the pelvis are divided into two general groups, the *internal iliac nodes,* which are associated with various branches of the internal iliac vessels, and *sacral nodes,* which lie on the front of the sacrum. These nodes are embedded in the general extraperitoneal connective tissue associated with the pelvic wall and floor and receive much of the lymphatic drainage from the pelvic viscera. Their removal, part of the treatment of some pelvic neoplasms, involves dissection of the nerves and vessels of the lateral pelvic wall, cleaning as much connective tissue as possible from around the nodes. The lymphatics from the viscera pass, in general, along the blood vessels. Not all, however, end in internal iliac or sacral nodes. Some may reach nodes along the brim of the pelvis (external and common iliac nodes); others from the ovary, the uterine tube, and the fundus of the uterus drain upward into lumbar nodes. The chief drainage from the rectum is upward along the superior rectal vessels to the inferior mesenteric nodes, and the drainage from the lowest part of the anal canal and the vagina is downward and forward into superficial inguinal nodes. These nodes also receive some lymphatics from the uterus, which accompany the round ligament.

Nerves

Nerves enter the pelvis through the superior pelvic aperture or through the pelvic foramina of the sacrum. They leave it by passing over the brim of the pelvic diaphragm or through the urogenital hiatus; some ascend out of the pelvis through the superior aperture. The entering **somatic nerves** include the lumbosacral trunk and the obturator nerve on the ala of the sacrum (Fig. 27-10) and the anterior rami of sacral nerves through the pelvic sacral foramina (the minute coccygeal nerves are inconsequential). Entering **autonomic nerves** include the two sympathetic trunks and the hypogastric nerves over the sacral promontory; the ovarian plexus around the ovarian vessels as they cross the pelvic brim; the superior rectal nerve plexus, descending with the superior rectal artery in the sigmoid mesocolon (see Fig. 27-10); and the pelvic splanchnic nerves, entering the pelvis with the anterior rami of the sacral nerves.

The branches of the sacral plexus leave the pelvis through the greater sciatic foramen, and the obturator nerve leaves through the obturator canal. Exiting autonomic nerves include the sympathetic fibers for the lower limb and perineum, running with the branches of the sacral plexus, and the *cavernous nerves,* extensions of the inferior hypogastric plexus through the urogenital hiatus for the supply of erectile tissue in the perineum. Autonomic nerve plexuses ascend through the superior pelvic aperture around the ductus deferens (deferential plexus) and along the superior rectal artery for the supply of the colon distal to the left flexure.

The Sacral Plexus

The sacral plexus is the lower part of the lumbosacral plexus, the nerve plexus of the lower limbs. The composition, formation, and main branches of the sacral plexus are described in Chapters 14 and 17, because an understanding of the plexus is essential for comprehending the innervation of the lower limbs (see Figs. 14-6 and 17-9).

The plexus takes form on the posterior wall of the pelvis, just lateral to the pelvic foramina of the sacrum, and most of it disappears in the buttock just as it gives rise to its branches (Fig. 27-11). The major part of the plexus lies on the anterior surface of the piriformis muscle, and all the larger branches pass through the greater sciatic foramen, most of them below the piriformis, to appear in the buttock.

The sacral plexus is formed by the union of the lumbosacral trunk, containing some of the fibers from the

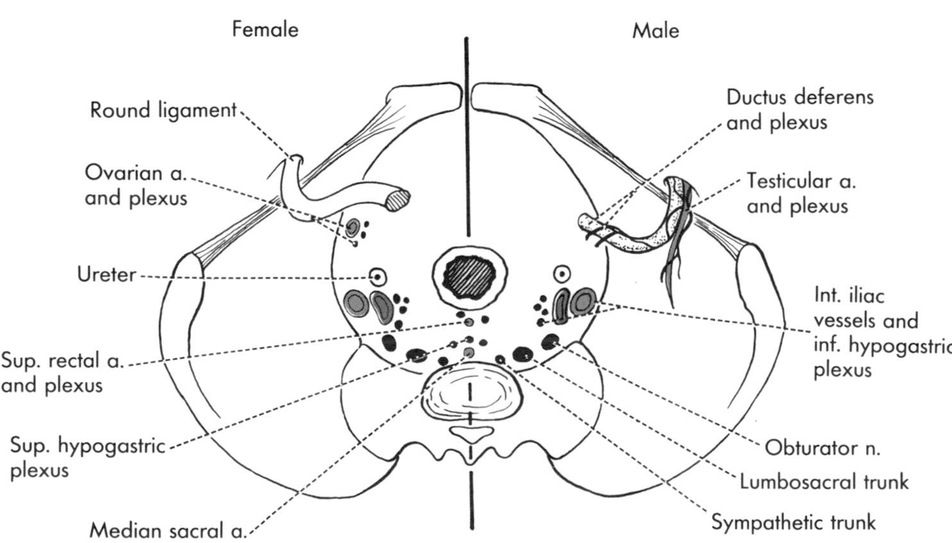

FIGURE *27-10.* **A schematic representation of nerves, vessels, and other structures that pass through the pelvic inlet: left side the female pelvis; right side, the male. Although the superior and inferior hypogastric plexuses are at different levels, both are included in the diagram.**

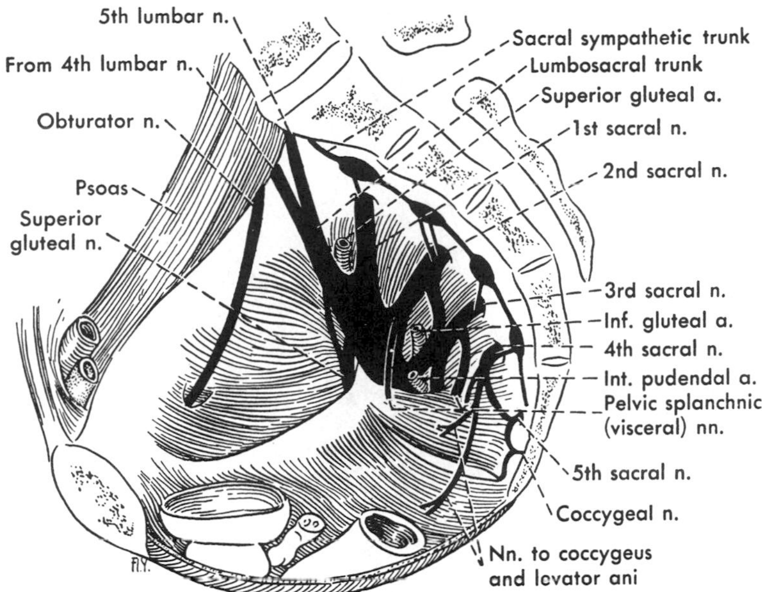

FIGURE *27-11.*
The sacral plexus in the pelvis: The muscle visible between the sacral nerves is the piriformis. The obturator nerve is a branch of the lumbar plexus, but traverses the pelvis.

fourth lumbar anterior ramus, all those from the fifth lumbar anterior ramus, and the anterior rami of the first three or four sacral nerves. The nerves formed by the plexus supply the musculature and skin of the buttock, the posterior compartment of the thigh, and the entire leg and foot below the knee, except for the cutaneous area medially, which is supplied by the saphenous nerve, a branch of the femoral nerve derived from the lumbar plexus. The sacral plexus also gives off the chief somatic nerve of the perineum called the pudendal nerve and sends branches to the pelvic diaphragm as well.

The lumbosacral trunk and the sacral anterior rami can be considered the *roots* of the plexus. Conforming to the general plan of the limb plexus, these roots divide into *anterior* and *posterior divisions.* Such a division, however, is more difficult to demonstrate by dissection than are the divisions in the brachial or lumbar plexuses. The *branches* of the sacral plexus, like those of the brachial and lumbar plexuses, are formed either by the anterior or by the posterior divisions of certain anterior rami and are then distributed to the skin and musculature over the original anterior and posterior compartments of the limb, respectively (Fig. 27-12).

After the sacral anterior rami have emerged from the pelvic sacral foramina and before they enter into the formation of the plexus, each root of the plexus receives a ramus communicans from the sacral sympathetic trunk; this brings into the nerves postganglionic sympathetic fibers to be distributed to the lower limb and the perineum.

Branches. The branches of the sacral plexus are difficult to recognize in a dissection of the pelvis, because many of them arise as the plexus leaves the pelvis. The largest branch of the plexus is the **sciatic nerve,** the largest nerve in the body. The sciatic nerve, however, is a composite nerve consisting of the *common fibular* (*peroneal*) *nerve,* formed by posterior divisions, and the *tibial nerve,* formed by anterior divisions. These two nerves separate from each other some distance above the knee (see Fig. 18-20). The **common fibular nerve** is formed by the posterior divisions of L-4 to S-2 and the other nerves derived from the posterior divisions are as follows (see Fig. 27-12): the *superior gluteal nerve* from L-4, L-5, and S-1; the *inferior gluteal* from L-5, S-1, and S-2; a lateral part of the *posterior femoral cutaneous* from S-1 and S-2; one or more nerves from S-1 and S-2 *to the piriformis muscle;* and often a *perforating cutaneous branch* from S-2 and S-3 to the skin of the buttock.

The nerves formed from the anterior divisions of the plexus are the **tibial nerve** from L-4 to S-3; two small nerves, the *nerve to the quadratus femoris* and *inferior gemellus* from L-4, L-5, and S-1 and the *nerve to the obturator internus* and *superior gemellus* from L-5, S-1, and S-2; the medial part of the *posterior femoral cutaneous* from S-2 and S-3; and the **pudendal nerve** from S-2 and S-3 or from S-2, S-3, and S-4. Twigs from the fourth sacral nerve also supply the coccygeus and levator ani muscles. The fifth sacral and coccygeal nerves, not considered a part of the sacral plexus, unite to form the *anococcygeal nerves,* which contribute to the innervation of the skin between the anus and the tip of the coccyx.

Branches of the sacral anterior rami that are not considered part of the sacral plexus are the **pelvic splanchnic nerves.** These nerves, given off by S-3 and S-4 anterior rami (and sometimes S-2 as well), contribute to the formation of the *inferior hypogastric* (or *pelvic*) *plexus,* taking into that plexus preganglionic parasympathetic fibers and conveying visceral afferents from the pelvic plexus to sacral segments of the spinal cord.

The superior gluteal nerve makes its exit from the pelvis above the upper border of the piriformis muscle in company with the superior gluteal vessels; all the other branches of the sacral plexus that leave the pelvis do so below the piriformis muscle. The plexus, as a whole, is covered on its pelvic surface by the internal iliac vessels. The superior gluteal vessels always, the inferior gluteal

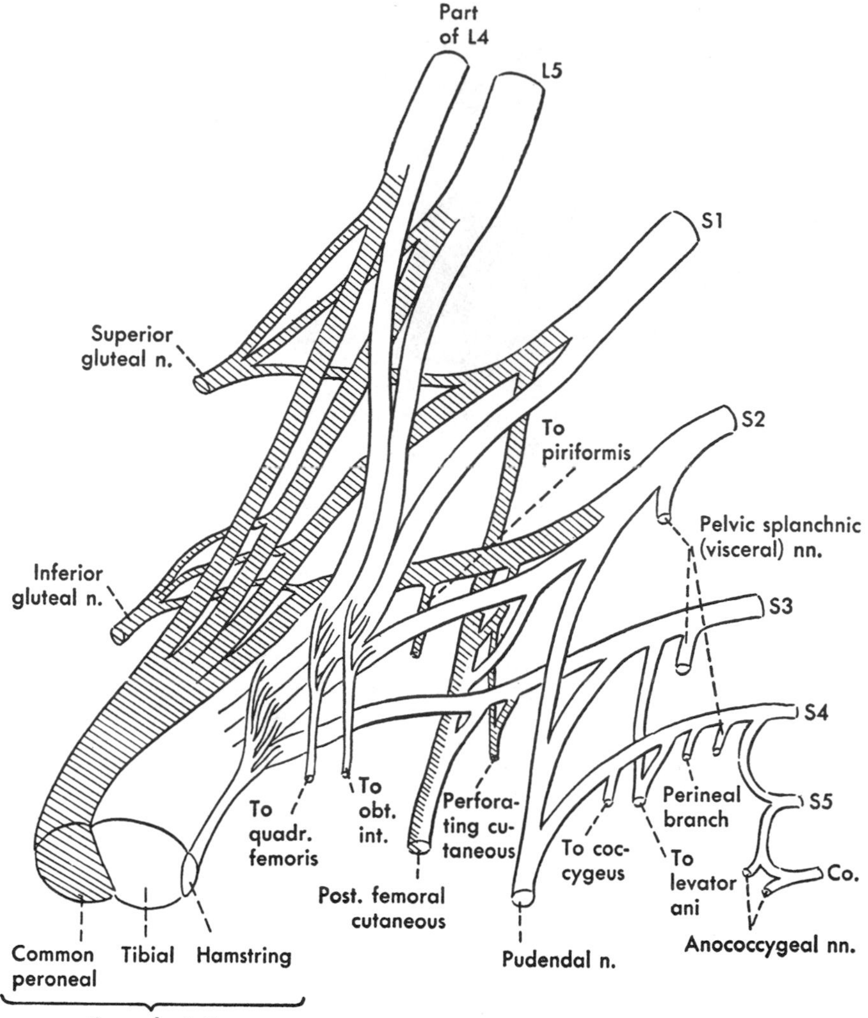

FIGURE *27-12.*
A diagram of the sacral plexus: The roots of the plexus, the anterior divisions of the roots, and the branches of the plexus composed of the anterior divisions are shown in *white* (*unshaded*); the posterior divisions of the roots and their branches are *shaded*.

and internal pudendal vessels often, pass through the plexus as they leave the pelvis. The precise distribution of the branches of the sacral plexus is described, for the most part, in chapters on the lower limb. The distribution of the pudendal nerve to the perineum is described in Chapter 28.

Variations. Of the many variations in the formation and branching of the sacral plexus, most important are prefixation and postfixation of the plexus. The prefixed type may receive all the fibers from L-4, L-5, and S-1 and sometimes fibers from L-3; it may or may not receive fibers from S-2 and S-3. In a postfixed plexus, fibers from S-4 enter the sciatic nerve, but its important characteristic is that it receives fewer fibers than normal from L-4 or that the highest nerve contributing to it may be L-5. The composition of various branches of the sacral plexus necessarily varies with the segments contributing to the plexus.

The Obturator Nerve

The obturator nerve is described in Chapters 14, 17 and 25. Having been formed by the anterior rami of L-2, L-3, and L-4, the obturator nerve emerges from the medial border of the psoas near the pelvic brim and descends into the pelvis on the ala of the sacrum, lying lateral to the lumbosacral trunk; lower down, it is on the lateral side of the internal iliac vessels (see Figs. 27-8 and 27-11). Keeping to the lateral pelvic wall, the nerve slopes forward and downward to meet the obturator artery and vein at the obturator canal, through which it leaves the pelvis. In the pelvis, it lies on the obturator fascia and does not give off any branches until it enters the thigh. Here it is distributed to some of the adductor muscles and an area of skin on the medial side of the thigh.

The Sympathetic Trunks

The sacral portions of the paired sympathetic trunks are the continuation of the lumbar trunks over the sacral promontory. The trunks enter the pelvis shortly after they have passed behind the common iliac vessels and descend on the sacrum, converging toward each other. They lie on the medial side of the sacral foramina (see Fig. 27-11). The two trunks may meet at the tip of the coccyx and fuse with each other to form a slight enlargement known as the *gan-*

glion impar. Each sacral sympathetic trunk tends to bear three or four ganglia, but the number may vary from one to six. The interganglionic portions of the trunk consist primarily of descending fibers that are mostly preganglionic. These fibers have entered the lumbar portion of the trunks through white rami communicantes given off by upper lumbar nerves. Most of them synapse in the sacral sympathetic ganglia and give off *gray rami communicantes* to the sacral nerves, thus furnishing these nerves with the postganglionic fibers they carry to the lower limbs and perineum.

The ganglia also have slender visceral branches (one might call them *sacral splanchnic nerves*) consisting presumably of preganglionic fibers that join the inferior hypogastric plexus. The precise function of these nerves is unknown. They may also convey some visceral afferent fibers to the trunks from the inferior hypogastric plexus that presumably terminate in lumbar segments of the spinal cord. There may be transverse or oblique connections between the two sympathetic trunks across the front of the sacrum.

The Autonomic Plexuses

The chief autonomic plexus of the pelvis is the **inferior hypogastric plexus**, also known as the **pelvic plexus**. All pelvic viscera receive visceral efferent and afferent nerves through this plexus. In addition to the nerves that form the pelvic plexus, the superior rectal and ovarian plexuses bring autonomic nerves to the rectum and ovary, respectively, but do not pass through the inferior hypogastric plexus. Both the superior rectal and ovarian plexuses consist chiefly of sympathetic fibers, but in the inferior hypogastric plexus, parasympathetic components predominate, although the plexus receives substantial contributions also from the sympathetic system.

The **superior rectal plexus** is a continuation of the inferior mesenteric plexus along the superior rectal vessels. As such, it is derived from the aortic plexus. Its sympathetic fibers are presumably concerned with vasoconstriction. The visceral afferents in the plexus ascend into the inferior mesenteric plexus and contain afferents from the sigmoid colon, but not the rectum.

The **ovarian plexus** is derived from the aortic and renal plexuses. This plexus contains sympathetic visceral efferents from T-10 and T-11 segments and is distributed to the ovary and the uterine tube. In the pelvis, the plexus communicates with the inferior hypogastric plexus. Apart from vasoconstriction, its effects on the ovary and uterine tube are unknown.

The **inferior hypogastric plexus** is formed by lateral extensions of the superior hypogastric plexus, known as the *hypogastric nerves*, and the *pelvic splanchnic nerves*. Each of these merit description before discussing the inferior hypogastric plexus itself.

The Superior Hypogastric Plexus and Hypogastric Nerves. The superior hypogastric plexus (presacral nerve) is the direct extension of the aortic plexus below the aortic bifurcation (Fig. 27-13). It lies immediately behind the peritoneum and descends over the anterior surface of the fifth lumbar vertebra in the retroperitoneal tissue that continues downward in front of the sacrum and is often referred to as "presacral fascia." Similar to the aortic plexus, the superior hypogastric plexus consists of a mixture of preganglionic and postganglionic sympathetic fibers, small ganglia, and visceral afferents that mediate pain sensation from the fundus and upper part of the uterus and follow the route of sympathetic efferents. The visceral efferents are from the T-10 to L-2 segments; the afferents also terminate in the same segments. In front of the fifth lumbar vertebra, these small fibers may form a true plexus or they may become condensed into one or two nerve trunks.

The superior hypogastric plexus ends by bifurcating into **right** and **left hypogastric nerves** (see Fig. 27-13). The two hypogastric nerves (in truth, plexuses) diverge from each other at about the level of the sacral promontory and run down and forward along the walls of the pelvis in the lamina of the pelvic fascia closest to the peritoneum. Slightly more anteriorly, the ureters enter the pelvis in the same lamina and, in a dissection, serve as a guide to the hypogastric nerves and the inferior hypogastric plexus, in which the hypogastric nerves terminate well below the level of the pelvic peritoneum.

The hypogastric nerves and the superior hypogastric plexus apparently do not contain any parasympathetic fibers. The sympathetic efferents are vasomotor.

> **Presacral Neurectomy.** Resection of the superior hypogastric plexus has been practiced for the relief of *dysmenorrhea* (excessive pain associated with menstruation) because of the presence of uterine pain afferents in the plexus. This operation has no detectable effect on the control of micturition or defecation, nor on uterine or ovarian function. It has been claimed that the superior hypogastric plexus conducts some sensation from the bladder, but the important sensory nerves from both the bladder and the rectum travel with the pelvic parasympathetic system.

The Pelvic Splanchnic Nerves. The pelvic splanchnic nerves represent the sacral parasympathetic outflow, and they are known also as the **nervi erigentes,** because they are the nerves capable of causing erection of the penis and clitoris. The pelvic splanchnic nerves are also the major pathway for visceral afferents for most pelvic organs. These nerves take origin from two or three sacral anterior rami just after they emerge from the pelvic sacral foramina (see Fig. 27-13). The largest contribution is from S-3, with a smaller one from S-4 and occasionally S-2. The pelvic splanchnic nerves run forward and medially between the branches of the internal iliac vessels and the lamina of the pelvic fascia that contains them, and on the medial surface of these vessels, they mingle with the hypogastric nerves, contributing to the formation of the inferior hypogastric plexus (see Fig. 27-13).

The **visceral efferents** in these nerves have their cell bodies in the intermediolateral column of S-2 to S-4 segments. These preganglionic fibers leave the spinal cord

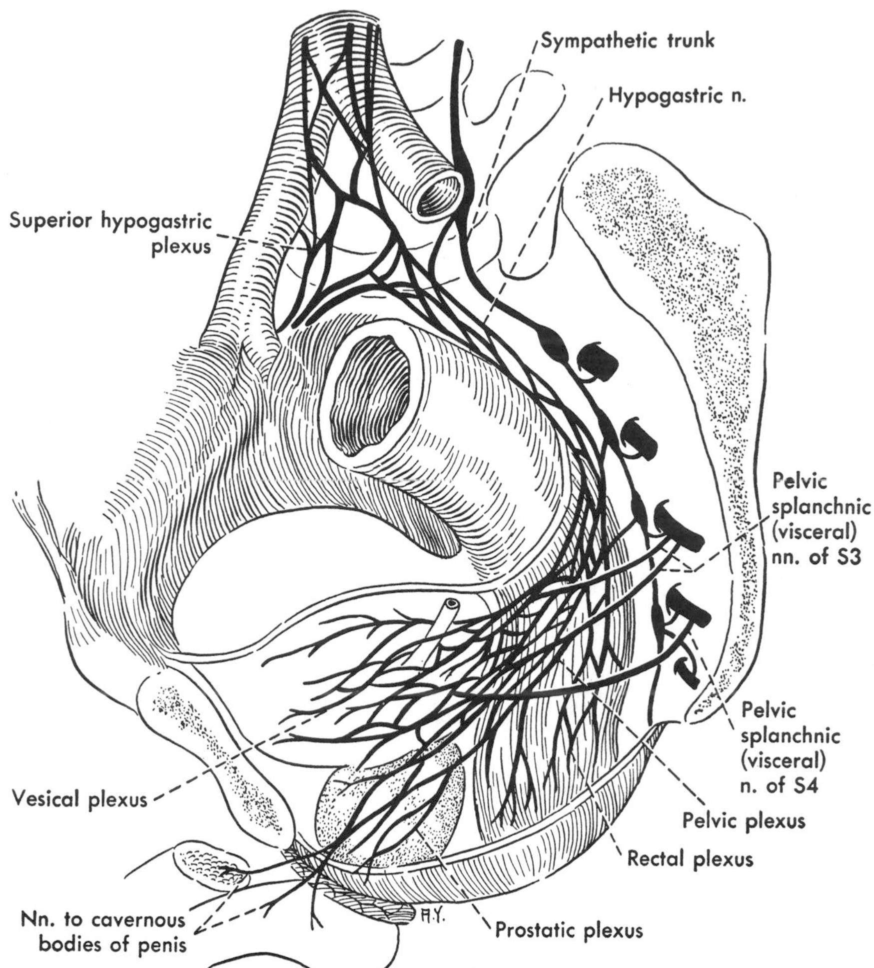

FIGURE 27-13.
The superior and inferior hypogastric plexuses and the sympathetic trunks in the male pelvis seen from the left side. The subsidiary plexuses of the inferior hypogastric plexus (the vesical, prostatic, and rectal in the male; the vesical, uterovaginal, and rectal in the female) run medially through the connective tissue below the peritoneal level to reach the viscera that they supply. The fibers that ascend in the sigmoid mesentery to reach the descending colon are not shown here.

along the anterior root, pass along the spinal nerve and its anterior division and, without passing through the ganglia of the sacral sympathetic trunk, they synapse either in ganglia located in the inferior hypogastric plexus or in the walls of the viscera they innervate (Fig. 27-14). They are motor to the muscle wall of the bladder and the rectum. **Visceral afferents** ascend through the posterior roots to cell bodies in the spinal ganglia of S-2 to S-4 spinal nerves. It is generally stated that they are not only general visceral afferents but they also mediate sensations of pain from all pelvic organs, which is noteworthy because pain sensation from thoracic and abdominal viscera in general follows the sympathetic pathway.

There is evidence, however, that the uterus is an exception to this generalization, as explained later.

The Inferior Hypogastric Plexus. The large, dense inferior hypogastric plexus is formed by the commingling of the hypogastric and pelvic splanchnic nerves (see Fig. 27-13). The small visceral branches of the sacral sympathetic ganglia (sacral splanchnics) also feed into this plexus, although their precise contribution is uncertain.

The inferior hypogastric plexus is 2.5 cm high and 3 to 5 cm long. It lies against the posterolateral pelvic wall, internal to the branches of the internal iliac vessels and lateral to the rectum, the vagina, and the base of the bladder. Its subsidiary plexuses, embedded in some of the ligaments formed by the subperitoneal connective tissue, extend medially toward the viscera.

Posteriorly, the inferior hypogastric plexus gives off the *middle rectal plexus* (often known simply as the rectal plexus); farther forward, in front of the rectum, it gives rise, in the female, to the *uterovaginal plexus*; anteriorly, in both sexes, it gives rise to the *vesical plexus*. Fibers from the lower part of the uterovaginal plexus form the vaginal nerves. In the male, a few fibers from the vesical plexus follow the ductus deferens and form the *deferential plexus*, and other fibers from the lower part of the vesical plexus form the *prostatic plexus*. Finally, fibers from the prostatic plexus in the male and the vesical plexus in the female follow the urethra through the urogenital hiatus to be distributed to the corpora cavernosa of the penis or the clitoris and to other erectile tissue. These fibers constitute the *cavernous nerves*. Except for the cavernous nerves, the various plexuses, in general, reach the viscera in company with the vessels to the viscera.

In addition to these branches, both inferior hypogastric plexuses give rise to ascending fibers that join behind the upper end of the rectum and run through the sigmoid mesocolon to be distributed to the sigmoid and the de-

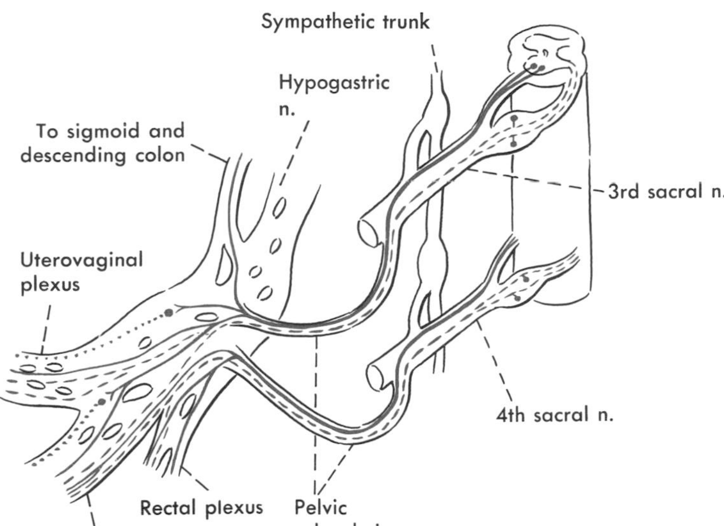

FIGURE 27-14.
Schema of the pelvic splanchnic nerves and their contribution to the pelvic plexus: Visceral afferents are indicated by *broken lines*, preganglionic fibers by *solid lines*, and postganglionic fibers by *dotted lines*. Many of the postganglionic parasympathetic cell bodies are in the wall of the viscera.

scending colon. These fibers have never been named, although they have been described by several investigators.

The pelvic plexus contains **pelvic ganglia,** in which both sympathetic and parasympathetic preganglionic fibers synapse. Usually, sympathetic and parasympathetic ganglia are separate. Thus, the plexus consists of preganglionic and postganglionic sympathetic and parasympathetic fibers and of visceral afferents. Presumably, most of the branches of the pelvic plexus transmit sympathetic, parasympathetic, and visceral afferent fibers. However, it is not known whether any sympathetic efferents pass into the nerves to the cavernous bodies of the penis and clitoris or whether any parasympathetic efferents pass into the uterovaginal plexus. Furthermore, the ascending pathway to the sigmoid and the descending colon apparently consists entirely of preganglionic parasympathetic fibers. They synapse in the enteric ganglia that lie in the subserous, myenteric, and submucosal plexuses. There is clinical evidence that the sensory fibers in the pelvic splanchnic nerves reach no higher than the rectum and that pain afferents from the descending and the sigmoid colon accompany the sympathetic system and run through the lumbar splanchnic nerves and the sympathetic trunks before reaching the spinal ganglia.

The paucity or absence of the enteric ganglia of the rectum or lower part of the colon creates difficulty in the passage of feces and usually leads to gross dilation of the large intestine above the inactive segment. This condition is known as **megacolon.**

Because the pelvic splanchnic nerves and the inferior hypogastric plexus long have been known to be responsible for contraction of the bladder, it has often been assumed that transient retention of urine following operations on the rectum (a common complication) is a result of injury to the inferior hypogastric plexus or the pelvic splanchnic nerves. There is evidence, however, that the pelvic diaphragm is the chief controller of bladder emptying, and spasm resulting from damage to this diaphragm, rather than to the inferior hypogastric plexus, may be the cause of urinary retention.

PELVIC VISCERA

The pelvic viscera developed equally in both sexes are the rectum, the urinary bladder, and the ureters. Although quite separate in their fully developed state, the rectum and bladder are derived from a common endodermal chamber called the *cloaca*. The reasons for the differences in the pelvic viscera of the two sexes are twofold: 1) the descent of the female gonad is arrested in the pelvis, whereas that of the male gonad proceeds to the perineum; and 2) the genital ducts that transport gametes develop from two distinct duct systems in the male and the female.

Both genital duct systems appear in association with the mesonephros and terminate in the dorsal wall of the ventral division of the cloaca, called the *urogenital sinus*. This interposes the genital ducts and their derivatives between the urogenital sinus, from which the bladder and urethra develop, and the *rectum*, derived from the dorsal division of the cloaca.

The purpose of the following section is to consider the development of pelvic viscera in sufficient detail to make their particular anatomy and topographical relations intelligible.

Developmental Considerations

The Cloaca and Its Divisions

The cloaca is formed in the tail of the embryo by the union of the hindgut with the allantois. The **allantois** appears very early as a diverticulum of the yolk sac into the body stalk. Its proximal segment becomes incorporated into the embryo as a consequence of the tail fold and forms the ventral portion of the cloaca (see Fig. 9-3). The ventral portion of the cloaca is broader than its dorsal portion, derived from the hindgut. The posterolateral wall of the ventral portion admits the two mesonephric ducts descending from the urogenital ridges (Fig. 27-15; see Fig. 25-29).

The cloaca is surrounded by intraembryonic mesoderm unsplit by the celomic ducts, and its floor, surfacing on the ventral aspect of the tail, is the *cloacal*

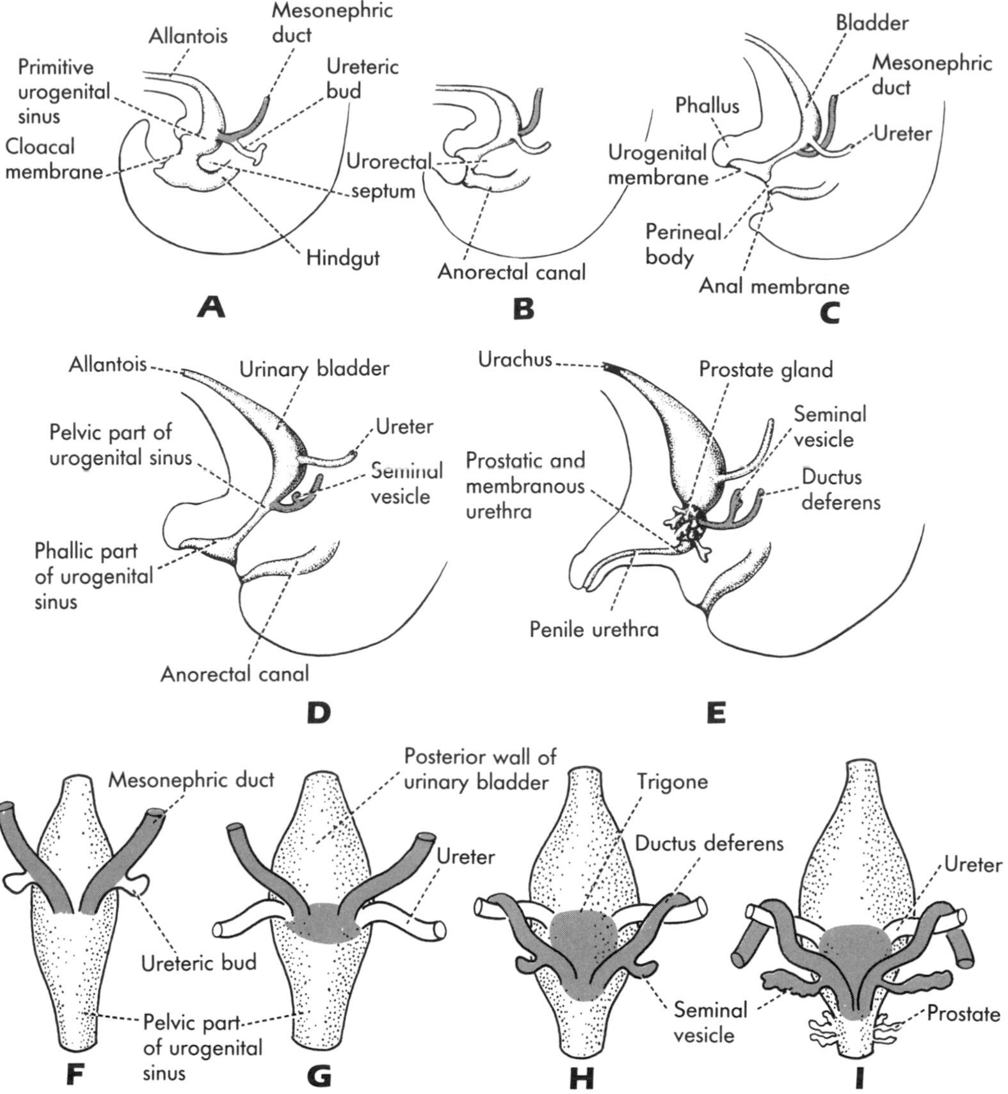

FIGURE *27-15.*
(A through C) Stages of embryonic development illustrated schematically to show the division of the cloaca into the urogenital sinus and the anorectal canal. (D through E) The development of the urogenital sinus, and (F through I) the absorption of the mesonephric ducts into the posterior wall of the urogenital sinus. Note the development of the prostate and the seminal vesicles. (Adpated from Langman J. Medical embryology. 3rd ed. Baltimore: Williams & Wilkins, 1975.)

membrane. After its expansion with the growth of the tail, the cloaca becomes partitioned into a ventral and a dorsal compartment, the urogenital sinus and the rectum, respectively. The partitioning is effected by the **urorectal septum,** formed by the proliferation of the mesoderm filling the sulcus between and above the broad ventral and narrow dorsal parts of the cloaca. The growth of the urorectal septum progresses toward the cloacal membrane, and when the septum contacts the membrane, it divides it into a posterior *anal* and an anterior *urogenital membrane* (see Fig. 27-15*A* through *C*). With the perforation of the anal membrane, the definitive anatomy of the rectum and anal canal is essentially established; however, there are several complex and rather poorly understood developmental steps required for transforming the urogenital sinus into the bladder, the various segments of the urethra, the prostate, and the vestibule of the vagina.

The Urogenital Sinus. The cranial, or **vesical part** of the urogenital sinus and the adjoining allantois expand to form much of the urinary bladder. The rest of the allantois becomes the **urachus,** later to be transformed into the median umbilical ligament. Caudally, the urogenital sinus is divided into two additional parts: a pelvic and a phallic portion. From the **pelvic portion** develops most of the urethra of the female or the prostatic urethra of the male. Buds arise on the wall of the pelvic portion of the sinus that form the prostate. The phallic portion of the sinus, to be discussed in Chapter 28, extends into the phallus to form the vestibule of the vagina in the female and the penile urethra in the male (see Fig. 27-15*D* and *E*).

After the metanephric diverticula (ureteric buds) have appeared on the mesonephric ducts (see Fig. 25-29), each ureter acquires a direct and independent opening into the bladder, it is thought by the absorption of the terminal segments of the mesonephric ducts into the posterior wall of the primitive bladder. Subsequently, the new openings of the mesonephric ducts are transferred to the pelvic portion of the urogenital sinus by an extension of this absorption process. It is believed that as the mesonephric ducts loop caudally between the ureteric openings, they contact the dorsal wall of the urogenital sinus and become incorporated into it (see Fig. 27-15*F* through *I*).

There are two consequences of this absorption process: 1) The triangular area (trigone) in the posterior wall of the urogenital sinus between the openings of the ureters and the mesonephric ducts is formed by mesoderm derived from the ducts, whereas the rest of the sinus lining is derived from endoderm. It is believed, however, that endoderm later overgrows this mesodermal component of the bladder and urethral wall. 2) The mesonephric ducts, which function as the male genital ducts, open into the pelvic portion of the urogenital sinus along with the glands of the prostate. The female genital ducts also contact the pelvic part of the urogenital sinus, and, at their point of contact, the posterior sinus wall gives rise to the vagina.

The Genital Ducts

As explained in Chapter 26, the male gonad connects its seminiferous tubules with the **mesonephric duct,** and along this duct, spermatozoa pass to the pelvic portion of the urogenital sinus. The female gonad does not connect directly with any duct system; the ova are discharged into the peritoneal cavity and are picked up and transported by a highly specialized duct system developed from the paramesonephric ducts.

The **paramesonephric ducts** develop in the urogenital ridges parallel with the mesonephric ducts and accompany them to the pelvic portion of the urogenital sinus (Fig. 27-16). In addition to transmitting gametes, the uterus and uterine tubes, derived from the paramesonephric ducts, provide the conditions necessary for fertilization and the development of the zygote into a viable offspring. The different functional requirements of the genital duct systems in the two sexes are instructively contrasted by comparing their development and later their anatomy.

The mesonephric duct is formed by the longitudinal anastomosis of the nephric ducts, originally located in the pronephros; it conducts urine to the cloaca. The paramesonephric ducts are formed by a longitudinal invagination of the celomic mesothelium on the urogenital ridges; they never convey urine. Cranially, the mesonephric ducts end blindly; the paramesonephric ducts are open because the fusion of the lips of the groove that forms the ducts stops short of sealing their cranial end, leaving an ostium through which the ducts communicate with the celom from the time of their inception.

Once the mesonephros disappears, both sets of ducts are suspended in the urogenital mesentery along the lateral side of the gonad. Because the female gonad remains in the pelvis, this mesentery persists as the broad ligament, but disappears in the male as the testis descends into the inguinal canal.

Each duct converges medially to approximate its counterpart of the opposite side. In so doing, both sets of ducts cross the caudal pole of the gonads, their genitoinguinal ligament, and the ureter. The paramesonephric ducts fuse with each other in the median plane, and their fused caudal tip makes contact with the urogenital sinus. The unfused, lateral parts of the ducts become the uterine tubes, their fused portions form the uterus, and from the tip of the tubes develops the uterine cervix. The mesonephric ducts open into the urogenital sinus on each side of the midline as the ejaculatory ducts; they remain unfused.

Both mesonephric and paramesonephric ducts become tethered to the genitoinguinal ligament as they cross it; this remains evident as the attachment of the gubernaculum to the cauda epididymidis as well as to the testis (a factor probably responsible for the alignment of the epididymis along the testis) and as the attachment of the ligament of the ovary and round ligament (together representing the genitoinguinal ligament) to the uterus. The attachment of the genitoinguinal ligament to the paramesonephric ducts, which persists in the female pelvis, is probably the chief factor for the retention of the ovaries in the pelvic cavity.

The mesonephric ducts regress and the paramesonephric ducts persist unless a male gonad is formed in the embryo. The testis secretes factors that suppress the paramesonephric ducts (which commence to atrophy at the point where they cross the testis) and promote the differentiation of the mesonephric ducts. The latter concerns the events of linking the seminiferous tubules to the mesonephric duct (see Chap. 26; Fig. 26-12) and, at the caudal end of the duct, the development of the seminal vesicles. The *seminal vesicles* appear as diverticula similar to the ureteric buds before the ducts enter the pelvic part of the urogenital sinus. The same factors promote the appearance of the prostatic buds on the wall of the pelvic urogenital sinus; the buds come to surround not only the urethra but the ejaculatory ducts as well. The suppressed paramesonephric duct system is represented in the male by the appendix testis and probably also the prostatic utricle. The vestigial mesonephric duct system in the female is represented by blind tubules in the mesentery of the ovary (*paraoophoron* and *epoophoron*) and a vestigial duct (*duct of Gärtner*) along the wall of the uterus.

Formation of the Vagina

As the tips of the fused paramesonephric ducts contact the urogenital sinus, they form an eminence known as the *sinus tubercle*, which evidently induces the endoderm on the dorsal wall of the pelvic part of the sinus to proliferate. This proliferation produces the **sinuvaginal bulb** or *vaginal plate*, a flattened cylinder of tissue composed of sinus endoderm, which, as it grows, causes the sinus tubercle to recede from the sinus lumen farther and farther in a craniodorsal direction, into the urorectal septum (Fig. 27-17). When the sinuvaginal bulb becomes canalized, the vagina is formed with a lumen. The tubercle differentiates into the cervix, and its canal links the vagina to the uterine cavity; the sinus wall separating the lumen of the vagina from that of the sinus forms the *hymen*. It is

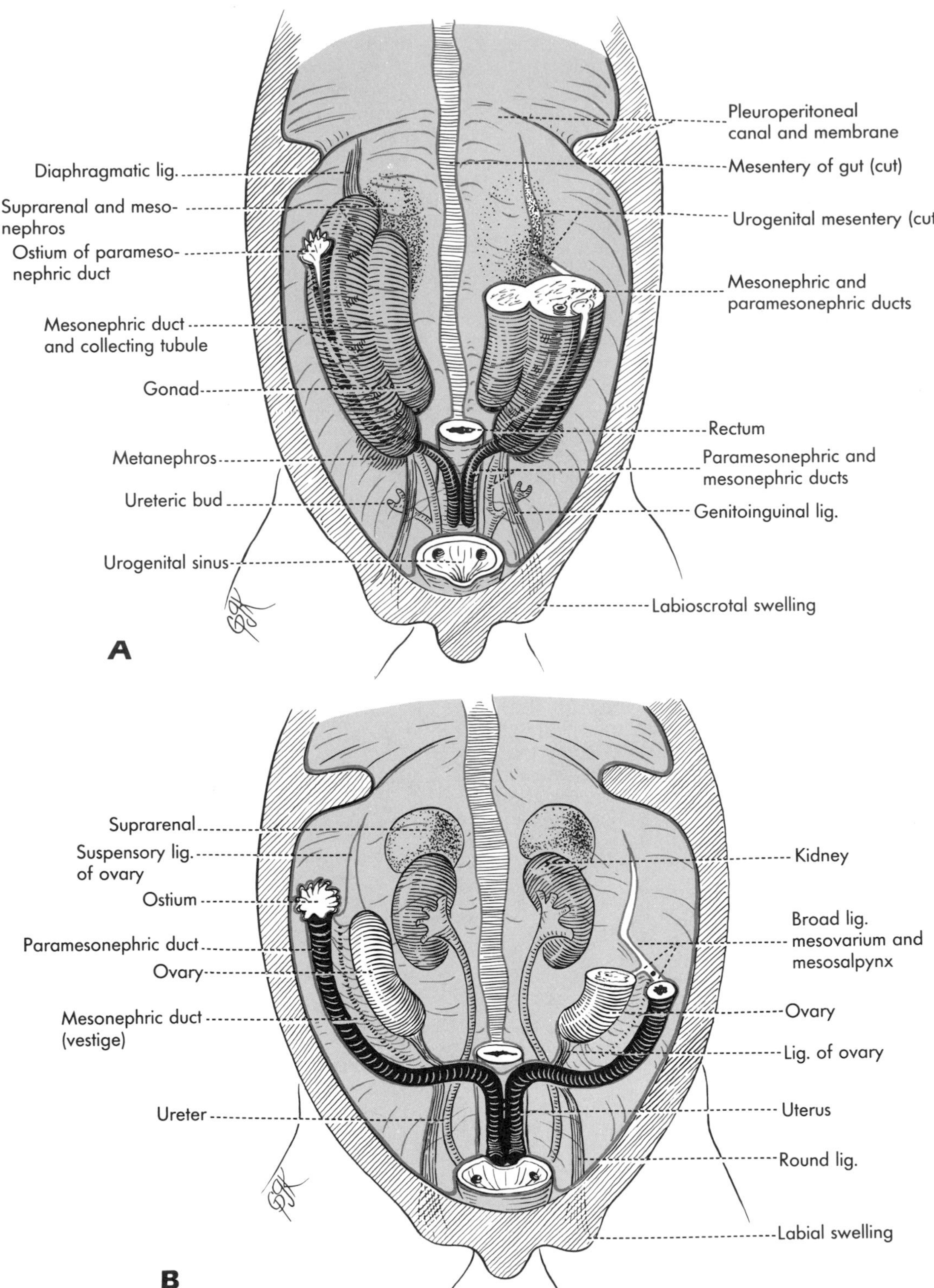

FIGURE *27-16.*
The development of the paramesonephric ducts in the urogenital ridges illustrated diagrammatically: Except for the rectum, the gut has been excised with its mesentery. The mesothelial lining of the celom is *pink*. Two successive stages of development are shown: (A) the mesonephros and the mesonephric ducts are present; (B) the mesonephros has regressed and its duct atrophied. On the *right side*, the ridges have been transected to reveal the urogenital mesentery. Compare with Figures 25-29 and 26-12, from which the paramesonephric ducts have been omitted.

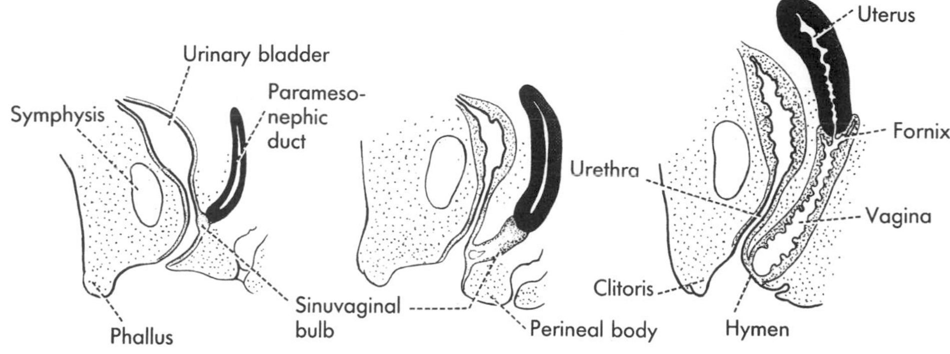

FIGURE 27-17.
Schematic sagittal sections showing the formation of the vagina. (Langman J. Medical embryology. 3rd ed. Baltimore Williams & Wilkins, 1975.)

controversial whether any contributions are made by the paramesonephric ducts to the formation of the sinuvaginal bulb.

The phallic part of the urogenital sinus, caudal and anterior to the hymen, becomes the vestibule of the vagina into which the urethra also opens.

The Rectum

Located in the pelvis, the rectum is the inferior segment of the large intestine, in which feces accumulate until their evacuation through the anal canal. The rectum begins at the rectosigmoid junction, in front of the third sacral vertebra, as the continuation of the sigmoid colon; it ends at the anorectal junction, in front of the tip of the coccyx, as the rectum, passing through the pelvic floor, leads into the anal canal. The rectum is about 12 cm long; its upper limit cannot be reached by an index finger inserted through the anus.

The **sigmoid colon** descends into the pelvis across the left sacroiliac joint, the attachment of its mesocolon crossing the left common iliac or external iliac artery and vein at the pelvic brim and sometimes the left ureter. The sigmoid mesocolon becomes shorter as it descends in front of the sacrum and is lost at the rectosigmoid junction. Although the transition between the sigmoid colon and the rectum is a gradual one, several external features identify the **rectosigmoid junction.** At this junction, the bowel loses its mesentery and becomes closely applied to the curve of the sacrum, so that it presents an anterior concavity, the *sacral flexure*, the commencement of which may make a definite angle with the sigmoid colon (Fig. 27-18). There is a gradual broadening of the teniae coli of the sigmoid colon to form broad anterior and posterior bands that meet laterally and form a complete layer of longitudinal muscle around the rectum. With this change, there is a disappearance of the haustra, sacculations that characterize most of the colon. The appendices epiploicae, another characteristic of the colon, are lost from the sigmoid colon after it enters the pelvis.

Contrary to what is implied by its name, the rectum is not straight; it presents not only the anteroposterior sacral flexure but also three lateral curves or bends that give it a sinuous profile in the anterior view, although both the beginning and the end of the rectum are retained in the midline. The upper and lower curves are convex to the right, the middle one to the left (Fig. 27-19). The part of the rectum in the region of the middle and lower curves is called the *rectal ampulla*, because it is somewhat dilated and is especially distensible. At its inferior end, the *perineal flexure* markedly angulates the anorectal junction; the anal canal bends posteriorly at the level of the puborectalis muscle (see Fig. 28-2).

As the rectum reaches the pelvic diaphragm, most of its longitudinal muscle continues downward along the anal canal, but a few fibers may reflect from it anteriorly and posteriorly on the upper surface of the diaphragm. In the male, the anterior fibers pass to the urethra and are known as the *rectourethral muscle*; the slips that pass backward to the coccyx form the *rectococcygeus muscle*.

On the **interior,** there is a change in the character of the mucosal lining in the region of the rectosigmoid junction. The fluffy, rugose mucosa of the colon gives rise to the smooth mucosa of the rectum. Three permanent semilunar folds project into the lumen of the rectum from its lateral walls, located in the depths of each of the lateral curvatures. These are the *transverse rectal folds*, formed by the reduplication of the mucosa, submucosa, and circular muscle coat.

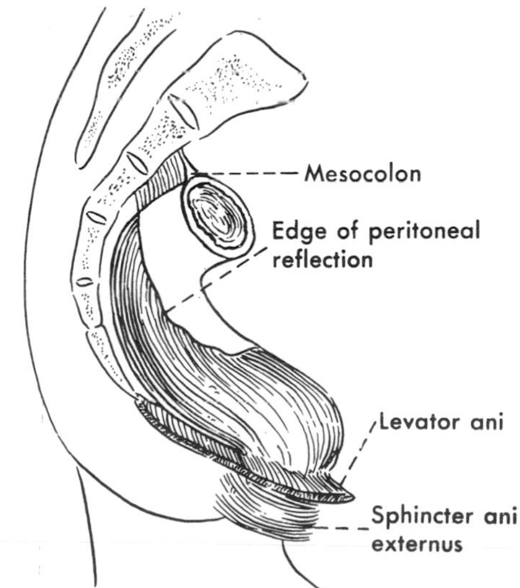

FIGURE 27-18.
Lateral view of the rectum and the lower end of the sigmoid colon. Both sacral and perineal flexures are clear.

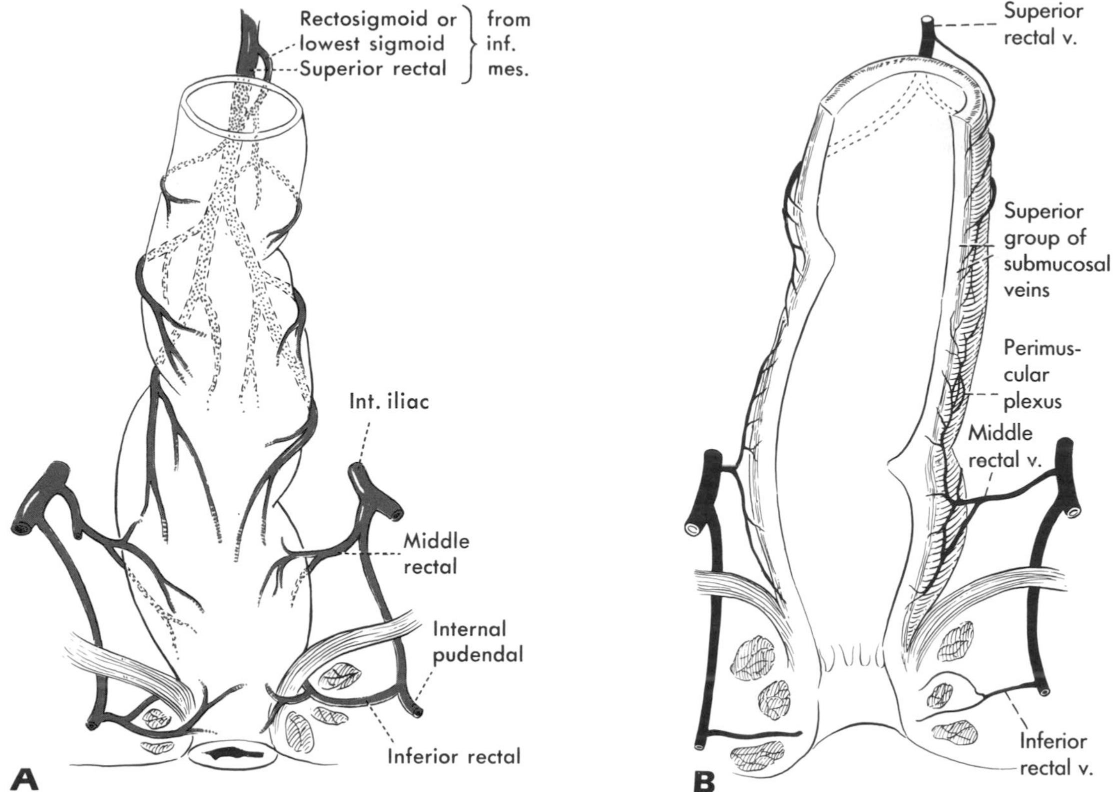

FIGURE *27-19.*
Blood supply of the rectum and anal canal: (A) arteries; (B) veins.

Relations

Peritoneum covers the front and sides of the rectum in its upper third, only the front in the middle third, and none of it in the lower third (see Fig. 27-22). The peritoneum sweeps forward from the rectum to the base of the bladder in the male or the posterior surface of the vagina and uterus in the female, creating the *rectovesical* and *rectouterine pouches*, respectively. In these peritoneal spaces, the rectum is related to loops of small bowel or sigmoid colon.

The *pararectal fossae* of the peritoneal cavity surround the rectum laterally and are limited on the sides by the sacrogenital folds in the male and the rectouterine folds in the female.

Except for its peritoneal surfaces, the rectum is surrounded by pelvic fascia. The *rectal fascia* is a filmy layer of areolar tissue that forms a tubular sheath for the rectum loose enough to allow distention of the ampulla. The condensations of subperitoneal pelvic fascia around the middle rectal vessels form the so-called *lateral ligaments of the rectum*. The anorectal junction is connected to the sacrum by an avascular condensation of fascia called the fascia of Waldeyer. Anteriorly, the *rectovesical septum* separates the rectum from the prostate, seminal vesicles, and bladder or the *rectovaginal septum* from the vagina. The deferent ducts and the terminal part of the ureters are also anterior to this peritoneoperineal fascia. The posterior surface of the rectum rests on the lower sacral vertebrae, the median sacral and superior rectal vessels, the pelvic sacral foramina filled by the sacral anterior rami, and the piriformis muscles. The inferior hypogastric plexuses are related to the lateral sides of the lower part of the rectum.

Blood Supply and Lymph Drainage

The rectum is supplied primarily by the **superior rectal artery.** This vessel, the continuation of the inferior mesenteric artery, reaches the rectum in the sigmoid mesocolon. At about the rectosigmoid junction, the superior rectal artery divides into right and left branches that run forward around the sides of the rectum in the rectal fascia, give off branches into the bowel, and disappear into its walls (Fig. 27-19*A*). They continue into the anal canal.

The lower part of the rectum also receives the *middle rectal arteries*, branches of the internal iliac arteries. These arteries are variable in size and in their place of origin; they anastomose freely with the superior rectals. The *inferior rectal arteries* supply the anal canal rather than the rectum.

The **venous drainage** of the rectum follows the arterial supply. The chief drainage from the *rectal plexus* is into the superior rectal veins. These are at first paired, as is the lower end of the artery, but unite at about the rectosigmoid junction into a single *superior rectal vein. Middle rectal veins* drain predominantly the musculature rather than the mucosa (see Fig. 27-19*B*).

The **lymphatic drainage** of the rectum is also primarily upward, paralleling the superior rectal blood vessels (Fig. 27-20). Numerous lymph nodes are associated with these lymphatics. The superior rectal lymphatics enter into the *inferior mesenteric nodes* around the origin of the inferior mesenteric artery. The lymphatics that parallel the middle rectal vessels on the upper surface of the pelvic diaphragm empty into the *internal iliac nodes*. Finally, the lymphatic plexus of the lower part of the rectum is directly continuous with that of the upper part of the anal canal and joins the lymphatics that accompany the inferior rectal and internal pudendal blood vessels below the pelvic diaphragm. Because this route follows the internal pudendal vessels, it passes with them through the buttock into the pelvis, where it ends in *internal iliac nodes* as the middle route.

Carcinomas of the rectum metastasize along the lymphatics. Those situated particularly low in the rectum or in the anal canal may metastasize by still another route: although the connections between the lymphatic plexus in the upper part of the anal canal and that in the lower part are few, a low-lying carcinoma may spread through these connections when other lymphatic pathways are blocked. The carcinoma may also grow across the "lymphatic divide" and involve the lymphatics of the lower part of the anal canal. The drainage of this part is into the *superficial inguinal nodes*.

Innervation

The rectal plexus receives its nerves from two plexuses: the superior rectal and the middle rectal. The *superior rectal plexus* descends along the artery of the same name and may supply rectal blood vessels, but it is not important in the physiology of the rectum. The motor fibers to the rectum appear to be entirely parasympathetic and are conveyed in the *middle rectal plexus*, derived from the inferior hypogastric plexus. Moreover, the afferent supply to the rectum, both the fibers concerned with pain and those that sense the presence of feces or gas in the rectum, belong to the parasympathetic system. Thus, the rectum receives both its afferent and efferent innervation through the *pelvic splanchnic nerves* in the rectal plexus.

Emptying of the bowel occurs as the result of the activity of the pelvic splanchnic nerves, which increase the peristaltic activity of the rectum. This, with the help of increased abdominal pressure, moves the feces through the anal canal. Reflex restraint of a bowel movement is brought about through the activity of the voluntary muscle around the anal canal. As peristaltic activity increases the pressure in the rectum, the afferent fibers in the lower part of the rectum are stimulated and bring about a reflex contraction of the voluntary musculature. This contraction lasts just long enough to resist the increasing pressure caused by peristalsis, disappearing as the peristaltic activity abates. The initiation of the reflex activity depends on the presence of a definite part of the rectum. If the entire rectum is removed and the colon anastomosed to the anal canal, the passage of gas or feces can be resisted only by the rather incompetent voluntary contraction of the external anal sphincter; thus, a large majority of persons with complete removal of the rectum suffer from anal incompetence. In contrast, if the lower 2 cm or so of the rectum can be retained, good control of the passage of gas and feces can be expected.

Anomalies

Congenital anomalies of the rectum include **imperforate anus** (discussed in connection with the anal canal in Chap. 28), which may involve an arrest in

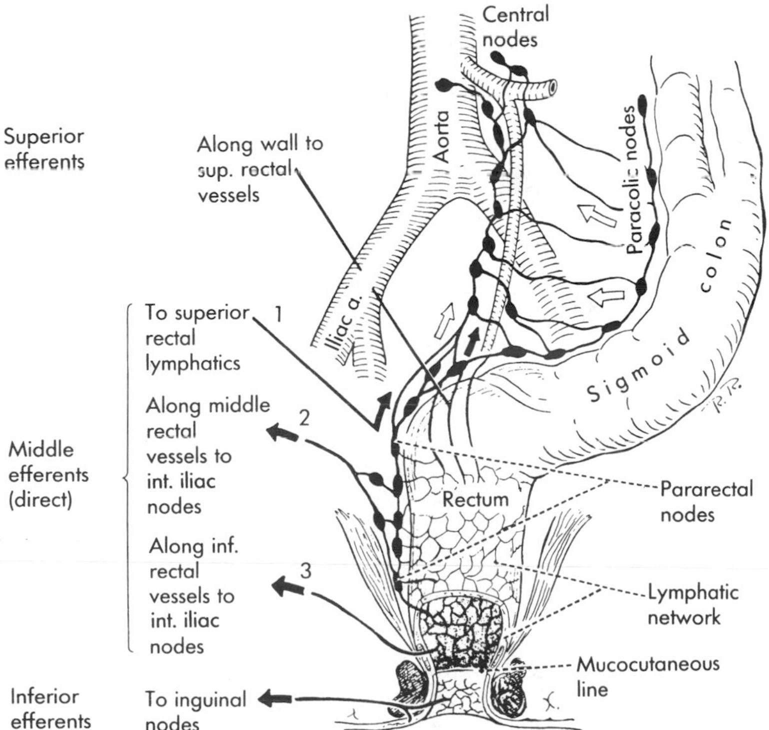

FIGURE 27-20.
The lymphatic drainage of the sigmoid colon, rectum, and anal canal: As indicated here, drainage from the sigmoid colon and from the rectum is in large part upward to nodes (central nodes) around the origin of the inferior mesenteric artery; however, there is also a lateral drainage of the rectum to internal iliac nodes. Below the levator ani, the anal canal drains in part laterally to internal iliac nodes, but that part below the mucocutaneous (pectinate) line drains to superficial inguinal nodes. (Best RR; Blair JB. Ann Surg 1949;50:538.)

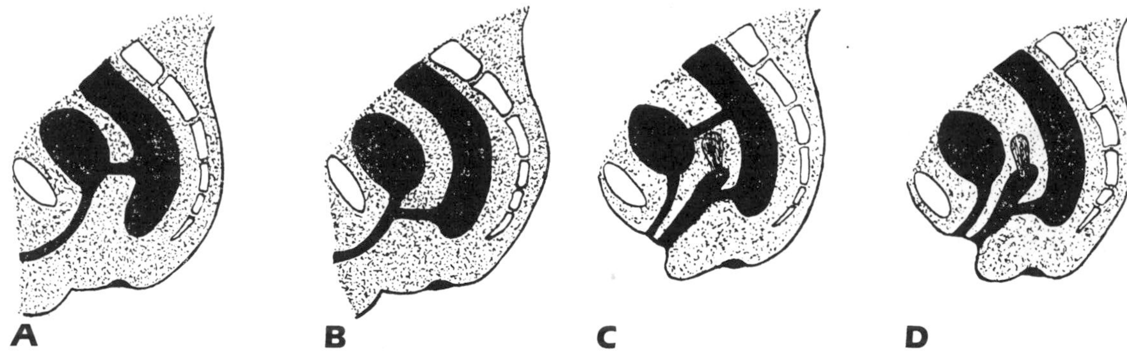

FIGURE *27-21.*
Some types of rectal fistulae associated with imperforate anus in the male (A and B) and female (C and D) (Ladd WE, Gross RE. Am J Surg 1934;23:167.)

the development of the rectum as well as the anal canal, and **fistulae** between the rectum and the viscera located anterior to it. These fistulous connections are readily explained on the basis of the division of the cloaca (described earlier). Defective growth of the urorectal septum may leave the bladder and the rectum in continuity below through a *persistent cloaca*. More common are narrow apertures between the rectum and the derivatives of the urogenital sinus, which constitute *rectovesical* or *rectourethral fistulae* (Fig. 27-21*A* and *B*). These communications persist owing to gaps in the urorectal septum. A *rectovaginal fistula* can be explained by the development of the vagina in the urorectal septum with a defect in the mesoderm between the vagina and the rectum (see Fig. 27-21*C* and *D*). Fistulae of the rectum are often associated with imperforate anus.

The Urinary Bladder, Ureters, Urethra, and Prostate

The Urinary Bladder

The urinary bladder (*vesica urinaria*) accumulates urine more or less continuously discharged into it by the ureters, until the bladder walls are sufficiently distended to activate the reflexes for micturition. The bladder is located behind the two pubes and the pubic symphysis; when empty, it is entirely within the pelvic cavity. As the bladder fills, it rises above the pelvic brim, coming in contact with the posterior surface of the anterior abdominal wall (Fig. 27-22); if fully distended, it may reach as high as the umbilicus. During infancy and early childhood, the dimensions of the pelvis are small and even the empty bladder is largely above the pelvic brim.

Although the distended bladder rises as a dome, the empty viscus is flat, presenting a roughly triangular superior and posterior surface, the latter called the *base*, or *fundus*, and two triangular inferolateral surfaces. The anterior angle of this tetrahedron is the *apex* with the median umbilical ligament attached to it; the inferior angle leads into the urethra and is called the *neck* of the bladder. The two posterolateral angles admit the ureters and are unnamed. The superior and inferolateral surfaces make up the *body* of the bladder.

Interior and Structure. The pink vascular mucosa of the bladder is loosely attached to the underlying muscular wall on the interior of the body, but is closely adherent over the fundus. Therefore, in the empty contracted bladder, the mucosa of the bladder base is conspicuously smooth, contrasting with the small irregular rugae over the body.

On the interior, the base of the bladder is defined by the two *ureteric ostia* and the *internal urethral orifice*. The smooth triangular area outlined by these three openings

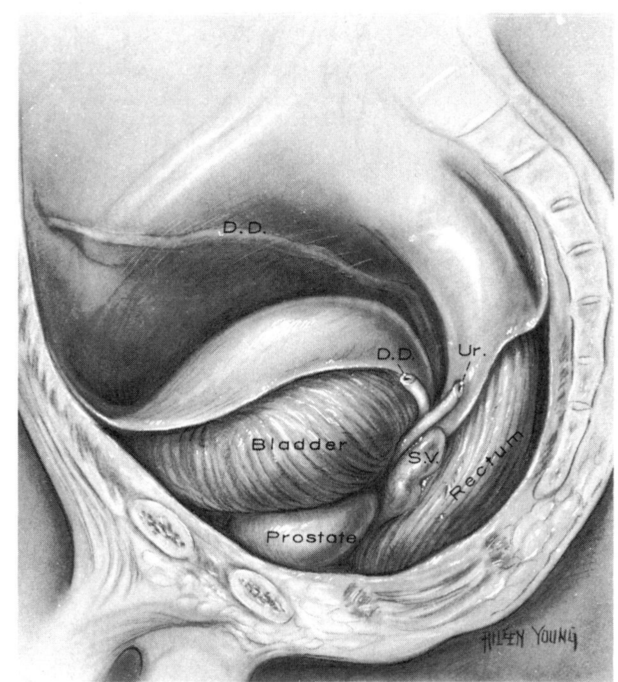

FIGURE *27-22.*
Pelvic viscera in the male: The peritoneum over the bladder and rectum was cut where it was reflected upon the lateral pelvic wall. *D.D.* identifies the right and left deferent ducts; *Ur*, the left ureter; and *S.V.*, the left seminal vesicle. The ureter here has been displaced somewhat forward from where it was running retroperitoneally on the lateral pelvic wall, and the lower end of the sigmoid colon is so close to the sacrum that the flexure between it and the rectum is almost obliterated.

is called the **vesical trigone** (Fig. 27-23). The *interureteric fold* is a ridge in the mucosa between the two ureteric ostia; in the male, the *uvula* is a smooth and small eminence at the inferior corner of the trigone just above the internal urethral orifice. With advancing age, the uvula becomes exaggerated, owing to the enlargement of the underlying median lobe of the prostate. The trigonal submucosa, especially that over the uvula, contains mucous glands or glands similar to those of the prostate. Hypertrophy of these glands may contribute to the factors causing urinary obstruction at the bladder neck.

The **musculature** of the bladder (*tunica muscularis*) as a whole is referred to as the *detrusor muscle*. It consists of an interlacing network of smooth muscle bundles that run longitudinally, transversely, and obliquely and that change their course from one direction to another. Many of the longitudinal fibers, both on the interior and exterior of the bladder, continue into the urethra. Some of the outer fibers that descend to the bladder neck reflect forward as the *pubovesical muscle* and mingle with the fibrous tissue of the puboprostatic and pubovesical ligaments. Similar muscle slips that diverge posteriorly from the bladder neck blend with the sacrogenital or rectouterine ligaments and constitute the *rectovesical muscle*.

Over the trigone, an innermost lamina of muscle is formed by the longitudinal muscle of the ureters, which passes with the ureters obliquely through the bladder wall. This *trigonal muscle*, spread out between the trigonal mucosa and the detrusor, connects the ureteric ostia to each other (beneath the interureteric fold) and each ostium to the internal urethral orifice. Many of the fibers descend into the posterior wall of the urethra. The function of the muscle has been controversial. There is evidence to suggest that it maintains the obliquity of the ureters through the bladder wall and helps close their ostia. At the same time, the contraction of the trigonal muscle contributes to opening the urethral orifice. Should the mechanism that closes the intramural part of the ureters fail, as the bladder contracts, urine will be forced retrogradely up the ureters during voiding. If there is infection in the bladder, it can reach the renal pelvis, eventually causing pyelonephritis.

Unlike the intestine, the bladder has no continuous circular muscle. Furthermore, several surveys have verified that there is no anatomically demonstrable *vesical sphincter* at the junction of the bladder and the urethra. The *internal sphincter of the bladder* is a functional entity that prevents urine from entering the urethra and the ejaculate from entering the bladder, but the mechanisms responsible for its maintenance are not understood completely.

Relations. Peritoneum covers the bladder on its superior surface and is continuous anteriorly with the median and medial umbilical folds and with the parietal peritoneum of the supravesical fossae (see Fig. 27-22). Posteriorly, the peritoneal continuities are different in the two sexes. *In the male*, the peritoneum descends onto the base of the bladder, lining the rectovesical pouch, the peritoneal recess that intervenes between the bladder and the rectum (see Fig. 27-22); posterolaterally, it continues as the sacrogenital folds. *In the female*, the peritoneum reflects onto the uterus without covering the base and lines the shallow vesicouterine pouch (see Fig. 27-36).

In the male, subjacent to the peritoneum, the ductus deferens descends in direct contact with the base of the bladder, having crossed to the medial side of the ureter (see Fig. 27-29). The bladder neck rests on the upper sur-

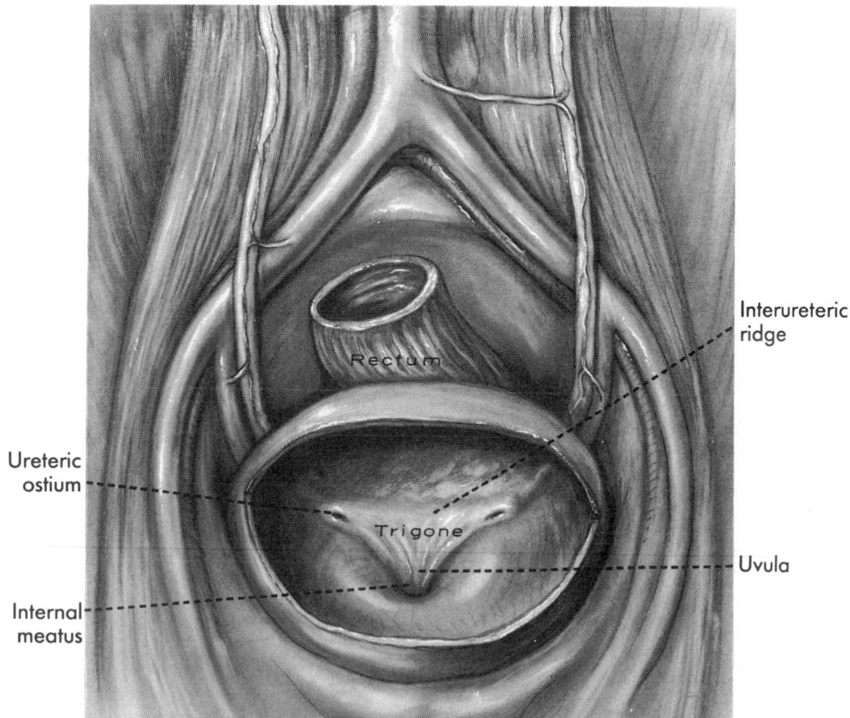

FIGURE 27-23.
The trigone of the urinary bladder, lying between the openings of the two ureters and that of the urethra.

face of the prostate. Posteriorly, between the prostate and the deferent ducts, the seminal vesicles rest against the base of the bladder.

In the female, the base of the bladder is bound to the supravaginal part of the cervix and the anterior wall of the vagina by the fusion of the fascial sheaths of the organs (see Fig. 27-36). Inferolaterally, the empty bladder rests on the pubic bones and the pelvic diaphragm with the areolar tissue and ligaments of the pelvic fascia intervening.

The neck and base of the bladder are relatively firmly fixed by their fascias and ligaments and move up and down with the contraction of the pelvic diaphragm. Their relations are not altered by distention of the bladder. As the body of the bladder distends, its superior surface rises, elevating the peritoneum and bringing its inferolateral surface more and more in contact with fascia on the anterior abdominal wall (Fig. 27-24).

Ligaments and Fascias. The neck of the bladder is connected to the pubis on the upper surface of the pelvic diaphragm by the puboprostatic ligaments in the male and the pubovesical ligaments in the female, and to the lateral wall by the lateral ligaments of the bladder (see Fig. 27-7). The latter blend posteriorly with the tissue of the sacrogenital folds of the male and the lateral cervical ligaments of the female. All these ligaments contain smooth muscle reflected into them from the bladder neck. Vessels, nerves, and the ureters reach the bladder embedded in the lateral and posterior ligaments. Posterolaterally, these ligaments form the floor of the perivesical spaces, which are roofed over by the peritoneum and contain loose connective tissue continuous with these ligaments. Anteriorly, the retropubic space is similarly limited below by the puboprostatic and pubovesical ligaments (see Fig. 27-24).

The *median umbilical ligament*, attached to the apex of the bladder, is the remnant of the embryonic urachus; at its base, the ligament usually retains a lumen communicating with the bladder. Rarely, urine will be discharged from the umbilicus because the patency of the urachus persists along its entire length.

Below the floor of the rectovesical pouch, the bladder base is separated from the rectal fascia by the rectovesical septum (Fig. 27-25). The connective tissue space anterior to the bladder is divided into two compartments by a similar lamina of fascia called the *umbilical prevesical fascia*, which connects the two medial umbilical ligaments to the median umbilical ligament and separates the immediate perivesical space from the retropubic space (see Fig. 27-24). This space provides an extraperitoneal approach not only to the bladder and prostate, as mentioned earlier, but also to the pregnant uterus which, similar to the distended bladder, elevates the peritoneum and contacts the anterior abdominal wall above the bladder. In a cesarean section, the uterus is opened through the retropubic space without incising the peritoneum.

The Ureters

The ureters are described from the kidney to the pelvic brim in Chapter 25. They cross the pelvic brim at approximately the level of the bifurcation of the common iliac artery. The left ureter is related to the base of the sigmoid colon. In the female, both ureters may also be closely related to the ovarian vessels, for these often cross the pelvic brim just lateral to the ureters. In surgical procedures on the ovaries, the ureter is prone to damage in securing the ovarian vessels at the pelvic brim, one of the common sites of iatrogenic injury to the ureter in the female.

In both sexes, after it crosses the pelvic brim, the ureter lies at first immediately deep to the peritoneum, medial to the internal iliac artery, passing downward and forward along the lateral pelvic wall. In the female, it tends to run just behind the ovary, forming the posterior

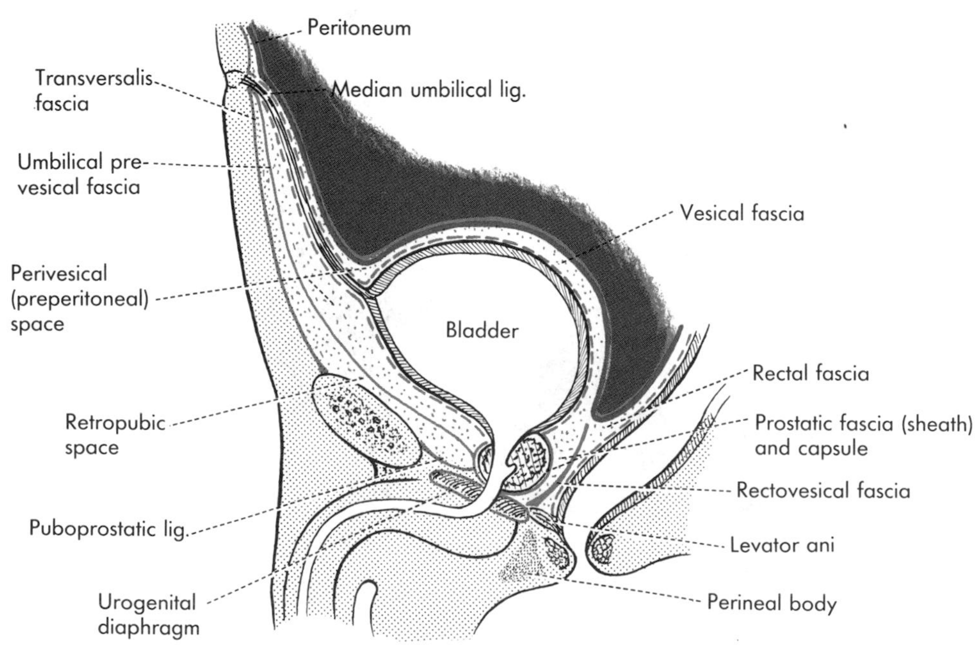

FIGURE 27-24. **Fascial spaces and laminae associated with the bladder, prostate, and rectum. The bladder is shown distended.**

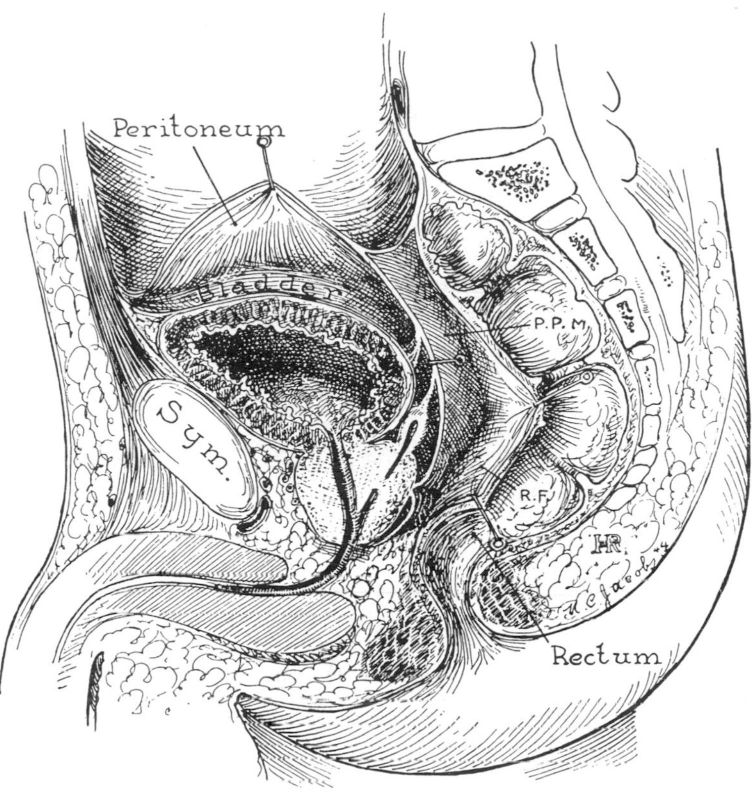

FIGURE 27-25.
A dissection of the rectovesical septum (*P.P.M.*, or peritoneoperineal membrane). *R.F.* is the rectal fascia, here retracted backward with the rectum. (Tobin CE, Benjamin JA. Surg Gynecol Obstet 1945;80:373.)

boundary of a shallow fossa, against which the ovary usually lies. As they reach the level of the peritoneal floor of the pelvis, the two ureters converge toward each other and enter the connective tissue of the sacrogenital folds or the rectouterine folds of the female, in which they continue medially with the vessels and nerves contained in these ligaments.

As it approaches the bladder, the ureter runs more deeply and, in the male, comes in contact with the ductus deferens. The ureter passes below the ductus and then in front of the seminal vesicles (see Fig. 27-29). It enters the posterolateral aspect of the bladder and courses obliquely through its wall.

In numerous gynecologic procedures, the relations of the ureter as it approaches the bladder are particularly important in the female pelvis. In the lateral cervical ligaments, the ureter is closely associated with the blood vessels and nerves of the uterus and vagina. It passes forward and medially at the base of the broad ligament and, in so doing, is crossed above and in front by the uterine artery as this vessel runs a more direct transverse course toward the uterus. The crossing of the ureter by the uterine artery occurs about 1.5 cm lateral to the uterus, but can vary markedly when pathologic conditions have distorted relations. This crossing is oblique; the two structures are in contact for approximately a centimeter or more. This is another common site of surgical injury to the ureter. The ureter may be injured by a clamp, or even ligated and divided, when the uterine vessels are clamped to control uterine bleeding, or it may be ligated and divided in the process of removing the uterus (hysterectomy).

After crossing behind and below the uterine artery, the ureter continues its course forward and medially and passes to the front of the vagina surrounded by the upper parts of the vesical nerve plexus. It enters the posterolateral aspect of the bladder just as it does in the male.

Ectopic Ureter. Interference with the normal process of the absorption of the mesonephric duct into the dorsal wall of the urogenital sinus may displace one or both ureteric ostia from their normal location. This condition is known as ectopic ureter.

The most common ectopia is one in which the ureter opens distal to the bladder into the prostatic urethra in the male or into the urethra or vaginal vestibule in the female. Openings into the ductus deferens or seminal vesicle or the vagina also occur sometimes. These ectopias can be explained by the embryonic derivation of these structures either from the mesonephric ducts or from portions of the urogenital sinus. Rarely, an ectopic ureter opens into the rectum, the explanation for which is not so obvious.

The Urethra

The urethra connects the bladder to the exterior. It commences at the internal urethral orifice of the bladder and terminates at the external orifice located at the tip of the penis or in the vestibule of the vagina. In the female, the urethra transmits only urine; in the male, it is the final passage for both urine and semen.

The **female urethra** is a simple tube, measuring barely 4 cm in length. It is closely fused to the anterior vaginal wall, runs with the vagina through the urogenital hiatus, and opens just anterior to the vagina into the vestibule (see Fig. 28-18). Its walls are simple, containing much elastic tissue as well as smooth muscle continuous with that of the bladder and voluntary muscle derived from the urogenital diaphragm.

The *urogenital diaphragm*, described with the perineum (see Chap. 28), consists of muscles that span the triangular space between the conjoint rami of the pubis and ischium and includes the sphincter urethrae.

The **male urethra** is approximately 20 cm long and is divisible into three portions (see Fig. 28-11): the part that leaves the bladder, called the *prostatic part*, because it is surrounded by the prostate; a part that passes through the urogenital diaphragm, called the *pars membranacea* or membranous urethra, because it is between the superior and inferior connective tissue membranes of the urogenital diaphragm; and the third, most distal part, enclosed by the corpus spongiosum of the penis and therefore called the *pars spongiosa*. The membranous and spongy parts of the urethra are located in the perineum and are described in Chapter 28. Only the prostatic urethra is in the pelvis.

The average length of the **prostatic urethra** is about 2.5 cm, and its lumen is spindle-shaped (Fig. 27-26). Its walls are formed by the prostate itself, for the ducts and glands that compose the prostate are outgrowths from the urethra (see Fig. 27-15), and the muscular fibrous tissue of the prostate is part of the original urethral wall.

On the posterior wall of the prostatic urethra is a longitudinal ridge, the *urethral crest*, raised up largely by the continuation of the trigonal muscle into the urethra. The crest is continuous above with the uvula of the bladder (see Fig. 27-26). A similar crest exists in the female urethra. In the male, the crest widens to form a smooth eminence, the *colliculus seminalis*, which urologists call the *verumontanum*. The colliculus is 2 to 4 mm long, and its center lies about two-thirds of the distance down the prostatic urethra. In the midline and usually just distal to its center, the *prostatic utricle* opens on the colliculus by a rounded or slitlike aperture. The utricle is believed by some to be the remnant of the fused paramesonephric ducts, which form the uterus, and is sometimes called the *uterus masculinus*. It is more likely that the utricle is a homologue of the vagina and should rather be called the *vagina masculina*.

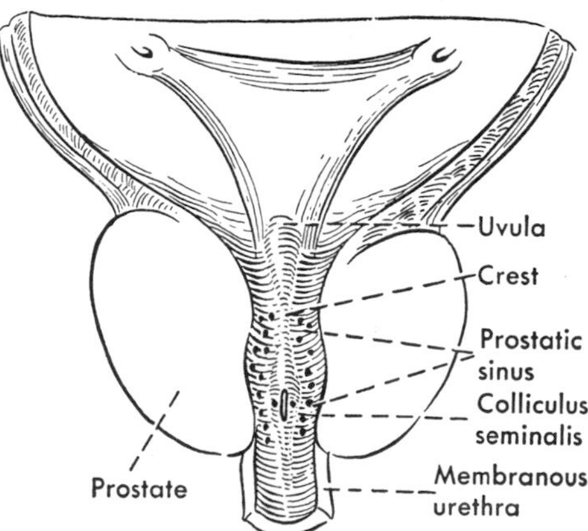

FIGURE *27-26.*
The posterior wall of the prostatic urethra: The relatively large midline opening on the colliculus seminalis is the utriculus; on each side of it is the small opening of an ejaculatory duct. The similarly small openings in the prostatic sinuses are those of prostatic ducts.

The *ejaculatory ducts* also open on the colliculus on each side of the utricle. Their openings are tiny and often cannot be seen in the cadaver, but in living persons it is possible to catheterize them and inject radiopaque contrast medium into the genital ducts (see Fig. 27-30).

On each side of the colliculus and the urethral crest is a sulcus called the *prostatic sinus*. In it, the 12 to 20 tiny orifices are the openings of the prostatic ducts (see Fig. 27-26).

The Prostate

The prostate is an encapsulated gland developed only in the male around the urethral lumen between the neck of the bladder and the pelvic floor. It is developmentally and actually the thickened wall of this part of the urethra. Its firm consistency is due to the significant amount of smooth muscle present in its stroma, which is continuous with the musculature of the bladder. Secretions of the glandular follicles of the prostate account for much of the seminal plasma.

The prostate is deeply placed, in contact with the gutter-shaped pelvic floor, directly behind the lower border of the symphysis pubis (see Figs. 27-22, 27-24, and 27-25). It is shaped like an asymmetric cone: its **apex** points inferiorly, resting on the pubococcygeus, and through the urogenital hiatus is in contact with the superior fascia of the urogenital diaphragm. The oval **base,** fused to the bladder neck, measures approximately 2 and 4 cm along its anteroposterior and lateral diameters, respectively. The vertical extent of the posterior surface is greater than that of the anterior surface, and the gland bulges posterolaterally, creating a shallow median sulcus on the posterior surface, which can be palpated by rectal examination. The two inferolateral surfaces are broad posteriorly and converge on the narrow **isthmus** that connects the two sides anteriorly in front of the urethra and may consist of only fibromuscular tissue.

Lobes. Behind the urethra, the prostate is traversed obliquely by the two ejaculatory ducts, which enter its posterosuperior margin behind the bladder and slope medially toward their orifices on the colliculus seminalis (Fig. 27-2; see Fig. 27-26). The two ducts, with the urethra, define a somewhat cone-shaped core of the gland, which is considered its **median lobe.** The base of the median lobe underlies the uvula of the bladder, and the blind prostatic utricle extends into it between the ejaculatory ducts.

Although no definite lobulation is evident on either the interior or the exterior of the prostate, the isthmus is designated as the **anterior lobe** and the two bulging posterolateral portions as the **lateral lobes.** The tissue joining the latter in the posteromedian sulcus is the **posterior lobe.**

Prostatic Enlargement. Benign hypertrophy (*prostatic*

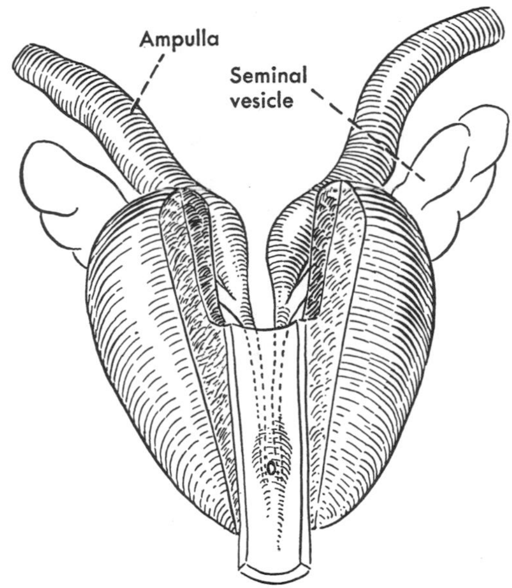

FIGURE 27-27.
The ejaculatory ducts seen from the front: A midsegment of the upper part of the prostate has been completely removed to the level at which the ejaculatory ducts enter the gland, and a corresponding segment of the anterior urethral wall and the associated part of the prostate has been removed below. The intraglandular portions of the duct are indicated by *broken lines*.

hyperplasia), common after middle age, affects preferentially the median lobe. The lobe may bulge into the prostatic urethra and obstruct it, or its base may bulge into the bladder and, acting as a ball valve, be forced into the internal urethral orifice by the vesical pressure developed for emptying the bladder and obstruct the flow of urine. Hyperplasia of the uvular submucosal glands contributes to this obstruction. The benign tumor may be pared away as it bulges into the prostatic urethra through a cystoscope (*transurethral resection*), or it may be shelled out after the urethra has been opened by transecting the isthmus of the prostate (*retropubic prostatectomy*). The prostate may also be approached surgically through the bladder or from the perineum. Malignant change (carcinoma of the prostate) most often affects the posterior lobe, and its treatment usually combines radiation and hormone therapy with some type of resection of the cancerous tissue.

Capsule and Ligaments. Outside its firm, white, shiny capsule, continuous with the fibromuscular trabeculae of the gland, the prostate is surrounded by a rather dense fascial sheath, with the rich prostatic plexus embedded in it. This prostatic fascia also contains nerves and lymphatics and is continuous above the level of the pelvic floor with the puboprostatic ligaments, the lateral ligaments of the bladder, and the connective tissue of the sacrogenital folds (see Fig. 27-7). Directly behind the prostate, the rectovesical fascia separates the prostatic sheath from the rectal fascia (see Fig. 27-25).

The fibers of the pubococcygeus insert into the prostatic fascia and the prostatic capsule, and these fibers are called the *levator prostatae muscle*.

Internal Structure. Inside the capsule, the major part of the prostate consists of numerous glands that have grown out from the posterolateral aspect of the urethra and expanded to form the glandular substance that is mixed with fibromuscular tissue of the urethral wall. An internal and peripheral zone have been defined histologically in the gland. It is the glands of the peripheral zone posteriorly that are prone to carcinomatous transformation and those of the internal zone that are prone to benign hypertrophy. The ducts of the glands combine to form the 12 to 20 prostatic ducts opening into the prostatic sinus of the urethra.

Blood Supply and Lymph Drainage

The **arteries of the urinary bladder** vary in number and have been variously named. Usually, two or three arteries arise from the umbilical artery as it runs anterolateral to the apex of the bladder and are distributed to the apex and the upper part of the body; these are the *superior vesical arteries* (Fig. 27-28). Close to its origin, the umbilical artery usually gives off a vessel, the *artery of the ductus deferens* (deferential artery), which has also been called the *middle vesical artery*. It is distributed to the body of the bladder as well as to the ductus and seminal vesicles. In the female, the middle vesical artery is a branch of the uterine artery.

There is, in addition, an *inferior vesical artery* on each side. This is inconstant in its origin, for it may arise from many different parts of the internal iliac system. It runs through the connective tissue close to the floor of the pelvis and is distributed to an inferior part of the bladder, including the vesical neck, and also sends branches to the prostate. In the female, the inferior vesical artery is a branch of the vaginal artery.

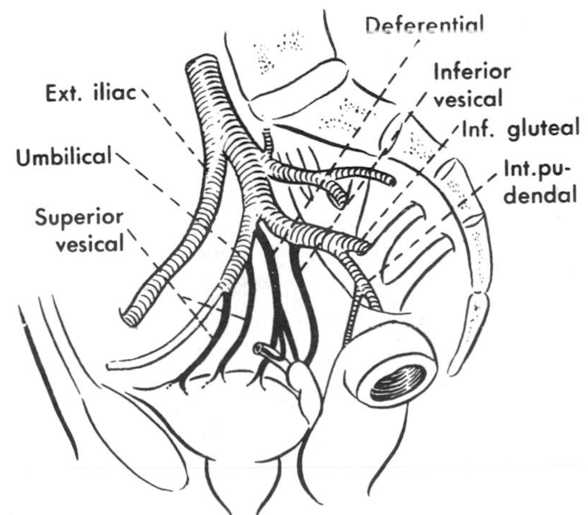

FIGURE 27-28.
Common origins of the chief arteries (*black*) that supply the bladder. (Redrawn from Braithwaite JL. Br J Urol 1952;24:64.)

In the pelvis, the **ureters** receive one or more arterial branches. There may be a branch from the common iliac artery, as the ureter crosses the pelvic brim, or from the internal iliac artery within the pelvis. A rather regular branch to the ureter is given off by the artery to the ductus deferens or by a vesical artery. This branch enters the ureter close to the bladder.

The **arteries of the prostate** are derived from the inferior vesical, middle rectal, and internal pudendal arteries.

The veins of the bladder, urethra, and prostate form fairly dense venous plexuses in the fascial sheaths. The **prostatic venous plexus** lies lateral to the gland and receives the dorsal vein of the penis. Superiorly, the prostatic plexus joins the **vesical venous plexus** around the neck of the bladder. The venous drainage from the plexuses is, in general, laterally and posteriorly along the inferior vesical arteries into the internal iliac veins. There is usually also some venous drainage anterolaterally into the lower ends of the external iliac veins. The internal iliac veins communicate freely with the veins draining the vertebral column and the coxal bone, explaining the metastases of prostatic carcinoma to the coxal bone and the rest of the vertebral column.

The female lacks a prostatic plexus, and the dorsal vein of the clitoris drains into the vesical plexus. This plexus drains, as in the male, into the internal iliac vein directly, but is also united to the vaginal plexus; therefore, it is drained, in part, by the uterine veins. Pelvic cancer in the female spreads primarily along lymphatics.

The **lymphatic drainage** of much **of the bladder** is laterally and upward across the pelvic brim into *external* and *common iliac nodes*. Some of the drainage is more posterior, into *internal iliac nodes* situated along the branches of these vessels, and these, in turn, drain into the common iliac nodes. In the female, some of the lymphatics of the bladder unite with vaginal and uterine lymphatics and drain to the internal iliac and sacral nodes, but others drain laterally into the iliac nodes as in the male.

The **lymphatic drainage of the prostate** is similar to that of the bladder, with which its lymphatics communicate. The prostatic lymphatics begin largely or entirely in the capsule of the prostate, not in the prostatic tissue. This may explain why metastases from the prostate are more likely to pass along veins than along lymphatics.

Innervation

The **vesical** and **prostatic nerve plexuses** are forward extensions of the inferior hypogastric plexus. In the female, the *vesical plexus* is less distinct, because it merges with the larger, *uterovaginal plexus* (to be described later).

The parasympathetic fibers in the vesical plexus are involved in reflex emptying of the bladder, but the role and even the distribution of the sympathetic fibers are disputed. It has been both claimed and denied that sympathetic fibers end only on the blood vessels and the trigonal muscle, rather than on the detrusor muscle. However, certain experimental evidence, including pharmacologic data, seems to indicate that the old and generally discarded concept that sympathetic innervation relaxes the detrusor may be true after all.

The prostatic musculature, as that of other parts of the genital duct system, is apparently innervated by sympathetic and not by parasympathetic efferents. Sympathetic excitation produces contraction of the smooth muscle of the gland, emptying the prostatic secretions into the urethra during ejaculation.

The **deferential plexus** around the ductus deferens is an offshoot of the vesical plexus. It leaves the pelvis along the deferent duct.

Some fibers of the prostatic plexus accompany the urethra through the urogenital hiatus into the perineum to the erectile bodies of the penis; these are the cavernous nerves. Similar nerves to the clitoris and bulb of the vestibule are derived from the vesical plexus in the female.

Visceral afferents from the bladder and the prostate are believed to reach the sacral spinal cord segments through the pelvic splanchnic nerves.

Neural Control of Micturition. Urine will flow from the bladder through the urethra when the vesical pressure is higher than urethral resistance. Contraction of the detrusor muscle is the usual way in which vesical pressure is raised. Although a few workers insist that the once widely held concept of voluntary control over the autonomic system innervating the bladder is valid, much evidence indicates that it is the somatic nerves that supply the voluntary muscles related to the bladder that start and stop micturition. The part of the pelvic diaphragm that directly supports the vesical neck (pubococcygeus) relaxes so that the vesical neck moves downward. This apparently decreases the resistance in the urethra and at the same time reflexly increases the activity of the detrusor, allowing urine to flow freely if the vesical pressure is high enough. If it is not, it can be increased by voluntary contraction of the abdominal muscles and the diaphragm. Cessation of urination is then brought about by contraction of the pubococcygeus. The voluntary muscle around the urethra (sphincter urethrae) is thought to relax and contract with the pelvic diaphragm, but is not generally considered to be essential to voluntary control.

In support of this concept, it has been claimed that malfunction of the pelvic diaphragm is a cause of loss of urinary control. Spasm of the diaphragm, for instance, has been said to be responsible for the urinary retention that complicates rectal operations. Similarly, it has been shown in women that strengthening the muscles of the pelvic outlet by exercise will often cure urinary incontinence, indicating that it is voluntary rather than involuntary muscle that primarily controls the emptying of the bladder.

The Male Genital Ducts

The ductuli efferentes and the epididymis and its duct are described in Chapter 26, and the ductus deferens is traced as far as the deep inguinal ring. The male genital ducts in the pelvis include the pelvic portions of the deferent ducts, the seminal vesicles, and the ejaculatory ducts.

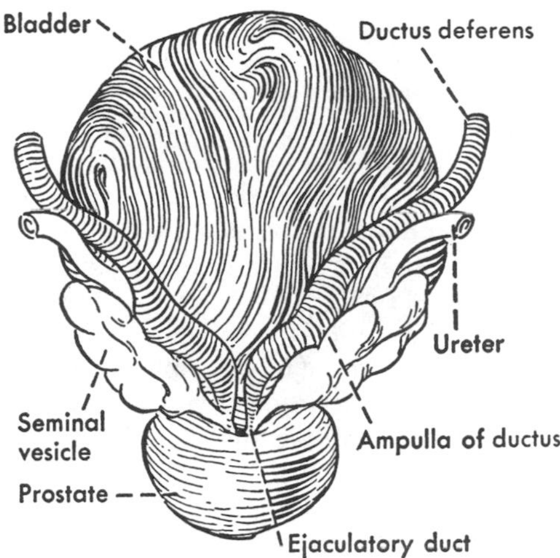

FIGURE *27-29.*
Posterior view of the bladder, prostate, and seminal vesicles.

The Ductus Deferens

The ductus, more commonly known by clinicians as the *vas deferens*, enters the abdominal cavity through the deep inguinal ring. At this ring, it leaves the testicular vessels by turning medially, soon passing the brim of the pelvis and running downward and backward along the lateral pelvic wall (see Fig. 27-22). In so doing, it enters the lateral ligaments of the bladder, crosses above and medial to the ureter, and turns medially to converge with the other ductus on the posterior aspect of the bladder (Figs. 27-29 and 27-30). It is retroperitoneal throughout its course.

Beyond the point of crossing the ureter, the ductus deferens enlarges to form the **ampulla.** The ampullae of the two ducts come close together in the midline, then each suddenly narrows, before uniting with the duct of the seminal vesicle to form the ejaculatory duct (see Figs. 27-27 and 27-29).

The Seminal Vesicles

Each seminal vesicle is a nearly 15-cm–long blind tube, folded upon itself. The coils of the tube are held together by connective tissue; therefore, each seminal vesicle appears as a compact, elongated, oval body less than a third of the length of its tube. Its coils give the vesicle a lobulated appearance (see Figs. 27-27, 27-29, and 27-30). The distal end of the duct of the seminal vesicle becomes narrow and, together with the ductus deferens, forms the ejaculatory duct. The secretions of the epithelium of the vesicle are discharged into the ejaculate by the contraction of the muscular walls of the vesicle. This adds fructose to the seminal plasma, necessary for maintaining the motility of the spermatozoa. Spermatozoa are stored in the ampulla, the ductus, and the epididymis, but not in the seminal vesicle.

The seminal vesicles lie below and lateral to the ampullae of the deferent ducts, resting against the base of the bladder (see Fig. 27-29). Posteriorly, both they and the ampullae of the ducts are separated from the rectum by the rectovesical fascia (see Fig. 27-4).

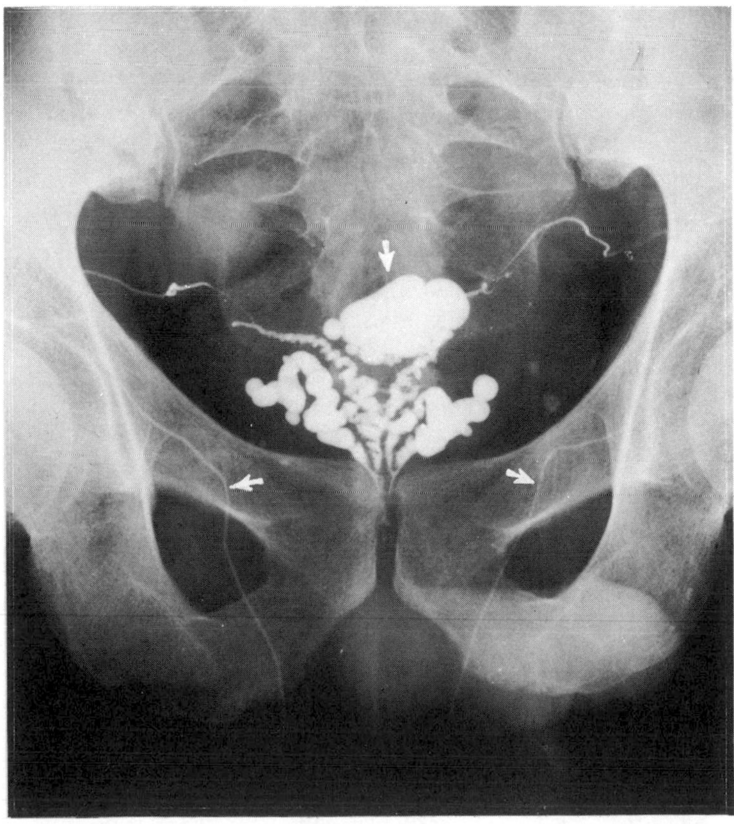

FIGURE *27-30.*
The genital duct system in the male: Both deferent ducts were injected with radiopaque material and show particularly well where they cross the pubes (*lateral arrows*) and their pelvic course. The larger convoluted lumina, as the two ducts converge, are the ampullary parts of the ducts; the still larger convoluted structures *lateral* to these are the seminal vesicles. On the *reader's right*, the junction of the ductus deferens and the seminal vesicle, and the origin of the ejaculatory duct at this junction, can be seen. Some of the injected medium has entered the bladder (*middle arrow*). (Braasch WF, Emmett JL. Clinical urography. Philadelphia: WB Saunders, 1951.)

The Ejaculatory Ducts

The thin-walled ejaculatory ducts are about 2 cm long. They taper from their origins to their termination and are about 0.5 mm in diameter when they end. They converge toward each other as they run through the prostate between the median and lateral lobes, so that they open close together on the colliculus seminalis just lateral to the utriculus (see Fig. 27-27).

Blood Vessels, Lymphatics, and Nerves

Close to its lower end, the ductus deferens receives the *deferential artery*, which is derived from the umbilical artery. It follows the duct to the testis. The seminal vesicles receive their blood supply from the deferential and inferior vesical arteries and often also receive branches from the middle rectal arteries.

The **veins** of the seminal vesicles join the vesical plexus of veins, and the **lymphatics** join those of the prostate and bladder.

The **innervation** of the smooth muscle of the seminal vesicles, deferent ducts, and ejaculatory ducts, similar to that of the prostate, is apparently exclusively by sympathetic fibers. Ejaculation is a function of the sympathetic nervous system. Unlike the testis, which receives its nerve supply from a higher level along the testicular artery, the nerve fibers in the *deferential plexus* are derived from the pelvic plexus and the superior hypogastric plexus.

Lumbar sympathectomy may interfere with ejaculation, either because it eliminates the efferent input into the plexus or because it affects the functional vesical sphincter, permitting the semen to be discharged from the prostatic urethra into the bladder rather than into the membranous and spongy urethra (retrograde ejaculation).

The Ovary and the Derivatives of the Female Genital Ducts

The ovary is the female gonad: its function is the production of ova and the secretion of estrogen and progesterone. Through these hormones, the ovary influences the cyclic maturation and discharge of the ova and the development and maintenance of the secondary female sex organs and secondary somatic sex characteristics of the female phenotype. Furthermore, these hormones establish the requirements for implantation of the embryo and maintain those necessary for retention of the embryo and fetus in the uterine cavity until the time of birth. As recounted in Chapter 23, the ova are transported to the uterus by the uterine tubes, which communicate with the peritoneal cavity. The uterine cavity communicates, in turn, with the vagina through the cervical canal. The uterus, its tubes, and the ovaries are associated with the *broad ligament*, which, acting as a mesentery, suspends the uterine tubes and the ovaries from the pelvic floor (Fig. 27-31).

The Ovary

Each ovary (*ovarium*) is a firm, almond-shaped organ, about 3 cm long, 1.5 cm wide, and 1 cm thick. Its surface, devoid of peritoneum, is smooth until puberty; thereafter, the scars left by the degenerating corpora lutea (discussed later) render it somewhat irregular.

The ovary is suspended from the posterior lamina of the broad ligament by its own mesentery, the *mesovarium*, and is embraced anteriorly and laterally by the uterine tube (Fig. 27-32). It is quite mobile, and its position in the pelvic portion of the peritoneal cavity may vary. However, in the young, nulliparous woman, the ovary lies against the lateral pelvic wall (see Fig. 27-36), held there by its suspensory ligament (see Fig. 27-31). It has a lateral and medial surface, a mesovarian and a free border, and a tubal and uterine extremity, or pole.

The *lateral surface* lies against the parietal peritoneum of the pelvic wall in the *ovarian fossa*, a depression bordered by the internal iliac artery and the ureter. In the fossa, the ovary is related to the obturator nerve and vessels. Its **medial surface** faces toward the pararectal fossae and the rectouterine pouch and is in contact with loops of bowel.

To appreciate the peritoneal and ligamentous attachments of the ovary, it needs to be lifted from its fossa and gently pulled upon. The fimbriated lateral end of the uterine tube is tethered to the pole of the ovary that points laterally and upward; hence, this pole is called its *tubal extremity* (see Figs. 27-31 and 27-32). This extremity is connected to the pelvic brim by the **suspensory ligament of the ovary,** a peritoneal fold draped over the ovarian vessels and nerves, representing the lateral continuation of the broad ligament beyond the uterine tube (see Figs. 27-31 and 27-32). The opposite pole of the ovary, pointing toward the uterus and downward, is its *uterine extremity*. This is attached to the uterus in the inferior angle of the uterotubal junction by a fibromuscular band, the **ligament of the ovary** (see Fig. 27-32). This ligament is within the broad ligament and raises a ridge in its posterior lamina.

The **mesovarium,** a reduplication of the posterior lamina of the broad ligament, is attached along the anterior, or *mesovarian, border* of the ovary (Fig. 27-33). The mesovarium contains the vessels and nerves of the ovary, which enter and leave the organ through its hilum, to which the mesovarium is attached.

Development and Structure. The ovary, as does the testis, develops in the urogenital ridges; during their initial phase of development, the two gonads are indistinguishable (see Fig. 25-29). The proliferation of celomic mesothelium forms the cortex of the ovary; its more vascular medulla is derived from the mesenchyme of the intermediate mesoderm. Primordial germ cells, derived from the yolk sac, invade the cortex. There they will develop into oogonia and oocytes, surrounded by cells of the cortex, which form a follicle around each developing egg.

The outer surface of the ovary is devoid of peritoneum. The so-called *germinal epithelium* (which

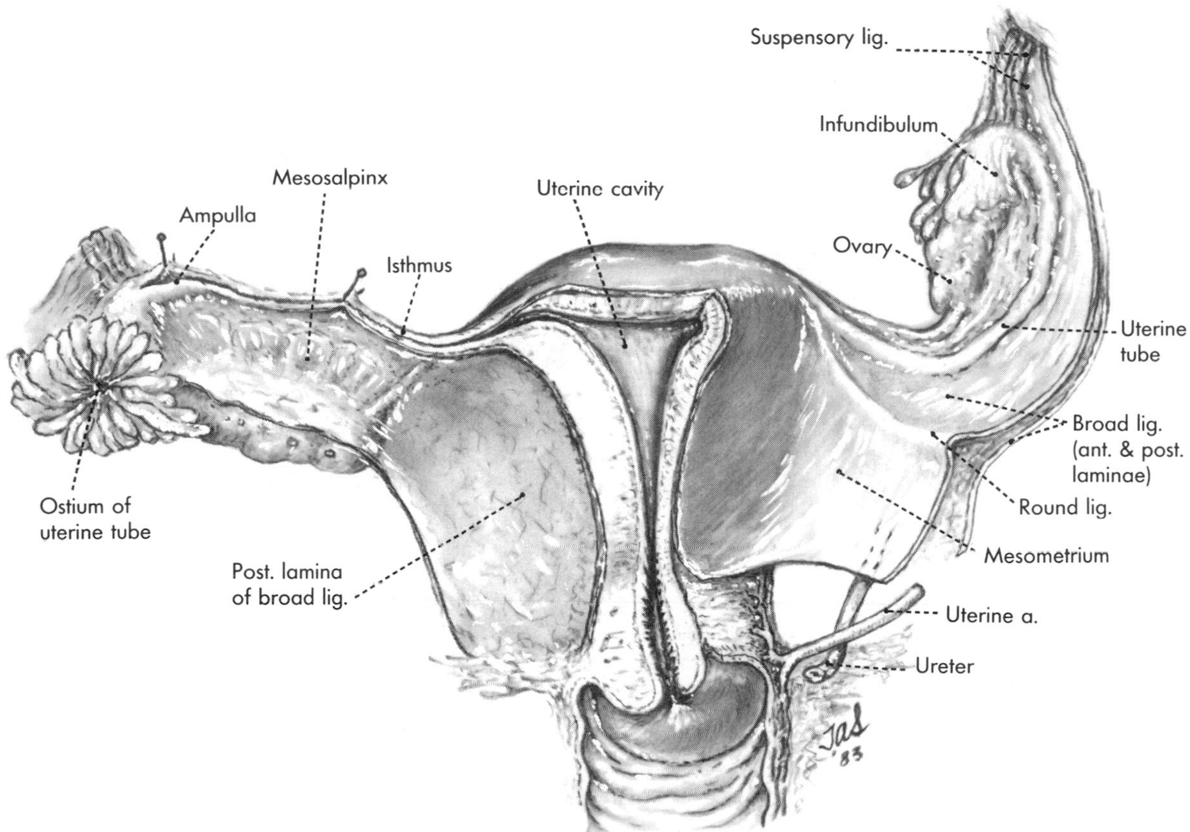

FIGURE 27-31.
The uterus and its adnexa viewed the front: The anterior leaf of the right broad ligament has been resected with the anterior wall of the uterus and uterine tube. (Adapted from Blandau RJ. The female reproductive system. In: Weiss I, ed. Histology: cell and tissue biology. 5th ed. New York; Elsevier Biomedical, 1983.)

does not give rise to oocytes) merges with the mesovarian mesothelium along the mesovarian border of the ovary. Subjacent to the germinal epithelium is the *tunica albuginea*, a collagenous stratum that surrounds the cortex and is breached by the *ovarian follicles* as they mature, enlarge, and burst on the surface of the ovary. The cortex contains such follicles in various stages of maturation. After the discharge of the ovum from the follicle (ovulation), the follicular cells are transformed into the *corpus luteum*, a yellow, glandular body that persists through most of pregnancy if the ovum has been fertilized and implantation has occurred. Otherwise, the corpus luteum degenerates before the next ovulation. A

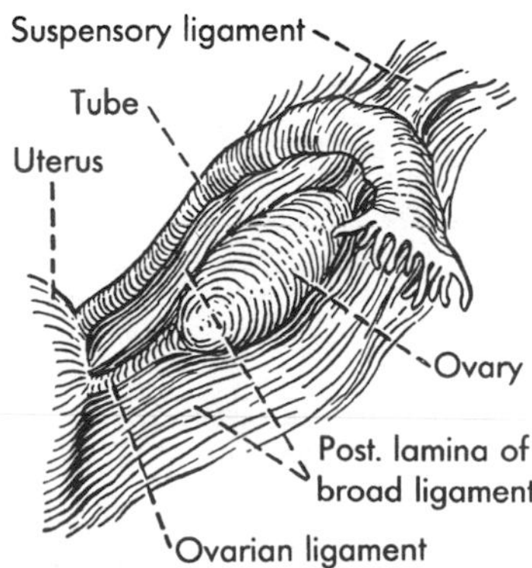

FIGURE 27-32.
The right ovary seen from behind.

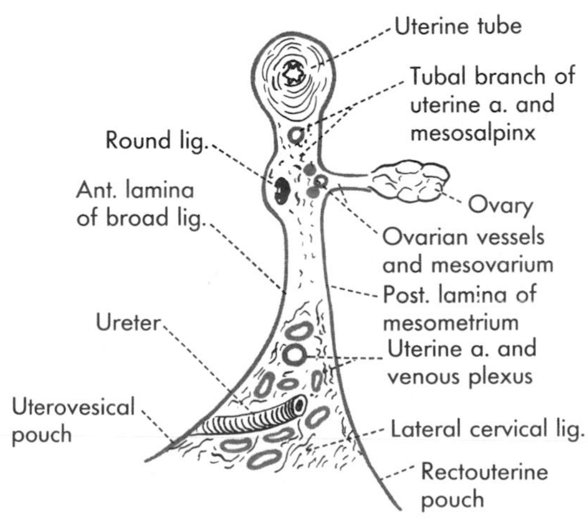

FIGURE 27-33.
A schematic sagittal section across the broad ligament, uterine tube, and ovary.

degenerated corpus luteum forms a small fibrosed body called a *corpus albicans,* also located in the ovarian cortex.

The Uterine Tube

The uterine tubes (*tuba uterina, salpinx uterina*), also known as fallopian tubes, are the bilateral ducts that extend from the uterus to the ovary and connect the uterine cavity to the peritoneal cavity (Figs. 27-34 and 27-35). Each tube is about 10 cm long and is almost completely surrounded by peritoneum along the superior margin of the broad ligament as the anterior and posterior laminae of the ligament become continuous with one another around the tube (see Fig. 27-33). The part of the broad ligament between the tube and the base of the mesovarium is called the **mesosalpinx.** The lateral part of the tube arches over the lateral pole of the ovary and turns posteriorly (Fig. 21-36; see Fig. 37-32). Its trumpet-shaped, expanded open end becomes closely applied to the ovary.

Parts. Four parts are recognizable on each tube: the infundibulum, the ampulla, the isthmus, and the uterine part (see Fig. 27-34). The **infundibulum** is the funnel- or trumpet-shaped lateral expansion of the tube (*infundibulum* meaning funnel; *salpinx* meaning trumpet). The wide circumference of the infundibulum presents numerous fingerlike processes called **fimbriae,** one of which, the *ovarian fimbria,* is attached to the ovary. The exterior of the infundibulum is completely peritoneal, but the internal surface of the fimbriae and the tapering cavity of the tube are covered by highly ciliated columnar epithelium thrown into irregular longitudinal folds that converge toward a small opening, the *abdominal ostium of the tube,* located at the bottom of the infundibulum. The **ampulla,** succeeding the infundibulum, is wide, thin-walled, and tortuous. It leads into the more narrow **isthmus.** The **uterine part of the tube,** also called the *intramural part,* traverses the thick uterine wall and, through the *uterine ostium* (or *uterotubal junction*), opens into the uterine cavity.

The uterine tube has a narrow lumen that is filled by the highly complex folds of its ciliated mucosa. Nevertheless, the patency of the tubes can be tested, as it is done in investigations of infertility, by filling the uterine cavity with radiopaque contrast medium through the cervix and

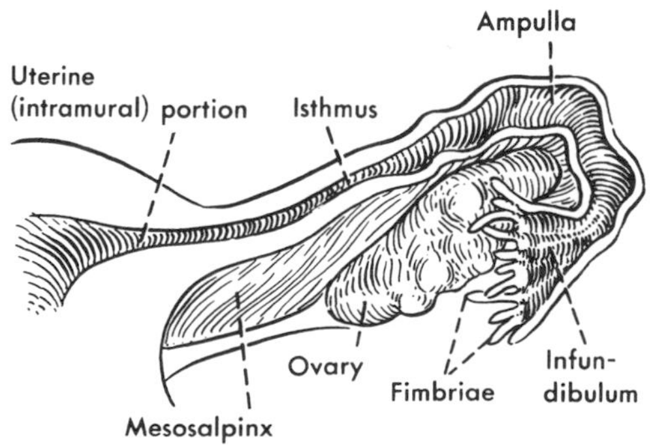

FIGURE *27-34.*
The right uterine tube, opened from behind.

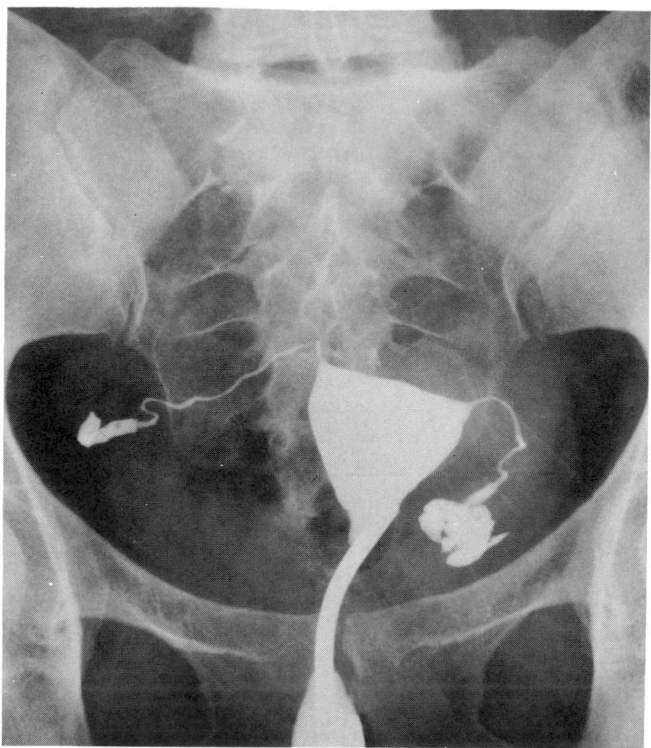

FIGURE *27-35.*
A uterosalpingogram: The catheter through which the radiopaque material has been injected extends through the vagina into the cavity of the body of the uterus; to the *left* of the upper part of the catheter can be seen part of the cavity of the isthmus and cervix. Both uterine tubes are clearly visualized, and from that on the *reader's right,* radiopaque material has entered the peritoneal cavity. (Courtesy of Dr. R. B. Wilson.)

observing on x-ray film the spillage of the medium into the peritoneal cavity through the tubes (see Fig. 27-35). This procedure is known as salpingography. In addition to the mucosa, the wall of the tube has the usual layers of submucosa, muscularis, and serosa.

Gamete Transport. The function of the uterine tubes in coordinating egg and sperm transport for fertilization to take place is highly complex and incompletely understood. Although there is evidence that an ovum discharged from one ovary can be transported through the peritoneal cavity and picked up by the uterine tube of the opposite side, under normal circumstances, ovum transport is less hazardous. The fimbriae are usually closely applied to the surface of the ovary. Aided by muscular contractions of the tube and the ligaments (all of which contain smooth muscle), the fimbriated infundibulum appears to sweep the surface of the ovary. The ovum discharged from the ripe follicle is surrounded by the *cumulus oophorus,* an aggregation of several thousand follicular cells held together around the egg rather tenaciously. The cilia of the fimbriae can effectively grasp the cumulus, and it may, in fact, be difficult to pull the cumulus away from the fimbriae with a pair of forceps. Thus, it is an irregular mass of cells, rather than a naked egg, that is swept into the abdominal ostium of the uterine tube.

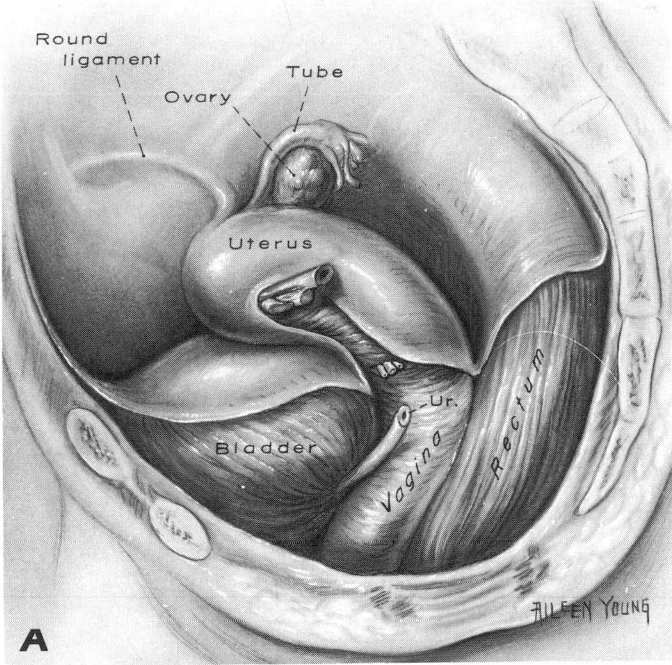

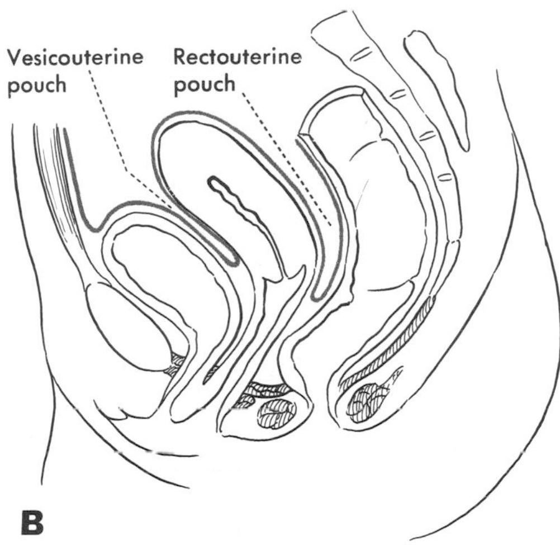

FIGURE 27-36.
(A) Pelvic viscera in the female: The cut edges of peritoneum indicate the reflection to the lateral pelvic wall. *Ur* is the left ureter. At the base of the broad ligament, above the ureter, are the stumps of the uterine vessels as they enter the uterus. Between the cut edges of the leaves of the uppermost part of the broad ligament are stumps of the left uterine tube, of the ovarian ligament just below this, and of the round ligament just anterior to the ovarian ligament. (B) A diagrammatic sagittal section of the female pelvis.

The cilia carry the cumulus to the ampulla, where the egg is liberated from the cumulus and its progress along the tube is held up for some time awaiting fertilization.

The passage of spermatozoa along the uterine and isthmic parts of the tube is believed to be aided by the muscular activity of the tube itself. Normally, fertilization takes place in the ampulla, and the descent of the fertilized egg into the uterus is delayed for about 3 days, during which several cell divisions occur. The conceptus then enters the uterus as a morula (a solid ball of cells) and completes its development into a blastocyst while lying free in the uterine cavity, a process that takes another 3 to 4 days. Thus, there is a delay of 6 to 7 days between fertilization and implantation. The factors responsible for this delay, necessary both for the completion of blastocyst development and for the uterine mucosa to become receptive to the conceptus, remain unknown.

Interference with the timing of this mechanism may result in the implantation of the conceptus in the tube (**tubal ectopic pregnancy),** inevitably leading to rupture of the tube, a major emergency. Should the fertilized egg be transported into the peritoneal cavity rather than the uterus, or should the egg be fertilized in the peritoneal cavity, an **abdominal ectopic pregnancy** may result. The embryo and fetus may develop outside the uterus and have to be delivered by laparotomy.

The most common cause of **infertility** in women is blockage of the uterine tubes. This usually results from pelvic inflammatory disease, often a consequence of the spread of infection along the initially patent tubes into the pelvis. Surgical interruption of the tubes is the procedure for permanent sterilization, a not infrequent method of contraception. The tubes are doubly ligated and divided between the two ligatures. Reanastomosis of the tubes and reestablishment of fertility has been achieved with microsurgical techniques.

The Uterus

The uterus, or womb, is the organ of gestation. It is a somewhat pear-shaped, hollow organ, slightly flattened anteroposteriorly (Fig. 27-37). Its thick muscular walls enclose a slitlike cavity, the triangular anterior and posterior walls of which are essentially in contact with one another (see Fig. 27-35).

The uterus is located behind the bladder and in front of the rectum, entirely below the plane of the pelvic brim. The vertical length of the uterus is about 8 cm. Its broadest part, between the attachment of the uterine tubes, measures 5 cm, and its anteroposterior thickness is about half that much. During pregnancy, the uterus undergoes an astonishing degree of enlargement. This involves hypertrophy of its walls, ligaments, and peritoneal coverings, as well as the growth of the vessels and nerves associated with it. No less astonishing is the involution of the organ after parturition.

Parts. The upper, broad, piriform part of the uterus

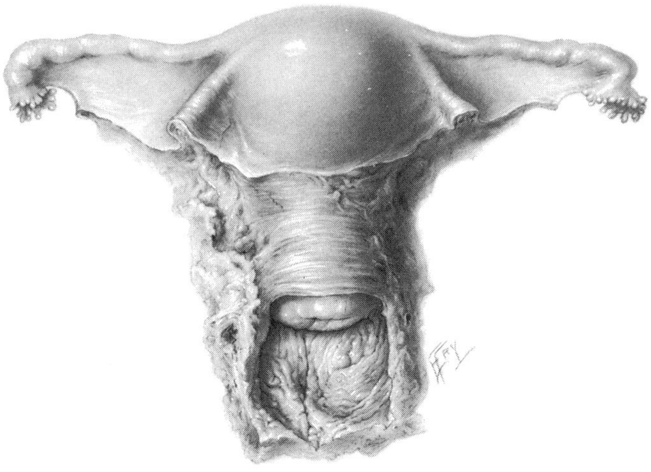

FIGURE 27-37.
Anterior view of the uterus and upper part of the vagina: Parts of the broad ligaments, enclosing the tubes and the upper ends of the round ligaments, have been left on the sides, and the vagina has been opened to show the lower end of the cervix uteri. Note the subperitoneal pelvic connective tissue (parametrium) along the side of the uterus and in between the laminae of the broad ligament.

is its **corpus,** or *body*; a narrow, more cylindrical inferior portion is the *neck*, or **cervix.** The dome-shaped part of the body, projecting above the level of the entrance of the uterine tubes, is the *fundus*. The tapering inferior part of the body leads into the cervix; the cervix projects into the vagina through the anterior wall of its vault, which demarcates the *supravaginal* and *vaginal parts of the cervix*. The vaginal lumen surrounding the cervix is called the **fornices of the vagina.** The lower part of the body adjoining the supravaginal cervix is designated as the **isthmus,** or the *lower uterine segment* (Fig. 27-38).

The posterior surface of the body and supravaginal cervix is covered with peritoneum and is convex (Fig. 27-39; see Fig. 27-36). It is in contact with coils of intestine; hence, it is called its intestinal surface. The concave anterior surface is peritoneal only as far down as the cervix; both peritoneal and bare parts are related to the bladder, and this surface, therefore, is called the *vesical surface of the uterus* (see Fig. 27-36). The rounded right and left borders give attachment to the two laminae of the broad ligament and superiorly receive the uterine tubes (see Figs. 27-36 and 27-39). The part of the broad ligament adjacent to the borders of the uterus is called the **mesometrium.**

Uterine Cavity. The triangular cavity of the uterus which, in comparison with the size of the organ, is surprisingly small, receives the uterine ostia of the uterine tubes and leads inferiorly through the **internal os** into the cervical canal (see Figs. 27-35 and 27-38). The **cervical canal** is somewhat spindle-shaped; it opens through the **external os** (*ostium uteri*) into the superior part of the vagina. The external os is a transverse slit guarded by the broad anterior and posterior lips, or the *labia of the cervix*.

The lumen of the cervical canal is normally filled by a viscous mucous plug, the consistency of which changes during the menstrual cycle. The strands of mucus are stabilized in the canal by the *palmate folds* of the cervical mucosa, which interlock as they project into the canal from its anterior and posterior walls. The cervical canal remains closed during pregnancy until the second stage of labor, and its premature dilation is a sign of imminent abortion. The isthmus, on the other hand, becomes dilated rather early in pregnancy and is incorporated into the expanding uterine cavity.

Orientation. The body of the uterus is normally bent anteriorly on the cervix. This relation is spoken of as *anteflexion*. The axis of the cervix is likewise bent forward on the axis of the vagina, so that the external os faces the posterior wall of the vagina. This relation is called *anteversion* of the uterus. Because of the anteversion, the depth of the posterior vaginal fornix is much greater than that of the anterior or lateral fornices.

The factors responsible for anteflexion are intrinsic to the fibromuscular walls of the uterine body and cervix. The factors responsible for anteversion are not completely understood, but probably relate to the pull exerted on the cervix by the rectouterine ligaments. A full bladder tends to eliminate to some degree the angles of both anteflexion and anteversion. Permanent reversal of these angles, called retroflexion and retroversion, has been suspected as a cause of infertility.

Structure. The mucous membrane lining the uterine cavity, called **endometrium**, is covered by a columnar, largely nonciliated epithelium. Its invaginations form simple glands extending into the cellular and vascular *endometrial stroma*. The cervical canal is lined by columnar cells; however, the exterior of the vaginal cervix facing into the fornices is covered by stratified squamous epithelium. The cervical glands secrete the cervical mucus.

During each *menstrual cycle*, the endometrium undergoes cyclic changes and is shed, with a variable quantity of blood; this constitutes the menstrual flow. The mucosa of the uterine tubes and the cervical canal are not shed.

The tunica muscularis, or **myometrium**, is more than a centimeter thick over most of the organ. It consists of interlacing bundles of smooth muscle, divisible into external, intermediate, and internal laminae, but these are rather indistinct. The smooth muscle is intermixed with fibrous and elastic tissue; fibrous tissue predominates in the cervix. The visceral pelvic fascia on the exterior of the body and cervix is called the **parametrium** and **paracervix,** respectively (*metra* is a Greek word meaning uterus). The paracervix is dense and continuous with the supporting ligaments of the uterus (see Fig. 27-37). The peritoneal covering of the uterus constitutes its serosa and reflects from its lateral borders as the **mesometrium,** the medial part of the broad ligament. The cervix is devoid of serosa, except for the supravaginal part posteriorly, where it forms the anterior wall of the rectouterine pouch.

Ligaments. Three types of ligaments are associated

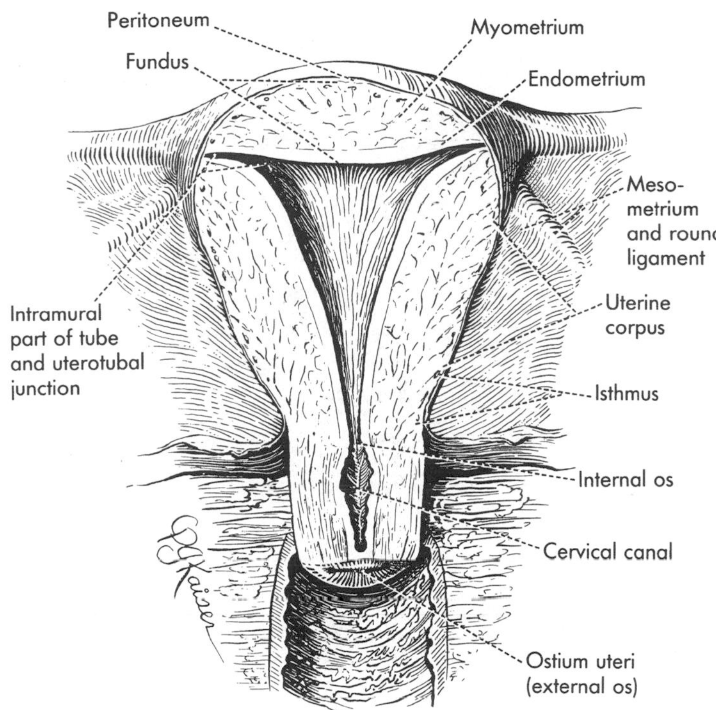

FIGURE *27-38.*
A coronal section of the uterus to show its parts.

with the uterus: a peritoneal ligament, two fibromuscular ligaments derived from the genitoinguinal ligament, and several ligaments formed by condensations of subperitoneal pelvic connective tissue.

The peritoneal ligament of the uterus is the **broad ligament**, consisting of three named parts: mesometrium,

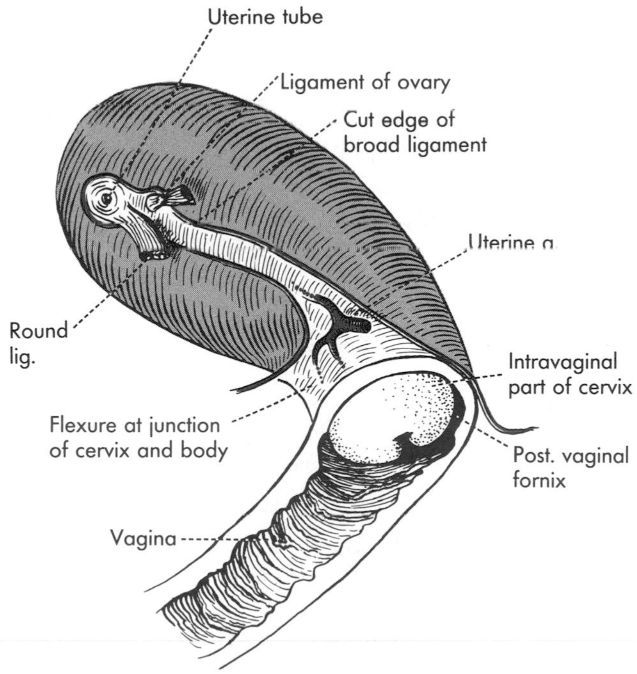

FIGURE *27-39.*
The uterus seen from the left side to show the relation of the cervix to the vagina. Note the relation of the peritoneum to the cervix and vagina anteriorly and posteriorly.

mesosalpinx, and mesovarium (see Figs. 27-31 and 27-33). Each has been described in preceding sections of this chapter.

The broad ligament is derived from the *urogenital mesentery* which, after the regression of the mesonephros and its duct in the female, supports the paramesonephric ducts and the ovary (see Fig. 25-29). It contains the vestiges of the mesonephric ducts, the epoophoron and its duct, the paraoophoron, and the duct of Gärtner, as well as the derivatives of the genitoinguinal ligament and blood vessels and nerves that supply the ovary, uterus, and uterine tubes.

The two broad ligaments, with the uterus between them, form a transverse septum in the pelvic part of the peritoneal cavity. The anterior lamina becomes continuous at the base of the ligament with the parietal peritoneum of the paravesical fossae; these fossae communicate with each other through the uterovesical pouch. The posterior lamina becomes continuous, at the base of the ligament, with the parietal peritoneum of the rectouterine folds and the pararectal fossae, which communicate with each other through the rectouterine pouch (Fig. 27-40). The base of the ligament is some distance above the pelvic diaphragm, and just below it run the lateral cervical ligaments, with the uterine vessels and the ureter embedded in them.

A transverse mesenterial septum, such as is formed by the broad ligament, is lacking in the male pelvis, because the descent of the male gonad into the scrotum and the regression of the paramesonephric ducts eliminate the urogenital mesentery in the male.

The **derivatives of the genitoinguinal ligament** in the female are the *ligament of the ovary* and the *round ligament of the uterus*. Both attach to the uterus (see Figs. 27-31

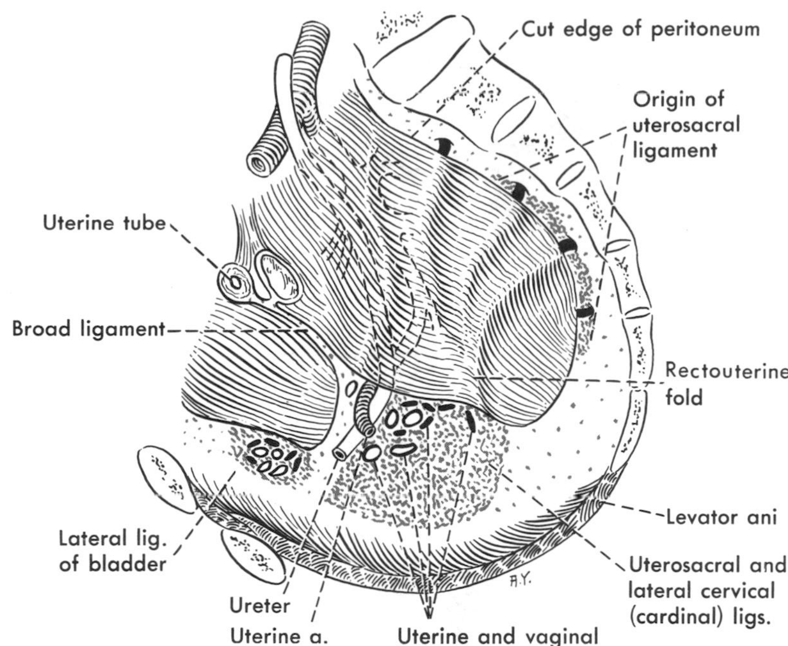

FIGURE 27-40.
Schema of the lateral cervical, or cardinal, and uterosacral ligaments in a section of the pelvis lateral to the uterus: The subperitoneal tissue that constitutes the ligaments is in *blue*. The course of the ureter and of some branches of the internal iliac artery is indicated by *broken lines*.

and 27-32). As already described, the ovarian ligament runs in the broad ligament from the uterine pole of the ovary to attach to the inferior angle of the uterotubal junction (see Fig. 27-32). The forward continuation of the ovarian ligament from its uterine attachment is the **round ligament of the uterus** (*ligamentum teres uteri*; see Figs. 27-31 and 27-39). The ligament raises a ridge in the anterior lamina of the broad ligament and in the floor of the paravesical fossa as it runs retroperitoneally from the uterotubal junction to enter the deep inguinal ring (see Fig. 27-36). Its fate in the inguinal canal has already been described (see Chap. 26).

Uterine **ligaments formed by pelvic fascia** occupy a pyramidal space on the lateral side of the cervix, bordered above by pelvic peritoneum and below by the sloping muscular pelvic floor (see Fig. 27-40). The ligaments that can be defined in this mass of connective tissue are continuous medially with the *paracervix*, the dense fascial sheath around the supravaginal part of the cervix, and the upper part of the vagina. Peripherally, they attach to the pelvic walls (see Fig. 27-7).

The posterior ligament of this mass of connective tissue is contained in the uterosacral folds and is called the *uterosacral ligament*, attached posteriorly more to the sacrum than to the rectum. Smooth muscle contained in these ligaments makes up the *rectouterine muscle*. The dense connective tissue below the base of the broad ligament is described as the *lateral cervical ligament*, also called by gynecologists Mackenrodt's ligaments or *cardinal ligaments of the uterus*, implying their importance in support of the uterus. Anteriorly, the *pubocervical ligaments* connect the cervix to the posterior surface of the pubes.

Support. It is believed that the tension of these ligaments keeps the uterus suspended in the pelvic cavity. It is also thought that the uterosacral ligaments are responsible for anteversion of the uterus. Although both pelvic and urogenital diaphragms are involved in the support of the uterus, stretching or tearing of the ligaments of the cervix is probably an important factor in producing prolapse. **Prolapse** is the protrusion of pelvic viscera through the pelvic floor into the vagina. In prolapse of the uterus, the cervix descends in the vagina and may appear at the vaginal orifice or even outside it, everting the vagina. The base of the bladder similarly may prolapse or bulge into the anterior vaginal wall, forming a *cystocele*, or the rectum into the posterior vaginal wall, forming a *rectocele*. A prolapse of the urethra into the anterior vaginal wall is a *urethrocele*.

The treatment of prolapse involves tightening the ligaments of the cervix, especially the lateral cervical ligaments, and repairing other damage, followed by strengthening of the muscles of the pelvic and urogenital diaphragms.

The Vagina

The vagina is the female organ of copulation; the word *vagina* means sheath. The entrance into the vagina (*ostium vaginae*) is in the vestibule between the labia minora and is described with the external genitalia in Chapter 28. The vagina passes upward with a posterior inclination through the urogenital diaphragm and the urogenital hiatus (see Fig. 27-36). Its major part is located in the pelvis, where it terminates by fusing around the cervix of the uterus.

The vagina is about 10 cm long and is greatly distensible. Normally, it is flattened anteroposteriorly, its anterior and posterior walls lying in contact with each other. At the upper end of the vagina, often called the *vaginal vault*, the lumen forms recesses, or *fornices*, around the vaginal part of the cervix. Because of the angle made between the vagina and the cervix, the posterior vaginal wall is longer than the anterior wall and the posterior fornix is deeper than the anterior and lateral fornices.

The anterior wall of the vagina is related to the urethra and the base of the bladder; the urethra is, in essence, embedded in the vaginal wall. The wall of the posterior fornix is covered by peritoneum of the rectouterine pouch, and below that, the vagina is separated from the rectum by the rectovaginal septum (peritoneoperineal septum). Its perineal portion is separated from the anal canal by the *perineal body* (see Fig. 28-9).

Structure. The bulk of the wall of the vagina consists of a tunica muscularis in which smooth muscle and dense connective tissue are mixed. There are many elastic fibers in this connective tissue. The outer part of the vaginal wall is largely connective tissue and contains the vaginal plexus of veins, the vaginal arteries, and the vaginal nerves. The mucosa is thrown into transverse folds (vaginal rugae) and a longitudinal fold called the *vaginal column*, on both the anterior and posterior walls. Its surface epithelium is stratified squamous, which undergoes cyclic changes that can be correlated with the ovarian cycle, but are much less pronounced than in many mammals. Nevertheless, a vaginal smear technique can give some information on the stage of the menstrual cycle. It was the study of vaginal smears that led to the technique of diagnosing early carcinomatous change of the cervix uteri through cervical smears.

Congenital Abnormalities of the Uterus and Vagina

Abnormalities of the paramesonephric ducts and their derivatives may be due to agenesis, noncanalization, and failure of fusion (Fig. 27-41). Failure of fusion of the paramesonephric ducts, the most common group of abnormalities, can result in complete duplication of the uterus and the vagina, or the body of the uterus may be split into two equal parts (bicornuate uterus) with a single or double cervix. The terminal part of one or both of the paramesonephric ducts may fail to canalize and consequently atrophy, resulting in a uterus unicornus or in the absence of the uterus or the uterine tubes or both.

The vagina may be absent because the sinuvaginal bulb failed to develop or the vaginal plate failed to canalize. The external genitalia in such cases may be normal. Incomplete canalization may leave septa in the vagina or result in an abnormally thick hymen. If a normal vagina is absent, an artificial vagina can be constructed surgically by creating a cleavage plane along the rectovesical fascia and lining it with skin.

Faulty development of the urorectal septum may result in rectovaginal fistulae (see Fig. 27-21).

Blood Supply and Lymph Drainage

The blood supply of the uterus and uterine tubes is derived from the uterine artery. This artery also contributes to the supply of the ovary and the vagina, although each of these relies to a large extent on the ovarian and vaginal arteries, respectively. Veins and lymphatics of the female genital tract largely follow the arteries.

Arteries. The blood supply of the uterus is through paired **uterine arteries.** These are branches of the internal iliac artery and run medially toward the uterus close to the upper surface of the lateral ligaments of the cervix along the base of the broad ligament. This connective tissue also contains the uterine veins and a uterovaginal plexus of nerves. The ureter also passes through this tissue, coursing posteroinferior to the uterine artery on its way to the bladder (see Fig. 27-33). Just above the lateral vaginal fornix, the uterine artery approaches the supravaginal part of the cervix as soon as it has crossed the ureter (Fig. 27-42). Here it gives off branches to the cervix and

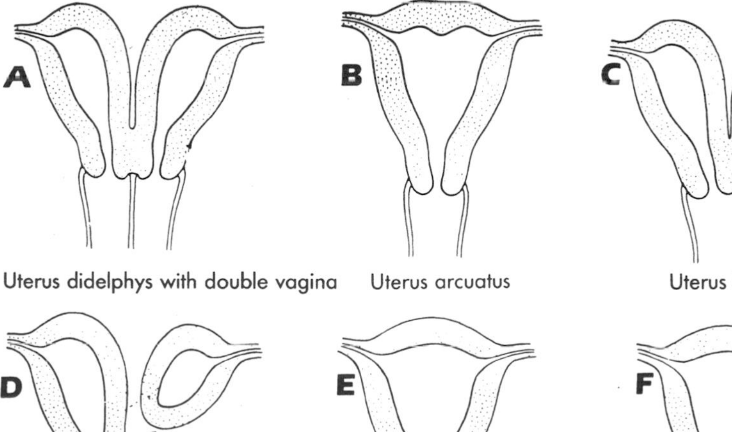

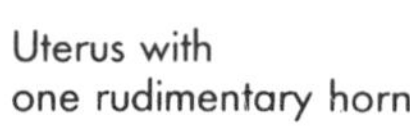

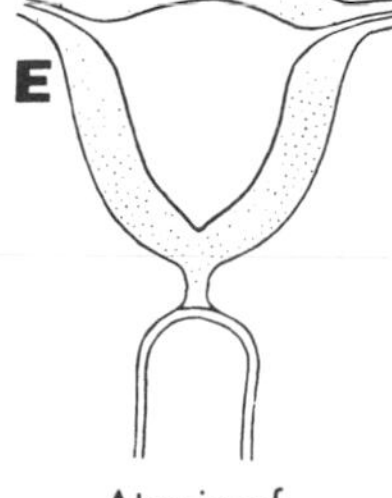

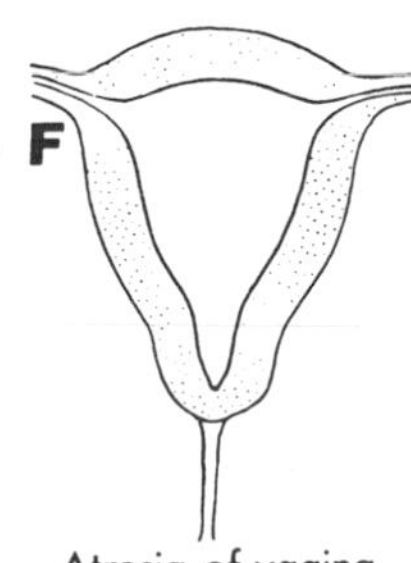

FIGURE *27-41.*
Schematic representation of the main abnormalities of the uterus and vagina, caused by persistence of the uterine septum or obliteration of the lumen of the uterine canal. (Langman J: Medical embryology. 3rd ed. Baltimore: Williams & Wilkins, 1975.)

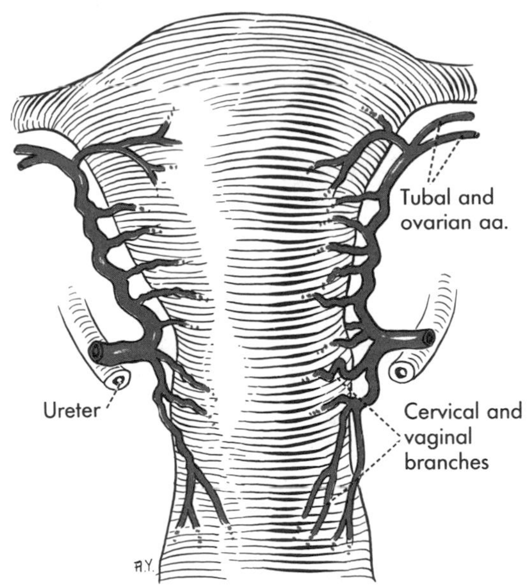

FIGURE 27-42.
The uterine artery.

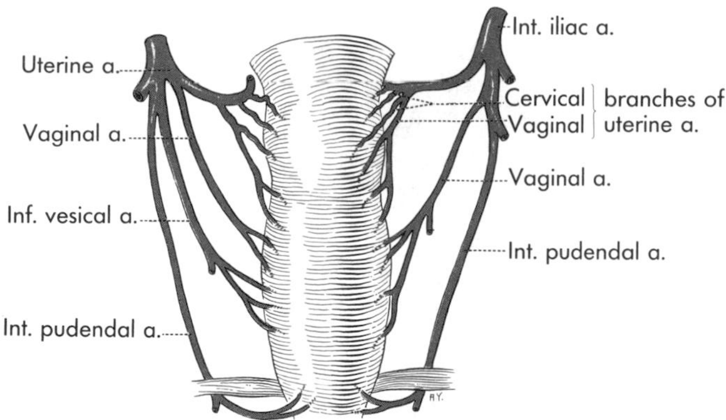

FIGURE 27-44.
Arteries to the vagina. On the *reader's right,* the vaginal artery arises from a stem common to it and other branches of the internal iliac; on the *left,* a vaginal artery arising from the uterine artery is supplemented by a branch arising from the inferior vesical artery, which is distributed mostly to the bladder.

also one or more to the vagina and then turns upward on the lateral aspect of the uterus, either between the leaves of the broad ligament or in the substance of the uterus. A little below the uterine fundus, the artery gives off tubal and ovarian branches, and the remainder of the vessel ends in the fundus.

The **tubal branch** of the uterine artery leaves the uterus close to the attachment of the uterotubal junction and runs laterally in the mesosalpinx to supply the whole length of the tube (Fig. 27-43). The **ovarian branch** enters the uterine pole of the ovary through the mesovarium and supplements the chief supply delivered through the ovarian artery. The **ovarian artery,** described in Chapter 25 as far as the pelvic brim, enters the mesovarium through the suspensory ligament of the ovary. During pregnancy, all these vessels become very much enlarged.

The chief blood supply of the vagina is through **paired vaginal arteries** (Fig. 27-44). These arteries arise from the internal iliac independently or are branches of the uterine arteries. They may be multiple. Branches of the uterine arteries to the cervix uteri help supply the upper part of the vagina. The lower part of the vagina is supplied by branches of the internal pudendal artery.

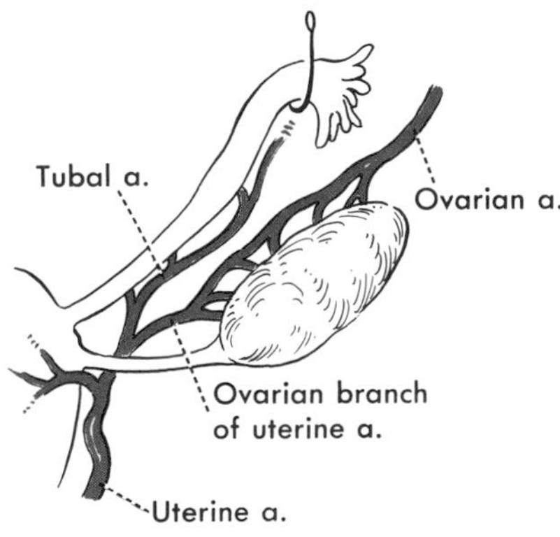

FIGURE 27-43.
The blood supply of the ovary.

Veins. A venous plexus surrounds the vagina and the uterus. These plexuses are located in the fascial sheaths of the organs. Although the **vaginal plexus** has connections with the vesical plexus, for the most part it drains upward into the **uterine plexus**. The uterine plexus also receives the veins from the uterine tubes. The **uterine veins** begin in the uterine plexus and drain laterally, usually as two trunks on each side, and join the internal iliac vein. The **ovarian veins** leave the mesovarium through the suspensory ligaments and ascend to the inferior vena cava on the right and the renal vein on the left.

Lymphatics. The distribution of lymphatics from the **uterus** is particularly important because of the relative frequency of uterine carcinoma, which spreads preferentially along lymphatics. The lymphatics diverge widely and empty into a number of differently situated nodes. A few from the **fundus** and upper part of the body drain along the round ligament into *superficial inguinal nodes* but most of the upper lymphatics pass laterally in the upper parts of the broad ligaments. They unite with lymphatics from the **uterine tube** and **ovary** and pass with the ovarian vessels over the pelvic brim. Instead of ending in iliac nodes at this level, they continue upward along the ovarian vessels and empty into nodes of the lumbar chain close to the level of the renal vessels. The drainage of the **lower part of the body** of the uterus and **cervix,** where carcinoma most frequently originates, is largely to nodes within the pelvis. The lymphatics of the lower part of the body and of the cervix pass laterally in the lower part of the broad ligament. Many end in *internal iliac nodes;* others reach the pelvic brim and end in *external iliac nodes;* still others run posteriorly and medially to empty into *sacral nodes* or nodes associated with the common iliac vessels.

Because of this wide area of lymph drainage from the cervix, successful treatment of cervical carcinoma usually requires resection of the entire uterus (hysterectomy; *ystera*, another Greek name for the uterus) plus thorough dissection of lymph nodes on the pelvic walls and in the inguinal region.

The **lymphatic drainage of the vagina** is in two directions. From about the upper three-fourths, the lymphatics run upward and laterally, joining those of the cervix uteri to empty into *internal iliac nodes*; the lower fourth drains downward to the perineum, and hence, into *superficial inguinal lymph nodes*.

Innervation

A dense **uterovaginal plexus** of nerves passes to the uterus with the uterine vessels through the lateral cervical ligament. The plexus reaches the uterus at about the junction of the cervix and body. The plexus gives off *vaginal nerves* and a particularly abundant supply to the cervix before it turns upward with the uterine artery to supply the rest of the uterus.

The uterovaginal plexus consists primarily of visceral afferent and sympathetic efferent fibers and contains few, if any, parasympathetic efferents. The physiology of the motor supply to the uterus is not understood. Innervation is not necessary to the functions of the uterus, not excepting its contractions during labor.

In contrast with the afferent innervation of most of the pelvic organs, that of the body of the uterus travels from the inferior hypogastric plexus with the sympathetic system through the superior hypogastric and aortic plexuses. Pain fibers from the body of the uterus evidently enter the spinal cord through the last two thoracic nerves. These are the nerves that mediate pain sensation during the first stage of labor, and this pain is referred to the lower thoracic and lumbar region in the back. The elimination of this pain requires that anesthetic be injected into the epidural space or into the thecal sac. This procedure blocks all nerves that leave and enter the lumbar and sacral parts of the spinal cord.

It has long been assumed that pain fibers from the cervix uteri do not follow those from the body; rather they were believed to pass from the inferior hypogastric plexus with the pelvic splanchnic nerves into S-2 to S-4 segments of the cord. Several clinical studies cast doubt on this assumption: paravertebral block of the 11th and 12th thoracic nerves, paravertebral block of the upper lumbar sympathetic trunks, or presacral neurectomy all eliminate pain caused by dilation of the cervix during the first stage of labor. This indicates that pain afferents from the cervix ascend from the inferior hypogastric plexus with pain afferents from the uterine body. Pain caused by dilation of the cervix may also be blocked by injecting anesthetic around the *paracervical plexus of nerves* (the uterovaginal plexus) through the lateral fornices of the vagina. Such a paracervical block is effective also when the cervix has to be dilated artificially for scraping out the uterus. The cervix, similar to the vagina, is insensitive to cutting and burning; pain is caused only by its dilation.

Nothing particularly is known of **nerves to the uterine tubes.** Presumably, they are derived from the uterovaginal plexus of nerves and from the ovarian plexus.

The **vaginal nerves** are mostly from the uterovaginal plexus, but little is known concerning their physiology. Presumably, most of the pain fibers from the vagina travel with the sacral parasympathetic fibers and therefore enter the spinal cord through S-2 to S-4 nerves. These nerves respond only to tension in the vagina. Large vaginal lacerations may remain painless unless they include the lower part of the vagina. Approximately the lower 2 to 3 cm of the vagina receives its innervation from the pudendal nerves that, although originating from the same sacral segments, are somatic rather than visceral nerves and convey somatic rather than visceral pain afferents.

The **nerves to the ovary** probably include sympathetic efferent and visceral afferent fibers, but ovarian function is not at all dependent on motor nerve supply. These nerves form a delicate plexus, not grossly visible except at the level of origin of the ovarian artery, where it can be seen to be derived from the aortic plexus.

RECOMMENDED READINGS

Bastian D, Lassau JP. The suspensory mechanism of the uterus. Anat Clin 1982;4:147.

Benoit G, Merlaud L, Meduri G, et al. Anatomy of the prostatic nerves. Surg Radiol Anat 1994;16:23.

Berglas B, Rubin IC. Study of the supportive structures of the uterus by levator myography. Surg Gynecol Obstet 1953;97:677.

Bonica JJ. Principles and practice of obstetric analgesia and anesthesia. Philadelphia: FA Davis, 1967.

Borell U, Fernstrom I. Radiologic pelvimetry. Acta Radiol 1960;181:3.

Braithwaite JL. The arterial supply of the male urinary bladder. Br J Urol 1952;24:64.

Braithwaite JL. Variations in origin of the parietal branches of the internal iliac artery. J Anat 1952;86:423.

Castellino RA, Marglin MI. Imaging of abdominal and pelvic lymph nodes: lymphography or computed tomography? Invest Radiol 1982;17:433.

Clegg EJ. The arterial supply of the human prostate and seminal vesicles. J Anat 1955;89:209.

Curtis AH, Anson BJ, Beaton LE. The anatomy of the subperitoneal tissues and ligamentous structures in relation to surgery of the female pelvic viscera. Surg Gynecol Obstet 1940;70:643.

Curtis AH, Anson BJ, McVay CB. The anatomy of the pelvic and urogenital diaphragms in relation to urethrocele and cystocele. Surg Gynecol Obstet 1939;68:161.

Flocks RH, Culp D, Porto R. Lymphatic spread from prostatic cancer. J Urol 1975;81:194.

Fritsch H, Hötzinger H. Tomographical anatomy of the pelvis, visceral pelvic connective tissue, and its compartments. Clin Anat 1995;8:17.

Gosling JA, Dixon JS, Lendon RG. The autonomic innervation of the human male and female bladder neck and proximal urethra. J Urol 1977;118:302.

Grabbe E, Lierse W, Winkler R. The perirectal fascia: morphology and use in staging of rectal carcinoma. Radiology 1983;149:241.

Haynor DR, Mack LA, Soules MR, Shuman WP, Montana MA, Moss AA. Changing appearance of the normal uterus during the menstrual cycle: MR studies. Radiology 1986;161:459.

Hollinshead WH. Anatomy for surgeons: vol 2, the thorax, abdomen, and pelvis. 2nd ed. New York: Harper & Row, 1971.

Hutch JA, Rambo ON Jr. A study of the anatomy of the prostate, prostatic urethra and urinary sphincter systems. J Urol 1970;104:443.

Kimmel DL, McCrea LE. The development of the pelvic plexuses and the distribution of the pelvic splanchnic nerves in the human embryo and fetus. J Comp Neurol 1958;110:271.

Koff AK. Development of the vagina in the human fetus. Contrib Embryol 1933;24:59.

Krantz KE. The anatomy of the urethra and anterior vaginal wall. Am J Obstet 1951;62:374.

Kuru M. Nervous control of micturition. Physiol Rev 1965;45:425.

Lepor H, Gregerman M, Crosby R, Mostofl FK, Walsh PC. Precise localization of the autonomic nerves from the pelvic plexus to the corpora cavernosa: a detailed anatomical study of the adult male pelvis. J Urol 1985;133:207.

Lowsley OS. The development of the human prostate gland with reference to the development of other structures at the neck of the urinary bladder. Am J Anat 1912;13:299.

McNeal JE. Anatomy of the prostate: an historical survey of divergent views. Prostate 1980;1:3.

Mildenberger H, Kluth D, Dziuba M. Embryology of bladder exstrophy. J Pediatr Surg 1988;23:166.

Milley PS, Nichols DH. A correlative investigation of the human rectovaginal septum. Anat Rec 1969;163:443.

Panici BP, Scambia G, Baiochi G, Matonti G, Capelli A, Mancuso S. Anatomical study of para-aortic and pelvic lymph nodes in gynecologic malignancies. Obstet Gynecol 1992;79:498.

Parks AG, Porter NH, Melzak J. Experimental study of the reflex mechanism controlling the muscles of the pelvic floor. Dis Colon Rectum 1962;5:407.

Roberts WH, Habenicht J, Krishingner G. The pelvic fasciae and their neural and vascular relationships. Anat Rec 1964;149:707.

Tobin CE, Benjamin JA. Anatomical and surgical restudy of Denonvilliers' fascia. Surg Gynecol Obstet 1945;80:373.

Uhlenhuth E, Hunter DWT, Loechel WE. Problems in the anatomy of the pelvis. Philadelphia: JB Lippincott, 1952.

Vanneuville G, Mestas D, Le Bouedec G, et al. The lymphatic drainage of the human ovary in vivo investigated by isotopic lymphography before and after the menopause. Surg Radiol Anat 1991;13:221.

Vinnicombe SJ, Norman AR, Nicolson V, Husband JE. Normal pelvic lymph nodes: evaluation with CT after bipedal lymphangiography. Radiology 1995;194:349.

Woodburne RT. Anatomy of the bladder and bladder outlet. J Urol 1968;100:474.

Hollinshead's Textbook of Anatomy, by Cornelius Rosse and Penelope Gaddum-Rosse.
Lippincott-Raven Publishers, Philadelphia, © 1997.

CHAPTER 28

The Perineum

The perineum is the most inferior region of the trunk, located between the thighs and the buttocks. It contains the anal canal with its external opening, the anus, and the associated sphincters; and the external genitalia, with the fascias and muscles that support and surround them. Superiorly, the perineum is limited by the pelvic diaphragm; inferiorly, it presents a free surface covered by skin. The lateral walls of the perineum are formed by the medial surface of the inferior pubic and ischial rami, the obturator internus below the attachment of the levator ani, and, posterolaterally, the medial surface of the sacrotuberous ligaments overlapped by the gluteus maximus.

The osseoligamentous frame of the perineum is the **inferior pelvic aperture,** described in Chapter 27 (Fig. 28-1). The area enclosed by this rhomboidal or diamond-shaped frame can be divided into two triangular regions by a line connecting the two ischial tuberosities: anteriorly, the *urogenital region* and posteriorly, the *anal region.* These regions are often spoken of as the urogenital and anal *triangles.* The **anal region** contains the anal canal and the ischiorectal fossae on each side of the anal canal. In the **urogenital region,** a muscular shelf stretches between the conjoint ischiopubic rami of the two sides; this is the *urogenital diaphragm.* It is pierced by the urethra and, in the female, also by the vagina. The diaphragm serves as a foundation for the attachment of the external genitalia. The external genitalia in the male include the penis, made up of three cavernous erectile bodies (two corpora cavernosa and the corpus spongiosum), and the scrotum. The female external genitalia include the labia majora, the labia minora, with the vestibule of the vagina in between them; the bilateral erectile bulbs of the vestibule; the clitoris; and the mons pubis. Fascias attached to the urogenital diaphragm define two spaces of considerable anatomic and clinical importance; these are the *superficial* and *deep perineal spaces,* or pouches. The superficial perineal space contains all the external genitalia and the superficial perineal muscles associated with them; the deep space is filled by the deep muscles of the perineum, which constitute the urogenital diaphragm.

The chief blood supply of the perineum is provided by the *internal pudendal artery.* Blood is drained from the perineum, in general, by the internal pudendal veins, but the blood from some of the erectile bodies of the external genitalia is returned to the prostatic or vesical plexuses by the *deep dorsal vein* of the penis or clitoris, respectively. Most of the perineal lymphatics do not follow the internal pudendal vessels; perineal structures drain to primarily the inguinal lymph nodes. The motor and sensory supply to somatic structures in the perineum is provided chiefly by the *pudendal nerve,* a branch of the sacral plexus; parasympathetic efferents responsible for erection enter the perineum through the urogenital hiatus in the *cavernous nerves,* branches of the prostatic or vesical plexuses; sympathetic nerves reach perineal structures in the pudendal nerves.

This chapter will first describe the anal region, followed by the urogenital region. The blood supply, lymphatic drainage, and innervation will then be considered for the perineum as a whole.

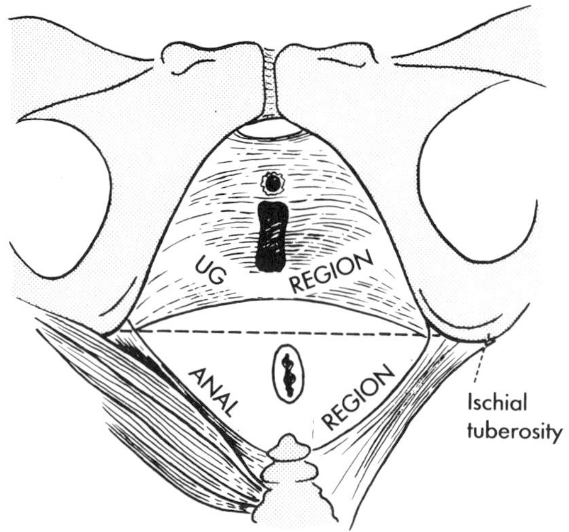

FIGURE *28-1.*
Schema of the regions of the perineum. The arbitrary division between the urogenital and anal regions (*triangles*) is indicated by a dashed line.

THE ANAL REGION

The Anal Canal

The anal canal is the terminal part of the alimentary tract. It commences at the *perineal flexure,* where it is continuous with the rectum, and terminates at the anus, its opening to the exterior. The anorectal junction at the perineal flexure is marked by the narrowing of the rectal ampulla and by the change of the forward inclination of the rectum to the backward inclination of the anal canal (Fig. 28-2). The flexure between the rectum and anal canal is chiefly due to the forward pull of the puborectalis as it swings around the anorectal junction in the posterior boundary of the urogenital hiatus. The anal canal, approximately 4 cm long, is thus directed posteriorly as well as downward. As the longitudinal muscle coat of the rectum continues down on the anal canal, it becomes gradually replaced by fibroelastic tissue. Fibromuscular contributions from the puborectalis reinforce this outer layer of the anal canal, which is then surrounded by the *sphincter ani externus,* formed by voluntary striated muscle. Fibromuscular and fatty bodies are related to the anal canal outside its external sphincter on all sides: anteriorly, the perineal body, or central tendon of the perineum (to be described later);

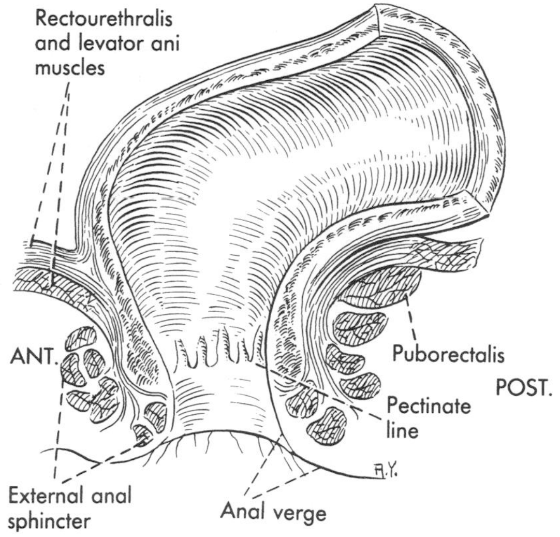

FIGURE 28-2.
The lower part of the rectum and the anal canal hemisected and viewed from the left.

posteriorly, the anococcygeal body, or ligament, which separates the anal canal from the coccyx; and laterally, the mass of fat in the ischiorectal fossae.

Sphincters

The circular muscle coat of the rectum becomes thicker as it continues below the anorectal junction to form the **internal anal sphincter,** which surrounds the upper two-thirds of the anal canal. Delicate septa from the outer longitudinal fibromuscular coat of the anal canal penetrate the internal sphincter and spread out in the submucosa; other septa fan out into the dermis of the perianal skin and the fibrous tissue of the ischiorectal fat pads. The thickest of these septa limits the internal sphincter inferiorly and is identifiable on the interior of the anal canal as the *intersphincteric groove.*

The **external sphincter** (*sphincter ani externus*) surrounds the entire length of the anal canal, and it has been described as consisting of three parts: subcutaneous, superficial, and deep (see Fig. 28-2). It is difficult to distinguish these three parts, and, in the opinion of some, only two parts can be recognized. The most inferior, **subcutaneous part** of the sphincter surrounds the lower third of the canal, below the internal sphincter; the **superficial** and **deep parts** overlap the internal sphincter, and the deep part fuses above with the puborectalis muscle.

There are truly annular fibers in the subcutaneous and deep parts of the sphincter; many other fibers, as well as most of those in the superficial part of the sphincter, run in parallel bundles along the sides of the anal canal and decussate in front and behind it as they attach to the anococcygeal ligament behind and the *central tendon of the perineum* (perineal body) in front of the anus (Fig. 28-3).

The tone of the external and internal sphincters keeps the lateral walls of the canal apposed to each other, except when the sphincters relax during defecation. Probably as a consequence of the anteroposterior direction of many of the fibers in the external sphincter, the anus is a longitudinal slitlike opening, rather than a circular one. The anal skin around the opening is puckered by the *corrugater cutis ani,* which consists of smooth muscle and elastic fibers derived from the septa of the external fibromuscular coat that have traversed the internal sphincter and submucosa of the canal. The same strands of tissue create tiny, circumscribed compartments in the perianal subcu-

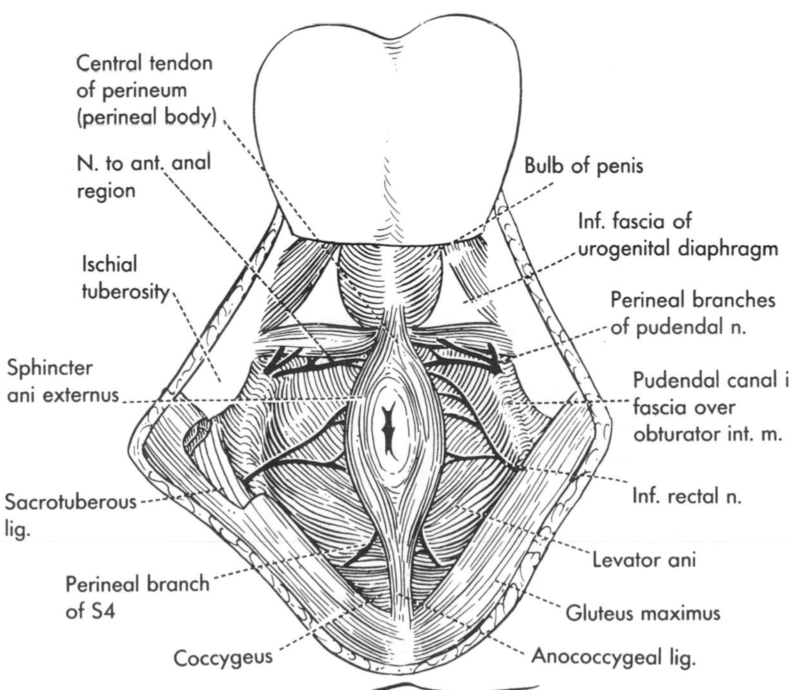

FIGURE 28-3.
Muscles and nerves of the anal region. Also shown is the posterior part of the urogenital region. The internal pudendal artery and its inferior rectal and perineal branches, although not shown here, accompany the pudendal nerve and its branches.

taneous tissue. Distention of these compartments by perianal abscesses or hemorrhage is particularly painful.

On rectal examination, the tone of the sphincters offers a definite resistance to the finger inserted into the anal canal. The intersphincteric groove can be palpated between the subcutaneous part of the external sphincter and the internal sphincter. The so-called *anorectal ring*, palpable above the intersphincteric groove, is formed by the fused fibers of the deep parts of the external sphincter and the puborectalis. Because of the slinglike puborectalis, the ring is strongest posteriorly and its tearing or division results in rectal incontinence.

The external sphincter is innervated by the inferior rectal branch of the pudendal nerve and the internal sphincter by autonomic nerves that descend from the superior rectal plexus.

Interior

For clinical reasons, it is useful to relate the internal features of the anal canal to its dual **embryologic derivation.** The upper part of the anal canal, like the rectum, develops from the dorsal compartment of the cloaca and is lined by endoderm. The lower part is derived from the *proctodeum*, a depression lined by ectoderm (see Fig. 9-2). The ectodermal and endodermal parts of the canal become confluent when the anal membrane breaks down.

Approximately halfway up the canal, the mucosa is raised up into a transverse row of six to ten folds that encircle the anal canal (Fig. 28-4). These folds are the *anal valves*, and the serrated line formed by them is called the *pectinate line* (dentate line). At the meeting of adjacent valves, the mucosa is raised up into longitudinal folds, the *anal columns*, that extend into the upper part of the anal canal. Below the pectinate line, a narrow band of mucosa, the *transitional zone*, also known as the *pecten*, encircles the anal canal and is limited below by the intersphincteric groove. The intersphincteric groove has long been known as the *white line*, described in 1863 by Hilton (despite the fact that it does not appear white in either the living body or the cadaver).

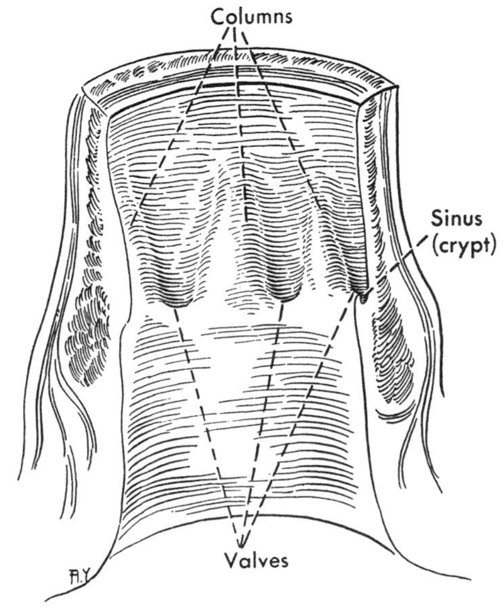

FIGURE *28-4.*
The anal columns.

There is no agreement from these anatomic features on the precise location of the anal membrane, which marks the junction of the endoderm- and the ectoderm-derived portions of the anal canal. The indiscriminate use of a number of terms for the description of this junction has further confused the issue. The ectodermal–endodermal junction, however, is somewhere in the region of the pecten; it certainly is not above the pectinate line and is not below the "white line." The pecten, therefore, represents the "watershed" or "divide" between the two types of epithelium lining the canal and also between the two sources of blood and nerve supply and the territories of lymphatic drainage.

The *mucous membrane* above the pectinate line is similar to that of the rectum, whereas below the pecten, it is nonkeratinized, stratified squamous epithelium devoid of hairs. There is a transition between these two types of epithelium across the pecten. Carcinomas arising in either region are distinct in their nature and clinical history. Above the pecten, the mucosa is supplied by branches of the superior rectal artery and drained by the superior rectal vein. The radicles of these vessels raise up the anal columns, and transverse anastomotic vessels run between them at the bases of the anal valves. This submucous venous anastomosis is the **internal "rectal" venous plexus.** The veins in three of these six to ten columns (two on the left and one on the right) are prone to distention, together with the plexus behind the valves. This causes them to bulge into the anal canal, forming *internal hemorrhoids*, or piles. The anal canal below the pecten is supplied and drained by the inferior "rectal" vessels, and the **inferior "rectal" venous plexus,** formed in the submucosa, can, when distended, give rise to *external hemorrhoids*. The mucosa above the pecten is innervated by autonomic nerves and, therefore, is insensitive to touching, pricking, and cutting. It is the site of choice for injecting hemorrhoids to promote their thrombosis and fibrosis. The mucosa over and below the pecten is extremely sensitive, being supplied by somatic nerves contained in the inferior rectal branch of the pudendal nerve. Fissures and tears in the lining of the anal canal, often commencing at the valves, are very painful.

Each of the valves shelters a small pocket, the *anal sinus*. Into the sinus open the *anal glands*, which extend into the submucosa and sometimes into the muscle coat. Suppuration in these glands results in abscesses and may lead to the formation of fistulae.

The lymphatic drainage of the anal canal above the pecten is upward along the superior rectal vessels and below the pecten into the superficial inguinal nodes.

Developmental Anomalies. The common congenital anomaly of the rectum and anal canal is failure of the bowel to open to the outside in the normal fashion. Regardless of whether the anomaly is primarily in the rectum or the anal canal, the condition is referred to as

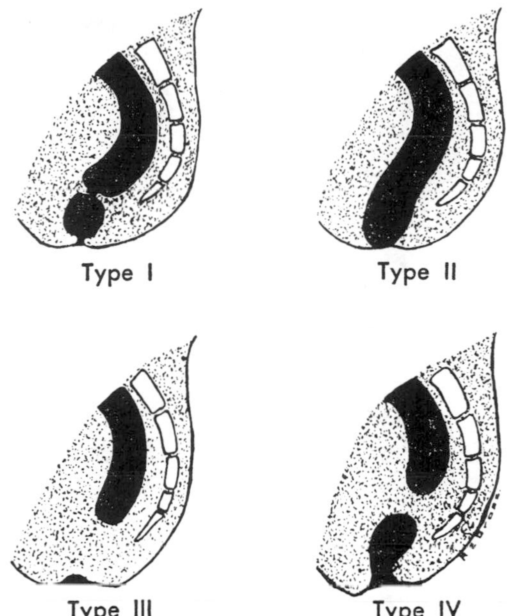

FIGURE *28-5.*
Some congenital anorectal anomalies: type I: a stenosis, here both at the anus and above; type II: a simple type of imperforate anus; type III: imperforate anus, in which the bowel ends blindly a considerable distance above the perineum; type IV: an atresia of the rectum. (Ladd WE, Gross RE. Am J Surg 1934;23:167.)

imperforate anus. Imperforate anus has been estimated to occur in 1 in every 1500 to 5000 newborns. There are several different types (Fig. 28-5) it may only consist of a marked stenosis, rather than a true lack of any opening; there may be little tissue between the bowel and the outside; or the bowel may end high on the inside. There may be no sign of an anus, or there may be a normal anus that leads into a blind anal canal or a blind rectum. Imperforate anus is often associated with fistulous connections between the rectum and the derivatives of the urogenital sinus (see Fig. 27-21).

The Ischiorectal Fossae

The ischiorectal fossae are roughly wedge-shaped spaces on each side of the anal canal (Fig. 28-6). The anal canal and the perineal body separate the fossae of the two sides; the only communication between them is posteriorly through a narrow potential space located deep to the fibers of the sphincter ani externus that attach to the coccyx.

The somewhat vertical **lateral wall** of each fossa is formed by the obturator internus, which covers the medial side of the obturator foramen and the fused bodies of the ilium and ischium above the ischial tuberosity; the **base** of the fossa is perineal skin, and its sloping **superomedial wall** is the levator ani. The fossa is sealed off above by the fusion of the inferior fascia of the pelvic diaphragm to the obturator fascia and medially by the fusion of the same fascia to the external anal sphincter, the outer longitudinal fibromuscular coat of the anal canal, and the perineal body. Anteriorly, the fossa is limited by the fusion of the perineal fascia to the posterior margin of the urogenital diaphragm (see Fig. 28-12*B*). Above the urogenital diaphragm, the *anterior recess* of the fossa extends forward. The **anterior recesses** are narrow spaces between the pelvic and urogenital diaphragms, limited laterally by the conjoint rami of the ischium and pubis and medially by the fusion of the inferior fascia of the pelvic diaphragm to the fascia of the urogenital diaphragm (see Fig. 28-8*A*). Posterolaterally, the ischiorectal fossae are continuous with a potential space in the buttocks located deep to the gluteus maximus, the inferior border of which overlaps the fossae posteriorly.

The subcutaneous connective tissue of the anal region expands to fill the fossa, forming an **adipose body** that adapts its shape to the fossa and permits distention of the anal canal during defecation. The adipose body is permeated by tough fibrous strands that do not form well-defined compartments and, therefore, permit the expansion and spread of abscesses in the fat without generating tension and pain.

In addition to the fat, the ischiorectal fossa contains the *pudendal nerve* and *internal pudendal vessels* in a fascial canal that runs along the lateral wall of the fossa, and the *inferior rectal nerve and vessels,* which cross from the lateral wall toward the anal canal.

The Pudendal Canal

The pudendal canal is a fascial sheath in which the pudendal nerve and the internal pudendal artery reach the perineum and the internal pudendal veins leave it. The **pudendal nerve,** a branch of the sacral plexus, and the **internal pudendal artery,** a branch of the internal iliac, leave the pelvis between the piriformis and coccygeus, passing over the upper margin of the pelvic diaphragm and entering the gluteal region through the greater sciatic foramen. Destined for the perineum, the nerve and artery run vertically downward and, in so doing, skirt the lateral side of the ischial spine. They attain the medial surface of the obturator internus just below the spine by passing through the lesser sciatic foramen, enclosed by the

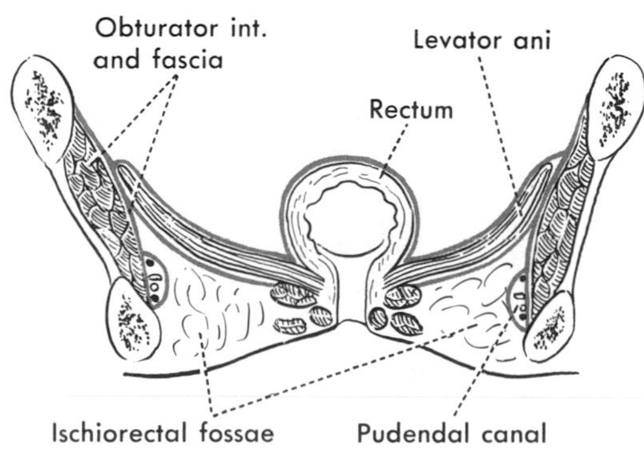

FIGURE *28-6.*
Coronal section through the ischiorectal fossae. The obturator fascia and the superior and inferior fascias of the levator ani are shown in *blue*.

sacrospinous and sacrotuberous ligaments. Clinging to the medial surface of the obturator internus, the vessels are in the lateral wall of the ischiorectal fossa. Some distance above the ischial tuberosity, they change their course forward, heading for the urogenital region. The fascial sheath of the nerve and vessels is fused to the obturator fascia and is called the *pudendal canal*. The canal extends forward, sheltered by the *falciform process* of the sacrotuberous ligament along the ischiopubic ramus. It terminates at the posterior border of the urogenital diaphragm, which the nerve and vessels penetrate. As they continue forward along the pubic ramus, they are surrounded by the attachment of the muscles of the urogenital diaphragm to that ramus.

The branches of the pudendal nerve and internal pudendal artery to the anal canal are given off just above the ischial tuberosity, and they run medially in the fat of the ischiorectal fossa; they are called the inferior rectal nerve and artery. The inferior rectal vein runs with the nerve and artery to join the internal pudendal veins in the pudendal canal.

THE UROGENITAL REGION

The Urogenital Diaphragm, The Perineal Fascias and Spaces

The Urogenital Diaphragm

The urogenital diaphragm is a continuous sheet of muscle spanning the triangular space bordered on each side by the conjoint rami of the ischium and pubis (Fig. 28-7). The fascias that cover the superior and inferior surfaces of the muscle are part of the diaphragm (Fig. 28-8). These fascias, called the **superior** and **inferior fascia of the urogenital diaphragm**, fuse with each other along the relatively short anterior and much longer posterior margins

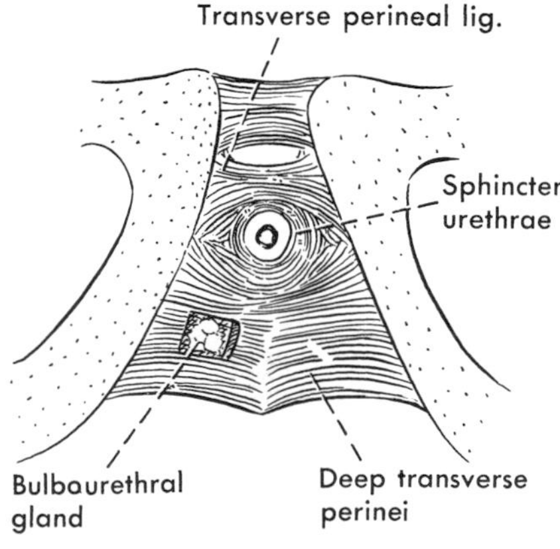

FIGURE 28-7.
The muscle of the urogenital diaphragm of the male seen from below after removal of the inferior layer of fascia (perineal membrane). A piece has been cut from the muscle on the *left* to show the bulbourethral gland.

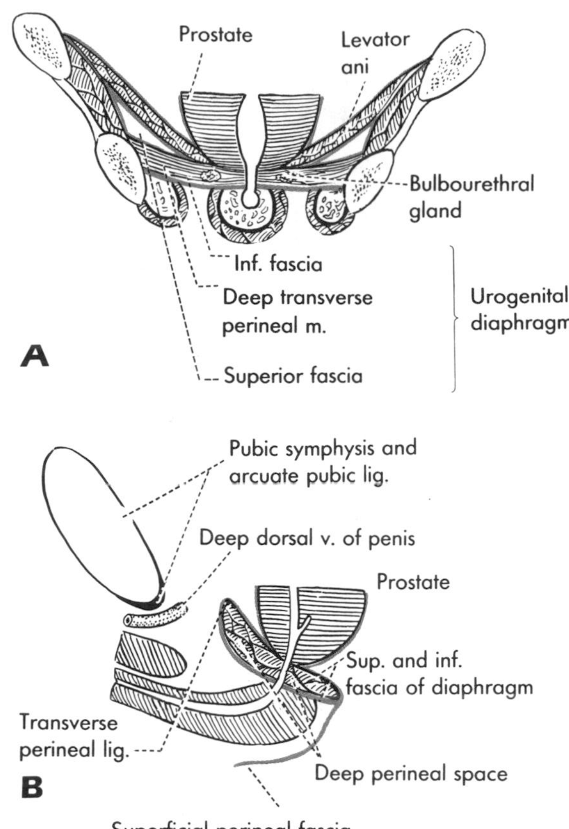

FIGURE 28-8.
The urogenital diaphragm and the deep perineal space: (A) in coronal section through the posterior part of the diaphragm and (B) in sagittal section. The fascial layers are shown in *blue*.

of the muscle. Along the anterior margin of the diaphragm, the fusion of its fascias creates the *transverse perineal ligament*, which is a short distance posterior to the *arcuate pubic ligament* lying along the inferior border of the symphysis pubis. The gap between the two ligaments transmits the deep dorsal vein of the penis or clitoris from the perineum into the pelvis. At the midpoint of the posterior margin of the diaphragm is a fibromuscular tendinous mass called the *central tendon of the perineum* or **perineal body**, described in the next section. The urogenital diaphragm lies below the anterior part of the pelvic diaphragm, and its central region forms the floor of the urogenital hiatus. In the female, the diaphragm is less distinct than in the male, because the vagina passing through it more or less splits the diaphragm into right and left halves. Its function as the foundation of the urogenital region is more obvious in the male, because it is uninterrupted except for the passage of the urethra.

The Deep Perineal Muscles. The muscle sheet of the urogenital diaphragm consists of the deep muscles of the perineum. For descriptive purposes, two main parts are distinguished in this muscle: anteriorly, the *sphincter urethrae,* and posteriorly, the *deep transversus perinei* (Fig. 28-9; see Fig. 28-7). The fibers of both muscles generally run

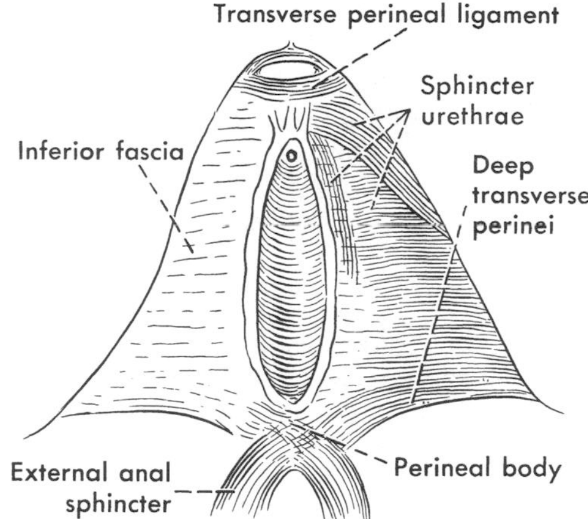

FIGURE 28-9.
The urogenital diaphragm of the female, from *below*. On the reader's *left*, the inferior fascia is intact; on the *right*, it has been removed to show the musculature.

transversely from each ischiopubic ramus toward the midline. Those in front arch around the urethra and make up the **sphincter urethrae;** those further posteriorly meet in the central tendon of the perineum and are called the **deep transverse perineal muscle.** It may be possible to define some intrinsic circular fibers around the urethra in the sphincter urethrae and others that run on each side of the urethra from the transverse perineal ligament to the perineal body.

In the female, the urethra is embedded in the anterior wall of the vagina, the sphincter urethrae arches around the vagina as well as the urethra, and some of its fibers blend with the vaginal wall (see Fig. 28-9). As in the male, the deep transversus perinei inserts into the perineal body, located behind the vagina.

Both deep muscles of the perineum are innervated by perineal branches of the pudendal nerve. Their contraction puts tension on the perineal body and elevates it; thereby, they presumably contribute to the support this body provides for the pelvic viscera. The sphincter urethrae compresses the urethra, especially when there is urine in the bladder. It can also interrupt the stream of urine.

The Perineal Body

More recently called the *central tendon of the perineum*, the perineal body is a pyramid-shaped mass of fibromuscular tissue, rather than a flat or round tendon, located between the anal canal and the vagina (or the bulb of the penis). A number of perineal muscles terminate in it. The perineal body is larger in the female than in the male, filling the space between the divergent vagina and anal canal (Fig. 28-10). It is of considerable importance in obstetrics and gynecology.

The base of the perineal body rests against the perineal skin between the anus and the vestibule of the vagina; its apex points into the urogenital hiatus, where it is continuous with the rectovaginal septum.

The muscle fibers that are interlaced in it include the pubovaginalis and pubococcygeus (parts of the pelvic diaphragm), both deep perineal muscles (the sphincter urethrae and deep transversus perinei), the sphincter ani externus, and, of the superficial perineal muscles, the bulbospongiosus and the superficial transversus perinei, which are described in a following section.

The perineal body permits a remarkable degree of stretching of the perineum as the presenting fetal head distends the vagina and the entire perineum. Overstretching may tear the perineal body, and such tears may or may not involve the perineal skin.

Deliberate division of the perineal body during delivery is called an **episiotomy.** A cut is made with a pair of scissors toward the anus, starting at the midpoint of the posterior margin of the vaginal orifice (the introitus). This is done to prevent an uncontrolled or concealed tear and to make suturing of the perineum easier than it would be to repair a tear. When the perineal body is torn, contraction of the perineal muscles attached to it will widen the gap in the tear and, rather than strengthening, will weaken the support of pelvic viscera.

The support provided by the perineal body for pelvic viscera is illustrated by the sequelae that develop should its integrity not be restored. These sequelae include various types of *prolapse*, discussed in Chapter 27.

The Deep Perineal Space

The superior and inferior fascias of the urogenital diaphragm enclose what is called the deep perineal space, or pouch. In truth, this is not a space, not even a potential one, because it is completely filled by the deep perineal muscles, the fibers of which attach to both fascial membranes that cover the surfaces of the diaphragm.

The deep perineal space is completely closed, and it does not communicate with other perineal or pelvic spaces. The rather thin **superior fascia of the diaphragm** forms the floor of the anterior recesses of the ischiorectal fossae and medially fuses with the inferior fascia of the

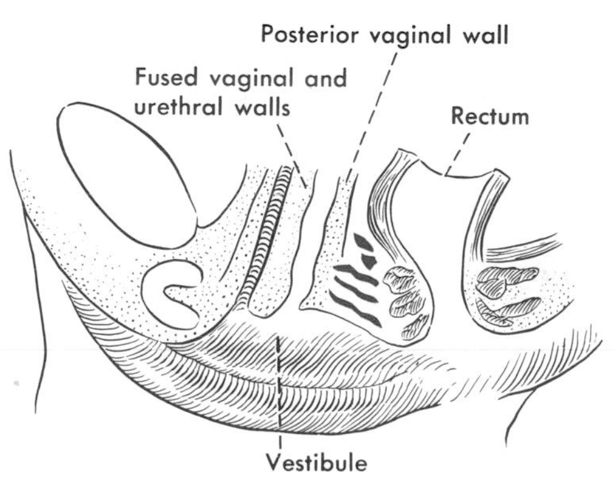

FIGURE 28-10.
The central tendon or perineal body (*red*) in sagittal section.

pelvic diaphragm (see Fig. 28-8). No communication exists between the pelvic cavity and the perineum around the urethra or vagina, which pass through the deep space, because the urogenital diaphragm is fused to the walls of these structures. The **inferior fascia of the urogenital diaphragm** is significantly thicker and is often called the **perineal membrane.** This fascia forms the roof of the superficial perineal space and to it are attached the external genitalia.

The deep perineal space contains, in addition to the deep perineal muscles and the urethra and vagina, the bulbourethral glands in the male. The branches of the pudendal nerve and internal pudendal artery entering the deep space from the pudendal canal are buried among the fibers of the deep perineal muscles as they attach along the inferior pubic ramus.

The Membranous Urethra. The part of the urethra between the superior and inferior fascias of the urogenital diaphragm is called the membranous urethra (*pars membranacea urethrae*). The sphincter urethrae that surrounds the membranous urethra extends above the diaphragm, especially in the anterior urethral wall, into the prostatic part of the male urethra or the pelvic part of the female urethra.

In the male, the membranous urethra is the shortest segment of the urethra and its walls are the thinnest. It connects the prostatic and spongy parts of the urethra, and as it penetrates the urogenital diaphragm, it is surrounded by the urethral sphincter. It is approximately 1 cm long, passing from the apex of the prostate into the bulb of the penis (Fig. 28-11). It enters not the back end but the upper surface of the bulb and, as it does so, turns forward in the corpus spongiosum.

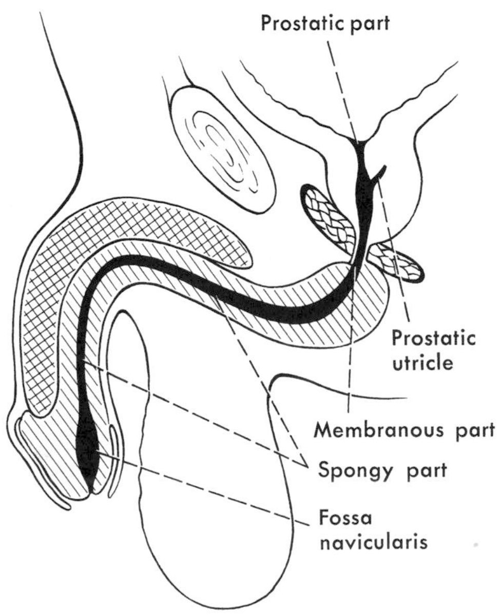

FIGURE 28-11.
Subdivisions of the urethra.

The **female urethra** terminates at the urethral orifice in the vestibule as soon as it has passed through the urogenital diaphragm. The **paraurethral glands,** considered by some to be the homologues of the prostate, are embedded in the wall of the urethra and their ducts open along the urethra into the vestibule. There are simple, small mucous glands opening into the lumen of both the male and female urethra.

> The membranous part of the urethra in the male is especially subject to damage through physical violence. It may be perforated by ill-advised attempts to force a probe through it, or it may be ruptured below the diaphragm as a result of a fall astride an object. Rupture above the diaphragm usually results from a fracture of the pelvis, with displacement of the prostatic part of the urethra. In crushing injuries of the pelvis, common in automobile accidents, the bladder and prostate are displaced upward and backward with such force that the urethra ruptures between the apex of the prostate and the pelvic diaphragm.

The Bulbourethral Glands. A small gland located on each side of the membranous urethra is embedded in the muscle of the urogenital diaphragm (see Fig. 28-16). The ducts of these bulbourethral glands descend through the diaphragm, piercing the perineal membrane, and terminate in the spongy urethra. The clear mucus they secrete during sexual excitation lubricates the urethral orifice and the glans penis. The female homologues of the glands are the greater vestibular glands, located below the inferior fascia of the urogenital diaphragm.

The Superficial Perineal Space

Deep to the skin of the urogenital region, a potential space surrounds the external genitalia; this space, called the superficial perineal space, or pouch, is limited by the superficial perineal fascia and the inferior fascia of the urogenital diaphragm. It is more extensive and clinically more important in the male than in the female, because, in the male, it surrounds the scrotum and penis, whereas in the female, it is split by the vestibule and is confined on each side to the labia majora and minora.

The **superficial perineal fascia** is a continuation of the membranous layer of the superficial fascia from the anterior abdominal wall into the perineum (see Fig. 23-2). Frequently known as Colles' fascia, the superficial perineal fascia is a thin membrane; the *superficial penile fascia* and the *tunica dartos* are two named parts of it. At the symphysis pubis, the membranous superficial fascia of the abdomen becomes the superficial penile fascia, which invests the penis. This fascia, doubling back on itself in the prepuce, attaches to the penis around the neck of the glans (Fig. 28-12). Below the penis, the superficial penile fascia invests the scrotum as the tunica dartos, acquiring a significant amount of smooth muscle. Posterior to the scrotum, the dartos continues as a fibrous membrane called the *superficial perineal fascia* and attaches to the posterior margin of the urogenital diaphragm. Lateral to the penis

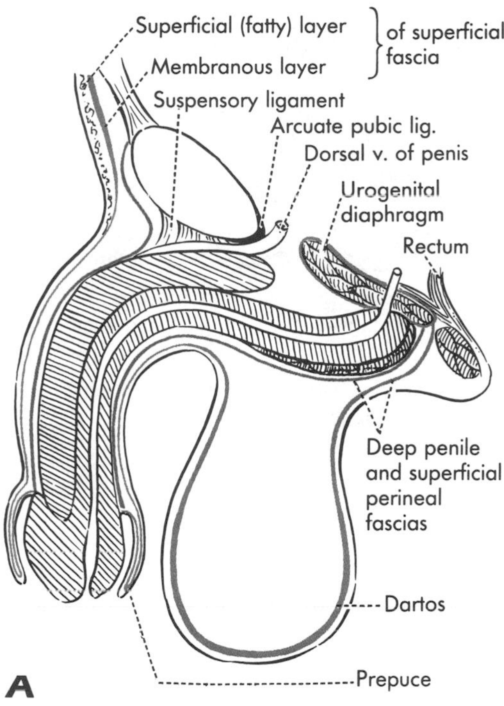

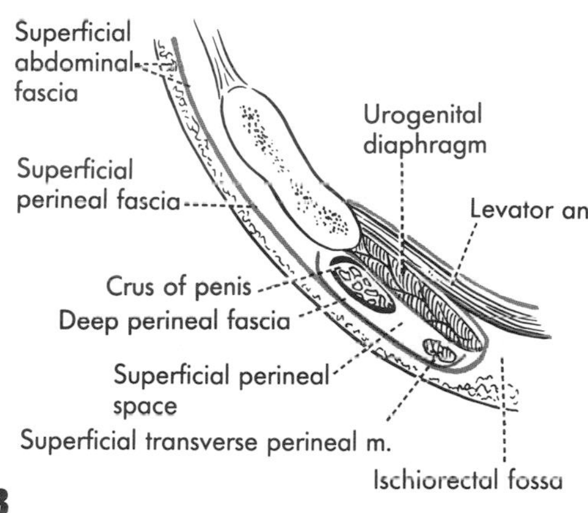

FIGURE *28-12.*
Continuities of the subcutaneous connective tissue (superficial fascia) and deep fascia of the abdominal wall with fascia of the penis, scrotum, and perineum. (A) a sagittal section close to the midline; (B) one lateral to the penis and scrotum. The fascias of the urogenital diaphragm and the levator ani are *blue*, as in previous illustrations; the membranous layer of the superficial abdominal fascia is also *blue*, as is its continuation, the superficial penile and superficial perineal fascias. The deep perineal fascia and its continuation, the deep penile fascia, are *red*.

and scrotum, the superficial perineal fascia is attached to the ischiopubic rami, thus sealing the superficial perineal space everywhere except anterosuperiorly. The lateral and posterior attachments of the superficial perineal fascia are similar in the female perineum, but medially, the fascia fuses with the margins of the vaginal orifice.

Another layer of membranous fascia can be defined in the urogenital region that is deep to the superficial perineal fascia. It surrounds more intimately the cavernous bodies that constitute the penis and clitoris and the superficial perineal muscles associated with them. This is the **deep perineal fascia,** which essentially divides the superficial perineal space into a superficial and deep compartment. The deep perineal fascia over the penis becomes the *deep penile fascia* and does not descend into the scrotum (see Fig. 28-12). At the root of the penis, it attaches laterally to the ischiopubic rami and posteriorly to the margin of the urogenital diaphragm, just deep to the attachments of the superficial perineal fascia (Fig. 28-13; see Fig. 28-12). Anteriorly, deep perineal fascia fuses to the symphysis pubis. Thus, the deep compartment of the superficial perineal space is closed anterosuperiorly, whereas the superficial compartment is continuous with the tissue space between the deep fascia of the external

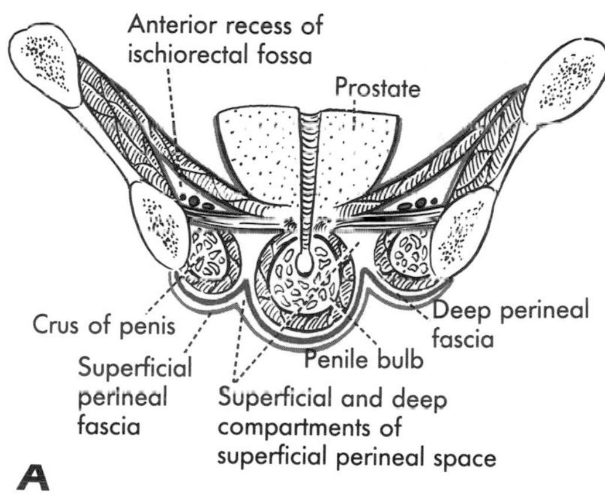

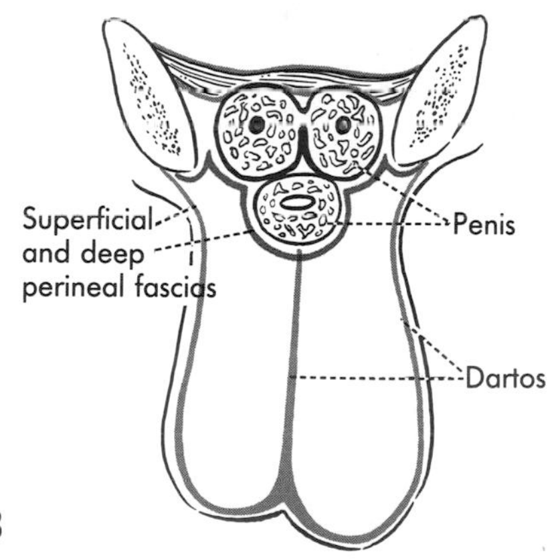

FIGURE *28-13.*
Diagram of the superficial and deep perineal fascias in coronal section through (A) the level of the penile bulb, and (B) the scrotum. In (B) the dartos replaces regions of the superficial perineal fascia. The nerve and vessels lying in the "anterior recess" of the ischiorectal fossa are the dorsal nerve of the penis and the pudendal vessels. The *color designation* of the fascias corresponds to that in Figure 28-12.

oblique and the membranous layer of the superficial fascia of the anterior abdominal wall.

> Injuries to the male urethra below the urogenital diaphragm are frequent and cause extravasation of urine in the perineum. The extravasated urine will be confined to the perineum if it is limited by the deep perineal fascia; it will distend the deep compartment of the superficial perineal space, causing swelling of the shaft of the penis and the perineum between the ischiopubic rami. If the deep perineal fascia is also injured, the urine will escape into the superficial compartment of the superficial perineal space, distending not only the perineum between the ischiopubic rami in front of the anus but also the scrotal sac and the shaft of the penis, including the prepuce, and will ascend into the anterior abdominal wall.

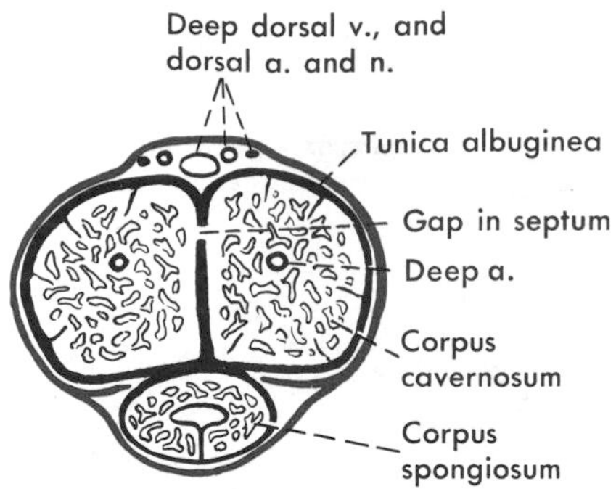

FIGURE *28-15.*
Cross section through the body of the penis. The deep penile fascia is shown in *red*.

The Male Genitalia and the Superficial Perineal Muscles

The Penis

The penis is the male organ of copulation, capable of becoming hard and erect due to its engorgement with blood, a requirement for its intromission into the vagina. The penis consists of two parts: the *body* (*corpus*, or shaft) and the *root* (*radix*).

In the flaccid state of the organ, the **body** hangs free below the symphysis pubis, anterior to the scrotum, and terminates in an acornlike enlargement, the *glans penis.* The body has a so-called *dorsal surface*, which faces anterosuperiorly when the penis is flaccid, and a *urethral surface*, which faces the scrotum (see Fig. 28-12). In the body of the penis, three parallel, cylindrical masses of erectile tissue are held together by the penile fascias and by the fusion of their capsules: along the midline of the urethral surface is the *corpus spongiosum*, containing the urethra, and along the dorsal surface are the two *corpora cavernosa* (Figs. 28-14 and 28-15).

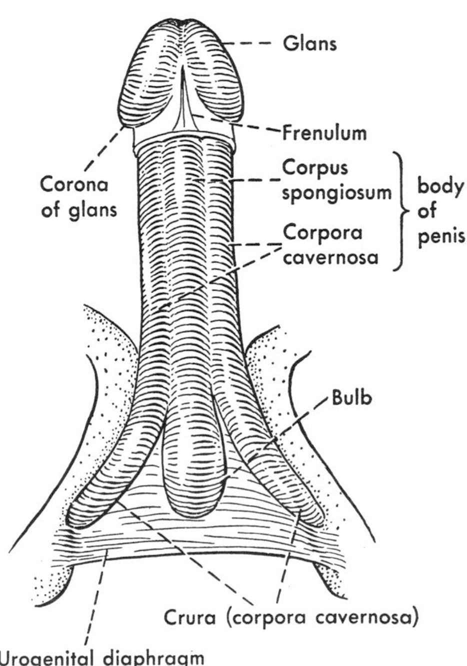

FIGURE *28-14.*
The urethral surface of the penis. The muscles in the superficial perineal space have been removed to show the crura and the penile bulb.

The **root of the penis** is deep to the scrotum, attached to the inferior fascia of the urogenital diaphragm. It consists of the divergent *crura of the penis,* continuous with the corpora cavernosa, and the *bulb of the penis* between them, continuous with the corpus spongiosum (see Fig. 28-14).

Each of the three corpora and their posterior extensions into the root of the penis are composed of spongy connective tissue with vascular sinuses, or *cavernae*, between the fibrous trabecular network. Their *tunica albuginea*, continuous with the trabeculae, forms the capsule of these cavernous bodies. The arteries of the penis penetrate the tunica albuginea, arborize in the trabeculae, and terminate in spiral branches called *helicine arteries*, which, in response to excitation of the cavernous nerves (derived from the "nervi erigentes"), pour arterial blood into the cavernae at a faster rate than it can leave through the cavernous veins. Erection is achieved by tumescence of the corpora with arterial blood. Thus, compression of veins or contraction of muscles plays no important part in erection; it is, in essence, an arterial phenomenon. The commingling of elastic fibers and smooth muscle with the predominantly collagenous trabeculae and tunics of the corpora permits the enlargement of the penis as it becomes erect and accounts also for the return to its smaller, flaccid state after excitation of the cavernous nerves ceases.

The Corpora Cavernosa. Each corpus cavernosum commences in the root of the penis as the **crus** attached to the everted medial surface of the conjoint ischiopubic ramus and to the perineal membrane along the bone. Reaching the inferior margin of the pubic symphysis, the two crura approximate each other, their tunicae albugineae fuse, and they continue forward into the body of the penis as the corpora cavernosa (see Fig. 28-14). The median **sep-**

tum (*septum penis*) that separates the corpora is penetrated by blood vessels and, posteriorly, is fenestrated, permitting communication between the vascular spaces in the two corpora (see Fig. 28-15). The corpus spongiosum is fused to the groove on the urethral surface of the corpora cavernosa without significant vascular connections. The blunt, distal ends of the corpora cavernosa stop short of the tip of the penis and are capped by the glans penis (Fig. 28-16).

The Corpus Spongiosum. Smaller in diameter along the body of the penis than the corpora cavernosa, the corpus spongiosum expands anteriorly as the glans and posteriorly as the bulb of the penis. It encloses along its entire length the spongy part of the urethra.

The base of the **glans** is wider than the circumference of the corpora cavernosa; its projecting margin, the *corona glandis,* shelters a groove at the junction of the glans with the corpora cavernosa called the *neck of the glans* (see Fig. 28-14). Extending from the tip of the glans to its urethral surface is the slitlike opening of the urethra, the *external urethral ostium.*

The posterior expanded end of the corpus spongiosum, the **bulb of the penis,** is tightly attached to the inferior fascia of the urogenital diaphragm between the crura (see Figs. 28-14 and 28-16). Its adherent upper surface, rather than its convex posterior end, is penetrated by the urethra, which turns forward as soon as it enters the bulb (see Fig. 28-11). The ducts of the bulbourethral glands, descending from the deep perineal space, also penetrate the bulb on each side of the urethra and terminate in it after traversing the bulb (see Fig. 28-16).

The Spongy Urethra. The terminal part of the urethra, called the spongy urethra (*pars spongiosa urethrae*), is continuous proximally with the membranous urethra. It extends within the corpus spongiosum from the perineal membrane through the bulb to the external urethral ostium on the glans penis (see Fig. 28-11). Within the glans, the urethra dilates to form the **fossa navicularis,** but the external ostium is the narrowest and the least dilatable part of the urethra. A small mucosal valve may be present at the proximal end of the fossa, and a mucosal pit, the *lacuna magna,* is in the roof of the fossa. There are numerous smaller lacunae in the mucosal lining of the spongy urethra, and several mucous glands also open into it.

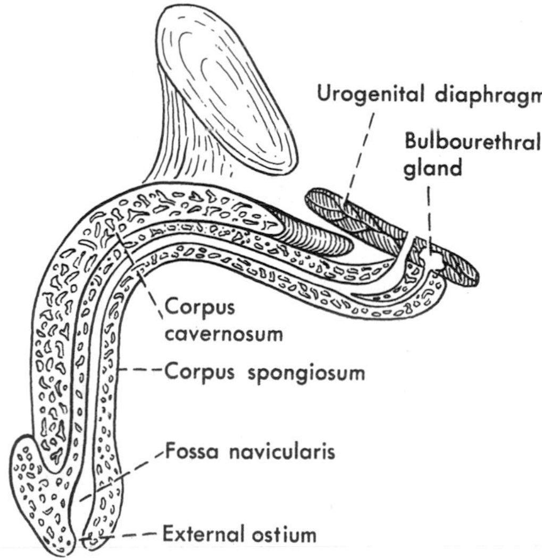

FIGURE *28-16.*
Diagrammatic sagittal section through the penis. The bulbourethral gland, shown here, actually lies lateral to the urethra (see Figs. 28-7 and 28-8) and, therefore, would not show in a section close to the midline.

Penile Fascias and Ligaments. The superficial fascia of the perineum over the penis is called the **superficial penile fascia.** It is subjacent to the skin, without any fat intervening between the two. It doubles back with the skin of the prepuce and is attached around the neck of the glans.

The **deep penile fascia** is continuous with the deep perineal fascia. It binds the corpora cavernosa and corpus spongiosum together in the body of the penis and also attaches around the neck of the glans. The apposition of these two fascias accounts for the mobility of the skin over the shaft of the penis. The superficial vessels and nerves of the penis run along the dorsum of the penis between superficial and deep penile fascias; they supply the skin. The deep dorsal vein, dorsal arteries, and dorsal nerves of the penis are enclosed by the deep penile fascia, and they penetrate the tunica albuginea of the corpora cavernosa and spongiosum (see Fig. 28-15).

The proximal end of the body is attached to the pubic symphysis by the triangular **suspensory ligament** of the penis, which fuses with the deep penile fascia (see Fig. 28-12). The **fundiform ligament** of the penis is a continuation of the median septum of the membranous layer of the superficial fascia attached to the linea alba. The ligament encircles the body of the penis below the pubic symphysis and blends with the superficial penile fascia.

The Penile Skin and Prepuce. The skin over the body of the penis is thin, hairless, and very mobile. On the urethral surface, it presents a midline raphe continuous with the raphe of the scrotum. Over the glans, the penile skin forms a redundant hood, called the **prepuce** (*preputium penis*), by doubling back on itself and attaching around the neck of the glans (see Fig. 28-12). The prepuce covers the glans to a variable extent and can be retracted from it completely. Over the urethral surface, the prepuce forms a small median fold called the *frenulum,* which leads to the posterior end of the external urethral ostium. Preputial glands are located along the frenulum, the corona, and the neck of the glans. These are visible to the naked eye through the transparent skin on the inside of the prepuce as tiny white granules. The glands secrete *smegma,* a white sebaceous material that accumulates in the preputial sac. The skin over the glans is so thin that it is semitransparent and firmly bound to the tunica albuginea of the glans. Over the lips of the urethral meatus, it is continuous with the urethral mucosa.

Circumcision. Resection of the prepuce, or circumcision, has been a ritual practiced by certain races and in certain cultures since time immemorial. It has been adopted for putative hygienic reasons in some modern societies. Two to three generations of Americans have been routinely circumcised during the newborn period. The adoption of this practice was largely based on apparent evidence for the pathogenic effects of smegma: the incidence of cervical carcinoma among Jewish women, whose consorts have for generations been circumcised, was found to be lower than in uncircumcised populations. The validity of the interpretation of the findings has now been called into question. Furthermore, the availability of modern amenities of personal hygiene argues against the necessity or advisability of routine circumcision, even if smegma should be shown to be carcinogenic. Circumcision may be indicated when the preputial sac becomes chronically inflamed (*balanitis*) and causes fibrosis and stricture. Stricture of the preputial skin (*phimosis*) prevents its retraction from the glans. Retraction of the prepuce is necessary for successful coitus.

The Scrotum

The anatomy of the scrotum and its contents are discussed in Chapter 26.

The Superficial Perineal Muscles

The muscles of the superficial perineal space are mostly associated with the root of the penis. They are rather insubstantial sheets of voluntary muscle wrapped around the crura and the bulb of the penis and a small transverse muscle along the posterior edge of the urogenital diaphragm (Fig. 28-17).

The **superficial transverse perineal muscle** passes from the front end of the ischial tuberosity to meet its fellow at the midline in the perineal body. Both perineal fascias turn around the posterior borders of these muscles to fuse with the posterior border of the urogenital diaphragm.

The **ischiocavernosus muscle,** on each side, surrounds the free surface of the crus of the penis and, like the penile crus, is attached to the ischiopubic ramus. The muscle ends by a tendinous insertion into the corpus cavernosum of its own side, just as the two corpora come together.

The **bulbospongiosus** arises, in part, from the central tendon of the perineum and raphe of the penis and wraps around the bulb and the posterior end of the corpus spongiosum. The muscle inserts into the upper surface of the bulb and the corpus spongiosum. The most anterior fibers of the muscle pass around the entire body of the penis to end on its dorsal aspect deep to the deep penile fascia. Through the central tendon, there may be a variable amount of continuity with the sphincter ani externus.

All these muscles are covered by the deep perineal fascia and are supplied by twigs from the perineal branches of the pudendal nerve. The bulbospongiosus aids the emptying of the urethra at the end of micturition and during ejaculation. The functions of the ischiocavernosus and superficial transverse muscles are not readily obvious.

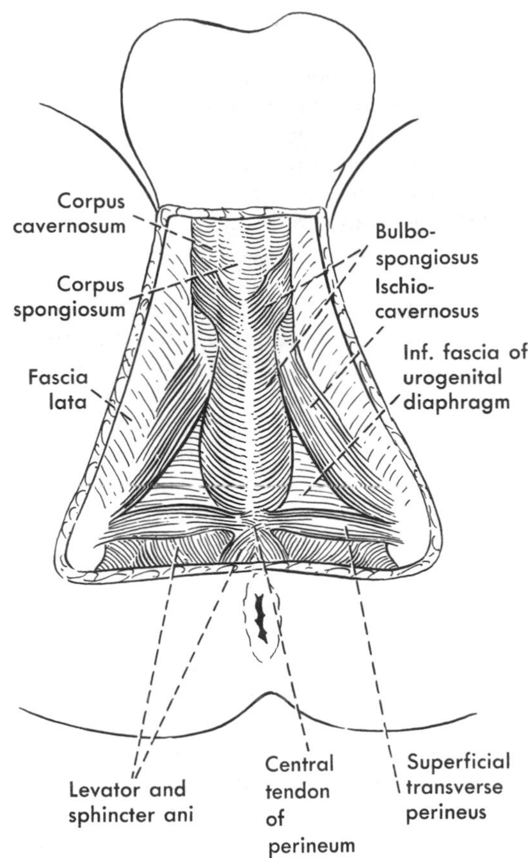

FIGURE *28-17.*
Muscles of the superficial perineal space in the male. The superficial perineal fascia has been removed.

The Female External Genitalia

The female external genitalia are collectively referred to as the **vulva.** The vulva consists of the mons pubis, the labia majora and minora, the clitoris, the bulbs of the vestibule and the vestibule of the vagina, into which open the orifices of the vagina, the urethra, and the ducts of the paraurethral and vestibular glands (Fig. 28-18).

The *mons pubis* is a conspicuous, subcutaneous fat pad over the pubic bones and symphysis. It is covered by pubic hair and is largely absent in the male. The other components of the vulva are homologues of the male external genitalia. Their anatomy will be discussed before considering the developmental relations between the respective parts.

The Labia Majora and Minora

Each **labium majus** is a broad, longitudinal fold of skin filled with subcutaneous fat and fibrous tissue, continuous anteriorly with the subcutaneous tissue of the mons

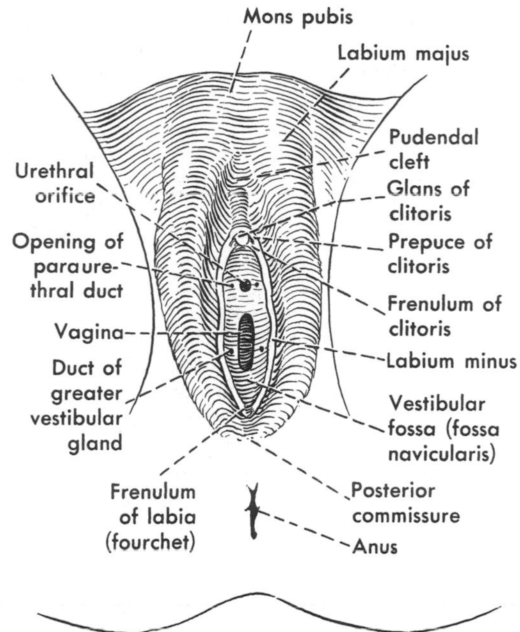

FIGURE *28-18.*
External genitalia of the female.

pubis and posteriorly with ischiorectal fat. The lateral surface of the labia facing the thighs is hairy; their smooth medial surface is studded with sebaceous glands and encloses the *pudendal cleft* (*rima pudendi*). The junction of the two labia anteriorly and posteriorly are the rather indistinct *anterior* and *posterior commissures.*

The labia majora are homologues of the two halves of the scrotal sac, and some subcutaneous smooth muscle in them, the homologue of the dartos. The fibromuscular strands of the round ligament of the uterus are interlaced in the connective tissue of the labia, and a patent processus vaginalis may extend into them.

Each **labium minus** is a smaller fold of skin in the pudendal cleft and, unlike the labia majora, contains no fat. Their lateral surfaces are in contact with the smooth, inner surface of the labia majora, and their medial surfaces are in contact with each other. Between them is the vestibule of the vagina, which is opened up by separation of the labia minora. Posteriorly, the labia minora are united by a fold, the *frenulum of the labia,* also called the "fourchette." Anteriorly, they approach the clitoris, and each labium divides into two tiny folds that fuse with their fellow of the opposite side around the clitoris. The two upper folds unite over the clitoris to form the *prepuce of the clitoris;* the two lower folds meet each other on the undersurface of the clitoris as the *frenulum of the clitoris.* Glands located along these folds secrete white sebaceous material.

The labia minora are homologues of the skin that covers part of the penis. Along the base, and partly in the substance of each labium minus, is located an oval-shaped mass of erectile tissue called the **bulb of the vestibule.** Each bulb is a homologue of half of the bulb of the penis and the posterior part of the corpus spongiosum. The bulb of the vestibule, however, does not surround the urethra. Each bulb is attached to the inferior fascia of the urogenital diaphragm and is enclosed by the deep perineal fascia. As they taper toward the clitoris, the bulbs are joined to one another and to the undersurface of the clitoris by the *pars intermedia* and the *commissure of the bulb* (Fig. 28-19).

The Clitoris

The clitoris is the homologue of the penis, but it consists of only two erectile bodies, the *corpora cavernosa clitoridis,* and is not traversed by the urethra. The corpora cavernosa commence as the *crura of the clitoris,* attached to the ischiopubic rami and the inferior fascia of the urogenital diaphragm. They unite in the midline to form the body of the clitoris, which is connected to the symphysis pubis by the *suspensory ligament.* The body ends in the tiny *glans* (see Fig. 28-19).

Similar to the penis, the clitoris and the bulb of the vestibule become tumescent during sexual excitation. The clitoris, richly supplied with sensory nerve endings, plays a dominant role in the excitatory phase of the sexual response.

The Vestibule of the Vagina

The space bordered by the labia minora and their frenulum is the vestibule of the vagina. The anterior part of the vestibule receives the **external urethral ostium,** the margins of which are rather raised and puckered. On each side of this ostium are the tiny openings of the *paraurethral glands* (of Skene). A short distance posterior to the urethral orifice is the **orifice of the vagina,** also known as the *introitus.* Although above the urogenital diaphragm the lumen of the vagina is a transverse slit, the vaginal orifice is elongated in the sagittal plane (see Fig. 28-19). It may be partially closed by the hymen. The **hymen** is a thin fold of mucous membrane of variable extent and shape; it is usually crescentic, covering the posterior margin of the vagi-

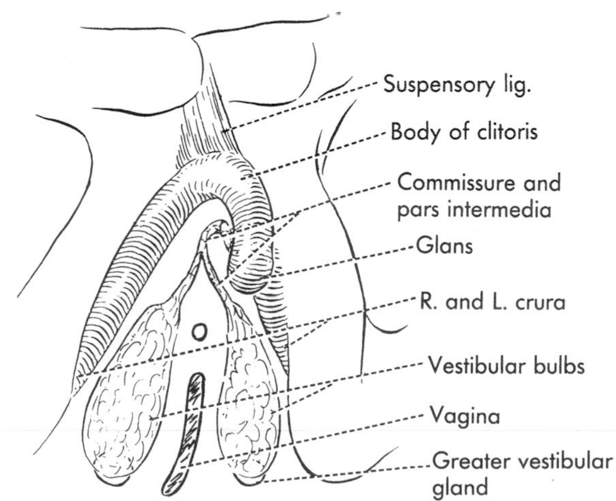

FIGURE *28-19.*
The clitoris: The connections of the vestibular bulbs with the glans clitoridis are shown.

nal orifice. If it is imperforate, it must be incised at the time of puberty to provide exit for the menstrual flow. After the hymen has been ruptured, by coitus or by other means, it is recognizable only as small tags of mucous membrane, the *carunculae hymenalis.*

The space in the vestibule posterior to the vaginal opening is the *vestibular fossa.* Into it open, on each side, the ducts of the greater vestibular glands. The **greater vestibular glands,** associated for a long time with the name of Bartholin, are roughly pea-sized, lobulated structures located at the posterior poles of the bulbs of the vestibule. They are the homologues of the bulbourethral glands. They, like the numerous *lesser vestibular glands,* which also open into the vestibule, secrete mucus and lubricate the vulva.

The Superficial Perineal Muscles

The superficial perineal space of the female contains essentially the same structures as that of the male. The muscles associated with the erectile bodies of the female external genitalia correspond to those of the male (Fig. 28-20). The **ischiocavernosus muscles** surround the crura of the clitoris; the **bulbospongiosus muscles** remain separate on the two sides, and, as they enclose the bulb of the vestibule, they surround the orifice of the vagina. Posteriorly, these are attached to the perineal body, as are the two **superficial transverse perineal muscles.** All these muscles are less well developed than in the male.

Development of the External Genitalia

As the urorectal septum reaches the ventral surface of the tail, it divides the cloacal membrane into the anal membrane posteriorly and the urogenital membrane anteriorly (see Fig. 27-15). The caudal edge of the septum contacting the cloacal membrane will form the perineal body. The primordia of the external genitalia develop as swellings around the cranial and lateral margins of the urogenital membrane: the *genital tubercle* in the midline cranially, and the *urogenital folds* and *labioscrotal swellings* laterally. The genital tubercle soon elongates into the *phallus* and along its caudal surface draws forward with it a narrow prolongation of the urogenital membrane, deep to which is the *phallic part of the urogenital sinus.* The margins of the urogenital membranes soon become prominent, forming the *urogenital folds* and causing the urogenital membrane to lie in a *sulcus.* Just lateral to the urogenital folds, a pair of swellings appear called the *labioscrotal swellings* (Fig. 28-21). The membrane in the urogenital sulcus breaks down, opening the phallic part of the urogenital sinus to the amniotic cavity and permitting urine formed by the mesonephros and metanephros to be voided. The urogenital folds, united by a commissure posteriorly, form the lips of the open phallic urogenital sinus, continuous above with the pelvic part of the urogenital sinus.

These events establish, in essence, the definitive anatomy of the female external genitalia. From the phallus develop the cavernous bodies of the corpora cavernosa and glans clitoridis; from the urogenital folds, the labia minora with the bulb of the vestibule within their substance; and from the labioscrotal swellings, the labia majora. The phallic urogenital sinus becomes the vestibule of the vagina into which open the urethra, representing the pelvic part of the urogenital sinus, and the vagina.

The establishment of the definitive anatomy of the male external genitalia requires three additional events that modify this simple arrangement: 1) The urogenital folds fuse along the phallus, resealing the phallic urogenital sinus, uniting the two parts of the bulb of the penis, which develop in the urogenital folds, and enclosing the spongy urethra. 2) The navicular fossa of the urethra is formed by the canalization of the glans

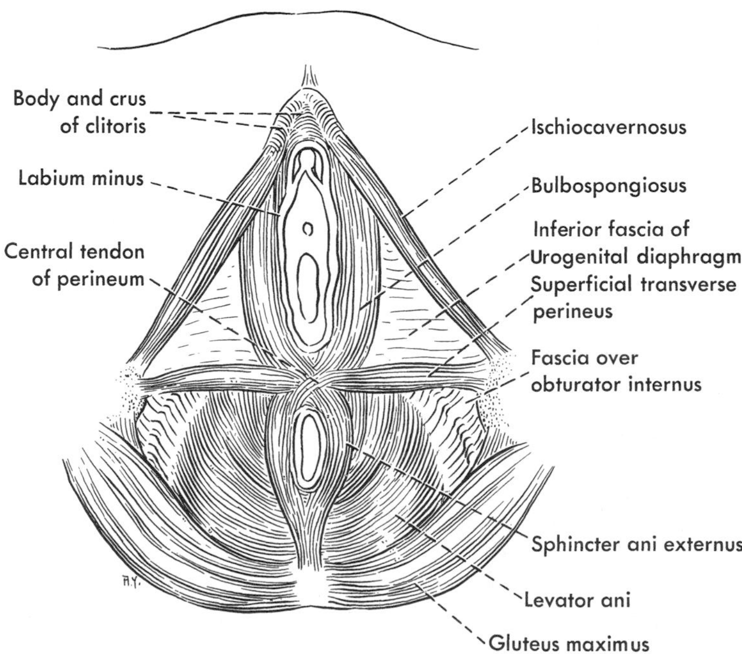

FIGURE *28-20.*
Muscles of the superficial perineal space in the female.

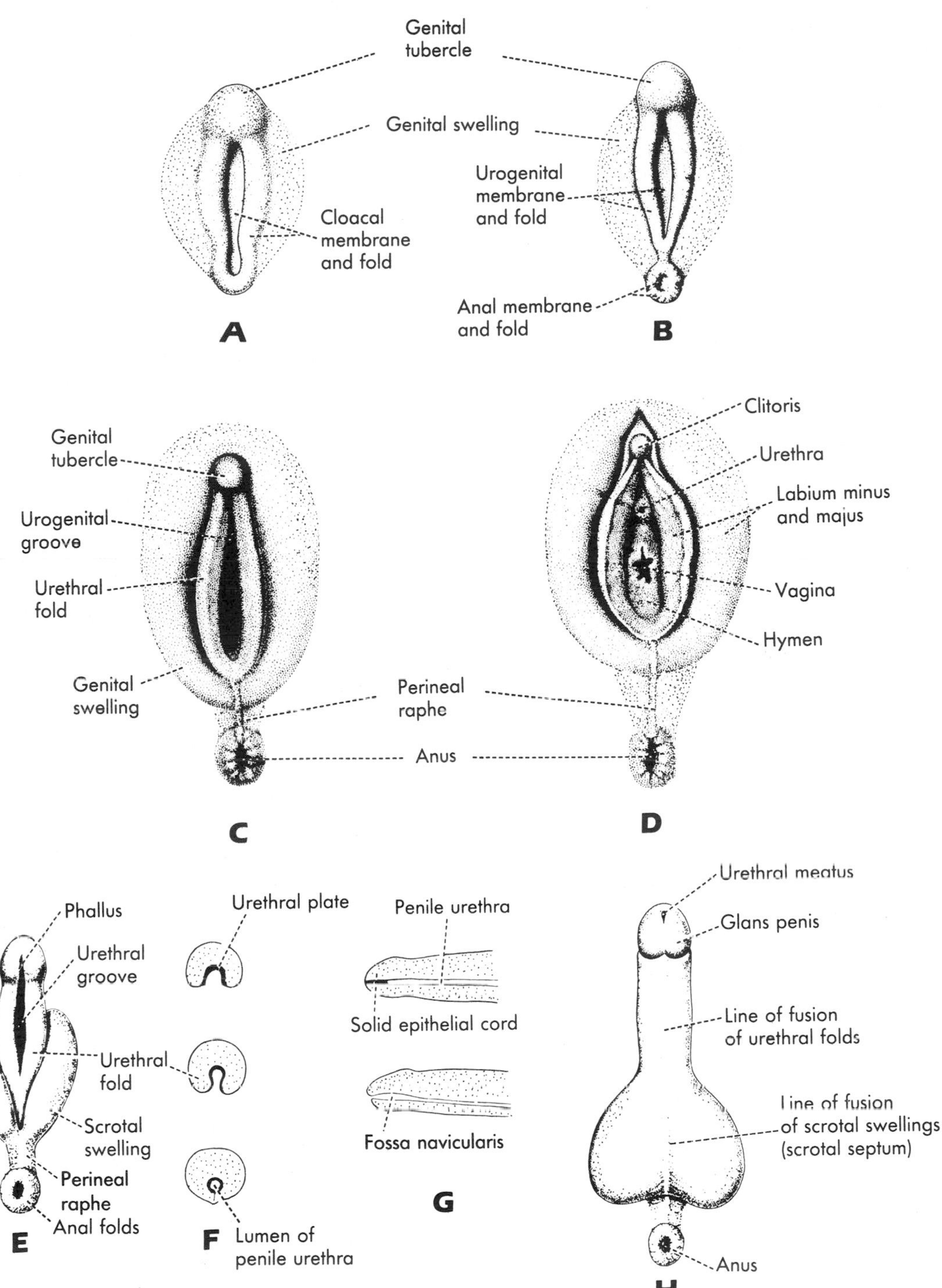

FIGURE *28-21.*
Development of the external genitalia: (A,B) indifferent stage; (C,D) female; (E-H) male. F and G show the development of the penile urethra. (Langman J. Medical embryology, 3rd ed. Baltimore: Williams & Wilkins, 1975).

penis. 3) The labioscrotal swellings approximate each other and fuse on the ventral surface of the root of the phallus and form the scrotal sac.

Anomalies. Congenital anomalies of the external genitalia are common. They may be minor, or they may make sex determination difficult and are often associated with maldevelopment of the gonads, the mesonephric and paramesonephric duct systems, and the kidneys.

Fusion of the urogenital folds and labioscrotal swellings may be arrested at various stages in the male.

In its most severe form, the perineum resembles the vulva. When the abnormality is limited to incomplete fusion of the urogenital folds, the urethra does not reach the glans and opens somewhere along the urethral surface of the penis. This is known as **hypospadias.** When the urethral opening is close to the glans, this imposes no disability. However, when the opening is more proximal on the body of the penis, the corpus spongiosum does not develop properly and, distal to the opening, is replaced by a fibrous band that causes a marked ventral flexure of the penis. A little boy so affected cannot urinate standing up, and in an adult, the penile flexure prevents coitus. In such cases, the penis must be straightened surgically and the urethra reconstructed.

Rarely, there may be a urethral opening on the dorsum of the penis. This is called **epispadias,** and the abnormality is related to **extrophy of the bladder.** When somatic mesoderm fails to migrate into the ventral body wall distal to the umbilicus, the surface ectoderm apposed to the endoderm of the vesical part of the urogenital sinus breaks down, and the trigone of the bladder becomes exposed on the anterior abdominal wall. This is extrophy of the bladder. The defect in the anterior abdominal wall may extend to the dorsum of the phallus, or it may be limited to the phallus. The latter condition is epispadias. Both extrophy and epispadias may occur in the male and in the female.

Congenital anomalies of the female external genitalia consist of various degrees of fusion between the urogenital folds (labia minora) and labioscrotal swelling (labia majora) usually associated with hypertrophy of the clitoris.

BLOOD SUPPLY, LYMPHATIC DRAINAGE, AND INNERVATION

The introduction to this chapter identified the internal pudendal artery and pudendal nerve as the chief sources of blood and nerve supply to the perineum. Earlier in this chapter the course of these structures was traced from the pelvis, through the pudendal canal, into the urogenital region. The purpose of this section is to deal, in particular, with the branches of distribution of this artery and nerve, as well as with others that supplement the supply of the perineum, and to enlarge on the general statements made in the chapter with reference to the venous and lymphatic drainage of the perineum.

Arterial Supply

The Internal Pudendal Artery

A branch of the anterior division of the internal iliac artery in the pelvis, the internal pudendal artery enters the perineum from the buttock through the lesser sciatic foramen and passes downward and forward in the lateral wall of the ischiorectal fossa enclosed with the pudendal nerve in the pudendal canal. Reaching the urogenital diaphragm, it passes along the ischiopubic ramus in the deep perineal space and terminates by dividing into a *deep* and a *dorsal artery of the penis* or *clitoris* before it reaches the transverse perineal ligament (Fig. 28-22).

In addition to its terminal branches and various small muscular branches distributed to the pelvic and urogenital diaphragms, the internal pudendal artery gives off several named branches: the inferior rectal, the perineal, and the urethral arteries and the artery of the bulb of the penis or the bulb of the vestibule.

The first branch of the artery, the **inferior rectal,** is given off just above the ischial tuberosity. It runs medially across the ischiorectal fossa to supply the muscles and the lining of the anal canal and the perianal skin. In the wall of the canal, it anastomoses with branches of the middle and superior rectal arteries and with those of the inferior rectal artery from the opposite side.

The **perineal artery** is given off in the vicinity of the posterior margin of the urogenital diaphragm. It almost immediately divides into *transverse perineal* and *posterior scrotal* or *posterior labial* branches (Fig. 28-23). These run through the superficial perineal space and supply perineal subcutaneous tissue in the scrotum or the labia, as implied by their name. They also give twigs to the lower part of the vagina along with twigs from other branches of the internal pudendal.

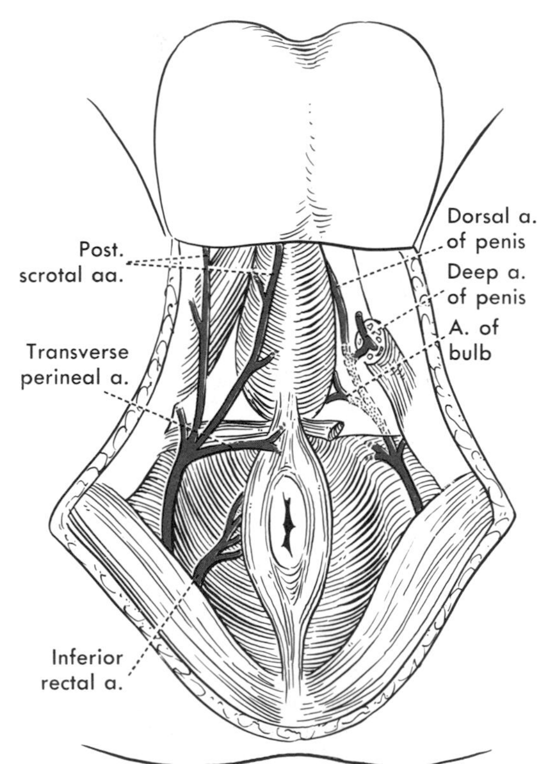

FIGURE 28-22.
The internal pudendal artery. The perineal artery and its branches are cut away on the *right*, as is most of the corpus cavernosum of the penis, to show the deep branches; the course of the artery through the urogenital diaphragm and the anterior recess of the ischiorectal fossa is indicated by *dotted outline*.

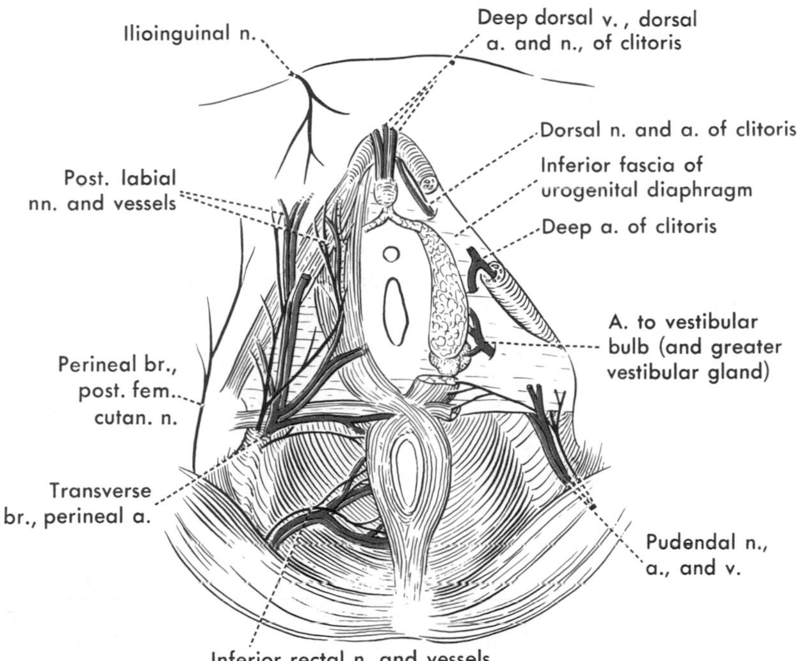

FIGURE *28-23.*
Nerves and vessels of the female perineum.

The **artery of the bulb** arises within the deep perineal space just lateral to the bulb and runs medially to pierce the inferior fascia of the urogenital diaphragm and enter the bulb. It also supplies the bulbourethral gland. In the female, it is distributed to the bulb of the vestibule and the greater vestibular gland.

The **urethral artery** arises distal to, or sometimes with, the artery of the bulb; it also pierces the inferior fascia and, after entering the corpus spongiosum, runs distally in this body to anastomose with branches of the dorsal artery. In the female, this branch is absent or inconspicuous.

The **deep artery of the penis** or **clitoris,** one of the terminal branches of the internal pudendal, leaves the deep perineal space by piercing the perineal membrane and entering the crus of the penis or the clitoris attached to that membrane. It continues along the axis of the corpus cavernosum, supplying the erectile tissue and anastomosing with branches of the dorsal artery of the penis or clitoris that pierce the tunica albuginea of the corpora cavernosa. The **dorsal artery of the penis** or **clitoris** pierces the inferior fascia of the diaphragm farther forward, in company with the dorsal nerve, medial to the crus. The two arteries and nerves reach the dorsal surface by passing between the corpora cavernosa and corpus spongiosum. The arteries run on each side of the centrally placed deep dorsal vein of the penis, and along the lateral side of the arteries run the dorsal nerves (Fig. 28-24). Over the body of the penis, the vessels and nerves are deep to the deep penile fascia, in contact with the tunica albuginea of the corpora cavernosa (see Fig. 28-15). As the arteries are traced forward on the penis, the vessels and nerves give off branches that run around the body of the penis. Their deep branches penetrate the corpora cavernosa and spongiosum. The artery terminates in the glans penis. The dor-

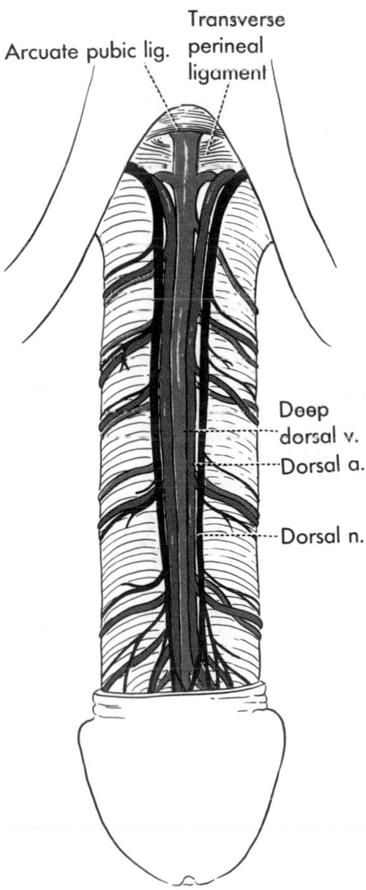

FIGURE *28-24.*
Dorsal nerves and vessels of the penis, after removal of the penile fascia.

sal artery of the clitoris pursues a similar course (see Fig. 28-23). In the corpora cavernosa and in the glans, these arteries anastomose with the deep artery of the penis or clitoris.

The External Pudendal Arteries

The blood supply to the skin and superficial fascia of the external genitalia is provided largely by the external pudendal arteries (Fig. 28-25). There are usually two on each side, a *deep* and a *superficial external pudendal artery.* They are branches of the femoral artery that emerge through the cribriform fascia and pass in the fatty subcutaneous tissue medially across the thigh and the spermatic cord or the round ligament. Their branches enter the scrotum or labia majora and the dorsum of the penis. They anastomose with the posterior scrotal or labial branches derived from the internal pudendal artery and with the branches of the dorsal artery of the penis.

Venous Drainage

Venous tributaries accompany all the branches of the internal and external pudendal arteries and receive names corresponding to their arterial branches (see Figs. 28-23 and 28-25). Veins from the bulb of the penis or vestibule, the scrotum or labia majora, and the anal canal join to form two venae comitantes of the internal pudendal artery, called the **internal pudendal veins,** which terminate in the internal iliac vein on reaching the pelvis through the pudendal canal and the buttock. The **external pudendal veins** are formed on each side by tributaries

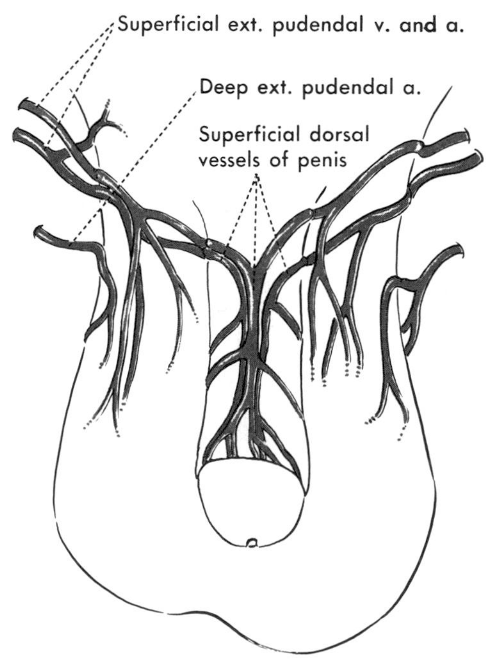

FIGURE 28-25.
The external pudendal vessels: Those on the penis supply the skin and subcutaneous tissue, not the erectile tissue.

from the skin of the penis, prepuce (*superficial dorsal vein of the penis*), and scrotum or labia majora and terminate in the great saphenous vein. (There is no vein along the deep artery of the penis or clitoris, and most of the blood from the cavernae of the corpora cavernosa and the glans penis or clitoris is drained by tributaries of the **deep dorsal vein of the penis** or **clitoris;** see Figs. 28-23 and 28-24). The deep dorsal vein is an unpaired vein that runs between the two dorsal arteries of the penis or clitoris deep to the deep fascia. It leaves the perineum through the gap between the transverse perineal ligament and the arcuate pubic ligament and joins the prostatic plexus in the male and the vesical plexus in the female. It communicates with tributaries of the internal pudendal veins.

Lymphatic Drainage

Most perineal structures send their lymphatics along the branches of the external pudendal vessels to the superficial inguinal nodes. A few lymphatics from the deep structures of the perineum pass with the internal pudendal vessels into the pelvis to end in the internal iliac nodes. Thus, lymphatics of the lower part of the anal canal, the perineal skin (including the scrotum as well as the glans penis), the spongy urethra, and the entire vulva drain to the inguinal nodes. Enlargement of these nodes may be the first sign of an infective or neoplastic lesion in the superficial tissues of the perineum. Lymphatics from the deep perineal space, the membranous urethra, and the vagina just above the hymen, as well as some part of the anal canal, drain along the internal pudendal vessels in the internal iliac nodes. The upper part of the anal canal drains upward along superior rectal vessels (see Fig. 27-20), and the upper part of the vagina has the same lymphatic drainage as the cervix uteri (see Chap. 27).

Innervation

The Pudendal Nerve

Formed by S-2 to S-4 anterior rami, the pudendal nerve is a branch of the sacral plexus. It reaches the perineum with the internal pudendal artery and gives off branches that correspond closely to those of the artery (Fig. 28-26; see Fig. 28-23). Approaching the posterior edge of the urogenital diaphragm, the nerve divides into its terminal branches, the *perineal nerve* and the *dorsal nerve of the penis* or *clitoris,* while it is within the canal. The pudendal nerve gives off the inferior rectal nerve in the posterior part of the ischiorectal fossa before it divides into its terminal branches.

The **inferior rectal nerve** crosses the ischiorectal fossa from its lateral wall to the anal canal, running with the vessels of similar name. It supplies the external anal sphincters, the lining of the lower part of the anal canal, and the perianal skin.

The **perineal nerve** breaks up into numerous muscular branches and two long cutaneous nerves, the *posterior scrotal* or *posterior labial* branches. The muscular branches

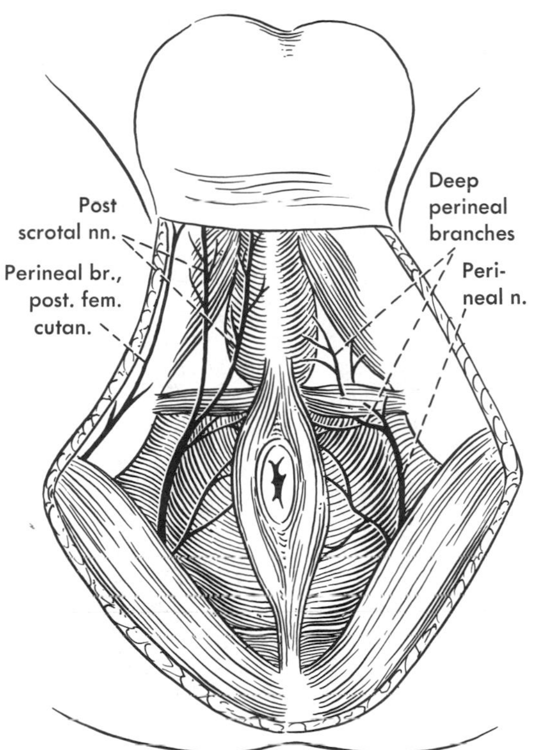

FIGURE 28-26.
Nerves in the superficial perineal space in the male: On the *reader's right,* the posterior scrotal nerves (superficial branches of the perineal nerve) have been cut away. In the ischiorectal fossa, the inferior rectal nerve, a branch of the pudendal nerve, is shown, but the dorsal nerve of the penis, lying above the perineal nerve, is omitted.

are distributed to all the deep and superficial muscles of the perineum, including the external anal sphincter and a part of the levator ani. One of the branches enters the bulb of the penis or vestibule. The posterior scrotal or labial branches pass forward in the superficial perineal space and are distributed to the scrotum or labia majora.

The **dorsal nerve of the penis** or **clitoris** continues forward along the ischiopubic rami with the dorsal artery of the penis or clitoris, running either in the deep perineal space or in the anterior recess of the ischiorectal fossa. The nerve gives a branch to the corpus cavernosum and then reaches the dorsum of the penis or clitoris running on the lateral side of the dorsal artery of the penis or clitoris (see Figs. 28-23 and 28-24). It terminates in the glans penis or clitoris.

Thus, in essence, the pudendal nerve is the sole somatic motor nerve of the perineum and it is sensory to most of the perineal skin Knowledge of the sensory innervation of the perineum is important in the female because of the frequent gynecologic and obstetric procedures that may require local anesthetics. The pudendal nerve conducts sensations from the prepuce and the penis; from the glans penis or clitoridis; from the vestibule of the vagina, including the lower part of the vagina; from part of the anal canal; and from the perianal skin, as well as from the posterior parts of the labia majora and the scrotum (Fig. 28-27). The areas of skin on the periphery of the perineum are supplied by other cutaneous nerves.

Other Cutaneous Nerves of the Perineum

Skin over the lateral portions of much of the ischiorectal fossa is supplied by the *perineal branches* of the **posterior femoral cutaneous nerves** (derived from the sacral plexus) that course forward superficially at about the level of the ischial rami. The mons pubis and the anterior portion of the labia are supplied by **anterior labial nerves** from the *ilioinguinal nerve* and by the *genitofemoral nerve.* Both these nerves are derived from the lumbar plexus and contain L-1 segments (see Fig. 28-27).

The *anterior scrotal nerves* are likewise branches of the ilioinguinal and genitofemoral nerves, and they supply the skin over the anterior surface of the scrotum and the root of the penis (Fig. 28-28).

Perineal Anesthesia

During some gynecologic and obstetric procedures, local anesthesia of the perineum can obviate a general anesthetic. The most important nerve to block is the pudendal nerve. A **pudendal block** is performed by palpating the ischial spine through the vagina and injecting local anesthetic around it through a needle inserted either through the perineal skin or through the vaginal wall. In addition, the anterior parts of the labia and the mons pubis may also need to be infiltrated with anesthetic. Because somatic afferents do not reach above the lower part of the vagina, the female genital tract may be cut, cauterized, and sutured after a pudendal block. The cervix is sensitive only to stretching and not to other stimuli. To eliminate the pain caused by dilation of the cervix, a paracervical block is required (see Chap. 27).

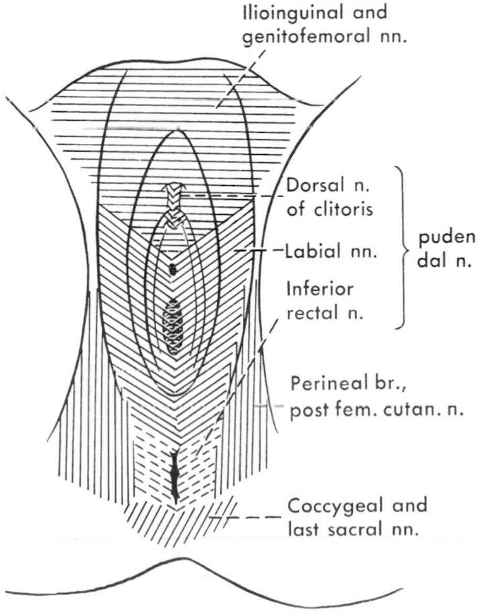

FIGURE 28-27.
General cutaneous distribution of nerves to the female perineum.

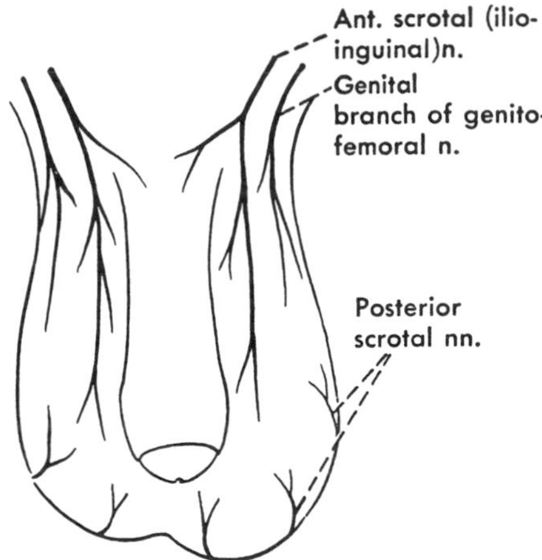

FIGURE *28-28.*
Cutaneous nerves of the scrotum; anterior view.

Pelvic Splanchnic Nerves

The visceral efferents required for erection of the penis or clitoris are derived from the pelvic splanchnic nerves. They reach the perineum along the urethra, passing through the urogenital hiatus and diaphragm. Fractures of the pelvis may damage these nerves and cause impotence.

RECOMMENDED READINGS

Alvarez-Morujo A. Terminal arteries of the penis. Acta Anat 1967; 67: 387.

Ayoub SF. Anatomy of the external anal sphincter in man. Acta Anat 1979; 105: 25.

Bennet RC, Duthie HL. The functional importance of the internal anal sphincter. Br J Surg 1964; 51: 355.

Benoit G, Delmas V, Gillot C, Jardin A. The anatomy basis of erection. Surg Radiol Anat 1987; 9: 263.

Bonica JJ. Principles and practice of obstetric analgesia and anesthesia, vol 1. Philadelphia: FA Davis, 1967.

Duthie HL, Gairns FW. Sensory nerve endings and sensation in the anal region of man. Br J Surg 1960; 47: 585.

Goligher JC, Leacock AG, Brossy JJ. The surgical anatomy of the anal canal. Br J Surg 1955; 43: 51.

Hollinshead WH. Anatomy for surgeons: vol 2, the thorax, abdomen, and pelvis. 2nd ed. New York: Harper & Row, 1971.

Juenemann KP, Lue TF, Schmidt RA, Tanagho EA. Clinical significance of sacral and pudendal nerve anatomy. J Urol 1988; 139: 74.

Kiesewetter WB, Nixon HH. Imperforate anus: its surgical anatomy. J Pediatr Surg 1976; 2: 60.

Ladd WE, Gross RE. Congenital malformations of anus and rectum: report of 162 cases. Am J Surg 1934;23: 167.

Lepor H, Gregerman M, Crosby R, Mostofl FK, Walsh PC. Precise localization of the autonomic nerves from the pelvic plexus to the corpora cavernosa: a detailed anatomical study of the adult male pelvis. J Urol 1985;133: 207.

Masters WH, Johnson VE. Human sexual response. Boston: Little, Brown, 1966.

McConnell J, Benson CS, Schmidt WA. The vasculature of the human penis: a reexamination of the morphological basis for the polster theory of erection. Anat Rec 1982; 203: 475.

McVay CB, Anson BF. Aponeurotic and fascial continuities in the abdomen, pelvis and thigh. Anat Rec 1940; 76: 213.

Mitchell GAG. The innervation of the ovary, uterine tube, testis and epididymis. J Anat 1938; 72: 508.

Moore KL, Persaud TVN. The developing human: clinically oriented embryology. 5th ed. Philadelphia: WB Saunders, 1993.

Oelrich TM. The urethral sphincter muscle in the male. Am J Anat 1980; 158: 229.

Roberts WH, Habenicht J, Krishingner G. The pelvic and perineal fasciae and their neural and vascular relationships. Anat Rec 1964; 149: 707.

Schmidt RA. Technique of pudendal nerve localization for block or stimulation. J Urol 1989; 142: 1528.

Shafik A, El-Sherif M, Youssef A, Olfat E-S. Surgical anatomy of the pudendal nerve and its clinical implications. Clin Anat 1995; 8: 110.

Stormont TJ, Cahill DR, King BF, Myers RP. Fascias of the male external genitalia and perineum. Clin Anat 1994; 7: 115.

Tobin CE, Benjamin JA. Anatomic and clinical re-evaluation of Camper's, Scapa's, and Colles' fasciae. Surg Gynecol Obstet 1949; 88: 545.

Tramier D, Argême M, Huguet JF, Juhan C. Radiological anatomy of the internal pudendal artery (a. pudenda interna) in the male. Anat Clin 1981; 3: 195.

Uhlenhuth E, Smith RD, Day ED, et al. A re-investigation of Colles' and Buck's fasciae in the male. J Urol 1949; 62: 542.

PART VIII

HEAD AND NECK

Hollinshead's Textbook of Anatomy, by Cornelius Rosse and Penelope Gaddum-Rosse.
Lippincott-Raven Publishers, Philadelphia, © 1997.

CHAPTER 29

Head and Neck in General

The head and neck are particularly complex and difficult to dissect, the former because of the bone of the skull and lower jaw, and the latter because so many important structures are crowded together in the front of the neck.

The head (*caput*) is roughly divisible into cranium, or brain case, and face. By definition, a *cranial nerve* is one that emerges through the cranium; therefore, all 12 cranial nerves must be sought in the head. Most of them are also distributed there, but two, the vagus and the accessory, have particularly long courses in the neck, and others appear where neck and head blend. Except for the skeleton, there is no clear demarcation between the head and neck; the floor of the mouth, for instance, can be considered part of the head or part of the neck. Similarly, muscles continue from one to the other, as do veins and arteries, so that it is only as the head is dissected that the upper parts of many of the soft structures of the neck can be seen. Thus, the pharynx (Fig. 29-1) into which both nose and mouth open, begins in the head but extends to the lower border of the larynx in the neck, before giving way to the esophagus; of the large vessels in the neck, the internal jugular vein receives most of its blood from the head, and the common carotid artery sends most of its blood to the head.

The neck (*collum*) consists of an anterior region, the *cervix*, and a posterior region, the *nucha*. The nucha consists primarily of the vertebral column and its associated muscles and is described in Chapter 12. It may be helpful to recall that although there are only seven cervical vertebrae, there are eight cervical nerves. The trapezius and levator scapulae muscles, also attaching to the cervical vertebral column, are described in Chapter 15 with other muscles of the shoulder, the group to which they belong. In this section of the text, therefore, we are primarily interested in the cervix rather than the neck as a whole. For practical purposes, the cervix can be thought of as extending from about the lower border of the mandible (lower jaw) to the level of the first rib and as extending posterolaterally behind the clavicular insertion of the trapezius.

Brief mention has already been made of the continuities between neck and head. Equally important are the continuities at the base of the neck between neck and thorax and neck and upper limb (Fig. 29-2). These continuities mean that in a regional dissection of the neck, neither the origin nor the destination of many of the most important structures can be seen, yet the student must know something of these matters if their functional significance is to be grasped.

The most obvious continuity at the base of the neck is the extension of the *trachea*, or windpipe, from the neck into thorax, where it is distributed to the lungs. Immediately behind it is the *esophagus*, which must pass through the thorax to reach the abdomen. Originating in the thorax from the arch of the aorta (just above the heart) are the great arterial stems found at the base of the neck. On the right side, a single stem, the *brachiocephalic artery*, enters the neck, but in the base of the neck, it divides into two arteries, the *right subclavian* and the *right common carotid*. The *left subclavian* and *left common carotid arteries* have separate

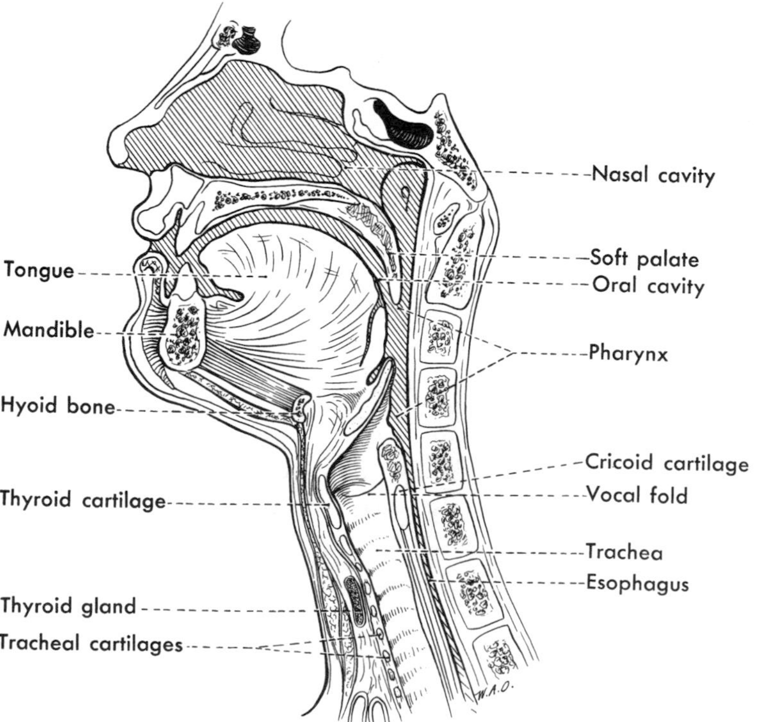

FIGURE *29-1.*
The respiratory and digestive systems in a sagittal section of the head and neck.

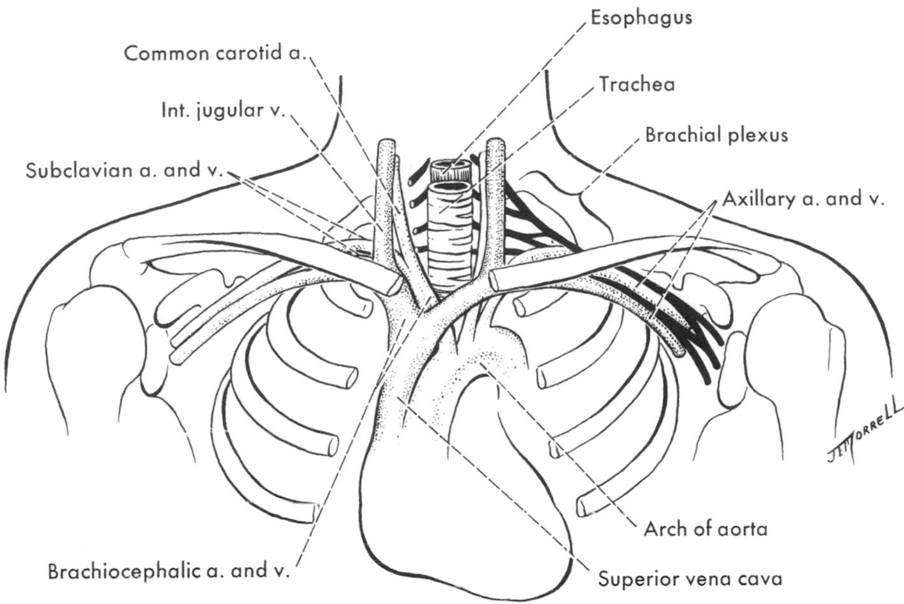

FIGURE 29-2.
Some of the more important continuities between structures in the base of the neck and those of the thorax and upper limb.

origins from the arch of the aorta and, therefore, appear separately in the neck. On both sides, the common carotid runs upward to be distributed mostly to the head, and the subclavian runs laterally at the base of the neck. The subclavian gives off branches to the neck and shoulder and to the thorax, but ends by crossing the first rib behind the clavicle, where, as the axillary artery, it is the chief artery of the upper limb.

In the same fashion, the two *subclavian veins* are continuations of the two axillary veins, the chief veins of the upper limb. On both sides, they unite with the *internal jugular vein*, from the head, to form a brachiocephalic vein. These two veins enter the thorax and then unite to form the superior vena cava, a short trunk that enters the heart.

The *brachial plexus*, which supplies the nerves to all except a few muscles of the upper limb, does originate in the neck. However, it extends into the axilla around the axillary artery and gives off most of its branches here, so that even its general form is not apparent in a dissection confined to the neck.

Besides smaller vessels that run into the thorax from the neck, and lymphatics, usually not dissectible, that enter the neck from the axilla, two other important structures should be mentioned. The *vagus nerves*, which descend through the length of the neck, continue into the thorax and, hence, to the abdomen. On the left side, the *thoracic duct*, the largest lymphatic channel in the body, joins the venous system close to the junction of the internal jugular and subclavian veins. The thoracic duct begins in the abdomen, where it receives lymph from the lower limbs and the abdomen and pelvis, and traverses the thorax before reaching the neck (Fig. 29-3).

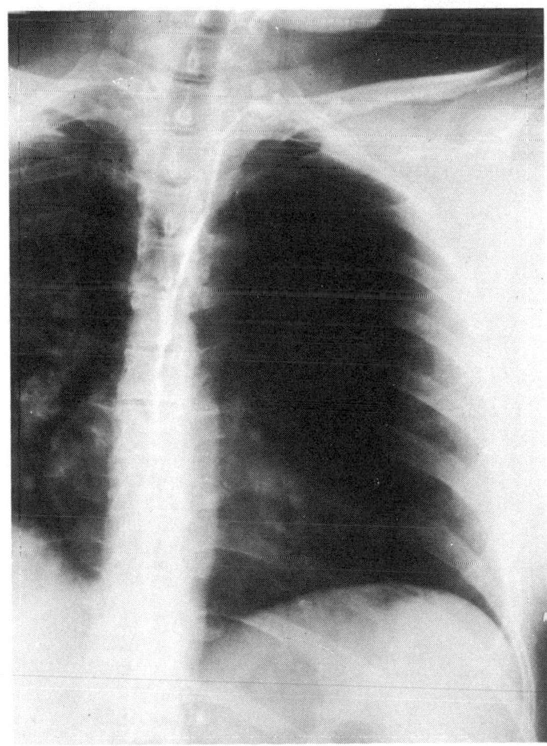

FIGURE 29-3.
Lymphangiogram of the upper end of the thoracic duct as it leaves the thorax and enters the neck. (Courtesy of Dr. W. E. Miller.)

RECOMMENDED READINGS

Cummings CW, ed. Otolaryngology—head and neck surgery. 2nd ed. St Louis: Mosby-Year Book, 1993.

Grodinsky M, Holyoke EA. The fascia and fascial spaces of the head, neck and adjacent regions. Am J Anat 1938; 63: 367.

Hollinshead WH. Anatomy for surgeons: vol 1, the head and neck. 3rd ed. Philadelphia: Harper & Row, 1982.

McMinn RMH, Hutchings RT, Logan BM. A colour atlas of head and neck anatomy. London: Wolfe Medical Publications, 1981.

Hollinshead's Textbook of Anatomy, by Cornelius Rosse and Penelope Gaddum-Rosse.
Lippincott-Raven Publishers, Philadelphia, © 1997.

CHAPTER 30

The Neck

The anterior part of the neck, or cervix, has two important landmarks: in the anterior midline is the *laryngeal prominence* (the hyoid bone is palpable just above the larynx), and on each side, extending obliquely upward and backward between the sternum and clavicle and the prominence (mastoid process) behind the ear is the *sternocleidomastoid muscle* (Fig. 30-1). The sternocleidomastoid divides the cervical region of its side into an anterior and a lateral part, usually called the *anterior* and *posterior triangles* (Fig. 30-2). Of these, the anterior triangle is bordered above by the mandible, medially by the cervical midline, and laterally by the anterior border of the sternocleidomastoid muscle. The posterior triangle is bordered by the clavicle below and by the posterior and anterior borders, respectively, of the sternocleidomastoid and trapezius muscles. Subsidiary triangles within the two major triangles also are described, as indicated in the figure, but become apparent only after reflection of overlying skin and fascia.

THE SKELETON AND SUPERFICIAL STRUCTURES

Skeleton, Fascia, Nerves, and Veins

Skeletal Structures

The **cervical vertebrae** are described in Chapter 12. Their bodies, largely covered by prevertebral muscles, are the deepest structures in the front of the neck, and their transverse processes give attachment to anterior and anterolateral muscles of the neck as well as to muscles of the back and shoulder. Of these processes, those of the atlas (first cervical) are palpable below the mastoid processes, but those of the others are too deeply buried in muscles to be felt distinctly. The cervical nerves run laterally and downward in the grooves between the anterior and posterior tubercles of the transverse processes and emerge between or through the muscles that attach to the tubercles.

The **thyroid cartilage** (shield-shaped cartilage) is a part of the skeleton of the larynx and, therefore, is described with that (Chapter 34). It also serves, however, for attachment of certain muscles of the neck. Its two laminae, facing anterolaterally, meet in the anterior midline at an angle that is especially prominent above and is surmounted by the superior thyroid notch.

The **cricoid cartilage,** also a part of the laryngeal skeleton, lies below the thyroid cartilage; unlike the latter, it completely encircles the larynx. Its anterior part, the arch, is palpable immediately below the thyroid cartilage. Below the arch are the smaller cartilages of the trachea.

The **hyoid bone,** above the larynx, is U-shaped. Its front part is its body, and its posterolateral free extremities are its **greater cornua** (horns). These can be felt easily in the living person if the hyoid bone is displaced manually to the side that is to be palpated. The junction of the body with each greater horn is marked on the upper surface by a small projection, the lesser cornu. The hyoid bone receives the attachments of anterior neck muscles on both its upper and lower borders and is highly mobile (note its movement during swallowing). It also gives attachment to certain muscles of the tongue, providing a stable or a mobile base, as necessary, for that organ.

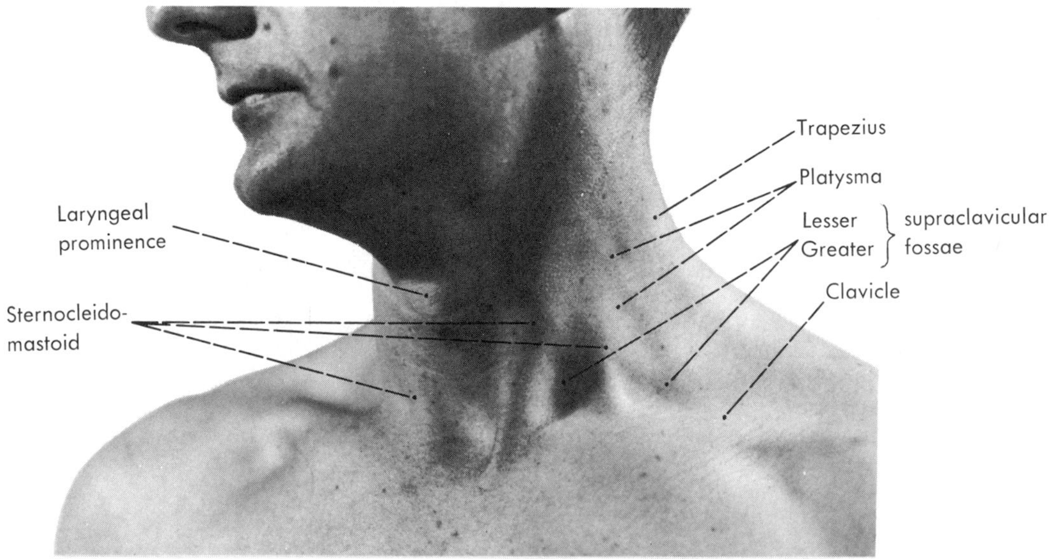

FIGURE *30-1.*
Surface anatomy of the neck.

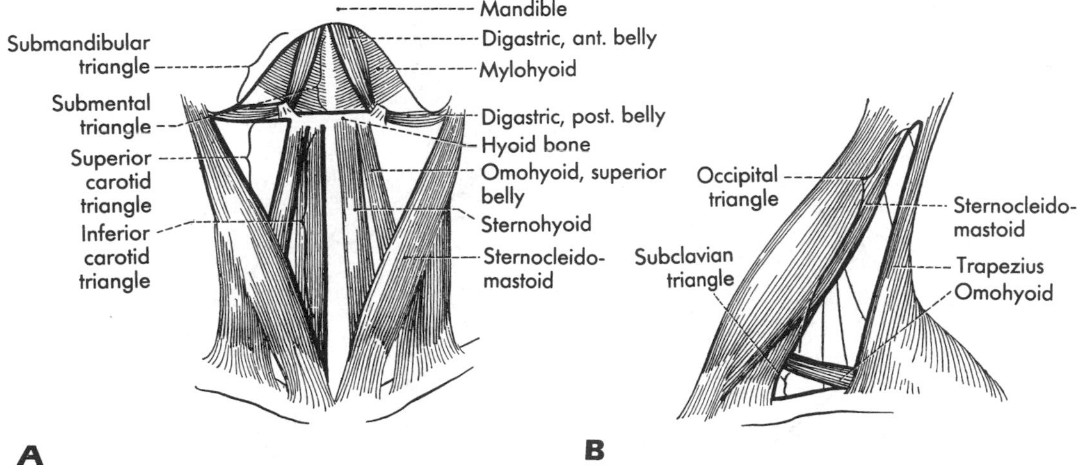

FIGURE 30-2.
(A) The anterior triangle of the neck; (B) the posterior triangle; subsidiary triangles into which they can be divided are also shown. The superior carotid triangle is often called "the carotid triangle," and the inferior one "the muscular triangle."

Ligaments and membranes fill the spaces between the thyroid cartilage and the hyoid bone, the thyroid and cricoid cartilages, and the latter and the upper tracheal cartilage. Of these, the **thyrohyoid membrane** is most extensive; nerves and vessels penetrate this membrane to enter the larynx.

The skin and the tela subcutanea (superficial fascia) of the cervix usually are rather thin, but there may be an appreciable amount of subcutaneous fat. Within the superficial fascia is an exceedingly thin muscle, the **platysma muscle,** that begins in the tela subcutanea over the upper part of the thorax, passes over the clavicle, and runs upward and somewhat medially in the neck and across the mandible to blend with superficially located facial muscles (see Fig. 31-16). Descending on its deep surface close to the junction of the posterior and inferior borders of the lower jaw (the angle of the mandible) is its nerve, the cervical branch of the facial nerve. Also deep to it, and then piercing it, are cutaneous nerves of the neck. The platysma muscle has no very important action, but will transversely wrinkle the skin of the neck and help open the mouth. It is the cervical equivalent of the facial muscles. Certain superficial veins of the neck lie immediately deep to the platysma in the superficial fascia.

Cervical Fascia

Removal of the tela subcutanea and the platysma does not clearly reveal the musculature and other structures of the cervix, for these are covered by the cervical fascia (often called deep cervical fascia). The cervical fascia is rather complicated, and the more complete descriptions of it include layers that are not named in the *Nomina Anatomica*. Furthermore, the looser connective tissue between layers is described as constituting fascial spaces of the neck. Opinions differ much among investigators on how some of the fascias are arranged, which fascial spaces communicate with each other, and which do not. However, there has been so much discussion of the fascia and fascial spaces of the neck that the student will undoubtedly be expected to be at least vaguely familiar with the question at the time of entry into clinical studies.

The cervical fascia is in three layers—a *superficial*, a *pretracheal* and a *prevertebral* (Fig. 30-3). In the anterolateral part of the neck, where these layers are fairly closely associated with each other, they form the *carotid sheath* around the great vessels of the neck: the internal jugular vein and common carotid artery. A simple concept is that the superficial layer surrounds all the important structures in the neck; the prevertebral layer surrounds the vertebral column and the muscles closely connected with it; and the pretracheal layer helps form a visceral compartment around the chief viscera, trachea, and esophagus, with the carotid sheath forming a neurovascular compartment.

The **superficial layer** of the cervical fascia can be traced posteriorly to the cervical spinous processes and the ligamentum nuchae. It passes both superficial and deep to the trapezius muscle; then, coming together to form a single layer, it passes forward across the posterior triangle of the neck to the posterior border of the sternocleidomastoid muscle. On reaching this muscle, the fascia again divides to pass on both sides of it and continue across the front of the neck, joining the layer of the other side in the anterior midline. It also gives off from its deep surface a special investment around the omohyoid muscle that runs from the scapula to the hyoid bone, but takes an abrupt turn in the anterior part of the neck (see Fig. 30-10). This fascial investment holds the muscle to the clavicle, so that it pulls the hyoid bone primarily downward, rather than laterally. Medial and deep to the sternocleidomastoid, the superficial layer gives off delicate laminae that pass between and behind the muscles in front of the trachea, and it blends with the connective tissue (carotid

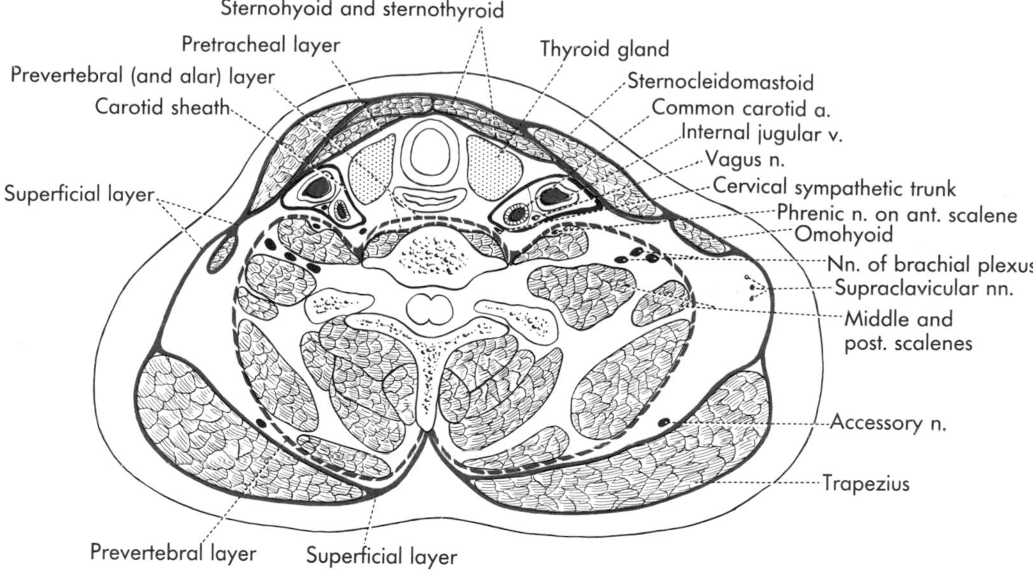

FIGURE *30-3.*
Diagram of the fascial layers of the neck, in a cross section below the level of the larynx.

sheath) around the great vessels lateral to the trachea and mostly behind the sternocleidomastoid.

Traced vertically, the superficial layer of cervical fascia over and posterior to the sternocleidomastoid simply blends with fascia of the head, forming a part of the scalp. Anteriorly, this layer is attached below to the clavicle and above to the hyoid bone (Fig. 30-4), after which it continues from the hyoid bone to the lower border of the mandible. Above and behind the hyoid bone, it runs upward to envelop muscles connected with the mandible, and between the mandible and the ear, it splits to envelop the parotid gland. Thereafter, it attaches to the skull. Between the sternocleidomastoid muscles, the superficial lamina attaches, below, to the anterior and posterior surfaces of the sternum; consequently, between these two attachments, there is a small blind *suprasternal space.*

The cutaneous nerves of the neck (see the following section) enter the superficial layer of cervical fascia at the posterior border of the sternocleidomastoid and thereafter run, in part, in it before entering the tela subcutanea. In cleaning the fascia from the external surface of the sternocleidomastoid muscle, care must be taken to isolate the nerves as they run around the posterior border of the muscle. Otherwise, removing the fascia will leave only

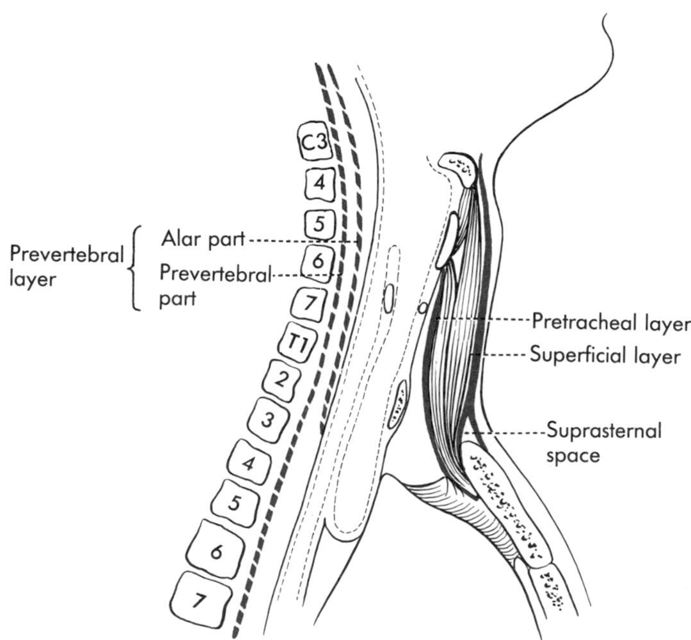

FIGURE *30-4.*
Diagram of the fascial layers of the neck in a longitudinal section. (Redrawn from Grodinsky M. Holyoke EA. Am J Anat 1938; 63: 367.)

their stumps. The major superficial veins of the neck lie largely external to the fascia, and there is often a communication between the two anterior jugular veins in the suprasternal space.

The **pretracheal lamina** of cervical fascia stretches across the front of the neck, immediately behind the infrahyoid muscles, and is usually described as continuous on both sides with that part of the superficial layer deep to the sternocleidomastoid muscles (see Fig. 30-3). (It also is described as surrounding the trachea, esophagus, and thyroid gland, or the trachea and esophagus; but not the thyroid gland.) It is attached above to the thyroid cartilage (see Fig. 30-4) and runs downward behind the infrahyoid or "strap" muscles to their origins from the posterior aspect of the sternum. Here, it blends with connective tissue between the pericardial sac and the sternum and with the adventitia of the great vessels as they leave or enter the pericardial sac. On its deep surface, the pretracheal layer blends laterally with the carotid sheath, just as does the superficial layer. The pretracheal layer of the cervical fascia is generally thin and probably of no great importance in itself; however, it is supported anteriorly by the infrahyoid muscles, such that it and these muscles, and the stronger carotid sheath laterally, bound the area in which the trachea, esophagus, and thyroid gland lie in loose connective tissue in front of the vertebral column. The space so enclosed is often known as the *visceral compartment*.

The **prevertebral lamina,** the third layer of cervical fascia, begins, as does the superficial layer, in the posterior midline (see Fig. 30-3). Here, it is closely adjacent to the superficial layer, but it covers the outer surfaces of the muscles of the back and, as it proceeds forward, it forms the floor of the posterior triangle of the neck. Particularly at the base of the neck, there is loose connective tissue between the superficial and prevertebral layers, through which run nerves and vessels to the upper limb. As the prevertebral layer continues forward from the superficial surface of the muscles of the back, it covers anterolateral muscles, the scalenes, connected with the vertebral column, and this part is often called **scalene fascia.** It then attaches to the transverse processes of the cervical vertebrae and splits into two layers that continue across the front of the vertebral column to fuse again on the other side as they attach to the transverse processes.

Only this most anterior part is truly prevertebral in position; sometimes the two layers here are given different names (see Fig. 30-4). Between them there is some loose connective tissue, constituting one of the fascial spaces of the neck. The two parts of the prevertebral layer in front of the vertebral column behave differently. Although both attach above to the skull, the *anterior lamina* ends below by blending with the fascia on the posterior wall of the esophagus in the upper part of the thorax, thus obliterating the posterior part of the visceral compartment, but the *posterior lamina* continues downward along the front of the thoracic portion of the vertebral column.

The cutaneous nerves of the neck penetrate the prevertebral fascia in their courses to a superficial position. However, the lower cervical nerves and the accompanying artery (subclavian), instead of penetrating this fascia, carry with them a sleevelike diverticulum of the fascia as they emerge from behind it. This accompanies them to the axilla, where it contributes to the *axillary sheath*.

The **carotid sheath** is a condensation of connective tissue around the great vessels of the neck and is particularly prominent because these vessels are so large. Superficially, it blends with, or is formed by, the superficial layer of the cervical fascia deep to the sternocleidomastoid muscle and the adjacent part of the pretracheal layer. The anteromedial and posterior layers of the carotid sheath come together medially to complete the sheath, and here looser connective tissue unites the posterior layer of the sheath to the prevertebral fascia (Fig. 30-5). The carotid sheath contains the internal jugular vein anterolaterally, the common carotid artery medially, and the main trunk of the vagus nerve posteriorly. The cervical sympathetic trunk lies behind the carotid sheath, between it and the prevertebral fascia.

Fascial Spaces. Accounts of the *fascial spaces* of the neck (the looser connective tissue between fascial layers) vary markedly, and there is little agreement among clinicians as to whether infections spread through spaces that are continuous with each other, thus making them of clinical importance, or whether they do not. None of the spaces have official names.

The potential space in front of the trachea and behind the infrahyoid muscles and pretracheal fascia (part of the visceral compartment) usually is called the **pretracheal space.** It is limited above by the attachment of fascia and muscles to the thyroid cartilage and below by the blending of the pretracheal fascia with connective tissue in the anterior mediastinum (Fig. 30-6). The space behind the esophagus, between it and the prevertebral fascia, is the **retrovisceral** or **retropharyngeal space.** It extends above to the base of the skull, behind the pharynx as well as the esophagus, and is limited below in the posterior mediastinum by the attachment of the anterior layer of the prevertebral fascia to the esophagus. According to most, but not all,

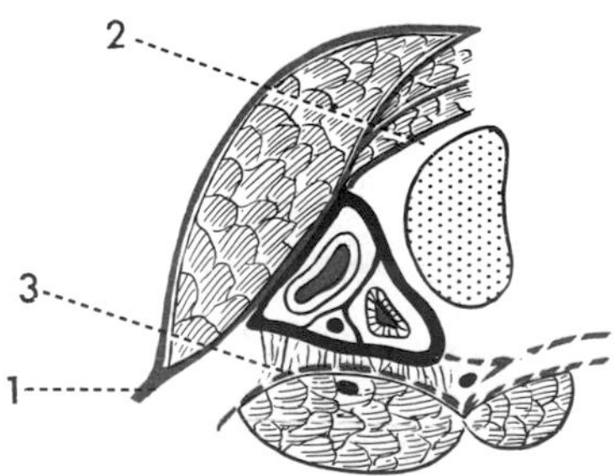

FIGURE *30-5.*
The carotid sheath. *1* is the part of the superficial layer that passes deep to the sternocleidomastoid; *2* is the pretracheal layer; and *3* is the prevertebral layer on the anterior scalene muscle. The internal jugular vein laterally, the common carotid artery, and the vagus nerve appear within the sheath; the phrenic nerve lies behind the prevertebral layer, and the sympathetic trunk lies in front of it, between it and the attachment it receives from the carotid sheath.

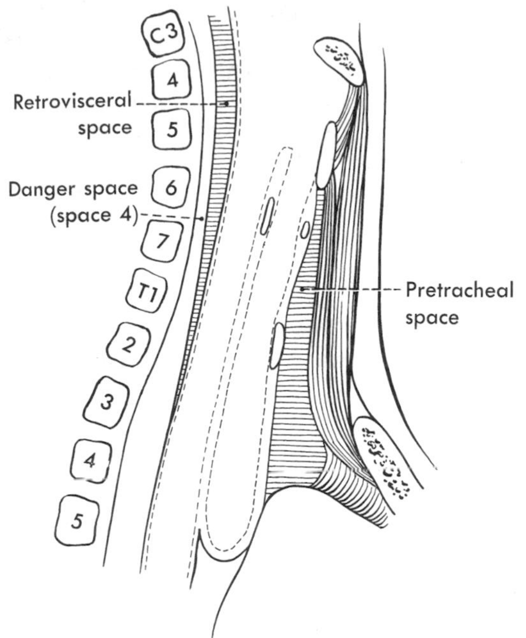

FIGURE 30-6.
The visceral compartment (*horizontally lined*) in a sagittal section of the neck. The "danger space" is also indicated. (Adapted from Grodinsky M, Holyoke EA. Am J Anat 1938; 63: 367.)

accounts, the two spaces are continuous with each other around the thyroid gland; thus, infections originating close to the pharynx have been described as descending in the retrovisceral space to the posterior mediastinum, or sometimes passing forward into the pretracheal space and involving the anterior mediastinum. The potential **space between the two layers of prevertebral fascia** in front of the vertebral column has been called the "danger space," because, although it also begins above at the base of the skull, it extends downward throughout the thorax. The **space of the carotid sheath** sometimes has been described as reaching the base of the skull and sometimes as being obliterated at the level of branching of the common carotid artery.

Superficial Nerves

The cutaneous nerves of the neck are all branches of the cervical plexus, and the upper three appear at the posterior edge of the sternocleidomastoid muscle (see Fig. 30-8). The highest, the **lesser occipital nerve,** appears at the upper part of the posterior border of the sternocleidomastoid and runs vertically upward toward the mastoid process, to be distributed to skin and scalp behind the ear. Below it, close to the middle of the muscle, is the **great auricular nerve.** This also runs vertically upward, usually accompanied by the external jugular vein, about in line with the front of the ear. It supplies much of the external ear and some skin of the face below and in front of the ear. A little below it is the **transversus colli** (or transverse cervical) **nerve.** As or soon after it rounds the posterior border of the sternocleidomastoid muscle, it divides into two major branches. One of these runs upward and forward, and one downward and forward, so that between them they supply most of the skin of the anterior part of the neck.

The lowest set of cutaneous nerves, not so intimately related to the posterior border of the sternocleidomastoid, consists of three **supraclavicular nerves.** They enter the superficial lamina of the cervical fascia in the posterior triangle, and the *medial supraclavicular nerve* then runs downward and anteriorly across the lower part of the sternocleidomastoid to supply anterior skin at the base of the neck and over approximately the upper two inter-

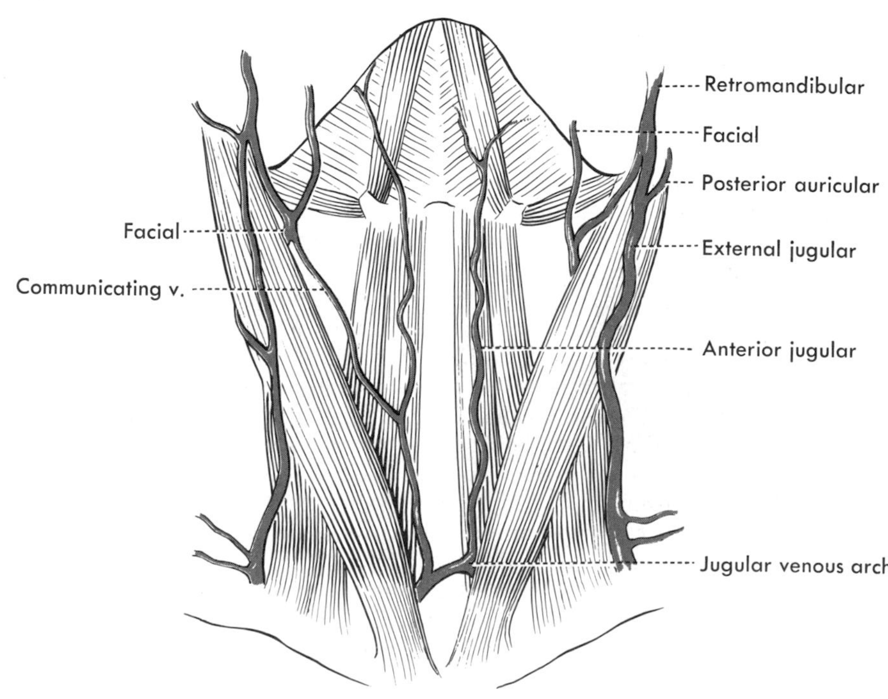

FIGURE 30-7.
Superficial veins of the neck.

costal spaces. The *intermediate* nerve descends through about the middle of the base of the posterior triangle and supplies skin of the base of the neck and the upper part of the thorax. The *lateral* (posterior) *supraclavicular nerve* runs over the anterior border of the trapezius muscle to supply skin toward and over the tip of the shoulder.

Superficial Veins

The superficial veins of the neck are the external and anterior jugulars (Fig. 30-7). The **external jugular** begins on the superficial surface of the sternocleidomastoid muscle at about the level of the angle of the mandible, where it usually is formed by the union of two veins: the posterior auricular vein, from skin and scalp behind and above the ear, and a branch from the retromandibular vein, from in front of the ear. The external jugular is closely paralleled by the great auricular nerve. At the base of the neck, just posterior to the sternocleidomastoid muscle, the external jugular turns more deeply to pierce the deep fascia and end in the subclavian vein. Close to its termination, it receives the anterior jugular vein and veins from the shoulder.

The variable **anterior jugular vein** typically begins by the union of small veins between the hyoid bone and the chin and may receive connections from the external jugular or the fascial vein; either of these connections may form its upper end, or it may be absent. It often sends a communication, the **jugular venous arch,** to the vein of the opposite side through the suprasternal space. It ends by passing deep to the sternocleidomastoid muscle and entering the external jugular vein.

Sternocleidomastoid Muscle

The sternocleidomastoid muscle arises by a tendinous head from the sternum and by a broader but thin muscular head from the medial part of the clavicle. The two heads unite, and the muscle extends obliquely upward and laterally across the neck to insert into the mastoid process behind the ear.

The **spinal accessory nerve** (Figs. 30-8 and 30-9) runs posteriorly and downward to enter the deep surface of

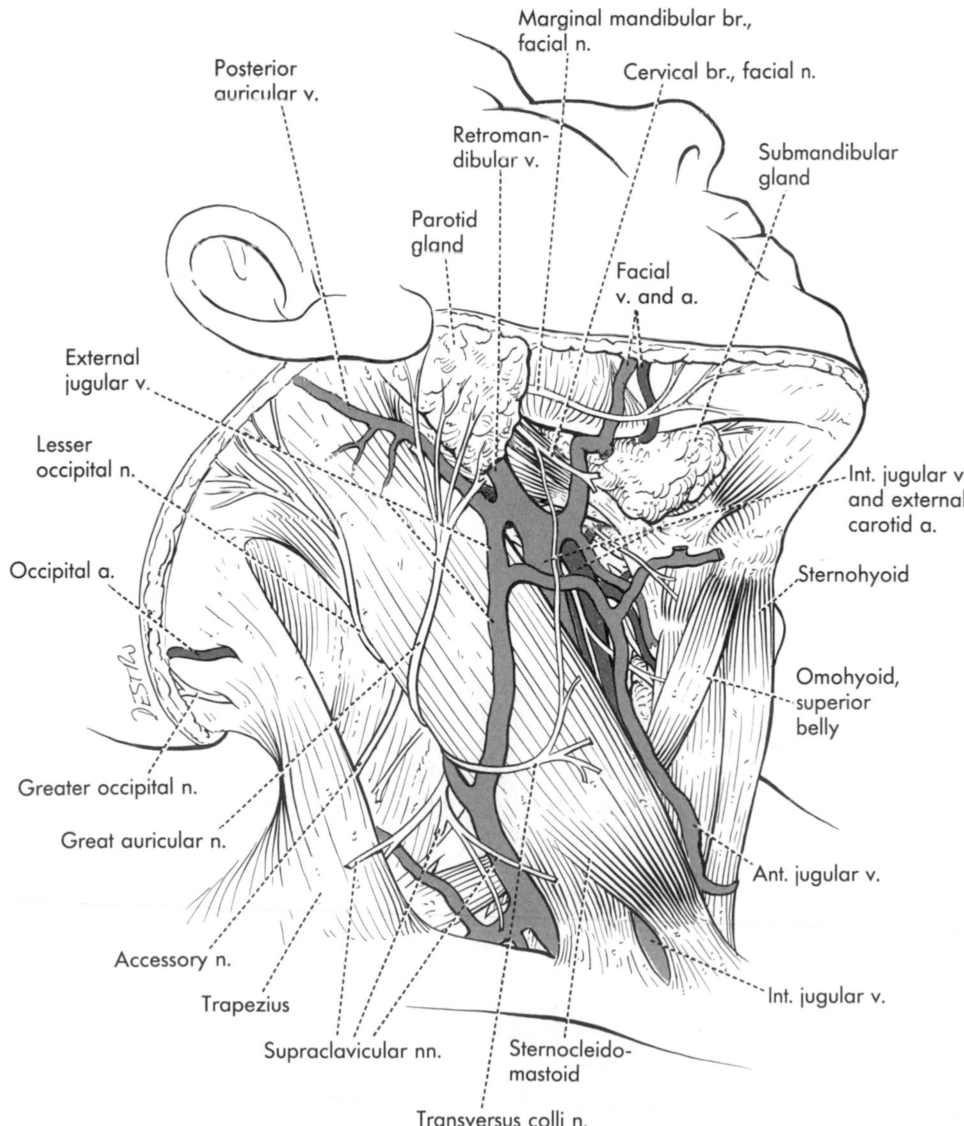

FIGURE *30-8.*
Superficial structures of the neck after removal of the platysma muscle and the cervical fascia: Further detail and identification can be found in following figures.

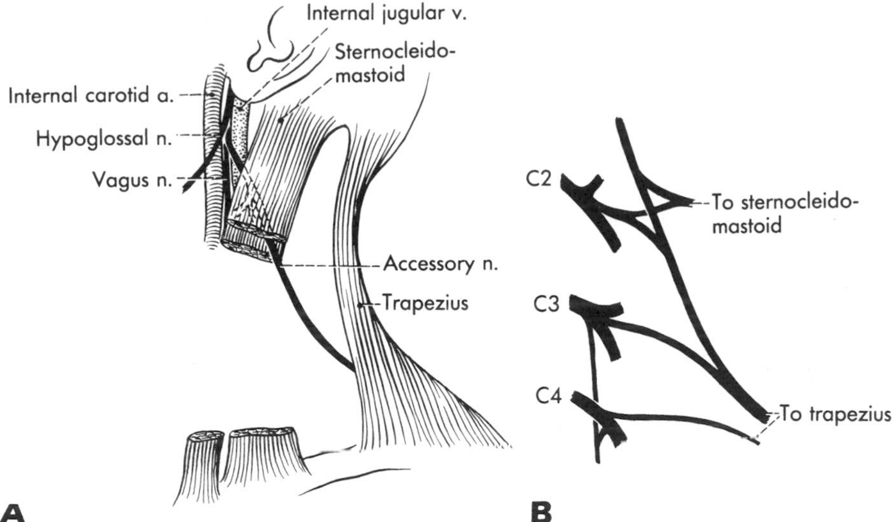

FIGURE *30-9.*
(A) Usual course and relations of the accessory nerve, and (B) its connections with the cervical plexus.

the sternocleidomastoid. It usually runs through the muscle, but sometimes, runs deep to it. After supplying the sternocleidomastoid, the nerve runs downward and laterally through the posterior triangle to disappear deep to the trapezius and supply that muscle also. The accessory nerve is joined by cervical nerve fibers, typically from C-2, that enter the muscle as a part of the accessory nerve and contribute afferent fibers.

The muscle receives two fairly prominent vascular twigs. The upper one is from the *occipital artery*, and the lower one is from the *superior thyroid artery*. It also receives a lesser blood supply from vessels at the base of the neck and from vessels related to its upper end.

Action. The sternocleidomastoid, acting alone, laterally flexes the neck and rotates the face to the opposite side. The two muscles acting together flex the head and neck forcibly. Spasm of the muscle, usually of unknown origin, but sometimes congenital, is one cause of a flexion deformity of the neck known as *wryneck* or *torticollis*; other muscles that rotate and flex the neck also may contribute to torticollis.

THE ANTERIOR TRIANGLE

Removal of the superficial lamina of the cervical fascia between the two sternocleidomastoid muscles allows identification of the subsidiary triangles in the anterior triangle. Two of these (see Fig. 30-2) are important: the submandibular triangle and the carotid (superior carotid) triangle; two others are not in the NA, but are usually called the submental triangle and the inferior carotid or muscular triangle.

The **submandibular triangle** lies below the border of the mandible and above the hyoid bone. It is bordered anteroinferiorly by the anterior belly of the diagastric muscle and posteroinferiorly by the posterior belly of the digastric and the associated stylohyoid muscle. It is filled largely by the submandibular gland, one of the major salivary glands. The **carotid triangle** lies below the submandibular triangle, and its upper border is the stylohyoid and the posterior belly of the digastric. Its posterior border is the anterior border of the sternocleidomastoid muscle. Its anteroinferior border is the superior belly of the omohyoid.

The **submental triangle** lies above the hyoid bone between the submandibular triangle and the anterior midline, and the **muscular** or inferior carotid **triangle** lies between the (superior) carotid triangle and the anterior midline below the hyoid bone. Both these triangles have muscular floors.

Muscles, Vessels, and Nerves

Carotid Sheath and Contents

The major structures in the carotid sheath are the internal jugular vein, the common carotid artery, and the vagus nerve. The carotid sheath begins at the base of the neck, where it is continuous with the connective tissue around the great vessels here, and usually is described as ending at about the upper border of the thyroid cartilage in the same manner, although some authorities claim to have traced it higher. In its lower part, it is covered by the sternocleidomastoid muscle, and it also is crossed anteriorly by the omohyoid muscle. Care must be taken in removing it from about the vascular structures, for nerves to the infrahyoid (strap) muscles traverse it; one part of the loop that supplies these muscles (*ansa cervicalis*) may run lateral and anterior to the vein in the carotid sheath to join the other part that runs between the artery and vein, or both may run deep to the vein (Fig. 30-10). Many of the deep lymph nodes of the neck lie in the carotid sheath, along the internal jugular vein and between it and the common carotid artery. These nodes may be small and scattered and not easily visible in the usual dissection, but they are important when there is carcinoma of the mouth, larynx, or other structures of the head and neck.

The **internal jugular vein** (see Fig. 30-10) emerges from deep to the posterior belly of the digastric muscle and receives one or more veins at about the level of the hyoid bone. The one vein regularly entering the internal jugular at this level is the facial, usually after it has been joined by part of the retromandibular vein. The *facial vein* runs downward superficially across the submandibular gland; but the *retromandibular vein* usually divides at the anterior border of the sternocleidomastoid muscle to contribute partly to the external jugular and partly to the facial. Other veins entering the internal jugular at about this level are from deeper structures and are difficult to identify until they have been traced to the region from which they come. Moreover, they may join together in various combinations to empty into the internal jugular, or they may join the facial vein and empty with it into the internal jugular. The largest vein here is typically the *lingual vein*, but also there may be *pharyngeal veins*, and there is a *superior thyroid vein*. Below this level, the internal jugular vein usually receives no tributaries until it is at the level of the middle of the thyroid gland, where it often receives a *middle thyroid vein*. Below this, it receives no other tributaries and ends by joining the subclavian vein at the base of the neck. The union of these two veins forms the brachiocephalic vein.

The dilated upper end of the internal jugular vein, the *superior bulb*, is located in the jugular fossa of the skull. It is primarily a continuation of the sigmoid venous sinus. The lower end of the vein, also dilated, is the *inferior bulb*.

The *thoracic duct*, the great lymphatic channel of the thorax, joins the angle of junction of the internal jugular and subclavian veins on the left side (see Fig. 30-27) or either of these veins close to their junction. The smaller *right lymphatic duct* or the several channels that may represent it, identifiable with more difficulty, empty in a corresponding position on the right side.

The internal jugular vein largely covers the **common carotid artery.** The right common carotid and the right subclavian separate from each other at the base of the neck, arising as the terminal branches of the brachio-

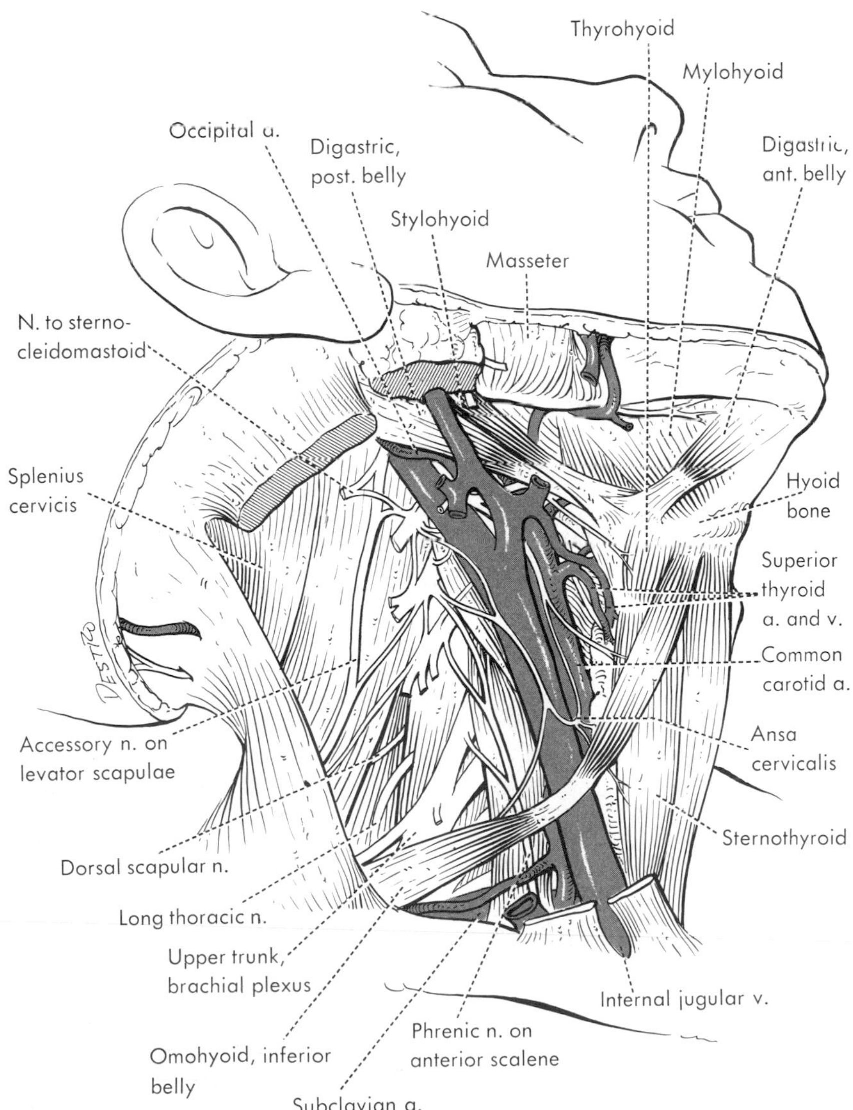

FIGURE *30-10.*
Structures in a deeper dissection of the neck. The superficial veins and the sternocleidomastoid muscle have been removed, as have the submandibular gland and a segment of the facial vein. The cutaneous nerves have been cut down to short stumps arising from the second, third, and fourth cervical nerves.

cephalic trunks, hence the origin of this carotid can be seen in a dissection of the neck. The left common carotid, however, is an independent branch from the arch of the aorta, and it enters the neck separately from and a little anteromedial to the left subclavian artery. The two common carotids run upward one on each side of the trachea (where the pulse can easily be felt) to about the upper border of the thyroid cartilage before they give off any branches. Here, each common carotid divides into its terminal branches, the internal and external carotids.

Each **vagus nerve** (Figs. 30-11 and 30-12) lies behind and somewhat between the common carotid artery and the internal jugular vein. Of its upper branches, given off while it is related to the internal carotid artery and the internal jugular vein, the *superior laryngeal nerve* descends into the neck (see Fig. 30-12), dividing into external and internal branches that are both distributed to the larynx. In the lower part of the neck, each vagus gives off slender *superior and inferior cardiac branches* that run downward and medially, usually passing behind the subclavian artery to disappear into the thorax and join the cardiac plexus. At the base of the neck each nerve passes in front of the subclavian artery (but behind the vein) before disappearing into the thorax. At the lower border of the artery, the right vagus gives off the **right recurrent laryngeal nerve,** which loops below and behind the artery to run upward and medially in the groove between the trachea and esophagus. The left recurrent laryngeal nerve originates in the thorax and runs below and behind the arch of the aorta. In the neck it follows a course similar to that of the right nerve. Each recurrent nerve gives twigs to the esophagus and trachea and ends as an *inferior laryngeal nerve.*

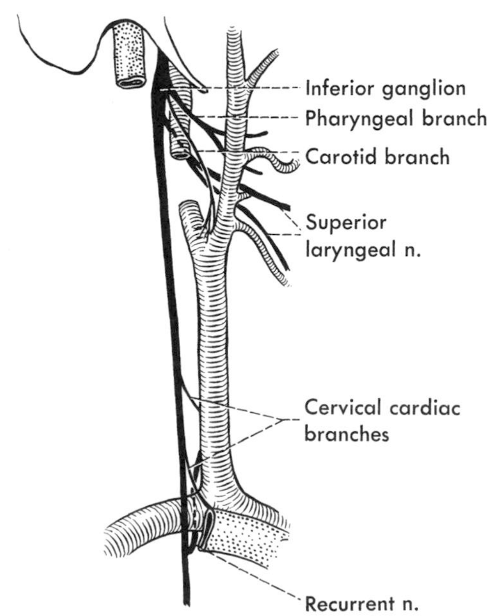

FIGURE *30-11.*
Course of the right vagus nerve in the neck.

Infrahyoid Muscles

The sternohyoid, omohyoid, sternothyroid, and thyrohyoid muscles are often referred to as "strap muscles" (Fig. 30-13; see also Figs. 30-8; 30-10). They cover the front and much of the sides of the larynx, trachea, and thyroid gland and, with a deeper-lying suprahyoid muscle (geniohyoid), represent a cervical continuation of the muscle mass that, in the abdomen, forms the rectus abdominis.

Most superficially and on each side of the midline, ascending from an origin on the posterior surface of the manubrium sterni and the sternal end of the clavicle, are the **sternohyoid muscles.** These thin, flat muscles attach above to the body of the hyoid bone. Lateral to the sternohyoid muscle is the *superior belly* of the **omohyoid muscle,** which attaches to the hyoid bone just lateral to the attachment of the sternohyoid. In the upper part of its course, this muscle almost parallels the sternohyoid, but it diverges somewhat laterally as it runs downward (passing in front of the carotid sheath and its contents). In the lower part of the neck, its muscle fibers usually give way to a tendon, through which it is joined to its inferior belly; the tendinous junction may or may not be obvious. The *inferior belly* of the omohyoid runs laterally, inferiorly, and posteriorly across the posterior triangle of the neck, dividing this triangle into an upper occipital and a lower subclavian triangle (see Fig. 30-2), and disappears deep to the trapezius. It attaches to the superior border of the scapula (*omo;* shoulder) just medial to the scapular notch.

Deep to the sternohyoid are the sternothyroid and the thyrohyoid. The **sternothyroid** takes origin from the posterior surface of the manubrium and attaches above to an oblique line on the thyroid cartilage. The **thyrohyoid** runs from this line to the hyoid bone. Its lateral border usually appears posterolateral to the omohyoid.

The infrahyoid muscles are *innervated* by fibers from upper cervical nerves, which reach them in a somewhat peculiar fashion (see Fig. 30-13). The nerves of the lower part of these muscles are given off from a loop, the **ansa cervicalis.** The inferior root of the loop is a direct branch from the cervical plexus, typically containing fibers from the second and third cervical nerves. It descends either deep or superficial to the internal jugular vein and passes medially to form a loop (*ansa* means loop) with the terminal part of the superior root from which branches are given off to the inferior belly of the omohyoid and to the lower parts of the sternohyoid and sternothyroid. Depending on the relation of the inferior root, the loop may be either around the internal jugular vein or deep to it. The superior root of the ansa cervicalis appears to take origin from the hypoglossal (12th cranial) nerve, usually just visible at about the level of the hyoid bone. It descends between the common carotid artery and the internal jugular vein, sends a branch to the superior belly of the omohyoid and one to the sternohyoid and sternothyroid muscles close to the level of the thyroid cartilage, and then, joins the inferior root to complete the loop. Actually, the superior root contains not hypoglossal, but cervical, nerve fibers that leave the first and second cervical nerves,

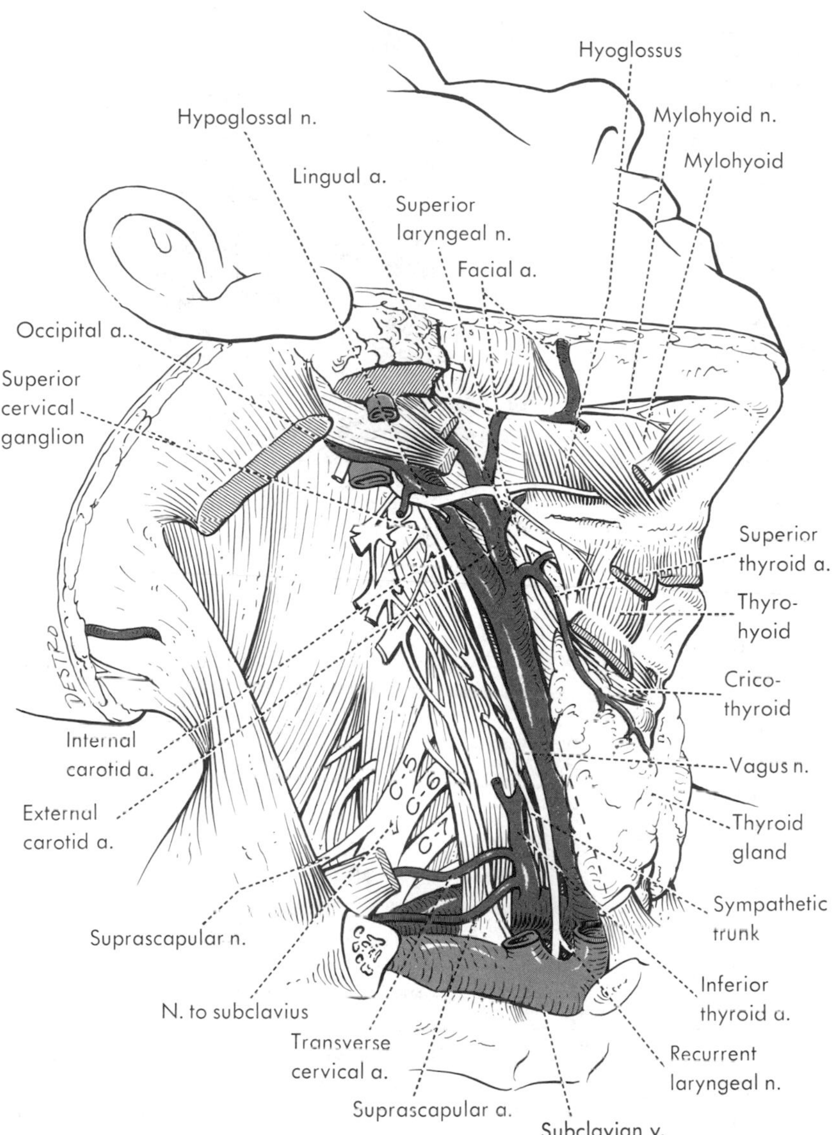

FIGURE 30-12.
A still deeper dissection of the neck. The internal jugular vein has now been removed, as have the long infrahyoid muscle and parts of the stylohyoid muscle, of both bellies of the digastric, and of the clavicle. The only remaining part of the ansa cervicalis is the stump of its superior root projecting downward from the hypoglossal nerve. The upper and middle trunks of the brachial plexus are recognizable; the nerve to the subclavius has been largely removed.

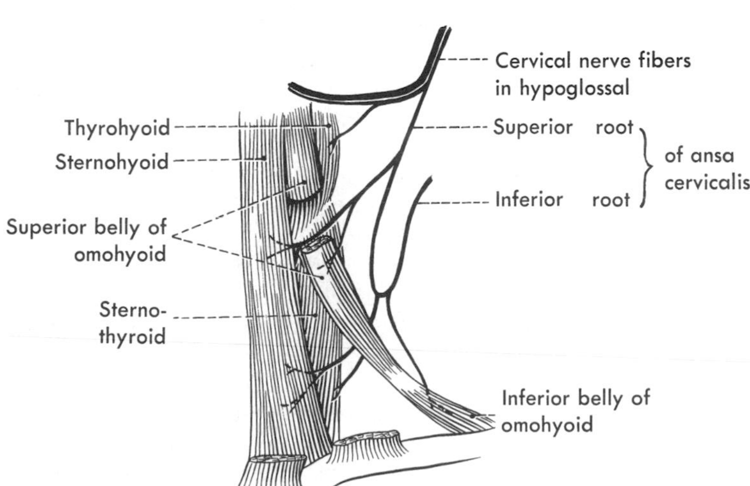

FIGURE 30-13.
The ansa cervicalis.

or the latter alone, and join the hypoglossal a little before they leave it by the superior root. Other cervical nerve fibers in the hypoglossal continue farther forward and give rise to a thyrohyoid branch that descends to enter the thyrohyoid muscle. (Still other cervical nerve fibers pass even farther forward with the hypoglossal and supply the geniohyoid.)

The infrahyoid muscles lower the larynx and the hyoid bone, a motion occurring in singing a low note and following elevation of these structures during swallowing. With suprahyoid muscles, they fix the hyoid bone, thereby providing a firm base upon which the tongue can move.

Superficial Suprahyoid Structures

Most of the suprahyoid structures related to the mandible are best examined during or after dissection of that part, but certain superficial ones should be noted early, even though they must be examined more carefully later (see Figs. 30-8, 30-10, and 30-12).

Extending downward and forward from deep to the sternocleidomastoid muscle, the lower end of the parotid gland, and the angle of the jaw are two closely associated muscles, the **stylohyoid** and the **posterior belly of the digastric.** Their origins are too deep to be observed at this time, but can be seen in Figure 31-36. A little above the hyoid bone, the deeper-lying stylohyoid divides to pass on both sides of the tendon of the digastric and attach to the hyoid bone. The tendon from the posterior belly of the digastric, after passing through the stylohyoid, is held to the hyoid bone by a fascial sling or by tendinous fibers; thereafter, it gives place to muscle fibers which, as the **anterior belly of the digastric,** run forward and slightly upward to attach to the inner surface of the lower border of the mandible just lateral to the midline.

Immediately above the anterior belly of the digastric is the **mylohyoid.** This arises from the inner surface of the mandible and inserts with its fellow of the opposite side into a midline raphe and, posteriorly, into the hyoid bone; it thus fills the space between the mandible and the hyoid bone and forms a movable floor for the mouth. It and the anterior belly of the digastric muscle are innervated by a branch of the trigeminal, or fifth cranial, nerve that lies on the lower surface of the mylohyoid muscle. A small artery accompanies the nerve.

The two bellies of the digastric may be overlapped superficially by the **submandibular gland,** a salivary gland that lies partly below and partly medial to the mandible and both below and behind the mylohyoid muscle. The duct of this gland lies above the mylohyoid muscle. Associated with the gland are **submandibular lymph nodes** that receive some of the lymphatic drainage from the face, jaws, and tongue. The **facial vein** leaves the face by crossing the mandible at the level of the submandibular gland and runs superficially across this gland to reach the internal jugular. The **facial artery,** a branch of the external carotid, crosses the lower border of the mandible just in front of the facial vein; however, it first runs deep to the submandibular gland and appears between it and the mandible. A branch (marginal mandibular) of the **facial nerve** runs forward toward muscles of the lower lip and chin at about the lower border of the mandible and typically crosses the facial vessels superficially. Sometimes this nerve is above the lower border of the mandible; sometimes it passes across the submandibular gland.

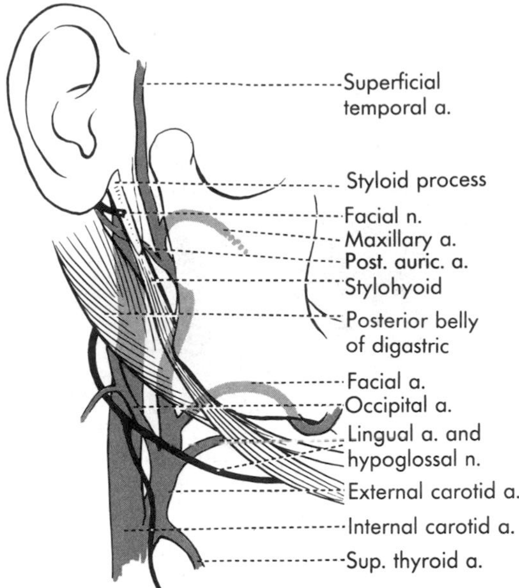

FIGURE *30-14.*
Relations of the carotid arteries and the external carotid branches in the upper part of the neck and the retromandibular region. The ascending pharyngeal artery is not shown.

Posteriorly, the external and internal carotid arteries, the internal jugular vein, and, more deeply, the vagus nerve can be traced upward until they disappear deep to the digastric. Running downward and forward lateral to the vessels and the occipital artery (the branch of the external carotid directed upward and backward) is the **hypoglossal** or *12th cranial* **nerve** (Fig. 30-14). This nerve usually turns forward lateral to the occipital artery and below its sternocleidomastoid branch, continuing forward a little above the level of the hyoid bone to disappear deep to the suprahyoid muscles. It gives off the superior root of the ansa cervicalis at about the point at which it makes its turn around the occipital artery.

Internal and External Carotids

Only parts of these vessels appear in the neck, but branches of the external carotid spread so widely to the neck and head that portions of them will be seen in various regions.

The **carotid bifurcation** lies at approximately the level of the upper border of the thyroid cartilage (see Fig. 30-12). At the bifurcation, the **internal carotid** usually is posterior or posterolateral to the external carotid, from which it can always be distinguished, because it gives off no branches in the neck, whereas the external does.

The common carotid at its bifurcation and the first part of the internal carotid are often somewhat dilated, and form the **carotid sinus.** This is a segment provided with nerve endings that are sensitive to pressure, and the sinus normally responds to increases in blood pressure within it by initiating impulses that reflexly lower the pressure. Behind the upper end of the common carotid, with its upper pole usually projecting into the angle between the vessels, is a flattened, somewhat ovoid body, the **glomus caroticum** (*carotid body*). This is a highly vascular epithelial body that also contains special nerve fibers. It responds to chemical changes in the composition of the blood, particularly to reduced oxygen, and reflexly increases the depth and rapidity of breathing. The pulse rate and blood pressure also rise. Both carotid sinus and body are innervated by nerve fibers (carotid sinus branch) that descend between the two carotid vessels to the bifurcation, primarily from the ninth (glossopharyngeal) cranial nerve.

Beyond its origin, the **internal carotid artery** is inclined somewhat more medially than the external carotid and, therefore, comes to lie more medially than posteriorly to that vessel. After the internal carotid disappears deep to the stylohyoid and the posterior belly of the digastric, it runs upward, deep to the mandible, to enter the skull and gives off no branches until it has done so.

The **external carotid artery** gives off some of its branches in the neck below or close to the level of the hyoid bone and some during its further course upward medial to the jaw. There are eight named branches, and most of those rebranch extensively, for the external carotid supplies most of the structures of the head, except the brain and the contents of the orbit, and helps supply structures in the neck. The branches of the external carotid are the superior thyroid, lingual, ascending pharyngeal, occipital, facial, posterior auricular, maxillary, and superficial temporal (Fig. 30-15; see Fig. 31-14).

Ligation of the external carotid artery, sometimes carried out to help control bleeding from a branch that is relatively inaccessible, cuts down the blood flow through the artery and its branches, but does not abolish it. Rather, blood flows retrogradely into the carotid from the other side through such anastomoses as those of the face and the scalp.

The first branch of the external carotid, arising anteriorly close to or even at the carotid bifurcation, is usually the **superior thyroid artery.** This descends obliquely downward and forward, disappearing deep to the infrahyoid muscles to reach the upper pole of the thyroid gland.

Above the superior thyroid artery, the external carotid gives off, also anteriorly, the **lingual artery.** This originates at about the level of the hyoid bone and runs forward or loops upward and forward to disappear deep to the suprahyoid muscles and the submandibular gland. If the lingual artery branches into two major stems before it disappears, one of the two stems probably is the facial artery, for sometimes lingual and facial arteries arise by a common **linguofacial trunk.** Sometimes the lingual artery is not visible because it arises deep to or above the posterior belly of the digastric.

The small **ascending pharyngeal artery** arises from the deep surface of the external carotid, usually between the levels of origin of the superior thyroid and lingual arteries. It has a deep course upward, on the posterolateral wall of the pharynx, to which it is largely distributed.

The **occipital artery** arises from the posterior aspect of the external carotid, usually a little below the level of the hyoid bone. It runs upward and posteriorly, gives off a branch to the sternocleidomastoid muscle (below which the hypoglossal nerve turns forward), and disappears deep to the posterior belly of the digastric. It later appears in the upper part of the posterior triangle of the neck.

The remaining branches of the carotid, with the possible exception of the facial (which may arise with a lingual of normal origin), arise from the external carotid af-

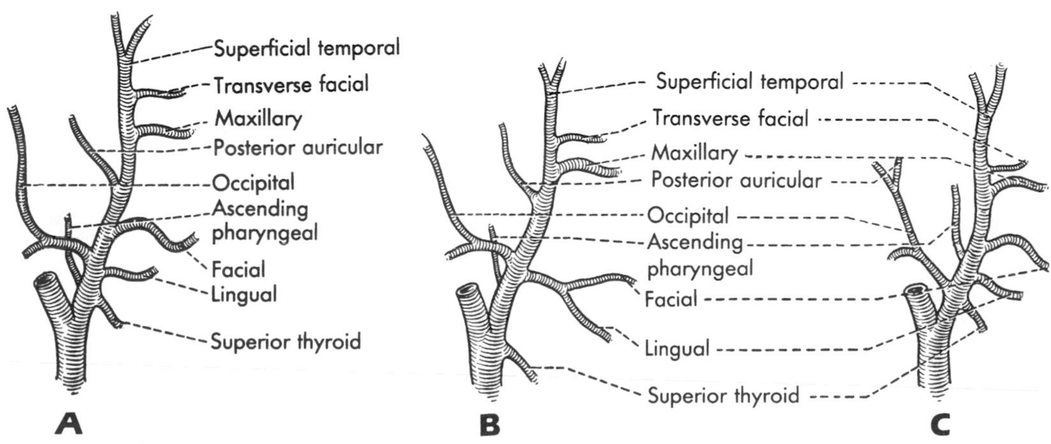

FIGURE *30-15.*
Some variations in the branching of the external carotid artery: (A) an approximately normal pattern; (B) the facial and lingual arteries arise by a common stem; (C) the posterior auricular arises from the occipital, rather than directly from the external carotid.

ter that artery has disappeared deep to the posterior belly of the digastric and the associated stylohyoid muscle. After doing so, the external carotid runs deep to the angle of the mandible and then just deep to the ramus of the mandible; therefore, deep to or through the parotid gland, which lies between the ear and the jaw. This gives it a course almost straight up in front of the ear.

Under cover of the suprahyoid muscles or of the mandible, the external carotid gives off its third anterior branch, the **facial artery.** This loops upward and forward and then downward over the submandibular gland. After giving off certain branches, it emerges between the gland and the lower border of the mandible and turns upward on the face.

The small **posterior auricular artery** arises below the ear from the posterior aspect of the external carotid and runs upward and backward to be distributed primarily behind the ear.

The **maxillary artery** is given off medial to the upper part of the jaw and runs forward. It is distributed particularly to the jaws, the palate, and the inside of the nose.

The **superficial temporal artery** is the upward continuation of the external carotid artery after the maxillary has been given off. It is primarily distributed to the side of the head (temple) and is easily palpable in front of the upper part of the ear.

Cervical Plexus

The cutaneous branches of the cervical plexus (see Fig. 30-8) are its largest ones. After reflection of the sternocleidomastoid muscle, under cover of which they lie, they can be traced to their origins, and the formation of the cervical plexus can be examined. The nerves contributing to the plexus are primarily the anterior rami of the second, third, and fourth cervical nerves (Fig. 30-16); see Fig. 30-12); the first cervical nerve frequently, but not always, reaches the plexus by forming a loop with some of the fibers of the second cervical nerve. From this loop, or from the second cervical nerve directly, fibers are given off to the hypoglossal nerve. It is these fibers that form the superior root of the ansa cervicalis, the nerve to the thyrohyoid muscle, and that to the geniohyoid.

In addition to the branch of the hypoglossal nerve, the second cervical also sends a branch to the spinal accessory nerve, to be distributed with it to the sternocleidomastoid and trapezius muscles (or this branch may enter the sternocleidomastoid independently). It contains afferent fibers to the muscle. Still another branch from the second cervical runs downward to join a branch from the third and form the inferior root of the ansa cervicalis.

The small muscular branches of the cervical plexus include twigs to the adjacent muscles of the neck—the longus muscles on the front of the vertebral column, the scalenus medius, more laterally, and the levator scapulae, which arises from the transverse processes of cervical vertebrae posterior to the scalene muscles.

An important muscular branch of the cervical plexus is the **phrenic nerve,** although this does not arise exclusively from the cervical plexus. It takes origin from the third, fourth, and fifth cervical nerves (the fifth cervical regularly contributes to the brachial plexus) and descends on the anterior surface of the anterior scalene muscle (Fig. 30-17) behind the fascia on this muscle. The roots contributing to the phrenic nerve may unite after only a short course, or they may be long. In some instances, therefore, two parts of the phrenic nerve parallel each other for a variable distance on the anterior scalene, in which case one of them, usually the lower, is called an *accessory*

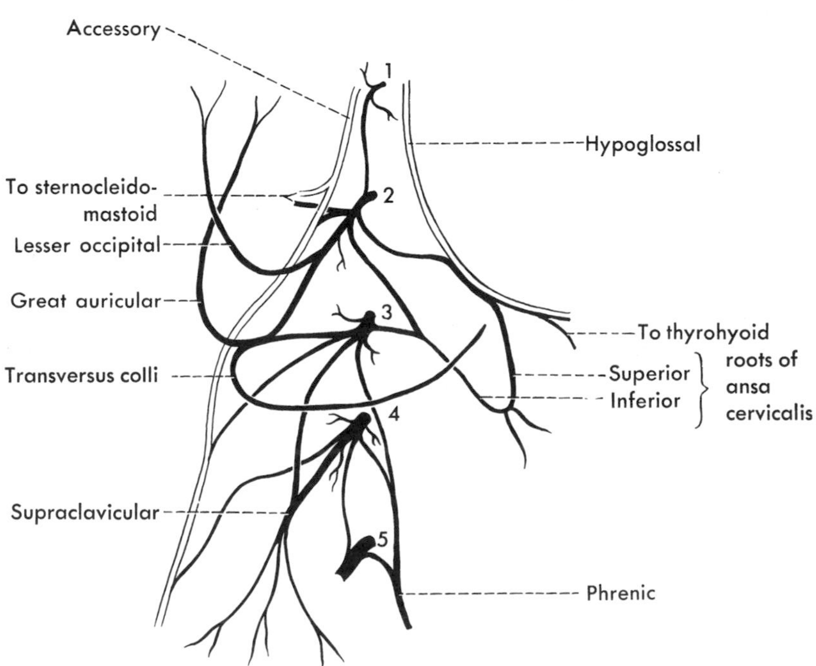

FIGURE 30-16.
Diagram of the cervical plexus: The small *unlabeled* branches are muscular ones.

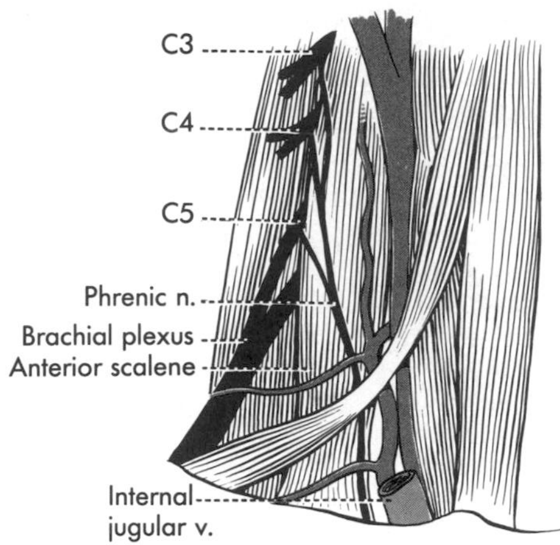

FIGURE 30-17.
The right phrenic nerve in the neck: The arteries crossing it are the transverse cervical, *above*, and the suprascapular, *below*.

phrenic nerve. They join either low in the neck or in the thorax. Typically the phrenic nerve enters the thorax by passing behind the subclavian vein, but sometimes it or an accessory phrenic will run in front of the vein.

The nerves of the cervical plexus receive (close to the level at which they appear) rami communicantes, most of which descend from the superior cervical ganglion, located high in the neck, but these may run through muscles and be difficult to identify.

The cutaneous branches of the cervical plexus arise in the following manner. The **lesser occipital nerve** usually is a direct branch from the main stem of the second cervical nerve. The larger remaining part of this stem then unites with a part of the third cervical nerve to form a trunk from which arise the **great auricular** and the **transversus colli** (transverse cervical) **nerves.** Another part of the third cervical nerve runs downward to unite with a major part of the fourth and form a common supraclavicular trunk, which then divides into the three **supraclavicular nerves.**

Finally, both the third and fourth cervical nerves typically send a branch to the spinal accessory nerve, or directly into the deep surface of the trapezius, to furnish sensory fibers to this muscle. The fourth cervical nerve may send a branch downward to join the fifth cervical and participate in the formation of the brachial plexus.

Thyroid and Parathyroid Glands

The thyroid and parathyroid glands are endocrine or ductless glands (see Chap. 11) that originate from the pharynx but "migrate" caudally (have their relative positions changed by growth) to assume their definitive position in the neck. The thyroid gland is the largest endocrine gland in the body and is unpaired. The parathyroid glands are small, and typically, there are four of them.

Thyroid Gland

The two large **lobes** of the thyroid gland lie anterolateral to the trachea and larynx. The **isthmus** unites the lobes across the front of the trachea, immediately below the larynx. Sometimes a pointed process, the pyramidal lobe, projects upward from the isthmus, usually close to the anterior midline, but occasionally asymmetrically. This may be attached by connective tissue to the front of the thyroid cartilage, or it may even extend to an attachment on the hyoid bone.

Developmentally, the thyroid gland grows out from the floor of the pharynx in the region in which the tongue (lingua, glossa) later develops, and its duct of origin is the **thyroglossal duct.** The duct normally disappears early in development, but a part of it may persist, usually close to the hyoid bone, as a *thyroglossal duct cyst;* or the duct may retain its connection to the pit on the tongue (the foramen cecum) where the gland originated and form a fistula. Sometimes, also, part or all of the thyroid gland fails to "migrate" into the neck and remains in close association with the tongue. This is called a "lingual thyroid."

The normally placed thyroid gland lies in the visceral compartment of the neck, in a space bordered anteriorly by the pretracheal fascia and the infrahyoid muscles, laterally by the two carotid sheaths, and posteriorly by the prevertebral layer of the cervical fascia.

The thyroid gland receives two pairs of arteries (Figs. 30-18 and 30-19) and is drained by two or three pairs of

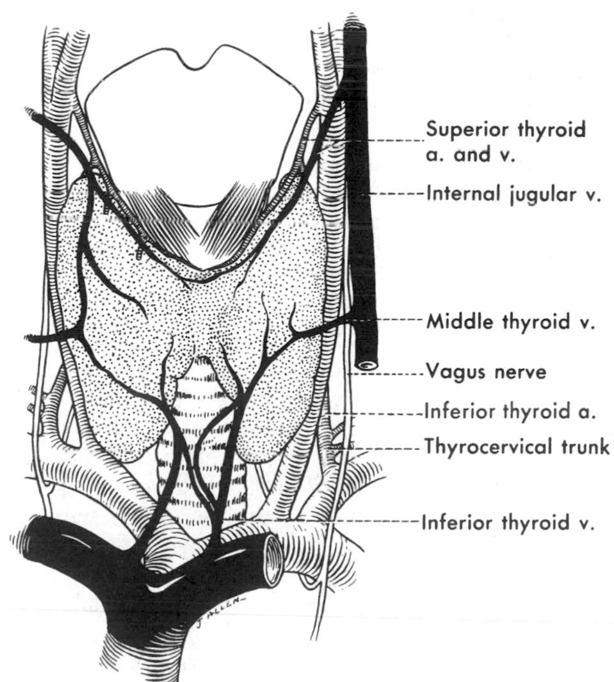

FIGURE 30-18.
Anterior view of the thyroid gland and its vessels. (Hollinshead WH. Surg Clin North Am 1952; Aug: 1115.)

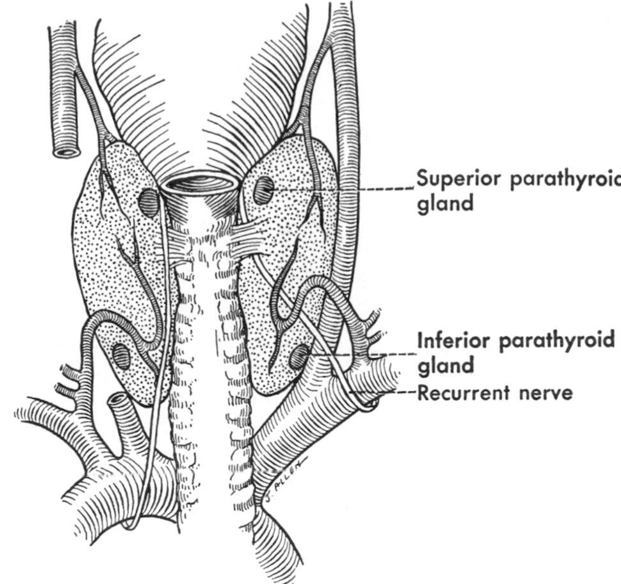

FIGURE *30-19.*
Posterior view of the thyroid and parathyroid glands: Superior and inferior thyroid arteries are shown. (Hollinshead WH. Surg Clin North Am 1952; Aug: 1115.)

veins. Close to its origin, the **superior thyroid artery** gives off three branches: an infrahyoid branch that runs along the lower border of the hyoid bone; a branch into the sternocleidomastoid muscle; and the transversely running superior laryngeal artery that disappears deep to the thyrohyoid muscle, (with the internal branch of the superior laryngeal nerve) to enter the larynx. It then descends, at first in close company with the external branch of the superior laryngeal nerve, gives off a cricothyroid branch that runs forward between the thyroid and cricoid cartilages, and, as it reaches the upper pole of the thyroid gland, divides into anterior and posterior branches. The posterior branch disappears into the posterior surface of the gland, but the anterior one usually runs along the upper medial border of the lobe and may anastomose with the vessel of the opposite side along the upper border of the isthmus.

The superior thyroid artery is accompanied by the **superior thyroid vein,** which joins the internal jugular either independently or after union with other veins that enter the same general region of that vessel. Venous anastomoses on the anterior surface of the thyroid gland are frequently fairly prominent and usually can be seen to unite the superior and inferior thyroid veins. There may or may not be a **middle thyroid vein** arising at about the midlevel of the gland and passing directly laterally to perforate the carotid sheath and end in the internal jugular vein.

The **inferior thyroid veins** are more obvious than are the inferior thyroid arteries, for they take form in part on the anterior surface of the gland (although they drain posterior parts also) and descend in front of the trachea. They may unite to form a single stem, in which case this typically ends in the left brachiocephalic vein, or the left vein may end in the left brachiocephalic and the right one in the right brachiocephalic. The two inferior thyroid veins may interchange numerous connections to form a **plexus thyroideus impar** in front of the trachea.

Tracheostomies are commonly done below the isthmus of the thyroid gland, by cutting approximately the third and fourth tracheal cartilages. In this approach, the inferior thyroid veins and, if the incision is carried too far toward the sternum, the jugular venous arch (and even, occasionally, an anomalous artery) are potential sources of bleeding. Some workers prefer to displace the isthmus and cut the trachea just below the cricoid cartilage.

The **inferior thyroid artery** is a branch of the thyrocervical trunk, which arises from the subclavian artery. It runs upward and medially behind the carotid sheath, pierces the prevertebral layer of fascia behind the thyroid gland, and then usually loops downward, commonly dividing into two or more branches as it nears the gland. While it lies behind the prevertebral fascia, it gives off the **ascending cervical artery,** which ascends on the anterior and lateral muscles of the vertebral column, gives branches into them, and also gives off spinal branches that pass through the intervertebral foramina to help supply the vertebral column and the spinal cord and its meninges. The inferior thyroid artery crosses the cervical sympathetic trunk behind the carotid sheath, usually behind this trunk, but sometimes in front of it or between two parts of a double trunk.

After penetrating the prevertebral fascia, the inferior thyroid artery gives off pharyngeal branches to the lower part of the pharynx, and esophageal and tracheal branches to the upper parts of these structures. As it passes medially behind the thyroid gland, it crosses the recurrent laryngeal nerve, which runs more vertically; it may cross in front of the nerve or behind it, or send branches on both sides of it. The small inferior laryngeal artery, from the inferior thyroid, runs upward with the recurrent nerve to help supply the larynx.

The lobes of the thyroid gland are attached to the cricoid cartilage and several of the upper tracheal rings by some fairly dense connective tissue, the adherent zone or **suspensory ligament of the gland,** and the recurrent laryngeal nerve passes close to or even through this on its way to the larynx. The nerve or one of its branches sometimes is injured at this level in thyroidectomy, or it may be injured at the level at which it crosses the superior thyroid artery.

Sometimes an abnormal artery to the thyroid gland (usually on only one side) arises from the arch of the aorta, the brachiocephalic trunk, or the lower end of a common carotid and supplements or replaces the inferior thyroid artery. This is called a *thyroidea ima* (lowest thyroid) *artery*.

Nerves to the thyroid gland accompany the thyroid vessels, lying in their adventitia. They probably are entirely vasomotor; neither the thyroid nor the parathyroid glands depend upon the nervous system to govern their secretory activity.

Parathyroids

The four parathyroid glands are small and particularly difficult to recognize in the cadaver because they are about the same color as the thyroid gland and the lymph nodes; however, in the living person their yellowish color contrasts fairly well with the deep red of the thyroid gland. Each slightly oval parathyroid tends to be approximately 4 to 6 mm in diameter and 1 to 2 mm thick. Normally, they all lie on the posterior and posteromedial surfaces of the lateral lobes of the thyroid (see Fig. 30-19). The two glands of one side are usually known as the superior and inferior parathyroid glands, or sometimes, in reference to their origin from branchial pouches, as parathyroid IV (the upper gland) and parathyroid III (the lower one). However, either parathyroid may not be in its proper position—for instance, one may lie on the superior thyroid artery or even as high as the carotid bifurcation, or one may lie on the inferior thyroid artery or even in the mediastinum. Also, one may lie laterally or anteriorly on the thyroid instead of posteriorly.

It is not always possible to distinguish between superior and inferior parathyroid glands or, indeed, to locate four glands. Removal of all parathyroid tissue has serious consequences (see Chap. 11): surgeons, therefore, take care to preserve at least some of the glands during thyroidectomy. The parathyroid glands typically receive their blood supply from the inferior thyroid arteries; when these are ligated, however, the glands can receive blood through the anastomoses that the thyroid arteries make with other vessels that supply the pharynx, larynx, and esophagus.

Trachea and Esophagus

The tubular **trachea** begins immediately below the larynx and is supported by a series of C-shaped cartilages united by elastic *annular ligaments,* with the incomplete part of the cartilaginous ring facing posteriorly. The posterior wall of the trachea is entirely membranous and muscular (*musculus trachealis*). Immediately behind it is the esophagus. The trachea descends in the anterior midline. In front of it lie the infrahyoid muscles, the isthmus of the thyroid gland, the inferior thyroid veins, and usually some pretracheal lymph nodes; on each side lie the lateral lobes of the thyroid gland and the carotid sheaths. The trachea disappears at the base of the neck behind the great vessels and the sternum. In the lateral grooves, between the upper part of the trachea and the esophagus, are the recurrent laryngeal nerves. They give off branches to the trachea and esophagus before they disappear into the larynx. The larynx is discussed in a later chapter.

The **pharynx** and the upper end of the **esophagus** are discussed also in a later chapter. The pharynx is somewhat funnel-shaped and the anterior wall of its small lower end is also the posterior wall of the larynx. Concerning the esophagus, it need only be noted here that it is a tubelike continuation of the pharynx arising at the lower border of the larynx and that, rather than remaining constantly open, it is collapsed anteroposteriorly except when something is being swallowed. Its cervical part is supplied by twigs from the recurrent laryngeal nerves and the inferior thyroid arteries. The muscle of the esophagus (outer longitudinal and inner circular) in the neck is typically striated muscle, being supplied by branchial efferent rather than visceral efferent elements of the vagus nerves.

THE SCALENES AND POSTERIOR TRIANGLE

The scalene (scalenus) muscles lie in part deep to the sternocleidomastoid, but appear also in the posterior triangle. There are three of them: anterior, middle, and posterior (Fig. 30-20). Each anterior scalene has the phrenic nerve on its anterior surface; each also is crossed anteriorly by arteries to the shoulder that arise from the thyrocervical trunk and by the subclavian vein of its side. The subclavian artery, however, passes behind the anterior scalene.

On the left side, the thoracic duct turns laterally in front of the anterior scalene to enter approximately the angle of junction between internal jugular and subclavian veins. The subclavian artery and most of the elements of the brachial plexus emerge between the anterior and middle scalene muscles; therefore, they partly hide the latter muscle. Two nerves, the dorsal scapular nerve (to the rhomboids) and the long thoracic nerve (to the serratus anterior), usually run through the middle scalene.

The **anterior scalene** muscle usually arises from the anterior tubercles of the transverse processes of approximately the third or fourth to the sixth cervical vertebra. It runs downward and somewhat laterally. The phrenic nerve on its anterior surface runs downward and slightly medially, at an angle to the fibers of the muscle. The muscle ends in a tendon that attaches to the first rib.

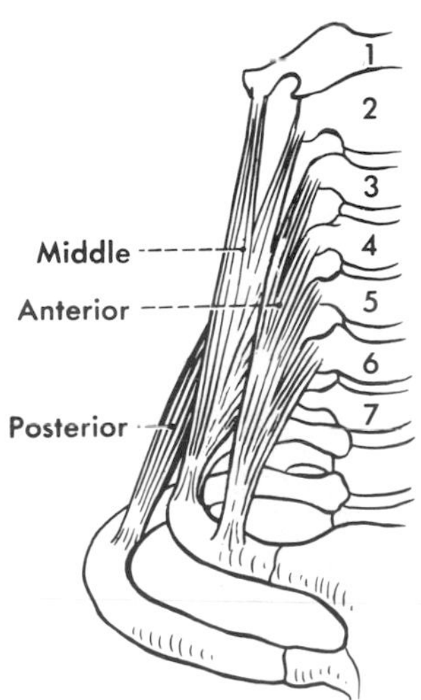

FIGURE *30-20.*
The scalene muscles.

The **middle scalene** muscle usually is the largest of the three. It originates from the transverse processes of all the cervical vertebrae, from all except the first or the first and second, or sometimes from all except the seventh. It also runs downward and laterally and inserts on the first rib. The gap between the anterior and middle scalenes is traversed by the brachial plexus and the subclavian artery, and those structures sometimes suffer damage here as they cross the first rib (see Chap. 15).

The **posterior scalene** usually is a small muscle. It arises from the posterior tubercles of the transverse processes of about the fifth and sixth cervical vertebrae and descends between the middle scalene and the levator scapulae to cross the first rib and insert upon the second or third.

The scalene muscles are innervated by twigs from nerves that contribute to the cervical and brachial plexuses. Because the particular segmental nerves concerned are those most intimately related to the muscle, they vary with the origin of the muscle. They are flexors and rotators of the neck and head, but also are respiratory muscles, for they usually take their fixed point from above and elevate the thorax.

In addition to the three scalene muscles named, there is fairly frequently, between the anterior and middle one, a small muscular bundle known as the **scalenus minimus.** This usually arises from the anterior tubercle of either the sixth or the seventh cervical vertebra and passes downward between the anterior and middle scalenes. It may attach entirely to the first rib or pass behind the rib to attach into the fascia over the lung, the suprapleural membrane, or it may attach to both structures. In attaching to the first rib, it may separate some elements of the brachial plexus from other parts or the subclavian artery from the brachial plexus. Presumably, a scalenus minimus sometimes is responsible for signs of compression of the brachial plexus.

Immediately behind the posterior scalene muscle is the **levator scapulae,** a muscle of the shoulder that arises from cervical transverse processes. The accessory nerve runs downward on it across the posterior triangle. Above and behind the levator scapulae, the splenius muscles, muscles of the back, form part of the floor of the triangle. The occipital artery usually appears in the uppermost part of the triangle as it passes from under cover of the sternocleidomastoid to disappear deep to the trapezius muscle, which it then pierces to turn upward in the scalp.

Brachial Plexus

The brachial plexus originates in the neck and terminates in the axilla as the main nerves that supply the upper limb (Fig. 30-21). Its smaller branches given off in the neck and axilla supply muscles of the pectoral girdle and the skin that covers parts of the shoulder region and the free upper limb. The composition, formation, and branches of the brachial plexus are described in Chapters 14 and 15, because understanding of the plexus is essential for comprehending the innervation of the upper limb. The plexus consists of roots, trunks, divisions, and cords (see Fig. 15-20). This section is concerned with the topographic relations of the plexus in the neck and those of its branches that are given off above the level of the clavicle. The roots, trunks, and divisions of the plexus are located in the neck; the cords are in the axilla.

The roots of the plexus are constituted by the anterior rami of C-5 through C-8 and T-1 spinal nerves. After they split off from the respective spinal nerves in the intervertebral foramina, the roots proceed laterally between the anterior and middle scalene muscles. Twigs arise from these roots for the scalene muscles and the longus cervicis muscles. The phrenic nerve, formed by C-3 and C-4 anterior rami, receives a branch from C-5 anterior ramus as the nerve winds its way onto the front of the anterior scalene (see Fig. 30-12). Two nerves are given off by the roots for the supply of the girdle musculature: the **dorsal scapular nerve** from C-5 root passes backward through the middle scalene to innervate the rhomboids and the levator scapulae; the **long thoracic nerve** is formed by twigs from C-5 through C-7 roots, which may

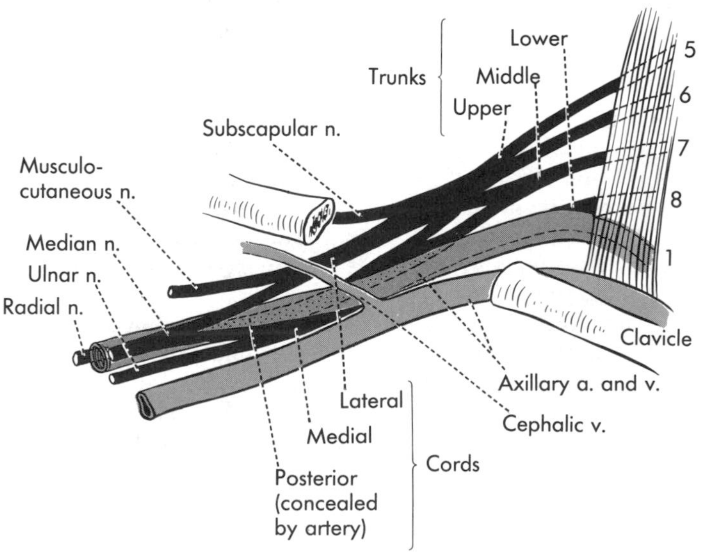

FIGURE *30-21.*
The relation of the brachial plexus to the subclavian and axillary arteries: The posterior cord is exaggeratedly prolonged to show its position.

come together in the substance of the middle scalene or may run separately within the muscle, or on its anterior or posterior surface. After the twigs come together, the long thoracic nerve descends vertically on the middle scalene to the serratus anterior, which it innervates (see Figs. 15-21 and 15-22).

The fifth and sixth cervical roots merge with each other on the anterior surface of the middle scalene and form the upper trunk of the plexus (see Figs. 30-12 and 30-17; also Fig. 15-21). Two nerves are given off from the upper trunk, the nerve to the subclavius and the suprascapular nerve. The **nerve to the subclavius** is small and runs downward in front of the plexus to end in the subclavius muscle (see Fig. 30-12; also Figs. 15-21 and 15-22). The **suprascapular nerve** is much larger, runs downward and laterally to join the suprascapular artery, and supplies the supraspinatus and infraspinatus muscles (see Fig. 15-21).

The middle trunk of the plexus formed by C-7 root, and the lower trunk formed by roots C-8 and T-1, also pass laterally on the anterior surface of the middle scalene (see Fig. 30-12). Neither of them gives off any branches. The formation of anterior and posterior divisions and their regrouping into cords is described in Chapter 15. No branches arise from the divisions. The cords of the plexus become associated with the subclavian artery as they lie behind the clavicle (see Fig. 30-21). Their relations to the axillary vessels are described in Chapter 15.

Vessels and Nerves

Arteries and Veins

Besides the occipital artery, already mentioned, the vessels that appear in the posterior triangle are largely the subclavian artery and its branches and the subclavian vein and its tributaries; lymphatics and lymph nodes, not very obvious, are arranged along these vessels.

The two subclavian arteries have different origin, but similar courses in the neck (Fig. 30-22). The **left subclavian,** a branch of the arch of the aorta, arises in the thorax behind the left border of the manubrium sterni. It ascends almost vertically on the left side of the trachea and adjacent to the parietal pleura of the left lung. At the base of the neck, it arches upward and laterally in front of the apex of the lung to disappear behind the left anterior scalene muscle. The **right subclavian artery,** in contrast, originates at the base of the neck behind the right sternoclavicular joint, where it and the right common carotid are the terminal branches of the brachiocephalic trunk. It then curves laterally across the anterior surface of the apex of the right lung and disappears behind the right anterior scalene muscle. The part of each subclavian artery between its origin and the medial edge of the anterior scalene muscle frequently is known as the first part of the artery; the second part lies behind the anterior scalene, and the third part lies between the lateral edge of the muscle and the first rib. At the latter level the subclavian artery enters the axilla, and its name changes to axillary artery.

The anterior scalene muscle separates the subclavian artery from the subclavian vein. The third part of the artery lies in front of the lower trunk of the brachial plexus and immediately behind the subclavian vein. The upper and middle trunks of the plexus and their continuations lie mostly above the level of the artery but become closely related to its upper (lateral) aspect close to the level of the first rib.

The usual description of the subclavian artery has been that it has four branches, all of which arise from the first part of the artery (medial to the anterior scalene), but frequently, a fifth branch arises from the second or third part of the subclavian. The branches of the subclavian artery that typically arise from the first part of the subclavian are the vertebral artery, the thyrocervical trunk, the internal thoracic artery, and the costocervical trunk. A branch arising from the second or third part of the subclavian may be the transverse cervical or the suprascapular artery, both of which are said to have a "normal" origin when they arise from the thyrocervical trunk; most frequently, it is an abnormally arising branch of the transverse cervical artery. An artery arising from the second or third part of the subclavian artery usually passes through, rather than in front of, the brachial plexus.

The **vertebral artery** (Fig. 30-23) typically arises from the posterosuperior aspect of the subclavian artery, although occasionally the left one may arise from the arch of the aorta. It runs upward and slightly posteriorly and

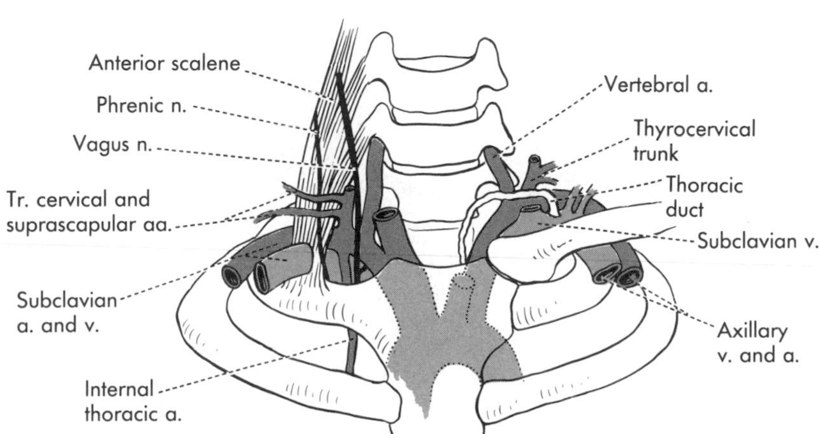

FIGURE *30-22.* Vascular relations at the base of the neck: The left common carotid is indicated as a *stump* behind the sternum, and the left anterior scalene is removed, so the fact that the thoracic duct runs behind the common carotid, but in front of the scalene, is not apparent here.

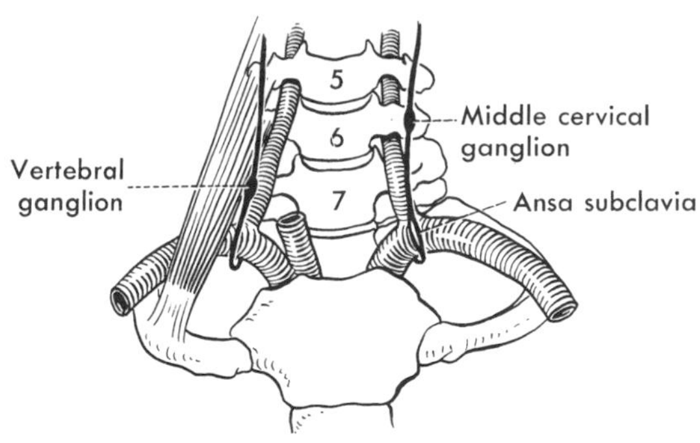

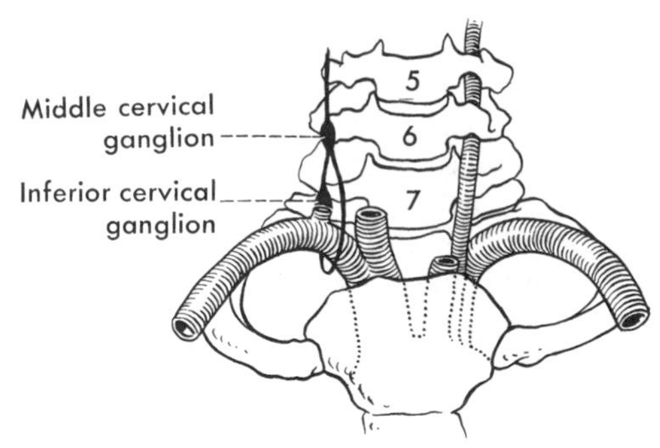

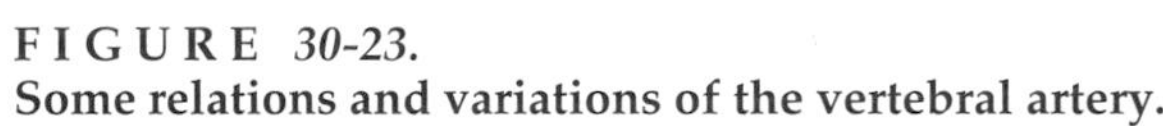
FIGURE *30-23.*
Some relations and variations of the vertebral artery.

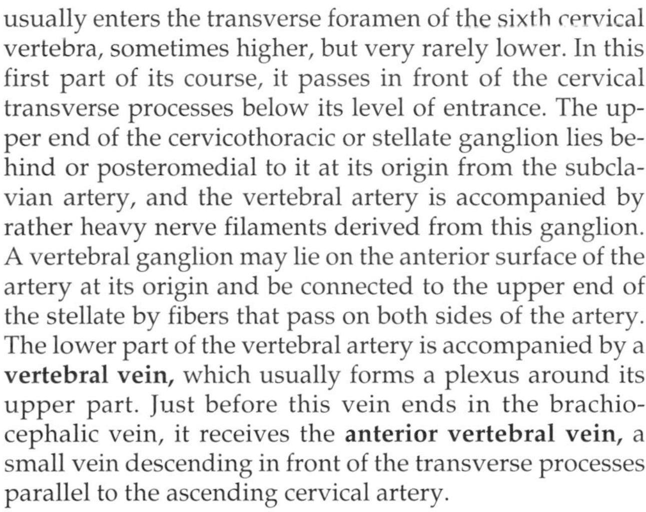

usually enters the transverse foramen of the sixth cervical vertebra, sometimes higher, but very rarely lower. In this first part of its course, it passes in front of the cervical transverse processes below its level of entrance. The upper end of the cervicothoracic or stellate ganglion lies behind or posteromedial to it at its origin from the subclavian artery, and the vertebral artery is accompanied by rather heavy nerve filaments derived from this ganglion. A vertebral ganglion may lie on the anterior surface of the artery at its origin and be connected to the upper end of the stellate by fibers that pass on both sides of the artery. The lower part of the vertebral artery is accompanied by a **vertebral vein,** which usually forms a plexus around its upper part. Just before this vein ends in the brachiocephalic vein, it receives the **anterior vertebral vein,** a small vein descending in front of the transverse processes parallel to the ascending cervical artery.

After entering a transverse foramen, the vertebral artery runs upward through successive transverse foramina to the base of the skull, accompanied by the vertebral vein. After emerging through the vertebral foramen of the first cervical vertebra, it turns dorsally and medially on the upper surface of this vertebra and enters the vertebral canal by penetrating the posterior atlantooccipital membrane. Its major distribution, to the brain, is described in Chapter 32. Its branches in the neck are small. They consist of some that supply adjacent deep muscles of the neck and spinal branches that pass through intervertebral foramina to enter the vertebral canal. In the suboccipital triangle, some of its branches anastomose with branches of the occipital and deep cervical arteries. The vertebral vein does not accompany the artery into the vertebral canal, but participates in the formation of the **suboccipital venous plexus.** This plexus receives the occipital veins, may receive emissary veins (from inside the skull), and gives rise to the vertebral and deep cervical veins.

The **thyrocervical trunk** (Fig. 30-24) arises from the upper anterior part of the subclavian artery, close to the medial border of the anterior scalene. After giving off the transverse cervical and suprascapular arteries, it ends as the inferior thyroid. The inferior thyroid artery ascends with a somewhat medial course and already has been described. The **transverse cervical artery,** the upper of the two branches to the shoulder, runs laterally and posteriorly across the front of the anterior scalene muscle and the brachial plexus. At the posterior border of the posterior triangle, it disappears deep to the trapezius muscle. Its further course has been described in Chapter 15 (see Fig. 15-31); it may divide into a superficial and a deep branch, which are distributed deep to the trapezius and deep to the rhomboid muscles, respectively. Commonly, the vessel corresponding to the superficial branch arises independently from the thyrocervical trunk and is then known as the **superficial cervical artery.** The vessel corresponding to the deep branch then arises from the subclavian artery and is known as the **dorsal** or **descending scapular artery.**

The other branch of the thyrocervical trunk, the **suprascapular artery,** is usually the first branch from the trunk. It runs transversely across the neck parallel to, but below, the transverse cervical artery and behind the clavicle. It passes in front of the anterior scalene muscle and the brachial plexus and, as it reaches the lateral border of the plexus, is joined in its course by the suprascapular nerve. Nerve and artery disappear together deep to the trapezius, and their further course is described with the shoulder. The suprascapular artery has been reported to arise directly from the subclavian in more than 20% of instances.

Single or paired **transverse cervical** and **suprascapular veins** accompany the arteries. These veins do not join

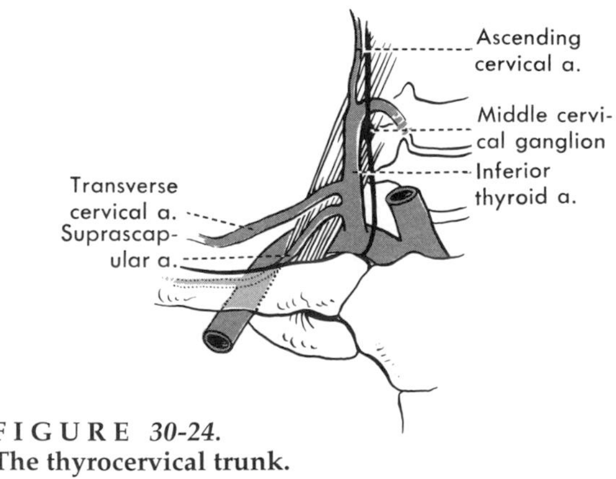

FIGURE *30-24.*
The thyrocervical trunk.

the inferior thyroid vein, however, but enter the lower end of the external jugular vein or the proximal part of the subclavian.

The **internal thoracic artery** (formerly internal mammary) arises from the anteroinferior aspect of the subclavian at about the same level as the thyrocervical trunk. It passes downward, forward, and somewhat medially, lying on the anterior aspect of the parietal pleura covering the apex of the lung, and behind the brachiocephalic vein and the sternal end of the clavicle. It enters the thorax behind the cartilage of the first rib. The **internal thoracic veins** do not quite parallel the uppermost parts of the arteries, for they enter the brachiocephalic veins, rather than the subclavians.

The **costocervical trunk** arises from the posterior aspect of the subclavian artery just medial to or behind the medial border of the anterior scalene muscle. It runs posterosuperiorly to divide into deep cervical and supreme intercostal arteries. The **supreme intercostal artery** supplies approximately the upper two intercostal spaces with posterior intercostal arteries. The **deep cervical artery** passes backward between the transverse process of the seventh cervical vertebra and the neck of the first rib, and below the eighth cervical nerve. It then ascends between two muscles of the back (semispinalis capitis and semispinalis cervicis), anastomosing as it does so with branches of the ascending pharyngeal and vertebral arteries and ending above by anastomosing with a descending branch of the occipital artery. Sometimes the deep cervical and the supreme intercostal arise separately from the subclavian, or the supreme intercostal may be lacking and supplanted by branches from the aorta.

Each **subclavian vein** is the direct, continuation of the axillary vein on its side and, therefore, begins at the upper border of the first rib. At the base of the neck, the vein runs at first in front of and partly below the subclavian artery and then is separated from that by the anterior scalene muscle and the phrenic nerve. In front of the medial border of the muscle, the vein ends by joining the internal jugular vein, thereby forming the upper end of the brachiocephalic vein. The two **brachiocephalic veins,** therefore, begin behind the medial ends of the clavicles and pass downward to enter the thorax.

The subclavian vein has only one constant named tributary, the **external jugular.** This enters the subclavian close to the posterior border of the sternocleidomastoid muscle. Through the external jugular, the subclavian receives blood from the suprascapular and transverse cervical veins. The veins corresponding to other branches of the subclavian artery empty into the brachiocephalic: the internal thoracic veins enter the brachiocephalic veins in the thorax; the vertebral veins empty into the upper ends of the brachiocephalics; and the supreme intercostal and deep cervical veins empty separately into either the vertebral or the upper end of the brachiocephalic.

Lymph Nodes and Lymphatics

Note has already been made that **deep cervical lymph nodes** lie in the connective tissue of the carotid sheath, particularly closely related to the internal jugular vein. Sometimes they are divided roughly into a superior and an inferior group, and two nodes usually are named (Fig. 30-25): the **jugulodigastric node** lies at about the level at which the digastric muscle crosses the internal jugular vein, and the **juguloomohyoid node** lies at the level of crossing of the omohyoid muscle and the vein. The deep cervical lymph nodes receive, directly or indirectly, most of the lymphatics from the head and neck. Among the nodes draining into them are the *submental nodes,* in the submental region; *submandibular nodes,* associated with the submandibular salivary gland; *retropharyngeal nodes* that lie posterolateral to the pharynx; and nodes that lie along the course of the facial vessels. Lymphatics from the face, tongue, and other parts of the head also bypass the regional nodes along their course and directly enter deep cervical nodes. In addition to the nodes mentioned, *occipital, retroauricular,* and *superficial* and *deep parotid nodes*

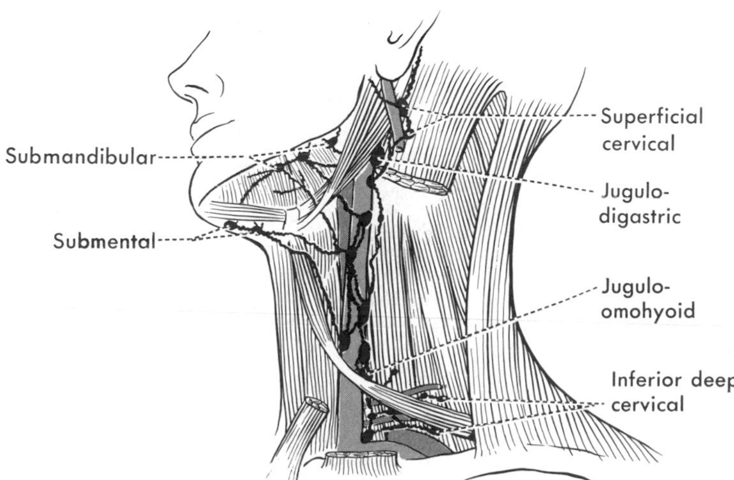

FIGURE *30-25.*
Superficial and deep lymph nodes of the submandibular region and neck.

drain into the deep cervical nodes. They also drain, in part, into a few superficial cervical nodes that lie along the course of the external jugular vein. There are also nodes and lymphatics along the accessory nerve and the suprascapular and transverse cervical vessels (the latter two sets usually included among the inferior deep nodes) in the posterior triangle and deep to the trapezius that drain into the nodes along the internal jugular vein.

> In the operation known as "radical neck dissection," carried out when carcinoma has reached some of the deep cervical nodes, the tissue containing them is removed as completely as possible and in one piece as far as that can be managed. The sternocleidomastoid muscle and the part of the omohyoid lying deep and medial to it, the internal jugular vein and the connective tissue around it and the carotid artery and the vagus nerve, and the connective tissue in the posterior triangle of the neck are dissected out from the base of the neck to the lower border of the jaw. The dissection includes the submandibular gland and the lower end of the parotid gland, both bellies of the digastric muscle, and the stylohyoid muscle. Often, the accessory nerve is resected and tissue is dissected from deep to the trapezius muscle. The major arteries, the vagus nerve, the brachial plexus, and the phrenic nerve are spared, but the cutaneous branches of the cervical plexus are sacrificed. The attempt is to remove in one block all the node-bearing tissue of one side of the neck.

The formation and thoracic course of the **thoracic duct** have been described. It enters the neck slightly to the left of the midline, lying on the vertebral column and behind the esophagus. As it diverges farther to the left, it passes behind the carotid sheath and its contents, but in front of the parietal pleura over the apex of the left lung and in front of the branches of the subclavian arising medial to the anterior scalene. As it runs laterally or arches laterally and downward to enter approximately the angle of union of internal jugular and left subclavian veins, it passes also in front of the anterior scalene muscle and the phrenic nerve (Fig. 30-26). It may run upward only high enough to reach the angle of junction of the two veins, or

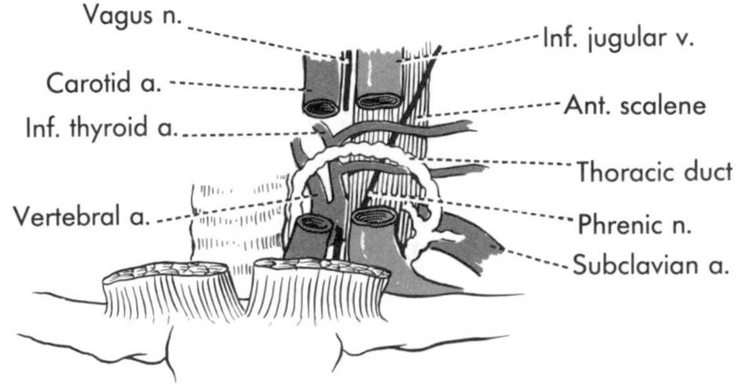

FIGURE *30-26.*
The thoracic duct in the neck: It passes behind the structures within the carotid sheath, and these are shown with a segment of each removed.

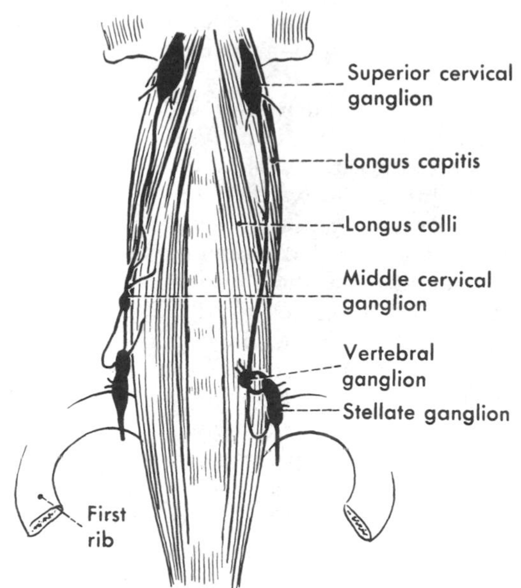

FIGURE *30-27.*
The cervical sympathetic trunks: The two trunks are not necessarily symmetric, and there may be both a middle cervical and a vertebral ganglion on one side.

it may run much too high and farther laterally than necessary and then loop downward and medially, thereby being exposed to injury in almost any operation at the base of the neck. Close to its ending, it usually receives a **jugular trunk** from the deep cervical nodes and a **subclavian trunk** from the axillary nodes on its side and may receive the **left bronchomediastinal trunk;** or these vessels may enter the venous system independently or in various combinations. These smaller lymphatic trunks are difficult to recognize in the usual dissection; indeed, even the thoracic duct may not be easily recognized, because its proximal end is frequently filled with blood in the cadaver.

A **right lymphatic** (right thoracic) **duct,** representing a vessel formed by a combination of jugular, subclavian, and bronchomediastinal trunks, may enter the angle of junction of the right subclavian and internal jugular veins, but frequently the vessels on the right do not combine to form a single trunk.

Sympathetic Trunks and Ganglia

The lowest ganglion of the **cervical sympathetic trunk** (Fig. 30-27) is the **stellate** or **cervicothoracic ganglion,** formed by fusion of the lowest cervical and first thoracic ganglion; sometimes these are separate, and there is then an **inferior cervical ganglion.** The ganglion is particularly large if it is truly cervicothoracic. It lies in front of the neck of the first rib and the transverse process of the seventh cervical vertebra, behind the upper end of the first part of the subclavian artery and the origin of the vertebral artery, and just above or partly behind the dome of the pleura. It receives one or more white rami communicantes (preganglionic fibers) from the first thoracic nerve and may receive one from the second. It gives off gray rami communicantes to the first thoracic and lower cervical nerves, thus contributing postganglionic fibers to the brachial plexus, and sends other rami (grouped to form the *vertebral nerve*) along the vertebral artery to the upper nerves of the brachial plexus.

The cervical sympathetic trunk passes upward on the front of the longus colli and longus capitis muscles, behind the common carotid artery while that is in the carotid sheath, and then behind the internal carotid. It is a rather slender strand of fibers and ends above in the **superior cervical ganglion.** This elongated ganglion lies in front of the upper two cervical vertebrae. It sends rami communicantes to the upper three or four cervical nerves and a small **external carotid nerve,** difficult to find by dissection, downward to the external carotid to form a delicate external carotid plexus that follows branches of that vessel. Its largest branch is a broad band of fibers from its upper end, the **internal carotid nerve.** This breaks up into the internal carotid plexus, which follows the artery into the skull.

Between the cervicothoracic and the superior cervical ganglia, there are one or two other ganglia. One, the **middle cervical ganglion,** lies on the trunk at the level of the transverse process of the sixth cervical vertebra. It typically is connected to the cervicothoracic ganglion both by fibers that pass in the trunk behind the subclavian artery and by fibers, constituting the **ansa subclavia** (see Fig. 30-23), that loop down in front of the subclavian artery and then turn below it to reach the cervicothoracic ganglion. A second ganglion, the **vertebral ganglion,** may lie anterior or anteromedial to the vertebral artery at its origin and, when present, may receive the ansa subclavia, in addition to being connected behind the subclavian artery to the cervicothoracic ganglion by fibers that usually pass on both sides of the vertebral artery.

The vertebral or middle cervical ganglia typically supply rami communicantes to about the fourth and fifth cervical nerves. There is considerable variation as to exactly which cervical nerves receive rami from which ganglia, and it is often difficult to determine this without extreme care in dissection, because many of the rami communicantes disappear into the longus muscles on their way to the spinal nerves. Superior, middle, and inferior **cardiac nerves** (the superior cardiac nerves are very tiny) arise from or close to the similarly named ganglia and run downward to join the cardiac plexus in the thorax.

The Prevertebral Muscles

The **longus colli** and **capitis** have been mentioned, but no complete view of them can be obtained until a great deal of dissection has been done on the neck and head. It should suffice to say here that they are complex in structure, closely bound to the front of the vertebral bodies and transverse processes, and consist of two overlapping muscles, the lower being the longus colli and the upper the longus capitis (see Fig. 30-27). They are primarily flexors of the neck and head.

Lying partly behind the upper end of the longus capitis is the **rectus capitis anterior,** which arises from the lateral mass of the atlas and inserts on the basilar part of the occipital bone. Lateral to it is the **rectus capitis lateralis,** arising from the transverse process of the atlas and inserting more laterally on the occipital bone.

RECOMMENDED READINGS

Bachhuber CA. Complications of thyroid surgery: anatomy of the recurrent laryngeal nerve, middle thyroid vein and inferior thyroid artery. Am J Surg 1943; 60: 96.

Barton JW, Margolis MT. Rotational obstruction of the vertebral artery at the atlantoaxial joint. Neuroradiology 1975; 9: 117.

Calen S, Pommereau X, Gbikpi-Benissan AM, Videau J. Morphologic and functional anatomy of the subclavian veins. Surg Radiol Anat 1986; 8: 121.

Coller FA, Yglesias L. The relation of the spread of infection to fascial planes in the neck and thorax. Surgery 1937; 1: 323.

Daseler EH, Anson BJ. Surgical anatomy of the subclavian artery and its branches. Surg Gynecol Obstet 1959; 108: 149.

Deslaugiers B, Vaysse PH, Combes JM, et al. Contribution to the study of the tributaries and the termination of the external jugular vein. Surg Radiol Anat 1994; 16: 173.

Dresser LP, McKinney WM. Anatomic and pathophysiologic studies of the human internal jugular valve. Am Surg 1987; 154: 220.

Fernando DA, Lord RSA. The blood supply of vagus nerve in the human: its implication in carotid endarterectomy, thyroidectomy and carotid arch aneurectomy. Ann Anat 1994; 176: 333.

Graney DO. Developmental anatomy of the neck. In: Cummings CW, ed. Otolaryngology—head and neck surgery. 2nd ed, vol 2, St Louis: Mosby-Year Book, 1993: 1517.

Graney DO, Hamaker RC. Anatomy of the thyroid/parathyroid. In: Cummings CW, ed. Otolaryngology—head and neck surgery. 2nd ed, vol 2. St Louis: Mosby-Year Book, 1993: 2403.

Grodinsky M, Holyoke EA. The fasciae and fascial spaces of the head, neck and adjacent regions. Am J Anat 1938; 63: 367.

Hollinshead WH. Anatomy for surgeons: vol 1, the head and neck. 3rd ed. Philadelphia: Harper & Row, 1982.

Huelke DF. A study of the transverse cervical and dorsal scapular arteries. Anat Rec 1958; 132: 233.

Kelly WO. Phrenic nerve paralysis: special consideration of the accessory phrenic nerve. J Thorac Surg 1950; 19: 923.

Lingeman RE. Surgical anatomy of the neck. In: Cummings CW, ed. Otolaryngology—head and neck surgery. 2nd ed, vol 2. St Louis: Mosby-Year Book, 1993: 1530.

Melnick JC, Stemkowski PE. Thyroid hemiagenesis (hockey stick sign): a review of the world literature and a report of four cases. J Clin Endocrinol Metab 1980; 52: 247.

Millzner RJ. The normal variations in the position of the human parathyroid glands. Anat Rec 1931; 48: 399.

Rath G, Anand C. Vagocervical complex replacing an absent ansa cervicalis. Surg Radiol Anat 1994; 16: 441.

Reed AF. The relations of the inferior laryngeal nerve to the inferior thyroid artery. Anat Rec 1943; 85: 17.

Schmidt CF, Comroe JH Jr. Functions of the carotid and aortic bodies. Physiol Rev 1940; 20: 115.

Smith JR. Lymphatic cannulation of the head and neck. Plast Reconstr Surg 1963; 32: 607.

Stockwell M, Lozanoff S, Lang SA, Nyssen J. Superior laryngeal nerve block: an anatomical study. Clin Anat 1995; 8: 89.

Vitti M, Fujiwara M, Basmajian JV, Iida M. The integrated roles of longus colli and sternocleidomastoid muscles: an electromyographic study. Anat Rec 1973; 177: 471.

Wiseman O, Logan B, Dixon A, Ellis H. Tortuosity in the cervical part of the vertebral artery. Clin Anat 1994; 7: 26.

Hollinshead's Textbook of Anatomy, by Cornelius Rosse and Penelope Gaddum-Rosse.
Lippincott-Raven Publishers, Philadelphia, © 1997.

CHAPTER 31

Skull, Face, and Jaws

Intelligent study of the soft tissues of the head is impossible without knowledge of the skull; therefore, a clean skull with a removable top should be studied before dissection of the head is undertaken.

THE SKULL

The skull consists of 22 bones, 21 of which are firmly bound together. One, the mandible, or bone of the lower jaw, is movable and articulates with the remainder of the skull through paired synovial joints. The term *cranium* has been used in several ways: strictly speaking, it is synonymous with the term *skull (nomina anatomica)* but it has also been used to imply the skull without its mandible. More commonly, however, *cranium* implies the parts of the skull that enclose the brain, the remainder of the skull being the *facial skeleton*.

Knowledge of the skull as a whole, of the way in which its bones fit together, and of the chief foramina through which structures enter or leave the cranial cavity is much more important than are details of each bone. If the latter are to be studied, individual bones, rather than the skull as a whole will prove more useful. In addition to facial skeleton and cranium, a few general terms that are applied to the skull should be understood. The skull contains five large cavities, four of which, the paired nasal cavities and the paired orbits (so called because the eyeballs rotate in them), open freely to the outside. The fifth and largest cavity, the cranial cavity, houses the brain and, except at the base of the skull where brain and spinal cord are continuous, it is a closed cavity during life.

The roof of the cranial cavity is referred to as the **calvaria.** The outer periosteum of the cranium is known as the **pericranium.** Most of the cranial bones have dense external and internal **laminae** (tables) separated by spongy bone known as the **diploë.** Relatively large venous channels, the *diploic veins*, run within canals in the diploë and empty their blood in some instances into veins outside the skull, in others into cranial venous sinuses. Some of the bones of the skull—particularly the frontal, ethmoid, sphenoid, and maxillary bones—have their diploë in part replaced by air-filled cavities, the **paranasal sinuses,** that grow from the nasal cavity into adjacent bones. Similarly, the paired temporal bones largely surround the middle ear cavity, from which other air-filled extensions (mastoid air cells) grow into adjacent bone.

The highest part of the skull when it is held in an approximately normal position (with the floor of the orbit at the level of the opening of the external ear) is the **vertex. Frontal** refers to the forehead; **occipital** to the back of the head; and **temporal** to the side of the head. The internal surface of the base of the skull (*basis cranii interna*) is the floor of the cranial cavity. It and the external base deserve particularly careful study. Although most of the bones of the skull are bound together by sutures, in a few locations the gap between bones is greater, and the articulation is a synchondrosis, rather than a suture.

The names of many of the sutures indicate the bones between which the suture in question lies—for instance, the frontozygomatic suture is between the frontal and zygomatic bones, the sphenoparietal between sphenoid and parietal bones—and for these sutures there is no necessity of learning their names. For others, however, the terms are not so obvious: one must learn, for instance, where the lambdoid suture is and that the suture between the temporal and parietal bones is considered to be two sutures, of which one is named the squamous suture and the other the parietomastoid suture.

Exterior of the Skull

The calvaria (Figs. 31-1 and 31-2; (see also 31-6) is formed anteriorly by the unpaired **frontal bone,** behind this by the paired **parietal bones,** and posteriorly by the unpaired **occipital bone**. The suture between the frontal bone and the two parietal bones is the **coronal suture** (hence, the coronal plane of the body is the same as the frontal plane); that between the two parietal bones is the **sagittal suture** (hence, the planes of the body through or parallel to it are sagittal planes). The sagittal suture is so called because in the infant, before the bones of the skull are firmly united, it and fontanels associated with it make it somewhat resemble an arrow (*sagitta*). Fontanels or fonticuli are the soft places in an infant's skull where the membrane in which the bones of the calvaria are formed has not yet been replaced by bone. The inverted V-shaped suture between the two parietal bones and the occipital bone is the **lambdoid suture** (see Fig. 31-2), so called because of its resemblance to the Greek letter lambda (λ). There may be small bones, sutural bones, in the sagittal or lambdoid sutures.

Lateral View

In a lateral view of the skull, in which the bones of the calvaria also can be seen, most of the bones visible (see Fig. 31-1) are those of the cranium; however, the bone forming the lateral rim of the orbit and the bony prominence of the cheek is the zygomatic bone, and below and medial to it is

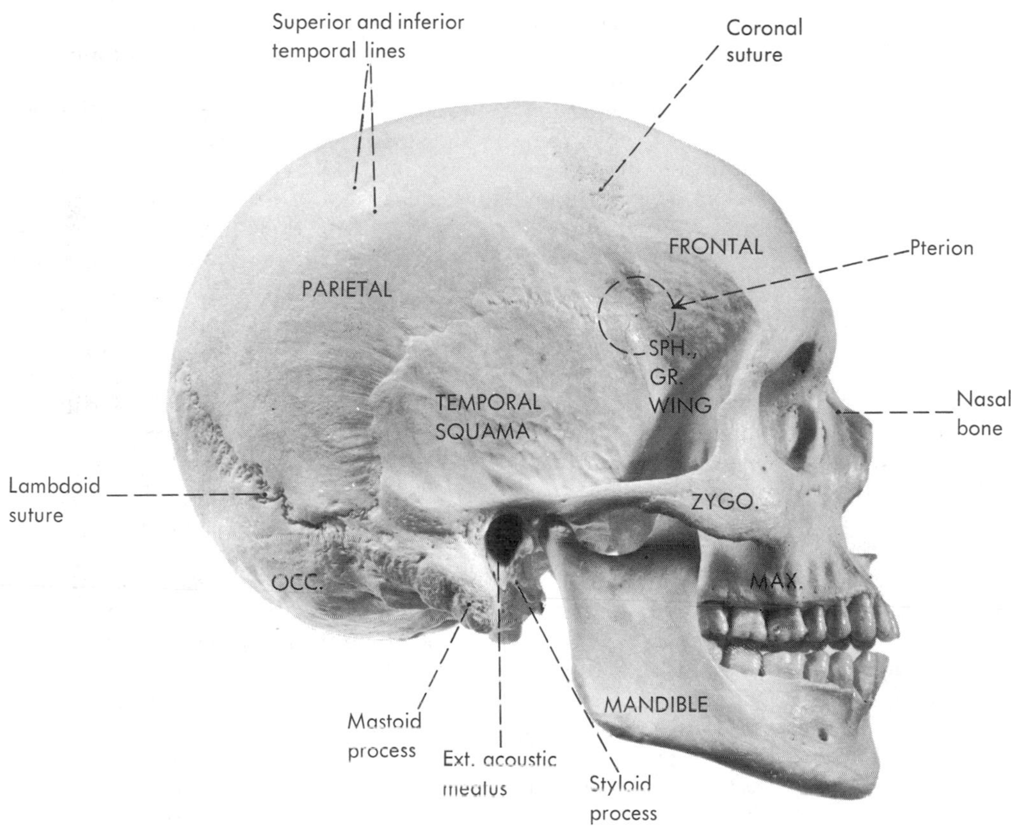

FIGURE 31-1.
Lateral view of the skull: *MAX., OCC., SPH., GR. WING,* and *ZYGO.* identify the maxillary and occipital bones, the greater wing of the sphenoid, and the zygomatic bone.

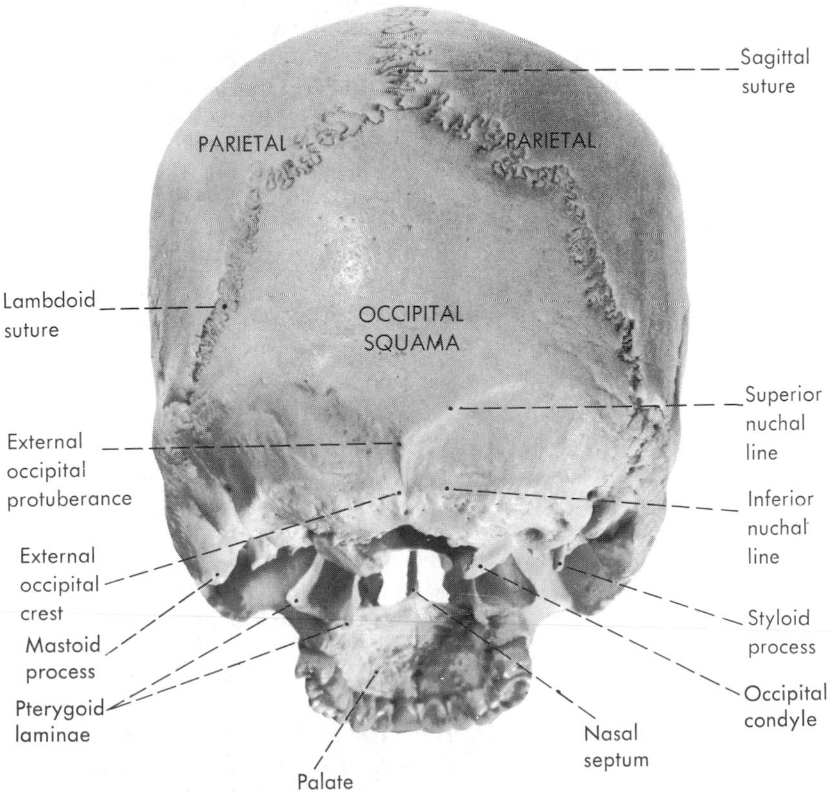

FIGURE 31-2.
Posterior view of the skull.

the maxilla, the tooth-bearing bone of the upper jaw. The mandible is described later; it is best removed while studying the rest of the skull.

The orbital surface of the **zygomatic bone** forms a part of the lateral wall of the orbit and is not visible from the side; the rounded lateral surface forms the prominence of the cheek; and the temporal surface is posterior and medial. The zygomatic bone sends a **frontal process** upward along the lateral border of the orbit to articulate with the frontal bone close to the roof of the orbit and a freely projecting **temporal process** almost horizontally backward to articulate with a similar forward projection from the temporal bone; together the two processes form the **zygomatic arch.** On its lateral surface, the zygomatic bone usually presents a small **zygomaticofacial foramen,** and on its temporal surface, a small **zygomaticotemporal foramen.** These two foramina communicate with one or two foramina in the orbital surface of the bone, and the canals through the bone transmit branches of the maxillary nerve. Sutures unite the zygomatic bone medially with the maxillary bone; above, at the lateral rim of the orbit, with the frontal; posteriorly, below the frontal, with the sphenoid bone (greater wing of this bone); and with the temporal through the zygomatic arch.

Below the zygomatic, and extending in front of and behind it, is the **maxilla.** Many of its features can best be seen in anterior and basal views of the skull, described in following sections. The **body** of the bone is hollow, containing the large **maxillary sinus.** There is a **zygomatic process** that extends upward to articulate with the zygomatic bone, and the tooth-bearing part of the maxilla is the **alveolar process.** (*Alveolus* means pit, and the term refers to the sockets or dental alveoli in which the teeth are set.) On the back end of the alveolar process is a small projection, the **maxillary tuber.** Behind and above this is a thin plate of bone, the lateral lamina of the pterygoid process of the sphenoid bone, described on a following page.

Just behind the zygomatic bone and largely below the frontal, forming part of the lateral wall of both the cranial cavity and the orbit, is the **greater wing of the sphenoid bone.** In addition to articulating with the zygomatic, frontal, and parietal bones, the greater wing shares a sphenosquamous suture with the squamous (flat) part of the temporal bone. The area where the frontal, parietal, sphenoid, and temporal bones are all close together is known as the **pterion.**

The somewhat concave outer surface of the greater wing of the sphenoid and the squamous part of the temporal bone together form the concavity on the side of the skull, deep to the zygomatic arch, known as the **temporal fossa.** At the lower border of the temporal fossa, the greater wing of the sphenoid presents a sharp ridge, the **infratemporal crest,** below which the bone is more horizontal, forming a part of the floor of the cranial cavity. The concavity below the crest, thus behind the maxilla and below the sphenoid and temporal bones, is the **infratemporal fossa** (see Fig. 31-5). The lateral lamina of the pterygoid process of the sphenoid bone forms much of the medial wall of this fossa.

Immediately behind the greater wing of the sphenoid bone, the part of that bone best studied in lateral view, is the **temporal bone.** This forms much of the lower lateral part of the skull, contributes to the base, and houses the middle and internal ears. It is particularly complicated. The **squamous part** (*pars squamosa*) of this bone has been identified as the flat plate articulating anteriorly with the greater wing of the sphenoid. Behind the *sphenosquamous suture* it shares the curved *squamous suture* with the parietal bone. The pars squamosa participates with the sphenoid in forming the medial wall of the temporal fossa and the roof of the infratemporal fossa. From its lower part, the **zygomatic process** projects laterally and forward to complete the zygomatic arch. Behind the zygomatic process is the **external acoustic** (auditory) **meatus,** or ear canal. The thin part of the temporal bone forming the anterior wall, floor, and part of the posterior wall of this canal is the **pars tympanica;** details of the pars tympanica can best be examined when the base of the skull is studied. Just posterosuperior to the canal, there is often a sharp crest, the *suprameatal spine.* Above this, leading toward the root of the zygomatic arch, is a triangle that marks a surgical approach to both the tympanic cavity and the mastoid air cells.

The bony prominence behind the external acoustic meatus is the **mastoid process,** the posterior end of the **petrous portion of the temporal bone** (*petrous,* because much of this part of the bone, with the exception of the mastoid process, is particularly dense, hence, somewhat rocklike—the meaning of petrous). Most of the petrous part of the temporal appears at the base of the skull and, therefore, is described later. The mastoid part articulates with the parietal bone through a *parietomastoid suture* and with the occipital bone through an *occipitomastoid suture.* These two sutures are continuous with each other, and the parietomastoid, in turn, is continuous anteriorly with the squamous suture. On the lateral surface of the bone above the mastoid process proper, there is usually a *mastoid foramen* through which a vein (emissary vein) leaves the skull. Projecting downward from the lower surface of the petrous portion of the temporal bone, in front of the mastoid process, is the more slender **styloid process;** this can be examined better in an external view of the base.

Only a little of the occipital bone can be seen from the lateral side; this is best examined in posterior and inferior views.

Posterior View

The chief bone of the posterior wall of the skull is the **occipital bone.** It consists of *basilar and lateral parts and the squama,* the part best seen in posterior view (see Fig. 31-2). The *lambdoid sutures* through which it articulates with the parietal bones, and at the back end of the sagittal suture, are both visible. The upper part of the squama may persist as a separate bone here, the *interparietal.* At its lower end, which may be indistinct, the lambdoid suture joins the parietomastoid and occipitomastoid sutures. The projection on the posterior surface of the squama is the **external occipital protuberance,** easily palpable in the living person. Its highest point is called the **inion.** There may be a ridge, the *external occipital crest,* extending downward in the midline from the protuberance. Extending laterally from it is the curved **superior nuchal line,** which may have a *supreme nuchal line* just above it. The *inferior nuchal line* is much lower, barely visible in a posterior view of the skull.

In a posterior view, also, the mastoid process again can be recognized. The deep groove on its inferomedial surface is the **mastoid incisure** or notch, the origin of the posterior belly of the digastric muscle. The styloid process may be visible anteromedial to the mastoid process.

Basal View

In external views of the base of the skull (Figs. 31-3 and 31-4), the **occipital bone** is the prominent posterior element. The large foramen that it surrounds is the **foramen magnum,** through which brain and spinal cord are continuous. Anterolateral to the foramen are the **occipital condyles** for articulation with the atlas (first cervical vertebra). Behind each occipital condyle is a depression, the **condylar fossa,** into which there usually opens an oblique **condylar canal** that transmits a vein from a cranial venous sinus inside the skull (sigmoid sinus) to the suboccipital plexus of veins outside the skull. Anteriorly, under cover of about the middle of each condyle and running almost horizontally, is the **hypoglossal canal** for the emergence of the nerve of that name (cranial nerve XII).

There are no distinct boundaries between the squama, the lateral parts, and the basilar part of the occipital bone, but in general, the **squama** lies behind and above the foramen magnum. On it, about halfway between the foramen and the external occipital protuberance, is the *inferior nuchal line.* Muscles of the back of the neck attach both below this line and between it and the

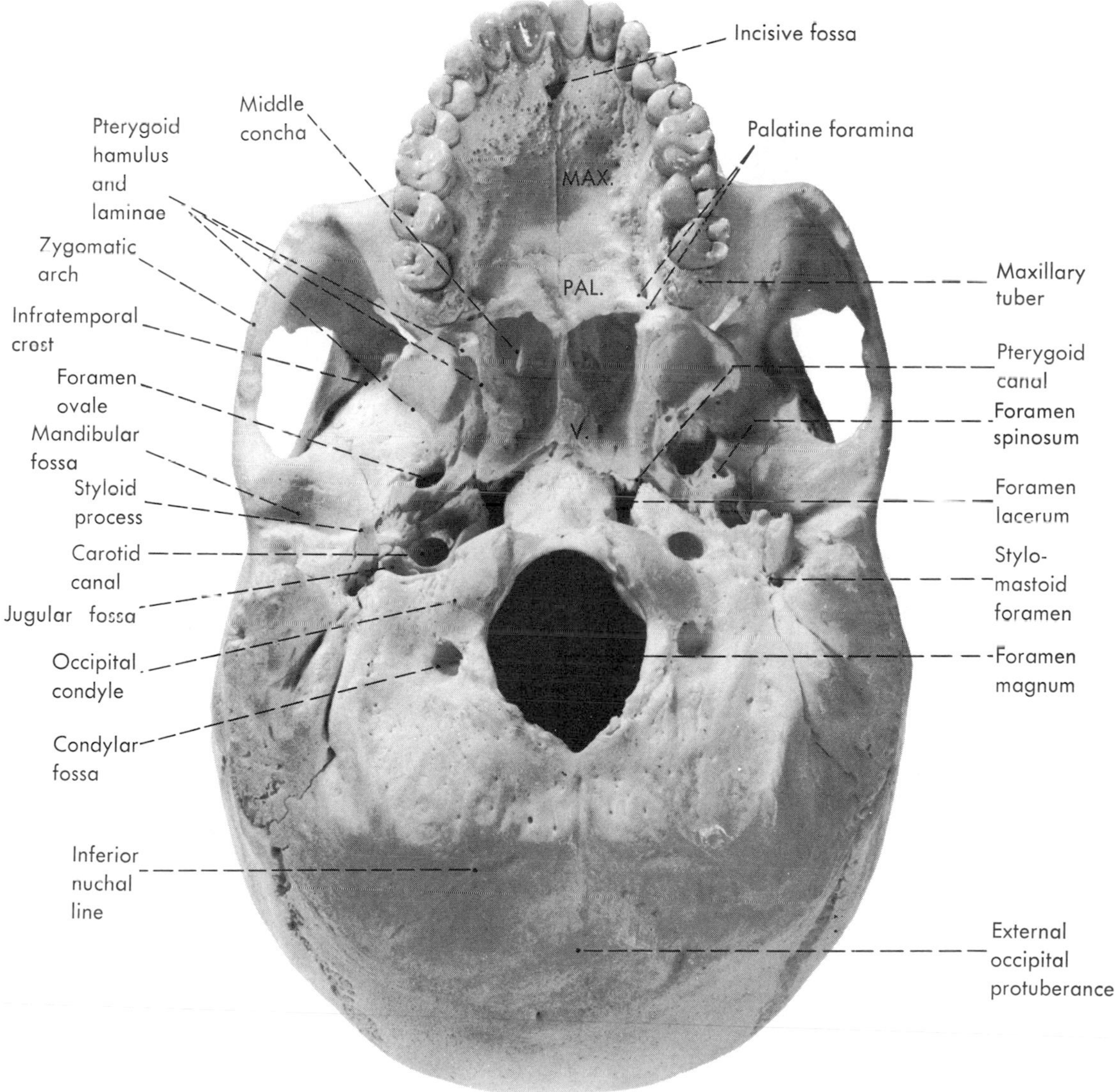

FIGURE *31-3.*
A view of the external surface of the base of the skull with the mandible removed: Here the view is at the same time slightly forward. See also the following figure. *MAX.* and *PAL.* identify the parts of the maxillary and palatine bones forming the hard palate; *V.* is the vomer.

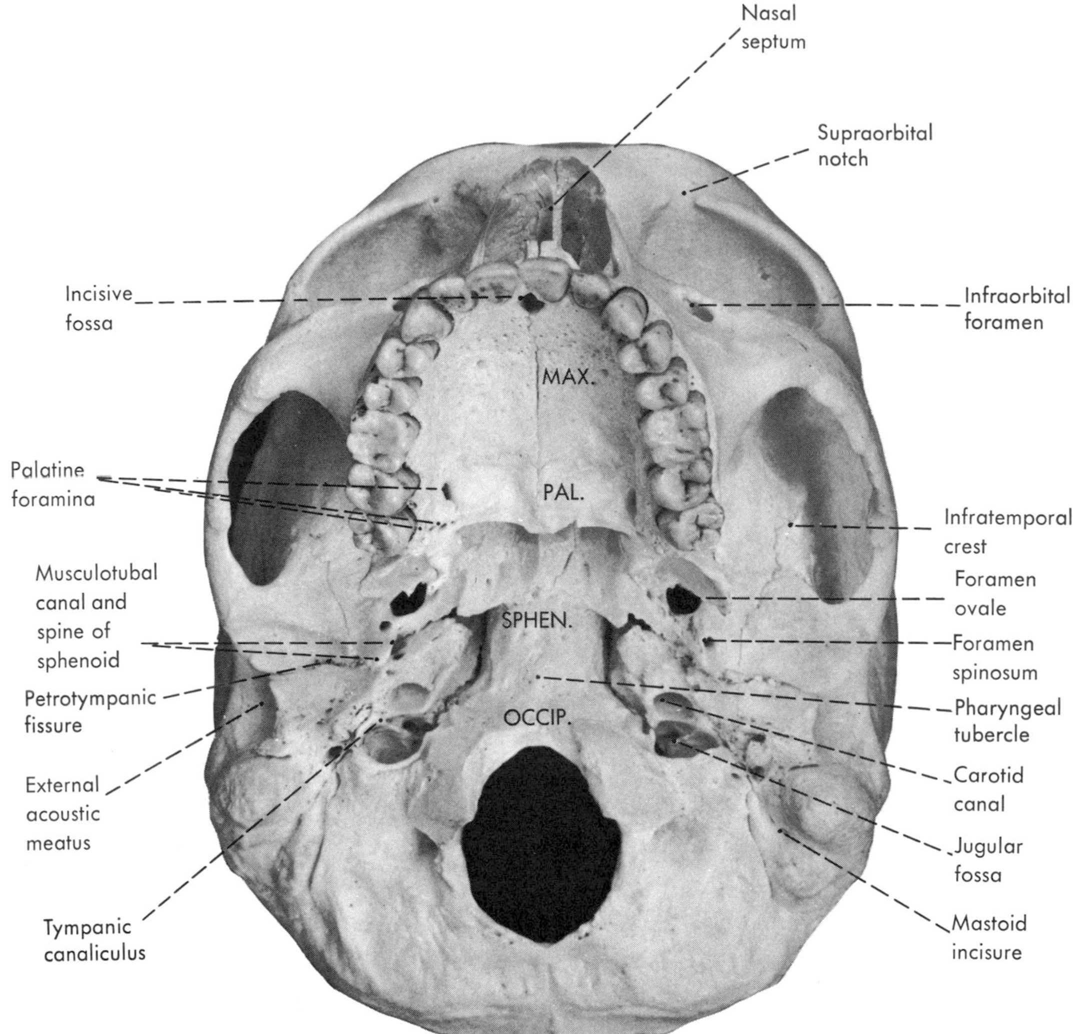

FIGURE *31-4.*
Another view of the external surface of the base of the skull, this time with the skull so tipped that one looks also slightly backward. Certain features are recognizable in both views, but each also shows structures not recognizable in the other: for instance, the jugular fossa in the present figure and the foramen lacerum in the preceding figure. ***MAX.*** **and** ***PAL.*** **are as in the preceding figure;** ***SPHEN.*** **and** ***OCCIP.*** **identify the bodies of the sphenoid and occipital bones.**

superior nuchal line. Each **pars lateralis** lies lateral to the foramen magnum and blends with the squama and basal part, and the **pars basilaris** extends forward as a midline bar of bone about an inch wide. Lateral to the lateral and basal parts are the petrous parts of the temporal bones, which include the mastoid processes.

Anteriorly, the basilar part of the occipital bone is fused, often indistinguishably, to the slanting posterior part of the body of the sphenoid bone; these parts together form the **clivus.** Laterally, there is a gap, the **foramen lacerum,** between the occipital, the sphenoid, and the petrous part of the temporal. This is occupied in life by cartilage and ligamentous tissue that unite the three bones and, therefore, constitute three *synchondroses*. The basal part of the occipital bone presents no other features of particular interest, except at about its middle, where there is a small **pharyngeal tubercle** to which the superior constrictor muscle of the pharynx is attached. In front of this tubercle, the mucous membrane of the upper part of the pharynx lies against the occipital bone.

The **petrous part of the temporal bone** forms the floor of the posterior part of the cranial cavity lateral to the occipital bone. Its mastoid process and notch have already been noted. Anteromedial to the mastoid process is the **styloid process,** of varying thickness and length and often broken in the prepared skull. Just behind the base of the styloid process is a prominent foramen, the **stylomastoid foramen,** through which the facial (seventh cranial) nerve leaves the skull. Medial to the styloid process, between it and the occipital condyle, the temporal bone presents a pronounced depression, the **jugular fossa,** bounded posteriorly by the **jugular process.** The fossa houses the upper end of the internal jugular vein and opens through the **jugular foramen** into the interior of the skull. In the lateral wall of the jugular fossa is the **mastoid canaliculus** for the auricular branch of the vagus nerve. In the ridge anterior to the fossa is the opening of the **tympanic canaliculus,** for the tympanic branch of the ninth nerve. The opening may be in a slight depression, the *fossula petrosa.* Anteromedial to the jugular foramen, the petrous part of the temporal bone is separated from the pars basilaris of the occipital by the *petrooccipital fissure,* which meets the *petrosphenoid fissure* (lateral to the petrous part of the temporal) at the anterior end of the pars petrosa to form the opening with jagged edges, the **foramen lacerum,** already noted.

The part of the petrous portion of the temporal bone in front of the ear is known as the **petrous apex.** It ends anteriorly at the foramen lacerum. On the external base of the skull, it is marked by the external opening of the **carotid canal,** which lies immediately in front of the jugular foramen. The carotid canal extends, first, vertically upward in the temporal bone, but then turns abruptly to run anteriorly and medially throughout the length of the petrous apex, emerging just above the foramen lacerum.

In front of the styloid process, closely fused to the petrous part of the temporal bone, is the **tympanic part.** This can be seen to form the anterior wall and floor of the external acoustic meatus and some of its posterior wall. It extends forward and medially, giving off an expansion or **sheath** to the base of the styloid process, to a level a little in front of the external opening of the carotid canal. In front of the lateral part of the pars tympanica is a small slit or fissure, the **tympanosquamous fissure,** that, traced medially, divides into two parallel and closely adjacent fissures. The posterior one, the **petrotympanic fissure,** important because the chorda tympani, a branch of the facial nerve that runs through the middle ear cavity, emerges through it. The fissure in front of the pars tympanica also lies just behind the **mandibular fossa,** the concavity of the inferior surface of the pars squamosa for articulation with the mandible. Anterior to the mandibular fossa is the rounded **articular tubercle.**

At the anteromedial end of the tympanic part, between it and the petrous part, is an opening that actually represents the bony anterior ends of two canals, an upper for the tensor tympani muscle (a muscle extending into the middle ear cavity) and a lower for the auditory tube that connects the middle ear cavity to the pharynx. This bony tube is the **musculotubal canal** and, in life, is divided into a small upper and a larger lower part by a thin bony septum.

Anterior to the base of the occipital bone, and anterior and lateral to the petrous apex, the **sphenoid bone** forms the major part of the floor of the skull. The body of the bone, in line with the basilar part of the occipital bone, contains paired **sphenoid sinuses,** but in an inferior view, it is largely covered by a bone, the **vomer;** that forms a part of the septum of the nasal cavity and by the **pterygoid processes** that form the lateral walls of the posterior openings of the nasal cavities. Each pterygoid process is also attached to a **greater wing** of the sphenoid bone. This wing, already seen in lateral view, extends backward medial to the temporal squama to the angle between that and the petrous part of the temporal. The fourth part of the sphenoid bone, the **lesser wing,** can best be seen in an inner view of the base of the skull (see Fig. 31-9).

The flattened inferior surface of the greater wing of the sphenoid bone is the **infratemporal fossa.** Laterally, it is separated from the temporal fossa on the side of the skull by the *infratemporal crest.* Posteromedially, between it and the adjacent part of the temporal bone, there is a groove that houses the cartilaginous part of the *auditory tube,* continued forward from the bony part of the tube in the musculotubal canal. The prominent **foramen ovale,** through which the mandibular branch of the trigeminal (fifth cranial) nerve makes its exit from the skull, opens into the posterior part of the infratemporal fossa. Posterolateral to the foramen ovale is the small round **foramen spinosum.** Through this the middle meningeal artery, the largest of the vessels to the coverings of the brain, enters the cranial cavity. The foramen spinosum obtains its name from the **sphenoid spine,** a small projection on the posterior tip of the greater wing of the sphenoid posterior to the foramen.

Anteriorly, the infratemporal fossa extends to the posterior (infratemporal) surface of the body of the maxilla, and here it is bounded medially by a thin plate of bone, the **lateral pterygoid lamina.** If one tilts the skull to obtain a view from below and laterally (Fig. 31-5); it can be seen that, although the lateral pterygoid lamina is fused to the maxilla below, it is separated above from that bone by a fissure, the **pterygomaxillary fissure,** that opens into the infratemporal fossa. The pterygomaxillary fissure is continuous anteriorly with a fissure (inferior orbital) that opens above into the orbit, but it also opens above and medially into a deep recess, the **pterygopalatine fossa.** This important fossa extends posteriorly, behind the maxilla, between the pterygoid part of the sphenoid bone and the perpendicular lamina of the palatine bone, which here is part of the lateral wall of the nasal cavity. Part of the maxillary artery enters the pterygopalatine fossa through the pterygomaxillary fissure, and the maxillary branch of the trigeminal nerve enters the fossa as it leaves the skull through the foramen rotundum, which opens into the posterior end of the fossa. From the fossa, both artery and nerve send small branches downward to the posterior surface of the maxilla, on which there are two or more **alveolar foramina** through which they enter the bone. They send large branches medially into the nasal cavity through the **sphenopalatine foramen,** which lies in the thin wall between the fossa and the nasal cavity, and can easily be seen through the posterior openings of the nose. They also send branches downward to appear on the posterior part of the bony palate through the several palatine foramina located here. Anteriorly, a major part of the maxillary nerve and a branch of the artery pass into the floor of the orbit through the inferior orbital fissure. Posteriorly, a small **palatovaginal canal** and a larger and more important **pterygoid canal,** both transmitting nerves and vessels (and described in a following paragraph), open into the pterygopalatine fossa.

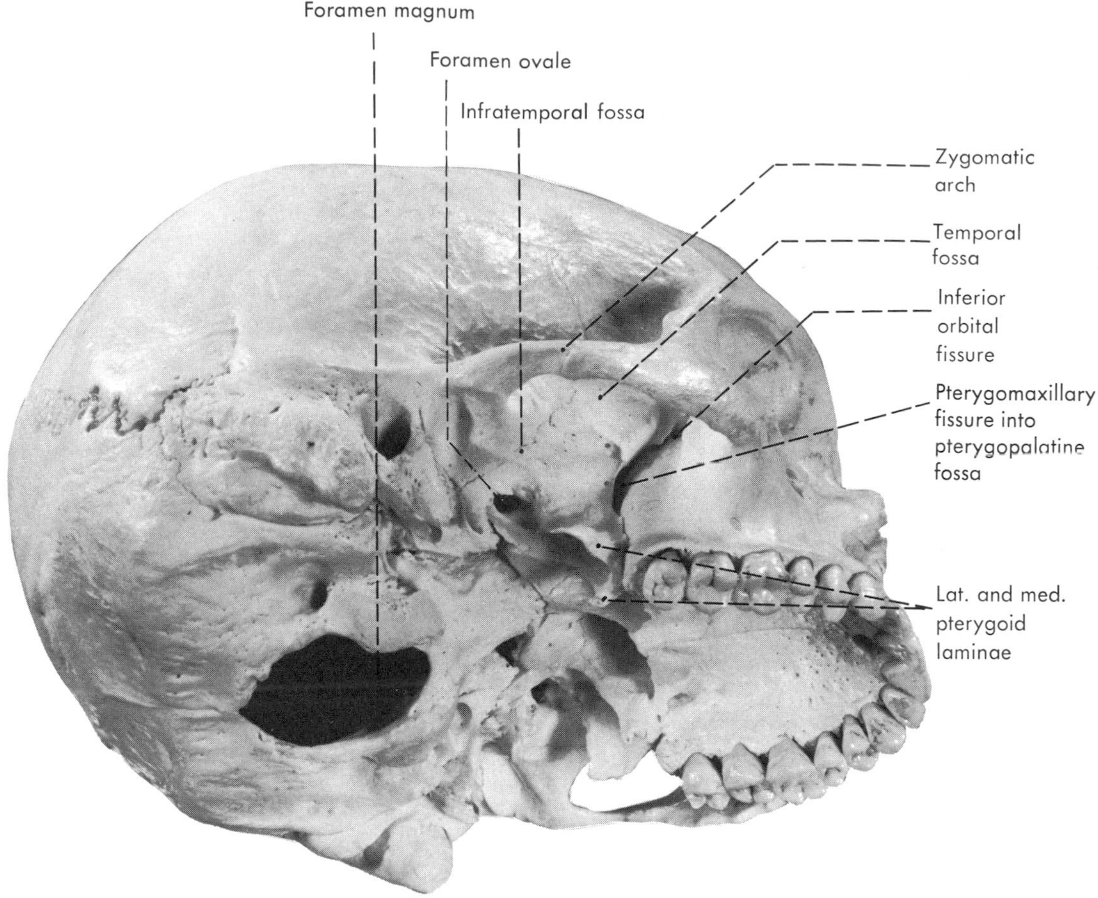

FIGURE *31-5.*
An oblique view of the base and lateral aspect of the skull, to show the pterygopalatine fossa; it and the inferior orbital fissure opening into it are seen through the pterygomaxillary fissure.

The **pterygoid processes** of the sphenoid bone, the lateral laminae of which have already been noted, have several important relations. Each pterygoid process, projecting downward from the body and greater wing of the sphenoid bone, has two laminae (plates), the *lateral and a medial lamina.* These are continuous with each other above and seem also to be continuous below. Here, however, the apparent continuity is brought about by the *pyramidal process of the palatine bone* (the small bone that forms the posterior edge of the bony palate). This process is fused to the maxilla and to both laminae of the pterygoid process. The concavity between the two pterygoid plates is the **pterygoid fossa.** At the lower end of the medial plate is a posteriorly projecting hook of bone, the **hamulus.** The tendon of one of the muscles of the palate (tensor veli palatini) passes downward lateral to the hamulus and then turns medially in a notch, the **pterygoid incisure,** on its lower surface. At its upper end, the thin edge of the medial pterygoid plate expands into two slight ridges that enclose between them a triangular flat area, the **scaphoid fossa;** the tensor of the palate, just mentioned, arises in part from this.

The process extending medially from the medial pterygoid plate over the inferior surface of the body of the sphenoid is the *processus vaginalis.* It meets the expanded upper end, or **ala, of the vomer** (the bone between the two nasal cavities). On the lower surface of the vaginal process there is frequently a small, but clear, groove that leads forward into a foramen. This foramen lies between the vaginal process and the perpendicular lamina of the palatine bone (which forms the lateral wall of the nose immediately in front of the medial pterygoid process) and, therefore, is called the **palatovaginal canal.** It transmits tiny nerve and arterial twigs from the pterygopalatine fossa to the roof of the pharynx. At the posterior end of the vaginal process, where it is joined by the medial side of the pterygoid plate, there is a small bulge, and immediately above that, opening into the anterior wall of the foramen lacerum, is the posterior end of the **pterygoid** (*vidian*) **canal.** The pterygoid canal transmits an important, but rather slender, nerve (nerve of the pterygoid canal) that typically leaves the interior of the skull at the foramen lacerum, enters the canal and, through this, runs forward into the pterygopalatine fossa, where it ends in an autonomic ganglion.

The posterior openings of the nose, already mentioned, are the **choanae.** Each is about twice as broad in the vertical diameter as it is in the transverse one. The bony septum extending between them is the **vomer.** The articulation of its expanded upper end, the **ala,** with the body of the sphenoid and the vaginal parts of the pterygoid processes has been noted. Inferiorly, the vomer articulates with the upper surface of the bony palate; anteriorly, it articulates with other bone and cartilage of the nasal septum (see Fig. 33-29).

The thin curved plates of bone projecting inward from the lateral wall of the nose are the **conchae;** three of these can be seen through the choana. The **inferior nasal concha** really is a separate bone, but is fused laterally to the palatine and maxillary bones (which form the lateral walls of the nasal cavity at the level of the concha). Above the inferior nasal concha is the **middle nasal concha.** The middle concha is almost as long as the inferior concha, but frequently appears thicker at its base, owing to the invasion of air cells from the ethmoid sinus. This is a part of the *ethmoid labyrinth,* a lateral part of the ethmoid bone that forms the upper lateral wall of the nasal cavity. Above the middle nasal concha, but primarily at its posterior end and, therefore, most easily visible posteriorly, is the **superior nasal concha,** also a part of the ethmoid labyrinth. The nasal cavities are described in more detail in Chapter 33. Concerning the bony wall, only one thing needs to be added at this time: just above the back end of the middle nasal concha is the **sphenopalatine foramen** that transmits important nerves and vessels from the pterygopalatine fossa to the nasal cavity.

The floor of the nasal cavities, the **bony palate** (*hard palate* when soft tissues cover the bone), is formed posteriorly by the **horizontal laminae** of the palatine bones. Each **palatine bone** is somewhat L-shaped: its horizontal lamina meets that of the other side in the midline, and its **perpendicular lamina** or plate runs upward as a posterior part of the lateral wall of the nasal cavity. The perpendicular lamina is fused posteriorly, through its pyramidal process, to the pterygoid process of the sphenoid bone, anterolaterally to the maxilla, and is almost hidden by the two. The sphenopalatine foramen, already noted, lies above an upper part of this lamina, between it and the body of the sphenoid. Behind the *sphenopalatine foramen,* the perpendicular plate articulates with the body of the sphenoid and the pterygoid process, and in front of the foramen, it extends into the floor of the orbit.

Anterolaterally, in the suture between the horizontal laminae of the palatine bones and the processes in front of them, are the paired **greater palatine foramina;** behind each of these, in the palatine bone, are one or two **lesser palatine foramina.** These foramina are the lower ends of the **greater** and **lesser palatine canals** through which nerves and vessels reach both the hard and the soft palate (the soft palate is attached to the posterior border of the hard palate). If bristles are passed up these canals, they will be found to converge above in the pterygopalatine fossa. Where the horizontal laminae meet in the midline, they form a posteriorly projecting **posterior nasal spine;** on their upper surfaces they send up a **nasal crest** for articulation with the vomer; and on their lower surfaces, a variable distance from the posterior edges, there may be a distinct ridge, the **palatine crest.**

The bony palate in front of the horizontal laminae of the palatine bone is formed by the fusion of the **palatine processes of the two maxillae.** Each blends laterally and anteriorly with the body of the maxilla and the alveolar process (the downward-projecting, tooth-bearing part) of the maxilla. Posterolaterally, there usually is a groove leading forward from the greater palatine foramen in the osseous palate. This transmits the large nerves and vessels of the hard palate. Sometimes there is a bony ridge, the *torus palatinus,* along the intermaxillary suture. In the anterior midline, where the palatine processes blend with the alveolar processes, there is a deep pit, the **incisive fossa.** In its walls, sometimes visible and sometimes not, are two to four **incisive foramina,** which are the lower openings of **incisive canals** that open above into the nasal cavity. There are most commonly four canals, two for blood vessels (one on each side) and two for nerves.

Anterior View

In an anterior view of the skull (Fig. 31-6), it is obvious that the two maxillae form a large part of the border of the anterior opening of the nasal cavities (**piriform aperture** in the bony skull) and also much of the inferior and medial border of the entrance to the orbit.

On inspection of the **nasal cavity,** the fused **nasal crests,** extending upward from the palatine processes to form the lowest part of the nasal septum, can be recognized. The crests end anteriorly in an **anterior nasal spine.** Posteriorly, they articulate with the vomer, but anteriorly, in the dry skull, their upper free borders are partly separated, thus presenting a cleft. Into this cleft, during life, there fits a cartilage that largely completes the nasal septum. The upper part of the bony septum is the **perpendicular plate** of the **ethmoid bone.** This bone also forms the narrow upper roof of the nose, the **cribriform plate,** best seen from inside the cranial cavity. It sends downward, on each side of the cribriform plate, the **ethmoid labyrinth** that separates the nose from the orbit. The ethmoid labyrinth appears on the medial orbital wall as the **orbital lamina** of the ethmoid bone and projects into the nasal cavity as the superior and middle nasal conchae, already seen through the choanae. The front ends of the inferior nasal conchae also are easily recognized in an anterior view of the nasal cavity. The middle conchae can be seen somewhat indistinctly above them, but the superior conchae are typically too far back and placed too high to be visible. Other features of the bony walls of the nasal cavity are best appreciated during dissection of this part.

Returning to the **maxilla,** the **alveolar process,** bearing the teeth, can be recognized again as it extends downward below the level of the palatine process. The body of the maxilla lies lateral to the lower part of the nasal cavity. Rather than being convex, as are its lateral and posterior surfaces, the anterior surface of the maxilla presents a concavity, the **canine fossa,** just below the prominence of the cheek and above the alveolar process. Above the canine fossa, a little below the lower border of the orbit, is the large **infraorbital foramen.** This transmits the largest branch of the maxillary nerve (a part of the trigeminal) as

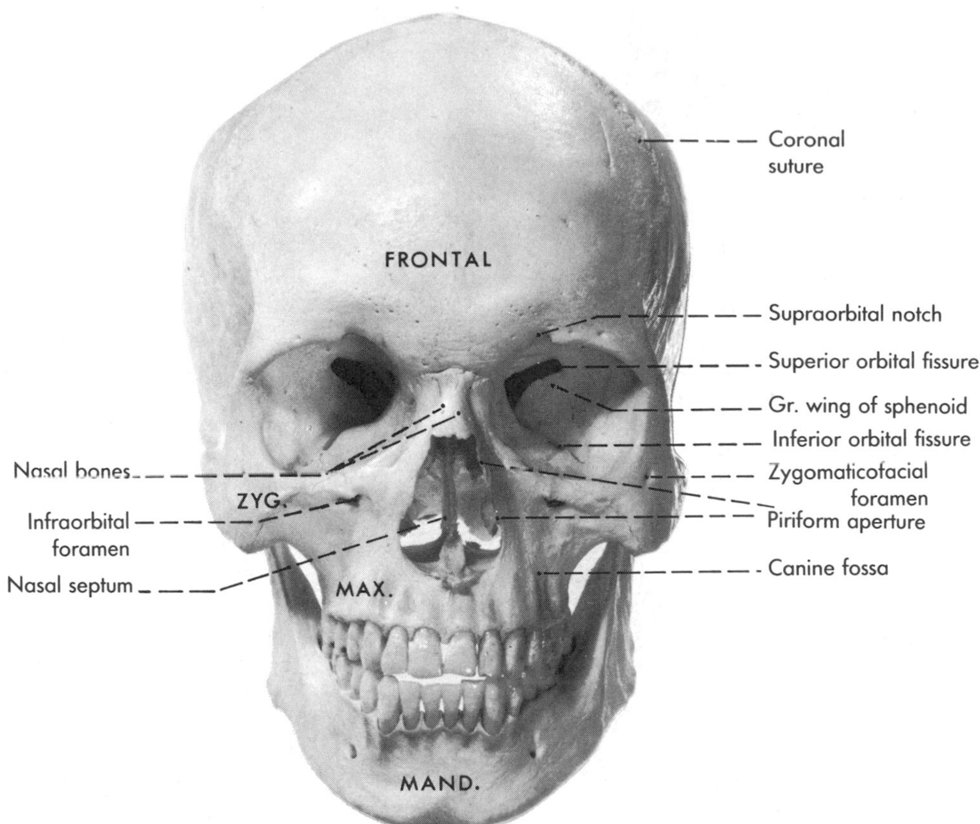

FIGURE *31-6*. Anterior view of the skull: *ZYG.* is the zygomatic bone; *MAX.* and *MAND.* are the maxilla and mandible.

it comes out onto the face to supply skin of the cheek, upper lip, and side of the nose. Laterally and above, the body of the maxilla articulates with the zygomatic bone and medial to and behind this forms a large part of the floor of the orbit (and the roof of the maxillary sinus). Most of the details of the bony orbit can be studied more profitably just preceding study of the soft tissues it contains and, therefore, are to be found in Chapter 33. It need only be noted that the **frontal process** of the maxilla extends upward between the nose and the orbit, forming a part of the lateral wall of the nasal cavity, to articulate with the frontal and nasal bones.

The two **nasal bones** articulate with each other in the midline, articulate laterally with the frontal processes of the maxillae, and articulate above with the frontal bone. Their lower free edges form the uppermost part of the piriform aperture. In life, they articulate with nasal cartilages that support the lower part of the nose. Posteroinferiorly, they articulate with the nasal septum. On the internal surface of each nasal bone there may be a slight groove, the *ethmoidal sulcus;* this accommodates a branch of the ophthalmic division of the trigeminal nerve, which leaves the nasal cavity to pass between the nasal bone and the nasal cartilage to a subcutaneous position.

The **frontal bone** has already been seen in superior and lateral views. The part of the frontal bone that forms the forehead is the **squama.** Just above and paralleling each supraorbital margin, the squama presents a ridge, the **superciliary arch.** Between the two superciliary arches in the midline, there is a slight protuberance, the **glabella,** in which some remains of the *frontal* or *metopic suture* (between the originally paired frontal bones) may be visible. The swellings of the squama that form the prominence of the forehead on each side are the *frontal tubers* or eminences. The supraorbital margin of the frontal bone is marked on its inner third by a **supraorbital foramen,** or supraorbital notch, that transmits the supraorbital nerve and vessels as these leave the orbit and turn up on the forehead. Sometimes, medial to the supraorbital foramen, there is a second notch or foramen, the **frontal notch** (foramen). It accommodates a medial branch of the supraorbital nerve that once was known as the frontal nerve.

Lateral to the orbit, the frontal bone sends a zygomatic process downward to articulate with the zygomatic bone and complete the lateral wall of the orbit. Between the two orbits, it also sends a short nasal process downward to articulate with the nasal bones and the frontal processes of the maxillae. Finally, the frontal bone has almost horizontal parts, each called a **pars orbitalis,** that extend backward from the supraorbital margins as major parts of the roofs of the two orbits.

The squama of the frontal bone is thick. It presents hard inner and outer laminae, between which lies diploë except in that part of the bone that is invaded by the **frontal sinuses.** These are paired sinuses, but vary greatly in size and often are asymmetric. They usually extend into both the squama and the orbital part of the frontal bone.

The orbital part contrasts greatly with the squama in strength, for it is a thin plate of bone or, where it contains a part of the frontal sinus, two very thin plates.

Mandible

The mandible (Figs. 31-7 and 31-8), the unpaired bone of the lower jaw, consists of the tooth-bearing **body** and the more vertically disposed **ramus** that receives the insertions of the chief muscles of the jaw and articulates with the temporal bone. Ramus and body meet posteriorly at the **angle.** The *body* of the mandible is divided into two parts; the lower is the *base*, and the upper part, bearing the teeth, is the *pars alveolaris* or alveolar process.

The base of the mandible shows a swelling on its anteroinferior surface where the two sides come together; this is the **mental protuberance.** The lower, lateral, part of the mental protuberance, the **mental tubercle,** is frequently more pronounced. Anterolaterally, about halfway between the upper border of the alveolar process and the lower border of the base, is the **mental foramen.** A large branch of the mandibular nerve emerges through this foramen, after having supplied the teeth, and supplies mucous membrane and skin of the lower lip and chin. The ridge running down from the front of the ramus onto the body of the mandible is the *oblique line*. It usually is traceable to the mental tubercle, but is not well marked except close to the ramus.

On the inner surface of the mandible in the midline, there is a roughened projection, the **mental spine.** This may be bilateral instead of in the midline, or it may be divided into an upper and lower spine, for one pair of muscles attaches to the lower part of the spine and another pair attaches to the upper part. Lateral to the mental spine on each side is a slight concavity, the **sublingual fovea**

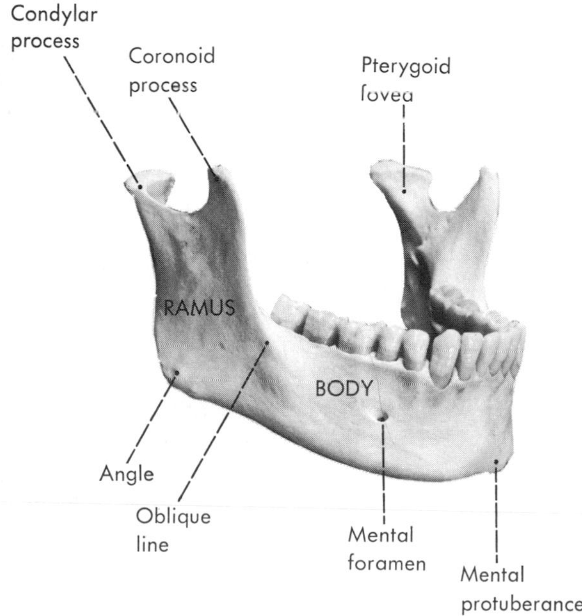

FIGURE *31-7.*
Anterolateral view of the mandible.

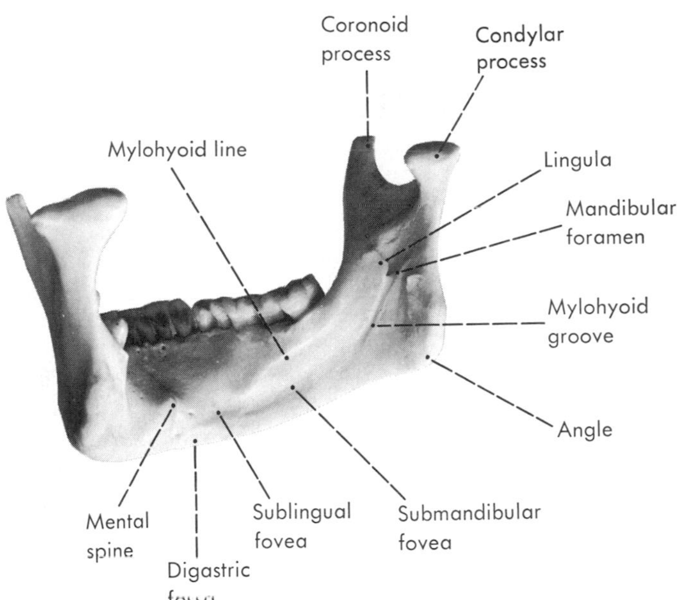

FIGURE *31-8.*
Inner surface of the mandible.

against which the anterior end of the sublingual salivary gland fits. Below each sublingual fovea, on the posteroinferior border of the mandible, is another slightly concave area, the **digastric fossa,** where the anterior belly of the digastric muscle is attached. Starting between the sublingual and digastric impressions, but not particularly marked until it is posterior to the former, is the **mylohyoid line.** This marks the attachment of the mylohyoid muscle, the muscle that forms the floor of the mouth. The mylohyoid line extends upward and backward for the entire length of the alveolar process. The long concave area below the major part of the mylohyoid line is the **submandibular fovea,** accommodating the salivary gland of the same name.

The almost perpendicular **ramus** of the mandible is continuous anteriorly with the alveolar process and base. Posteriorly, it ends below at the angle and above it presents two processes. Of these, the anterior, sharper **coronoid process** serves for the attachment of a muscle, and the *head* of the posterior **condylar process** helps form the temporomandibular joint. Below the head is the *neck,* and anteromedially, at the junction of the head and neck, is the **pterygoid fovea,** representing the attachment of part of the lateral pterygoid muscle. The concavity between the coronoid and condylar processes is the **mandibular notch** (*incisure*).

On the inner surface of the ramus of the mandible is the **mandibular foramen.** It is the entrance to the **mandibular canal,** which runs forward in the mandible deep to the roots of the teeth and carries to them their nerves and vessels. Parts of these nerves and vessels emerge on the outer surface of the mandible through the mental foramen. Anterior to and above the mandibular foramen is a thin projection of bone, the mandibular **lingula.** It somewhat overlaps the foramen and is a landmark for injection of the nerve here. Leading downward from the mandibular foramen is a small groove, the **mylohyoid groove,** which indicates the course of the mylohyoid nerve and vessels. The mylohyoid nerve and vessels leave the nerve and vessels that enter the mandible and run downward on the inner surface of the bone.

Not only the size but the shape of the mandible varies much with age and the condition of the dentition. At birth, the ramus of the mandible makes an obtuse angle with the body, because the condylar process projects more posteriorly than upward (see Fig. 31-13). As the teeth appear and the child uses them for chewing, the body of the mandible increases in size; the ramus grows particularly fast posteriorly and becomes more nearly vertical, so the angle becomes less obtuse. As the teeth are lost in old age, the alveolar part of the mandible is absorbed, and if dentures are not regularly worn, the altered muscular pull during attempted occlusion results in the condylar process being gradually displaced backward, so that the angle returns toward the infantile condition.

Interior of the Skull

Roof

The inner surface of the calvaria presents little of interest. The only structures worthy of note are the grooves that blood vessels leave here. In the sagittal plane, most marked in the region of the sagittal suture between the parietal bones, but extending also downward on the inner surface of the occipital and on the inner surface of the frontal, is the **sulcus of the superior sagittal sinus.** This great venous sinus becomes larger as it is traced backward, because it receives the veins from the upper surface of the adjacent brain. On each side of the sulcus of the superior sagittal sinus, usually on the inner surface of the parietal bone, but sometimes also on the frontal, there may be two or three depressions, the *foveolae granulares.* Laterally, extending upward from the cut lower edge of the calvaria, are a variable number of grooves that accommodate the meningeal vessels; almost all these markings are caused by the middle meningeal artery and its accompanying veins and can be seen better when the base of the skull is examined.

Base of the Skull

The interior of the base of the skull, the **cranial floor,** presents three levels (Fig. 31-9). The anterior part, the highest, is largely also the roof of the two orbits and of the nasal cavities and is the **anterior cranial fossa.** The middle part, the **middle cranial fossa,** lies at a lower level. Its deeper lateral parts are separated from the anterior fossa by sharp ridges of bone, often known as the "sphenoid ridges," but are united across the midline by a narrower and higher portion (the *sella turcica*). The whole fossa roughly resembles a butterfly. Finally, the most posterior part of the floor, surrounding the foramen magnum and largely separated from the middle fossa by the ridges ("petrous ridges") formed by the converging petrous parts of the two temporal bones, is the **posterior cranial fossa.** The internal anatomy of the skull is easier to learn if it is studied in terms of the cranial fossae.

Anterior Cranial Fossa. The **crista galli** (cock's comb), a part of the **ethmoid bone,** is the sharp projection of bone anteriorly in the midline of the floor of the anterior cranial fossa. Attached to the crista is the anterior end of a sheet of dura (*falx cerebri*) that partly separates the two cerebral hemispheres. In front of the crista, on the inner surface of the frontal bone, is the **frontal crest** (also for the attachment of the falx). This crest, sharp below, widens above and gives place to the *sulcus for the superior sagittal sinus.* There may or may not be, between the frontal crest and the crista galli, the small **foramen cecum** that leads into the nasal cavity. A small vein, often lacking in the adult, runs through this foramen and connects the veins of the nose with the intracranial sinuses. On each side of and behind the crista galli, the lowest part of the floor of the anterior fossa is formed by a part of the ethmoid bone that presents numerous holes that lead from the nasal cavity (transmitting filaments of the olfactory nerve); this is the **cribriform plate** (*lamina cribrosa*) of the ethmoid. Lateral to the cribriform plates and arching gently upward are the orbital parts of the frontal bone, which form major parts of the roofs of the orbits.

On the sides of the cribriform plates, between these and the frontal bone, are the medial ends of the small *anterior* and *posterior ethmoidal canals.* These medial ends are often difficult to observe but their other ends, the *ethmoidal foramina,* can be seen on the medial wall of the orbit. Through each of these canals, a blood vessel enters the cranial cavity, runs forward along the lateral border of the cribriform plate, and then turns downward into the nose. A nerve accompanies the anterior artery.

Behind the cribriform plates and the orbital parts of the frontal bone, the floor of the anterior fossa is formed by the **body** and the **lesser wings of the sphenoid bone.** The anterior border of a groove, the *chiasmatic sulcus,* across the body of the sphenoid, demarcates the anterior fossa from the middle part of the middle fossa. As the lesser wings project laterally, they form the sharp boundaries between the lateral parts of the anterior and middle cranial fossae, and it is these that often are referred to as the "sphenoid ridges." At their medial ends, the lesser wings project posteromedially as free processes, the **anterior clinoid processes,** that serve for the attachment of a part of the cranial dura mater.

Middle Cranial Fossa. The middle cranial fossa is particularly complex, because of its shape and because of the numerous foramina and grooves related to it. Between the body and the lesser wings of the sphenoid, anterior to the anterior clinoid processes, are the **optic canals,** opening anteriorly into the orbits and each transmitting an optic nerve and an accompanying (ophthalmic) artery. The **chiasmatic sulcus** unites the two canals and is bordered posteriorly in the midline by a small rounded elevation, the **tuberculum sellae.** The remaining small midline part of the middle cranial fossa, behind the optic canals and the chiasmatic sulci, is the **sella turcica** (Turk's saddle); it

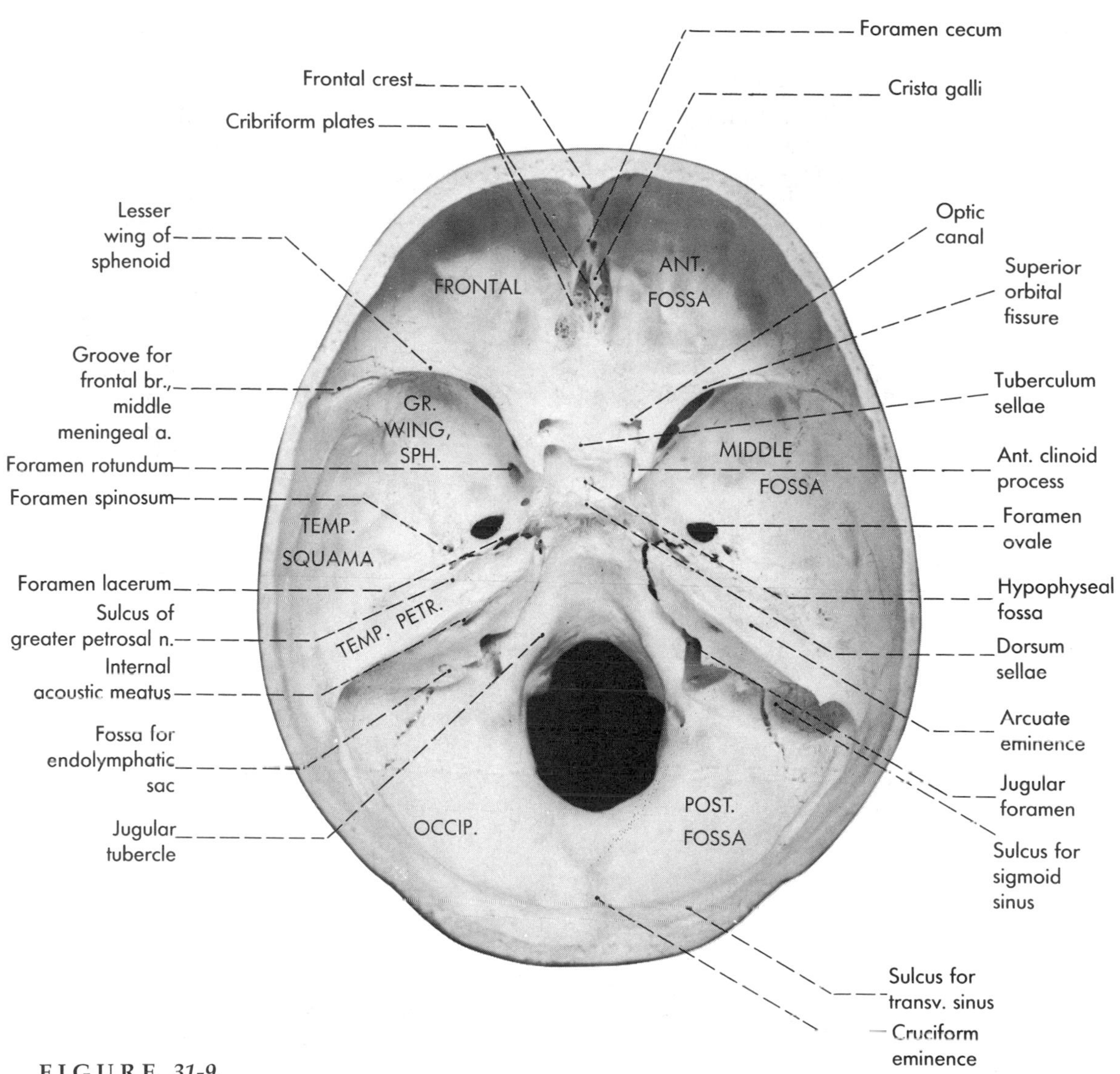

FIGURE *31-9.*
Interior of the base of the skull. ***GR. WING, SPH.*** **is the greater wing of the sphenoid bone;** ***TEMP. SQUAMA*** **and** ***TEMP. PETR.*** **are the squamous and petrous parts of the temporal bone; and** ***OCCIP.*** **is the occipital bone.**

is higher than the lateral parts and is formed by the body of the sphenoid bone. The anterior part of the sella turcica is the tuberculum. Posteriorly, the sella is bounded by the **dorsum sellae,** a ridge of bone that projects upward like the back of a saddle. Projecting forward from each side of the dorsum is a **posterior clinoid process,** usually not so marked as the anterior clinoid process. The deepest part of the sella is the **hypophyseal fossa,** so called because it houses the hypophysis. Tumors of the hypophysis, or long-standing increased intracranial pressure, produces decalcification, erosion, and expansion of the sella turcica, which can be detected in radiographs.

On each side, posterolateral to the dorsum sellae, is a jagged foramen, the **foramen lacerum,** already noted on the external surface of the skull. Here the tip of the petrous portion of the temporal bone fits in between the body and the greater wing of the sphenoid and presents the anterior end of the carotid canal. Leading upward from just above the foramen lacerum is the **carotid sulcus.** The internal carotid artery leaves the petrous tip to run in this sulcus to the undersurface of the anterior clinoid process, where it turns medially toward the tuberculum sellae and then leaves the cranial floor by turning superiorly to penetrate the dura and distribute branches to the brain. Just at the point where the carotid artery turns superiorly on the side of the sella turcica, there may be a *middle clinoid process.* Sometimes this is so marked that it meets or almost meets the anterior clinoid process, thus converting the terminal part of the carotid sulcus into a foramen.

Much of the floor of each lateral expanded part of the middle cranial fossa is formed by a **greater wing of the sphenoid bone** (see Fig. 31-9). Anteriorly, lateral to the anterior clinoid process, this wing is separated from the lesser wing by the **superior orbital fissure.** Lateral to this fissure the greater and lesser wings fuse. Behind the base of the superior orbital fissure, and at about the level of the middle of the sella turcica, there is a rounded foramen that is directed anteriorly and slightly laterally. This is the **foramen rotundum.** It opens into the pterygopalatine fossa and transmits the maxillary nerve, the second branch of the trigeminal nerve (the first or ophthalmic branch makes its exit through the superior orbital fissure). Behind the foramen rotundum is a larger oval foramen that is directed downward. This is the **foramen ovale,** which opens into the infratemporal fossa and transmits the third or mandibular branch of the trigeminal nerve. The trigeminal and other nerves in the middle cranial fossa are shown in Figure 31-10.

Posterolateral to the foramen ovale is the **foramen spinosum,** also opening below into the infratemporal fossa. This foramen transmits the middle meningeal artery, the largest of the arteries supplying the cranial dura and adjacent skull. Leading laterally from the foramen spinosum is a groove that marks the course of the middle meningeal artery. At a variable distance lateral to the foramen, this groove divides into two, to accommodate the frontal and parietal branches of the artery.

The upwardly bulging posteromedial walls of the middle cranial fossa are formed by the petrous parts of the temporal bones (*pars petrosa;* see Fig. 31-9). The anterior part or **petrous apex** (in front of the part containing the internal ear) usually presents, immediately above the foramen lacerum, a **trigeminal impression** that marks the position of the ganglion of the trigeminal nerve in the middle fossa.

Extending backward and laterally from the foramen lacerum, there usually is visible a slight groove that enters a foramen on the anterior surface of the petrous part. This groove is the **sulcus of the greater petrosal nerve,** and the foramen is the *hiatus of the canal of the greater petrosal nerve.* Anterolateral to the sulcus and usually ending in a small foramen just medial to the foramen spinosum, there may be visible a second groove, the **sulcus of the lesser petrosal nerve,** transmitting the nerve of that name. The tiny opening at the upper end of this groove is the *hiatus of the canal of the lesser petrosal nerve.* Both petrosal nerves arise in the temporal bone and make their exits through its anterior surface to appear inside the cranial cavity before they leave the skull. The most lateral part of the petrous part of the temporal bone on the anterior surface is the **tegmen tympani,** the roof of the middle ear cavity; the bone here is fairly thin. Anteromedial to the tegmen tympani is a protrusion of the bone, the **arcuate eminence,** that marks the position of the anterior semicircular canal of the internal ear.

The upper edge (superior margin) of the pars petrosa separates the middle cranial fossa from the posterior fossa; it may show a groove, the **sulcus for the superior petrosal sinus.**

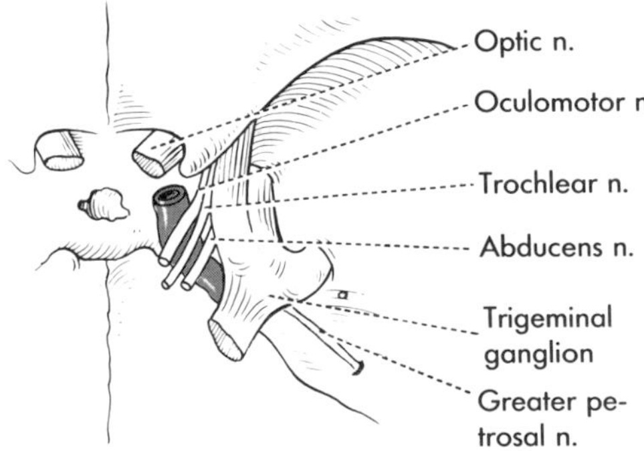

FIGURE *31-10.*
The trigeminal and other nerves in the middle cranial fossa.

Posterior Cranial Fossa. The anterior wall of the posterior cranial fossa is the dorsum sellae in the midline and the petrous parts of the temporal bones ("petrous ridges") laterally. The lateral parts of the fossa are, during life, roofed by the *tentorium cerebelli,* a layer of dura mater that is attached anterolaterally to the superior margins of the two petrous bones and posteriorly to the occipital bone. The tentorium presents a central notch extending backward from the two posterior clinoid processes. On the posterior surface of the petrous temporal is the opening of a canal, the **internal acoustic meatus,** that passes laterally into the bone. This opening is the *porus acusticus internus,* more often called the internal acoustic or auditory foramen. The seventh and eighth (facial and vestibulocochlear) nerves enter the internal acoustic meatus (Fig. 31-11).

Medial to, behind, and below the internal acoustic meatus, the temporal bone is separated from the occipital by the elongated **jugular foramen.** The deep, curved groove at the junction of temporal and occipital bones, extending downward and then medially and forward to the back end of this foramen, is the **sulcus for the sigmoid sinus.** This large venous sinus empties through the posterolateral part of the foramen into the upper end of the internal jugular vein. A variably developed projection, or *intrajugular process,* partially separates this part of the jugular foramen from the middle part, which transmits the vagus and accessory nerves (cranial nerves X and XI). The anteromedial part of the jugular foramen transmits the glossopharyngeal nerve (cranial nerve IX) and the inferior petrosal sinus.

On the posterior surface of the petrous part of the temporal bone, just lateral to and above the opening of the internal acoustic meatus, is a shallow depression, the *subarcuate fossa,* with one or two small vascular foramina opening into it. Below and lateral to that, extending almost to the groove for the sigmoid sinus, is a larger shallow depression that houses a flat sac (*endolymphatic sac*) from the internal ear. On the lower border of the bulge between these two depressions, at about the level of the internal meatus, but often hidden by the bulge or a projecting scale of bone, is a crevice that represents the **external aperture of the vestibular aqueduct.** This aqueduct trans-

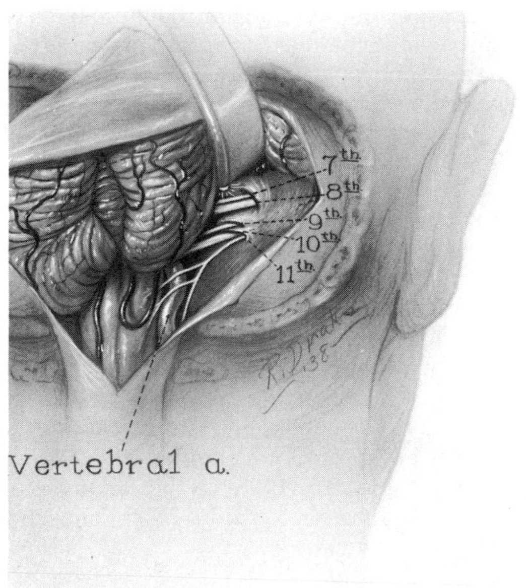

FIGURE *31-11.*
The 7th through the 11th nerves as they leave the posterior cranial fossa, with the cerebellum retracted. An enlarged vertebral artery here bulges laterally against them. (Craig WM. Am Heart J 1939; 17: 40.)

mits the endolymphatic duct that connects the endolymphatic sac to the internal ear.

In the anterior midline, the body of the sphenoid bone behind the dorsum sellae is fused to the basal portion of the occipital bone. This part of the floor of the posterior cranial fossa that slants downward and backward is the **clivus** (that is, the declining part). It is limited posteriorly by the foramen magnum and has already been seen in an external view. The *sulci for the inferior petrosal sinuses,* ending posteriorly at the jugular foramina, are along the sides of the clivus. Just medial to each jugular foramen, the occipital bone presents a rounded eminence called the **jugular tubercle.** Under cover of this tubercle, directed laterally and somewhat anteriorly, is the **hypoglossal canal** through which the hypoglossal nerve leaves the cranial cavity; The **condylar canal** opens posterolateral to the jugular tubercle into the floor of the last part of the groove for the sigmoid sinus, or into the posterior wall of the jugular foramen.

Behind and lateral to the foramen magnum, and posteromedial to the sigmoid sinuses, the floor of the posterior cranial fossa is concave where it accommodates the cerebellar hemispheres. The two concavities are separated from each other by a ridge placed in the sagittal plane. This ridge intersects a transverse ridge that bounds the posterior cranial fossa above, and the cross so formed is the **cruciform eminence.** The most prominent portion of the cruciform eminence is the **internal occipital protuberance.** It usually lies at about the level of the external occipital protuberance. The upper border of the transverse part of the cruciform eminence is the lower border of the **sulci for the transverse sinuses;** these two sulci lead laterally into the **sulci of the sigmoid sinuses,** for transverse and sigmoid sinuses are two parts of the same vascular channel. The tentorium cerebelli, the fold of dura covering the cerebellum and roofing the posterior fossa, is attached on both sides of the grooves for the transverse sinuses. The part of the skull above these sulci is occupied by the occipital lobes of the cerebral hemispheres of the brain.

Running downward on the inner surface of the occipital bone above the internal occipital protuberance, usually to the right of the midline and joining particularly the groove for the right transverse sinus, is the back end of the **sulcus for the superior sagittal sinus,** much of which is visible on the inner surface of the calvaria.

Summary of Foramina of the Skull

The foramina of the skull are so numerous that a summary of the important ones and the structures that they transmit should be useful. This summary is based on the description of the internal surface of the base of the skull. In reviewing it, it would be wise to note also the relations of the external openings.

In Anterior Fossa

The important openings into the anterior cranial fossa are those of the **cribriform plates.** The numerous foramina in each plate lead from the cranial cavity into the uppermost part of the nose, and most of them transmit filaments of the olfactory or first cranial nerve, the nerve of smell. On the sides of the cribriform plates are the openings of the two ethmoidal canals.

In Middle Fossa

The **optic canals,** situated in the most anterior part of the middle cranial fossa just anteromedial to the anterior clinoid processes, transmit two structures each. One is the optic or second cranial nerve, the nerve of sight, and the other, the ophthalmic branch of the internal carotid artery, which supplies structures within the orbit.

Lateral to the optic canal, situated lateral to the body of the sphenoid between that bone's greater and lesser wings, is the somewhat triangular gap of the **superior orbital fissure.** This, like the optic canal, leads into the back of the orbit. The structures traversing this fissure are the ophthalmic vein, the ophthalmic or first division of the trigeminal nerve, and all three nerves that supply muscles of the orbit: the oculomotor or third cranial nerve, the trochlear or fourth, and the abducens or sixth.

The **foramen rotundum,** in the floor of the middle cranial fossa behind the superior orbital fissure, opens into the upper posterior part of the pterygopalatine fossa. It transmits only one structure, the maxillary or second branch of the trigeminal nerve. Behind it is the **foramen ovale,** opening into the infratemporal fossa and transmitting the mandibular or third branch of the trigeminal nerve. A small artery, the accessory middle meningeal artery, may enter the skull by running retrogradely along the nerve. The ganglion of the trigeminal nerve, from which spring all three of its major branches, is located posteromedial to these three openings, lying against the anterior surface of the petrous portion of the temporal bone.

In the floor of the carotid groove, below the anterior end of the carotid canal in the petrous part of the temporal bone, can be seen the **foramen lacerum.** It should be obvious that the internal carotid artery, since it enters the middle fossa above the foramen, *does not* run through the foramen lacerum, which during life is almost completely filled by cartilage. (Sometimes the foramen lacerum is defined as including the upper border of the front end of the carotid canal, so the upper part of the foramen is then described as containing the internal carotid.) The groove for the greater petrosal nerve usually leads to the lateral part of the foramen lacerum. This nerve, together with a twig from the nerve plexus around the carotid artery, leaves the cranial cavity at the anterior lip of the foramen, where the posterior end of the pterygoid canal presents itself. The only structures actually passing through the foramen between the outside of the skull and the middle cranial fossa, or vice versa, are a meningeal twig of the ascending pharyngeal artery and some small veins and meningeal lymphatics.

Just posterolateral to the foramen ovale is the **foramen spinosum.** This transmits the middle meningeal artery and accompanying veins.

In Posterior Fossa

The largest foramen here is the **foramen magnum,** through which the brain and the spinal cord are continuous with each other. The two vertebral arteries ascend through this foramen to reach the brain; the venous channels of the cranial dura communicate through it with the vertebral venous plexuses around the spinal cord; and the spinal roots of the accessory nerves, which arise from the spinal cord, ascend through it.

Although all the cranial nerves except the first two are connected with those parts of the brain that lie in the posterior cranial fossa, the three to the muscles of the orbit (third, fourth, and sixth) run forward in the dura to the superior orbital fissure, and, therefore need no foramina for exit from the posterior fossa. Similarly, the fifth crosses the depression on the anterior part of the petrous apex, and the foramina for exit of its three branches have been noted in the description of the middle cranial fossa. Thus, the nerves that need foramina for leaving the posterior cranial fossa are the seventh through the 12th. The **internal acoustic meatus,** on the posterior surface of the petrous portion of the temporal bone, serves for the exit of both the seventh and eighth nerves (facial and vestibulocochlear). Both the vestibular (balance) and the cochlear (hearing) parts of the eighth nerve end in the internal ear, which is entirely enclosed within the temporal bone; therefore, they need no external openings. The facial nerve, however, leaves the temporal bone by turning downward to make its exit through the stylomastoid foramen. The seventh and eighth nerves are accompanied in the internal acoustic meatus by the labyrinthine artery, a branch to the internal ear from one of the arteries to the brain.

The **jugular foramen** transmits veins and nerves and usually also small meningeal branches of arteries. Anteriorly, the glossopharyngeal (ninth cranial) nerve leaves the skull, and the inferior petrosal sinus leaves to join the internal jugular vein; posteriorly, the sigmoid sinus leaves to form the internal jugular, and meningeal arteries enter; between these the 10th (vagus) and 11th (accessory) cranial nerves make their exits from the skull. Finally, the **hypoglossal canal,** under cover of the jugular tubercle, transmits the hypoglossal (12th cranial) nerve and opens externally just anterolateral to and above the occipital condyle.

These, then, are the particularly important foramina of the skull and the structures that they transmit. Other foramina, such as the condylar foramina and the mastoid foramina, can be grouped together as *emissary foramina.* They transmit connections between the venous sinuses inside the skull and the veins outside. These connections are known as emissary veins.

Development and Growth of the Skull

Development of the Skull as a Whole

The bones of the skull develop in part as cartilage bones, in part as membrane bones (see Chap. 5). Formation of cartilage begins during the second month at the base of the skull and is almost complete by the end of the third month of fetal life. In general, the **chondrocranium** (cartilaginous cranium) supports the brain and protects the internal ear and the nose. Cartilage surrounds the foramen magnum, giving rise to most of the occipital bone; it surrounds the internal ear on each side, giving rise to the petrous parts of the temporal bones; it extends forward below the brain, giving rise to most of the body, the lesser wing, and a small part of the greater wing of the sphenoid; and it surrounds the nasal cavities, giving rise to the ethmoid bone, the inferior nasal conchae, and a front part of the body of the sphenoid bone. Parts of the nasal chondrocranium persist as the nasal cartilages of the adult. The nasal bones and the maxillae develop in the membrane adjacent to the cartilaginous nasal capsule.

Besides these cartilages, those of the upper two **pharyngeal** or **branchial arches** also are connected with the skull (Fig. 31-12). The upper end of the first or mandibular branchial cartilage becomes enclosed in the developing middle ear cavity and gives rise to parts of two bones in this cavity (malleus and incus). The lower part does not give rise to the mandible, but disappears as membrane bone is formed around it. Similarly, the upper end of the hyoid or second cartilage, also presents itself in the middle ear cavity and subsequently forms the stapes. Another part fuses with the temporal bone to form the styloid process. The lower part of the hyoid cartilage unites with the third branchial cartilage to form the hyoid bone, and the part connecting the styloid process and hyoid bone typically is replaced by the stylohyoid ligament.

From this brief account, it should be clear that many of the bones of the skull are formed in part or entirely as membrane bones. Details of ossification are too complicated to be entered into at any length here, but in general the earliest centers of ossification both in

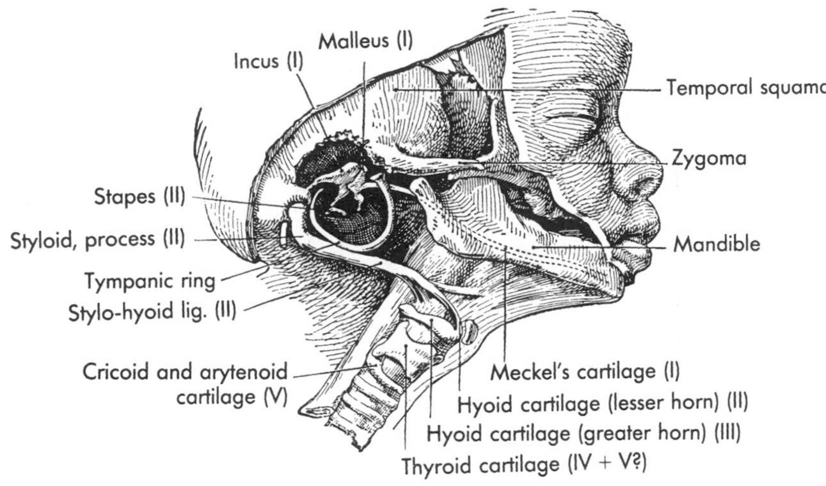

FIGURE *31-12.*
Skeletal derivatives of the branchial arches (identified by *Roman numerals*) as seen in a lateral dissection of the fetal head. (After Kollmann. Arey LB. Developmental anatomy, 6th ed. Philadelphia; WB Saunders, 1954)

cartilage bones (for example, the occipital) and in membrane ones (for example, the squama of the temporal) appear during the sixth and seventh weeks. Ossification is not complete at the time of birth; the bones forming the sides and roof of the skull still are united by membrane; and some of those of the base of the skull are united by cartilage (both of these permitting further growth of the skull).

The largest areas of membrane at birth are 1) at the junction of frontal and parietal bones and the sagittal

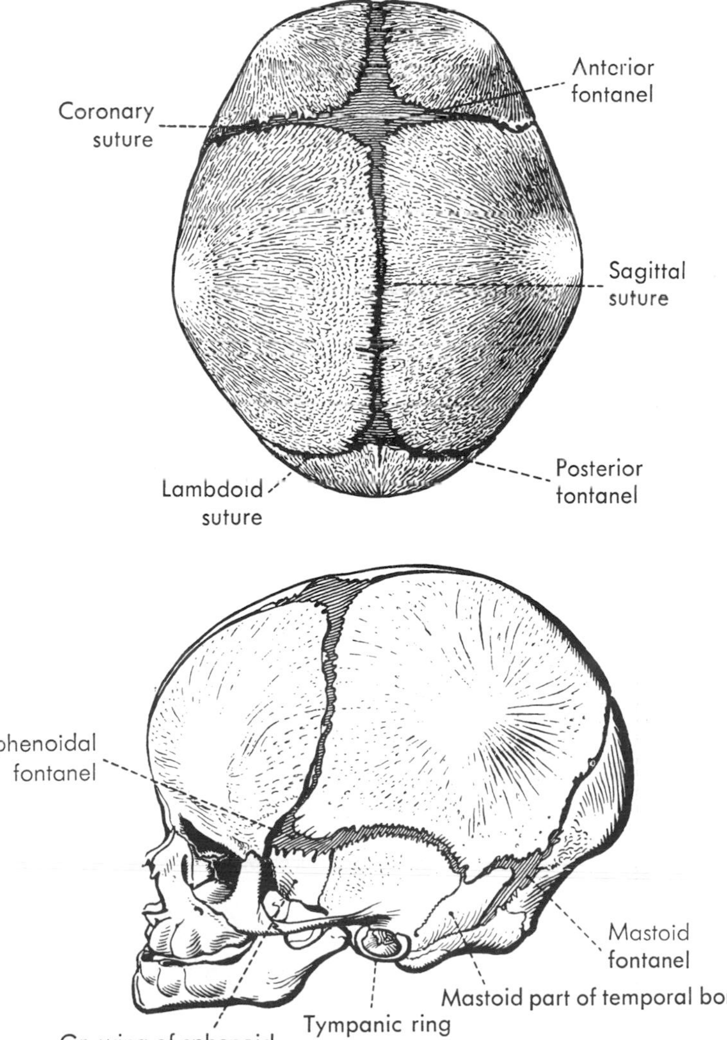

FIGURE *31-13.*
Superior and lateral views of the skull of a newborn, showing the sutures and fontanels. (Benninghoff A. Lehrbuch der Anatomie des Menschen, vol 1. Berlin. Urban & Schwarzenberg, 1949).

suture, this forming the **anterior fontanel** (fonticulus anterior; Fig. 31-13) 2) posteroinferiorly, between the parietal, temporal, and occipital bones, this forming the **mastoid fontanel** (fonticulus): 3) posteriorly, in the angle between the two parietal bones and the occipital one at the sagittal suture, this forming the **posterior fontanel;** and 4) laterally, in the angle between sphenoid, parietal, and frontal bones, this forming the **sphenoidal fontanel.** The mastoid and sphenoidal fontanels lie deep to muscle, but the anterior and posterior lie deep to only the scalp and constitute the "soft spots" of an infant's head. As the bones continue to grow in the membrane, they meet; the posterior fontanel closes approximately 2 months after birth, the sphenoidal and mastoid ones at approximately 3 months and 1 year, respectively, and the anterior one sometime during the second year.

Growth of the cranium is particularly rapid during the first year, and growth of the skull as a whole continues fairly rapidly to about the age of 7. Thereafter, the skull grows more slowly until the age of puberty, at which time growth again is accelerated. The rapid growth of the face is especially associated with a rapid enlargement of the paranasal sinuses. Until the bones of the skull begin to interlock, their growth occurs in the membrane separating them. Thereafter, growth probably is through absorption on the inner surface of the skull and addition to the outer surface. Although most of the cartilage of the skull is replaced by bone, cartilage persists in connection with the nasal cavity, as already noted, to form a part of the adult skeleton. Cartilage also persists between the sphenoid and the ethmoid bones and at the foramen lacerum between the occipital bone, the sphenoid, and the petrous portion of the temporal.

Development of Individual Bones

Following is a brief resumé of the development of the bones of the skull. The **occipital bone** ossifies in cartilage from five centers, one for the base of the bone, one each for the lateral (condylar) parts, and two (that quickly fuse) for the squama below the superior nuchal line. The part of the squama above the superior nuchal line develops in membrane from two centers that soon fuse with each other and subsequently with the lower part of the squama. At birth, there usually is some incomplete fusion laterally between upper and lower parts.

Each **parietal bone** is developed from two centers that appear in the membrane and spread to form a single continuous mass of bone. The **frontal bone,** originally paired, develops likewise in membrane. There is one chief center for each half of the bone, but secondary centers for smaller parts of it appear later. These centers fuse together several months before birth, but the frontal bone at birth is still paired, and fusion in the midline is not complete until the fifth or sixth year. Traces of the frontal or metopic suture may remain in the adult skull, especially in the region of the glabella.

The **temporal bone** has a particularly complicated developmental history, for, similar to the occipital bone, it is formed partly as a membrane bone and partly as a cartilage bone. The squama, including the zygomatic process, is a membrane bone and ossifies from a single center; the petrous portion of the temporal bone, including the mastoid process, is ossified about the internal ear from four centers that fuse together (but at birth, although most of the petrous part of the temporal bone is well formed, the mastoid process is a mere nubbin; it develops as an inferior projection at the time of puberty, when the mastoid air cells develop). The styloid process also develops in cartilage (of the hyoid arch) from two centers, one above the other; sometimes these fail to fuse. The tympanic part, like the squama developed in membrane, arises from a single center and at birth consists of a ring of bone (*annulus tympanicus,* or tympanic ring) incomplete above (see Fig. 31-12). After birth, the lower part of the ring expands medially, laterally, and downward to form the tympanic plate visible on the base of the skull.

The **sphenoid bone** also presents several centers of ossification, most of which are in cartilage and form the body, the lesser wing, and the pterygoid plates; most of the greater wings are formed in membrane. At least seven pairs of centers are described as contributing to the ossification of the sphenoid bone. At birth, this bone has three unfused parts; the middle one consists of the body, lesser wings, and medial pterygoid plates; the lateral ones consist of the greater wings and lateral pterygoid plates.

The **ethmoid bone** and the **inferior nasal conchae** ossify from the cartilage of the nasal capsule. Each inferior concha is ossified from a single center. Several centers contribute to the ethmoid, the ossification of which is not completed until after birth.

The remaining bones—the lacrimals, vomer, nasals, maxillae, palatines, zygomatics, and mandible—are ossified in membrane. Each **lacrimal bone** is ossified from a single center, the **vomer** is ossified from two centers, and each **nasal bone** is ossified from a single center. All these appear in membrane associated with the cartilaginous nasal capsule. The major part of each **maxilla** is ossified from a single center that spreads to form all the bone except that lying in front of the incisive fossa. In many animals, the latter part, bearing the incisor teeth, is a separate bone (the premaxilla) and, even in humans, develops as a separate one. Each premaxillary portion develops from at least two centers that usually fuse together. Traces of fusion between the premaxillary and maxillary portions, in the form of an indistinct suture that runs from the posterior border of the incisive fossa to the interval between the canine and lateral incisor teeth, are common in young adults. It is along this line that the cleft of unilateral cleft palate lies.

Each **palatine bone** is usually ossified from a single center, as is each **zygomatic bone;** apparently, either bone may sometimes have a second center: The **mandible** is ossified from paired centers of ossification, one for each half. It develops primarily in the membrane overlying the cartilage of the mandibular arch (**Meckel's cartilage**), but a small part of it is sometimes said to develop from this cartilage.

THE FACE AND SCALP

The subcutaneous connective tissue of the **face** blends with the deeper fascia surrounding the muscles, but the skin is particularly mobile because most of the muscles insert into it. Over the lips (labia), the external openings of the nose (nares), and the margins of the eyelids (palpebrae), the skin becomes continuous with the mucous membranes that line the oral and nasal cavities and (as the conjunctiva) the inner surfaces of the eyelids. The skin of the face varies considerably in thickness and is exceedingly thin in the eyelids; because of this, and the insertion of facial muscles into it, considerable care must be exercised in removing the skin if the underlying muscles are to remain relatively intact.

The **scalp** consists of three layers, firmly united (Fig. 31-14). The outer layer is the skin proper, normally provided with abundant hairs; the deepest layer is the strong **galea aponeurotica** (epicranial aponeurosis), a tendinous layer that covers the calvaria; and the intermediate or subcutaneous layer is composed of rather dense connective tissue that binds the skin to the galea and also contains an appreciable amount of fat. The nerves and blood vessels run in this intermediate layer, between the galea and the skin. The arteries of the scalp anastomose freely with each other both on the same side and across the midline, and they are so held by the dense connective tissue around them that they tend to remain open after they are cut; for both these reasons, bleeding from wounds of the scalp is particularly free.

In contrast to its firm attachment to the skin, the galea aponeurotica is separated from the **pericranium** (the periosteum on the outer side of the calvaria) by a layer of loose connective tissue that allows movement of the scalp over the skull.

The pericranium, not a part of the scalp, possesses little osteogenic capacity as compared with most periosteum. Except over the sutures, it is rather loosely attached to the bones of the calvaria.

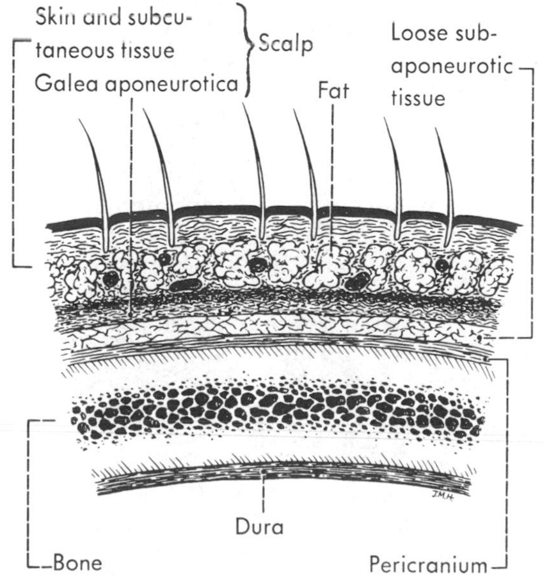

FIGURE *31-14.*
The layers of the scalp.

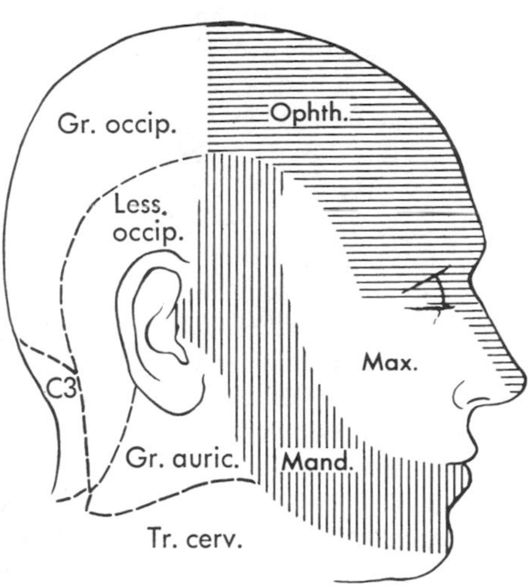

FIGURE *31-15.*
The distribution of cutaneous nerves to the face and scalp: The distributions of each of the three great divisions of the trigeminal nerve—the *ophthalmic, maxillary,* and *mandibular*—are shown as a whole rather than in terms of the distribution of their several named branches.

A few additional terms must be understood in studying the face. The upper and lower **lips** (labium superius, labium inferius) and the angle of the mouth (angulus oris) are easily understandable and need no comment. The depression in the center of the upper lip that extends down from the nose is the *philtrum.* The **nose** will be studied in some detail later; at the moment, it should be noted only that the *nares* (the anterior openings) are separated from each other by the midline *septum nasi* and that the flared part of the nose lateral to each naris is the *ala.* The tip of the nose is the *apex,* the *root* is the attachment of the nose to the forehead, and the *dorsum* is the free border between. Extending downward on each side from the ala toward the corner of the mouth is a groove, the *nasolabial sulcus.*

The **external ear** also will be studied more fully later. All that need be noted now is that the part of the external ear that projects from the side of the head is the *auricle,* that the dependent soft portion of the auricle (devoid of cartilage) is the *lobule,* and that the little part projecting backward over the external opening of the external acoustic meatus or auditory canal is the *tragus.*

Most of the names applied to the **regions** of the face are self-explanatory: the *nasal* and *oral regions* are those about the nose and mouth; the *mental region* is that of the chin; the *orbital and infraorbital* regions are about and below the orbits, respectively; the *buccal region* is that of the soft part of the cheek; the *zygomatic region* is that of the prominence of the cheek—of the zygomatic bone; and the *masseteric* and *parotid regions* are those of the ramus of the mandible (covered by the masseter muscle) and the parotid gland that lies between this ramus and the external ear. None of these regions is sharply defined.

The **innervation** of the skin of the face is largely through the three branches (ophthalmic, maxillary and mandibular) of the trigeminal nerve (Fig. 31-15), although some skin over the angle of the mandible and the back part of the ramus is supplied through ascending branches of cervical nerves. The cutaneous branches of the trigeminal nerve necessarily must pierce facial muscles or fascia to reach the skin, and because only their terminal twigs do so, they cannot be traced in the subcutaneous tissue; after the muscles of the face have been dissected, the nerves must be sought close to the bones of the skull in their regions of emergence. For the face, therefore, its innervation cannot be determined by dissection only; rather, this has been determined largely by clinical means. The branches of the facial nerve, which is the motor supply to all the facial muscles, also run deep to the muscles.

The cutaneous nerves of the scalp include some of those that supply the face, some branches of the cervical plexus (greater auricular and lesser occipital), and, posteriorly, posterior rami of upper cervical nerves that include the large greater occipital nerve. Most of them are closely associated with blood vessels.

Cutaneous vessels to the face, similar to cutaneous nerves, are tiny; the larger vessels run deep to the facial muscles. Therefore, if care is taken to remove only the skin and fascia from the outer surface of the superficial facial muscles and not to undercut the muscles, the nerves and vessels of the face can be left intact for study after the muscles have been studied. The vessels of the scalp are superficially placed, but the layer in which they are embedded is so tough that they are difficult to dissect. They are continuations of vessels, mostly branches of the external carotid, that supply the face or upper structures in the neck. It is the pulsating distention of the arteries of the scalp that accounts for most of the pain in migraine headache.

Facial Muscles

All the facial (mimetic) muscles are differentiated from a premuscle mass that originates from the hyoid arch, as do also the platysma muscle in the neck and a few deeper-lying muscles. They vary a good deal in development from one person to the next, and there may be some blending between muscles. Most of them are thin and flat and need little description other than a reference to their shapes and attachments. They are named primarily from their actions.

Damage to the facial nerve or its branches produces variable amounts of weakness or paralysis of facial muscles, sometimes called "Bell's palsy." Weakness is particularly noticeable about the mobile mouth, where it may be evidenced even in repose by a sagging corner and becomes obvious as a result of the asymmetry attending an attempt to show the teeth or to smile. Upper facial weakness can be similarly brought out by having a patient attempt to frown, raise his or her eyebrows, or close the eyes tightly. Paralysis of an entire side of the face is an indication that the facial nerve, as a whole, has been damaged, the level of injury being either in the brain, at the level of origin of the nerve, along the course of the nerve in the skull (for instance, as it runs through the temporal bone), or between its exit from the skull and its dispersion into diverging branches as it emerges from the parotid gland.

Weakness, rather than complete paralysis, of a group of muscles typically results from injury to facial nerve branches, because of the overlap in their distribution. A peculiarity of the voluntary control over the facial muscles is that only a lower, rather than a complete, unilateral facial paralysis results from the usual cerebral stroke that in general, paralyzes half the body; the part of the facial nucleus controlling the muscles of the forehead is bilaterally controlled from the cerebral cortex; therefore, these muscles are spared in a unilateral lesion above the level of the nerve's origin.

Muscles about the Mouth

Beginning below, on the mandible, there are several muscles that are attached to it and to skin of the chin or to skin and mucosa of the lower lip (Fig. 31-16). The somewhat triangular muscle arising close to the lower border of the mandible, at about the level of the corner of the mouth, is the **depressor anguli oris.** From a broad base, where it is partly blended with fibers of the platysma, it tapers as it proceeds toward the corner of the mouth to blend with other muscles here. Medial to it, and in part covered by it, is the **depressor labii inferioris** muscle. This somewhat quadrilateral muscle runs upward to blend with the muscle about the mouth (orbicularis oris) and insert also into the lower lip. It and the depressor anguli oris cover the mental foramen. The fibers of the depressor labii inferioris almost meet those of the opposite side as they reach their insertion, but the origins of the two muscles are some distance from the midline. Appearing between these, arising also from the mandible, but running downward to insert into the skin of the chin, are the two **mentalis** muscles, one on each side of the midline.

The muscle encircling the mouth and forming the muscular substance of the lips is the **orbicularis oris.** Some of the fibers of this rather complex muscle arise from the maxilla above the incisor teeth, but many of them are continuations from adjacent muscles, particularly from the buccinator (in the cheek), the depressor of the angle of the mouth, and the levator of the angle of the mouth. Some of the fibers of the upper and lower lips decussate at the angle of the lips. The muscle fibers insert into the skin and mucous membrane of the lips, particularly medially.

Extending medially, and usually somewhat upward to its insertion into the angle of the mouth, is the **risorius** (*risus* meaning "laughter" or "grin"), a rather straplike muscle that arises from the fascia over the parotid gland, but blends in its lower part with the platysma. Above the risorius, partly and covered by the fat pad that lies in the cheek, is the **buccinator** muscle (the bugler's muscle). This is the muscular part of the cheek. It arises in part from both the maxilla and the mandible, and posteriorly, deep to the mandible, it arises along the pterygomandibular raphe, a line that extends from the medial pterygoid plate to the mandible (see Fig. 34-3). The duct of the parotid gland pierces the buccinator to reach the oral cavity. As the muscle passes forward to the angle of the mouth, it is partly covered by the other muscles inserting here. Some of its fibers run into the upper lip and some into the lower

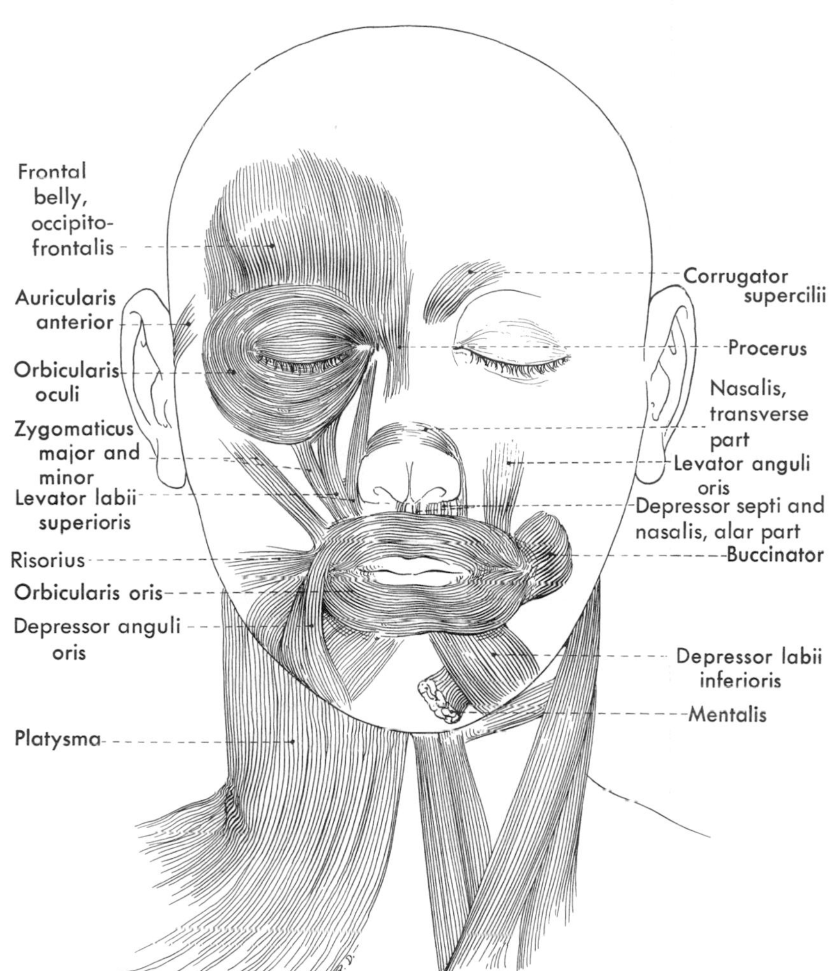

FIGURE *31-16.*
Muscles of the face, and the platysma muscle: The facial muscles shown on the *reader's left* are the more superficial ones; on the *right*, most of these have been removed to show the deeper-lying muscles. The medial muscle labeled *levator labii superioris* is the levator labii superioris alaeque nasi.

lip without crossing, becoming continuous here with the orbicularis oris. Others cross each other to reach the upper and lower lips, respectively.

Extending downward and forward toward the angle of the mouth from an origin on the zygomatic arch or the fascia over the upper part of the parotid gland is the **zygomaticus major.** This inserts into skin at the angle of the mouth and becomes, in part, continuous with the orbicularis oris. It pulls the angle of the mouth laterally and upward, as in a smile.

There are three muscles running downward into the upper lip, and a fourth, deeper-lying, related to the angle of the mouth. The **zygomaticus minor** arises from the zygomatic bone (where it is often continuous with the muscle around the eye, the orbicularis oculi) and runs downward and forward to insert into the upper lip; the **levator labii superioris** arises from the maxilla just above the infraorbital foramen and inserts into the upper lip; and the **levator labii superioris alaeque nasi** (levator of the upper lip and of the ala of the nose) arises from the frontal process of the maxilla alongside the nose and descends with a slightly lateral course. The labial part of the levator labii superioris alaeque nasi inserts into the skin of the lip, but a medial part inserts into the ala of the nose. The last of the muscles connected with the upper lip is the **levator anguli oris.** This arises from the maxilla below the infraorbital foramen and under cover of the three superficial muscles. It inserts partly into skin of the mouth and, in part, is continuous with fibers of the lower part of the orbicularis oris.

Nasal Muscles

The muscles connected with the nose are usually poorly developed. As already noted, a part of the levator labii superioris alaeque nasi inserts into the ala. Of the nasal muscles proper, the **depressor septi** is a somewhat quadrilateral muscle that arises from the maxilla under cover of the orbicularis oris and passes upward, in contact with its fellow at the midline, to insert into the lowest part of the septum of the nose. It draws the septum downward. Just lateral to it is the **nasalis,** also arising from the maxilla. One part of this muscle inserts into the lower margin of the ala of the nose, and another part crosses the dorsum of the nose to be united to its fellow of the opposite side by a tendon.

The **procerus,** a thin, bandlike muscle blended with the one on the other side, arises from the nasal bone and runs upward to insert into skin of the forehead. The two muscles pull the skin down, forming horizontal wrinkles between the eyebrows.

Muscles of the Eyelids, Ear, and Scalp

The large muscle of the eyelids is the **orbicularis oculi.** It surrounds the orbit and extends into both lids. Of the three parts of this muscle, one is placed deeply and can be seen only when the orbit is dissected. The parts visible in a superficial dissection are the *pars orbitalis* and the *pars palpebralis*; the latter, thinner and paler, is the portion in the lids. Both parts work together in closing the lids, but the orbital part is much heavier and, therefore, closes them more forcibly. These fibers arise at the medial side of the orbit, in part from a heavy ligament (*medial palpebral ligament*) that holds parts of the eyelids against the medial wall, and in part from the bone above and below this ligament. From these origins, the fibers originating above the medial palpebral ligament and those originating below it usually become continuous with each other around the lateral border of the orbit, with no obvious intersection; some of the fibers here may be continuous with the zygomaticus minor. The upper and lower palpebral fibers, in contrast, usually intersect in a more or less distinct line, the *lateral palpebral raphe*, at the lateral angle of the lids.

The other muscle of the lid, which raises it, is not really a facial muscle, but an orbital one, and is described with the orbit.

Originating deep to the upper part of the orbicularis oculi, from the frontal bone just above the nose, are two rather stout bundles of fibers that run laterally to insert into the skin of the eyebrows. These are the **corrugator supercilii** muscles. They draw the eyebrows together such that they produce vertical wrinkles in the forehead above the nose.

There are three extrinsic muscles of the ear: anterior, superior, and posterior (Fig. 31-17). They are variably developed. The **anterior auricular** muscle arises from the temporal fascia in front of and above the auricle and runs downward and backward to insert into it. The **superior auricular,** the best developed of the three, also arises from the temporal fascia above the ear and converges, such that it is fan-shaped, to insert into the upper medial side of the auricle. The **posterior auricular,** a small muscle, arises behind the ear from the mastoid process of the temporal bone and inserts into the medial side of the auricle, running approximately horizontally.

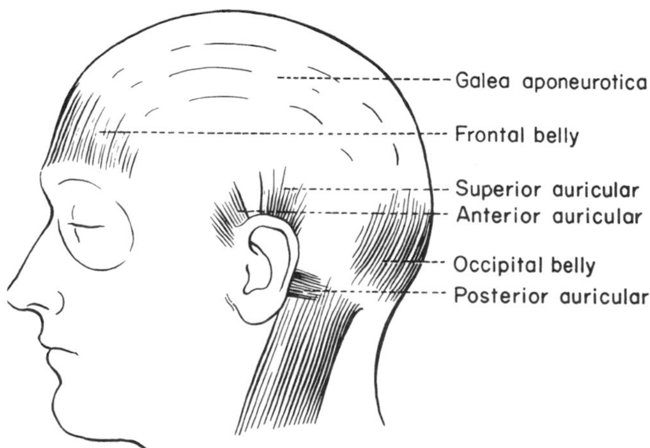

FIGURE *31-17.*
The occipitofrontalis and auricular muscles.

The paired muscles of the scalp are referred to as the **epicranius muscles.** Their parts insert into the tendinous galea aponeurotica that forms the deepest layer of the scalp and is separated from the calvaria by looser connective tissue so that the scalp, as a whole, is movable. The chief components of the epicranius muscles are the **occipitofrontalis** muscles, with frontal and occipital bellies. The frontal belly begins above the orbit where it is attached to the skin of the eyebrow (and can thus draw this upward to produce horizontal wrinkles in the forehead). It blends with the orbicularis oculi muscle, extending up through most of the height of the forehead to attach above into the galea aponeurotica. The two muscles together usually cover the entire forehead, meeting in the midline. The occipital belly is smaller, forming a flat band that arises from the lateral half or more of the superior nuchal line on the occipital bone. Its fibers run upward to end, as does the frontalis, in the galea. Alternating contraction of the occipitofrontalis bellies produces forward and backward movement of the scalp. It is the tense, involuntary, sustained contraction of the epicranius muscles that accounts for most of the pain of tension headache, probably the most common headache seen in clinical practice.

Parotid Gland and Facial Nerve

Parotid Gland

The parotid gland, largest of the three most important paired salivary glands (the others being the submandibular and the sublingual), is an outgrowth from the mouth. Its duct empties through the cheek, piercing the buccinator muscle. The gland itself is lodged partly superficial to and partly behind the ramus of the mandible and the masseter muscle that covers it (Figs. 31-18 and 31-19). The gland extends from about the inferior border of the mandible to the level of the zygomatic arch, but varies considerably in size and shape. Superficially, it overlaps a posterior part of the masseter muscle, and it largely fills the space between the ramus of the mandible and the anterior border of the sternocleidomastoid muscle. Deeply, it extends between the ramus of the mandible anteriorly and the sternocleidomastoid muscle, mastoid process, and external acoustic meatus posteriorly. Because of this relation, the deep part of the gland is compressed between the mandible and the posteriorly lying bone when the mouth is opened; hence, this movement may be painful when the gland is swollen by stored secretion and may be highly painful or impossible when it is greatly swollen, as in mumps.

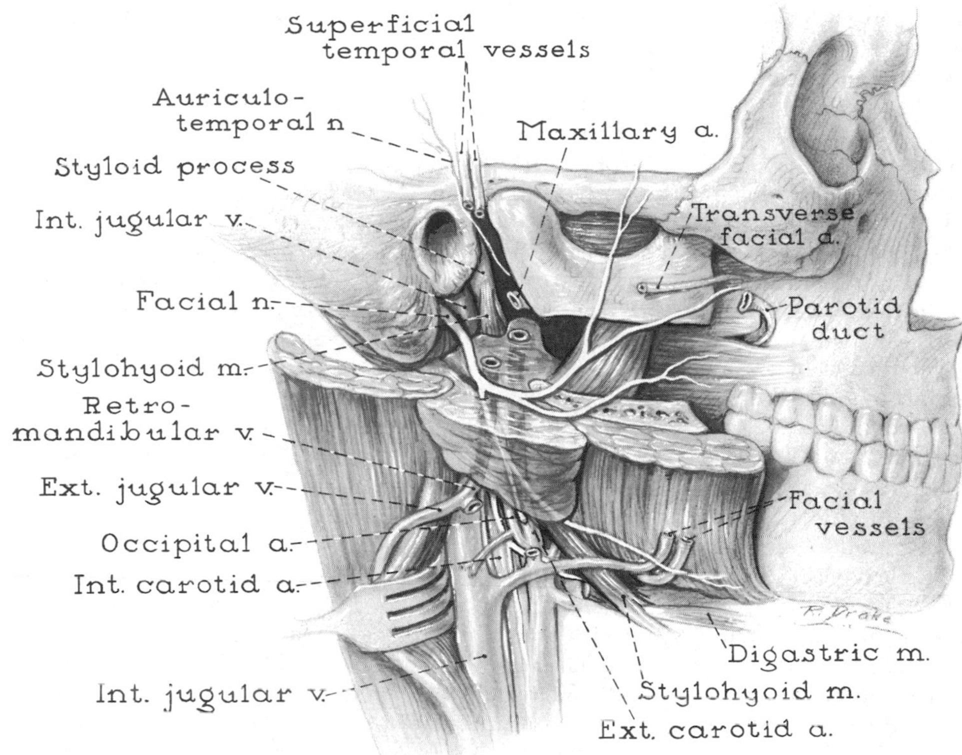

FIGURE 31-18.
Relations of the parotid gland: Upper parts of the sternocleidomastoid muscle, the parotid gland, and the mandible with the overlying masseter muscle have been removed to show deep relations of the gland and the courses of the facial nerve, external carotid artery, and retromandibular vein through it. (Beahrs OH, Adson MA. Am J Surg 1958; 95: 885.)

Several structures traverse or lie just deep to the parotid gland. Most important of these is the **facial nerve,** the branches of which emerge at the anterior, upper, and lower borders of the gland. The facial nerve enters the deep surface of the gland as a single stem, passing posterolateral to the styloid process as it does so. Within the substance of the gland, it may at first divide into two stems, or it may rebranch and anastomose to form a **parotid plexus.** Regardless of the presence or absence of a parotid plexus in the gland, the facial nerve usually leaves the shelter of the gland as five or more branches.

In its course through the parotid gland, the facial nerve runs superficial to those chief blood vessels that traverse the gland, but is interwoven with the glandular tissue and its ducts. Thus, removal of part or all of the parotid gland demands the most meticulous dissection if the nerve is to be spared.

At the upper pole of the gland, the **superficial temporal vein and artery** appear immediately in front of the ear. The vein runs deep to the upper pole of the gland and then through the deeper part of the gland, where it unites with the maxillary vein (which runs transversely medial

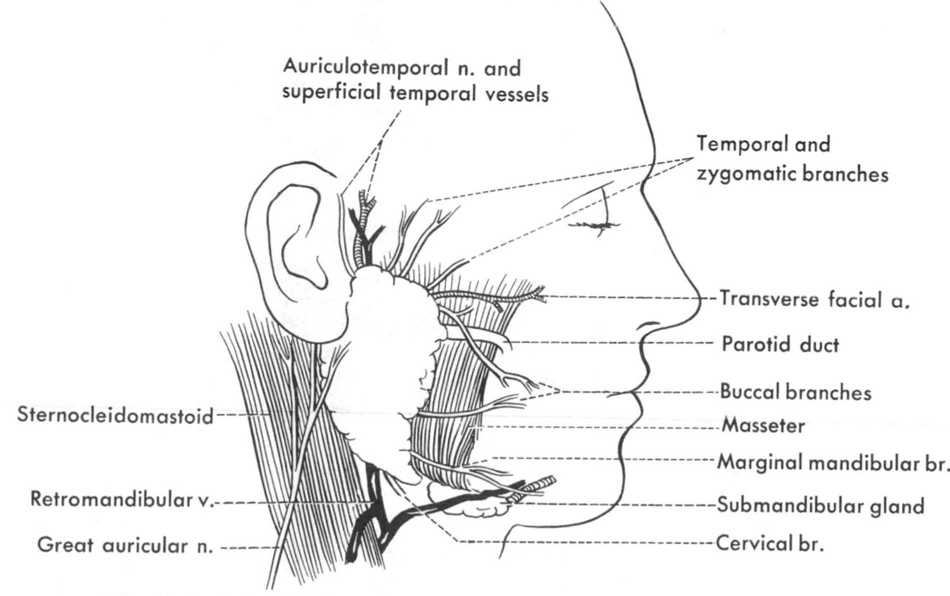

FIGURE 31-19.
Superficial relations of the parotid gland and the branches of the facial nerve on the face and in the neck.

to the mandible) to form the **retromandibular vein.** This descends through the substance of the gland and usually divides into two parts before or just after emerging at its lower pole. The posterior part joins the posterior auricular vein to form the external jugular, and the anterior part joins the facial vein and empties with it into the internal jugular. The retromandibular vein may be small, or it may empty exclusively into the external or internal jugular or the facial vein.

The upper end of the **external carotid artery** ascends deep to or through the deep part of the parotid gland, although it is separated from the lower part of the gland by the digastric muscle and other muscles attached to the hyoid bone. Above this level, the external carotid runs along the posterior aspect of the ramus of the mandible, deep to the retromandibular vein. It gives off twigs to the gland and, a little below the ear, divides into maxillary and superficial temporal branches. The maxillary artery passes almost horizontally forward deep to the mandible, and the superficial temporal artery ascends in a groove on the deep surface of the gland. One of its branches, the **transverse facial artery,** emerges from under cover of the gland and runs forward across the face a little below the zygomatic arch. Accompanying the superficial temporal vessels above the parotid gland is the **auriculotemporal nerve,** a branch of the mandibular.

The *posterior belly of the digastric muscle*, close to its origin, lies posterior to the parotid gland and as it runs downward comes to lie medial to the gland. Also, the *styloid process* lies just deep to the gland, the muscles originating from this process being fairly intimately related to it; the large *internal jugular vein* lies close to or against the deep part of the gland. Of these various structures, it is the facial nerve that is most likely to be injured in removing a part or all of the gland (as when tumors arise in its substance). The possibility of injury to the nerve usually is minimized by identifying the nerve before it enters the gland and following it or its branches forward through the gland, dissecting glandular tissue away from its superficial surface. However, it is often easier in the cadaver to trace branches of the facial nerve as they emerge from the parotid gland back into the substance of the gland to their union with other branches.

The **duct of the parotid gland** is formed within the glandular substance and emerges at its anterior border. It runs almost horizontally forward across the superficial surface of the masseter muscle, at about the level of the tip of the lobule of the ear (therefore, below the transverse facial artery). At the anterior border of the masseter, it turns deeply to penetrate the buccinator muscle and open on the inside of the cheek at about the level of the crown of the second molar tooth of the upper jaw. Sometimes the part of the duct closest to the gland has along its upper border a bit of glandular tissue known as the **accessory parotid gland.**

Sensory twigs from the great auricular and the auriculotemporal nerves end in the parotid gland. The auriculotemporal branches also contain secretory fibers to the gland, derived from the otic ganglion through that ganglion's *communicating branch* with the auriculotemporal.

Facial Nerve

Before the facial nerve enters the parotid gland, it gives off several branches, and in the gland it gives rise to five named branches or sets of branches that appear on the face: temporal, zygomatic, buccal, marginal mandibular, and cervical (see Fig. 31-19). These are named according to their general course and distribution. They all are distributed to voluntary muscle and consist largely of motor fibers. They do contain sensory fibers, however, which have been considered as proprioceptive to the muscles of the face (just as the motor fibers are motor to these muscles) or as being concerned with pain. Although there is no evidence that the facial nerve is concerned with cutaneous pain, many authors have attributed deep pain from the face to conduction by the facial nerve.

Of the branches of the facial nerve, the temporal, zygomatic, and buccal branches often are double or triple as they leave the parotid gland, or divide soon thereafter; the marginal mandibular branch and the cervical branch (ramus colli) usually are single, although sometimes the former is double. As these diverging branches are traced farther distally, they subdivide further and there may be communicating loops between similarly named branches or adjacent, differently named branches; thus, the pattern of the facial nerve on the face is variable.

In general, the **temporal branches** supply the frontal belly of the occipitofrontal muscle, the corrugator supercilii, the orbicularis oculi, and the anterior and superior auricular muscles; a temporal branch to the auricular muscles may join the auriculotemporal branch of the mandibular nerve and be distributed with that. The **zygomatic branches,** similarly, typically help supply the orbicularis oculi and supply all the muscles connected with the upper lip and the external aperture of the nose, as well as a part of the buccinator muscle; some of these branches anastomose with the cutaneous branches of the infraorbital nerve (maxillary division of the trigeminal) as this emerges from the infraorbital foramen.

Buccal branches of the nerve, at first, may run with zygomatic ones and then diverge downward toward the angle of the mouth, or they may come off the lower part of the facial nerve and run approximately horizontally across the masseter toward the angle. They supply the muscles converging on the angle of the mouth, including the buccinator and the levators of the upper lip and angle of the mouth that are also innervated by zygomatic branches, and the depressors of the lower lip and angle of the mouth that are also innervated by the marginal mandibular branch. They anastomose with the buccal branch of the mandibular nerve that supplies skin and mucous membrane of the cheek. The **marginal mandibular branch** passes across the masseter and the external surface of the mandible close to the lower border of the mandible; hence, its name. Occasionally, it may run lower, across the superficial surface of the submandibular gland. Similar to the other branches of the facial nerve, it runs deep to most of the superficial facial muscles, and it is also deep to the platysma muscle. However, it typically crosses superficial to the facial vein and artery, being most easily identified by the surgeon as it crosses the vein. It supplies muscles connected with the lower lip and those that run upward to the corner of the mouth. The marginal mandibular branch anastomoses with the mental nerve (a branch of the trigeminal) as this emerges to go to skin of the chin. Finally, the **cervical branch** of the facial nerve leaves the parotid gland close to its lower end and runs downward and then forward, just behind and below the angle of the mandible, to enter the deep surface of the platysma muscle, which it supplies. It usually anastomoses with the transversus colli (transverse cervical) nerve, the cutaneous nerve of this region.

Vessels

The arteries of the face and scalp, except the forehead, are branches of the external carotid. The veins drain into the jugular system.

Facial Vessels

The chief artery of the face is the **facial artery.** This appears at the lower border of the mandible between that bone and the submandibular gland, just in front of the masseter muscle, for after its origin from the external carotid, it at first lies deep to some of the suprahyoid muscles. However, the **facial vein,** which lies immediately behind the artery at the lower border of the mandible, has a different course below that; it passes downward over the superficial surface of the submandibular gland to enter the internal jugular, usually being joined before it does so by that part of the retromandibular vein that does not go to the external jugular and, variably, by pharyngeal, lingual, and superior thyroid veins. Where the facial artery and vein lie against the submandibular gland, they are connected to it by small twigs. The artery gives off a **submental artery** that runs forward beneath the chin, and the vein receives a corresponding tributary.

At the lower border of the mandible, the facial vessels lie deep to the platysma muscle and, at about the same level, are crossed superficially by the marginal mandibular branch of the facial nerve. Above this, they lie deep to most of the facial muscles along their course and deep to the branches of the facial nerve that supply these muscles. The facial artery may be tortuous or fairly straight, but in any event, the course of the facial vessels is an oblique one past the corner of the mouth and along the side of the nose to the angle between the eye and the nose (Fig. 31-20).

Before the artery reaches the corner of the lip, it gives off an **inferior labial artery** that runs medially in the lower lip and anastomoses with its fellow of the opposite side; this artery may be double. It next gives off the **superior labial artery** to the upper lip. Thereafter, it runs along the side of the nose toward the medial angle of the eye, as the **angular artery.** Instead of ending by breaking up into small branches, the angular artery may anastomose with a terminal branch of the ophthalmic artery (the dorsalis nasi) that leaves the orbit and runs downward to supply the nose. Sometimes, also, the angular artery is very poorly developed or is absent. The **angular vein,** the up-

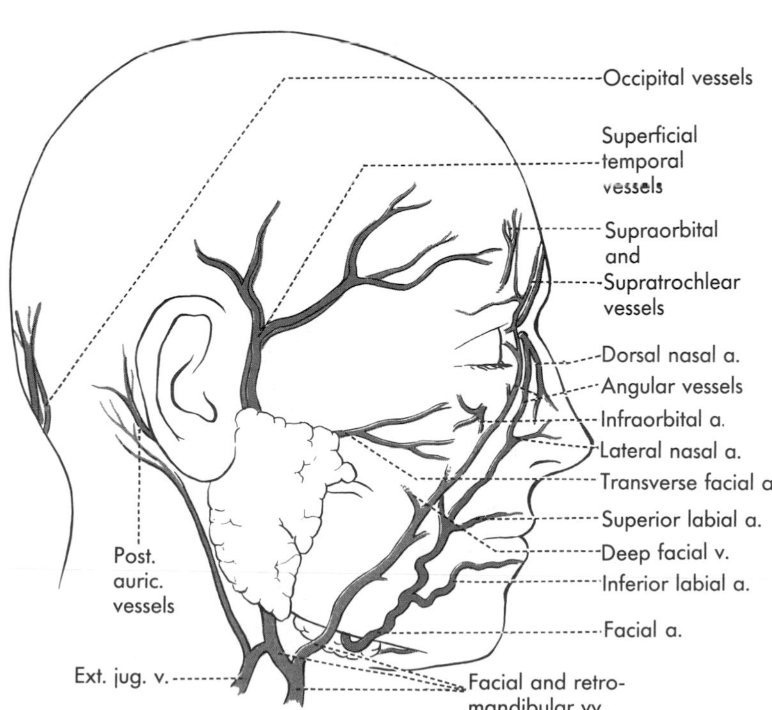

FIGURE 31-20.
Blood vessels of the face and scalp.

per end of the **facial vein,** lies immediately adjacent to the angular artery. It often has no obvious beginning, however, for when traced upward, it is usually continuous with veins of the forehead, usually sends a connection through the upper lid to enter the orbit and join the ophthalmic vein there, and may also send a communication through the lower lid.

Because the veins in the orbit drain blood into intracranial venous sinuses, the angular vein, when well developed, is one of the important extracranial veins having anastomotic connections with the intracranial venous system. As it lies beside the nose, the angular vein receives small veins from the nose and from both eyelids; as the facial vein descends past the mouth, it receives superior and inferior labial veins. In addition to tributaries corresponding to the branches of the artery, the facial vein also receives, as it lies on the buccinator muscle, the **deep facial vein.** This emerges from deep to the ramus of the mandible and its covering muscles in company with a small artery and nerve (buccal artery and buccal branch of the mandibular nerve). Above this, it also may receive the front end of the infraorbital vein as this emerges from the infraorbital foramen.

Through the deep facial vein and veins in the orbit, and also often through the infraorbital vein, the facial vein is connected to the cavernous sinus within the cranial cavity (Fig. 31-21). Because none of these veins is provided with valves, blood from the face either may drain down through the facial vein or, when conditions of pressure are different, may run through the connections of this vein to the cavernous sinus. If infectious material from the face is carried along the latter course, thrombosis of the cavernous sinus and ensuing meningitis are likely to occur; serious neurologic damage or even death may result. Infection and thrombosis of the cavernous sinus commonly are initiated by squeezing pustules around the upper lip or side of the nose and even by careful surgical opening of such pustules; thus, this region is often known as the "danger area" of the face.

Branches of the Ophthalmic Artery

In addition to the facial vessels, branches of the ophthalmic vessels (the vessels within the orbit) also appear close to the medial angle of the eye, where they pierce the upper lid. The **dorsalis nasi** artery emerges through the upper lid and runs downward on the side of the nose to supply that, often anastomosing with the upper end of the angular artery. Another branch of the ophthalmic, the **supratrochlear artery,** appears just above or with the dorsal nasal branch, to turn upward on the forehead. Here, it runs close to the midline, in company with the supratrochlear vein and a correspondingly named nerve (a branch of the ophthalmic division of the trigeminal). Lateral to the supratrochlear vessels and nerve are the **supraorbital vessels** and nerve. They round the upper border of the orbit by passing through the supraorbital foramen or notch. The nerve is the largest cutaneous branch of the ophthalmic division of the trigeminal nerve. Both supratrochlear and supraorbital vessels and nerves round the upper rim of the orbit immediately against the bone, under cover of the orbicularis oculi and frontalis muscles. They then enter the scalp to lie in its tough subcutaneous or middle layer. Here the vessels anastomose freely with the other vessels supplying the scalp.

The other branches of the ophthalmic artery to appear on the face are small **palpebral arteries** that supply the eyelids and are described with these parts.

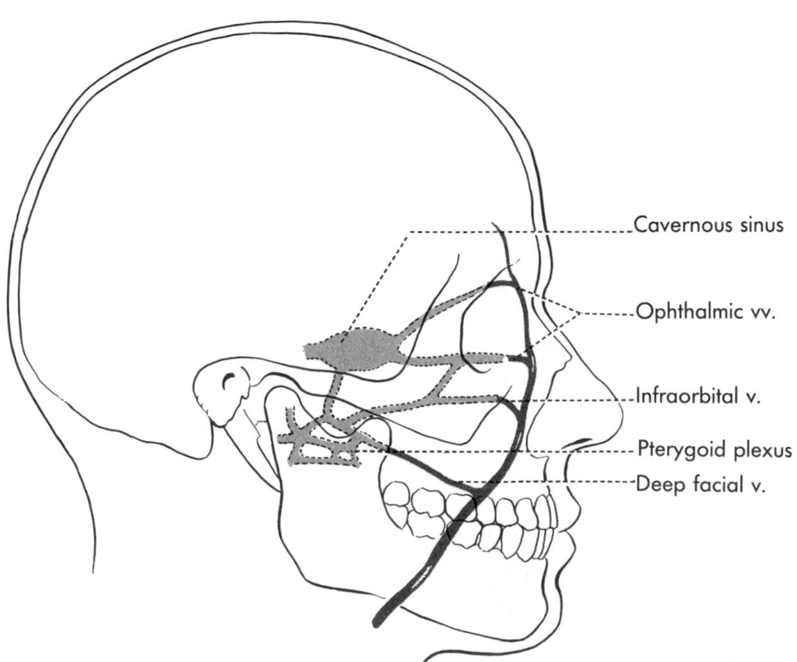

FIGURE *31-21.*
Chief connections of the facial vein to the cavernous sinus.

Other Blood Vessels

The remaining arteries, all branches of the external carotid, chiefly supply the scalp, although the superficial temporal also helps to supply the face. The **superficial temporal vessels** appear above the parotid gland as they cross the zygomatic arch. Each soon divides into a *frontal* and a *parietal branch.* Both branches enter the dense connective tissue of the scalp, where they anastomose with each other, with vessels of the opposite side, and with the supraorbital and other vessels that supply the scalp. The auriculotemporal nerve runs with the superficial temporal vessels as they lie in front of the ear. Before dividing into its terminal branches, the superficial temporal artery gives off small *anterior auricular* and *parotid branches,* the *transverse facial,* a *zygomaticoorbital artery,* and, usually just below the level of the zygomatic arch, a *middle temporal branch.* The zygomaticoorbital artery, which may arise from the middle temporal, runs forward toward the orbit along the upper border of the zygomatic arch enclosed in the temporal fascia. The middle temporal crosses the arch deep to the superficial temporal and then pierces the temporal fascia to reach the deep surface of the temporal muscle.

The tributaries of the **superficial temporal vein** accompany the branches of the artery. The vein ends by joining the maxillary vein, thus forming the retromandibular vein.

The small **posterior auricular artery** arises from the posterior aspect of the external carotid at about the point at which that artery emerges from deep to the posterior belly of the digastric, or sometimes it arises from the occipital artery. It runs upward and backward behind the ear to help supply the external ear and scalp behind the ear. It also gives off *stylomastoid* and *posterior tympanic arteries,* which contribute to the supply of the temporal bone and the middle ear cavity. The **posterior auricular vein,** usually much larger than the artery, leaves the artery at the upper border of the sternocleidomastoid muscle and runs superficial to this muscle to join the external jugular vein.

The **occipital artery** emerges from under cover of the sternocleidomastoid to cross the uppermost part of the posterior triangle of the neck and turn upward, piercing the deep fascia and usually the trapezius muscle, into the scalp. Here it is accompanied by the greater occipital nerve and the occipital vein, and it anastomoses with the posterior auricular and superficial temporal arteries. Just before it turns upward, it gives off a descending branch that anastomoses with the transverse cervical, deep cervical, and vertebral arteries. The **occipital vein** accompanies the artery only on the scalp. Where the artery turns upward, the vein ends in the suboccipital venous plexus, drained by the deep cervical and vertebral veins, but it may communicate with the posterior auricular vein and help form the external jugular.

Lymphatics

The lymphatics of the face and scalp are fairly simple (Fig. 31-22). Those from the anterior part of the face accompany the facial blood vessels or, for the lower lip, drain directly downward. A few tiny lymph nodes (*buccal* and *mandibular*) occur along the facial vessels, but most of the anterior lymphatics drain into nodes associated with the **submandibular gland,** into **submental nodes,** or, beyond these, into upper nodes of the **deep cervical set.** Lymphatics from more laterally on the face, including parts of

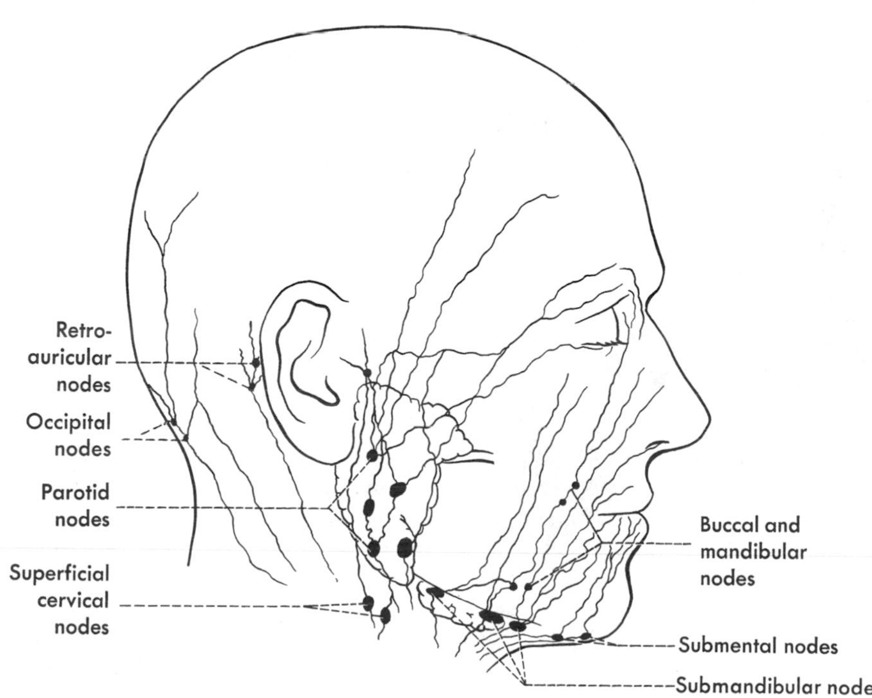

FIGURE *31-22.* Lymphatics of the face and scalp.

the eyelids, drain diagonally downward and posteriorly toward the parotid gland, as do the lymphatics from the frontal region of the scalp. Associated with this gland, some lying superficially and some more deeply, are **parotid nodes.** These, in turn, drain downward along the retromandibular vein to empty in part into the superficial lymphatics and nodes along the outer surface of the sternocleidomastoid muscle and in part into upper nodes of the deep cervical chain. Lymphatics from the parietal region of the scalp drain, in part, into the parotid nodes in front of the ear and in part into **retroauricular nodes** in the back of the ear that, in turn, drain into upper deep cervical nodes. The largest retroauricular node frequently is palpable as it lies over the mastoid process, especially in children. Lymphatics from the occipital region end, in part, in **occipital nodes** (which, in turn, drain into upper deep cervical ones) and, in part, directly in upper deep cervical nodes.

Cutaneous Nerves

The face and scalp are supplied largely by the trigeminal nerve and the upper cervical nerves (Fig. 31-23). The chief exception to this is a bit of skin behind the ear that is supplied mostly by a small twig from the vagus (tenth cranial) nerve.

Trigeminal Distribution

The larger cutaneous nerves of the face already have been noted, for they anastomose with branches of the facial nerve, and those on the forehead accompany the arteries.

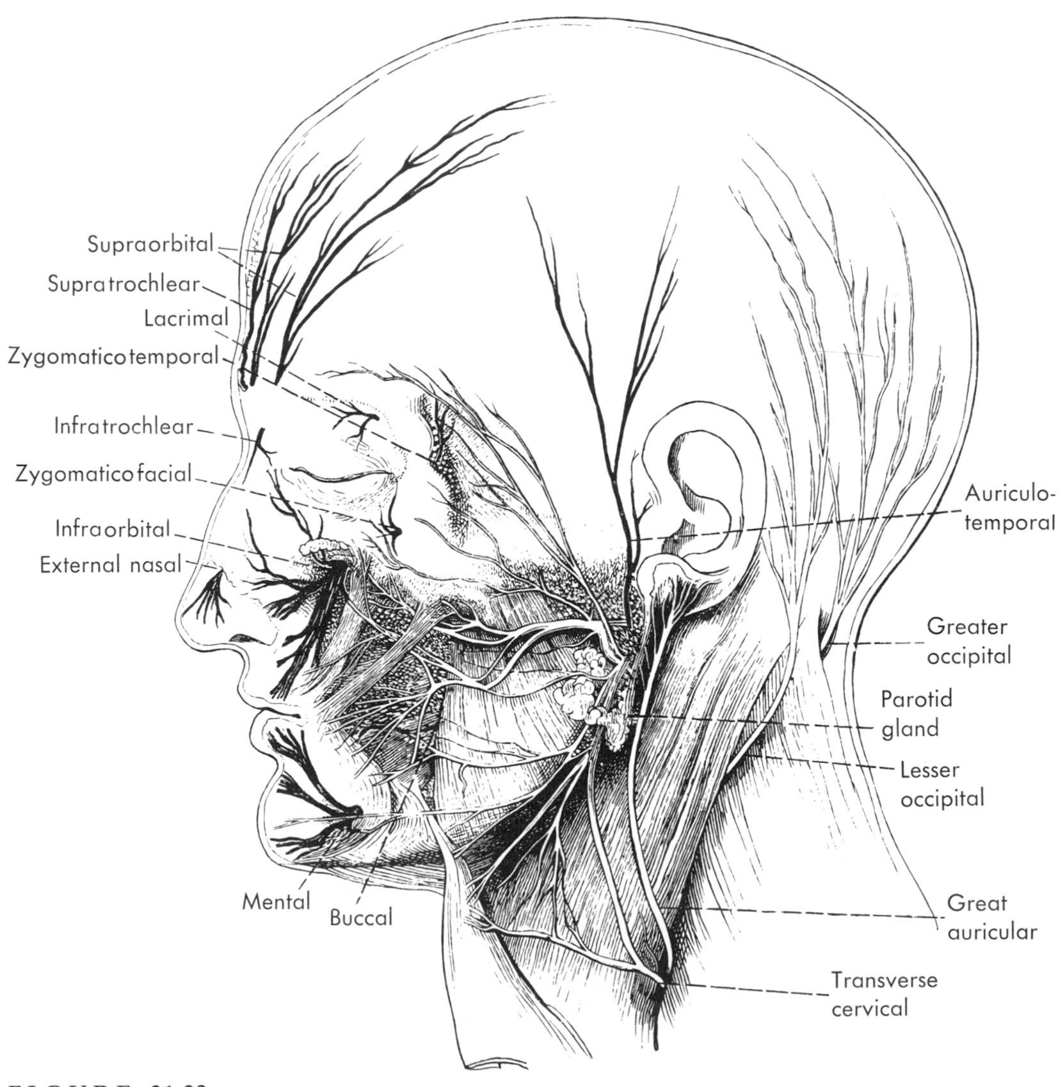

FIGURE *31-23.*
The cutaneous branches of the trigeminal nerve, *black*: Shown in *outline* are upper branches of the cervical plexus and branches of the facial nerve. The parotid gland has been partly removed. (Henle J. Handbuch der systematischen Anatomie des Menschen, vol 3, pt 2. Braunschweig: Vieweg und Sohn, 1868.)

The trigeminal or fifth cranial nerve provides the sensory supply to the skin of most of the face, except for much of the ear, some skin immediately in front of this, and that over the angle of the jaw, which are innervated by fibers from upper cervical nerves.

All three divisions of the trigeminal nerve supply the face. In general, the **ophthalmic** or upper division supplies the upper eyelid, the entire dorsum, and the upper parts of the sides of the nose the forehead, and the scalp about as far back as the interauricular line (see Fig. 31-15). The **maxillary** or second division supplies the lower eyelid, the side of the lower part of the nose, the skin on and above the prominence of the cheek, and that of the upper lip. The **mandibular** nerve supplies an anterior part of the lateral surface of the external ear, as well as much of the skin of the external acoustic canal and the eardrum or tympanic membrane; skin extending up in front of the ear onto the scalp; the skin of the cheek lateral to the lips; and the lower lip and chin. Each division of the trigeminal nerve is represented on the face by several branches, and most of these branches appear on the face by running close against the skull or emerging from foramina in the skull. Therefore, they are deep-lying branches and are most easily found in their deep positions. Traced superficially, they anastomose with branches of the facial nerve and penetrate the overlying facial muscles; therefore they cannot really be traced accurately to their distribution.

Five **branches of the ophthalmic nerve** reach the skin of the face. The largest of these is the **supraorbital nerve,** running through the supraorbital foramen or notch and turning up on the forehead, where it usually divides into a medial and a lateral branch and is distributed to the forehead and to the scalp about as far back as the interauricular line. Medial to it is the smaller **supratrochlear nerve,** distributed to a medial part of the skin of the forehead. Each of these accompanies the similarly named blood vessels. Also leaving the orbit close to the medial angle of the eye, but lying below the supratrochlear nerve and, therefore, not against the upper bony rim of the orbit, is the **infratrochlear nerve.** This gives off twigs to the lateral side of the nose and to the upper eyelid. About halfway down the dorsum of the nose there emerges from between the nasal bone and the nasal cartilage a small branch of the ophthalmic, the **external nasal branch of the anterior ethmoidal nerve,** that then runs subcutaneously down the nose to the tip, supplying the distal part of the dorsum. The fifth cutaneous branch of the ophthalmic is a twig that is difficult, or often impossible, to find by dissection; it is the **lacrimal nerve,** which pierces the lateral part of the upper eyelid and is distributed to this lid and the immediately adjacent skin.

Three **branches of the maxillary nerve** reach the skin of the face. The **infraorbital,** the largest, emerges from the infraorbital foramen with a small artery and vein. It anastomoses with zygomatic branches of the facial nerve and spreads out toward skin of the ala of the nose, the upper lip, and the lower eyelid. A small branch, the **zygomaticofacial,** emerges from the zygomatic bone on the anterior surface of the prominence of the cheek and supplies skin here and on up toward the lateral angle of the eye. The third cutaneous branch, the **zygomaticotemporal,** emerges from the skull through the anterior wall of the temporal fossa, but then penetrates the temporal fascia anterior to the temporal muscle to supply skin of the anterior part of the temple just lateral to the eye.

There also are three cutaneous **branches of the mandibular nerve.** The largest of these is the mental, a continuation of the nerve (inferior alveolar) that supplies the teeth of the lower jaw. The **mental nerve** emerges from the mental foramen, anastomoses with the facial nerve, and distributes branches to the chin and lower lip. The second cutaneous branch is the **buccal nerve.** This small nerve emerges from deep to the ramus of the mandible and appears on the external surface of the buccinator muscle, where it anastomoses with buccal branches of the facial nerve. It sends branches through the buccinator muscle to supply the mucous membrane on the inside of the cheek, and its superficial branches supply the skin of the outer surface. The third cutaneous branch is the **auriculotemporal.** This emerges from deep to the upper end of the parotid gland and crosses the back end of the zygomatic arch immediately in front of the ear in company with the superficial temporal vessels. As the nerve passes behind the temporomandibular joint, it gives a twig to this; as it passes the external acoustic meatus, it gives off a nerve to the meatus that supplies most of this and most of the tympanic membrane; it gives twigs to the parotid gland; and it supplies a small anterior part of the upper lateral surface of the ear before continuing to the skin and scalp of the posterior part of the temporal region. The auriculotemporal nerve often receives the facial nerve fibers to the anterior and superior auricular muscles.

That small part of the skin of the face that is not supplied by the trigeminal nerve—some of that over the angle of the jaw and extending up to include much of the skin of the external ear—is supplied from the cervical plexus through the **transverse cervical** (transversus colli) and **great auricular nerves** (see Fig. 31-15). Skin of the upper part of the posterior or medial surface of the ear and skin and scalp just behind the ear are supplied largely by the **lesser occipital nerve** from the cervical plexus. Finally, the scalp posterior to the interauricular line, and behind the distributions of right and left auriculotemporal and lesser occipital nerves, is supplied by dorsal branches of cervical nerves. The **greater occipital nerve,** primarily the cutaneous branch of the posterior ramus of C-2, runs with the occipital artery and reaches the posterior distribution of the supraorbital branch of the ophthalmic. A branch from the posterior ramus of C-3, the **third occipital nerve,** may run upward to supply scalp close to the midline about as high as the external occipital protuberance.

THE MOUTH AND JAWS

Oral Cavity

The mouth or oral cavity (Fig. 31-24) is bounded externally by the cheeks (*buccae*) and the lips (*labia*), above by

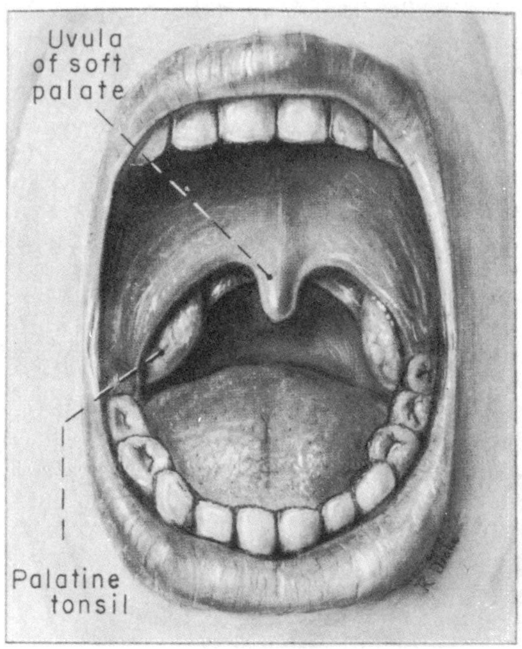

FIGURE 31-24.
The oral cavity, soft palate, and palatine tonsils. The palatoglossal arch partly hides the tonsil; the palatopharyngeal arch, visible above, is hidden by the tonsil below.

the palate, and below by mucous membrane that connects the floor of the mouth to the tongue. The major part of the tongue projects into the oral cavity, as do the teeth. The **rima oris** is the opening between the lips, and the cavity is divided into two parts: the **vestibule,** the part lying between the cheeks and lips on the one hand and the teeth and gums on the other, and the **oral cavity proper,** that part within the arches of the teeth. In the vestibule, a small midline fold, the **frenulum,** can be seen connecting the upper lip to the gum; there usually is a similar frenulum of the lower lip. Except at the frenula, the transition between the mucosa of the lips and cheek and that of the gums is generally smooth.

The parotid gland, the largest of the salivary glands, opens through the substance of the cheek, its point of opening being indicated by a **parotid papilla** that is situated at about the level of the upper second molar (next to last or last) tooth. The parotid papilla, as are most of the other features of the soft tissues of the mouth, is best seen in the living individual. Adequate examination of the mouth of the cadaver is difficult.

Numerous small glands also open into the vestibule. Sebaceous glands of the lips are especially concentrated at approximately the mucocutaneous junction. They are superficial and often appear as a series of small yellowish bodies close to the free borders of the lips. Fewer sebaceous glands occur in the cheeks close to the teeth.

Mixed or seromucous labial glands are closely packed in the submucosa of the lips, where they can be palpated easily. Buccal glands are less numerous; most lie in the submucosa of the cheek, but in the region of the molar teeth a few usually lie on the outer surface of the buccinator muscle and are called molar glands.

The muscles, nerves, and vessels of the lips and cheek have been described with the face.

Within the oral cavity proper there is a **frenulum** on the lower surface of the tongue (*lingua*) in the anterior midline. On each side of this frenulum is a projection of the mucous membrane, the **sublingual caruncle** (papilla), that contains the termination of the duct of the submandibular salivary gland as this opens into the mouth. Running backward from the caruncle, there may be in the floor of the mouth a bulge, the **sublingual fold,** produced by the sublingual salivary gland that lies immediately below the mucosa here. Small sublingual ducts open through the mucosa in this position, and a sublingual duct usually joins the submandibular duct to open on the sublingual caruncle.

The roof of the mouth is largely formed by the hard palate, which consists of the bony palate and the mucosa and glands associated with this. The smaller posterior part of the roof is formed by the soft palate, which also projects downward to separate the oral cavity partially from the nasal part of the pharynx. The palate and the tonsillar region, where the oral cavity opens into the pharynx, are described in Chapter 34. The margins of the hard palate are continuous with the alveolar processes of the maxillae, which bear the upper teeth.

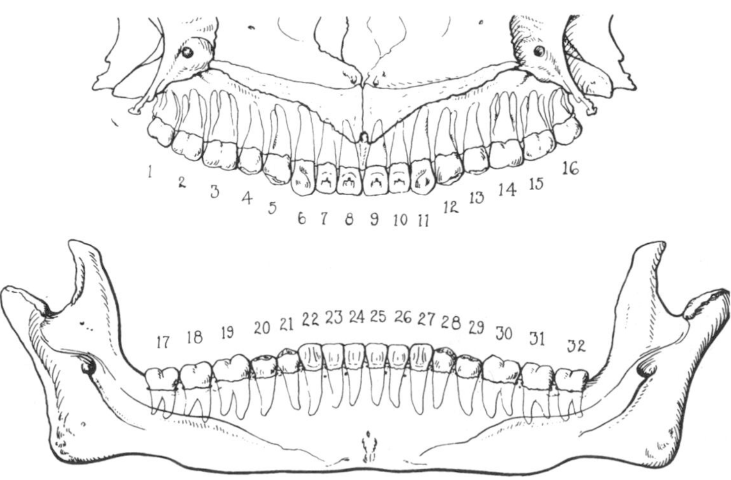

FIGURE 31-25.
Lingual aspect of the upper and lower teeth, with both dental arches widely spread. The method used here for numbering the teeth is only one of several.

Teeth

The anatomy of the gums and teeth should be examined in preparation for the dissection of the jaws. The **gums** (*gingivae*) are layers of mucous membrane that cover the alveolar processes of the upper and lower jaws. The inner and outer gums are continuous with each other in the spaces between the teeth, and those of the upper jaw are continuous with the mucosa of the lips and cheek and with that of the hard palate, respectively. Those of the lower jaw are similarly continuous with mucosa of the lips and cheek and the floor of the mouth lateral to and below the tongue.

The teeth (**dentes**) of the upper and lower jaws form **superior** and **inferior dental arches.** The **permanent teeth,** beginning in the anterior midline and proceeding laterally and posteriorly to the end of the arch, are similarly named on each side and in both upper and lower jaws. In this order, there are two incisive teeth (**incisors**), one **canine,** two **premolars,** and three **molars.** The last of these is slow to erupt, often does so imperfectly, and is a "wisdom tooth" (*dens serotinus*). A complete set of permanent teeth consists of 32, eight on each side of each jaw (Fig. 31-25; see also Figs. 31-3 to 31-8); however, many adults do not have their third molars, either because these failed to erupt or because they were removed. (They may push against the second molar and lie at such angles that they cannot erupt.) In contrast, the **deciduous** (baby) **teeth** are only 20. There are two incisors and a single canine on each side, as with the permanent teeth; the canines are followed by two molars that lie in the positions of the permanent premolar teeth (Fig. 31-26).

There are certain obvious differences among the teeth, but all of them have the same basic structure. A

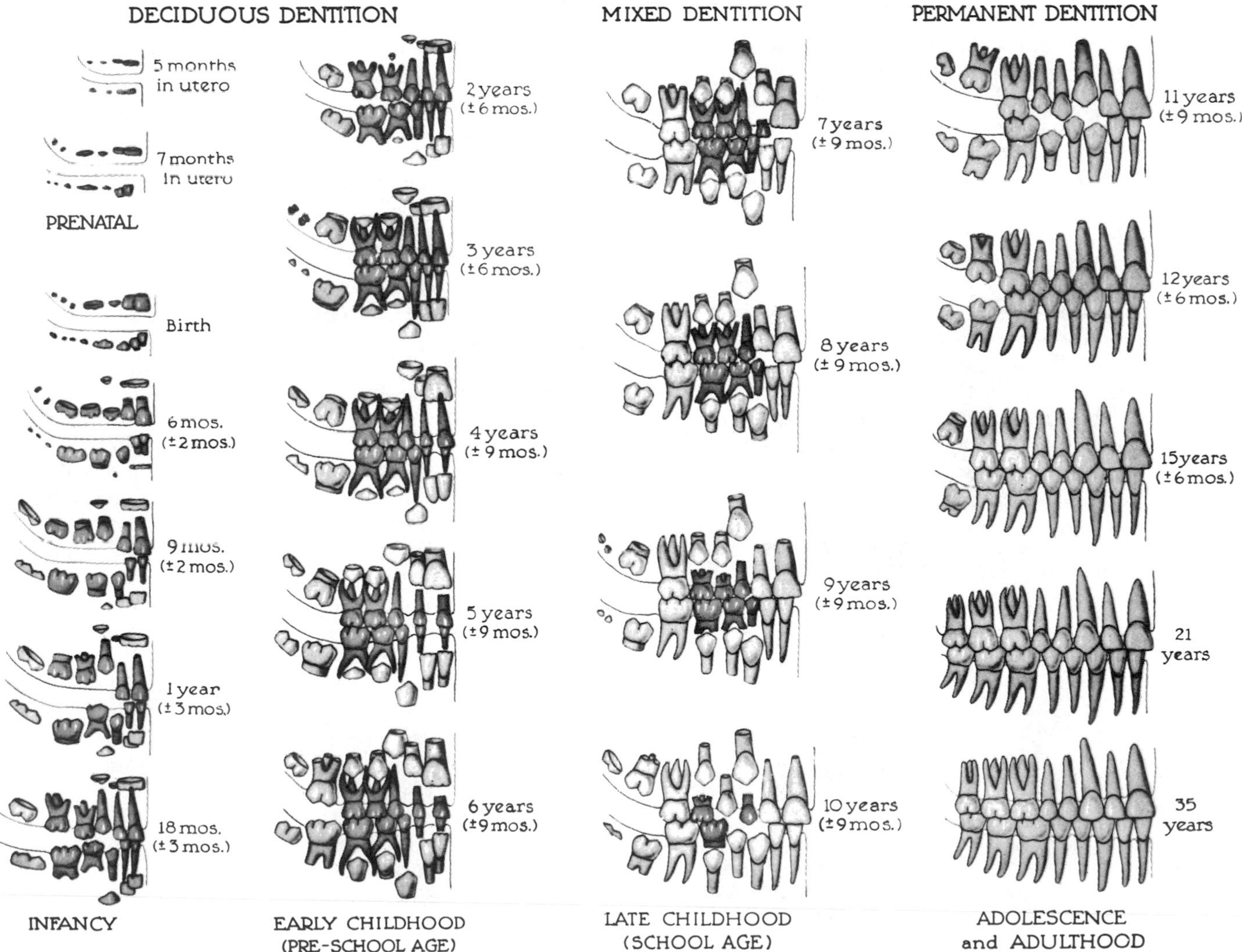

FIGURE *31-26.*
Development of dentition in the human. The deciduous teeth are *dark*, and the permanent ones are *lighter*. Note that the full quota of deciduous teeth is shown present and erupted at the ages of 2 and 3 years. (Schours I, Massler M. A chart prepared for and distributed by the American Dental Association, 2nd ed, 1944.)

tooth is largely formed of modified bone known as *dentine*, but the dentine of the **crown** (*corona dentis*) is covered by *enamel*. This thins out and disappears at the **neck** (*collum*), and the dentine of the root or roots is covered instead by *cementum*, which anchors the root in its alveolus or socket. Normally, the gum attaches at the neck of the tooth so that the crown is exposed and the root is enclosed in bone. If the gingivae and bone recede to uncover part of the bony root, that and the enamel-covered crown then are known as the **clinical crown;** the remainder of the root is known as the **clinical root.** The **surfaces** of the teeth are described as *occlusal* (masticatory), those that meet during chewing: *vestibular* or *facial* (outer), and *lingual* (inner); and surfaces of contact, which are designated as *mesial* (toward the center of the dental arch) and *distal* (towards the ends of the arch).

Each **incisor tooth,** designed for biting and cutting, presents an *incisal edge* (margo incisalis). The upper incisors, and particularly the upper canines, often show a marked thickening, the **cingulum,** on their lingual surfaces close to the gum. The canines end in blunted points instead of incisal edges. The **premolar** and **molar teeth,** designed for grinding and chewing, have their occlusal surfaces roughened by raised *cusps* (tubercles) that assist in the grinding process. There are typically two cusps on the premolars (hence, these are frequently called "bicuspids"), either three or four on the upper molars, and four or five (often the latter) on the lower molars. In the posterior teeth, a ridge, or *crista triangularis*, extends toward the center of the occlusal surface from the apex of each cusp, and if two crests meet, they form a *crista transversalis*.

The **cavum dentis,** or cavity within a tooth, is divided into the cavity of the crown (cavum coronale) and a **root canal,** both filled with **dental pulp.** When there are several roots to a tooth, the root canals fuse to form the cavum of the crown. The nerves and vessels in the dental pulp enter through an **apical foramen** at the tip of each dental root.

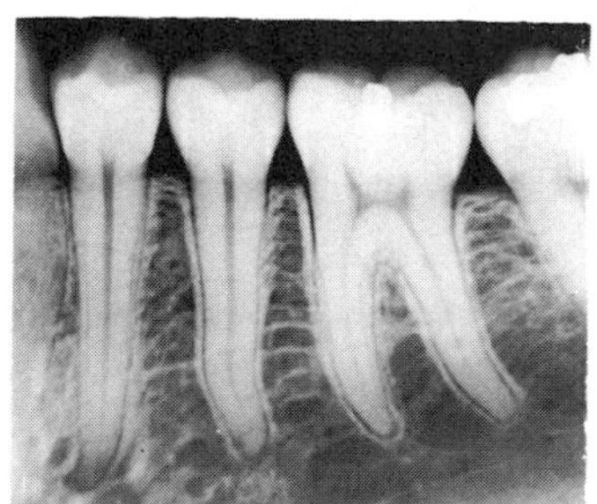

FIGURE *31-27.*
A radiograph of the two premolar teeth and the first molar tooth of the lower jaw. The root canals within the teeth show clearly. The periodontium (periodontal membrane) is the *thin dark line* immediately adjacent to the root or roots of each tooth. The thin layer of dense bone that lines the alveolus is known to dentists as the "lamina dura." The crown of the first molar contains a filling, as does the part of the second molar that is visible. (Stafne EC. Oral roentgenographic diagnosis. Philadelphia: WB Saunders, 1958.)

The **roots** of the teeth are most easily examined in radiographs (Fig. 31-27). Their great density makes them stand out plainly against the bone of the alveolar process. In such radiographs, the periosteum lining the alveolus, the **periodontium** (periodontal ligament or membrane), is also visible as a dark line just outside the tooth, and the cavum dentis is similarly visible. The incisor and canine teeth regularly each have a single root. The premolar teeth do also, but the root sometimes is grooved, and that of the upper first premolar, particularly, may be bifid. The molar teeth of the lower jaw usually have two roots each, and those of the upper, three roots, but the third molar (wisdom tooth) in either jaw may show fusion between its roots.

A few nerve twigs and blood vessels reach the outside of the tooth by penetrating the bone of the alveolar process. They are derived from the vessels and nerves of the gingivae. However, the major nerves and vessels of the teeth run in the bone of the jaws; at the apex of each root some branches enter the root canal to ramify in the pulp, but others extend into the periodontium to end there or pass through the bone to reach the gingivae.

The nerves and blood vessels of the gingival mucosa are largely those that supply the teeth; however, the labial and buccal gingivae also receive twigs from the nerves that supply the lips and cheek. The lymphatics from the lingual gingiva drain between the teeth to join those of the vestibular gingiva; these drain into buccal, mandibular, and submandibular glands.

Muscles, Joints, Nerves, and Vessels of the Jaws

Muscles

The muscles concerned primarily with chewing attach to the mandible and are often known as the muscles of mastication or as mandibular muscles. They are responsible not only for the bite, but also for the side-to-side movement of chewing. They are all innervated by the mandibular nerve, the lowest division of the trigeminal nerve and the only branch of the nerve that contains voluntary motor fibers. The mandibular nerve also innervates the teeth of the lower jaw, but the maxillary nerve, the second or middle division of the trigeminal, innervates those of the upper jaw. The blood supply to both the upper and the lower jaw is through the maxillary artery, which, with the superficial temporal, is one of the terminal branches of the external carotid.

The suprahyoid muscles attaching to the mandible usually are not considered to be muscles of mastication, although they may assist in movements of the jaw. Some of them may be identified without further dissection (Fig. 31-28), but they can be examined more thoroughly as the mandible is removed (see Figs. 31-36 and 31-40). The four muscles of mastication are the masseter, the temporal, and two pterygoid muscles. The masseter and temporal muscles (Fig. 31-29) are superficial ones covered on their superficial surfaces by deep fascia. The masseteric fascia

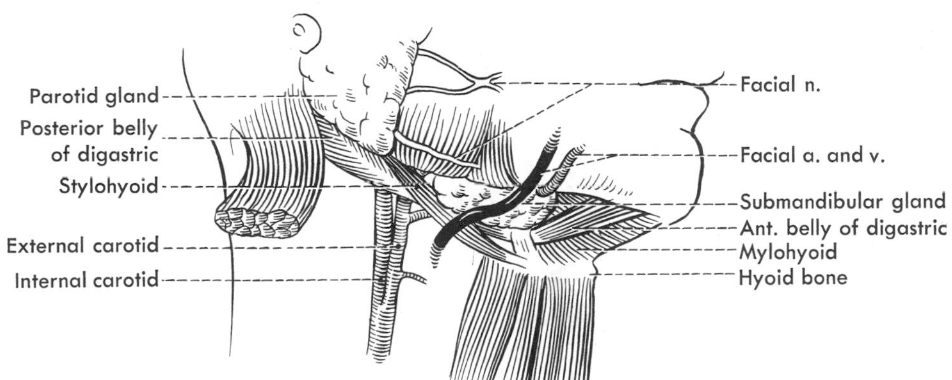

FIGURE 31-28.
Some suprahyoid structures after reflection of the sternocleidomastoid.

is thin and is continued posteriorly as the thicker parotid fascia around that gland. The temporal fascia is much thicker and hides that muscle. The temporal fascia blends above with the tendinous galea aponeurotica. Below, it attaches to the zygomatic arch, dividing as it does so into two layers, a superficial and a deep one.

The Masseter. The muscle is largely covered by the parotid gland posteriorly and by facial muscles anteriorly. Deep to the facial muscles, it is crossed superficially by the parotid duct, above this by the transverse facial artery, and both above and below the duct by branches of the facial nerve (see Fig. 31-19). The facial vessels lie just in front of its lower end as they cross the lower border of the mandible.

The masseter muscle largely covers the ramus of the mandible. It consists of two blended parts, of which the superficial arises from about the anterior two-thirds of the lower border of the zygomatic arch and extends downward and somewhat posteriorly. The deep part arises from the whole deep surface of the zygomatic arch and extends vertically downward. The muscle inserts on almost the entire lateral surface of the ramus of the mandible, including a lower part of the coronoid process; there is, however, no insertion on the condylar process. The *masseteric nerve and vessels* enter the deep surface of the masseter by passing through the mandibular notch.

The Temporalis. The large, fan-shaped temporal muscle covers much of the side of the head, arising from the temporal fossa and the deep surface of the temporal fascia and converging onto the coronoid process. The anterior fibers run almost vertically downward; the posterior fibers run both forward and downward. The muscle is thick as it reaches the coronoid process. The insertion is into the upper and anterior border of the coronoid process externally and along the whole internal surface of that process and the ramus of the mandible below it almost as far as the alveolar process.

The masseteric nerve and vessels pass behind the muscle to reach the masseter muscle. The buccal nerve and vessels pass downward and forward medial to the temporal, or sometimes through some of its fibers, to reach the cheek. Its nerve supply is usually two deep *temporal nerves,* the posterior commonly being larger, that run upward between the muscle and the bone of the temporal fossa. Each nerve typically is accompanied by a deep temporal artery from the maxillary. These supply both the muscle and the adjacent bone of the skull.

The Pterygoid Muscles. The remaining structures connected with the jaw are best examined after the zygomatic arch and the masseter have been reflected downward, the temporal muscle and the coronoid process have been reflected upward, and the upper part of the ramus of

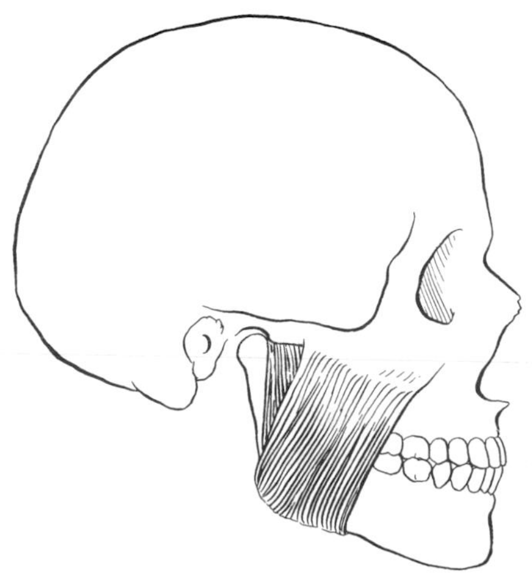
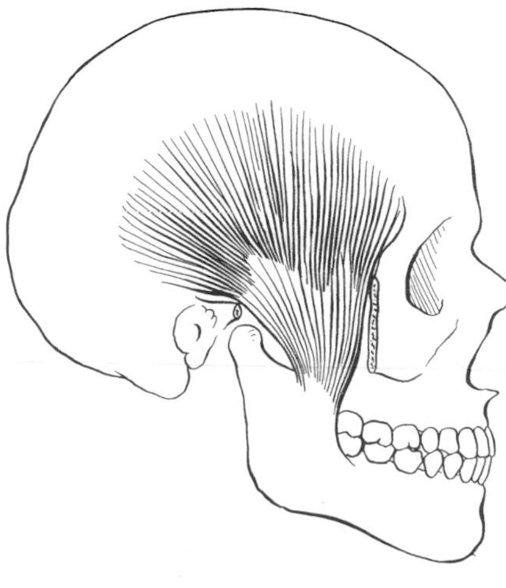

FIGURE 31-29.
Masseter and temporal muscles.

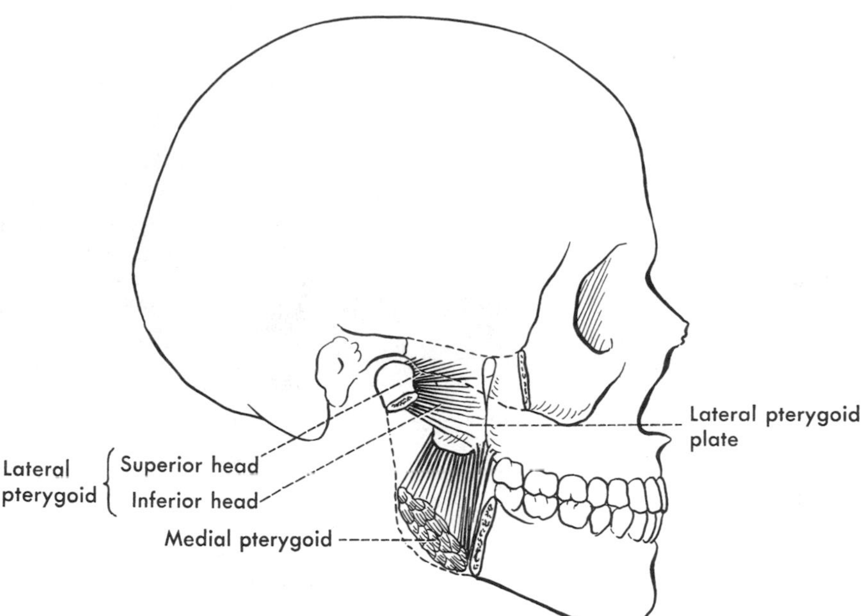

FIGURE *31-30.*
The pterygoid muscles after removal of the temporal and masseter muscles, the zygomatic arch, and most of the posterior part of the mandible.

the mandible has been removed (Fig. 31-30). The **lateral pterygoid muscle** runs almost horizontally backward to its insertion on the mandible. It arises by two heads, a small upper one from the infratemporal fossa and a larger lower one from the lateral surface of the lateral pterygoid plate. It inserts into the neck of the mandible, the capsule of the temporomandibular joint, and the articular disk that lies within the joint. The two heads are immediately adjacent and blend as they are traced toward the mandible. They are largely covered by a dense pterygoid plexus of veins that surrounds them and the maxillary artery.

Because the *mandibular nerve* lies deep to the lateral pterygoid, most of the branches of the nerve are intimately related to the muscle (Fig. 31-31). Thus, the anterior deep temporal and the buccal nerves usually pass between the two heads of the muscle. The posterior deep temporal and the masseteric nerve usually pass between the upper head and the infratemporal fossa. Two of the largest branches of the mandibular nerve, the lingual and the inferior alveolar, emerge below the lower border of the lateral pterygoid and run downward and forward; the third large branch, the auriculotemporal, passes posteriorly deep to the muscle and then continues deep to the

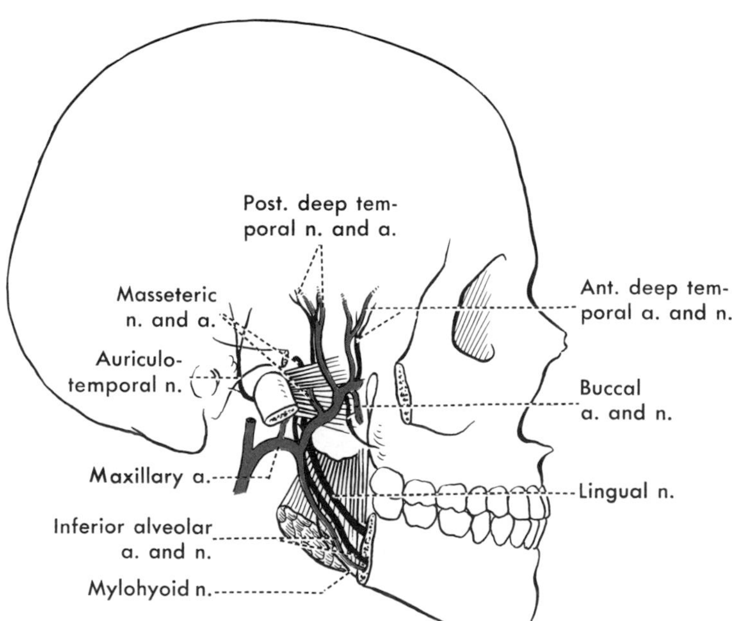

FIGURE *31-31.*
Relations of nerves and vessels to the pterygoid muscles: The middle meningeal artery arises just above the leader to the maxillary artery.

neck of the mandible before turning upward just behind the temporomandibular joint.

The **medial pterygoid muscle** partly covers, and is partly covered by, the inferior fibers of the lateral pterygoid. A small part of the muscle arises from the tuber of the maxilla and overlaps the lowest fibers of the lateral pterygoid at their origin. The major part arises from the medial side of the lateral pterygoid plate and from the pyramidal process of the palatine bone (in the lower part of the anterior wall of the pterygoid fossa); therefore, it appears at the lower border of the lateral pterygoid. The fibers of the medial pterygoid muscle run downward, posteriorly, and laterally to insert on the inner side of the ramus of the mandible below and behind the mylohyoid groove down to the lower border of the angle. It is innervated by a branch into its deep surface that leaves the mandibular nerve before that nerve gives off most of its other branches.

The masseter, temporal, and medial pterygoid muscles are powerful closers of the jaw, accounting for the strength of the bite. The temporal muscle abducts (deviates) the jaw to the same side, but the masseter and pterygoid abduct to the opposite side. With proper synchronization, therefore, these muscles can produce the grinding movement of chewing. The tongue and the buccinator muscle also aid mastication, but in a different way; the tongue positions the food on the teeth, and the buccinator muscle helps to maintain it there during chewing. The posterior fibers of the temporal muscle are the chief retractor of the mandible (pulling it back after it has been jutted forward) and also are primarily responsible for maintaining the resting position of closure of the mouth. Although both heads of the lateral pterygoid apparently aid in protracting (pulling forward) the mandible and thus deviating it to the opposite side when they act unilaterally, the superior head is said to become active only when the mouth is closed or being closed. The inferior head, however, pulls the condyle forward and downward and is active in opening the mouth—the function once assigned to both heads. When the mandible is protracted, the **sphenomandibular ligament** and a thickening of the deep cervical fascia called the **stylomandibular ligament** (extending from the styloid process to the posterior border of the angle of the jaw) have been said to act to keep the angle of the mandible from sliding as far forward as the condyles. This permits the jaw to rotate around a line that joins the centers of right and left rami; as the condyles go forward, the chin thus goes downward. The anterior belly of the digastric, and the geniohyoid and mylohyoid muscles, also help open the mouth.

The Masticator Fascial Space. The loose connective tissue deep to the ramus of the mandible and around the lower part of the temporal muscle is described as forming the masticator fascial space. It is this space that contains the pterygoid muscles, most of the branches of the mandibular nerve, and the branches of the maxillary artery. Although the masticator space lies lateral to the lateral pharyngeal space, there is no communication between the two. As the *superficial lamina* of the **cervical** (deep cervical) **fascia** reaches the lower border of the mandible, a part of it attaches to the mandible and then continues upward superficial to the masseter and the parotid gland, attaching also to the zygomatic arch and then blending with the fascia over the temporal muscle. A second *deep layer* of the cervical fascia splits off, however, and runs deep to both pterygoid muscles to reach the skull, thus separating the masticator and lateral pharyngeal spaces (Fig. 31-32). The masticator space is subdivided into a number of subsidiary spaces by fascia around the various muscles. It also extends forward superficially

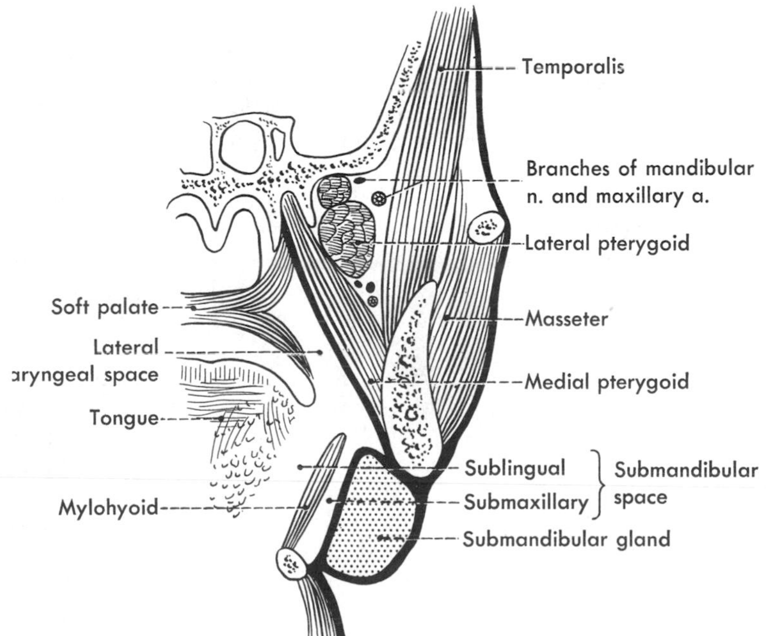

FIGURE *31-32.*
Schema of half of a frontal section close to the angle of the jaw, showing the disposition of the superficial layer of the deep fascia (*heavy lines*) above the level of the hyoid bone. After splitting to surround the submandibular gland, it attaches to the mandible and, thence, is reflected up both external and internal to the muscles of mastication. The spaces among the muscles of mastication together form the masticator space; also shown here is the submandibular space, lying both above and below the mylohyoid muscle, and its posterior communication with the lateral pharyngeal space, lying lateral to the pharynx and in part medial to the medial pterygoid muscle.

to include the **buccal fat pad** (overlying the buccinator muscle) and deeply to include the connective tissue and neurovascular structures in the pterygopalatine fossa.

In the masticator space the medial pterygoid muscle is crossed externally by the lingual and inferior alveolar nerves, which emerge below the lateral pterygoid muscle. The inferior alveolar nerve runs to the mandibular foramen on the medial side of the ramus. The lingual nerve passes farther forward, to the tongue. Inferior alveolar vessels, the artery a branch of the maxillary and the vein joining the pterygoid plexus, accompany the inferior alveolar nerve. The back part of the muscle is also crossed superficially by the **sphenomandibular ligament,** a thin band that runs from the sphenoid spine and the tympanosquamous fissure to the lingula and the adjacent inner surface of the mandible. The inferior alveolar nerve and vessels run between it and the mandible. The ligament represents remains of the cartilage of the mandibular arch (Meckel's cartilage) between the mandible and the skull.

Temporomandibular Joint.

The temporomandibular articulation is fairly simple, but it differs from many joints in that there are two synovial cavities, separated by an articular disk. Although it is reinforced externally by a **lateral ligament,** the capsule generally is lax between the disk and the temporal bone and much stronger both medially and laterally between the disk and the mandible. The **articular disk,** partly fibrocartilage but largely dense fibrous connective tissue, is loosely attached to the capsule posteriorly, but strongly attached anteriorly, where part of the tendon of the lateral pterygoid muscle blends with it. It moves forward with protraction of the mandible, but hinge movements—opening and closing—of the jaw take place between the disk and the mandible.

Because of the protraction when the mouth is opened widely, in some persons a great yawn or other excessively wide opening of the mouth will be accompanied by so much forward movement that the disk and condyle slide across the articular tubercle into the infratemporal fossa. The muscular pull is so altered by this dislocation that the jaw then is held open by the masseter and medial pterygoid. The dislocation must be reduced by forcing the condyle downward and then slipping it back into place.

The pressure produced by the closers of the jaw is normally borne almost entirely by the molar teeth and the synovial membrane of the joint, which extends in part over the articular surfaces and contains numerous nerves and vessels. Thus, malocclusion, or any factor that leads to spastic contraction of the muscles (*trismus*), may bring pressure to bear on the sensitive synovial membrane and cause pain. The spasm of the muscles may also be a cause of pain. Moreover, degenerative changes in the joint may be produced by pressure on the blood vessels of the membrane.

Vessels and Nerves Related to Jaws

The **inferior alveolar nerve and vessels**—the nerve from the mandibular, the artery from the maxillary—appear below the lateral pterygoid muscle and run downward across the medial pterygoid, passing between the mandible and the sphenomandibular ligament to reach the mandibular foramen. Just before they enter the foramen, each gives off a **mylohyoid branch** that runs downward on the medial side of the mandible, in the mylohyoid groove, and onto the lower surface of the mylohyoid muscle. Within the mandibular canal, nerve and vessels give off branches to the teeth until they reach the level of the mental foramen. Here a large branch of the nerve, and twigs of the artery and its accompanying vein, emerge as the **mental nerve and vessels.** The remaining parts of the nerves and vessels continue forward to supply teeth anterior to the mental foramen. The incisors, the canine, and the first premolar lie anterior to this foramen in about 50% of sides, for the most common location of the foramen is at the level of the second premolar tooth. Within the mandibular canal, the branches of the inferior alveolar nerve form an **inferior dental plexus,** which gives rise to both dental and gingival branches.

Some of the branches of the maxillary artery and most of those of the mandibular nerve already have been described.

The **maxillary artery** arises as one of the terminal branches of the external carotid artery at the posterior border of the ramus of the mandible, adjacent to or in the deep part of the parotid gland. It passes forward almost horizontally medial to the ramus of the mandible, at or a little below the level of the neck (see Figs. 30-14 and 31-31). Its branches are particularly numerous (Fig. 31-33). Close to its origin, it gives off a small **deep auricular artery** that passes upward in the parotid gland to supply the temporomandibular joint and the external acoustic meatus, and it may give off a tiny **anterior tympanic artery** that helps supply the tympanic cavity and the inner surface of the tympanic membrane.

Farther forward, the artery gives rise to two larger branches, the middle meningeal artery and the inferior alveolar. The inferior alveolar and its terminal branch, the mental, have already been noted. The **middle meningeal artery** runs upward deep to the lateral pterygoid muscle, passes between the two roots of origin of the auriculotemporal nerve, and enters the skull through the foramen spinosum. It may give off, or there may be given off directly from the maxillary, an **accessory meningeal artery.** This artery gives off branches to extracranial structures adjacent to it and often enters the skull through the foramen ovale (by which the mandibular nerve leaves the skull) to reach the meninges around the trigeminal ganglion.

As the maxillary artery reaches the lower border of the lateral pterygoid muscle, it may run deep or superficial to it. At about this level it gives off the **masseteric artery,** and if it runs deep to the lateral pterygoid, it then emerges between the two heads of the muscle to give off the **deep temporal** and **buccal arteries.** There are also branches to the pterygoid muscles.

The last part of the maxillary artery passes deeply, through the pterygomaxillary fissure into the pterygopalatine fossa. As it does so, it gives off one or more

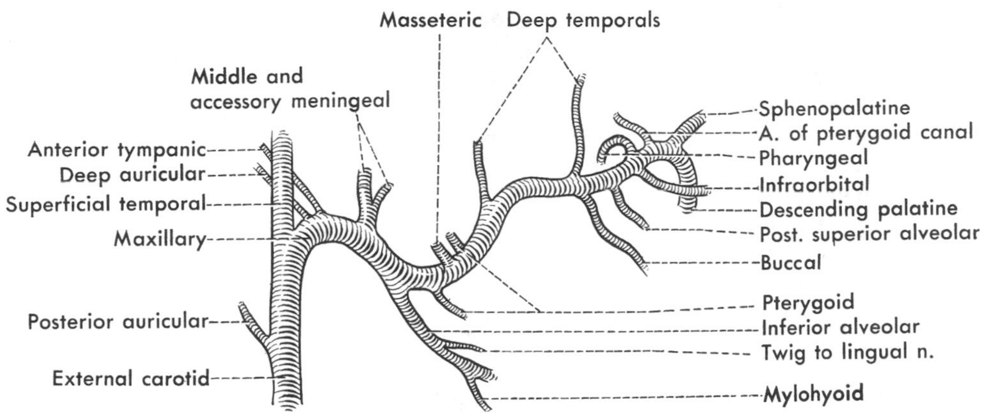

FIGURE *31-33.* Branches of the maxillary artery.

posterior superior alveolar arteries that run downward on the posterior surface of the maxilla, accompanied by posterior superior alveolar nerves. These arteries enter foramina on the posterior surface of the maxilla and run downward and forward in the alveolar process, supplying dental branches to the more posterior upper teeth (Fig. 31-34). Other terminal branches of the maxillary artery can be identified only with difficulty, if at all, at this time. Most of them will be seen in deeper dissections. They are a tiny **artery of the pterygoid canal** and a **pharyngeal branch** (entering the palatovaginal canal) to the pharynx; a larger **infraorbital artery,** a part of which emerges at the infraorbital foramen but which supplies through **anterior superior alveolar** branches (one of which is sometimes called the middle) the anterior teeth of the upper jaw; a large **descending palatine** that appears on the palate as greater and lesser palatine arteries; and a **sphenopalatine** that passes straight medially from the pterygopalatine fossa into the nasal cavity.

The **pterygoid plexus** of veins is a venous plexus around the maxillary artery and both superficial and deep to the lateral pterygoid muscle. It is drained posteriorly by the maxillary vein, but also has other connections: in addition to receiving veins corresponding to the branches of the maxillary artery, it is connected to the facial vein by the deep facial vein, accompanying the buccal branch of the maxillary artery; to the cavernous sinus in the skull by veins that travel with the mandibular nerve through the foramen ovale; and to the middle meningeal veins inside the skull through veins that travel through the foramen spinosum with the middle meningeal artery.

As the **mandibular nerve** (see Figs. 31-31 and 32-22) emerges from the foramen ovale, it consists of two roots: a large superficial (lateral) *sensory root* and a small, deeper-lying *motor root.* These join almost immediately outside the foramen ovale to form the mixed nerve. In this position, deep to the lateral pterygoid muscle, it gives off a tiny **meningeal branch** that runs backward to join the middle meningeal artery and accompany it into the skull, and it gives rise to the **medial pterygoid nerve.**

On the medial side of the mandibular nerve, sometimes closely applied to it, sometimes slightly farther out on a nerve stem to the medial pterygoid and tensor veli palatini muscles, is the **otic ganglion.** This ganglion is one of the four parasympathetic ganglia of the head. It receives its preganglionic fibers through a nerve that reaches it from posteriorly, the *lesser petrosal nerve,* a branch of the glossopharyngeal nerve. It gives off its post-

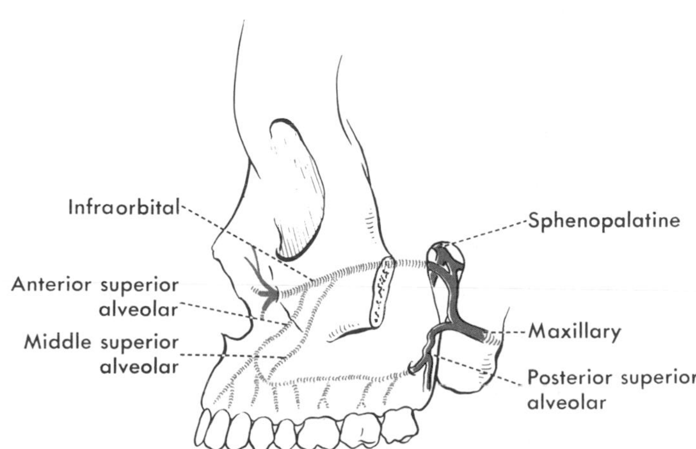

FIGURE *31-34.* Blood supply of the upper teeth.

ganglionic fibers into the auriculotemporal branch of the mandibular nerve (through its *ramus communicans with the auriculotemporal*); whence they pass into that nerve's parotid branches as the secretory pathway to the parotid gland. The **nerve of the tensor veli palatini,** the latter being the only muscle of the soft palate supplied by the mandibular, is described as a branch of the ganglion, as is the tiny **nerve to the tensor tympani** that parallels the lesser petrosal, proceeding posteriorly toward the middle ear. Actually, these nerves contain no fibers from the otic ganglion, for they go to voluntary muscles; it is simply that they are so small that, as they pass by the ganglion, they seem to be branches of it.

After giving off these branches, the mandibular nerve usually divides into a smaller anterior part and a larger posterior part. From the *anterior part* arise the masseteric, the two deep temporal, the lateral pterygoid, and the buccal nerves, so that this part of the nerve is largely to muscles. From the *posterior part* arise the auriculotemporal, the inferior alveolar, and the lingual. The **masseteric nerve** usually passes between the upper head of the lateral pterygoid muscle and the infratemporal fossa and reaches the muscle through the mandibular notch. The **deep temporal nerves** (there may be more than two) may both turn upward deep to the temporal muscle by passing between the lateral pterygoid muscle and the infratemporal fossa, or the posterior nerve may take this course, and the anterior emerge between the two heads of the lateral pterygoid to cross the muscle. The **lateral pterygoid nerve** usually arises with the buccal and enters the deep surface of the muscle. The **buccal nerve** emerges between the two heads of the lateral pterygoid muscle and runs forward and downward to supply skin and mucous membrane of the cheek.

The **auriculotemporal nerve** arises by two roots, between which the middle meningeal artery passes. These roots come together behind the artery, and the nerve passes posteriorly just deep to the mandible, turning upward behind the temporomandibular joint and deep to the parotid gland and joining the superficial temporal vessels in their course above the parotid gland.

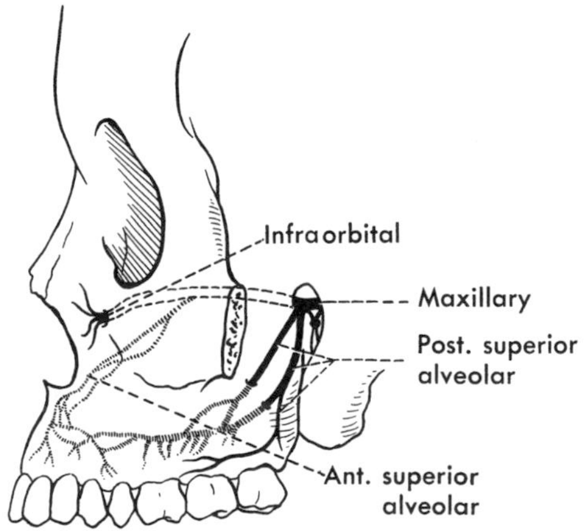

FIGURE *31-35.*
The superior alveolar nerves. A middle superior alveolar appears in Figure 32-21.

The inferior alveolar nerve already has been described. The **lingual nerve** at first almost parallels it, running downward above and in front of it but gradually diverging from it. After the lingual nerve leaves the lateral surface of the medial pterygoid muscle, it runs between the mandible and the uppermost muscle of the pharynx, the superior pharyngeal constrictor; its further course to the tongue is described with that organ.

Close to its origin, the lingual nerve receives the **chorda tympani,** a branch of the facial nerve that brings into it parasympathetic preganglionic fibers for the **submandibular ganglion** with which this nerve is connected, and taste fibers that this nerve conducts to the anterior two-thirds of the tongue. The chorda tympani emerges from the petrotympanic fissure, just behind and medial to the temporomandibular articulation. It runs downward and forward, passes deep to the middle meningeal artery and the inferior alveolar branch of the mandibular nerve, and joins the posterior border of the lingual nerve. It receives a twig *(ramus communicans with the chorda tympani)* from the otic ganglion.

Branches of the **maxillary nerve,** the **posterior superior alveolar nerves,** leave the nerve while it is in the pterygopalatine fossa and descend along the posterior surface of the maxilla with the corresponding vessels to run forward and supply the posterior teeth (Fig. 31-35). There usually are three of these nerves. One usually simply supplies the gums rather than entering the bone, and the other two enter the bone. Apparently, they never run any farther forward than the canine tooth and often supply only the molar teeth. There also are **anterior superior alveolar nerves** that are given off farther forward from the maxillary nerves. They run downward in the bone of the anterior wall of the maxilla to supply the more anterior teeth and usually spread back as far as the second premolar; apparently, they frequently cross the midline to help supply the medial incisor of the other side. There also is a less constant **middle superior alveolar nerve** to the premolars, so that these teeth apparently can be supplied by any combination of posterior, middle, and anterior nerves. The superior alveolar nerves form a **superior dental plexus** above the roots of the teeth; this gives rise to both dental and gingival branches. Because of their minute size, it is difficult to trace any of the superior alveolar nerves through the bone.

Suprahyoid Structures

The suprahyoid muscles are the digastric, the stylohyoid, the mylohyoid, and the geniohyoid. They are classified as muscles of the neck, but the mylohyoid is also considered as forming the floor of the mouth, for it fills much of the space between the two sides of the body of the mandible. The digastric and the stylohyoid lie below the mylohyoid (Fig. 31-36), but the geniohyoid lies above it.

A little connective tissue and some lymph nodes lie between the mylohyoid muscle and the fascia that covers it superficially (the superficial lamina of the cervical fas-

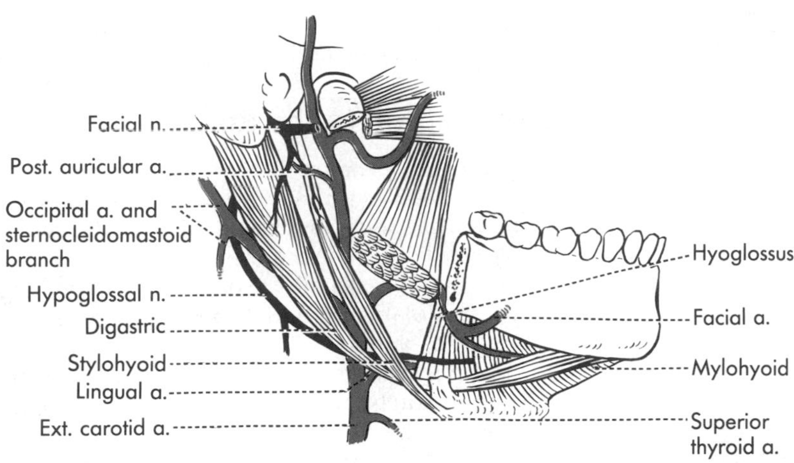

FIGURE 31-36.
The more superficial suprahyoid muscles after removal of the sternocleidomastoid muscle, the parotid and submandibular glands, and the posterior part of the mandible.

cia, attached below to the hyoid bone and above to the mandible). The potential space here communicates around the posterior border of the mylohyoid muscle, with the greater amount of loose connective tissue deep to the tongue (sometimes called the sublingual space): hence, the spaces above and below the mylohyoid are conveniently grouped together as the **submandibular fascial space** (see Fig. 31-32).

The *mylohyoid muscle* and the superficial relations of the **submandibular gland** are described in Chapter 30 (see Figs. 30-8 and 30-10). The gland largely fills the triangle between the two bellies of the digastric and the lower border of the mandible and extends upward deep to the mandible. It lies partly on the lower surface of the mylohyoid and partly behind that muscle against the lateral surface of a muscle of the tongue, the hyoglossus. Its duct, and often a process of glandular tissue, run forward above the mylohyoid (see Figs. 31-38 and 31-39). The hypoglossal nerve lies deep to it or below it, against the hyoglossus muscle and close to the hyoid bone, before disappearing above the mylohyoid. Posteriorly, the lingual artery lies deep to it for a short distance. The artery then goes deep to the hyoglossus muscle (see Fig. 31-36).

The **digastric** and **stylohyoid** muscles can be seen more fully after the parotid gland and part of the mandible have been removed. The **posterior belly of the digastric,** innervated by a branch of the facial nerve, arises from the mastoid notch on the medial side of the mastoid process. The *tendon* connecting the two bellies passes through the stylohyoid and is held to the hyoid bone by fascia or tendon or both. The **anterior belly of the digastric,** proceeding forward and medially from the connecting tendon, attaches on the inner surface of the mandible just lateral to the midline. The mylohyoid nerve, a branch of the inferior alveolar that reaches the lower surface of the muscle, also supplies the anterior belly of the digastric. The **stylohyoid,** the most lateral muscle arising from the styloid process, is innervated by a branch of the facial nerve. It runs downward and forward, superficial to the external carotid, facial, and lingual arteries, splits to pass on both sides of the digastric tendon, and inserts into the hyoid bone.

After the mylohyoid muscle is reflected, the **geniohyoid** can be seen from below and can be examined more completely after various structures lying lateral to it and the tongue muscles have been reflected (see Fig. 31-40). It extends from the lower part of the mental spine backward and downward to the body of the hyoid bone, the muscles of the two sides being adjacent at the midline. The geniohyoid is a suprahyoid strap muscle and is innervated by fibers from the first cervical nerve These fibers join the hypoglossal nerve and travel with it.

The suprahyoid muscles raise the hyoid bone and, therefore, the tongue and the floor of the mouth, or, acting with the infrahyoid ones, steady the hyoid bone so that it can provide a firm base for movements of the tongue. When the hyoid bone is fixed by the infrahyoid muscles, the suprahyoid ones can assist in opening the mouth. During swallowing, these muscles move the hyoid bone up. When high notes are sung, they also move the hyoid bone and, therefore, the larynx up, but when low notes are sung the infrahyoid muscles lower the hyoid bone and larynx.

THE TONGUE

The attached part of the tongue, through which muscles reach it deep to the mucous membrane, is its **root,** and the upper surface is its **dorsum.** The dorsum bounds part of the oral cavity, but the most posterior part faces posteriorly and is part of the anterior wall of the epiglottic valleculae and adjacent parts of the pharynx. The major part of the tongue is the **body,** extending to the **apex** or tip. Anterior to the root, the body and tip have also an inferior surface, and it is to this surface that the frenulum linguae is attached. On the lower surface of the tongue on each side of the frenulum, the deep lingual vein usually is obvious through the mucosa.

The dorsum of the oral part of the tongue is velvety because it is covered by numerous small **papillae,** the *filiform papillae,* among which can be seen occasional larger *fungiform papillae* (Fig. 31-37). The latter are provided with a few taste buds; the former have none. At the back end of

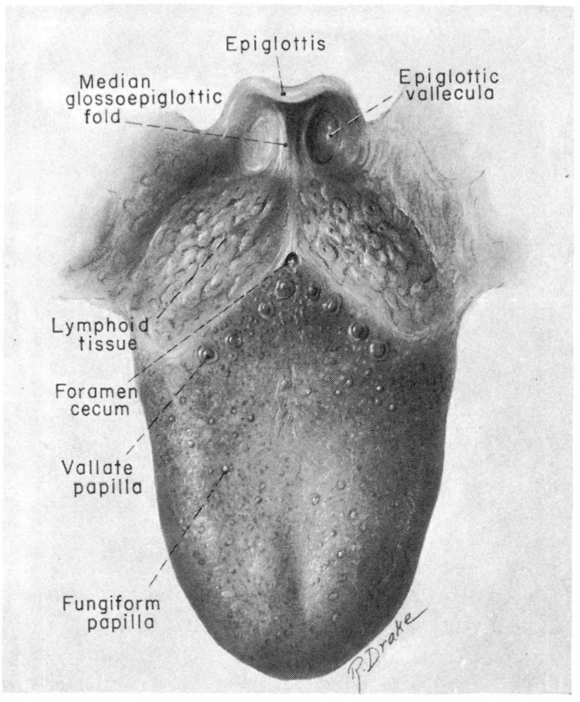

FIGURE 31-37.
The dorsum of the tongue. The folds forming the lateral boundaries of the epiglottic valleculae are the lateral glossoepiglottic folds. (Rankin FW. Crisp NW: West J Surg Obstet Gynecol 40: 105, 1932)

the oral part, arranged in a V with the apex pointed posteriorly, are large *vallate papillae* that are studded with numerous taste buds. Each papilla is deeply encircled by a groove. Immediately behind the vallate papillae is a V-shaped groove, the **sulcus terminalis.** This usually is described as separating the oral from the pharyngeal part of the dorsum. At the apex of the sulcus lies the **foramen cecum,** a tiny blind pit that indicates the point of origin of the thryoglossal duct. A shallow median sulcus that extends from the apex of the tongue toward the foramen cecum marks the attachment of the septum linguae. The pharyngeal part of the dorsum linguae is best examined in connection with the pharynx (see Chap. 34).

The musculature of the tongue lies above the hyoid bone and largely medial to the mandible and, therefore, it and the associated nerves and vessels can best be examined by removing most of the body of the mandible almost as far forward as the midline.

Structures Lateral to the Root

The **sublingual gland,** the smallest of the three chief salivary glands, lies between the mucous membrane of the floor of the mouth above, the mylohyoid muscle below, the mandible laterally, and muscles of the tongue medially. It varies in size, but usually is some 35 to 45 mm long. It is flattened mediolaterally, and its posterior end is slender, but it expands vertically at its anterior end (Fig. 31-38). From its upper surface, a series of small ducts, the **minor sublingual ducts,** empty through the mucous membrane of the the floor of the mouth immediately above the gland. There are commonly about a dozen of these. A duct at the anterior end of the gland may open into the submandibular duct. Called the **major sublingual duct,** it may be lacking or no larger than the minor sublingual ducts.

The **duct of the submandibular gland,** frequently accompanied by a process of the gland, runs above the mylohyoid muscle to disappear deep to the sublingual gland. The lingual nerve, descending and running forward, crosses lateral to the submandibular duct and also disappears deep to the sublingual gland; and the hypoglossal nerve, lying at a lower level, likewise passes forward between the gland and the muscles of the tongue before dividing into branches and extending deeper into the tongue. When the sublingual gland is elevated or removed, the submandibular duct can be traced forward to its ending on the sublingual caruncle, and the course of the lingual nerve into the tongue can be seen: after crossing the submandibular duct laterally, the nerve passes under the duct and then turns up medial to it into the tongue, thus making a loop around the duct (Fig. 31-39).

The **lingual nerve** has already been described as leaving the mandibular nerve, receiving the chorda tympani, and running downward and forward across the lateral surface of the medial pterygoid muscle. Beyond this, it runs adjacent to the superior constrictor muscle of the pharynx, medial to the mandible, and deep to the mucous membrane of the floor of the mouth lateral to the tongue. As it curves forward on the side of the tongue, it bears the **submandibular ganglion** (see Fig. 31-39). This parasympathetic ganglion is connected to the lingual nerve by

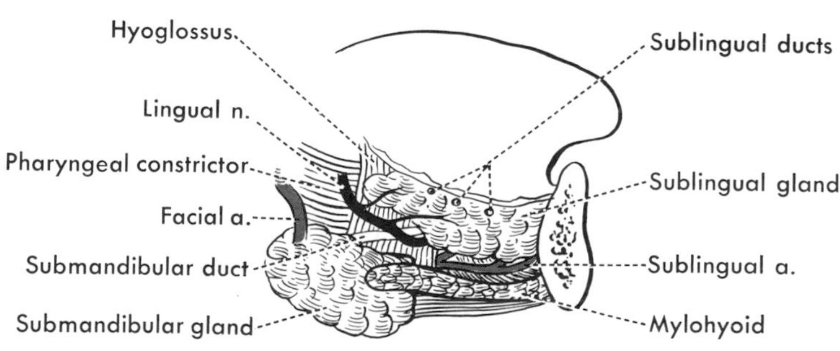

FIGURE 31-38.
Submandibular and sublingual glands from the lateral aspect after removal of the mandible.

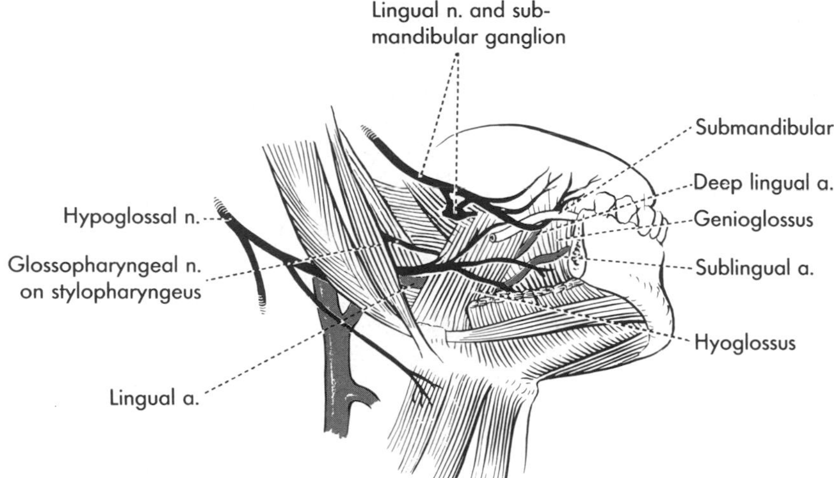

FIGURE 31-39.
Nerve and arterial relations above the mylohyoid muscle; the submandibular and sublingual glands have been removed.

rami communicantes and gives off into the submandibular gland one or more nerves that are formed of postganglionic fibers from the ganglion. The preganglionic fibers are furnished by the *chorda tympani,* a branch of the facial. The submandibular ganglion also sends fibers to the lingual nerve to be distributed to the sublingual gland and small glands of the oral cavity. As the nerve runs forward deep to the sublingual gland, it gives off fibers to the floor of the mouth and to the sublingual gland and breaks up into branches to the mucous membrane of the anterior two-thirds of the tongue. Postganglionic, secretomotor fibers from the submandibular ganglion are distributed to glands; the fibers of trigeminal origin, representing a great majority of its fibers, furnish general sensation to the tongue—touch, pain, heat, and cold—and the fibers of facial origin are for taste alone.

The **hypoglossal nerve** runs forward above the hyoid bone, crossing lateral to the hyoglossus muscle, supplying this muscle, and then branching as it continues forward deep to the sublingual gland. It supplies all the muscles of the tongue, and one branch, which contains cervical nerve fibers, supplies the geniohyoid muscle.

The largest part of the **lingual vein,** here called the *vena comitans of the hypoglossal nerve,* runs with the hypoglossal nerve, but the lingual artery runs deep to the hyoglossus muscle. Much of it turns up into the tongue, but the **sublingual artery** continues forward and appears anterior to the hyoglossus in the floor of the mouth, medial to the sublingual gland.

Muscles

The tongue consists largely of muscle fibers. Its **intrinsic muscles** are so arranged that they can, by appropriate action, change the shape of the tongue—flatten it, curl it, point it, and the like. Superior and inferior *longitudinal muscles,* and *transverse* and *vertical muscles,* are named, although both of the latter are somewhat oblique. The muscles of the two sides are separated, except at the tip, by a fascial **septum linguae,** and this also almost completely separates the branches of the two lingual arteries; in midline sectioning of the tongue, therefore, there is little bleeding. The "transverse" and "vertical" muscles form the major part of the tongue. The longitudinal muscles are arranged in two relatively narrow bands, one on the dorsum of the tongue immediately beneath the mucous membrane and one toward the lower surface.

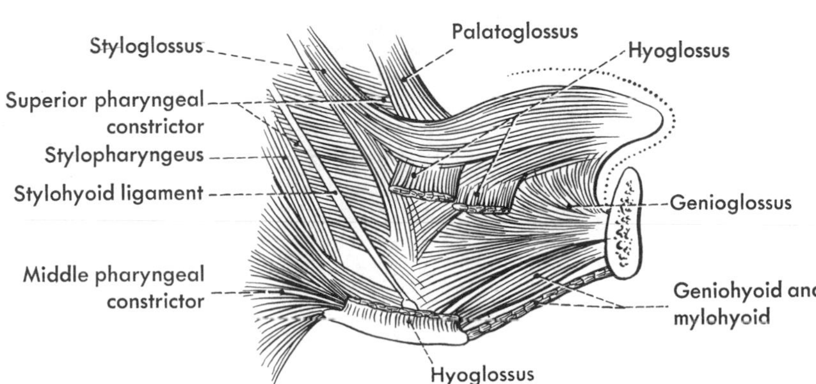

FIGURE 31-40.
Muscles of the tongue.

The **extrinsic muscles** of the tongue are three on each side; hyoglossus (with its subdivision, the chondroglossus), the styloglossus, and the genioglossus (Fig. 31-40).

The **hyoglossus** is a flat, quadrilateral muscle that arises from the body and the greater cornu of the hyoid bone, partly above and partly behind the mylohyoid muscle, and passes upward and forward into the tongue. The lingual nerve, the submandibular duct, and sublingual gland, and the hypoglossal nerve, with its accompanying vein, lie lateral to the muscle, and the lingual artery runs deep (medial) to it. The muscle ends in the tongue by becoming interlaced with the other muscle fibers there. The **chondroglossus** is a small bit of muscle that arises from the lesser cornu of the hyoid bone, passing into the tongue with the hyoglossus. It really is a slip of the latter muscle and is not always present.

The **styloglossus** arises from the anterior border of the styloid process and from the *stylohyoid ligament*, a slender band extending from the tip of the styloid process to the lesser cornu of the hyoid bone. The muscle runs forward, downward, and medially, to insert into the side of the tongue, mingling with fibers of the other muscles.

The **genioglossus** arises from the mental spine immediately above the geniohyoid. From this origin, it fans out as it runs backward: the lowest fibers insert into the body of the hyoid bone; the greater number of fibers run obliquely upward and posteriorly to blend with other muscles throughout the whole body of the tongue; and the most anterior fibers curve up and then forward to extend to the tip of the tongue.

The three extrinsic muscles, similar to the intrinsic muscles, are **innervated** by the hypoglossal nerve. They act with the intrinsic muscles in moving the tongue, and their chief actions are obvious from their positions and directions: the hyoglossus flattens the tongue, approximating the dorsum to the hyoid bone; the styloglossus pulls the tongue upward and backward; and the genioglossus pulls the body of the tongue forward and downward and the hyoid bone forward, thus helping to protrude the tongue (or, through action of its anterior fibers, can retract the tip of the protruded tongue). Since the tongue can be protruded in the midline only if the muscles of both sides work together, a hypoglossal nerve paralysis can be easily diagnosed by having the patient protrude the tongue as far as possible; the tongue is protruded only by the action of the muscles on the sound side and, therefore, deviates to the paralyzed side.

Another muscle, smaller than those just described, also attaches to the tongue. This, the **palatoglossus,** is described with the muscles of the soft palate. It enters the tongue anterior to and above the styloglossus, but it is improbable that it contributes to movements of the tongue.

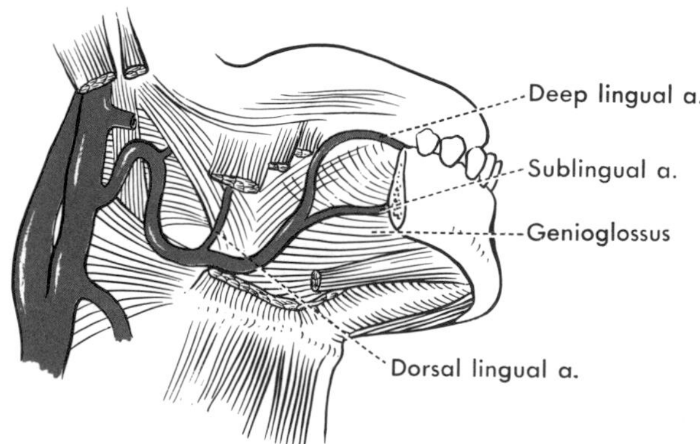

FIGURE *31-41.* The lingual artery.

Lingual Vessels

After its origin from the external carotid, the **lingual artery** runs forward above the hyoid bone and deep to the hyoglossus muscle (Fig. 31-41). It has a small suprahyoid branch that runs along the upper border of that bone, superficial to the hyoglossus muscle, but its other branches arise while it lies deep to that muscle.

In addition to a twig to the tonsillar region, the lingual artery gives off one or two **dorsalis linguae** rami, which pass upward between the hyoglossus and genioglossus muscles to the dorsum of the tongue. They supply the posterior part of the tongue, especially its pharyngeal part. The **sublingual artery** arises close to the anterior border of the hyoglossus muscle and continues forward between the mylohyoid and genioglossus muscles to supply these, the geniohyoid, and the sublingual gland. The remainder of the lingual artery, larger than the sublingual, is the **deep lingual** (*profunda linguae*). This runs forward on the lower surface of the tongue, between the inferior longitudinal muscle and the genioglossus, and when it reaches the free lower surface of the tongue, it is immediately adjacent to the mucous membrane. It is accompanied here by the **deep lingual vein**, usually easily recognizable through the mucous membrane in the living person. The deep lingual and sublingual veins form the **vena comitans nervi hypoglossi**, running with that nerve lateral to the hyoglossus muscle. The dorsal lingual veins accompany the lingual artery in its course deep to the hyoglossus.

The **lymphatics** of the tongue are of particular importance because of the relative frequency of carcinoma of that organ. Those from the *anterior part* of the tongue run downward among the lingual muscles, penetrate the mylohyoid, and end in part in *submental nodes* (see Fig. 30-26), in part in *submandibular nodes,* and in part, bypassing these nodes, in nodes of the *deep cervical chain* as low as the juguloomohyoid one (where the omohyoid muscle crosses the internal jugular vein). Lymphatics from a more *posterior part* of the tongue run behind the edge of the mylohyoid and join *deep cervical nodes,* and those from about the posterior third of the tongue penetrate the lateral pharyngeal wall to end in deep cervical nodes. Further, lymphatics from the *central portion* of the tongue, in contrast to those from the margin, drain both to the same and to the opposite side.

In consequence of this drainage, metastatic carcinoma from the tongue may be widely disseminated through the submental and submandibular regions and along the internal jugular

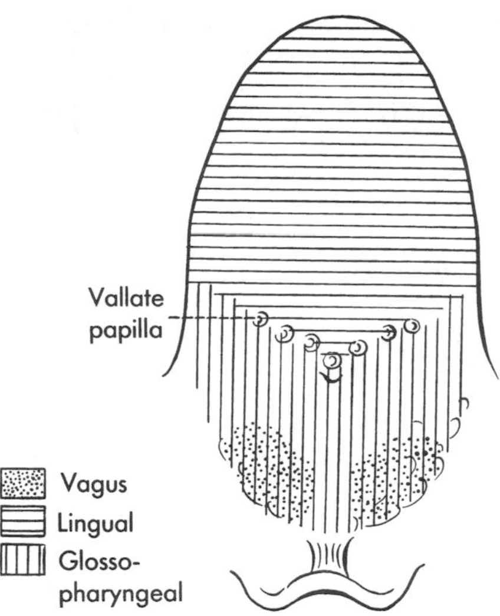

FIGURE 31-42.
Sensory innervation of the tongue.

vein. The operation designed to remove such metastatic lesions is called "radical neck dissection" or "block dissection of the neck".

Nerves

The courses of the **lingual** and **hypoglossal** nerves to the tongue have already been described. The hypoglossal nerve supplies all the lingual muscles, extrinsic and intrinsic. The lingual nerve is distributed to the mucous membrane in front of the vallate papillae, thus to about the anterior two-thirds of the tongue (Fig. 31-42). The afferent fibers that the lingual nerve receives from the chorda tympani branch of the facial nerve are distributed to the taste buds of the anterior two-thirds of the tongue and mediate only taste. The fibers in the lingual nerve that are of trigeminal origin mediate only general sensation from the mucous membrane.

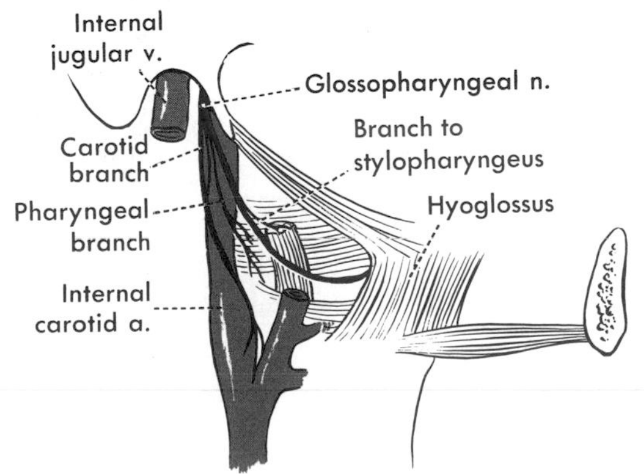

FIGURE 31-43.
The glossopharyngeal nerve after it leaves the jugular fossa.

The **glossopharyngeal nerve** (Fig. 31-43) supplies most of the mucous membrane of the posterior third of the tongue both with fibers for taste, ending especially in the vallate papillae, and with fibers of general sensation. This innervation is supplemented on the most posterior part of the tongue by twigs from the *vagus nerves*. The glossopharyngeal nerve runs downward and forward between the external and internal carotid arteries, giving off a carotid branch (*ramus sinus carotici*), which supplies both the carotid sinus and the carotid body, and one or more pharyngeal branches that join the vagus in forming the pharyngeal plexus. It then runs downward and forward, lying first below and then lateral to the most medial muscle (stylopharyngeus) that arises from the styloid process and giving off to that muscle its only *muscular branch*. In its course to the tongue, it runs along the lateral pharyngeal wall immediately lateral to the tonsil, giving off one or more *tonsillar branches* to the pharynx. It then turns upward into posterior part of the tongue, coursing deep to the styloglossus and hyoglossus muscles, and breaks up into its terminal branches.

RECOMMENDED READINGS

Basmajian JV, DeLuca CJ. Muscles of mastication, face, and neck. In: Muscles alive: their functions revealed by electromyography. 5th ed. Baltimore: William & Wilkins, 1985.

Bernick S. Innervation of teeth and periodontium after enzymatic removal of collagenous elements. Oral Surg Oral Med Oral Pathol 1957; 10: 323.

Birou G, Garcier JM, Guillot M, Vanneuville G, Chazal J. A study of the lateral pterygoid muscle: anatomic sections and CT appearances. Surg Radiol Anat 1991, 13. 307.

Carter RB, Keen EN. The intramandibular course of the inferior alveolar nerve. J Anat 1971; 108: 433.

Cavézian R, Iba-Zizen M-T, Pasquet G, Cabanis EA. Computed tomography: 3D reconstructions and colour coded discrimination of the dental groups. Surg Radiol Anat 1995; 17: 77.

Chandler SB, Derezinski CF. The variations of the middle meningeal artery within the middle cranial fossa. Anat Rec 1935; 62: 309.

Curtin HD. Separation of the masticator space from parapharyngeal space. Radiology 1987; 63: 195.

Gasser RF. The development of the facial muscles in man. Am J Anat 1966; 120: 357.

Gaughran GRL. Fasciae of the masticator space. Anat Rec 1957; 129: 383.

Graney DO, Baker SR. Anatomy of the face. In: Cummings CW, ed. Otolaryngology—head and neck surgery. 2nd ed. vol 1. St Louis: Mosby-Year Book, 1993: 305.

Graney DO, Petruzzelli GY, Myers EN. Anatomy of the oral cavity/oropharynx/nasopharynx. In: Cummings CW, ed. Otolaryngology—head and neck surgery. 2nd ed. vol 2. St Louis: Mosby-Year Book, 1993: 1101.

Hillen B, ed. Temporal bone and posterior cranial fossa [computer software program]. New York: Elsevier Science, 1994.

Hollinshead WH. Anatomy for surgeons: vol 1, the head and neck. 3rd ed. Philadelphia: Harper & Row, 1982.

Jamieson JK, Dobson JF. The lymphatics of the tongue: with particular reference to the removal of lymphatic glands in cancer of the tongue. Br J Surg 1920; 8: 80.

Jenkins DB, Spackman GK. A method for teaching the classical inferior alveolar nerve block. Clin Anat 1995; 8: 231.

Jiménez-Castellanos J, Carmona A, Castellanos L, Catalina-Herrera CJ. Microsurgical anatomy of the human ophthalmic artery: a mesoscopic study of its origin, course and collateral branches. Surg Radiol Anat 1995; 17: 139.

Johnstone DR, Templeton MC. The feasibility of palpating the lateral pterygoid muscle. J Prosthet Dent 1980; 44: 318.

Lang J. Anatomy of the posterior cranial fossa and its foramina. Paris: Thieme, 1991.

Lewis D, Dandy WE. The course of the nerve fibers transmitting sensation of taste. Arch Surg 1930; 21: 249.

Libersa C, Laude M, Libersa JC. The pneumatization of the accessory cavities of the nasal fossae during growth. Anat Clin 1981; 2: 265.

Mason DK, Chisholm DM. Salivary glands in health and disease. London: WB Saunders, 1975.

McKenzie J. The parotid gland in relation to the facial nerve. J Anat 1948; 82: 183.

McNamara JA Jr. The independent functions of the two heads of the lateral pterygoid muscle. Am J Anat 1973; 178: 197.

Moffett BC Jr. Johnson LC, McCabe JB, et al. Articular remodeling in the adult human temporomandibular joint. Am J Anat 1964; 115: 119.

Orliaguet T, Dechelotte. P, Scheye T, Vanneuville G. Relations between Meckel's cartilage and the morphogenesis of the mandible in the human embryo. Surg Radiol Anat 1993; 15: 41.

Rhoton AL Jr. Microsurgical anatomy of the jugular foramen. J Neurosurg 1975; 42: 541.

Schmolke C. The relationship between the temporomandibular joint capsule, articular disc and jaw muscles. J Anat 1994; 184: 335.

Sicher H. Masticatory fat pad and fasciae of the masticatory muscles. In: Sicher H, ed. Oral anatomy. 3rd ed. St. Louis: CV Mosby, 1960.

Szolar D, Preidler K, Ranner G, et al. The sphenoid sinus during childhood: establishment of normal developmental standards by MRI. Surg Radiol Anat 1994; 16: 193.

Tostevin PMJ, Ellis H. The buccal pad of fat: a review. Clin Anat 1995; 8: 403.

Watson C, Vijayan N. The sympathetic innervation of the eyes and face: a clinicoanatomic review. Clin Anat 1995; 8: 262.

Weddell G, Harpman JA, Lambley DG, et al. The innervation of the musculature of the tongue. J Anat 1940; 74: 255.

Weiglein AH, Anderhuber W, Jakse R, Einspieler R. Imaging of the facial canal by means of multiplanar angulated 2-D-high-resolution CT-reconstruction. Surg Radiol Anat 1994; 16: 423.

Hollinshead's Textbook of Anatomy, by Cornelius Rosse and Penelope Gaddum-Rosse.
Lippincott-Raven Publishers, Philadelphia, © 1997.

CHAPTER 32

The Cranial Parts of the Nervous System

The cranial parts of the nervous system consist of the brain, lodged within the cranial cavity; the 12 pairs of nerves that leave the cranial cavity; and the parts of the autonomic system, sympathetic and parasympathetic, that reach the head or arise there.

The interior of the bony cranium is described in Chapter 31. It should be studied again in connection with the following description, where the importance of the various markings on the interior of the skull, and of the foramina at the base of the skull, will become clearer. The contents of the cranial cavity are the brain and its meninges, associated blood vessels, and parts of the cranial nerves.

BRAIN AND MENINGES

After the calvaria has been cut by a circular incision, it can be pried loose from the underlying membrane, the dura mater, with no great difficulty, for it is only in the midline that there is a strong attachment between the dura and the overlying bone. The outer part of the dura actually is periosteum, but this periosteum is, like the pericranium, not very potent in forming bone. Within the dura mater, the brain is surrounded by the arachnoid and the pia. Both of these membranes are continuous with and structurally similar to the arachnoid and pia that surround the spinal cord.

Some basic knowledge of the anatomy of the brain is necessary to develop an understanding of the meningeal relations and of the relations of various parts of the brain to the bony walls of the cranial cavity. This basic knowledge is best obtained by study of a whole or half brain removed from the cranial cavity and properly hardened and the following description is based on such brains. Because neuroanatomy, which is usually studied separately, is beyond the province of this book, this description is a general one designed merely to introduce the student to gross aspects of the subject.

Cerebral Hemispheres

The great bulk of the brain, and all of that visible after removal of the skull cap, is formed by the two large paired cerebral hemispheres. Each hemisphere is described as having three surfaces: a convex one; a base, the slightly concave inferior surface; and a flat medial surface. The cleft between the medial surfaces of the two hemispheres is the **longitudinal cerebral fissure.** At the bottom of this fissure, the hemispheres are connected by a large bundle of transverse fibers, the **corpus callosum.**

Lobes

Each hemisphere is divided into four lobes, which are named from their chief bony relations (the frontal lobe next to the frontal bone, the temporal lobe next to the temporal bone, and so forth). The lobes are divided from each other by certain arbitrarily determined lines based on the folds and grooves (*gyri* and *sulci*) of the hemisphere.

The **frontal lobe** extends from the *frontal pole* of the brain to the **central sulcus** (Figs. 32-1 and 32-2). Because it lies mostly in the anterior cranial fossa, its lower surface is shallowly concave to fit the orbital roof. Some distance behind the frontal pole a prominent fissure, the **lateral sulcus,** begins below the frontal lobe and runs backward and

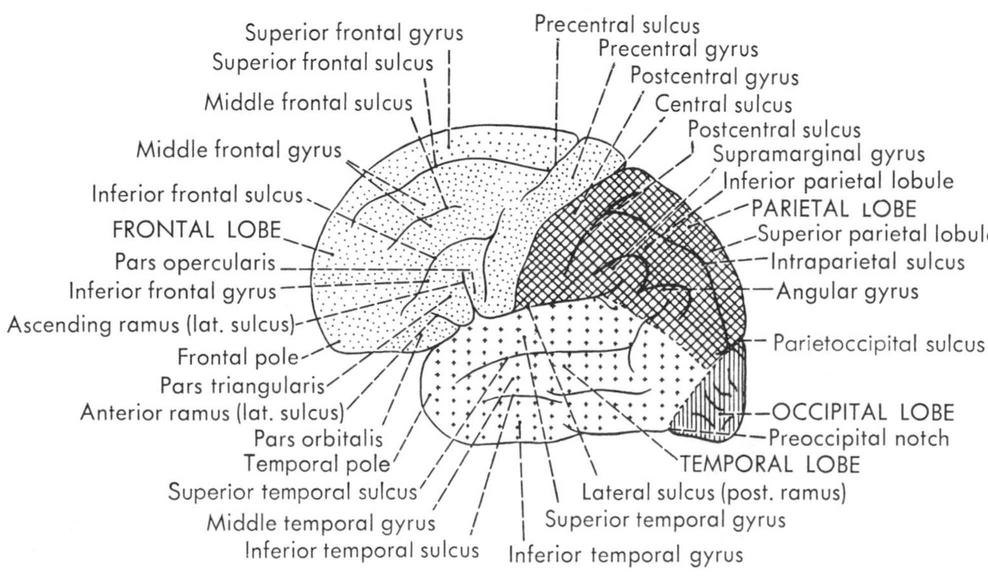

FIGURE *32-1.*
Lobes, gyri, and sulci of the lateral surface of the cerebral hemisphere. (DeJong RN. The neurological examination, 2nd ed. New York: Paul B Hoeber, 1958.)

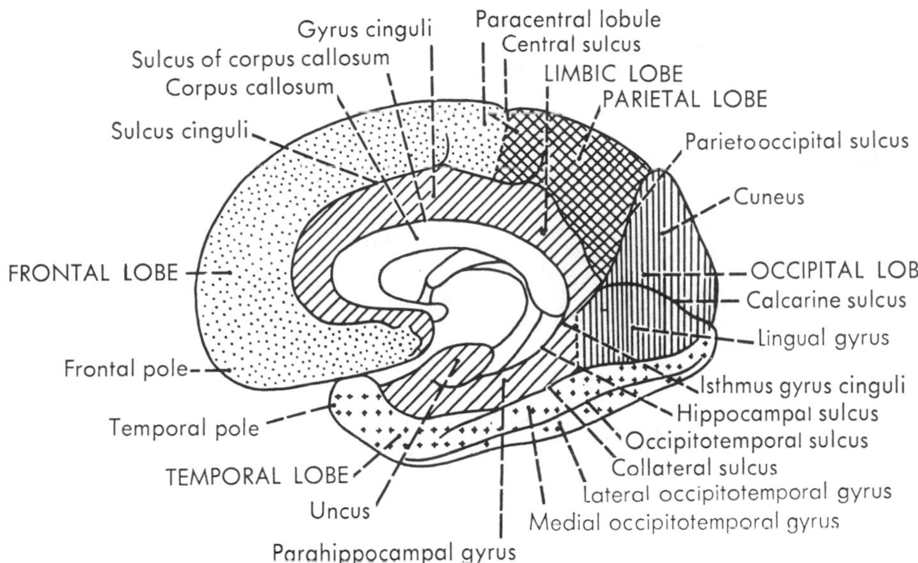

FIGURE 32-2.
Lobes, gyri, and sulci of the medial surface of the cerebral hemisphere. The "limbic lobe," indicated by the *oblique parallel lines,* is not an anatomic lobe in the sense that the other lobes are, but is thought to constitute a functional unit; its parts frequently are assigned to the frontal, parietal, occipital, and temporal lobes, according to their positions. (DeJong RN. The neurological examination. 2nd ed. New York: Paul B Hoeber, 1958.)

upward into the substance of the hemisphere. The part of the hemisphere below this sulcus is the **temporal lobe.** Its convex anterior end, the *temporal pole,* fits into the large lateral part of the middle cranial fossa. The back end of the cerebral hemisphere, the **occipital lobe,** is continuous with the temporal lobe and, like the posterior part of that lobe, lies on a shelf of dura, the *tentorium cerebelli,* that separates it from the posterior cranial fossa. The tentorium lies in the **transverse cerebral fissure,** below the cerebral hemispheres and above the cerebellum. The part of the cerebral hemisphere that lies between frontal, temporal, and occipital lobes is the **parietal lobe.** It is separated from the frontal lobe by the central sulcus. Similarly, it is largely separated from the temporal lobe by the lateral sulcus, but at the back end of this sulcus, parietal, temporal, and occipital lobes are confluent on the lateral surface of the hemisphere. The boundary between the parietal and occipital lobes, and the occipital and the temporal lobes, is best seen on the medial surface of the hemisphere. Here the **parietooccipital sulcus** is its upper part, and the division is completed by a line drawn from that sulcus to the *preoccipital notch* on the base of the hemisphere.

Although the gyri and sulci vary somewhat in different cerebral hemispheres, many are constant enough to be named, and most of them usually are recognizable in all cerebral hemispheres. Some knowledge of them is necessary if important craniocerebral relations are to be grasped.

Sulci and Gyri. Of the sulci visible **on the convex surface** of the brain, the *central* and *lateral sulci* are the most important. Immediately in front of the central sulcus is the *precentral gyrus,* and the frontal lobe anterior to this gyrus is composed of superior, middle, and inferior *frontal gyri.* Behind the central sulcus and above the transverse one is the *postcentral gyrus,* part of the parietal lobe. This lobe also has superior and inferior *parietal lobules.* The *supramarginal* and *angular gyri,* at the level of transition between parietal, temporal, and occipital lobes, are considered to be parts of the parietal lobe. There are three gyri, superior, middle, and inferior *temporal,* on the lateral surface of the temporal lobe. No individual gyri are named on the lateral surface of the occipital lobe.

On the medial side of the hemisphere, the *gyrus cinguli* lies immediately above the corpus callosum. Above it, proceeding from anterior to posterior, are the medial or superior frontal gyrus, the *paracentral lobule* (a fusion of the precentral and postcentral gyri), and the *precuneus.* The *cuneus,* behind and below the precuneus, is separated from that by the parietooccipital sulcus and is bounded below by the *calcarine sulcus.* Below the calcarine sulcus is the *lingual gyrus.* Gyri of the medial and inferior parts of the temporal lobe include the *parahippocampal gyrus,* an anterior continuation of the lingual gyrus that bears the hooklike *uncus* anteriorly; the *medial occipitotemporal gyrus* lateral to the lingual and parahippocampal gyri; and the *lateral occipitotemporal gyrus,* continuous with the inferior temporal gyrus on the lateral surface of the hemisphere.

The approximate relations of the lobes and important sulci of the hemispheres to some of the sutures of the skull are shown in Figure 32-3. These relations vary somewhat among heads, both because of variations in skulls and because of variations in hemispheres. Of importance is that the central sulcus, the division between frontal and parietal lobes, does not at all correspond to the coronal suture. It is not in the coronal plane, and even its most anterior part (its lower end) is behind the coronal suture, whereas its upper end is usually behind a vertical line erected from the external opening of the ear.

The cranial nerve connected with the cerebral hemisphere is the *olfactory,* or first cranial nerve. It consists of such tiny filaments that it is not visible after the brain has been removed. These filaments end in the **olfactory bulb,**

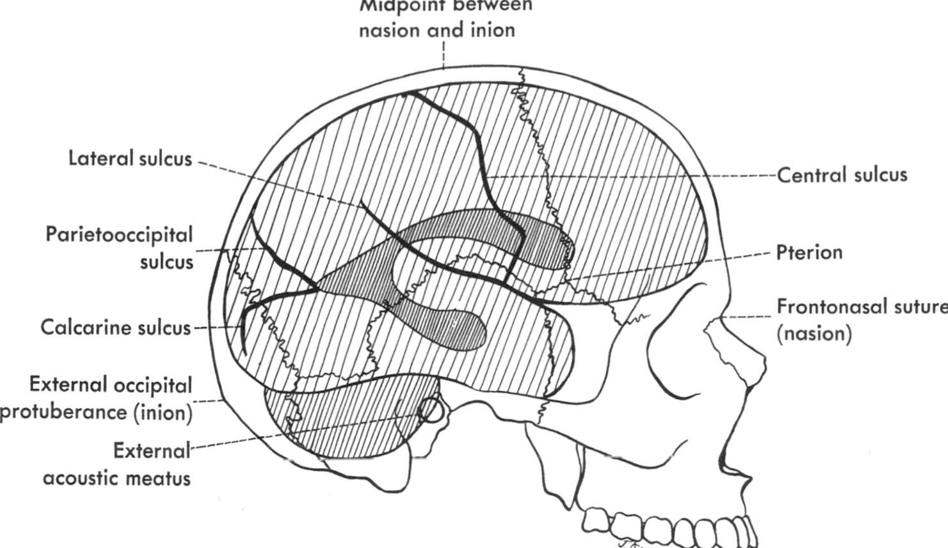

FIGURE 32-3.
Some relations of the brain to the skull: The lateral ventricle is indicated by the *heavily shaded area* in the cerebral hemisphere. The relations of the sulci to the skull are those found in a radiograph of a hemisected head in which the chief sulci had been marked with lead.

an elongated mass of gray matter lying in a groove on the lower surface of the frontal lobe and connected to the base of the hemisphere by the slender olfactory tract. The olfactory bulb lies in the anterior cranial fossa on the cribriform plate. Apertures in the cribriform plate transmit the olfactory nerve.

Interior

The cerebral hemispheres are outgrowths from the upper end of the hollow neural tube (see Chap. 7) and are themselves hollow: each contains a cavity, called a **lateral ventricle** (see Fig. 32-7), which has its *anterior horn* in the frontal lobe, continues back through the frontal and parietal lobes as the *body*, and sends a *posterior horn* toward the occipital lobe and an *inferior horn* curving downward and forward into the temporal lobe. The lateral ventricles do not communicate with each other, but each opens into a centrally placed **third ventricle** that lies between the right and left thalamus.

Most of the thickness of the wall of a cerebral hemisphere is composed of white matter (nerve fibers), but on the inner surface of the wall, close to the lateral ventricle, are some deeply placed masses of gray matter (nerve cells), the largest of which forms the *corpus striatum*. The corpus striatum consists of the *caudate* and the *lenticular* (lentiform) *nucleus* and is traversed by a large fiber bundle, the *internal capsule* (Fig. 32-4).

Cortex

In contrast with the spinal cord, many nerve cells of the cerebral hemisphere have migrated to the outer surface where they completely cover the white matter with a layer of gray matter. This gray matter is the *pallium* or **cerebral cortex,** and its thickness varies from a little more than 1 mm to as much as 4.5 mm. The cortex covers the outer surfaces of the gyri and dips down into the sulci. About two-thirds of the cortex is in the sulci.

Functional Aspects. The fibers in the walls of the cerebral hemispheres connect different parts of the same hemisphere with each other, including not only adjacent gyri, but also, for instance, the frontal and temporal lobes. They connect the two hemispheres, by way of the corpus callosum, and they connect the cerebral hemispheres to lower parts of the brain and to the spinal cord. These fibers include both fibers coming

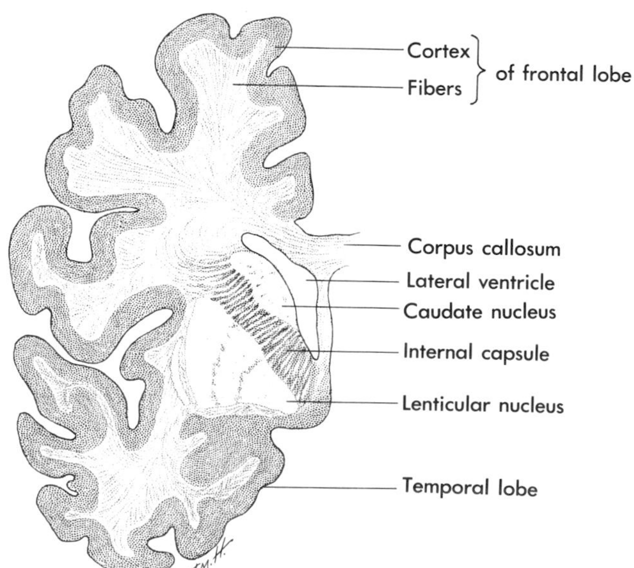

FIGURE 32-4.
A frontal section through the front part of an entire cerebral hemisphere of a child.

into a hemisphere and ones originating in the hemisphere and then leaving it to run downward.

The corpus striatum and certain associated masses, often grouped together as the **basal ganglia,** are reflex centers concerned particularly with voluntary muscle. Injury to them may result in changes in muscle tone and in the appearance of unwanted repetitive movements that interfere with the carrying out of desired movements.

Different parts of the cerebral cortex have specific functions, and within an area of given function, there may be smaller areas that are concerned with different parts of the body. Thus, the precentral gyrus is largely concerned with initiating voluntary movement (hence, it is known as the **motor area**). The adjacent postcentral gyrus is mostly concerned with the recognition of sensations from skin, muscles, and joints; therefore, it is known as the **sensory area.** In both motor and sensory areas, the lower limb is represented toward the top and onto the medial side of the hemisphere (paracentral lobule), the upper limb is represented lower on the lateral surface, and the face, tongue, and larynx are represented on the lowest part. The body is thus represented essentially upside down. It is necessary to remember also that each cortex controls primarily the opposite side of the body, for most ascending impulses cross before they reach the hemisphere, and most descending ones cross after they leave it.

Other important sensory areas include that of sight, centered around the calcarine sulcus, and that of hearing, below the lateral sulcus on the upper surface of the temporal lobe. More posterior parts of the parietal lobe have to do with particularly complex judgments and syntheses, such as recognition of an object placed in the hand through its shape, weight, and texture, or understanding language spoken or written. In one hemisphere, usually the left in right-handed persons, there is, at the back end of the inferior frontal gyrus, a "motor speech area" the function of which is to coordinate the muscles used in speaking. When it is injured, there is no paralysis of muscles, yet the patient says words only with great difficulty (ataxic or motor aphasia).

Parts of the frontal and parietal lobes assist the motor area in controlling voluntary movement, but the larger anterior part of the frontal lobe (called prefrontal cortex), much of the temporal lobe, and much of the medial surface of the hemisphere anterior to the visual area have to do largely with mental activity, rather than movement or sensation.

Because of the specialization in the brain, injuries to it, resulting, for instance, from wounds, tumors, or occlusion of blood vessels, may produce a great variety of symptoms. Sometimes it is possible to localize the area of injury accurately from the symptoms, but in other cases, the lesion is diffuse or involves a part of the brain the function of which is not well understood. Because functional areas of the cerebral cortex are relatively large, lesions of it may affect only one function primarily, or the function of only a part of the body. For instance, there may be a partial loss of sight or paralysis of one limb only. However, many of the fibers going to and from the broad expanse of cortex are collected in the **internal capsule,** and damage to this bundle may affect many motor and sensory activities of a hemisphere. Damage to the internal capsule from infarction or hemorrhage is a common form of stroke, resulting in loss of or decrease in sensation and movement of the opposite side of the body.

Cerebellum

Immediately below the posterior portions of the cerebral hemispheres, and separated from them, when in situ, by the tentorium cerebelli, is the cerebellum (little brain). It consists of paired lateral parts, the **cerebellar hemispheres,** and a smaller midline portion, the **vermis.** The vermis is continuous with both hemispheres, but it is so much smaller that it occupies a notch between them posteriorly and inferiorly. The cerebellum lies in the posterior cranial fossa. The convexity of the hemisphere fits into the concavity of the occipital bone and the adjacent petrous part of the temporal bone.

The cerebellum resembles the cerebral hemisphere in having a cortex that covers a much larger center of white matter. It also has certain masses of gray matter, the **cerebellar nuclei,** embedded deeply in it. The **cerebellar cortex** presents folia and fissures, names that correspond to the sulci and gyri of the cerebral hemisphere. Unlike the cerebral hemisphere, the cerebellum is solid, rather than hollow. It forms, however, a part of the roof of the cavity in the brain at this level (called the fourth ventricle).

No cranial nerve is directly attached to the cerebellum, although the eighth (vestibulocochlear) nerve, which is attached to the brain close to the cerebellum, has intimate connections with this part.

The cerebellum has to do, in part, with the maintenance of balance, and injuries to it of the type sometimes seen in children from tumors may primarily affect balance. However, the largest portion of the cerebellum, in conjunction with the cerebral hemispheres and other parts of the brain, is concerned with helping control the contraction of voluntary muscles and especially with controlling the time and strength of contraction of various muscles so that a desired movement is carried out smoothly and accurately. Damage to the cerebellum, therefore, may result in disturbances of voluntary movement.

Brain Stem

The remaining parts of the brain are so hidden by the cerebral hemispheres and cerebellum that, unless dissected specimens are available, they must be examined largely from below and in sagittal sections of the brain (Figs. 32-5 and 32-6). These parts are collectively called the brain stem and contain the third and fourth ventricles and the aqueduct, cavities derived from that of the neural tube. As in the spinal cord, the gray matter of the brain stem is, for the most part, placed centrally, close to the ventricles and aqueduct, whereas the white matter lies largely on the exterior. There is, however, more mixing of gray and white matter in the brain stem than there is in the spinal cord, and the gray matter, instead of forming continuous masses similar to the gray columns of the spinal cord, is separated into numerous smaller masses known as **nu-**

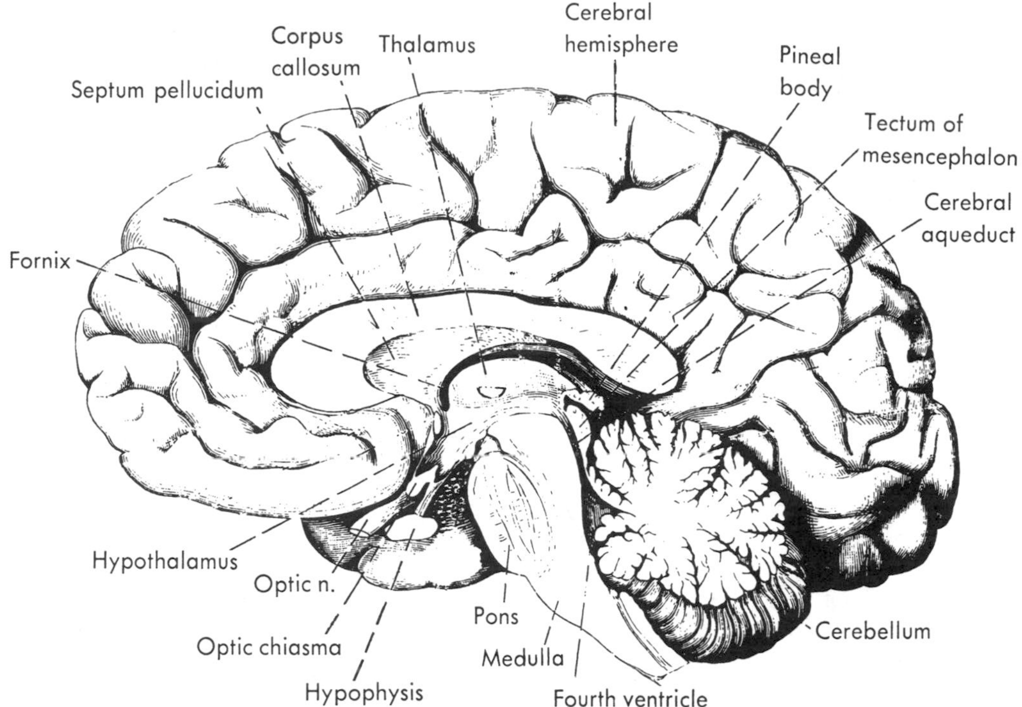

FIGURE *32-5.*
The medial side of a hemisected brain: The cerebral hemispheres have been separated from each other along the longitudinal cerebral fissure; the corpus callosum, brain stem, and cerebellum have been cut. (Henle J. Handbuch der systematischen Anatomie des Menschen, vol 3, pt 2. Braunschweig: Vieweg und Sohn, 1868.)

clei. Many of the nuclei are motor or sensory nuclei of the cranial nerves.

The uppermost part of the brain stem is the **diencephalon.** Only a little of this can be seen from the ventral surface, for the mesencephalon and cerebral hemispheres are close together here. The part visible ventrally is the **hypothalamus,** the region above and posterior to the **optic chiasma** (a prominent cross band of fibers composed of some of the fibers of the optic or second cranial nerve that cross to the opposite side). The nerves coming into the optic chiasma are the **optic nerves.** Leaving the chiasma and running posterolaterally are the two **optic tracts.** They also are part of the diencephalon. Behind the optic chiasma is a grayish protuberance, the **tuber cinereum,** that gives rise to a funnellike **infundibulum.** The **hypophysis,** which lies in the concavity of the sella turcica, normally is attached to the infundibulum. The little rounded eminences **(mammillary bodies)** behind the infundibulum also belong to the hypothalamus.

The **thalamus** is the largest part of the diencephalon, but much of it is buried in the cerebral hemispheres and cannot be seen, except in a hemisected brain. The thick right and left thalami are separated from each other by a slitlike cavity, the **third ventricle.** The ventricle's roof is thin, like that of the fourth ventricle, and usually has been torn away in prepared specimens. Its floor and the lower part of its walls are the hypothalamus. Posteriorly, the third ventricle is connected to the fourth ventricle by the narrow cerebral aqueduct that traverses the mesencephalon. Anterolaterally, it communicates by an *interventricular foramen* with each of the lateral (first two) ventricles in the cerebral hemispheres.

The diencephalon lies anterior to the tentorium cerebelli, and the hypothalamus lies directly above the narrow midline part of the middle cranial fossa, the sella turcica, that contains the hypophysis. Because the hypothalamus and the optic chiasma, nerves, and tracts are so close to the hypophysis, tumors of this gland may affect the visual system, causing partial blindness (commonly in both eyes), or may affect the functions of the hypothalamus. Operations on tumors of the gland are particularly delicate because of the vascular relations here, the presence of the optic system, and the hypothalamus. The hypothalamus is concerned with many basic functions of the body, including temperature regulation, appetite, and the control of the hypophysis, the "master gland" of the endocrine system. Therefore, operations in its region are sometimes attended by alarming or even fatal disturbances of these basic mechanisms—for instance, a transient period of extremely high fever often follows removal of tumors here.

The only nerves attaching to the diencephalon are the optic nerves, already noted. These, originating in the eyeballs, enter the cranial cavity through the optic canals, just at the anterior end of the sella turcica.

The diencephalon is followed by the **midbrain** or **mesencephalon.** On its ventral surface are two heavy

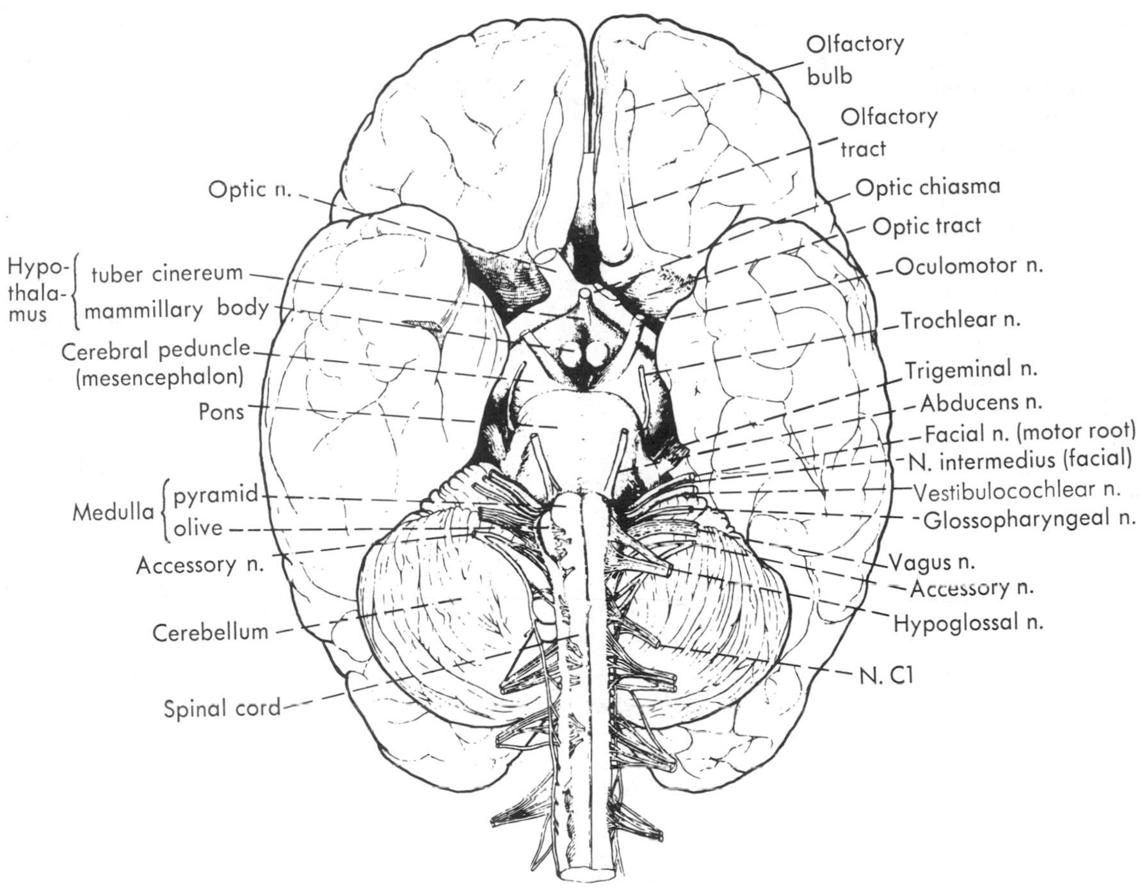

FIGURE *32-6.*
View of the base of the brain and the ventral surface of the brain stem and an upper part of the spinal cord. (Henle J. Handbuch der systematischen Anatomie des Menschen, vol 3, pt 2. Braunschweig: Vieweg und Sohn, 1868.)

fiber bundles, the **cerebral peduncles,** that converge as they run inferiorly and disappear into the pons. On the dorsal surface of the midbrain are two swellings on each side, the superior and inferior **colliculi** (little hills). Running through it is a cavity, usually somewhat smaller than the lead of a pencil, which is the **cerebral aqueduct,** the mesencephalic part of the ventricular system.

The mesencephalon lies at the junction of the posterior and middle cranial fossae, partly in both. Because the central part of the middle cranial fossa above the concavity of the sella turcica is almost horizontal, and the central part of the posterior cranial fossa, the clivus, slopes markedly downward, the brain stem is angulated here; thus, the mesencephalon is longer dorsally, where the colliculi are, than it is ventrally at the acute angle of the bend.

Two pairs of cranial nerves arise from the mesencephalon. The **third cranial nerve (oculomotor)** leaves it close to the medial edge of the cerebral peduncle, at the upper border of the pons. It runs laterally and forward to enter the dura mater just anterolateral to the posterior clinoid process. The **fourth cranial nerve (trochlear)** is the only one that attaches to the dorsal aspect of the brain. It leaves the brain at the lower border of the inferior colliculus. At first it runs laterally and then bends forward around the colliculus, passing through the posterior cranial fossa immediately below the tentorium cerebelli to enter the lower surface of this dural shelf just behind the dorsum sellae.

The **pons** or **metencephalon** succeeds the mesencephalon. All that is visible from the surface is a band of fibers of considerable superoinferior width, when viewed anteriorly, but narrower and more cordlike when viewed from the side. This band resembles a bridge between the two cerebellar hemispheres and gives the part its name (*pons* meaning bridge). Actually, the pontine fibers do not connect the two cerebellar hemispheres; rather, each side of the pons is part of the connection between the opposite cerebral hemisphere and the cerebellar hemisphere into which it can be traced. Dorsal to the transverse pontine fibers is a mixture of nuclei and fibers that makes this part of the pons essentially similar in structure to the upper part of the medulla. The upper part of the fourth ventricle lies in the pons, largely covered by the cerebellum.

The pons lies in the most anterior part of the posterior cranial fossa, against the upper part of the clivus and the posterior wall of the dorsum sellae. Only one cranial nerve, the **fifth** or **trigeminal,** attaches to it. This leaves laterally, through the narrower lateral part, and has two roots: a large *sensory root* and a small *motor root*. The two roots run anterolaterally from the posterior into the middle cranial fossa by passing across a notch on the upper border of the anterior end of the petrous part of the temporal bone. This notch is converted into a foramen by the attachment of the tentorium cerebelli above it. The *trigeminal ganglion* lies in the middle cranial fossa, and its branches leave the skull by foramina in this fossa.

The last part of the brain stem, obviously an upward continuation from the spinal cord, is the **medulla oblongata (myelencephalon).** Although the upper end of the medulla differs markedly in both size and structure from the cord, the lower end is very much like the cord, and there is no sharp transition between the two. The medulla usually is described as beginning at the level of the foramen magnum or at the uppermost rootlet of the first spinal nerve (these being at about the same level). The medulla expands, particularly laterally, as it is traced upward. Its upper border is the level at which it disappears deep to a heavy bundle of transversely placed fibers, the pons. The lowermost end of the medulla contains a tiny central canal, the upward continuation of the central canal of the spinal cord. As the medulla expands laterally, however, the central canal widens rapidly into the **fourth ventricle,** which is eccentrically placed in the medulla. Instead of lying centrally, it lies dorsally, and much of its roof is a thin membrane that stretches between the thicker lateral walls. It is frequently torn away from the specimen so that one can look into the fourth ventricle. The dorsal surface of the medulla lies against the lower and anterior surface of the cerebellum, which forms a major part of the roof of the fourth ventricle. At its upper end, above the cerebellum, the fourth ventricle tapers again to a small canal, the cerebral aqueduct.

The medulla lies in the posterior cranial fossa, as does the cerebellum, with its lower surface against the clivus. The last seven cranial nerves are attached to the medulla. Of these, the sixth nerve arises ventrally (anteriorly) at the caudal border of the pons; the seventh and eighth arise laterally just caudal to the lateral part of the pons and partly under cover of the cerebellar hemisphere; the ninth, 10th, and a part of the 11th arise by a series of small filaments from the lateral side of the medulla; and the 12th leaves the medulla anteriorly or ventrally, as does the sixth, arising by a number of rootlets that lie in a groove just medial to a smooth ovoid enlargement (the olive) that is present anterolaterally on the medulla.

The **sixth (abducens) nerve** has a short course downward and forward from the medulla to the dura over the clivus. After entering the dura, it runs forward in it as far as the superior orbital fissure, through which it enters the orbit.

The **seventh (facial) and eighth (vestibulocochlear) nerves** run laterally together from their origin, and both enter the internal acoustic meatus, on the posterior surface of the petrous part of the temporal bone.

The **ninth (glossopharyngeal), 10th (vagus),** and **11th (cranial accessory) nerves** run laterally and slightly forward to enter the anterior and middle compartments in the jugular foramen. The cranial roots of the accessory nerve are joined by spinal roots that leave the spinal cord and ascend alongside it to enter through the foramen magnum.

The last cranial nerve, the **12th (hypoglossal),** runs laterally to the hypoglossal canal.

Ventricles and Cerebrospinal Fluid

The cerebrospinal fluid fills the subarachnoid space and, therefore, surrounds the brain and spinal cord. Most of this fluid is formed in the ventricles of the brain where plexuses of blood vessels, the choroid plexuses, project into the ventricles by invaginating the medial walls of the lateral ventricles and the roofs of the third and fourth ventricles. The fluid formed within the lateral ventricles passes through the

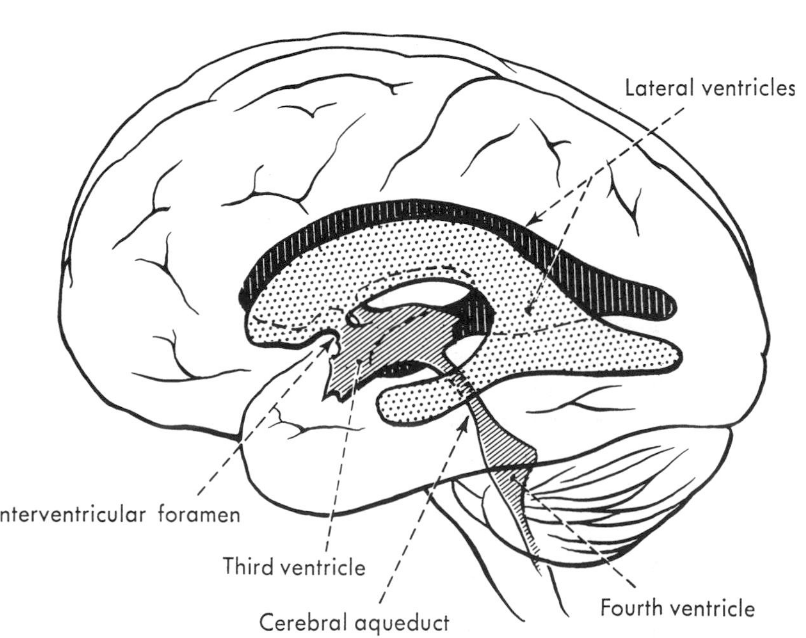

FIGURE *32-7.*
Diagram of the ventricular system of the brain. (Rushton JD. Neurology for nurses. Minneapolis: Burgess Publishing Co, copyright Mayo Association, 1959.)

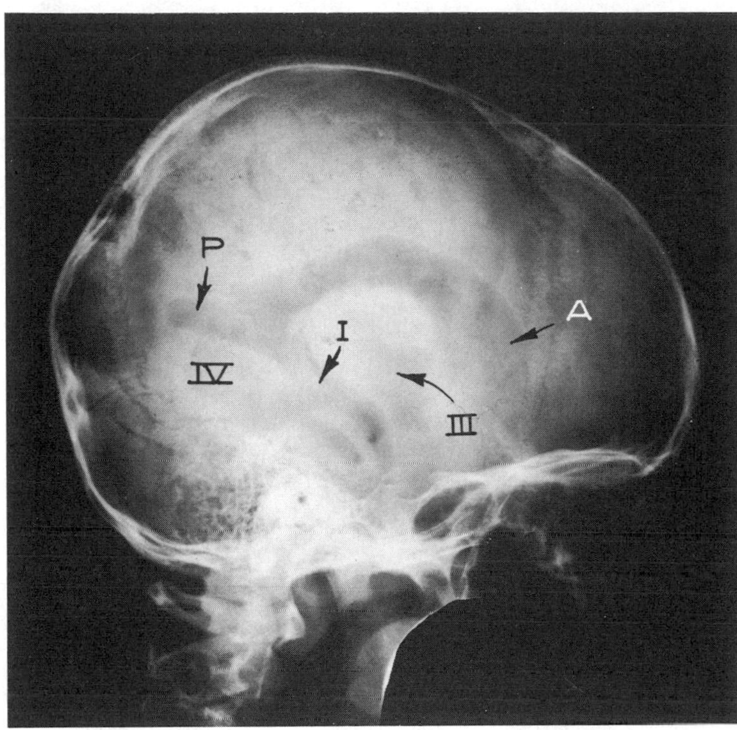

FIGURE 32-8.
A lateral ventriculogram in which the ventricular system has been fairly well filled with air. *A*, *P*, and *I* identify the anterior, posterior, and inferior horns, respectively, of the lateral ventricle, and *III* and *IV* identify the third and fourth ventricles. Some of the ventricular system of the other side also shows faintly. (Courtesy of Dr. D. G. Pugh.)

interventricular foramina into the third ventricle (Fig. 32-7), which adds additional fluid. It then passes through the narrow aqueduct into the fourth ventricle, where more fluid is added, and escapes from the fourth ventricle into the subarachnoid space through paired *lateral apertures* on the sides of the roof, which open close to the cerebellum and the ninth nerve, and through a *median aperture* in the caudal part of the roof. Cerebrospinal fluid continues to be formed in the lateral ventricles, sometimes at an unreduced rate, after complete ablation of the choroid plexuses. The source of its formation under these circumstances is unknown.

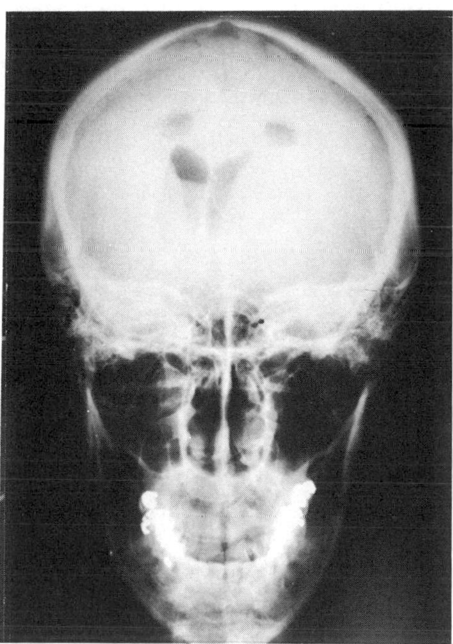

FIGURE 32-9.
An anteroposterior ventriculogram showing displacement of the left lateral ventricle to the right by a tumor. The *round areas* above the ventricular system are the burr holes through which air was introduced into the ventricles. (Courtesy of Dr. D. G. Pugh)

Meningitis (inflammation of the membranes of the brain) may result in the formation of scar tissue that closes the foramina of the fourth ventricle, or a tumor in the mesencephalon may occlude the aqueduct, preventing the escape of cerebrospinal fluid into the subarachnoid space. The result of this occlusion is *hydrocephalus*. The pressure in hydrocephalus dilates the ventricles of the brain and exerts pressure on the cerebral hemispheres, which are damaged in an adult by being squeezed between the fluid inside and the unyielding skull outside. In infants and young children, in whom the bones of the cranium are not yet joined, the internal pressure enlarges both the brain and the skull, widening the sutures and the fontanels. When the condition is not relieved, the cranium may become exceedingly large and the brain substance so stretched that it may be no more than a thin membrane. Such extreme conditions necessarily result in idiocy. It is, however, possible in some cases to remove the obstruction by operation and in others to devise a drainage system that allows escape of the fluid.

Air can be injected into one or both lateral ventricles to demonstrate them for radiographic examination (Fig. 32-8) Proper views of an air ventriculogram may show distortion or displacement of a ventricle (Fig. 32-9) and thus aid in diagnosing or localizing a tumor within the cranial cavity.

After the cerebrospinal fluid has escaped into the subarachnoid space, some of it circulates downward around the spinal cord, but that which remains in the cranial cavity around the brain circulates upward to the dorsal midline. Here **arachnoid villi** project into the lateral lacunae alongside the superior sagittal sinus, and through these thin-walled villi, the cerebrospinal fluid is returned to the bloodstream.

Small amounts of cerebrospinal fluid are apparently added from the tissue spaces, which drain to the surface of the brain along minute perivascular spaces. These apparently act in place of lymphatics in the central nervous system, which has no true lymphatics.

Cranial Meninges

The meninges of the brain (Fig. 32-10) are continuous with those about the spinal cord, receive the same names—dura mater, arachnoid, and pia mater—and are generally similar in structure and arrangement save in one respect: the cranial dura mater, instead of being separated from the bone and its covering periosteum by an extradural (epidural) space, as is that of the spinal cord, is fused to the periosteum on the inner surface of the skull. The strongest points of attachment are along venous sinuses and, at the base of the skull, to projecting ridges of bone and about the foramina. Elsewere the dura is not so tightly attached. Thus the calvaria may be readily separated from the dura, thus facilitating removal of bone for an operation on the brain. The **epidural space** (Fig. 32-11) in the cranial cavity is actually subperiosteal, between the periosteal layer of the dura and the bone of the skull. It is therefore, a potential space that becomes real when, for instance, there is an accumulation of blood between the dural and the bone as a result of a fractured skull.

Dura Mater and Venous Sinuses

Except for certain shelf-like projections, the dura mater conforms accurately to the shape of the cranial cavity. The projections that partially subdivide the cranial cavity (Fig. 32-12) are the falx cerebri (cerebral fold) and the tentorium cerebelli (tent of the cerebellum); there also are two smaller projections, the falx cerebelli and the diaphragma sellae.

The **falx cerebri** is a crescentic fold that projects downward between the two cerebral hemispheres. At its attachment to the convexity of the dura, the falx is divided into right and left layers, between which lies the *superior sagittal sinus.* In its free lower border, above the corpus callosum, is the small *inferior sagittal sinus.* At its front end, the falx is attached below to the crista galli and frontal crest, and at its back end, it is attached to and blends with the upper surface of the tentorium cerebelli.

The **tentorium cerebelli** is a layer of dura that intervenes between the lower surfaces of the cerebral hemispheres and the upper surface of the cerebellum and roofs the posterior cranial fossa. It is attached posteriorly to the occipital bone along the grooves for the *transverse sinuses,* which it partly encloses, and laterally to the uppermost part of the petrous portions of the temporal bones and to the posterior clinoid processes. The center of the tentorium, where it meets the falx cerebri, is higher than its sides, giving it a tentlike appearance. Its anterior free border is likewise highest in the midline and from this midline curves downward and forward to the posterior clinoid process on each side. Thus, a somewhat oval aperture is left between the free edge of the falx and the posterior surface of the dorsum sellae. This aperture, the *tentorial incisure* or notch, is occupied by the upper end of the mesencephalon.

The **falx cerebelli** is a small fold in the posterior mid-

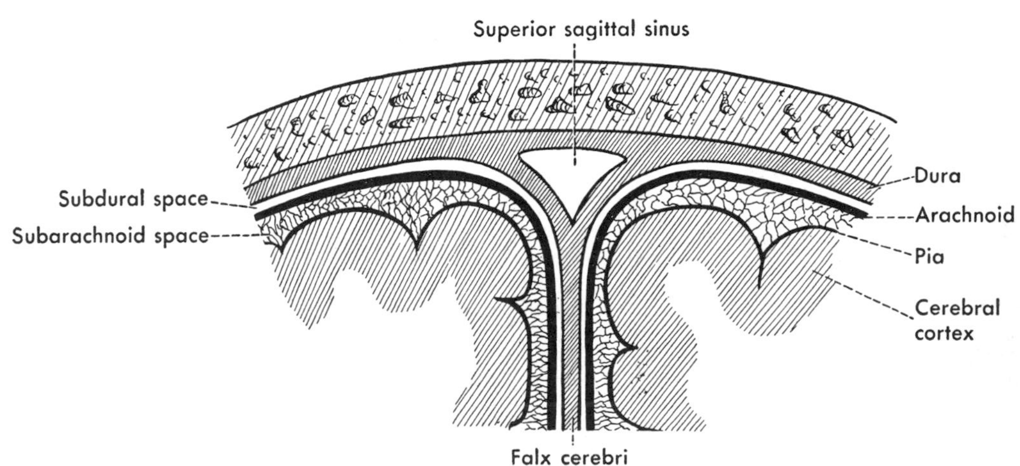

FIGURE *32-10.*
A small part of the skull and the meninges close to the upper medial surface of the cerebral hemispheres. The slitlike subdural space is much exaggerated.

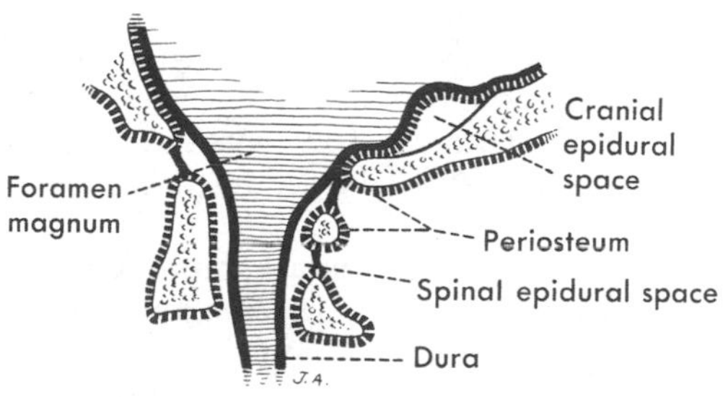

FIGURE 32-11.
Difference between the spinal and cranial epidural spaces. The cranial dura has been elevated to form an epidural space.

line of the posterior cranial fossa, running upward to the lower surface of the tentorium cerebelli. Its free edge projects between the two cerebellar hemispheres.

The **diaphragma sellae** is a layer of dura that largely covers the hypophyseal fossa in the sella turcica, but has in its middle an aperture, of variable size, through which passes the hypophyseal stalk connecting the hypothalamus and the hypophysis. Hypophyseal tumors, to affect the hypothalamic region or the optic system above them, must either expand through the opening in the diaphragm or bulge it upward.

The tentorial incisure is a little larger than is necessary to accommodate the brain stem; hence, when the pressure above the tentorium is markedly greater than that below (as may be true when there is a tumor), a part of the adjacent temporal lobe may herniate through the incisure. Tentorial herniation may lacerate the temporal lobe against the tough edge of the tentorium or, more seriously, stretch or compress various cranial nerves and compress blood vessels and the brain stem.

The dura mater has relatively little blood supply, for the middle meningeal arteries, the largest, supply the skull more than they do the dura. If these arteries are injured, as they may be in skull fracture, they can give rise to serious bleeding either epidurally or into the subarachnoid space. Tiny branches from several other arteries, including the internal carotid, also usually help supply the dura of the middle fossa at the base of the skull.

After the **middle meningeal artery** enters the skull through the foramen spinosum, it runs laterally and divides into a *frontal* and a *parietal branch,* the courses of which are indicated by grooves on the inner surface of the skull. Smaller branches of the middle meningeal include a *petrosal branch* that enters the canal of the greater petrosal nerve, a *superior tympanic artery* that enters the tympanic cavity from above, and a *communicating branch* with the lacrimal artery in the orbit.

Anterior meningeal arteries are small twigs from the ethmoidal arteries to the floor of the anterior cranial fossa. **Posterior meningeal arteries** usually are two, a branch of the ascending pharyngeal and one of the occipital artery, which enter the skull through the jugular foramen and supply dura in the posterior fossa.

Sensory nerve filaments are distributed to the dura, especially along the courses of the venous sinuses and the middle meningeal artery. Although the dura is relatively insensitive, stimulation along the vessels, particularly, gives rise to pain that is "referred to" (localized by a conscious patient as coming from)

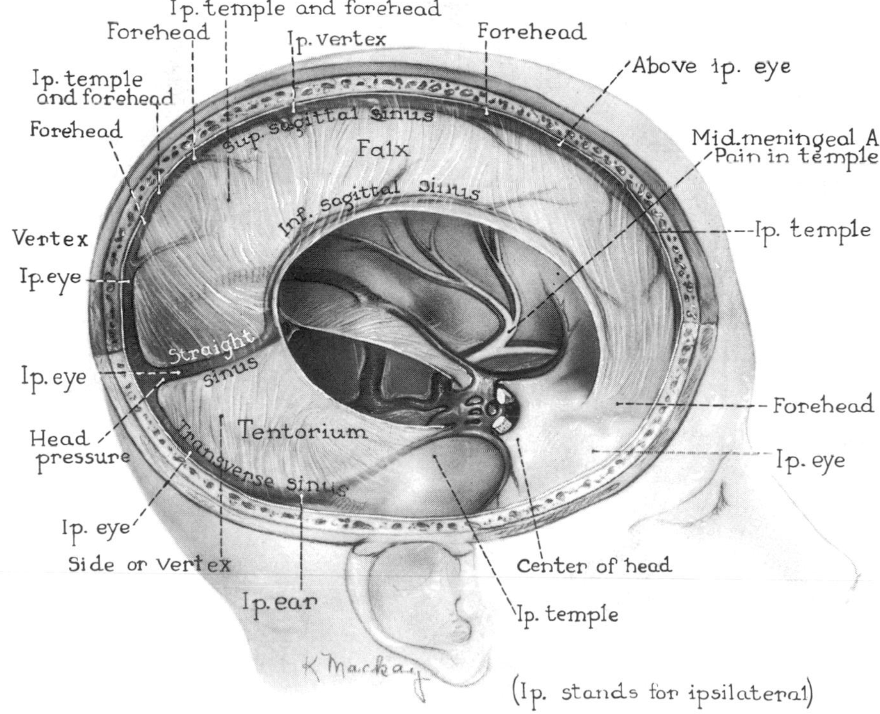

FIGURE 32-12.
The falx cerebri and tentorium cerebelli, the venous sinuses related to them, and the areas of the head to which pain is referred by the patient when the dura is stimulated. Behind the cut ends of the optic nerves is the diaphragma sellae with its central aperture. (Baker GS, Adson AW. Minn Med 1943, 26:282.)

various parts of the head. The **meningeal nerves** to the anterior and middle cranial fossae and to the supratentorial dura are all derived from the trigeminal nerve: the anterior ethmoidal branch of the ophthalmic division gives twigs to the floor of the anterior cranial fossa, and just before it leaves the middle cranial fossa, the stem of the ophthalmic gives off a tentorial branch that sweeps backward and upward over the tentorium cerebelli and the falx cerebri; the maxillary and mandibular divisions both give rise to meningeal branches that supply the floor of the middle fossa and otherwise largely follow the middle meningeal artery. In the posterior fossa are meningeal branches of the vagus and hypoglossal nerves. Both branches apparently consist largely of fibers from upper cervical nerves that have joined the main nerves extracranially, and the hypoglossal branch, at least, consists entirely of such fibers.

Most of the venous sinuses that lie within the dura are rather simply arranged. The **superior sagittal sinus** lies in the midline at the junction of the upper border of the falx cerebri with the dura over the convexity of the hemispheres (see Figs. 32-10 and 32-12). It begins at the front end of the crista galli and ends at the back end of the junction of the upper border of the falx with the tentorium cerebelli, where it is the largest of the several sinuses that come together here to form the **confluence of the sinuses.** Lateral to the main channel of the superior sagittal sinus, there are a variable number of expansions, the **lateral lacunae,** of otherwise tiny meningeal veins that enter the sinus.

The **inferior sagittal sinus** runs in the free edge of the falx cerebri. As the falx joins the tentorium, the sinus and the *great cerebral vein,* draining deeper parts of the brain, unite to form the **straight sinus** (sinus rectus). This runs posteriorly, still in the midline, at the junction of falx cerebri and tentorium cerebelli and also ends in the confluence of the sinuses. The **occipital sinus** often is small, but is sometimes very large . It begins in paired parts, usually called **marginal sinuses,** around the foramen magnum and runs upward at the attached border of the falx cerebelli, to join the confluence of the sinuses (Fig. 32-13). It and the marginal sinuses communicate with the internal vertebral venous plexuses.

From the confluence of the sinuses, there proceed laterally, at the posterior border of the attachment of the tentorium to the skull, two **transverse sinuses** (see Fig. 32-13). Usually the right one is larger, for the superior sagittal sinus often turns primarily to the right, giving only a small communication to the left transverse sinus. When this occurs, the occipital and straight sinuses usually join the left transverse sinus. The transverse sinuses run laterally in the attached edge of the tentorium to the posterior ends of the petrous parts of the temporal bones. Here their names change to **sigmoid sinuses,** each of which courses downward, medially, and forward, in a deep groove situated at the junction of occipital and temporal bones, and leaves the skull through the posterior part of the jugular foramen. Outside the skull, the sigmoid sinus is continued as the internal jugular vein.

The **superior petrosal sinus** is relatively small and

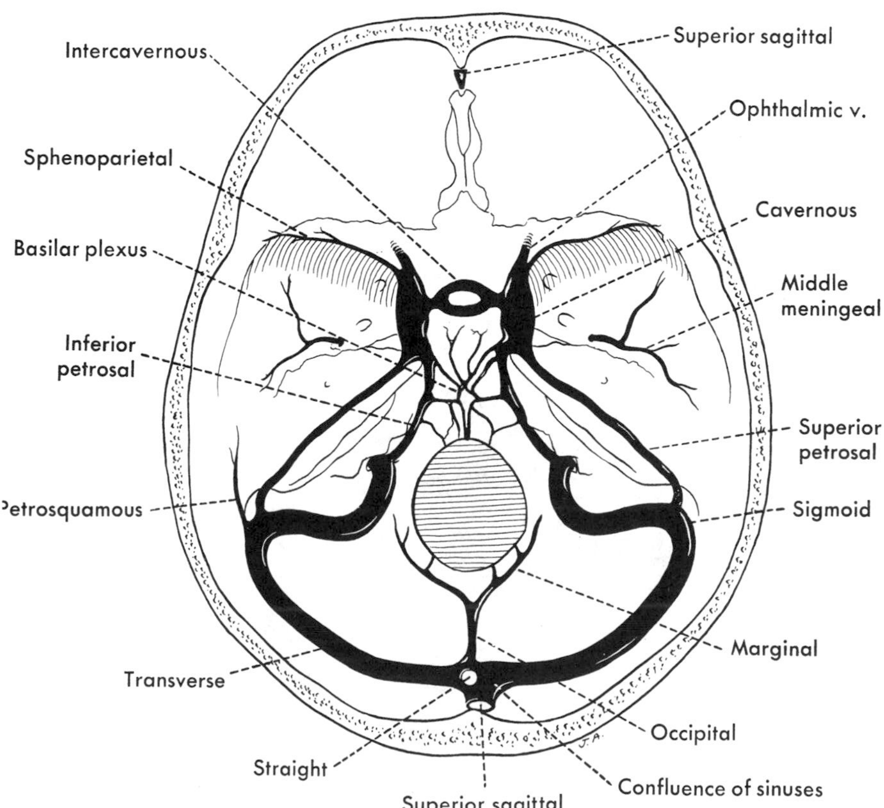

FIGURE *32-13.*
The chief venous sinuses at the base of the skull. The petrosquamous sinus, shown here on the *left side* only, is variable in its presence.

runs along the upper border of the petrous part of the temporal bone. Posteriorly, it joins the upper end of the sigmoid sinus. Anteriorly, it joins the cavernous sinus. The **inferior petrosal sinus,** usually larger than the superior, runs along the sphenoid and occipital bones at their junction with the petrous portion of the temporal. It originates from the cavernous sinus and leaves the skull through the anterior part of the jugular foramen, joining the internal jugular vein just outside the foramen. Between the two inferior petrosal sinuses, extending downward on the clivus to the foramen magnum, is a plexus of small veins, the **basilar plexus.**

The **cavernous sinuses** lie on each side of the sella turcica, where each surrounds the internal carotid artery of its side and is traversed also by the nerves that go to the orbit. Instead of containing a single large cavity, as do most of the cranial venous sinuses, the cavity of the cavernous sinus is broken up into numerous communicating chambers and therefore blood flow through it is slow. The cavernous sinuses of the two sides communicate with each other through an *intercavernous sinus* situated in the diaphragma sellae. They drain posteriorly through the superior and inferior petrosal sinuses. Anteriorly, each receives the ophthalmic vein or veins and also the small **sphenoparietal sinus** that lies along the posterior edge of the lesser wing of the sphenoid bone.

Although most of the blood from the brain leaves the skull by way of the internal jugular veins, into which the sigmoid and inferior petrosal sinuses empty, some can leave by other routes. The basilar plexus and the occipital sinus anastomose through the foramen magnum with the internal vertebral venous plexuses, and since neither these nor the cranial venous sinuses have any valves, blood can leave by this route. The superior or both ophthalmic veins, through their connections with both the cavernous sinus and the angular vein, likewise can conduct blood in either direction. There also are a number of fairly constant **emissary veins** through which blood can escape from the skull.

There are approximately six paired communications between vessels inside and those outside the skull that can be termed emissary veins, and there may be unpaired ones. The three pairs that are named emissary veins are the *parietal emissary veins,* which penetrate the parietal bones posterior to their middles, only a little on each side of the midline, and connect the superior sagittal sinus to tributaries of the two occipital veins; one or more *mastoid emissary veins,* which emerge through the mastoid processes to connect the sigmoid sinuses to the occipital or posterior auricular veins; and the *condylar emissary veins,* not always present, which pass through the condylar canals and connect the lower ends of the sigmoid sinuses with the suboccipital plexus just below the base of the skull. There may also be an unpaired *occipital emissary vein* passing through the occipital protuberance and connecting the confluence of the sinuses to a tributary of one of the occipital veins. The front end of the superior sagittal sinus in the child, although not often in the adult, is connected to veins of the nose through emissary veins in the foramen cecum.

There also are three plexuses that are really emissary veins: an *internal carotid venous plexus* around the artery connects the cavernous sinus with the internal jugular vein or the pharyngeal plexus (which empties into the internal jugular); a *venous plexus of the foramen ovale,* accompanying the mandibular branch of the fifth nerve, connects the cavernous sinus to the pterygoid plexus of veins; and a *venous plexus of the hypoglossal canal* accompanying the hypoglossal nerve, connects the lower part of the occipital sinus with the upper end of the internal jugular vein or the terminal part of the inferior petrosal sinus.

The emissary veins generally cannot be much enlarged because their size is limited by the surrounding bone; however, they, and particularly the connections to the vertebral venous plexuses, apparently can carry a great deal of blood. It was long held that simultaneous occlusion of both internal jugular veins would necessarily be fatal, because they receive by far the major amount of blood leaving the cranial cavity; however, it is possible to ligate and remove both internal jugular veins (in a radical dissection of the neck for carcinoma) in one operation.

Arachnoid, Pia, and Subarachnoid Space

The smooth outer surface of the **arachnoid** lies against the inner surface of the dura, separated from it only by a slitlike subdural space that contains enough fluid to keep the adjacent surfaces moist. From the inner surface of the arachnoid extend the cobwebby trabeculae that give the membrane its name. These cross the subarachnoid space and become continuous with the pia (see Fig. 32-10). Along the superior sagittal sinus, the arachnoid is tightly attached to the dura by *arachnoid granulations* (macroscopic collections of arachnoid villi) that it sends through the dura to project into the lateral lacunae of the sinus and that provide drainage for the cerebrospinal fluid. The positions of the largest granulations often are marked on the inner surface of the skull by *foveolae granulares* that result from absorption of the adjacent bone.

The **pia mater** consists of a thin layer of connective tissue covered by flattened cells continuous with those of the arachnoid. It is closely attached to the substance of the brain and follows its every contour. Thus, in contrast with the arachnoid, it dips into the sulci of the cerebral cortex, and it closely invests the roots of the cranial nerves as they leave the brain. Because the pia follows the contours of the brain, whereas the arachnoid follows those of the dura, the subarachnoid space is larger at some levels than at others. For instance, it is larger over the sulci than over the gyri of the hemispheres.

The larger expansions of the subarachnoid space are known as **cisterns** because they contain the largest accumulations of cerebrospinal fluid (Fig. 32-14). Those named by anatomists are the *cisterna cerebellomedullaris,* often called the cisterna magna, in the angle between the inferior surface of the cerebellum and the posterior surface of the medulla; the *cistern of the lateral cerebral fossa,* above the temporal pole; the *cisterna chiasmatis,* anterior to and above the optic chiasma; and the *cisterna interpeduncularis,* between the cerebral peduncles. The boundaries of none of these are really distinct, and the last-named two

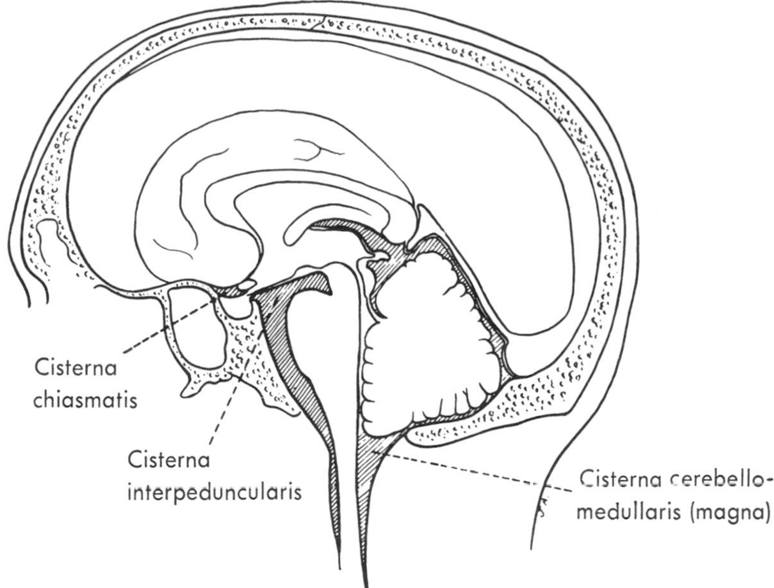

FIGURE 32-14.
Subarachnoid cisterns in a median sagittal section of the head. The labeled ones are those recognized in the official terminology, but those over the cerebellum and midbrain, and one ventral to the pons, can also be seen.

have been grouped together as the *cisterna basalis*. Clinicians use a variety of names to identify not only these, but many others, including dorsolateral extensions from the cisterns at the base of the brain, extensions from the cisterna cerebellomedullaris over the cerebellum and midbrain, and a cistern between the two cerebral hemispheres just above the corpus callosum. They can be studied by injecting air or radiopaque material into them (*encephalography*).

Blood Supply of the Brain

There are two sets of arteries to the brain, the paired internal carotids and the paired vertebrals (see Fig. 32-16). From its origin in the neck, the **internal carotid** ascends posterolateral to the wall of the pharynx to enter the carotid canal in the lower surface of the petrous portion of the temporal bone. This canal turns forward in the bone, and the internal carotid leaves the canal at the apex of the petrous part, just above the foramen lacerum. It runs upward and forward on the side of the sella turcica, through the cavernous sinus. It then turns upward and medially just medial to the anterior clinoid process, penetrating the dura and giving off a branch, the **ophthalmic artery,** that follows the lower surface of the optic nerve to reach the orbit. The part of the carotid artery close to the sella is often referred to as the "carotid siphon." The chief branches of the carotid are to the brain and, therefore, are best examined on a brain that has been removed from the skull, as are also the branches of the vertebral arteries.

Vertebral Arteries

The vertebral arteries reach the interior of the skull by ascending through the transverse foramina of the cervical vertebrae, turning medially along the upper surface of the posterior arch of the atlas and then penetrating the posterior atlantooccipital membrane and the underlying dura to enter the subarachnoid space and pass through the foramen magnum into the cranial cavity.

Although the vertebral arteries lie somewhat lateral to the lower end of the medulla, each gives off a small **posterior spinal artery** that runs down the spinal cord at about the point of attachment of the posterior nerve roots. Before the vertebral arteries come together on the ventral surface of the medulla, each gives off a root of the **anterior spinal artery** (Fig. 32-15). These two roots unite to form an artery that runs down in the anterior median fissure of the cord. These spinal branches are small and by no means sufficient to supply the length of the spinal cord. They are reinforced at irregular intervals by segmental arteries that pierce the dura and run along the spinal nerve roots to join them. Each vertebral artery also gives off branches to the medulla and a **posterior inferior cerebellar artery** to the posteroinferior surface of the cerebellum. The vertebral arteries end by fusing to form the **basilar artery.**

The basilar artery runs forward on the lower surface of the pons, gives off branches to that, and gives rise to

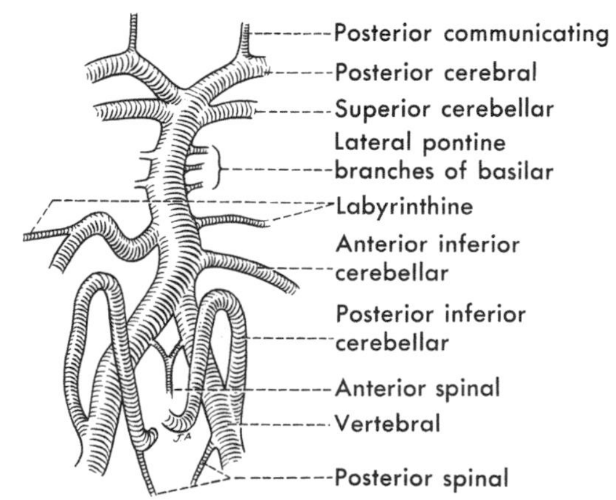

FIGURE 32-15.
The vertebral arteries and their intracranial branches.

two pairs of arteries to the cerebellum. Each **anterior inferior cerebellar artery** arises at about the level of the eighth nerve and often loops laterally along the nerve. It usually gives off the **labyrinthine artery** (to the internal ear), which follows the seventh and eighth nerves into the internal acoustic meatus, and it is distributed to the anterior or ventral surface of the cerebellum. The **superior cerebellar arteries** arise just before the basilar artery ends. They run laterally around the brain stem, which they help to supply, to reach the superior surface of the cerebellum.

Just beyond the origin of the superior cerebellar arteries, the basilar artery bifurcates into the **posterior cerebral arteries.** These also run laterally around and help to supply the brain stem. They then pass above the tentorium cerebelli and are distributed to the lower surface of the back part of the temporal lobe and to the occipital lobe. On the surface of the cortex, the cerebral arteries (there are three on each hemisphere) anastomose with each other; their central branches that pass into the brain do not anastomose, however.

Arterial Circle

The *circulus arteriosus cerebri* (circle of Willis) is a somewhat hexagonal formation of blood vessels at the base of the brain close to the sella turcica. It connects the vertebral and internal carotid arteries to each other and to the vessels of the opposite side (Fig. 32-16). Anteriorly, the circle is formed by the *internal carotid arteries*, their *anterior cerebral* branches, and an *anterior communicating artery* that connects the two anterior cerebrals. Each internal carotid also sends a *posterior communicating artery* to connect with the *posterior cerebral* of its side, and the origins of the posterior cerebrals from the basilar complete the circle posteriorly. Parts of the circle, particularly the posterior communicating arteries, vary much in size. Depending on this, blood may or may not be easily shunted from one side of the brain to the other, or from the carotid to the basilar system, or vice versa.

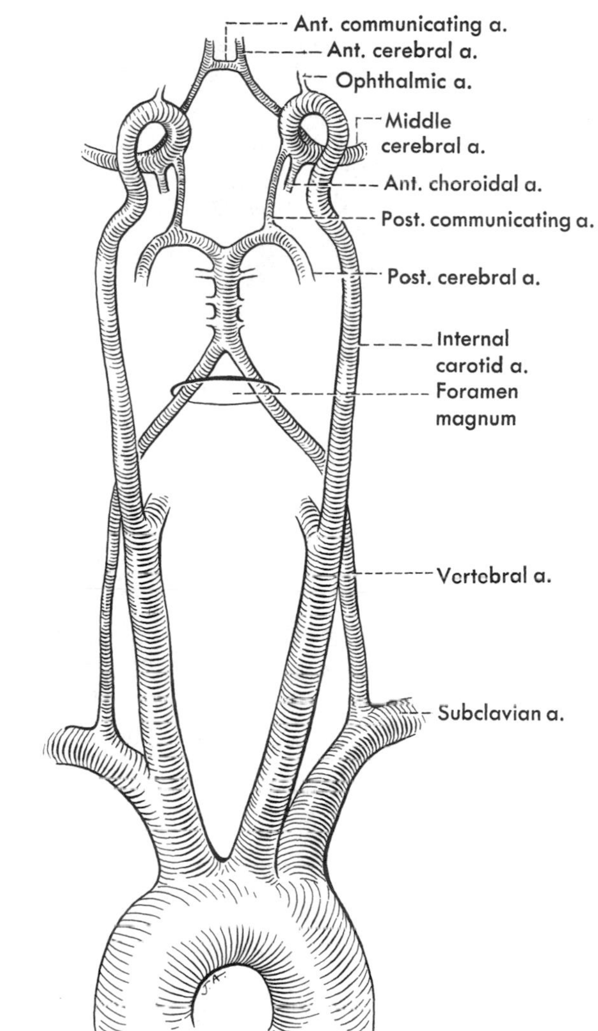

FIGURE *32-16.*
Formation of the circulus arteriosus cerebri.

Internal Carotid

The internal carotid gives rise to an **anterior choroidal** (the chief blood supply to the choroid plexus in the lateral ventricle, but also supplying brain tissue) and the **posterior communicating artery** before dividing into the anterior and middle cerebral arteries. The **middle cerebral artery** runs upward and laterally in the lateral cerebral fissure (between the temporal and frontal lobes) and spreads out to supply the lower and lateral surface of the cerebral hemisphere as far back as the distribution of the posterior cerebral artery on the lateral surface (Fig. 32.17). In addition to cortical branches, it and other branches of the internal carotid give off, close to that vessel, central or perforating branches that pierce the base of the brain. Some of these supply the important internal capsule (the bundle of fibers leading from and to the cerebral hemisphere) and part of the adjacent corpus striatum and are called **striate arteries.** Occlusion of or hemorrhage from some of these vessels is a common type of stroke.

The **anterior cerebral arteries,** after communicating with each other, proceed forward, upward, and then backward in the longitudinal fissure, each supplying the medial surface of its cerebral hemisphere back to the distribution of the posterior cerebral. Branches of the anterior cerebral run onto the upper lateral part of the cerebral hemisphere, helping supply this and anastomosing with branches of the middle and posterior cerebrals.

Venous Drainage

The venous drainage of the brain is through the venous sinuses in the dura mater. The drainage from the convex and most of the medial surface of the cerebral hemisphere is into superficial veins. **Superior cerebral veins,** from the upper part of the hemisphere, run upward to empty into the superior sagittal sinus (Fig. 32-18). **Inferior cerebral veins,** from the lower part of the hemisphere, join venous sinuses situated at the base of the skull. Running horizontally between the superior and inferior cerebral veins,

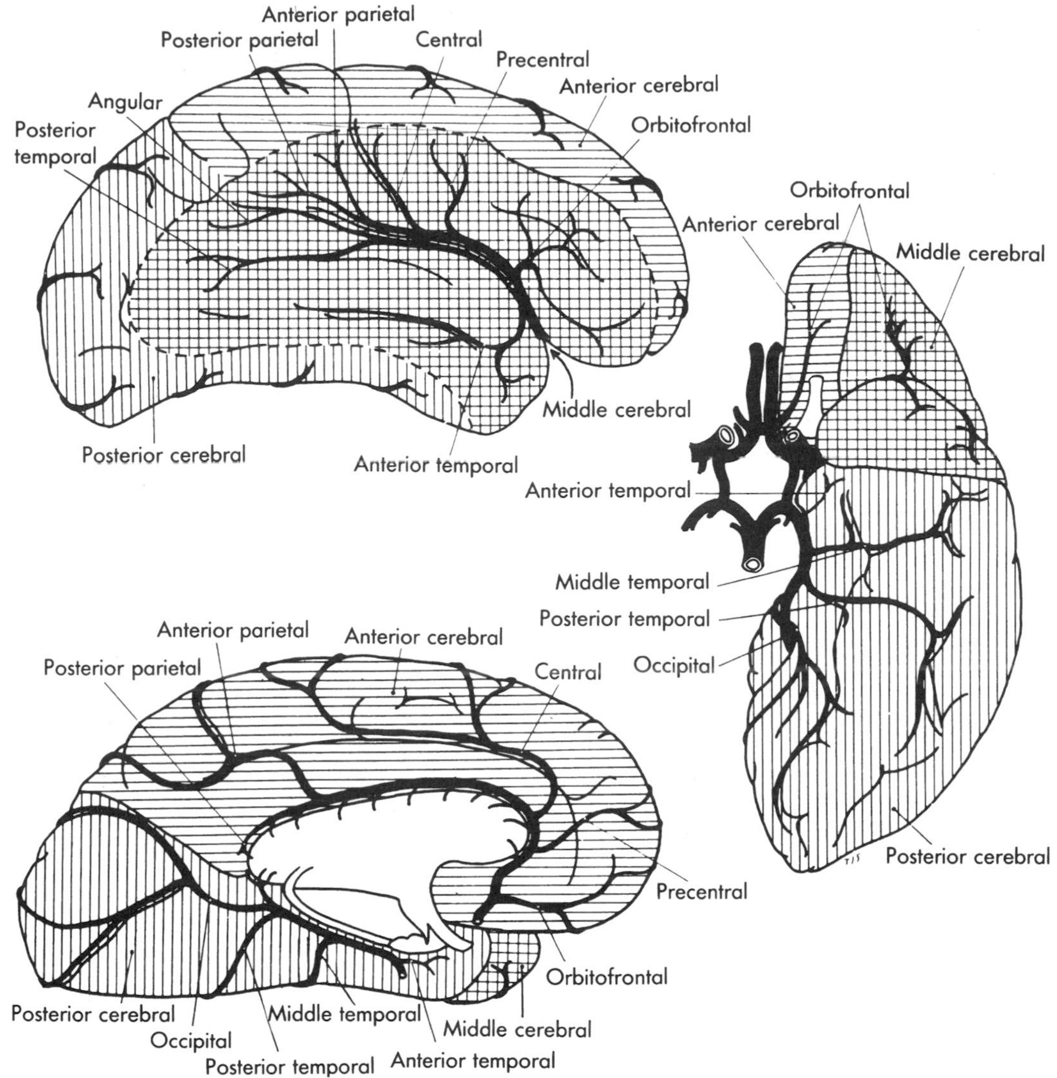

FIGURE *32-17.*
Distribution of the three cerebral arteries in *lateral, medial,* and *inferior* views of the cerebral hemisphere. The cortical branches are named here in more detail than in official anatomic terminology. (Mettler FA. Neuroanatomy, 2nd ed. St Louis, CV Mosby, 1948)

over the lateral sulcus, is the **superficial middle cerebral vein.** This drains anteriorly into the cavernous sinus or the superior petrosal sinus and is connected posteriorly to the transverse sinus by a vein known as the *inferior anastomotic vein.* Usually also it is connected to one or more superior cerebral veins and thus to the superior sagittal sinus by several channels, the largest of which is called the *superior anastomotic vein.*

The **deep middle cerebral vein** lies in the depth of the lateral sulcus, on the hidden cortex (the insula) that here connects the frontal, parietal, and temporal lobes. This vein unites lateral to the hypothalamus with veins from the inferior and medial surfaces of the anterior part of the hemisphere and with striatal veins to form the **basal vein** (vein of Rosenthal). The basal vein then runs laterally and dorsally around the cerebral peduncle to end in the **great cerebral vein.**

Veins from the deeper parts of cerebral hemisphere begin as the **thalamostriate vein** in the floor of the lateral ventricle, the **vein of the septum pellucidum,** on part of the medial wall of the ventricle, and the **choroidal vein** that drains the choroid plexus of the ventricle. These unite to form the **internal cerebral vein.** The two internal cerebral veins run posteriorly side by side in the roof of the third ventricle and, at about the level of the posterior end of the corpus callosum, unite to form the **great cerebral vein** (of Galen). The great cerebral vein receives the basal veins and veins from the midbrain as it runs backward in the transverse fissure just above the midbrain. It enters the dura at the point where the lower free edge of the falx cerebri joins the tentorium cerebelli and here joins the inferior sagittal sinus to form the straight sinus.

Superior cerebellar veins enter the great cerebral vein and the transverse and superior petrosal sinuses. **Inferior cerebellar veins** enter the straight or a transverse sinus and the inferior petrosal and occipital sinuses.

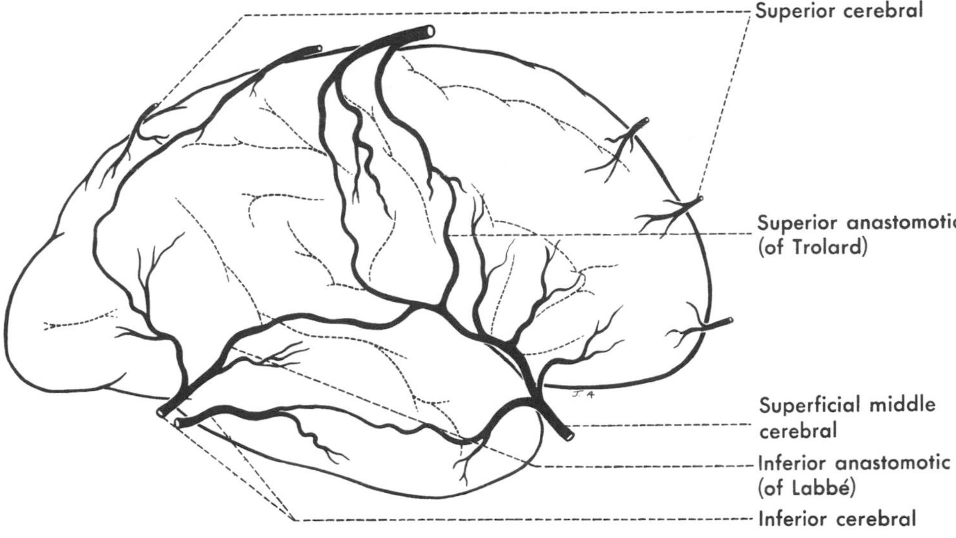

FIGURE 32-18. **The chief veins on the lateral surface of the cerebral hemisphere.**

CRANIAL NERVES

The extracranial courses and branches of most of the cranial nerves are described later; only their intracranial courses and the composition and distribution of each nerve are summarized here. Their attachments to the brain are shown in Figure 32-6, and their positions at the base of the skull and certain vascular relations are shown in Figure 32-19.

Among the 12 pairs of cranial nerves, some are sensory only, some supply only skeletal muscle, some are mixed nerves, and some contain autonomic fibers in addition to motor fibers to skeletal muscle (see Chap. 7). The cranial nerves that contain sensory fibers typically have ganglia, collections of nerve cells located outside the cen-

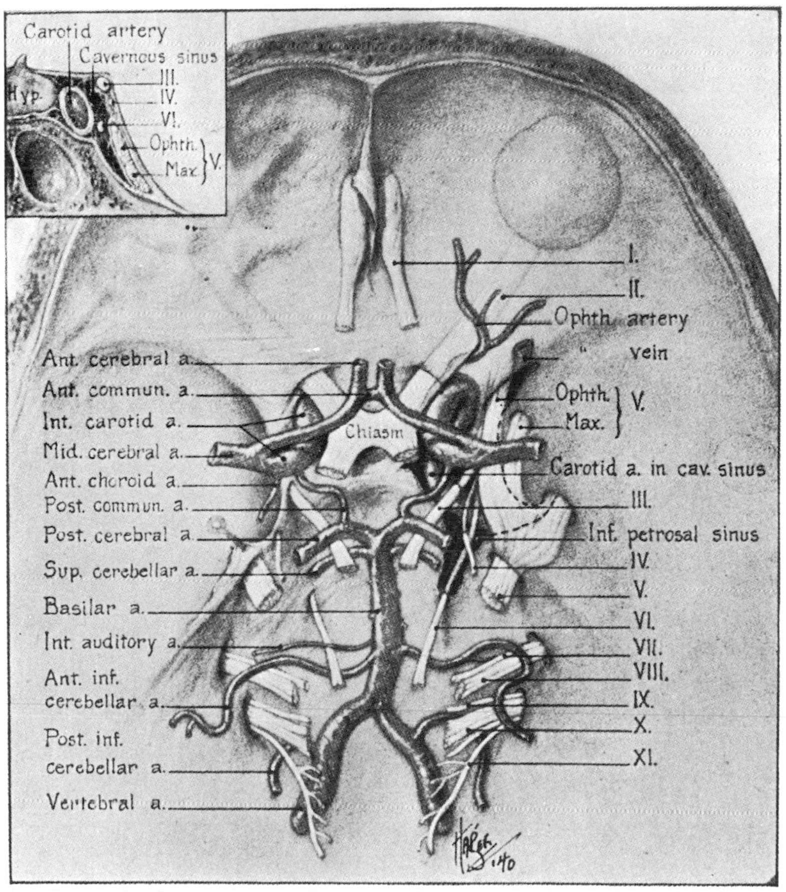

FIGURE 32-19. **Nerves and arteries at the base of the skull. On the *right side,* the floor of the anterior cranial fossa is shown as semitransparent, so that within the orbit the eyeball, optic nerve, and ophthalmic artery can be seen. The *broken line* over the ganglion and branches of the fifth nerve indicates the approximate posterior and lateral extent of the cavernous sinus in relation to this nerve, and the small inset is a frontal section to show relations within this sinus. *I,* the olfactory bulb and tract; the other *Roman numerals* identify the cranial nerves. *Int. auditory a.* is the name by which the artery now called the labyrinthine has long been known. (Dandy WE. Intracranial arterial aneurysms. Ithaca NY. Comstock, 1944.)**

tral nervous system, that give rise to these sensory fibers and are the cranial equivalent of the spinal (sensory) ganglia of spinal nerves. The voluntary motor and preganglionic autonomic fibers arise from cell bodies, grouped together as cranial nuclei, that lie inside the central nervous system and correspond collectively to the anterior and lateral gray columns of the spinal cord. Unlike spinal nerves, however, the motor and sensory fibers of the cranial nerves do not necessarily form different roots, but may be mixed together in a single root.

Olfactory Nerve

The olfactory nerve, or nerve of smell, is purely sensory. Its cell bodies are located in the mucosa of the uppermost part of the nasal cavity. The fibers from these cells unite to form several small filaments that enter the skull through the cribriform plate to end in the olfactory bulb.

Optic Nerve

The optic or second cranial nerve, the nerve of sight, usually is said to be sensory only, but may contain efferent fibers of unknown origin and function. However, it actually is neither developmentally nor anatomically a nerve: the ganglion cells giving rise to the fibers of the nerve constitute a layer of the retina of the eyeball, and the retina is an outgrowth from the central nervous system. Furthermore, the optic nerve is surrounded by meninges, as is the central nervous system, and contains neuroglia throughout its length. The optic "nerve" really is a tract of the brain, connecting two parts.

After it leaves the back of the eyeball, the optic nerve has a slightly sinuous course backward through the orbit, thus allowing for movement of the eyeball. It enters the cranial cavity through the optic canal, and the two optic nerves converge toward each other. They join to form the **optic chiasma,** attached to the hypothalamus, and in the chiasma exchange fibers: the fibers from the medial half of each retina cross to the opposite side; those from the lateral half of each retina remain uncrossed. The fibers behind the chiasma are a continuation of those in the optic nerves and the chiasma, but are called the **optic tracts.** Because of the chiasma, an optic tract differs fundamentally from an optic nerve in composition; an optic nerve contains all the fibers from one eye; whereas an optic tract contains fibers from the lateral half of the eye on its own side and from the medial half of the other eye. Because these halves of the two eyes receive impulses from the opposite side (for instance, the right half of each retina receives light that originates to the left of the body), the optic system behaves like most other sensory systems: impulses originating on one side of the body cross to end in the cerebral cortex of the opposite side. The right optic tract, transmitting impulses evoked in the right half of each retina by light waves from the left, relays these to the right cerebral cortex (Fig. 32-20).

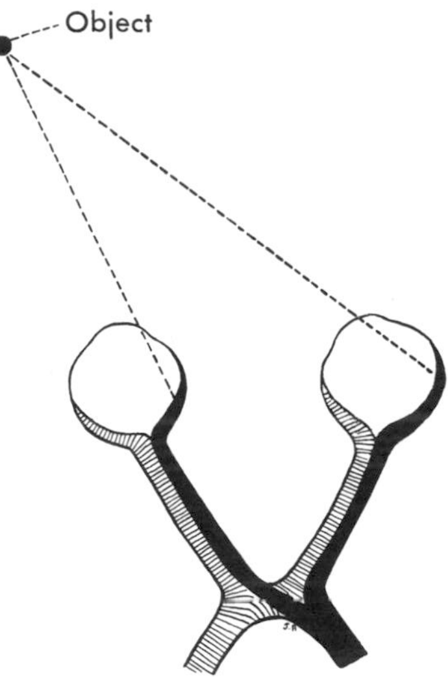

FIGURE *32-20.*
The manner in which visual stimuli on one side are conducted from both eyes to the opposite cerebral hemisphere.

Oculomotor and Trochlear Nerves

The third and fourth cranial nerves are two of the three nerves that supply the voluntary muscles in the orbit, which are concerned with moving the eyeball and raising the upper eyelid. The **oculomotor** supplies five of the seven muscles (all except the superior oblique and the lateral rectus) and is composed largely of somatic motor fibers. However, it also contains preganglionic autonomic fibers that synapse in a small ganglion, the ciliary ganglion, located within the orbit. Through this ganglion, the oculomotor nerve controls the smooth muscle that is responsible for constriction of the pupil of the eye and for accommodation of the lens to close vision.

The oculomotor nerve leaves the floor of the midbrain just in front of the pons, through the medial part of the cerebral peduncle. It runs forward through the subarachnoid space and pierces the dura over the cavernous sinus just anterolateral to the posterior clinoid process. It then runs forward in the wall of the sinus and enters the orbit through the superior orbital fissure.

The **trochlear nerve** supplies only one voluntary muscle (superior oblique) in the orbit, and no smooth muscle. It leaves the dorsal surface of the brain stem just below the inferior colliculus and runs forward against the lower surface of the tentorium cerebelli. Just behind the posterior clinoid process, it pierces the lower surface of the tentorium close to its free edge and runs forward in the dura of the lateral wall of the cavernous sinus, leaving the skull through the superior orbital fissure.

Muscle spindles (sensory organs, see Chap. 7) are in those muscles supplied by the oculomotor and trochlear nerves, and the sensory fibers ending in the spindles are in these nerves for at least a part of their course. However, neither nerve has a sensory ganglion (corresponding to a spinal ganglion of a spinal nerve), and the cell bodies giving rise to these sensory fibers most likely lie in the trigeminal ganglion.

Trigeminal Nerve

The trigeminal (fifth cranial) nerve is so named because it has three major branches. It contains both sensory and motor fibers. The sensory fibers are distributed particularly to the skin of the face and to the upper and lower teeth, and the motor fibers to muscles associated with the jaws. It is attached to the side of the pontine region of the brain stem and has two roots, a large sensory root and small so-called motor root that does contain all the motor fibers, but also proprioceptive (afferent or sensory) fibers. The two roots run close together across the upper surface of the tip of the petrous portion of the temporal bone to enter the middle cranial fossa, where the sensory root bears the **trigeminal ganglion.** This ganglion is covered by the dura of the middle cranial fossa, but its proximal part is surrounded by cerebrospinal fluid: the subarachnoid space around the pons continues across the petrous bone around the roots of the nerve and expands over the proximal part of the ganglion. This expansion into the middle fossa is the *trigeminal* (Meckel's) *cave.* When the sensory root of the nerve is cut to alleviate the painful *trigeminal neuralgia* (tic douloureux), this is often done in the subarachnoid space of the trigeminal cave.

From the trigeminal ganglion arise the three branches of the trigeminal nerve, the ophthalmic, maxillary, and mandibular. These leave the skull through three separate apertures. The **ophthalmic nerve** runs forward in the dura of the lateral wall of the cavernous sinus and enters the orbit through the superior orbital fissure. It contributes branches to the eyeball and the upper part of the nasal cavity, but for the most part leaves the orbit to supply skin of the upper eyelid, the dorsum of the nose, the forehead, and the scalp about as far back as the interauricular line (see Figs. 31-15 and 31-23).

The **maxillary nerve** (Fig. 32-21) leaves the skull by way of the foramen rotundum, which opens into the pterygopalatine fossa. Suspended from it at this point is the pterygopalatine ganglion, which sends fibers into the branches of the maxillary nerve that go to the interior of the nose and to the palate. While it is in the pterygopalatine fossa, the maxillary nerve gives off palatine and nasal branches, branches to the posterior upper teeth, and the zygomatic nerve, which runs with the remaining part of the maxillary into the orbit. The major continuation of the maxillary nerve, the infraorbital, leaves the pterygopalatine fossa by passing through the inferior orbital fissure into the orbit. Here it runs first in a groove and then in a canal in the floor of the orbit. It gives off superior alveolar nerves and then emerges to go to skin of the lower lid, side of the nose, upper lip, and upper part of the cheek (see Fig. 31-23). The zygomatic nerve divides within the orbit into zygomaticotemporal and zygomaticofacial branches, which also emerge to become cutaneous.

The **mandibular nerve** leaves the skull through the foramen ovale as two roots, a sensory root from the ganglion and the motor root, which join just outside the skull. The mandibular is the only branch of the trigeminal containing motor fibers to skeletal muscle. They are distributed to the muscles of mastication and to the mylohyoid, the anterior belly of the digastric, the tensor veli palatini, and the tensor tympani muscles (Fig. 32-22). In addition, the mandibular nerve has large

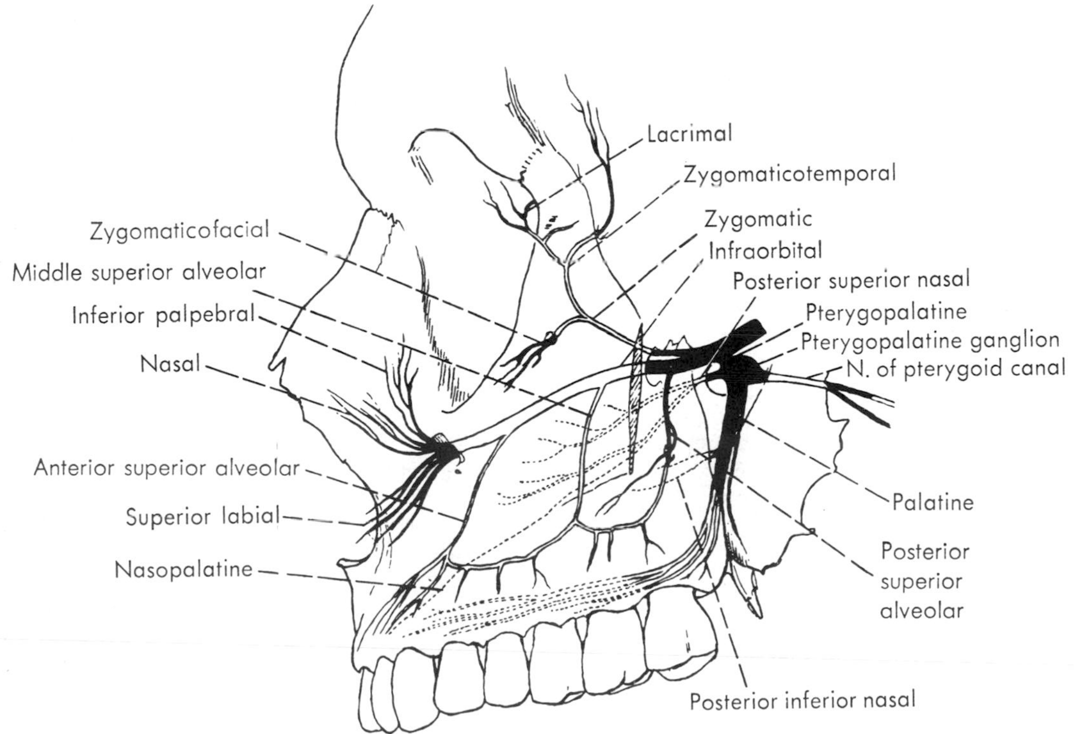

FIGURE *32-21.*
Diagram of the maxillary nerve. (Henle J. Handbuch der systematischen Anatomie des Menschen, vol 3, pt 2. Braunschweig: Vieweg und Sohn, 1868.)

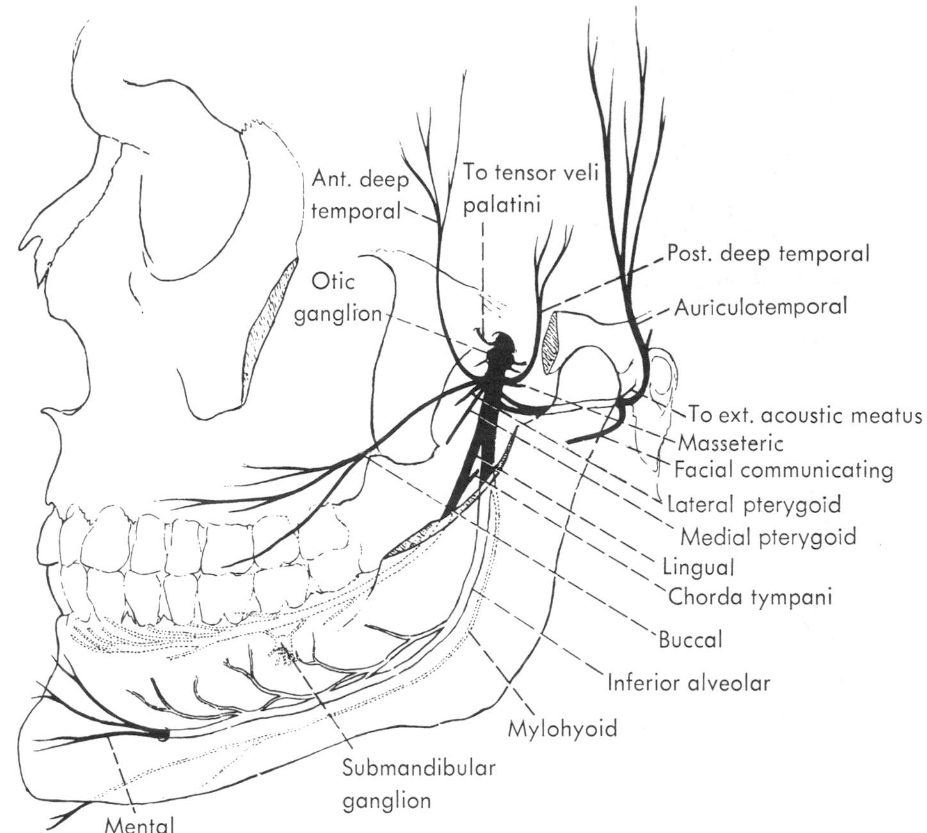

FIGURE 32-22.
Diagram of the mandibular nerve. (Henle J. Handbuch der systematischen Anatomie des Menschen, vol 3, pt 2. Braunschweig: Vieweg und Sohn, 1868.)

sensory branches: the lingual nerve, to the anterior two-thirds of the tongue; the inferior alveolar, to the lower teeth and the skin of the chin; the auriculotemporal nerve; and the buccal nerve. The otic ganglion is on the medial surface of the mandibular nerve immediately outside the foramen ovale. The submandibular ganglion, another parasympathetic ganglion of the head, is suspended from the lingual branch of the mandibular nerve.

Whereas all four of the cranial parasympathetic ganglia are located close to or on some branch of the trigeminal nerve, the preganglionic fibers to these ganglia, although they may run in a branch of the trigeminal, actually come from other nerves—the third, seventh, or ninth. The roots of the trigeminal nerve contain no autonomic fibers. The postganglionic fibers from the ganglia, however, typically join and are distributed with peripheral branches of the trigeminal.

Abducens Nerve

The abducens or sixth cranial nerve is like the trochlear in supplying only one voluntary muscle of the orbit (the lateral rectus). As do the third and fourth nerves, it contains afferent fibers to muscle spindles. All three of the eye muscle nerves frequently are classed as purely motor.

The abducens leaves the floor of the brain stem just behind the pons and has a short course downward and forward into the dura of the floor of the posterior cranial fossa. After entering the dura, it runs forward through the cavernous sinus and the superior orbital fissure into the orbit.

Facial Nerve

The facial or seventh cranial nerve (Fig. 32-23) is so known because it supplies the muscles of the face. It leaves the lateral surface of the medulla just caudal to the pons and anterior to the cerebellum, in company with the eighth nerve, and runs laterally with this nerve to the internal acoustic meatus. At the distal end of the meatus the facial nerve enters the facial canal in the petrous part of the temporal bone. This canal lies partly in the wall between the internal and middle ears and opens below at the stylomastoid foramen on the base of the skull. The ganglion of the nerve is located where the nerve makes a sharp turn in the facial canal, and because it is located at this bend (geniculum), it is called the **geniculate ganglion.**

Outside the stylomastoid foramen, the facial nerve passes lateral to the styloid process and into the parotid gland. Before passing into the gland, it gives off a branch to the posterior belly of the digastric and to the stylohyoid muscle and a *posterior auricular* branch that runs upward behind the ear to supply the posterior auricular muscle and the occipital belly of the occipitofrontal muscle. Its distribution on the face has already been described.

The **nervus intermedius** is the smaller sensory and parasympathetic motor root of the facial nerve. It is called nervus intermedius because it often lies between the seventh and eighth cranial nerves. It joins the facial

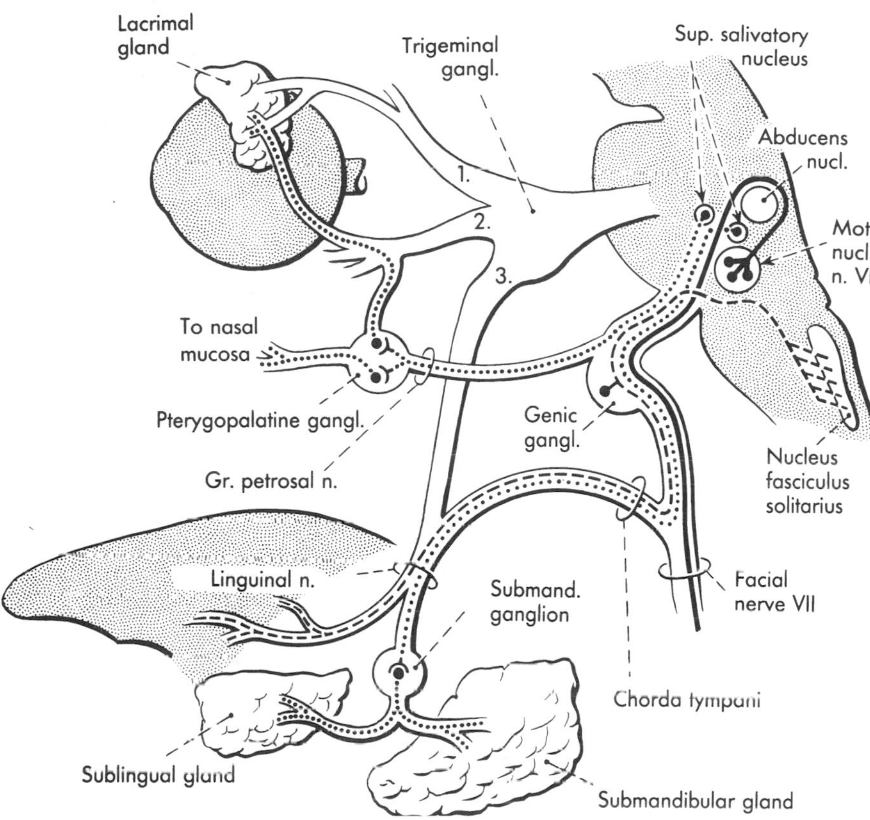

FIGURE 32-23. **Diagram of the facial nerve: motor fibers to skeletal muscle are indicated by *solid lines*; parasympathetic ones, both preganglionic and postganglionic, by *dotted lines*; and sensory fibers by *broken lines*. The only sensory fibers shown here are the best-known ones, those of taste that are distributed to the tongue. (Sections of Neurology and Section of Physiology, Mayo Clinic and Mayo Foundation. Clinical examinations in neurology, 2nd ed. Philadelphia: WB Saunders, 1963. After Strong OS, Elwyn A. Human neuroanatomy, 3rd ed. Baltimore: Williams & Wilkins, 1953.)**

nerve proximal to the geniculate ganglion and contributes fibers to both branches of the nerve that contain parasympathetic fibers (greater petrosal and chorda tympani).

The larger root of the facial nerve is composed of motor fibers that go to all the muscles of the face, including those of the scalp, and to the platysma, the posterior belly of the digastric, the stylohyoid, and the stapedius muscle. The autonomic fibers go to the pterygopalatine and submandibular ganglia through the greater petrosal and chorda tympani nerves. The exact distribution and function of many of the sensory fibers of the facial nerve are unknown, but some are thought to be concerned with deep pain from the face; some of them apparently are distributed to a small part of the soft palate; a few may reach the middle ear cavity; and the few cutaneous fibers that the nerve contains are distributed to skin on the posterior surface of the ear, along with similar fibers from the ninth and tenth nerves. The best-known sensory fibers in the facial nerve are those for taste on the anterior two-thirds of the tongue. These reach the tongue through the chorda tympani branch of the facial and the lingual branch of the mandibular, which the chorda tympani joins.

Vestibulocochlear Nerve

The eighth cranial nerve (n. vestibulocochlearis, or octavus) has two parts. At its origin from the upper lateral surface of the brain stem, the nerve consists of two roots, a cochlear and a vestibular, but these can be separated only by dissection. The nerve proceeds laterally into the internal acoustic meatus, in company with the facial nerve. Toward the lateral (distal) end of the meatus, it divides into its two parts, vestibular and cochlear. Each part has its own ganglion, and the **vestibular ganglion** is in turn divided into two parts. From the two parts of the vestibular ganglion, fibers go to the parts of the ear connected with balance, but from the cochlear or **spiral ganglion** fibers go to the part connected with hearing. Both parts of the eighth nerve, therefore, end in the petrous part of the temporal bone, instead of emerging from the skull as do all the other cranial nerves. Efferent fibers have been demonstrated in both branches of the eighth nerve. They end in the sense organs to which these nerves are distributed and apparently influence the sensitivity of these organs.

Glossopharyngeal Nerve

The glossopharyngeal or ninth nerve is a small one, arising by two or more rootlets from the side of the medulla dorsal to the olive, in line with the rootlets of the vagus nerve. It runs laterally to the front part of the jugular foramen and penetrates the dura separate from the vagus nerve. As it emerges through the jugular foramen, it bears two ganglia close together; the **superior ganglion** is particularly small, but the **inferior ganglion** is a little larger. Outside the jugular foramen, the glossopharyngeal nerve gives off a tympanic branch, sends a branch of communication to the auricular branch of the vagus, gives rise to a large carotid sinus branch that also supplies the carotid body, and sends one or more pharyngeal branches to the pharynx (see Fig. 31-43). These branches are all sensory. The only voluntary motor branch of the ninth nerve is to the stylopharyngeus muscle. Beyond these branches, the ninth nerve runs forward along the side of the pharynx, to which it gives off one or more tonsillar branches, and then continues into the tongue to end in the mucosa and taste buds of the posterior third, supplying both general sensation and taste. The preganglionic fibers that lie in the ninth nerve end in the otic ganglion and are described with that.

Vagus Nerve

The vagus or tenth cranial nerve arises by several rootlets emerging from the lateral border of the medulla dorsal to the olive. As these run laterally, they join to form the vagus nerve, which passes through the middle part of the jugular foramen, with the accessory nerve just behind it. At this point, the accessory nerve divides into two branches, an internal and an external. The internal branch then joins the vagus and is distributed with it. It is properly a part of the vagus, not of the accessory. The vagus, similar to the glossopharyngeal, typically bears a **superior** and an **inferior ganglion;** the inferior ganglion is large, and the superior one small. It is the wide distribution of the vagus that gives it its name, which means wandering.

The vagus sends a small meningeal branch to the dura of the posterior cranial fossa and a small auricular branch to a part of the external acoustic meatus and tympanic membrane and to skin behind the ear. The branches of the vagus in the neck (see Fig. 30-11) are one or more pharyngeal branches, motor to the muscles of the pharynx and most of the muscles of the soft palate; the superior laryngeal nerve, sensory to the larynx and motor to one muscle, an external one on the larynx (cricothyroid); superior and inferior cardiac branches, to the heart; and the right recurrent laryngeal nerve (the left one arises in the thorax). In the thorax, the vagus contributes fibers to the heart, lungs, and esophagus and descends on the esophagus to the abdomen. In the abdomen, it is distributed to the stomach and the liver and, after joining the celiac plexus, to the digestive tube about as far distally as the beginning of the descending colon. Branches of the vagus nerve in the neck and thorax contain motor fibers to skeletal muscle, autonomic fibers, and sensory fibers including those for pain. The abdominal part of the vagus consists of preganglionic parasympathetic fibers that end in the enteric ganglia located in the walls of the intestinal tract, and visceral afferent fibers.

Accessory Nerve

The accessory nerve arises by two sets of rootlets: **cranial** rootlets that are in line with the vagal rootlets on the side of the medulla, and **spinal** rootlets that ascend alongside the spinal cord, between the posterior and the anterior roots. These may come from as low as the fifth cervical segment and join each other as the nerve ascends. The cranial and spinal roots come together briefly as the nerve passes through the jugular foramen immediately behind the vagus, but then the fibers of the cranial root separate as the *internal ramus* and join the vagus (Fig. 32-24) to be distributed with that. The *external ramus* of the nerve, the spinal accessory nerve, then supplies only two voluntary muscles, the sternocleidomastoid and the trapezius. Afferent fibers in the accessory nerve are from cervical nerves.

Hypoglossal Nerve

The hypoglossal or 12th cranial nerve apparently is a purely motor nerve, containing no afferent fibers. It arises from the anterior surface of the medulla, just ventral to the olive. Its rootlets come together and it pierces the dura mater at the hypoglossal canal to leave the skull, sometimes as two filaments, sometimes as a single nerve. After the nerve leaves the hypoglossal canal and runs downward, it receives a communication from upper cervical nerves that helps form the ansa cervicalis. The hypoglossal nerve itself is motor to the extrinsic and intrinsic muscles of the tongue.

AUTONOMIC SYSTEM IN THE HEAD

The autonomic system in the head consists of both sympathetic and parasympathetic fibers, but the main autonomic ganglia in the head are parasympathetic. Two of these, the otic and the submandibular, have been described with the jaw; two others yet to be described lie within the orbit or adjacent to the nose.

Cranial Sympathetic System

Most of the postganglionic sympathetic fibers to the face and head are derived from the **superior cervical ganglion** in the upper part of the neck. This ganglion sends fibers along both external and internal carotid arteries. An **external carotid nerve** or several nerves

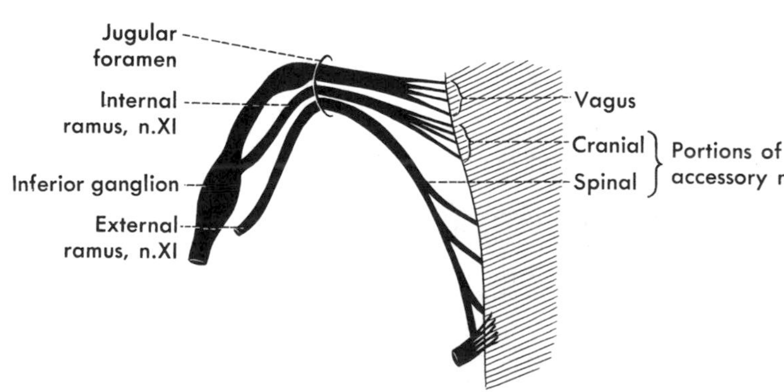

FIGURE *32-24.*
The grouping of the cranial rootlets of the cranial accessory nerve as the internal ramus that joins the vagus, and the continuation of the spinal rootlets as the external ramus, or spinal accessory nerve.

run downward from the ganglion to the base of the external carotid artery. These form a plexus along the external carotid and its branches, sending a smaller plexus downward along the common carotid. The **common carotid plexus** ends on the artery. The **external carotid plexus** ends in part on the branches of this artery, but also in the salivary glands and in the sweat glands of the lower part of the face. A tiny **jugular nerve** from the superior cervical ganglion divides to join the glossopharyngeal and vagus nerves.

The largest branch from the superior cervical ganglion to the head is the **internal carotid nerve,** which passes onto the internal carotid artery and forms an internal carotid plexus about this. The **internal carotid plexus** follows the carotid artery through its extracranial course and onto the part of the artery lying in the cavernous sinus. Here, many of the sympathetic fibers leave the internal carotid, but some of them follow the vessel and its cerebral branches (although autonomic fibers exert relatively little effect on cerebral blood vessels). It is believed also that sensory fibers run with the motor fibers in the carotid plexuses, just as they do in many other sympathetic branches.

While it is close to the middle ear cavity, the internal carotid plexus gives off twigs that join the tympanic plexus on the medial wall of the cavity, but the two main groups of sympathetic fibers leaving the plexus do so in the cavernous sinus. One, the *sympathetic branch to the ciliary ganglion,* runs forward through the cavernous sinus to the superior orbital fissure to enter the orbit and join the ciliary ganglion. However, its postganglionic sympathetic fibers do not end in this parasympathetic ganglion, but pass through it and help form the short ciliary nerves that the ganglion sends to the eyeball.

The other large group of sympathetic fibers forms the **deep petrosal nerve.** This leaves the internal carotid artery while that vessel lies on the side of the sella turcica and passes to the anterior lip of the foramen lacerum, as does the greater petrosal, to join the greater petrosal nerve and form the nerve of the pterygoid canal (Fig. 32-25). This runs forward to the pterygopalatine fossa, where it ends in the pterygopalatine ganglion. This ganglion is attached to the lower border of the maxillary nerve, and its apparent branches of distribution (primarily to the nose and the palate) contain more fifth nerve fibers than they do sympathetic or parasympathetic fibers. The sympathetic fibers contributed by the deep petrosal nerve do not synapse within the pterygopalatine ganglion, but simply pass through it to be distributed with its branches.

Because the preganglionic sympathetic fibers to the face and head arise from thoracic nerves and traverse the cervical sympathetic trunk to reach the superior cervical ganglion, interruption of this trunk denervates the glands and smooth muscle supplied by the ganglion. The resultant ptosis (drooping) of the eyelid and pupillary constriction (the smooth muscle of the upper lid and the dilator pupillae are both supplied by the sympathetic system) are known as *Horner's syndrome.*

Cranial Parasympathetic System

The parasympathetic system consists of both cranial and sacral fibers, but only the cranial ones are to be considered here; the sacral parasympathetic system is described in connection with the pelvis.

There are four major pairs of parasympathetic ganglia in the head: the ciliary, the pterygopalatine, the submandibular, and the otic. There also are four cranial nerves that contain preganglionic fibers: the oculomotor, the facial, the glossopharyngeal, and the vagus. However, the last-named nerve sends its parasympathetic fibers to structures in the thorax and abdomen, those of the thorax ending in small ganglia in the pulmonary and cardiac plexuses, and those of the abdomen ending upon the enteric ganglia in the walls of the digestive tract. Thus, although the vagal parasympathetic fibers belong to the cranial system,

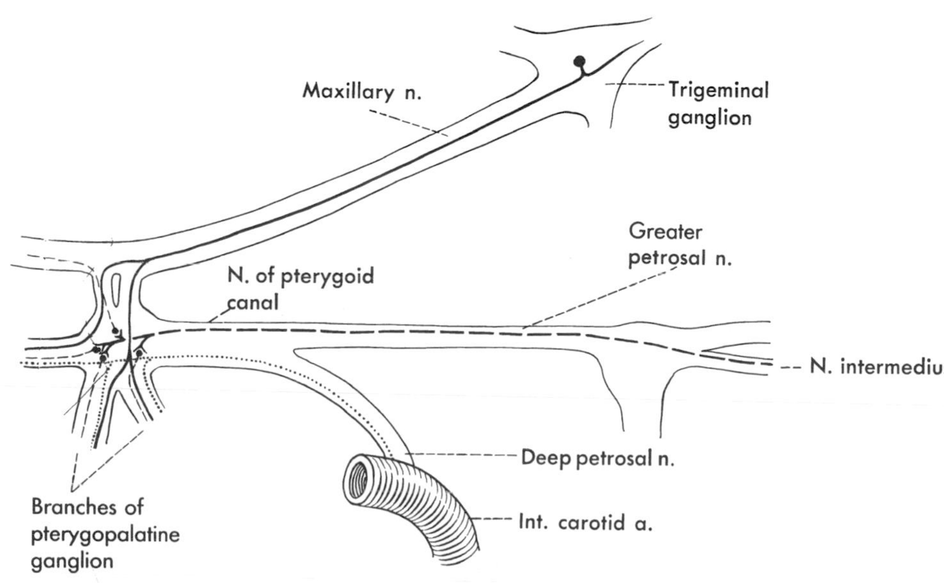

FIGURE 32-25.
Diagram of the connection of the pterygopalatine ganglion: Preganglionic parasympathetic fibers (which synapse in the ganglion) are indicated by *long broken lines*; postganglionic parasympathetic fibers arising from the ganglion by *short broken lines*; and postganglionic sympathetic fibers by *dotted lines*. The only afferent fibers (*solid lines*) shown are those of the fifth nerve, although the deep petrosal nerve is said to contain a few (of spinal origin) and the greater petrosal has afferent fibers of facial origin that are distributed to the back part of the soft palate and, sometimes, probably also fibers for taste from the tongue.

they are not connected with cranial parasympathetic ganglia.

Of the four ganglia, the oculomotor nerve supplies preganglionic fibers to the ciliary only, the facial supplies fibers to both the pterygopalatine and the submandibular, and the glossopharyngeal supplies fibers to the otic (Table 32-1). Most of the ganglia also have sympathetic and sensory fibers closely associated with them. The sympathetic fibers are derived from the superior cervical ganglion and pass through or close against the ganglion; similarly, the sensory fibers pass through or adjacent to the ganglion and are for the most part derived from the branches of the trigeminal nerve with which the cranial parasympathetic ganglia are closely connected.

Ciliary Ganglion

The ciliary ganglion is a small ganglion situated toward the back of the orbit on the lateral side of the optic nerve. It receives its preganglionic fibers through a short stout *oculomotor root* that arises from the oculomotor nerve; it also receives a *communicating branch* from the nasociliary branch of the ophthalmic nerve, which carries sensory fibers; and it usually receives a *sympathetic branch* from the internal carotid plexus. The postganglionic fibers from the ciliary ganglion, mixed with sensory and sympathetic fibers that bypass the ganglion, form short ciliary nerves that enter the eyeball to control the smooth muscle there.

Pterygopalatine Ganglion

The pterygopalatine ganglion lies in the pterygopalatine fossa, immediately adjacent to the lateral nasal wall at the level of the back end of the middle nasal concha. In the pterygopalatine fossa the ganglion lies immediately below the maxillary branch of the trigeminal nerve and is attached to it by *two pterygopalatine nerves*; most of the fibers of these nerves run past the ganglion and form a major part of the so-called branches of the ganglion (orbital, posterior nasal, nasopalatine, palatine, and pharyngeal). The pterygopalatine ganglion receives its preganglionic parasympathetic fibers from the facial nerve; it is joined also by sympathetic fibers (that run past it, but are distributed with its branches) from the internal carotid plexus. The sympathetic and parasympathetic fibers reach the ganglion in the same nerve, the *nerve of the pterygoid canal*; this is formed by the union of the *deep petrosal nerve*, carrying sympathetic fibers from the internal carotid plexus, and the greater petrosal nerve from the facial (see Fig. 32-25). As the greater and the deep petrosal nerves reach the anterior lip of the foramen lacerum, they unite and enter the pterygoid canal, which lies in the floor of the sphenoid sinus and opens anteriorly into the pterygopalatine fossa. (The canal is also known as the vidian canal, whence the nerve gets its alternative name, *vidian nerve.*)

The *greater petrosal nerve* leaves the facial nerve in the pars petrosa of the temporal bone at the level of the geniculate ganglion; it runs forward and medially through the pars petrosa in a small canal, escaping through the hiatus of this canal to run in the middle cranial fossa to the foramen lacerum, when it is joined by the deep petrosal. The greater petrosal nerve carries not only parasympathetic fibers, but also sensory ones, both running in the nervus intermedius part of the facial nerve.

The postganglionic fibers derived from the pterygopalatine ganglion run for the most part in the nasal and palatine nerves; although these are listed as branches of the ganglion, it should be emphasized again that they consist of a mixture of sensory fibers derived from the maxillary nerve, sympathetic fibers brought in by the deep petrosal, and only in part of postganglionic parasympathetic fibers. The sensory fibers derived from the facial nerve probably run with the palatine nerves to reach a small part of the soft palate.

The postganglionic parasympathetic fibers to the nose and soft palate are both vasodilatory and secretory; their activity accounts for some of the speed with which the nose can become stuffed up. The pterygopalatine ganglion also sends postganglionic fibers to the maxillary nerve by way of the pterygopalatine nerves; these travel with the maxillary nerve and then with its zygomatic and zygomaticotemporal branches to reach the lacrimal gland, to which they are secretory.

TABLE *32-1* Autonomic Ganglia of the Head

Ganglion	Preganglionic Fibers Via:	Postganglionic Fibers Distributed To:
Ciliary	Oculomotor nerve and its inferior division	Ciliary muscle, sphincter pupillae
Pterygopalatine	Nervus intermedius part of facial, greater petrosal, and nerve of pterygoid canal	Nose, palate, and lacrimal gland
Submandibular	Nervus intermedius part of facial, chorda tympani, and lingual nerve	Submandibular and sublingual salivary glands and smaller glands of oral cavity
Otic	Glossopharyngeal nerve, its tympanic branch, and lesser petrosal	Parotid salivary gland

Otic Ganglion

The otic ganglion lies on the medial side of the mandibular branch of the trigeminal nerve, just outside the foramen ovale and deep in the infratemporal fossa. It may be adherent to the medial side of the mandibular nerve or may be on some of its motor branches. Indeed, the nerves to the tensor veli palatini and to the tensor tympani muscles are listed as branches of the otic ganglion, although so far as is known they contain no fibers from this ganglion but consist, rather, of fibers derived from the mandibular nerve. The otic ganglion receives its preganglionic fibers from the *lesser petrosal nerve*. This is a derivative of the glossopharyngeal, but the fibers have a

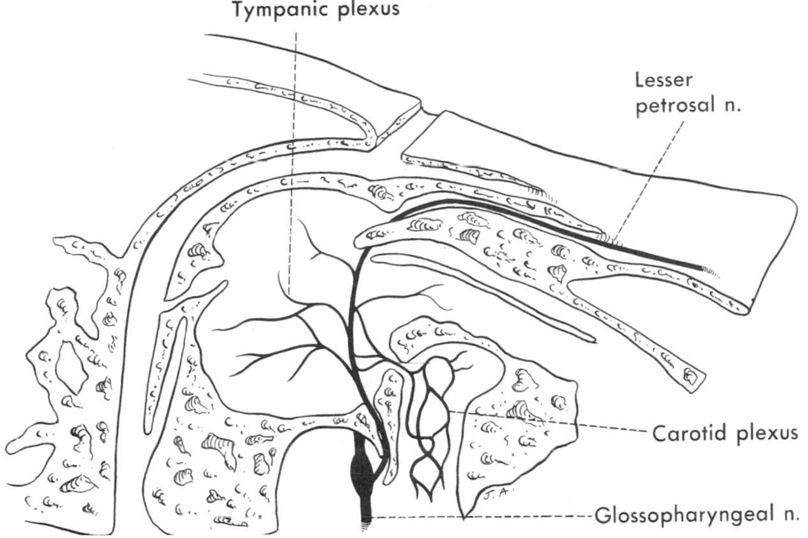

FIGURE 32-26.
The tympanic plexus and the origin of the lesser petrosal nerve.

somewhat circuitous course. The glossopharyngeal nerve gives off a *tympanic branch* that enters the middle ear cavity and there, with sympathetic twigs from the internal carotid plexus, and usually a twig from the facial nerve, forms a tympanic plexus; the preganglionic fibers of the glossopharyngeal that are destined for the otic ganglion run through the plexus, however, and as they leave it form the lesser petrosal nerve (Fig. 32-26). This emerges into the middle cranial fossa, runs just lateral to the greater petrosal nerve, and leaves the skull close to or through the foramen ovale to join the otic ganglion. There also may be in the lesser petrosal nerve some fibers derived from the facial nerve that reach it through communications between the greater and lesser petrosal nerves; these are too tiny to be found in the usual dissection. The ganglion has a *communicating ramus* with the *chorda tympani* nerve through which it also can receive facial fibers or send glossopharyngeal fibers toward the submandibular ganglion. The postganglionic fibers of the otic ganglion are believed to go entirely into the auriculotemporal branch of the mandibular nerve and to be distributed, with sensory fibers of this nerve, to the parotid gland.

Submandibular Ganglion

The submandibular ganglion lies medial to the mandible, suspended from the lingual nerve and close to the upper border of the submandibular gland. It is attached to the lingual nerve by *communicating branches* that represent both preganglionic fibers coming into the ganglion and postganglionic fibers that leave it. Its preganglionic fibers reach the lingual branch of the trigeminal through the *chorda tympani* (see Fig. 32-23). This leaves the facial nerve in the petrous part of the temporal bone, traverses the middle ear cavity, and leaves the skull through the petrotympanic fissure. It soon joins the posterior border of the lingual nerve. The preganglionic fibers then form a part of the lingual nerve until they leave it to end in the submandibular ganglion. Some authorities believe that the ganglion receives some preganglionic fibers from the glossopharyngeal nerve also, through the ramus communicans with the otic ganglion.

The submandibular ganglion gives off some of its postganglionic fibers as secretory fibers to the submandibular gland. Other postganglionic fibers return to the lingual nerve and are distributed through branches of this nerve to the sublingual salivary gland and to smaller glands of the oral cavity.

Nervus Terminalis

The nervus terminalis, seldom seen in the dissecting laboratory, now is thought to contain both autonomic and sensory fibers, although little is known about it. It consists of a few fibers that lie in the pia mater on the lower surface of the frontal lobe of the brain, just medial to the olfactory tract. Its fibers join olfactory nerve fibers and are distributed to the nasal mucosa. Along the course of the nerves there are small groups of ganglion cells, constituting the terminal ganglia; thus, these nerves seem to contain both preganglionic and postganglionic fibers, as well as afferent ones. Their function is unknown.

RECOMMENDED READINGS

Afifi AK. Basal ganglia: functional anatomy and physiology. Part 1. J Child Neurol 1994; 9: 249.

Barr ML, Kiernan JA. The human nervous system: an anatomical viewpoint. 6th ed. Philadelphia: JB Lippincott, 1993.

Basek M. Anomalies of the facial nerve in normal temporal bones. Ann Otol Rhinol Laryngol 1962; 71: 383.

Devinsky O, Feldmann E. Examination of the cranial and peripheral nerves. New York: Churchill Livingstone, 1988.

Dollenc VV, ed. Anatomy and surgery of the cavernous sinus. New York: Springer-Verlag, 1989.

Gillilan LA. Blood vessels, meninges, cerebrospinal fluid: blood supply to the central nervous system. In: Crosby EC, Humphrey T, Lauer EW, eds. Correlative anatomy of the nervous system. New York: Macmillan, 1962: 550.

Haines DE. Neuroanatomy: an atlas of structures, sections, and systems. 2nd ed. Baltimore: Urban & Schwarzenberg, 1987.

Hollinshead WH. Anatomy for surgeons: vol 1, the head and neck. 3rd ed. Philadelphia: Harper & Row, 1982.

Kerr FWL. The divisional organization of afferent fibres of the trigeminal nerve. Brain 1963; 86: 721.

Kullman GL, Dyck PJ, Cody DTR. Anatomy of the mastoid portion of the facial nerve. Arch Otolaryngol 1971; 93: 29.

Leblanc A. The cranial nerves: anatomy, imaging, vascularization. 2nd ed. Berlin: Springer, Verlag, 1995.

McCullough AW. Some anomalies of the cerebral arterial circle (of Willis) and related vessels. Anat Rec 1962; 142: 537.

Parkinson D, Johnston J, Chaudhuri A. Sympathetic connections to the fifth and sixth cranial nerves. Anat Rec 1978; 191: 221.

Penfield W, McNaughton F. Dural headache and innervation of the dura mater. Arch Neurol Psychiatry 1940; 44: 43.

Ray BS, Hinsey JC, Geohegan WA. Observations on the distribution of the sympathetic nerves to the pupil and upper extremity as determined by stimulation of the anterior roots in man. Ann Surg 1943; 118: 647.

Seeger W, ed. Atlas of topographical anatomy of the brain and surrounding structures. New York: Springer, 1978.

Streeter GL. The development of the venous sinuses of the dura mater in the human embryo. Am J Anat 1915; 18: 145.

Sundsten JW. The digital anatomist: interactive brain atlas (CD-ROM). Seattle: University of Washington School of Medicine, 1994.

Johnston JA, Parkinson D. Intracranial sympathetic pathways associated with the sixth cranial nerve. J Neurosurg 1974; 39: 236.

Tarlov IM. Sensory and motor roots of the glossopharyngeal nerve and the vagus–spinal accessory complex. Arch Neurol Psychiatry 1940; 44: 1018.

Villain M, Segnarbieux F, Bonnel F, Aubry I, Arnaud B. The trochlear nerve: anatomy by microdissection. Surg Radiol Anat 1993; 15: 169.

Waltner JG. Anatomic variations of the lateral and sigmoid sinuses. Arch Otolaryngol 1944; 39: 307.

Yilmaz E, Ilgit E, Taner D. Primitive persistent carotid–basilar and carotid–vertebral anastomoses: a report of seven cases and a review of the literature. Clin Anat 1995; 8: 36.

Hollinshead's Textbook of Anatomy, by Cornelius Rosse and Penelope Gaddum-Rosse.
Lippincott-Raven Publishers, Philadelphia, © 1997.

CHAPTER 33

The Ear, Orbit, and Nose

The ear, orbit, and nose constitute or contain the three major organs of special sense—the ear that of hearing, the orbit that of sight, and the nose that of smell. Taste, also a special sense, is mediated through taste buds that are primarily on the tongue. Unlike the nerve fibers from the larger organs of special sense, fibers for taste are incorporated in several of the cranial nerves—the facial and glossopharyngeal primarily, and in small degree, the vagus—along with fibers of other functions. In contrast, the ear, the eye, and the olfactory part of the nose have their own nerves. Associated with the organs of sense are other parts, such as a transmission system by which sound reaches the inner part of the ear, muscles and nerves that are responsible for movements of the eye and the nerves and vessels to parts of the nose other than the small area that is concerned with smell.

EAR

The ear is divided for purposes of description into the external ear, which includes not only the part projecting from the side of the head but also the canal leading inward (Fig. 33-1); the middle ear separated from the external ear canal by a membrane, but opening into the pharynx through a narrow tube; and the internal ear, which receives sound vibrations transmitted to it through the middle ear and has to do also with the balance of the head and body.

External Ear

The two parts of the external ear are the auricle (auricula), the projecting part of the ear, and the external acoustic meatus, the ear canal.

The chief named parts of the **auricle,** as seen in a lateral view, are shown in Figure 33-2. As can be determined by palpation, the *lobule*, consisting of skin and intervening connective tissue, is the only part of the auricle that is not supported by cartilage. Elsewhere, the skin of the auricle is firmly attached to the perichondrium that covers the auricular cartilage, and the shape of the cartilage can be largely seen in the intact ear. The one feature of this cartilage that cannot be so appreciated is that a part of it projects inward, from the *tragus* and the notch between it and the *antitragus*, to form the anterior and inferior wall of a part of the external acoustic meatus. The medial side of the ear has few named parts, and these are eminences corresponding to the depressions on its lateral surface—the eminence of the *concha*, for instance. The auricular muscles have already been described with the facial ones.

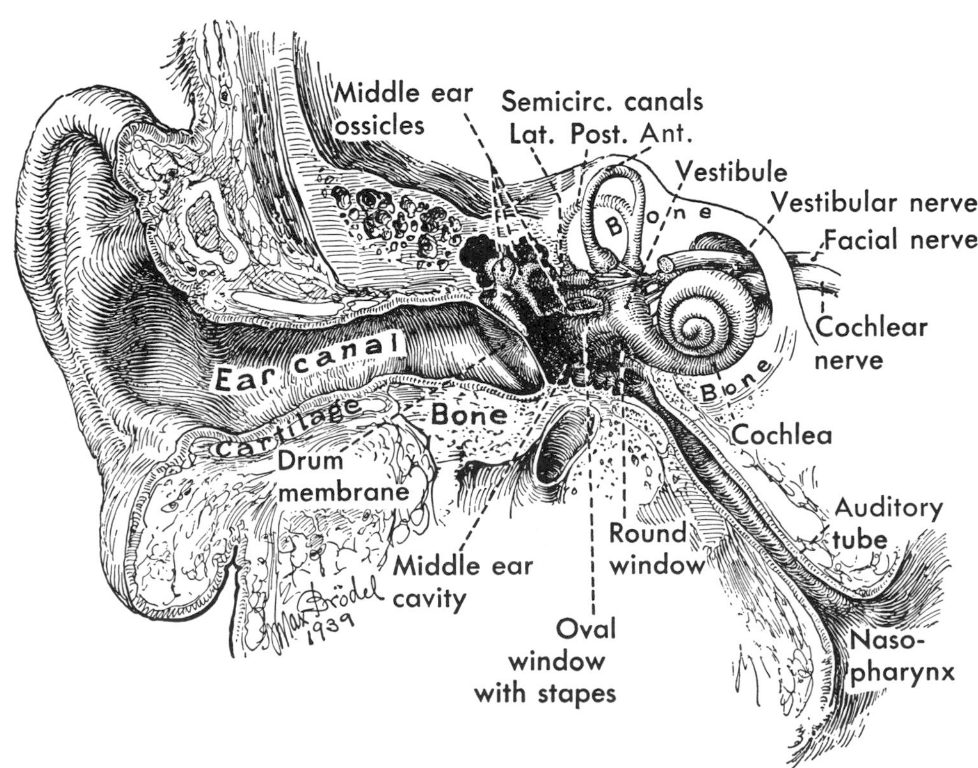

FIGURE *33-1.*
The external, middle, and internal ear. (Brödel M. Three unpublished drawings of the anatomy of the human ear. Philadelphia: WB Saunders, 1946.)

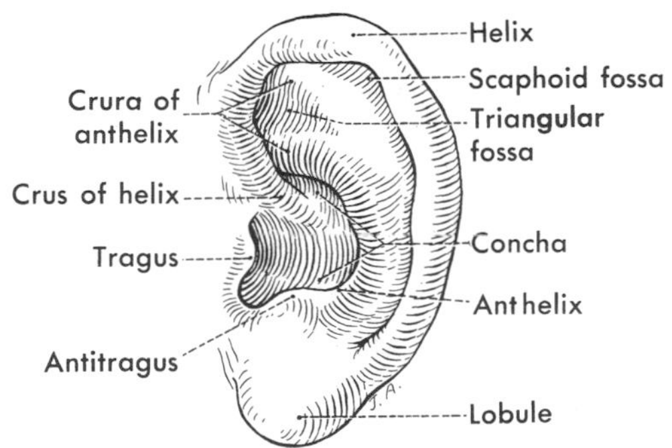

FIGURE 33-2.
Parts of the auricle.

The **external acoustic meatus** (external auditory meatus, external ear canal) leads from the deepest part of the concha to the tympanic membrane or eardrum. It is not straight, nor is it of uniform diameter throughout; as it is traced inward, a first part is directed somewhat forward and upward, the second part is directed slightly backward, and the third and longest part turns again to run forward and slightly downward.

A lateral part of the meatus, about 8 mm in length, has for its walls the troughlike cartilage of the meatus that extends inward from the cartilage of the auricle. The deficiency in the roof is completed by dense fibrous tissue, which converts the trough into a canal. Anteriorly and inferiorly, the cartilage extends farther medially, so that there is a part of the canal that has a bony roof and posterior wall, but a cartilaginous floor and anterior wall. The cartilage is firmly attached to the bony part of the canal by dense connective tissue. In the newborn, the bony canal has almost no length, for it is formed primarily by the small piece of bone known as the **tympanic ring** (see Fig. 31-12), to which the eardrum is attached. The term "tympanic ring" sometimes is used to designate that part of the temporal bone to which the eardrum is attached in the adult. Because the tympanic ring and the tympanic part of the temporal bone in the adult are incomplete above (where there is a gap called the *tympanic incisure*), the roof of the bony external meatus is completed here by the petrous part of the temporal bone.

The **tympanic membrane** or eardrum membrane (Fig. 33-3; see Fig. 33-1) is at the medial end of the acoustic meatus and separates this from the middle ear or tympanic cavity. In the newborn, it faces almost inferiorly and only slightly laterally, but with growth of the tympanic ring, its position changes. Even in the adult, however, it is still oblique, sloping medially from top to bottom and medially from posteriorly to anteriorly, so that the anterior wall and floor of the external meatus are longer than its roof and posterior wall. The tympanic membrane consists of a central fibrous core, composed of radial and circular fibers, interposed between a thin layer of skin on the side of the acoustic meatus and one of mucosa on the side of the tympanic cavity. At its periphery, it is attached by a fibrocartilaginous ring into a groove, the *sulcus tympanicus*, in the tympanic part of the temporal bone, and at its center, it is attached to the handle of the malleus (a bone of the middle ear). At this attachment, the *umbo*, the membrane is drawn inward so that it is somewhat cone shaped. Above and slightly anterior to the umbo, another part of the malleus (lateral process) is likewise attached to the inner surface of the membrane. Extending forward and backward from this *mallear prominence* are anterior and posterior *mallear folds* on the inner surface of the membrane. The part of the membrane above the mallear prominence and folds is attached peripherally at the tympanic incisure and is devoid of the central layer of fibrous tissue that forms the major part of the eardrum. This thin part is the *pars flaccida*, and the major remaining part is the *pars tensa*.

The tympanic membrane responds to air vibrations that are collected by the auricle and concentrated upon it through the acoustic canal. As it moves in response to such vibrations, it necessarily also moves the malleus, which is connected to it. The malleus in turn articulates with a second bone, and this articulates with a third (see Fig. 33-6). Through the movement of this chain of bones, vibrations are transmitted across the middle ear cavity to the internal ear.

The **blood supply** of the lateral surface of the auricle is from twigs (anterior auricular branches) of the superficial temporal artery. These help supply the meatus, which is supplied also by the deep auricular artery (a branch of the maxillary that runs through the parotid gland to the meatus and continues to the external surface of the eardrum). The medial side of the auricle is supplied by the auricular branch of the posterior auricular artery, a branch of the external carotid.

The **nerve supply** to most of the auricle is through the great auricular nerve. The auriculotemporal branch of the mandibular also contributes to the lateral surface of the auricle, as does the lesser occipital nerve to the medial surface. The major part of the external meatus and outer surface of the tympanic membrane is innervated through the auriculotemporal, but a posterior and lower part of both meatus and membrane is supplied by the tiny auricular branch of the vagus.

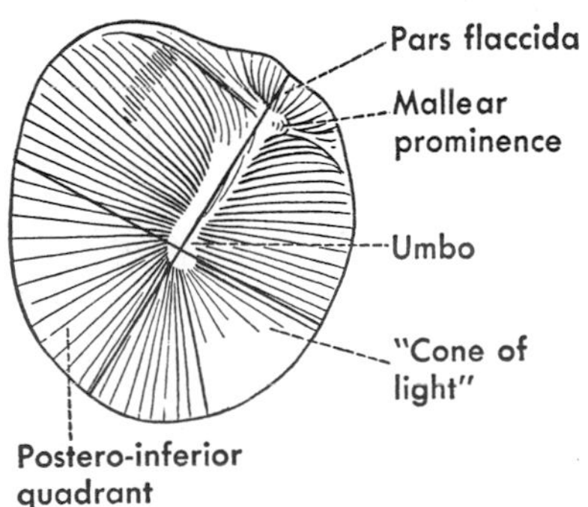

FIGURE 33-3.
The right tympanic membrane as it might appear through an otoscope, but with its quadrants indicated on it. Because the quadrants are determined by a line through the handle (manubrium) of the malleus and one at right angles to this, these lines are not perpendicular and horizontal. The "cone of light" is a reflection of light from the membrane.

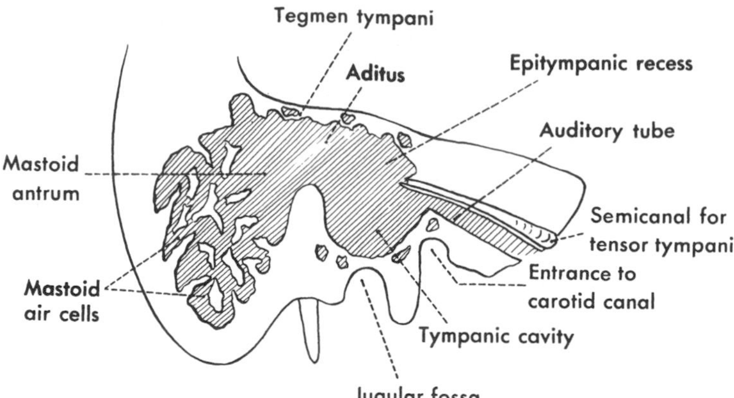

FIGURE 33-4.
Diagram of the middle ear cavity and its connecting air spaces, in a sagittal section.

This may contain fibers from the glossopharyngeal and facial nerves in addition to vagal fibers and supplies also a small bit of skin where the ear is attached over the mastoid process.

Middle Ear

The middle ear or tympanic cavity (see Figs. 33-1 and 33-4 through 33-7) lies in the temporal bone and is separated from the external acoustic meatus by the tympanic membrane. It has a greater height than the meatus and the tympanic membrane. Its floor is a little below the level of the inferior border of the membrane, and it extends well above the upper border. This upper extension of the tympanic cavity is the **epitympanic recess,** often referred to by clinicians as the "attic."

The tympanic cavity is wider above than it is below, and the epitympanic recess is still wider; however, the inward slant of the tympanic membrane to the umbo considerably narrows the cavity at the umbo's level. The floor of the cavity, called its *jugular wall* because it is also the roof of the jugular fossa seen on the outside of the skull, is exceedingly thin unless it is invaded by mastoid air cells. It presents a tiny **tympanic canaliculus** through which the *tympanic branch of the glossopharyngeal nerve* enters the middle ear. The anterior or *carotid wall* of the tympanic cavity is incomplete. Below, a thin layer of bone intervenes between the cavity and the internal carotid artery. The bone presents small *caroticotympanic foramina* through which caroticotympanic rami of the internal carotid artery, and one or more nerve twigs from the internal carotid plexus, enter the tympanic cavity. Above this partial wall is the relatively large *opening of the auditory tube.* The *roof* of the cavity is the **tegmen tympani** or tegmental wall; it also is thin and forms a small posterolateral part of the floor of the middle cranial fossa.

The posterior or *mastoid wall* of the tympanic cavity is, like the anterior wall, incomplete above. Below, there is a bony wall between the mastoid air cells and the tympanic cavity, but above this, the cavity extends back, as the **aditus** (*aditus ad antrum,* or entrance to the antrum), into the mastoid part of the bone. As it reaches the mastoid part, the aditus gives way to the larger cavity of the **mastoid antrum.** From the mastoid antrum a series of connecting air-filled and mucosa-lined spaces extend through most of the mastoid process; these are the **mastoid air cells.** They may extend forward into the roof, floor, or walls of the tympanic cavity and may come to partly surround some of the particularly hard bone that encloses the internal ear.

It is because of the sinuosity of the connections among the mastoid air cells that mastoiditis, before the advent of antibiotics, was regularly treated by exenteration (removal) of the mastoid cells. Necrosis of bone as a result of mastoiditis can easily lead to fatal infection, for the internal jugular vein is adjacent to the floor of the tympanic cavity, and the sigmoid sinus is adjacent to the mastoid air cells posteromedially and may be separated from them by only a thin lamina of bone.

Because of the close relations of the middle ear to great vessels and to the brain, severe bleeding or the escape of cerebrospinal fluid through a ruptured tympanic membrane may occur following an accident or blow on the head. Either is evidence of a dangerous fracture.

The medial or *labyrinthine wall* of the tympanic cavity (Fig. 33-5) is of special interest. The prominent bulge of this medial wall is the **promontory,** formed by the large basal coil of the cochlea, the part of the internal ear concerned with hearing. On the promontory there is a delicate **tympanic plexus** (see Fig. 32-26), contributed to mostly by the *tympanic branch of the glossopharyngeal nerve,* but joined also by twigs from the internal carotid plexus (*caroticotympanic nerves*) and usually by a *twig from the facial nerve* or its greater petrosal branch. Extensions from this plexus supply the mucous membrane of the tympanic cavity, the tympanic antrum and mastoid air cells, and the auditory tube. In addition, a part of the tympanic branch of the ninth nerve leaves the promontory to travel forward as the *lesser petrosal nerve* to the otic ganglion. Above the promontory in a depression, the *fossula fenestrae vestibuli,* is the opening into which the base of the stapes fits. This is the **fenestra vestibuli** (vestibular window, or oval window because of its shape). Below this, posteroinferior to the promontory, is another depression, the *fossula fenestrae cochleae* or cochlear fossula, that leads to a second opening into the internal ear, the **fenestra cochleae** (cochlear window, also called round window). This open-

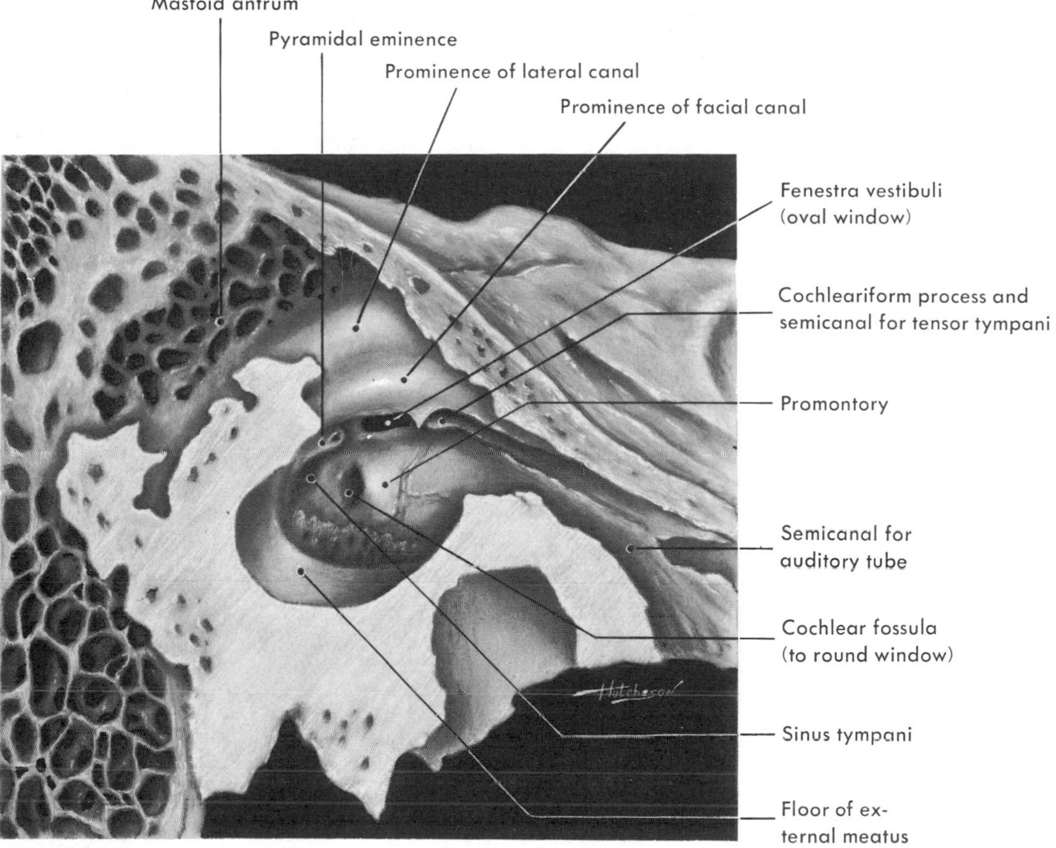

FIGURE 33-5.
The medial wall of the tympanic cavity.

ing is sealed during life by the **secondary tympanic membrane.**

Above and anterior to the fenestra vestibuli is the **cochleariform process** through which the tendon of the *tensor tympani muscle* enters the tympanic cavity. A little posterior to this fenestra is the tiny **pyramidal eminence** through which the tendon of the *stapedius muscle* enters the tympanic cavity. Above the vestibular window, directed posteriorly and somewhat downward, is the **prominence of the facial canal;** the *facial nerve* produces this, bulging the bone here after it has left the geniculate ganglion. Above and somewhat posterior to the prominence of the facial canal, on the medial wall of the aditus, is a broader bulge, the **prominence of the lateral semicircular canal,** caused by the enlarged anterior or ampullary end of this canal (and the adjacent ampullary end of the superior canal). These canals are part of the portion of the ear having to do with balance.

Recognition of the prominence of the facial canal and of the prominence of the lateral semicircular canal is critical in attempts to restore hearing by making an additional opening into the internal ear (fenestration), because the opening must be made into the lateral semicircular canal at its ampullary end. This operation is done to afford a second movable window between the middle and internal ear when, because of ossification of the membrane by which it is held in the fenestra vestibuli, the stapes becomes immovable (*otosclerosis*). It is also particularly important in operations for mastoiditis to recognize the course of the facial nerve.

A second way of restoring hearing after otosclerosis is to mobilize or replace the stapes. Stapes operations have certain advantages over fenestration in restoring hearing and are currently more often employed as the primary operation for otosclerotic deafness.

The **auditory tube** (pharyngotympanic tube, eustachian tube) opens through the anterior wall of the tympanic cavity. It originally was an outgrowth from the pharynx, representing the first pharyngeal pouch, and the middle ear cavity and mastoid air cells are expansions from it. From the ear, it extends forward, medially, and downward in a bony tube, called a **semicanal,** that lies in the temporal bone and opens on the external base of the skull between the foramen spinosum and the carotid canal. During life, however, the tube has also a cartilaginous part: the medial wall and the upper part of the lateral wall are composed of a folded piece of cartilage. The remainder of the tube is completed by membrane. The cartilage extends to the wall of the pharynx, where the opening of the tube and the elevation (torus) above and medial to this opening can be seen on the interior of the pharynx.

Immediately above the auditory tube, opening into the tympanic cavity through the cochleariform process, is the tube or "semicanal" for the **tensor tympani muscle.** The muscle arises in part from this canal and in part from the cartilage of the auditory tube and the greater wing of the sphenoid dorsolateral to the tube. As it enters the tympanic cavity, the tendon of the muscle turns sharply laterally to attach to the malleus.

The tympanic cavity and inner surface of the tympanic membrane, the mastoid antrum and cells, and the auditory tube are **innervated** by the tympanic plexus; therefore, primarily through the tympanic branch of the glossopharyngeal nerve. There are several **arteries,** all of them too tiny to be recognizable in an ordinary dissection. They include caroticotympanic branches from the internal carotid, parts of the stylomastoid and posterior tympanic arteries from the posterior auricular, the inferior tympanic artery from the ascending pharyngeal, the superior tympanic artery from the middle meningeal, and the anterior tympanic artery from the maxillary.

The auditory tube is normally closed at its pharyngeal end, but on occasion, must be opened if the pressure in the tympanic cavity is to be equalized with atmospheric pressure. The **tensor vell palatini,** which arises in part from the cartilaginous part of the tube, is primarily responsible for opening it. The fact that this muscle contracts when one yawns or swallows explains the effect these actions have in alleviating the discomfort arising from unequalized pressure.

Auditory Ossicles

The three bones of the middle ear cavity (Figs. 36-6 and 33-7) are the malleus (hammer), incus (anvil), and stapes (stirrup). They extend across the cavity (covered by mucous membrane) from the tympanic membrane to the internal ear.

The round upper end of the **malleus** is its *head* (caput). This fits into the concavity of the body of the incus,

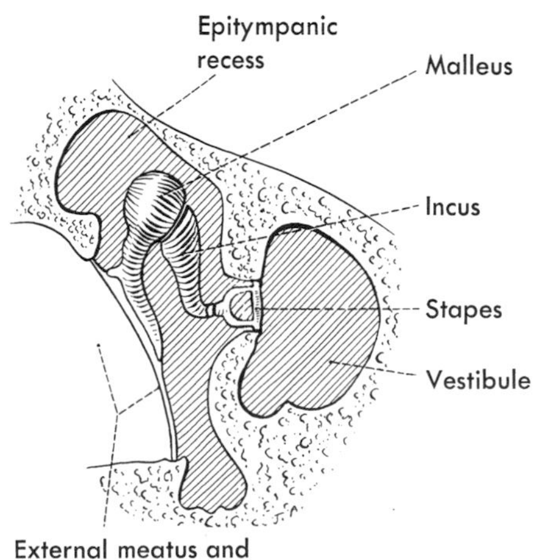

FIGURE 33-6.
Diagram of the three bones of the middle ear cavity as they extend between the tympanic membrane and the vestibule of the internal ear. In this figure, to show its form, the stapes has been rotated 90°—its crura actually are anterior and posterior, rather than superior and inferior.

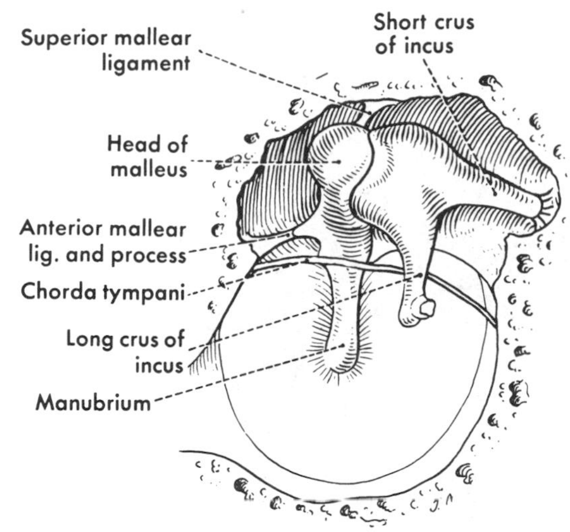

FIGURE 33-7.
The malleus, incus, and tympanic membrane seen from the medial side.

which lies behind it; both bones lie in part in the epitympanic recess. Below a slight neck, the malleus has a short *anterior process* and a more prominent *lateral process* that is attached to the inner surface of the tympanic membrane. The long lower part of the malleus is the *manubrium* (handle), attached at its lower end to the umbo. The tendon of the **tensor tympani muscle** attaches to the upper part of the manubrium. The tensor tympani muscle is innervated by a branch of the mandibular nerve and by its reflex contraction tends to check too great movement of the eardrum in response to loud noises. The malleus is attached to the eardrum by both the manubrium and the lateral process; it is suspended by ligaments, including one that comes down from the tegmen tympani; and it has a synovial joint, provided with ligaments of elastic tissue, between it and the incus.

Below the posterior mallear fold of the tympanic membrane, and passing upward and forward medial to the malleus to blend with the anterior fold, is a fold of mucosa that contains the *chorda tympani nerve.* This slender nerve leaves the facial nerve in the posterior wall of the tympanic cavity and traverses the *canaliculus of the chorda tympani* between the facial canal and the cavity. It then arches upward and forward between the incus and the malleus and leaves the tympanic cavity through a second canaliculus to emerge at the petrotympanic fissure. Beyond this, it joins the lingual branch of the mandibular nerve.

The body of the **incus** is concave anteriorly, where it articulates with the head of the malleus. From the body extend two *crura,* of which the upper, the short crus, extends almost horizontally backward to be attached by a ligament to the upper part of the posterior wall of the tympanic cavity. The long crus projects downward into the tympanic cavity, almost paralleling the manubrium mallei but lying posteromedial to it. At its lower end, this crus suddenly bends medially to articulate with the third bone, the stapes, through a nodule of cartilage called the *lenticular process.*

The **stapes,** shaped like a stirrup, has a head that receives the articulation of the long process of the incus. From the head proceed two limbs (crura), which join the *base* of the stapes, the footplate of the stirrup. The base is approximately oval and fits into the vestibular window on the medial wall of the tympanic cavity. Its inner surface is in contact with fluid in the inner ear, such that when the stapes is removed, one can look from the middle into the inner ear. The stapes is held in place by an *annular ligament* that not only seals the fluid within the inner ear, but also allows the stapes to move back and forth as vibratory impulses are transmitted to it from the eardrum by the malleus and the incus. The tendon of the small **stapedius muscle** emerges from the posterior aspect of the tympanum through an aperture at the end of the pyramidal eminence and attaches to the head of the stapes. This little muscle, innervated by a twig of the facial nerve, reflexly contracts to prevent too great oscillation of the stapes.

Facial Nerve

As evidenced by the prominence of the facial canal, the facial nerve is closely related to the middle and internal ears during a part of its course. Therefore, the relations and branches of this part of the nerve are best examined during dissection of the ear.

The facial nerve enters the petrous part of the temporal bone through the internal acoustic meatus (Fig. 33-8) in company with the eighth (vestibulocochlear) nerve and the labyrinthine artery. It lies above the eighth nerve and has two roots, a large voluntary motor root and a smaller nervus intermedius that consists of sensory and parasympathetic fibers and lies between the motor root and the eighth nerve or is attached to the latter. The two roots join in the acoustic canal. At the lateral end of the acoustic canal, the facial nerve enters the **facial canal,** in which it runs to the stylomastoid foramen. In this course, it first passes laterally between the upper parts of the bony vestibule and the bony cochlea, where it bears its sensory ganglion, the **geniculate ganglion,** and gives off the greater petrosal nerve. This nerve enters the middle cranial fossa through the hiatus of the canal of the greater petrosal nerve. At the geniculate ganglion, the facial nerve makes an abrupt turn (the *geniculum*) posteriorly and, as it passes across the lateral wall of the vestibule (medial wall of the tympanic cavity), just below the lateral semicircular canal, it raises the prominence of the facial canal (see Fig. 33-5). Behind the vestibule, the nerve turns somewhat more gradually to run downward in the bony wall between the middle ear cavity and the mastoid antrum and air cells.

Before it emerges at the stylomastoid foramen, the facial nerve gives off three small branches: a twig to the stapedius as it passes that muscle; the chorda tympani, already described; and a tiny branch that joins the auricular branch of the vagus.

In the lower part of its course in the facial canal, the facial nerve is accompanied by the **stylomastoid artery,** a branch of the posterior auricular that runs retrogradely along the nerve, helping to supply it and the middle ear cavity.

Internal Ear

The internal ear consists of a series of cavities in the petrous part of the temporal bone (these have particularly dense bony walls and give the name *petrous*—rocklike—to this part of the bone) and a series of membranous ducts and sacs that lie within the bony cavities. The bony part of the internal ear is known as the **osseous labyrinth,** and the membranous ducts and sacs are known as the **membranous labyrinth.** The membranous labyrinth does not fill the bony one (Fig. 33-9), although it is in places closely attached to the inner wall of this and in other places is attached by delicate trabeculae. The space between the membranous and bony labyrinths is filled with **perilymph** or perilymphatic fluid. Similarly, the membranous

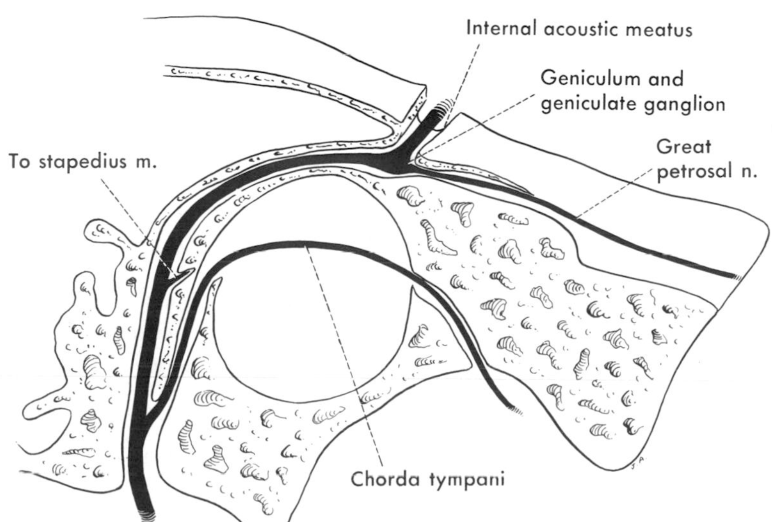

FIGURE 33-8.
The facial nerve in the temporal bone: The relation of the chorda tympani to the malleus and incus is shown in Figure 33-7.

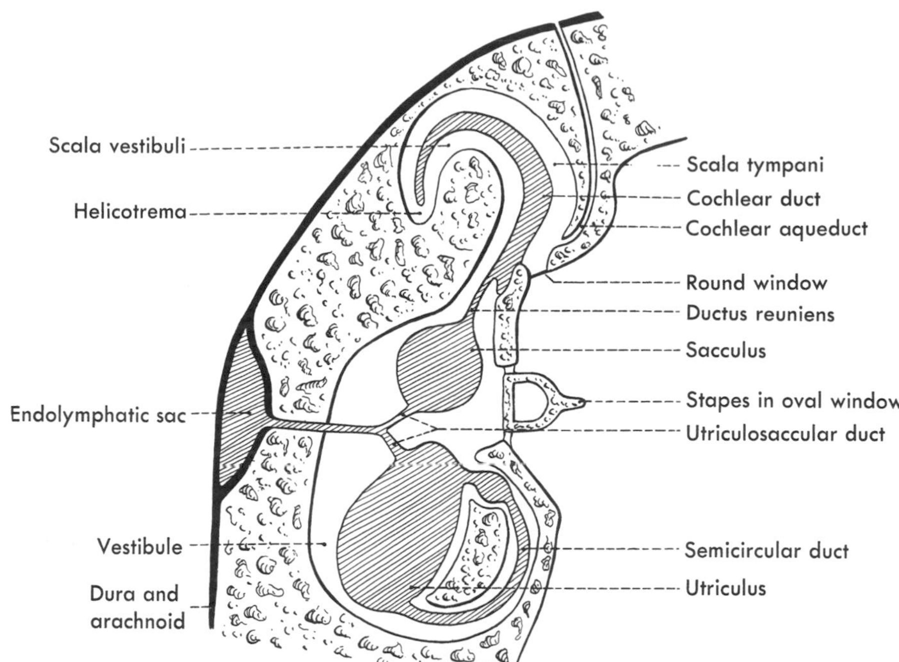

FIGURE 33-9.
Diagram of the perilymphatic and endolymphatic spaces; the latter, in the membranous labyrinth, is *shaded*.

labyrinth is filled with **endolymph** or endolymphatic fluid. The bony labyrinth forms a continuous mass, and the cavity within it is one continuous cavity. Similarly, all parts of the membranous labyrinth are connected together. However, both bony and membranous labyrinths are divisible into anterior and posterior parts, with different functions. The anterior part, the **cochlea,** is concerned with hearing, and the bony cochlea contains a membranous **cochlear duct.** The posterior part is concerned with balance. Its osseous parts are the **vestibule** and three **semicircular canals.** The vestibule contains two membranous parts, the **utriculus** and the **sacculus,** and each bony semicircular canal contain a membranous canal, called a **semicircular duct.**

Descriptions of the internal ear are easier to follow if emphasis is placed on its functional divisions, rather than on the differences between the bony and membranous parts. The following description is necessarily partly based on histologic studies, because in gross dissection of the ear little more can be done than to ascertain the position of the chief bony parts and display the perilymphatic cavity by removing a part of the wall of the bony labyrinth. Because of the small size of the internal ear, this dissection is a tedious and time-consuming one.

Vestibule and Semicircular Canals

The **vestibule** is the central chamber of the bony labyrinth. The bony cochlea is continuous with it anteriorly, and the bony semicircular canals, lying largely above and lateral to it, each are continuous with it at both their ends. Its relation to the middle ear cavity can best be observed by noting that the fenestra vestibuli, into which the stapes fits, opens from the tympanic cavity into the vestibule when the stapes is removed, and that a cavity within the promontory of the middle ear (produced by the large basal turn of the cochlea) also opens into the vestibule. (Another part of the perilymphatic cavity in the basal turn of the cochlea is separated from the middle ear cavity by the secondary tympanic membrane of the round or cochlear window.)

The vestibule (Fig. 33-10; see Fig. 33-9) is a small oval chamber approximately 6 mm long anteroposteriorly, 1 or 2 mm less in vertical diameter, and perhaps 3 mm wide. The facial nerve lies first anterior and dorsal to the vestibule and then in the lateral wall of the vestibule. The medial wall of the vestibule, between this cavity and the internal acoustic meatus, presents three small areas with minute perforations that transmit branches of the vestibular nerve from the meatus to the sense organs in the vestibule.

The sense organs are within two membranous sacs: the posterior sac, somewhat oval, is the **utriculus,** and the anterior sac, more rounded, is the **sacculus.** Each makes an impression on the medial wall of the vestibule, and they are united only by a tiny **utriculosaccular duct.** From the utriculosaccular duct, the **endolymphatic duct** runs posteriorly to emerge through the bone of the posterior cranial fossa (posterior surface of the petrous bone) and expands into a blind pouch, the **endolymphatic sac,** in the dura just above the sigmoid sinus. The utricle and saccule usually are destroyed in gross dissection; however, the endolymphatic sac can be found and opened by incising the dura in the fovea for this sac (see Fig. 31-9). The bony canal through which the endolymphatic duct runs necessarily opens at its proximal end into the vestibule and is called the **vestibular aqueduct.**

Abnormal increase in the endolymph, termed hydrops of the internal ear or Ménière's disease, produces distressing symptoms and may eventually destroy the

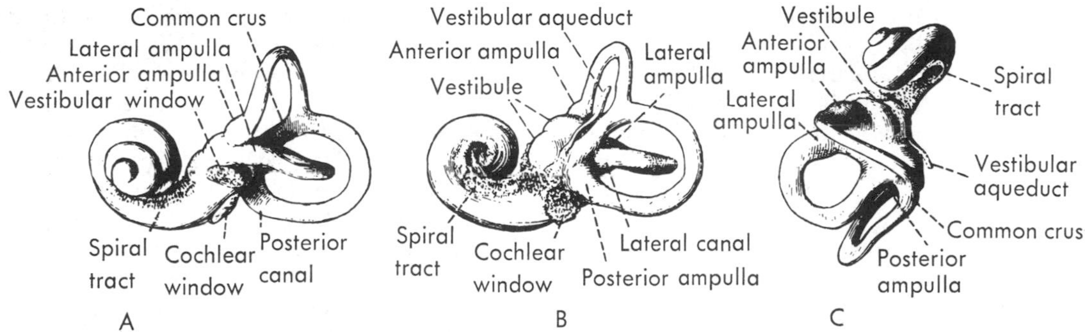

FIGURE *33-10.*
Casts of the bony labyrinth (perilymphatic space): (A) a lateral view of the left labyrinth; (B) a medial view of the right one; (C) a view of the left one from above. (Henle J. Handbuch der systematischen Anatomie des Menschen, vol. 2 Braunschweig: Vieweg und Sohn, 1868.)

sense organs of the ear. An operation to alleviate this condition takes advantage of the position of the endolymphatic sac to create an opening between it and the subarachnoid space, and thereby, relieve the endolymphatic pressure.

The sense organs within the utricle and saccule are essentially similar. They are called **maculae,** and there is a utricular and a saccular macula. A macula consists of a thick layer of epithelium, called neuroepithelium because its important functional component consists of "hair cells" that receive the stimulation. These cells have tiny processes projecting from their free surfaces, and the processes are embedded in a membrane in which are also embedded tiny crystals of calcium carbonate, called **statoconia** (otoconia) or otoliths. The neuroepithelial cells are innervated by fibers of the vestibular division of the eighth nerve. They are stimulated by the statoconia acting on their hairs.

The utriculus and sacculus are generally believed to be concerned entirely with balance (although some authorities think the sacculus may also have something to do with hearing) and are known to respond to gravity—that is, they initiate reflexes in response to the position of the head (the relation of the maculae to gravity), the statoconia either pulling or pushing upon the hairs. As a simple example of some of the complicated reflexes related to the position of the head, lowering the nose of a cat properly prepared to show these reflexes changes the relation of the maculae of the utriculus and sacculus to gravity and brings about a reflex response consisting of flexion of the anterior limbs and extension of the hind limbs—an appropriate reflex if one imagines that the cat, in lowering its head, wants to get its nose and mouth closer to a rat hole.

The bony canals necessarily move with the head, of which they are a part, and the ducts are so attached to the canals that they also move. The canals and ducts are so arranged that movement in any direction will necessarily move one or more somewhat along its long axis, with the result that fluid within the duct will exert a pressure in the direction opposite the movement (just as water in a drinking glass first stands still when the glass is rotated). In the ampulla of each semicircular duct there is a large projection, the **ampullary crest,** that contains neuroepithelial cells the hairs of which project into a gelatinous mass (*cupula*) that occludes the lumen of the membranous ampulla. Apparently, the pressure of the endolymph bends the cupula and this, in turn, stimulates the hair cells.

An important reflex connection of the semicircular ducts is with the muscles that move the eyes; when the head is moving, the eyes can move in the opposite direction to allow fixation of gaze—as in watching objects from a moving train. Each canal apparently controls certain muscles of the eyeball, so that stimulation of one will produce movement of the eyes in one direction and stimulation of another canal will produce movement in another direction. This movement, relatively slow, is followed by a quick movement in the opposite direction, and this combination of slow and quick movements is **nystagmus.** Clinically, the semicircular ducts can be tested by putting cold or warm water in the external ear canal or by rapidly revolving the patient with the head in different positions. The nystagmus that normally results is then described according to the direction of the quick movement (because it is easier to observe than the slow movement).

The **semicircular canals and ducts** have a somewhat different function from the utriculus and sacculus, for although they also are connected with balance, it is apparently movement alone, not position, that stimulates them. Each bony semicircular canal is much larger than the membranous canal (semicircular duct) that it contains, but one end of each duct is dilated to form a structure known as the **ampulla,** and the bony canal is also somewhat dilated here.

In the dissecting room one rarely sees the semicircular ducts, for they are of such size as to be barely visible grossly, are almost transparent, and frequently are destroyed in opening the bony semicircular canals. However, a good concept of the arrangement of the ducts can be obtained by examining a dissection of the canals. The three semicircular canals are called anterior, posterior, and lateral. Each canal opens at both its ends into the cavity of the vestibule, and each semicircular duct opens at both its ends into the utriculus; each has at one end an enlargement that identifies the ampullary end.

The **anterior semicircular canal** is placed vertically, and its position is indicated on the upper surface of the petrous part of the temporal bone (in the posterior part of the floor of the middle cranial fossa) by the arcuate eminence. Its anterior end, which bears the ampulla, is both anterior and lateral, for this canal lies at an angle of about 45° to the sagittal plane. The ampulla lies at the lower part of the curve at the anterior end, just before the canal joins the vestibule. The posterior end of the anterior canal curves downward and unites with the anterior end of the posterior canal, the two forming a **common crus** that opens into the upper and medial part of the vestibule. The **posterior semicircular canal** also is vertical, similar to the anterior one, but from the common crus that it shares with the anterior canal, it is directed posteriorly and laterally, such that although it also makes an angle of about 45° with the sagittal plane, it makes one of about 90° with the anterior canal. From the common crus, the posterior canal curves posteriorly, laterally, and downward, and its ampulla is on its posteroinferior end. Beyond the ampulla, the canal opens into the lower posterior part of the vestibule. The **lateral semicircular canal,** shorter than the anterior and posterior canals, has its ampullary end situated just below the ampulla of the anterior canal and opens into the vestibule immediately above the fenestra vestibuli. The lateral canal arches laterally, backward, and slightly downward (it is not quite horizontal) to pass through the loop of the posterior canal and open into the vestibule between the openings of the common crus and the ampullary end of the posterior canal.

The **semicircular ducts** need little further description. Because they lie within the canals, they have the same orientation; the anterior ends of the anterior and lateral ducts, and the posterior end of the posterior duct, have the membranous ampullae, and the posterior end of the anterior duct unites with the anterior end of the posterior duct to form a common crus. In short, just as there are only five openings for the three semicircular canals into the vestibule, there are only five openings of the semicircular ducts into the utriculus. Furthermore, each duct of one ear lies in a plane at almost right angles to each other duct, but in the two ears, the lateral semicircular ducts are approximately parallel, and the anterior duct of one ear is approximately parallel with the posterior one of the other.

Cochlea

The cochlea, concerned with hearing, consists of a bony cochlea and a membranous cochlear duct. Endolymph fills the cochlear duct, and perilymph largely surrounds this and fills the rest of the bony cochlea. The cochlea somewhat resembles the shell of a snail and presents about 2¾ turns, or, disregarding the turns, it takes the form of a short cone. The wide base of the cone is the **base** of the cochlea, and the apex is the **cupula.** Part of the basal turn of the cochlea protrudes into the middle ear cavity as the promontory and bears the cochlear window, and the base lies against both the vestibule and the distal end of the internal acoustic meatus. Where it abuts against the vestibule, part of the cavity within it is continuous with the vestibule. The part of the base lying against the meatus presents apertures through which the cochlear division of the eighth nerve leaves the cochlea.

The cochlea is most easily described as if it so sat upon its base that the line between the center of the base and the cupula were vertical. Actually, this axis of the cochlea (usually called its long axis, although it is only about 5 mm long and the base measures almost twice that across) runs anteriorly, laterally, and slightly upward.

Within the center of the cochlea is a central piece of bone extending from its base toward the cupula. This, the **modiolus,** forms a bony core around which the cochlear turns are arranged (Fig. 33-11). Through its hollow center, it transmits the branches of the cochlear nerve to the internal acoustic meatus. Between the turns of the cochlea, the modiolus is continuous with the outer bone of the cochlear wall. Projecting laterally from the modiolus at about the center of each turn, similar to the threads of a screw, is a thin lamina of bone, the **spiral osseous lamina.** At its upper end, instead of attaching the modiolus to the cupula, the spiral lamina ends freely in a little hook, the **hamulus.** The lamina contains tiny canals for nerve fibers. At the attached end of the lamina, these canals unite to form a larger one, the **spiral canal** of the cochlea, which houses the **spiral** (cochlear) **ganglion** and opens into the hollow of the modiolus.

The spiral bony lamina only partly subdivides the perilymphatic space of the cochlea into two passages, but this division is completed by the **cochlear duct.** This duct is somewhat triangular in cross section and is attached centrally at its apex to the osseous spiral lamina and peripherally to the outer wall of the bony canal. The cochlear duct will be described in more detail shortly. At the moment, the point to be made is merely that the osseous spiral lamina and the cochlear duct together divide the perilymphatic space within a single turn into two parts (Fig. 33-12). Of these parts, one (the upper one when the cochlea is placed upon its base) opens below into the vestibule; hence, it is known as the **scala vestibuli.** Through its opening, perilymph can be freely interchanged between the vestibule and the cochlea. The other, the **scala tympani,** opens below into the tympanic cavity through the fenestra cochleae in the dried condition. During life, the perilymph is prevented from escaping here by the **secondary tympanic membrane** that occludes this window.

Although separate elsewhere, the scala vestibuli and the scala tympani are continuous with each other at the cupula (their junction is called the *helicotrema*). Thus, each turn of the cochlea contains a perilymphatic space, the scala vestibuli, that is coiling upward from the base to the cupula and a continuation of this space, the scala tympani, that is coiling downward from the cupula to the base. Because they are continuous, movement of perilymph in the vestibule, induced by movement of the stapes, can induce movement of the fluid up the scala vestibuli to the cupula, then down the scala tympani to the cochlear fenestra (or pressure can be transmitted from one scala to the other through the membranous cochlear duct). Because fluid is essentially

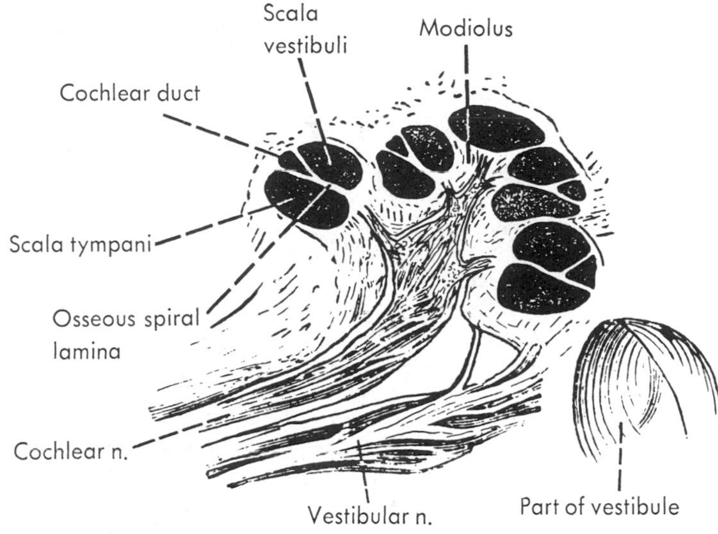

FIGURE 33-11.
A longitudinal section through the cochlea. (Modified from Henle J. Handbuch der systematischen Anatomie des Menschen, vol 2. Braunschweig: Vieweg und Sohn, 1868.)

incompressible, an inward movement of the stapes is accompanied by an outward movement of the secondary tympanic membrane and vice versa, and mobility of the two windows is thought to be essential for proper function of the ear. Although sound waves can enter the internal ear through the cochlear window, they can have little effect if the stapes or some other part of the wall cannot move. This is the rationale on which fenestration, providing a second opening into the perilymphatic space and sealing it with a thin and movable membrane, is done.

The origin of the perilymph, the few drops of fluid that fill the perilymphatic spaces of the vestibule, semicircular canals, and cochlear scalae, is not known. A tiny **cochlear aqueduct** (*perilymphatic duct*) extends from the lower end of the scala tympani to the anterior border of the jugular foramen and usually is described as opening into the subarachnoid space of the posterior cranial fossa. However, the much argued concept that perilymph is derived entirely from cerebrospinal fluid, which circulates through the aqueduct, seems to be untenable in view of reports that destruction of the aqueduct has no effect on the ear. Another concept is that it is partly derived from cerebrospinal fluid, partly from blood, and partly by secretion.

The **cochlear duct,** the membranous part of the cochlea, is attached to the saccule by a tiny canal, the *ductus reuniens* (see Fig. 33-9), below which the cochlear duct ends blindly. After winding around the modiolus attached to the spiral lamina, the cochlear duct ends at the cupula, and the helicotrema, connecting the two scalae passes around this blind end.

The peripheral or *external wall* of the cochlear duct is the lining of the bony cochlea (periosteum, to which is attached the lining epithelium of the duct), greatly thickened to form the **spiral ligament.** Deep to the epithelium over the upper part of the spiral ligament are numerous small blood vessels forming the **stria vascularis.** This stria and its associated epithelial cells are believed to be largely responsible for the formation of the endolymph, and it has been suggested that its part in the scala vestibuli may be concerned with the formation and reabsorption of the perilymph. Other markings on this wall are of less importance.

The thin *roof* of the cochlear duct intervening between the endolymphatic and the perilymphatic

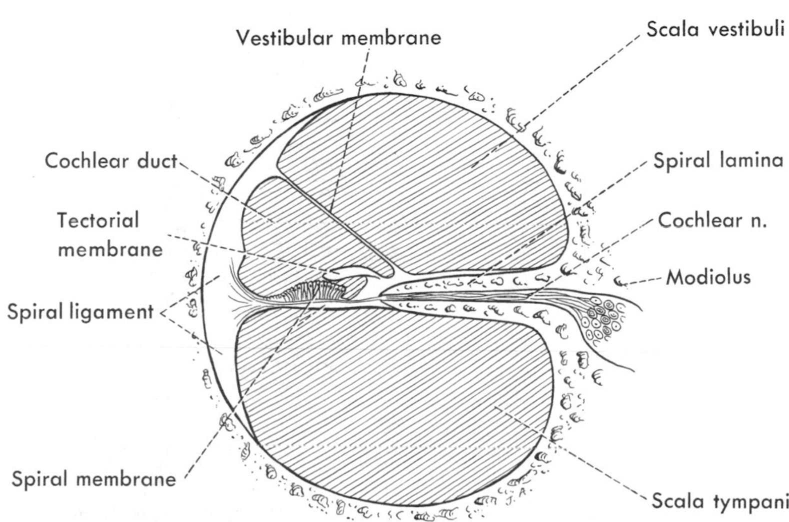

FIGURE 33-12.
Section through a single turn of the cochlea.

cavities of the scala vestibuli is the **vestibular membrane.** It has a thin core of connective tissue between two very thin layers of flattened epithelium, and it stretches between the upper part of the spiral ligament and the upper surface of the bony spiral lamina. Perilymph and endolymph differ markedly in their chemical makeup, and the vestibular membrane allows no free mixing between the two. Endolymph is believed to be absorbed largely through the endolymphatic sac, a part of which is very vascular. Both perilymph and endolymph are, according to some authorities, resorbed as well as formed at the **stria vascularis.**

The third or **tympanic wall** of the cochlear duct (between the duct and the scala tympani) is in part formed by the upper surface of the bony spiral lamina; the remainder is formed by the **spiral membrane.** The spiral membrane consists of a fibrous base of connective tissue, the **basilar lamina,** more often known as the basilar membrane, and the *spiral organ*, epithelium of the cochlear duct that is supported by the basilar lamina. The fibers of the basilar lamina or membrane are attached peripherally to a prominent projection (*basilar crest*) of the spiral ligament and centrally to the lower (tympanic) lip of the free edge of the osseous spiral lamina. The anatomy and vibratory properties of the basilar membrane have been extensively investigated.

The histology of the complicated **spinal organ** (of Corti) need not be described in detail here. Suffice it to say that among its tall epithelial cells are some neuroepithelial hair cells, from the outer surface of which project tiny hairlike processes. Nerve fibers end around these epithelial cells, and some of their hairlike processes are attached, in the living condition, to a fibrogelatinous mass, the **tectorial membrane**, that lies against the otherwise free surface of the spiral organ. This membrane is attached to the upper or vestibular lip of the spiral lamina, and its free edge extends just beyond the outermost neuroepithelial cells.

Vibration of the perilymph or endolymph stimulates the neuroepithelial cells; however, the exact way in which nerve impulses are set up in the cochlear nerve as a result of such vibration is beyond the scope of this text.

Blood and Nerve Supply

The bony labyrinth is supplied by the same vessels that supply adjacent parts of the temporal bone (for instance, the anterior tympanic branch of the maxillary, the stylomastoid branch of the posterior auricular, and the petrosal branch derived from the middle meningeal), but the membranous labyrinth has its own blood supply, distinct from this. The artery supplying it is the **labyrinthine artery.** It arises from the anterior inferior cerebellar artery or from the basilar and travels the length of the internal acoustic meatus with the facial and eighth nerves. The pattern of branching of the labyrinthine artery apparently varies among ears. However, there is regularly a *cochlear branch*, running in the modiolus and distributed to the cochlear duct and especially the stria vascularis, except a proximal part of the basal coil, and usually there are two *vestibular branches*, one distributed partly to the basal cochlear coil but primarily to the utriculus, sacculus, and semicircular ducts, and the other supplying only these parts.

The veins include vestibular veins and a spiral vein in the modiolus. The chief drainage is through a **labyrinthine vein** formed at the lateral end of the internal acoustic meatus and opening into either the inferior petrosal or the sigmoid sinus. There are two other small veins, a **vein of the vestibular aqueduct** that passes through that channel to enter the superior petrosal sinus, and a **vein of the cochlear aqueduct** that parallels the aqueduct and opens into the inferior petrosal sinus or the internal jugular vein.

The **eighth nerve** has already been largely described, both in the preceding description of the internal ear and in Chapter 32. Therefore, its distribution to the ear (Fig. 33-13) can be summarized briefly. At the distal (lateral) end of the internal acoustic meatus, the eighth nerve divides into a vestibular and a cochlear part. The **vestibular part,** in turn, divides into a superior and an inferior part, each of which bears a part of the **vestibular ganglion.** From the superior part, a short stem divides into branches that penetrate the bony wall between the end of the acoustic meatus and the cavity of the vestibule, ending in the ampullae of the anterior and lateral ducts, the macula of the utriculus, and a part of the macula of the sacculus. The inferior part of the ganglion gives a branch to the major part of the macula of the sacculus and one to the ampulla of the posterior semicircular duct. (The branch that passes from the inferior division of the vestibular nerve to the spiral ganglion of the cochlea apparently contains efferent or olivocochlear fibers that influence the sensitivity of the cochlea; the function of a twig from the cochlear ganglion to the saccule is not known.)

The ganglion cells of the **cochlear part** of the eighth nerve form the **spiral ganglion,** lying within the spiral canal of the cochlea. These cells send their fibers distally through the canals of the bony spiral lamina to reach the spiral organ. They send their fibers proximally into the modiolus, those from the upper (apical) part running through a central canal in the modiolus, those from lower parts through a series of spiral canals, and all of them opening through foramina at the lateral end of the internal acoustic meatus, where they unite to form the cochlear division of the nerve. As this is traced proximally, it unites with the vestibular division.

ORBIT AND EYE

The orbit largely surrounds and protects the eyeball and the nerves and vessels concerned with it. It lies below the anterior cranial fossa and mostly in front of the middle cranial fossa. Branches from the ophthalmic artery (from the internal carotid within the cranial cavity) supply the structures in the orbit, and some of them continue to the face and forehead, in company with similarly named branches of the ophthalmic nerve (a branch of the trigeminal). The optic nerve, originating from the eyeball, has its chief course within the orbit; it ends soon after it enters the cranial cavity. There are seven voluntary muscles, six of which move the eyeball. The remaining one is the levator

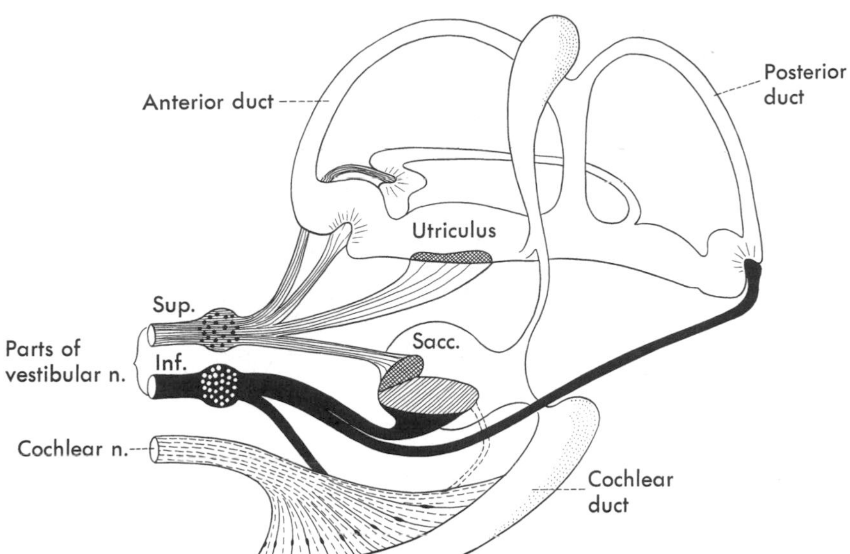

FIGURE *33-13.*
Schema of the distribution of the eighth nerve. (Redrawn from Hardy M: Anat Rec 1934;59:412.)

of the upper lid. These seven muscles are supplied by three nerves (oculomotor, trochlear, abducens), none of which has a cutaneous distribution, and all of which end in the orbit.

Bony Orbit

The orbit is somewhat pyramidal in shape and has superior, medial, inferior, and lateral walls. However, its long axis does not parallel the sagittal plane; rather, the medial walls of the two orbits are approximately parallel (see Fig. 33-19), and their lateral walls slope medially as they run posteriorly. The base of the pyramid is the anterior opening or aditus of the orbit. It has prominent supraorbital and infraorbital margins that meet laterally to give it a well-defined lateral border but are separated from each other medially by the more gradual transition between the medial wall of the orbit and the lateral side of the nose. At the back end, or *apex*, of the orbit there are two apertures: a large, somewhat triangular one, the **superior orbital fissure,** that opens into the front end of the middle cranial fossa; and just medial to this, visible when the orbit is inspected somewhat from the lateral side, a rounded aperture, the **optic canal,** that also opens into the middle cranial fossa (Fig. 33-14).

In the lateral part of the floor (inferior wall) of the orbit, separating it from the lateral wall, is a long fissure, the **inferior orbital fissure.** Its back end opens into the pterygopalatine fossa, its front end into the temporal fossa, and its middle into the most anterior part of the infratemporal fossa. Proceeding forward in the floor of the orbit from the junction of about the anterior third and the posterior two-thirds of the inferior orbital fissure is the **infraorbital groove.** This houses the largest branch of the maxillary nerve, which at the front end of the groove enters the infraorbital canal that opens onto the face below the infraorbital rim.

The **roof** of the orbit is composed almost entirely of the frontal bone. At the very back end, a little of the roof, medial to the upper part of the superior orbital fissure, is formed by the lesser wing of the sphenoid bone, which, with the body of the sphenoid medially, surrounds the optic canal. The roof intervenes between the orbit and the anterior cranial fossa. It is thin enough to be translucent and is readily penetrated, so that even such a thing as a pencil brought forcibly in contact with it may penetrate the brain. A part of the frontal sinus usually lies in the roof of the orbit, particularly anteromedially; the extent of the sinus in the roof varies. Anterolaterally, in the roof and lateral wall, is a large smooth depression, the **fossa for the lacrimal gland** (the tear gland). Anteromedially, at the junction of roof and medial wall, there is a small depression on the frontal bone, or a small spine, or both. These are, respectively, the **trochlear fovea** or **spine** and represent the attachment of a pulley (trochlea) through which one of the muscles to the eyeball runs. On the medial side of the supraorbital margin is the prominent **supraorbital foramen** or **notch** for transmission of the supraorbital nerve and vessels to the forehead, and medial to that there may be a less prominent **frontal notch** or **foramen** for a medial branch of the nerve.

The **medial wall** of the orbit is formed largely by the orbital lamina of the ethmoid bone. The orbital lamina contains ethmoid air cells and is so thin that the intercellular walls and, therefore, the pattern of some of the air cells can usually be seen without difficulty on examination of a dry skull. At about the junction of roof and medial wall, on or close to the frontoethmoid suture, are two small **ethmoidal foramina,** the orbital ends of the anterior and posterior ethmoidal canals; through them arteries and nerves leave the orbit.

Anterior to the ethmoid bone is the small lacrimal bone. This also is usually invaded by ethmoid air cells. Toward its anterior border is a fairly sharp margin, the *posterior lacrimal crest,* in front of which is a concavity, the **fossa for the lacrimal sac.** The frontal process of the max-

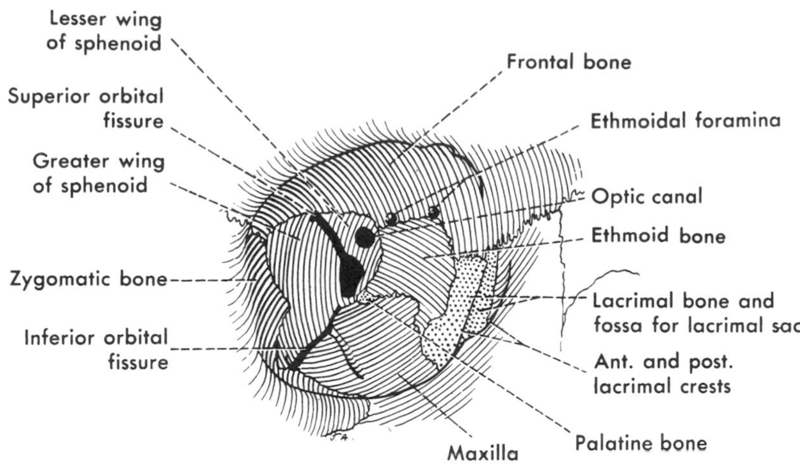

FIGURE *33-14.*
The bony orbit, in anterolateral view.

illa extends upward in front of the lacrimal bone and forms the *anterior lacrimal crest* that bounds the fossa anteriorly. The fossa for the lacrimal sac becomes deeper as it is traced downward and ends in the **nasolacrimal canal,** which opens below into the nasal cavity and houses the nasolacrimal duct.

The **floor** of inferior wall of the orbit is formed largely by the maxilla, which articulates medially with the lacrimal and ethmoid bones and, except anteriorly, is separated from the lateral wall by the inferior orbital fissure. The floor here also is the roof of the maxillary sinus. Anterior to the inferior orbital fissure, the zygomatic bone, which forms part of the lateral wall of the orbit, also contributes to its floor. Posteriorly, just in front of the back end of the inferior orbital fissure, at the point at which the maxilla, the ethmoid, and the lesser wing of the sphenoid seem to come together, the orbital process of the palatine bone forms a tiny part of the floor; this is not recognizable as a separate bone in some skulls.

A major part of the **lateral wall** of the orbit anteriorly is formed by the zygomatic bone, but the frontal bone curves downward to meet it. Behind the zygomatic bone, lateral to the inferior orbital fissure, is the greater wing of the sphenoid bone. The anterior part of the lateral wall separates the orbit from the temporal fossa (through which the orbit can be approached at operation), and a small posterior part separates it from the middle cranial fossa.

The orbit is lined by periosteum that is given the special name **periorbita.** It is continuous over the rim of the orbit and through the inferior orbital fissure with the periosteum of the outer surface of the skull, and through the superior orbital fissure and the optic canal with the periosteal or outer layer of the dura mater.

Eyelids: Lacrimal Apparatus

The skin of the eyelids or **palpebrae** (Fig. 33-15) is very delicate, and careless removal of it will remove also the thin layer of muscle deep to it. There is only a little connective tissue between the skin and muscle and deep to the muscle. Because it is particularly loose tissue, it allows ready accumulation of fluid—as, for instance, the minor hemorrhage resulting in a "black eye."

The muscle in the lid is the **palpebral portion of the orbicularis oculi;** the *orbital* part surrounds the orbit, and both these parts are described with the facial muscles (see Fig. 31-16). It need only be noted here that the palpebral portion is delicate and extends to the margin of the lid and that at the medial corner of the eye, many of the fibers of both palpebral and orbital parts attach to a ligamentous structure, the **medial palpebral ligament.** This ligament is attached medially to the anterior lacrimal crest. Laterally, under cover of the orbicularis, it bifurcates and attaches to the heavy structures (tarsi) that produce the curved shape of the upper and lower lids. Lateral to the corner of the eye, a **lateral palpebral raphe** may mark the intersection of fibers in the upper and lower lids, but this is not a palpebral ligament—the **lateral palpebral ligament** lies behind the muscle and gives no attachment to it.

A third part of the muscle is also demonstrable on careful dissection, for some of the fibers close to the free borders of the lids pass deeply as they near the medial corner of the lids, run behind the lacrimal sac, and attach to the posterior lacrimal crest. These form the **pars lacrimalis of the orbicularis oculi.** This part of the muscle surrounds two tiny tubes (the lacrimal canaliculi) that lead from the medial ends of the eyelids to the lacrimal sac (Fig. 33-16), carrying into it the tears that accumulate between the lids and the eyeball.

On the posterior surface of each lid is the thin **conjunctiva,** continuous at the margin of the lid with the skin. In the upper lid, it is reflected upward on the posterior surface of the lid and then turns down to run in front of the eyeball and attach to it close to the periphery of the cornea (the transparent front of the eyeball). Thus, there is a *palpebral* and a *bulbar* (eyeball) *layer* of conjunctiva; the angle that they make with each other is the **superior conjunctival fornix.** Similarly, the lower part of the conjunctiva is divisible into palpebral and bulbar parts and forms an **inferior conjunctival fornix.**

Ducts of the lacrimal gland open into the superior conjunctival fornix, primarily its lateral part, and blinking

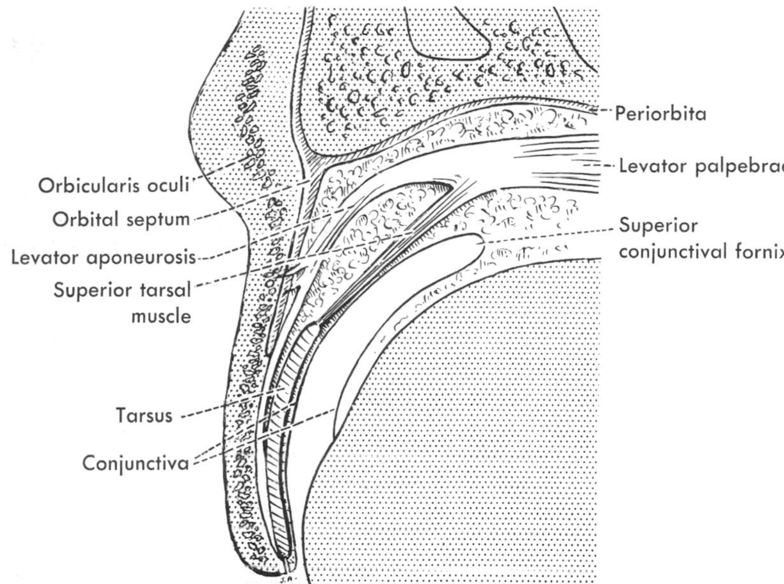

FIGURE *33-15.*
Structure of the upper eyelid: The space around the levator and its continuations into the lid is greatly exaggerated here.

movements keep the tears spread evenly over the eyeball. In the medial corner of the lids, on the posterior surface of each, is a little projection, the **lacrimal papilla,** that contains the opening or punctum of the **lacrimal canaliculus.** This drains excess tears. The two lacrimal canaliculi run medially, converging toward each other and usually joining, to empty into the lacrimal sac. The **lacrimal sac** is blind above (see Fig. 33-16), but below, it opens into the **nasolacrimal duct,** the lower opening of which can be seen when the nasal cavity is examined. The sac as a whole is lodged in the fossa for the lacrimal sac, between the anterior and posterior lacrimal crests (on the maxillary and lacrimal bones, respectively). It lies largely behind the medial palpebral ligament (although its upper end protrudes above that), but in front of the lacrimal part of the orbicularis oculi muscle. It also is surrounded by a special layer of **lacrimal fascia** that blends at the lacrimal crests with the periosteum in the fossa of the sac.

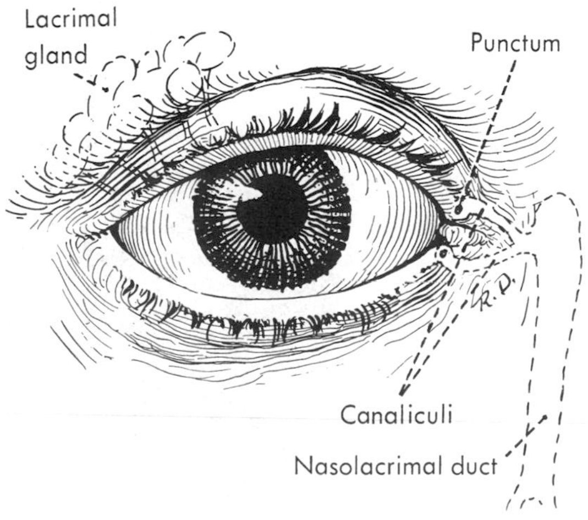

FIGURE *33-16.*
The lacrimal apparatus. (Wakefield EG. Clinical diagnosis. New York: Appleton, 1955.)

The major part of the thickness of each lid is formed by several **tarsal glands** that are embedded in dense connective tissue and form a plate, the **tarsus,** that is almost cartilaginous in appearance and maintains the shape of the lid (Fig. 33-17; see Fig. 33-15). The tarsi extend to the free margin of the lids, where their glands open. They are attached to the sides of the orbit by the palpebral ligaments. The medial palpebral ligament has already been noted. The *lateral palpebral ligament* lies behind both the orbicularis oculi muscle and some connective tissue and blends with other connective tissue behind it. Each palpebral ligament is bifid at its palpebral end and attaches to both the superior and the inferior tarsus. The superior tarsus is larger than the inferior, and its upper border is much more arched than is the lower border of the inferior tarsus. Until they are dissected free, however, neither has a free edge except at the edges of the lids, for they are overlapped by connective tissue that extends from the margin of the orbit into the lids and blends with the front of the tarsi.

The connective tissue extending over the front of both tarsi is derived from the periosteum at the margin of the orbit and simply projects down or up into the lid, as the case may be. It is known as the **orbital septum** and at its origin forms the most posterior part of the lid; its posterior surface is adjacent to the fat and connective tissue within the orbit.

In the upper lid, but not the lower, the tissue in front of the tarsus is also contributed to by tendinous fibers from the **levator palpebrae superioris** that run down behind the orbital septum to blend with it on the front of the tarsus and, according to some accounts, pass in part through the septum toward the skin. Behind the levator, a voluntary muscle, is a layer of smooth muscle that arises from its inferior surface and attaches below into the upper border of the superior tarsus; this is the **superior tarsal**

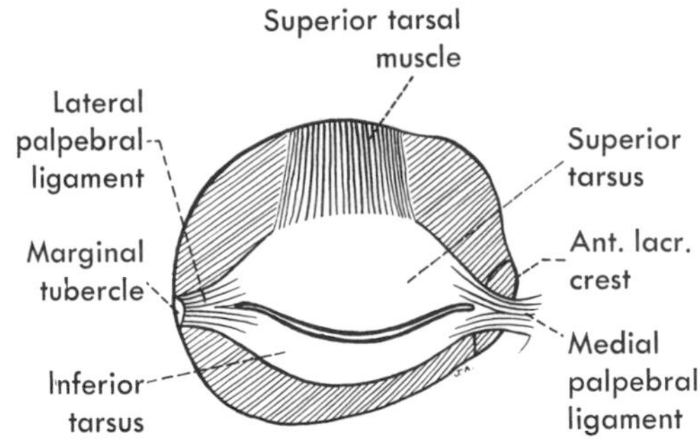

FIGURE *33-17.*
The tarsi and the palpebral ligaments.

muscle (see Figs. 33-15 and 33-17). An **inferior tarsal muscle** attaching to the lower edge of the inferior tarsus cannot be demonstrated by dissection.

Two **fascial spaces** are described in the lid: one, the *preseptal space,* lies in front of the orbital septum, between that and the orbicularis oculi; the other, the *pretarsal space,* lies behind the tendon of the levator palpebrae and is bounded posteriorly by the tarsus and the superior tarsal muscle and superiorly by the origin of that muscle from the levator palpebrae.

The **lacrimal gland** is located in the lateral part of the orbit behind the orbital septum. Its anterior part is deeply indented, and thus divided into two parts, by the tendon of the levator. The larger part, lying above the levator in the fossa for the gland, is the *pars orbitalis.* A slender *palpebral part* of the gland extends behind the levator into the upper lid, where it lies just deep to the conjunctiva on the posterior surface of the lid. The nerves and vessels of the lacrimal gland are described later.

The **cutaneous innervation of the lids** is through tiny branches of the large nerves that appear close to the rim of the orbit. The lower lid is supplied by branches from the *infraorbital nerve.* At the lateral corner of the eye, tiny twigs of the *lacrimal nerve* emerge to supply skin here but are difficult to find, for this nerve ends mostly in the lacrimal gland. In the upper medial corner of the orbit, three nerves, branches of the ophthalmic nerve, as is the lacrimal, penetrate the orbital septum and give twigs to the upper lid before continuing to the forehead and the side of the nose. The largest of them is the *supraorbital nerve,* which runs through the supraorbital foramen or notch to turn upward on the forehead close against the frontal bone. The smaller *supratrochlear nerve* likewise turns upward on the forehead a little medial to the supraorbital, and the still smaller *infratrochlear nerve* appears below the supratrochlear, running medially and downward to supply the upper part of the nose.

Associated with the nerves as they emerge from the orbit are **branches of the ophthalmic artery** (Fig. 33-18). The *supraorbital branch* turns up on the forehead with the supraorbital nerve, and the *supratrochlear* runs with the supratrochlear nerve. Similarly, the *dorsal nasal artery,* much larger than the infratrochlear nerve, turns downward to supply the upper part of the external nose. At the medial corner of the eye, between it and the nose, and in front of the medial palpebral ligament, are the angular artery and vein, upper parts of the *facial vessels.* The artery may inosculate with the dorsal nasal; consequently, it is impossible to say at what point the vessels join. Part of the *angular vein* enters the lid, above the medial palpebral ligament, to help form the superior ophthalmic vein. Above this level, the angular vein is formed by the junction of the supratrochlear and a part of the supraorbital vein. Lateral to and below the orbit are the *transverse facial vessels,* and lateral to and above the orbit are the frontal branches of the *superficial temporal vessels,* which may anastomose broadly with the supraorbital vessels. Part of the supraorbital vein joins the supratrochlear vein to form the *angular vein,* but another part turns into the orbit to help form the *superior ophthalmic vein.*

All these vessels about the orbit have twigs to or from the lids, but these supply primarily the skin of the lids and the orbicularis oculi; the blood supply to the deeper structures of the lids, particularly the tarsi, is mainly through the **medial palpebral arteries.** These, like the supraorbital and supratrochlear, are branches of the ophthalmic artery. The **superior medial palpebral** appears above the medial palpebral ligament and runs laterally, usually dividing into an upper and lower branch as it does so. The

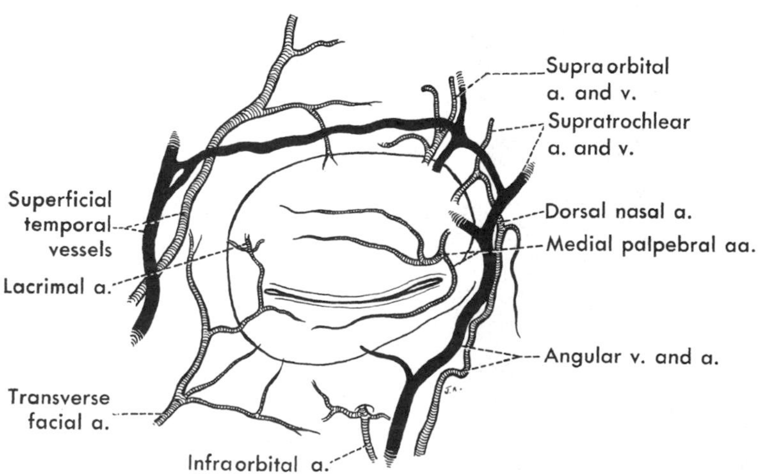

FIGURE *33-18.*
Chief vessels around the margin of the orbit and in the lids.

lower branch runs at first on the front of the tarsus and usually disappears into it, and the upper branch runs above the tarsus. The lower branch is described as anastomosing with a *lateral palpebral branch of the lacrimal artery* (also a branch of the ophthalmic) that appears at the lateral corner of the eye, to form the **superior palpebral arch.**

The *inferior medial palpebral artery* passes downward behind the medial palpebral ligament and then turns laterally to run on the anterior surface of the inferior tarsus. It usually disappears into this tarsus, but is described as anastomosing with a *lateral palpebral branch of the lacrimal artery* to form the **inferior palpebral arch.** The comparable **medial palpebral veins** drain into the angular vein.

Most of the lymphatic drainage of the lids is downward and backward toward the parotid nodes, but some of it, particularly from the medial corner of the eye, is downward along the angular and facial vessels to the submandibular lymph nodes.

Muscles and Associated Structures

The contents of the orbit are best studied by removing its roof, that is, much of the floor of the anterior cranial fossa. In doing this, the frontal sinus usually is opened, for it commonly sends an extension of varying size into the roof of the orbit, and some of the mucosa of the ethmoid cells may be exposed medially. The bone of the roof of the orbit strips off easily from the periorbita (periosteum lining the orbit), and the latter can be incised carefully without damaging the underlying structures. When this is done, the muscles will be seen to be partly concealed by fascia and connected to each other by intervening connective tissue that has a smooth outer surface where it was in contact with the orbital roof and walls. Because most of the muscles arise close together at the posterior end of the orbit and diverge to surround the eyeball as they are traced forward, they and the connective tissue connecting them form a cone. Most of the nerves and vessels of the eyeball lie within this muscular cone, but several appear peripheral to it and can be seen as soon as the periorbita of the roof of the orbit has been reflected.

Peripheral Nerves and Vessels

The largest peripheral structure is the **frontal nerve,** which enters the orbit through the superior orbital fissure above the origin of the bulbar muscles, therefore, it never lies within the muscle cone (Fig. 33-19). It is the largest branch of the ophthalmic nerve and is given off by this nerve in the cavernous sinus. As it runs forward, it divides into the lateral supraorbital and medial supratrochlear nerves, which round the upper rim of the orbit. Before the supraorbital nerve leaves the orbit, it is joined by the supraorbital artery, which emerges from the connective tissue and fat among the muscles to run forward in a superficial position.

Lateral to the frontal nerve, running along the upper part of the lateral wall of the orbit, is the **lacrimal nerve.** It likewise is given off from the ophthalmic within the cavernous sinus and passes, with the frontal nerve, through the superior orbital fissure above the origins of the bulbar muscles. As it runs forward, it is joined by lacrimal vessels that emerge from the muscle cone. Finally, the **trochlear nerve,** which, like the ophthalmic, traverses the cavernous sinus, enters the orbit with the frontal and lacrimal nerves and turns medially across the uppermost muscle here (the levator palpebrae) to reach the upper border of the muscle that lies highest on the medial wall of the orbit; this is the superior oblique muscle, which the trochlear nerve supplies.

The remaining vessels and nerves of the orbit lie within the cone formed by the muscles, embedded in the fat that occupies most of the space between the muscles. They are best seen, therefore, after the upper muscles have been reflected and the fat and connective tissue carefully dissected out.

Annulus Tendineus

Six of the seven voluntary muscles of the orbit arise from its posterior end. Four are rectus muscles and run forward to insert into the eyeball in the positions implied by their names: **superior rectus, medial rectus, inferior rectus,** and **lateral rectus.** These four muscles are blended at their origin to form a common tendon in the form of a ring, the **annulus tendineus communis,** that is attached to the body and lesser wing of the sphenoid bone medial to, above, and below the optic canal and laterally runs across the superior orbital fissure such that a part of this is enclosed within the ring (Fig. 33-20). The nerves that lie outside the muscle cone traverse the superior orbital fissure above the annulus, but the remaining nerves enter the orbit through that part of the superior orbital fissure enclosed by the annulus. The optic nerve and the ophthalmic artery also lie within the annulus, because this encloses the optic canal. The ophthalmic vein passes through the superior orbital fissure in a variable position, either above, through, or below the annulus.

Arising immediately adjacent to the annulus, but not forming a part of it, are two other muscles. One is the **levator palpebrae superioris,** the other the **superior oblique.** The seventh muscle of the orbit, the **inferior oblique,** arises from the floor of the front of the orbit and also runs obliquely to the eyeball. Therefore, it has no particular relation to the annulus.

Fascia

All the muscles of the orbit are surrounded by fascial sheaths that become thicker as they are traced forward toward the eyeball. Where the four recti and the two oblique muscles become applied to the eyeball, the fascia on them becomes continuous with a layer of fascia about the eyeball (Fig. 33-21). This layer ensheathes a major part of the eyeball, being attached to the sclera (the white part of the eyeball) posteriorly, close to the optic nerve and, anteriorly, just behind the cornea or transparent part of the eyeball. This is the sheath of the eyeball (**vagina bulbi** or **bulbar sheath**), also known as "Tenon's cap-

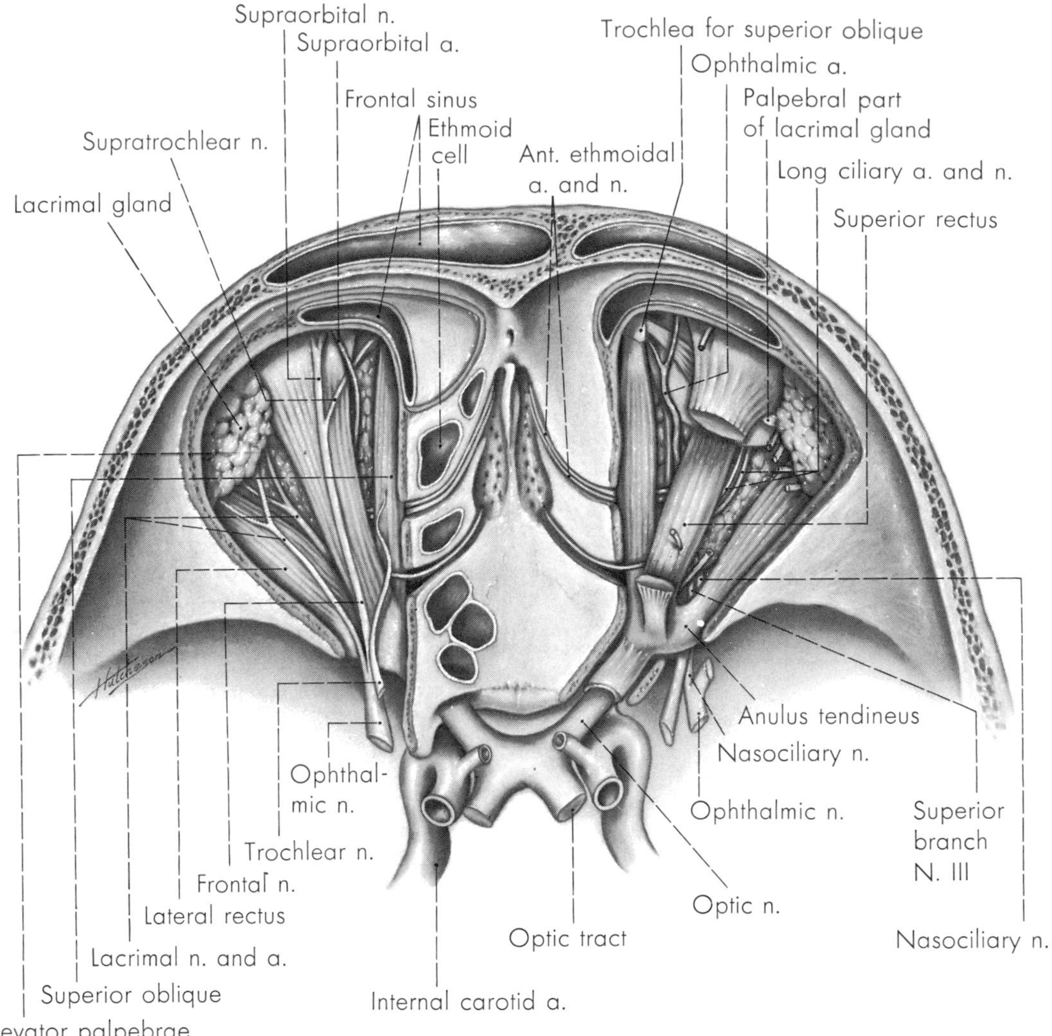

FIGURE *33-19.*
General anatomy of the orbit: On the *left*, bone and periorbita have been removed; on the *right*, the more superficially lying nerves and vessels have been removed, as has a part of the levator palpebrae, and the proximal part of the nasociliary nerve within the orbit has been moved laterally and anteriorly to bring it into view.

sule." As the sheaths of the muscles blend with it, their tendons pass between it and the eyeball to reach their points of insertion. Here, therefore, the bulbar sheath is separated from the sclera, although elsewhere it is bound to it by rather delicate connective tissue trabeculae, so that there is, between the sheath and the eyeball, an **episcleral space.**

Just before the fascial sheaths of the four rectus muscles blend with the bulbar sheath, they expand laterally to fuse with each other, thus forming what is usually called the **intermuscular membrane.** Tumors or other masses lying internal to this membrane and the rectus muscles may not be visible unless the space among the muscles is explored; therefore, the orbit is frequently described as being subdivided into two spaces, one inside and one outside the muscle cone.

Muscles and Their Nerves

Of the seven voluntary muscles of the orbit (see Figs. 33-19 and 33-21) (Fig. 33-22), the superior oblique is innervated by the trochlear nerve, and the lateral rectus by the abducens; all the others are innervated by the oculomotor.

The **levator palpebrae superioris** arises just above the superior rectus and follows that muscle forward, but instead of attaching to the eyeball, it continues into the lid. As it approaches the lid, its tendon widens rapidly and sends expansions ("horns") to attach to the medial and lateral walls of the orbit, but its major part attaches to the front of the superior tarsus (see Fig. 33-15). From the fascia between the levator and the superior rectus, there arises a thin lamina that attaches to the superior conjunctival fornix, so that these muscles also pull this up as they

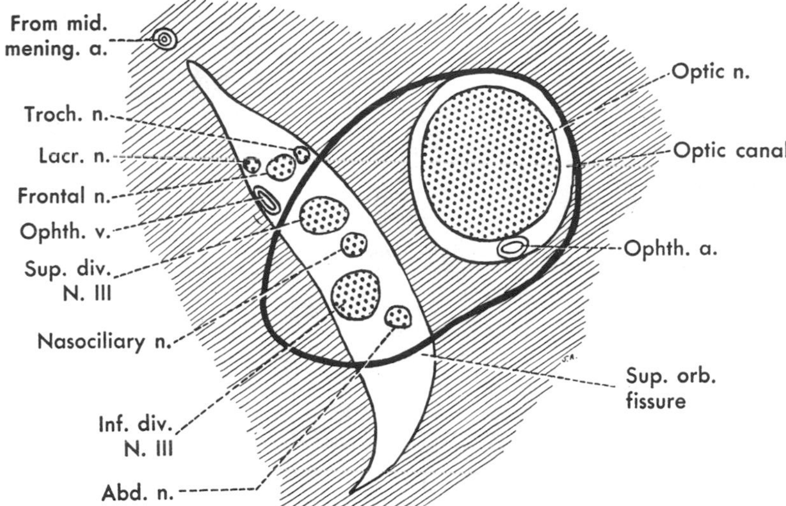

FIGURE 33-20.
Diagram of the annulus tendineus and relation of nerves and vessels of the orbit to it.

elevate the lid and turn the eyeball up. Fascia from the upper surface of the levator turns upward to attach to the superior orbital margin behind the orbital septum and often is described as forming a check ligament for the muscle. The levator palpebrae is innervated by the *superior branch of the oculomotor nerve* (the nerve divides into superior and inferior branches just before it enters the orbit), which first innervates the underlying superior rectus and then passes through this muscle to end in the levator palpebrae.

The **superior tarsal muscle,** often called "Mueller's muscle" by clinicians, arises from the lower surface of the levator palpebrae and inserts into the upper border of the superior tarsus. It is smooth muscle, innervated by *sympathetic fibers from the superior cervical ganglion*, and its denervation produces the ptosis or drooping of the lid that is characteristic of *Horner's syndrome* (see Chap. 32).

The **superior oblique muscle** arises medial to and a little below the origin of the levator palpebrae and, like it, just outside the annulus. Although it is straight at first, it runs obliquely to the eyeball. As it runs forward, it lies along the upper medial part of the wall of the orbit, above the upper edge of the medial rectus muscle. It becomes tendinous before it reaches the front of the orbit and thereafter is tendinous to its insertion on the eyeball. At the upper medial corner of the front of the orbit, its fascial sheath thickens and blends with a loop of dense fibrous connective tissue that contains a bit of cartilage and is attached at both ends to the frontal bone such that it forms a pulley (**trochlea**). At the trochlea, the tendon turns sharply backward, downward, and laterally, surrounded by a synovial sheath. Beyond the trochlea, the fascial sheath is thick.

It fuses with the bulbar sheath medial to the entrance

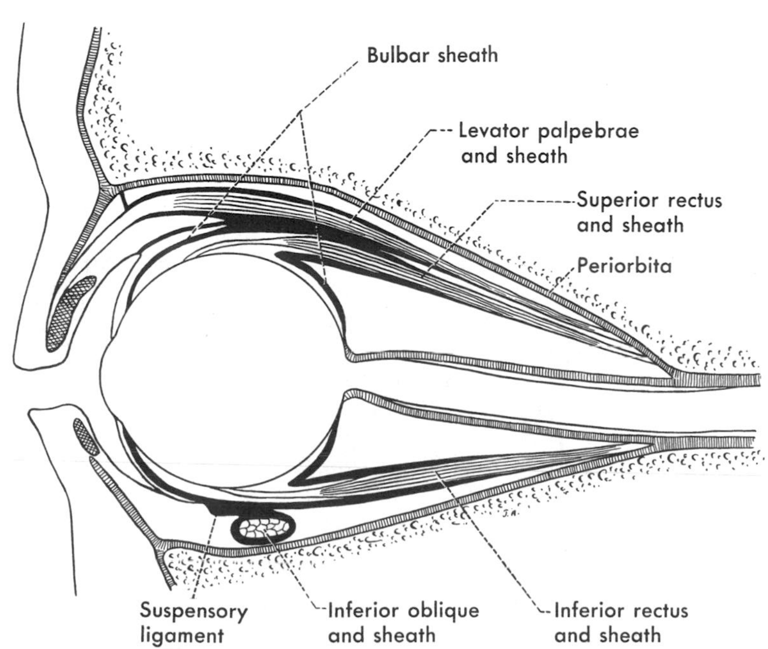

FIGURE 33-21.
Fascia of the orbit in sagittal section.

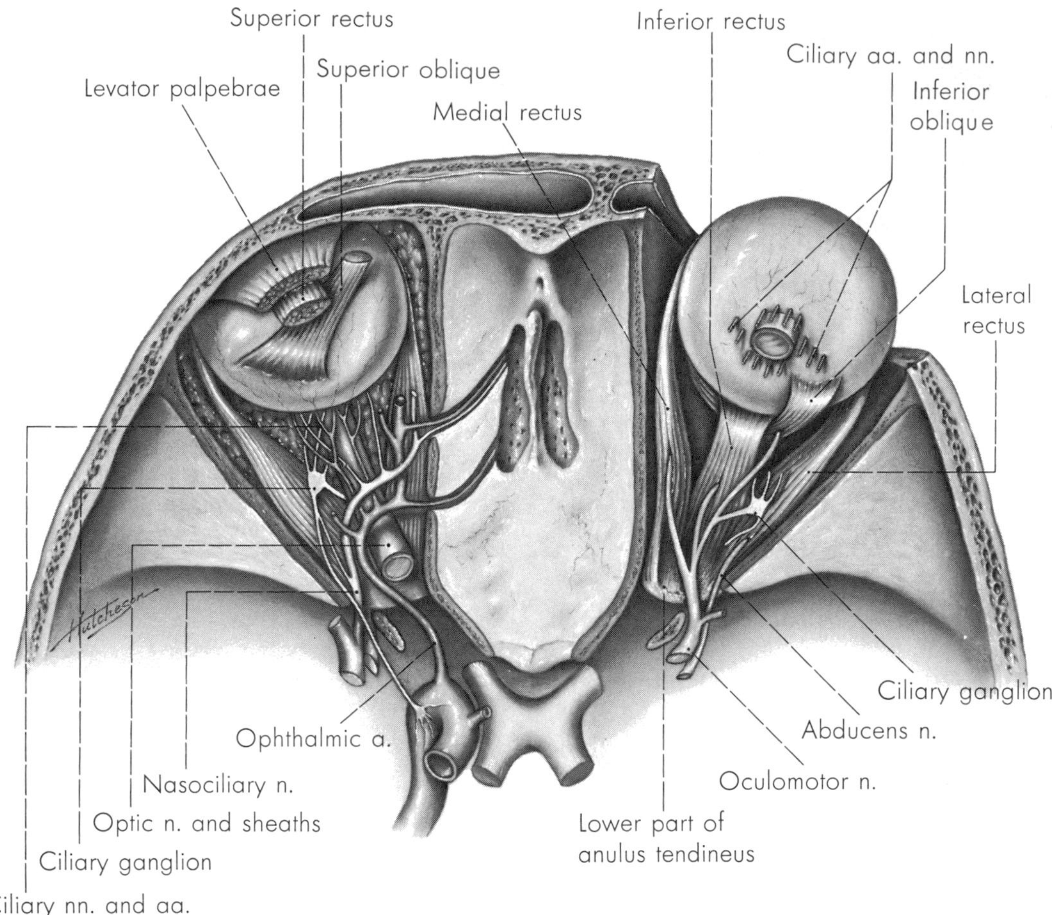

FIGURE *33-22.*
Further anatomy of the orbit: On the *left* the levator palpebrae, superior rectus, and superior oblique have largely been removed, and a segment has been taken from the optic nerve; on the *right*, most of the nerves and vessels of the orbit have been removed to show the abducens nerve and the inferior branch of the oculomotor nerve.

of the superior rectus into this sheath, but the superior oblique tendon continues posteriorly, laterally, and downward close against the upper and posterior surface of the eyeball. In this part of its passageway through the episcleral space, it passes deep to the superior rectus, between that muscle and the eyeball. As it nears its insertion lateral to and above the optic nerve (therefore, in the upper lateral quadrant of the posterior half of the eyeball), the tendon of the superior oblique expands from a cord to a thin membrane; hence, the insertion of the tendon is into a variably curved line on the sclera.

The superior oblique muscle is innervated by the *trochlear nerve,* which enters its upper border. When it contracts, it turns the eyeball so that the pupil is directed downward and outward.

The **superior rectus muscle** arises from the lesser wing of the sphenoid immediately above the optic canal; therefore its tendon forms the highest part of the annulus. As it runs forward, it is also directed somewhat laterally, as it must be to remain in the center of the orbit, and just before it reaches the eyeball, its fascial sheath separates from the sheath of the overlying levator. After its sheath has fused with the bulbar sheath, the muscle continues forward in the episcleral space, passing above the tendon of the superior oblique and inserting into the sclera above and behind the sclerocorneal junction. It is supplied by the *superior branch of the oculomotor nerve,* which is the uppermost nerve passing through the superior orbital fissure within the annulus. Shortly after it has entered the orbit, this stout branch turns upward to enter the proximal part of the superior rectus and continue into the overlying levator palpebrae.

The tendon of origin of the **lateral rectus** forms a lateral part of the annulus, particularly the upper and lateral limb of that part of the ring that crosses the superior orbital fissure. The nerves entering the orbit through this part of the fissure, therefore, are particularly intimately related to the lateral rectus muscle. The muscle runs forward against the lateral wall of the orbit. Just before its fascial sheath fuses with the bulbar sheath, it gives off an expansion that attaches to the lateral wall of the orbit to form a *check ligament* (*lacertus of the lateral rectus*) that limits the action of the muscle. After a course within the bulbar sheath, the muscle inserts into the sclera on the lateral side of the eyeball. The *abducens nerve* enters the orbit closely applied to the medial side of the lateral rectus and runs forward in this position only a short distance before entering the muscle.

The **medial rectus muscle** contributes the upper medial part of the annulus. Like the superior rectus, it is closely applied to the sheath of the optic nerve. It runs forward along the medial wall of the orbit, below the levator, and enters the episcleral space to attach to the medial side of the sclera. Its sheath, like that of the lateral rectus, gives off a *check ligament* that attaches to the medial wall of the orbit. The medial rectus is supplied by the *inferior branch of the oculomotor nerve;* this nerve lies just above the inferior rectus muscle, and its branch to the medial rectus runs medially below the optic nerve.

The **inferior rectus** contributes the inferior part of the annulus. It runs forward and laterally, as does the superior rectus. After it penetrates the bulbar sheath, it passes above the inferior oblique and inserts anteriorly on the eyeball. It is innervated by a branch from the *inferior division of the oculomotor nerve.*

The remaining voluntary muscle of the orbit, the **inferior oblique,** arises from the floor of the orbit anteromedially, just behind the orbital septum and often with some attachment to the fascia covering the lacrimal sac. It runs laterally and posteriorly to curve around the lower surface of the eyeball and insert into the lower lateral quadrant of the posterior half of the sclera: therefore, below the insertion of the superior oblique. As the muscle reaches the eyeball, its surrounding fascia contributes to the bulbar sheath, which is particularly thick below (where it is contributed to by the fascia of both the inferior rectus and the inferior oblique; see Fig. 33-21), and forms a sort of hammock that stretches upward to the fascia contributed by the medial and lateral rectus muscles. (This lower thickened part of the bulbar sheath is known to clinicians as the *suspensory*, or Lockwood's, *ligament.*) The inferior oblique passes below the inferior rectus muscle as it enters the bulbar sheath. It, like the medial and inferior recti, is innervated by the *inferior branch of the oculomotor nerve.* This muscle directs the pupil upward and laterally.

> All four rectus muscles insert on the anterior half of the eyeball, and their actions can be deduced from this. The medial and lateral rectus muscles direct the pupil medially and laterally, respectively. The superior rectus directs the pupil upward, and the inferior rectus directs it downward, but because neither pulls in a direction parallel to the long axis of the eye, both muscles also tend to direct the pupil medially. It is this medial pull of the superior and inferior recti that normally is overcome by the pull of the obliques. The inferior oblique directs the pupil laterally and upward, and therefore, when it and the superior rectus work together, a pure upward movement of the pupil can be obtained. Similarly, the superior oblique directs the pupil downward and laterally; therefore, when it and the inferior rectus work together, a pure downward movement can be obtained. Because of their attachments to the eyeball, the superior oblique and the superior rectus have long been described as rotating the eyeball medially, and the inferior oblique and inferior rectus as rotating it laterally. Rotation, however, is not a normal movement, and the superior and inferior recti actually prevent the rotation that the obliques produce when acting alone.

Other Nerves and Vessels

The frontal and lacrimal branches of the ophthalmic nerve, and the motor nerves to the orbit, now have been largely described. However, there is an additional branch from the inferior division of the oculomotor nerve that has not yet been mentioned; this is an *oculomotor root of the ciliary ganglion* that brings into it preganglionic fibers. It is a short, stout trunk, arising from the inferior branch just before that ends by branching into the nerves to the inferior rectus and inferior oblique, or arising from the first part of the nerve to the inferior oblique.

The **ciliary ganglion** (Fig. 33-23; see Fig. 33-22) lies well back in the orbit, just lateral to the optic nerve and between that and the lateral rectus muscle. It is a small ganglion, not much larger than the head of an ordinary pin. Sometimes it is double. In addition to its oculomotor root, the ganglion also receives a slender *ramus communicans from the nasociliary nerve* (a branch of the ophthalmic). This may leave the nasociliary nerve while that is in the cavernous sinus or after it has entered the orbit, but, in any case, runs forward just lateral to the optic nerve to end in the upper part of the ciliary ganglion. There also may be a third delicate root to the ciliary ganglion, a *branch from the sympathetic plexus on the internal carotid artery,* or the sympathetic fibers may reach the ganglion with the branch of the nasociliary nerve or follow the ophthalmic artery.

The branches given off by the ciliary ganglion are **short ciliary nerves** and consist of postganglionic parasympathetic fibers originating in the ganglion, afferent fibers from the nasociliary nerve that run through the ganglion, and postganglionic sympathetic fibers that do the same thing. They proceed forward toward the eyeball, accompanied by a number of small branches of the ophthalmic artery, and, although they originate lateral to the optic nerve, they spread out and branch as they run forward so that as they enter the eyeball close to the optic nerve, they almost surround that nerve.

The **nasociliary nerve** (see Figs. 33-19 and 33-22) leaves the rest of the ophthalmic nerve in the cavernous sinus and, unlike the frontal and lacrimal branches of that nerve, enters the orbit through the annulus, passing medially between the superior and inferior divisions of the oculomotor nerve as it does so. It runs above the optic nerve toward the medial wall of the orbit, giving off two delicate **long ciliary nerves** that run forward to enter the eyeball medial and lateral to the optic nerve, outside the general circle formed by the short ciliary nerves. They contain afferent fibers for the eyeball and, usually, sympathetic fibers derived from the internal carotid plexus.

When the nasociliary nerve reaches the medial wall of the orbit, it runs forward between the superior

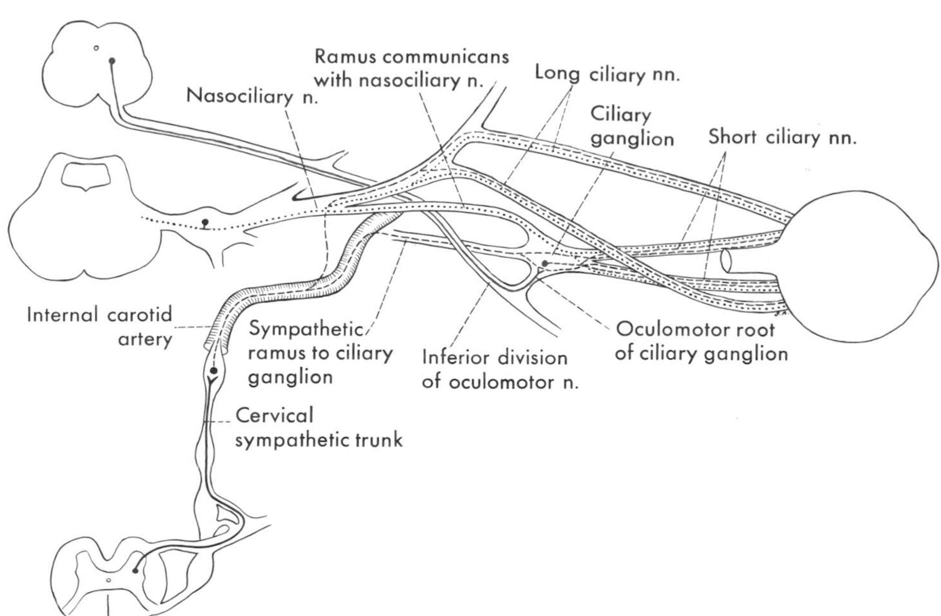

FIGURE 33-23.
The ciliary ganglion and nerves: Parasympathetic fibers are *red*, the preganglionic fibers (in the oculomotor nerve) being indicated by *solid lines*, the postganglionic ones (in the short ciliary nerves) by *broken lines*. Trigeminal sensory fibers are indicated by the *black dotted lines*. Sympathetic fibers are also *black*, with preganglionic fibers (from the thoracic part of the spinal cord) indicated by *solid lines* and postganglionic fibers (from the superior cervical ganglion) indicated by *broken lines*.

oblique and medial rectus muscles, giving off either one or two ethmoidal nerves. The small **posterior ethmoidal nerve,** if present, enters the posterior ethmoidal canal and supplies sensory twigs to the sphenoid sinus and perhaps posterior ethmoid cells. The **anterior ethmoidal nerve,** larger and constant, enters the anterior ethmoidal foramen or canal, which opens into the anterior cranial fossa just at the lateral edge of the cribriform plate. The nerve then runs forward on the lateral edge of the plate and at the anterior end turns downward to enter the nose. Its nasal branches are described in a following section. The ethmoidal nerves are accompanied by ethmoidal arteries.

After giving off its anterior ethmoidal branch, the nasociliary continues as the **infratrochlear nerve,** which passes just below the trochlea of the superior oblique muscle, penetrates the orbital septum, and gives branches to the side of the nose and the medial corner of the lids.

The largest nerve in the orbit, and the central structure in the muscle cone, is the **optic nerve.** This leaves the back of the eyeball and takes a somewhat sinuous course to the optic canal. In the orbit, the optic nerve is surrounded by a heavy sheath, the *external sheath* of the nerve, that is continuous with the dura and arachnoid within the skull. On the surface of the nerve is a thin layer of pia mater, the *internal sheath*, and between these two layers is an *intervaginal space* that is a continuation of the subarachnoid space. The optic nerve is the only nerve that is related to meninges throughout its length, and that is because it really is not a nerve, but a tract of the brain.

The **ophthalmic artery** (Fig. 33-24; see Figs. 33-19, 33-22) enters the orbit through the optic canal, where it lies below the optic nerve. As it emerges into the orbit, it deviates to lie lateral to the nerve and here gives off the **lacrimal artery.** This runs forward at first within the muscle cone, but then it emerges to run in the upper lateral part of the orbit with the lacrimal nerve and supply the lacrimal gland. Small twigs, the *lateral palpebral arteries*, continue into the lid to complete the superior and inferior palpebral arches. The lacrimal artery usually receives a tiny *anastomotic branch* from the middle meningeal artery that enters the orbit through or just lateral to the upper end of the superior orbital fissure. Sometimes this branch is larger, in which case it may form the origin of the lacrimal, and, very rarely, it gives rise to the whole ophthalmic artery.

After the ophthalmic artery has given off the lacrimal artery, it turns medially, usually above the optic nerve. As it does so, it gives off several branches that, in turn, subdivide as they run forward and become mingled with the short ciliary nerves from the ciliary ganglion. Most of these branches are **short posterior ciliary arteries** and enter the eyeball close to the optic nerve, along with the short ciliary nerves. One branch on each side is a **long posterior ciliary artery** that enters the eyeball medial or lateral to, respectively, the entrance of the short arteries.

Among the ciliary vessels is the **central artery of the retina.** This passes onto the inferior surface of the optic nerve penetrates its sheaths, and passes to the center of the nerve, in which position it enters the eyeball. It divides into four retinal arterioles, one to each quadrant, which run in the superficial or vitreous surface of the retina. It is accompanied by a central vein that, after leaving the optic nerve, enters the cavernous sinus. The retinal vessels can be clearly seen with the aid of an ophthalmoscope, and engorgement of the veins, swelling of the disk of the optic nerve (papilledema), or both commonly indicate arterial disease or increased intracranial pressure.

After the ophthalmic artery has crossed the optic nerve, it gives off its **supraorbital** branch, which runs for-

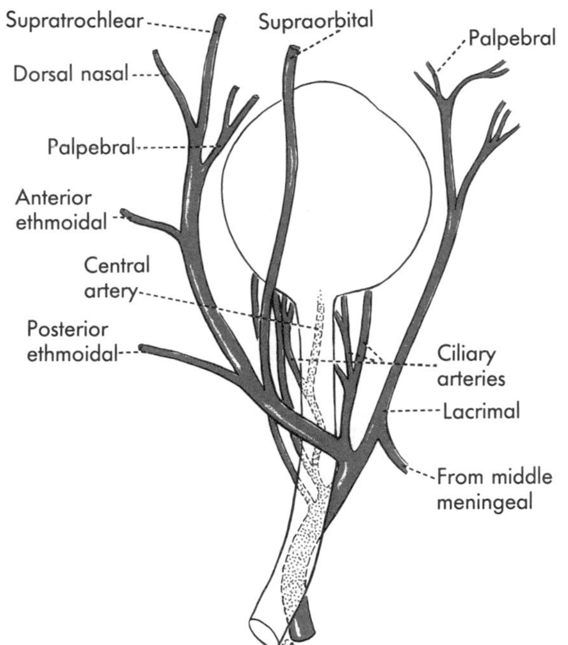

FIGURE 33-24.
Diagram of the ophthalmic artery.

ward at first within the muscle cone, but then emerges to join the supraorbital nerve and appear with that on the forehead. The artery then runs forward, in company with the nasociliary nerve, along the medial wall of the orbit and gives off **posterior** and **anterior ethmoidal arteries.** Both arteries enter the anterior cranial fossa, and the anterior ethmoidal usually gives rise to an **anterior meningeal artery.** Both also enter the nose and supply an upper part of it.

Beyond the anterior ethmoidal artery, the ophthalmic artery leaves the orbit, usually first giving off a **medial palpebral artery** that subdivides into superior and inferior medial palpebrals, and then dividing into terminal **dorsal nasal** and **supratrochlear arteries.** The palpebral arches that the medial and lateral palpebral arteries form supply the deeper structures of the lids and most of the bulbar conjunctiva. Again, because of the anastomoses between the branches of the ophthalmic artery and the branches of the external carotid on the face and forehead, the ophthalmic artery can conduct blood of external carotid origin to orbital structures.

In addition to the branches already mentioned, the ophthalmic artery also gives rise to muscular branches that enter all the muscles arising from the posterior part of the orbit, usually close to the entrance of the nerve into the muscle. These arteries run forward in the muscles, and usually two tiny twigs emerge on the surface of the tendons of the rectus muscles. These are the **anterior ciliary arteries,** which supply the sclera and conjunctiva closest to the cornea and then penetrate the sclera and anastomose inside the eyeball with posterior ciliary vessels.

There are two ophthalmic veins, superior and inferior (Fig. 33-25). As a rule, dissection of these is unsatisfactory because they are fragile and the nerves and arteries are more important. The **superior ophthalmic vein** begins within the orbit by the union of a stem from the supraorbital vein with one from the upper end of the angular vein. As the superior ophthalmic runs back in the upper medial part of the orbit, it receives branches corresponding to most of those of the ophthalmic artery—**anterior** and **posterior ethmoidal, lacrimal, muscular,** and a part of the **central vein of the retina.** Behind the eyeball, it also receives the upper two of the four **vorticose veins,** which are veins that leave the posterior aspect of the eyeball some distance from the optic nerve and penetrate the sheath of the eyeball to end in the ophthalmic veins. The superior ophthalmic vein usually also receives the inferior ophthalmic vein just before the venous drainage leaves the orbit.

The **inferior ophthalmic vein,** smaller than the superior, begins by the union of small veins in the floor of the orbit. It may receive a communication from the angular vein through the lower lid and, as it runs back, also has communications with the superior ophthalmic vein. It receives the veins from the lower bulbar muscles and the two inferior vorticose veins, which are placed below and on each side of the optic nerve in positions corresponding to those occupied by the superior vorticose veins above the nerve. The inferior ophthalmic vein also communicates through the inferior orbital fissure with the pterygoid plexus of veins, and often with the infraorbital vein.

The common stem formed by the two ophthalmic veins usually leaves the orbit through the part of the superior orbital fissure that lies above the annular tendon, but it may pass through the annulus, or occasionally, even below to enter the cavernous sinus. When the two veins do not join, but empty independently into the sinus, one may have one position, the other another.

The **central vein of the retina** is said to empty independently into the cavernous sinus always, but usually to have a branch that joins the superior ophthalmic vein.

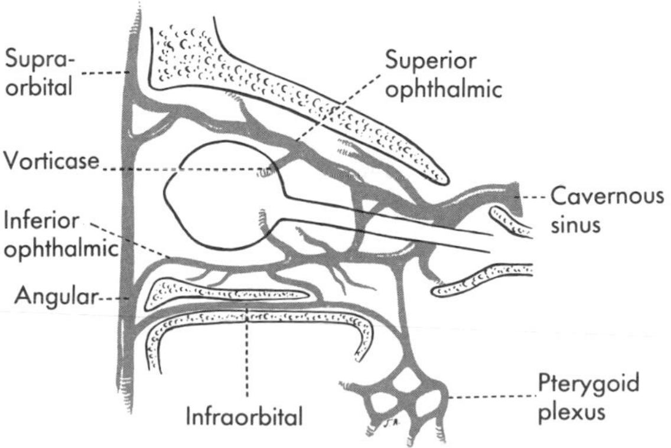

FIGURE 33-25.
Diagram of the ophthalmic veins.

In the floor of the orbit, the inferior orbital fissure is bridged by connective tissue and by smooth muscle, the **orbitalis muscle.**

Just deep to the orbitalis muscle in the posterior part of the orbit is the **maxillary nerve** as it runs forward in the pterygopalatine fossa. As the nerve enters the orbit to run along its floor in the infraorbital groove, it gives off the **zygomatic nerve.** The zygomatic nerve runs upward and forward in the periosteum of the lateral wall of the orbit and divides into **zygomaticofacial** and **zygomaticotemporal** branches. These both penetrate the bony lateral wall of the orbit to become subcutaneous, but before the zygomaticotemporal branch does so, it sends a twig upward to join the lacrimal nerve. It is this branch that brings secretory fibers to the lacrimal gland. The secretory fibers are postganglionic and arise from the pterygopalatine ganglion (the preganglionic fibers of which are from the seventh nerve). They join the maxillary nerve, immediately below where the pterygopalatine ganglion lies, and run forward with it into its zygomatic and zygomaticotemporal branches.

Accompanying the infraorbital nerve—the continuation of the maxillary—in the floor of the orbit are the infraorbital artery and vein. These may help supply structures of the floor.

Eyeball

The eyeball (*bulbus oculi*) usually cannot be satisfactorily examined in the dissecting room, and it is described here only in enough detail to give a general concept of its structure and function. Histologic and more advanced texts should be consulted for details.

Chief Layers

The major part of the eyeball consists of three layers (Fig. 33-26) an outer **fibrous tunic,** the *sclera* (white of the eye) and *cornea;* **a vascular tunic,** the *choroid* and its anterior extensions that form most of the *ciliary body* and *iris;* and a **tunica interna,** the sensory part or *retina.* The inner surface of the back part of the eyeball usually is called the **fundus.**

The **sclera** is composed of connective tissue and forms about five-sixths of the surface of the eyeball. It is continuous anteriorly with the transparent **cornea,** which allows light to enter the eyeball and is commented upon further in a following section. The cornea is part of a smaller sphere than is the sclera and, because of its greater curvature, protrudes in front of the sclera, so that the anteroposterior axis of the eye is its longest one.

The **choroid** consists primarily of blood vessels that are fed by the short posterior ciliary arteries and recurrent arteries from the front of the eyeball and drained by the four vorticose veins. Its smallest blood vessels form a choroidocapillary layer adjacent to the retina, but the largest ones lie peripherally; the long ciliary arteries, which supply more anterior structures, run between the choroid and the sclera. The choroid is nutrient to the retina, primarily to the outer part that is adjacent to the choroid.

For some 6 to 7 mm behind the sclerocorneal junction (*limbus* of the cornea) the choroid is thickened and tightly

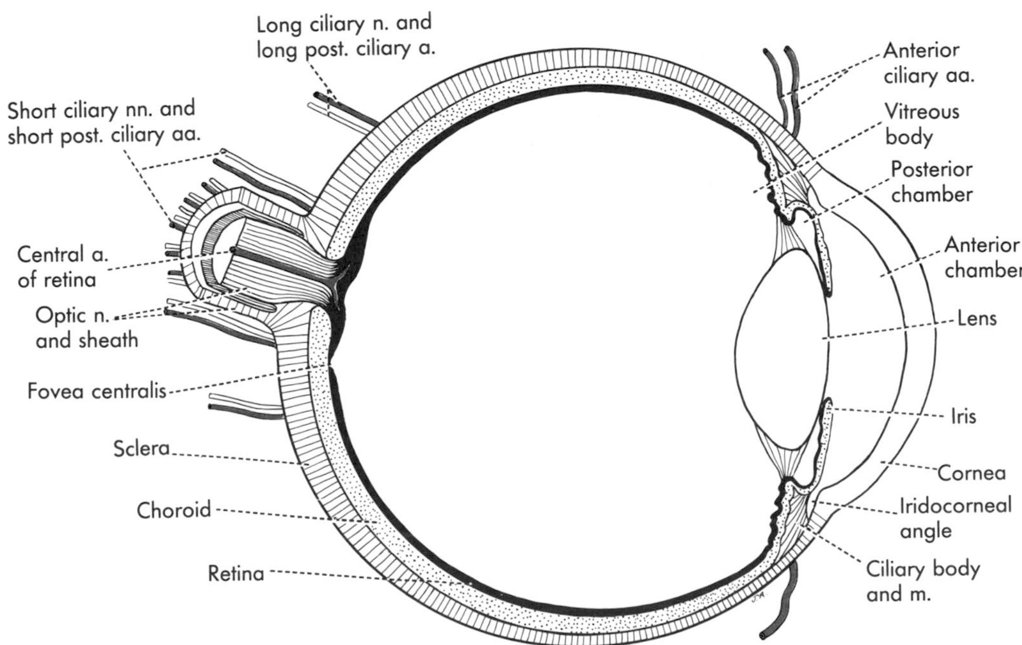

FIGURE *33-26.*
Schema of the eyeball in horizontal section.

attached to the sclera. This part is the **ciliary body** (so-called because of the numerous fine folds on its inner surface). To the posterior part of the ciliary body are attached fibers that suspend the lens (zonular fibers, often referred to collectively as the *suspensory ligament of the lens*), and anteriorly, a continuation of the choroid leaves the sclera to extend almost transversely across the eye and form most of the iris. Much of the bulk of the ciliary body is formed by the vascular layer of the choroid, but this body also contains smooth muscle fibers that form the **ciliary muscle.** Most of these muscle fibers are longitudinal (meridional) and radial fibers, but some of them are circular. They all, presumably, function to narrow the diameter of the ring formed by the ciliary body, thus releasing tension on the zonular fibers (suspensory ligament). The ciliary muscle is innervated by parasympathetic fibers through the oculomotor nerve and the ciliary ganglion.

The thick part of the **retina,** the innermost layer of the eyeball, can be easily stripped off as far forward as the posterior border of the ciliary body; here it tears away in an irregular line (*ora serrata*). Anterior to the retina is a thin layer closely attached to the posterior surfaces of the ciliary body and the iris. The *ciliary* and *iridial parts* of the retina are not sensitive to light. The part that is sensitive to light is called the *pars optica*.

The optic part of the retina consists of two layers, an outer pigmented layer and an inner nervous or cerebral stratum. The *pigmented layer* is a single layer of heavily pigmented cuboidal cells. It is this layer only that is continued as the ciliary and iridial parts of the retina, and it is tightly adherent to the choroid everywhere. The *cerebral stratum* or nervous layer is attached to the pigmented one only around the optic nerve as that leaves the eyeball and at the ora serrata. Therefore, it is only this layer that can be stripped off the eyeball; and when retinal detachment occurs as a result of accident or disease, the separation is between the two layers. The layers represent the outer and inner layers of an optic cup, developed by invagination of one side of a hollow, ball-like optic vesicle and are, therefore, adjacent to each other, rather than closely attached.

A little medial to the posterior pole of the eye there is, in the retina, a whitish circle about 1.5 mm in diameter; this, produced by the optic nerve as it leaves the retina, is the **optic disk,** or disk of the optic nerve. (It also has been called the "nerve head" and the "papilla of the optic nerve.") It is the thickest part of the retina except where close to its middle, it presents a depression, the excavation of the disk. The sensory elements that are affected by light are lacking in the optic disk; hence, this represents a **blind spot** in the retina. The blind spot must be differentiated from other blind spots or areas that may be brought about by disease. The central artery of the retina branches as it enters the retina at the optic disk, and the central vein is formed here by the convergence of its tributaries. Examination of the vessels is an important part of examination of the fundus through the ophthalmoscope.

Lateral to the optic disk, almost exactly at the posterior pole of the eye, is a region that is slightly yellow and is known as the **macula** (formerly macula lutea, or yellow spot). In its center is a depression, the **fovea centralis,** where the nervous part of the retina is thinnest and vision is most accurate. The fovea centralis and macula represent the area of central vision, and most movements of the eyes are attempts to bring light to focus on the macula.

The retina has been described as having from eight to ten layers including the pigmented part, but there actually are only three layers of nerve cells. The outermost or neuroepithelial layer, adjacent to the pigmented stratum, is composed of cells, the processes of which are shaped somewhat like rods and cones and, therefore, are so named. The **rods** have associated with them visual purple and are sensitive only to varying degrees of light (usually described as being for "night vision"); **cones,** employed in more accurate vision ("day vision," including color vision), are most numerous at the macula, where there are no rods. They become less numerous as the retina is traced toward the ora serrata, and the more peripheral parts of the retina contain none at all. Next is a layer formed primarily but not exclusively by **bipolar cells** that connect the rods and cones to the third layer of cells. This third or innermost layer is made up of the **ganglion cells** that give rise to the fibers of the optic nerve. These fibers, lying most superficially (that is, they are the first part of the retina to be reached by light entering the eyeball), converge at the optic disk to form the optic nerve. In this layer also, located superficially among the nerve fibers, are the branches of the central vessels of the retina.

The precise manner in which the retina functions is not yet understood. The layers of the retina are perfectly transparent, for light must penetrate them to reach the processes of the rods and cones.

Although the central vessels of the retina send delicate twigs into the deeper part of the retina, these do not reach the layer of rods and cones. This layer is dependent on the closer-lying capillary network of the choroid. Thus, retinal detachment produces blindness by depriving the receptive elements of adequate nutrition.

Iris

The iris, with its central aperture, the **pupil,** projects from the anteromedial surface of the ciliary body as a thin perforated disk, similar to the diaphragm of a camera. Its major bulk is a continuation of the choroid, and the anterior ciliary vessels enter it to anastomose with the posterior ones. In the white infant, all the pigment of the iris is in its posterior part at birth, and although the pigment actually is dark, it appears blue when seen through the other layers. In other races the pigment is deposited more generally through the iris; hence, the eye does not appear blue. During infancy the more anterior part of the iris may become heavily pigmented, and the blue eyes turn to brown; if the anterior pigmentation is less, the eyes turn to gray or remain blue.

The most important feature of the iris is its ability to change the diameter of the pupil, in a fashion somewhat similar to the change in the aperture of a camera diaphragm. This change is brought about by smooth muscle lying in the iris. Most of the muscle is circularly arranged and constitutes the **sphincter pupillae.** When the sphincter pupillae contracts, it reduces the size of the pupil, thus protecting the retina from excessive or unneeded light. It is innervated through the oculomotor nerve by way of the ciliary ganglion and the short ciliary nerves. Radially arranged fibers constitute a **dilator pupillae** innervated by the sympathetic system. The preganglionic fibers leave the spinal cord through the upper thoracic nerves, especially T-1, and run upward in the cervical sympathetic trunk to synapse in the superior cervical ganglion. The postganglionic fibers from the superior cervical ganglion join the internal carotid plexus and reach the iris either by joining the ophthalmic nerve and its long ciliary branches or by joining the sympathetic ramus to the ciliary ganglion and mingling with other fibers of the short ciliary nerves. Among the fibers to the iris there also are many sensory ones, particularly concerned with pain; fibers for pain also end in the ciliary body.

Refracting Media

In reaching the retina, light must travel through several transparent substances intervening between the retina and the outside air. Because these all have a tendency to bend or refract light rays that pass through them, they are grouped collectively as the refracting media of the eye. They consist of the cornea, aqueous humor, lens, and vitreous body.

The cornea is the anterior transparent continuation of the sclera, although its curvature is sharper. It consists mostly of connective tissue. Epithelium on its anterior surface is continuous with the epithelium of the bulbar conjunctiva; epithelium on its posterior surface is called the *endothelium of the anterior chamber*.

The **anterior chamber** of the eye lies behind the cornea, between that and the iris and lens. It is filled with fluid, the **aqueous humor,** that apparently is formed, probably from the epithelium of the ciliary body, in the small **posterior chamber** behind the attachment of the iris. After passing through the pupil into the anterior chamber, the aqueous humor, which constantly is being produced, is drained off through spaces that permeate a structure at the iridocorneal angle called the *pectinate ligament* and open into a circular venous channel, the **sinus venosus sclerae,** or *canal of Schlemm* (Fig. 33-27). If the rates of formation and absorption become out of balance, the amount of aqueous humor and, therefore, its pressure, may be increased above normal. This is known as *glaucoma* and, when it is severe, results in degeneration of the retina and blindness.

The **lens** lies immediately behind the iris, attached to the ciliary body by the gelatinous **ciliary zonule,** which consists of **zonular fibers** and intervening spaces. Between the lens and zonule and the iris is the posterior chamber of the eye.

The lens is a biconvex disk measuring about 9 to 10 mm in diameter and about 4 to 5 mm in anteroposterior thickness. Its posterior surface is more highly curved than is its anterior. It is made up of anucleate cells, which are normally perfectly transparent; an opacity of the lens is known as a *cataract*. The lens is the only refracting medium of the eye for which refracting ability can be varied from moment to moment to maintain visual acuity: the lens is elastic, but is so held under tension by the zonular fibers that it is somewhat flattened. When the ciliary muscle contracts and thereby relaxes the zonular fibers, the lens becomes more convex.

The large **vitreous chamber** behind the lens and the posterior chamber is filled with a gelatinous transparent mass known as the **vitreous body,** frequently referred to as the vitreous humor. In contrast to the aqueous humor, the vitreous body does not undergo constant replacement; it is formed early in development and cannot be replaced thereafter.

Some Functional Aspects

Certain functional aspects of bringing light rays to a focus on the retina can now be briefly considered. In the resting normal eye (with the ciliary muscle relaxed), the refraction of the flattened lens is just enough to bring into sharp focus on the retina an object seen at a distance, from which the light rays are traveling approximately parallel by the time they reach the eye. Because it is in the resting eye that the lens is most flattened, the resting eye is adapted for distance vision, not near vision. The closer an object is to the eye, the more the light rays from that object diverge as they approach the eye hence, the more refraction there must

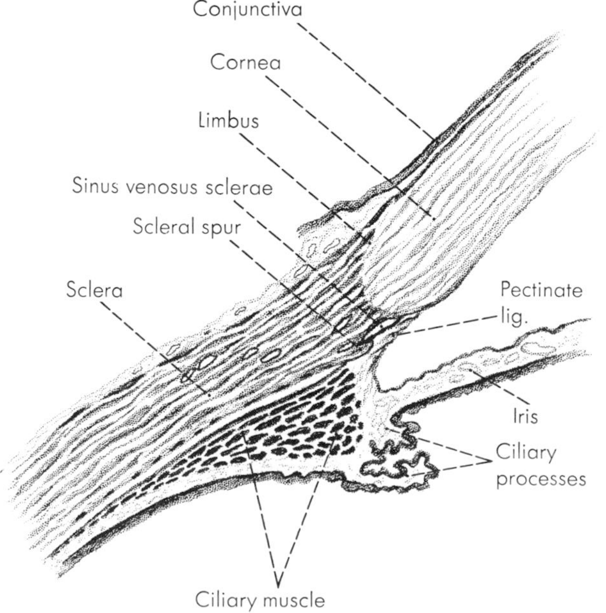

FIGURE 33-27.
The iridocorneal angle.

be to bring these rays to a focus on the retina. This greater refraction is brought about by change in the shape of the lens (*accommodation*). For near vision, the ciliary muscle contracts, releasing the tension on the zonular fibers and allowing the lens to become more convex. Although the increased thickness of the lens is a passive process, brought about by the elasticity of this body, near vision requires muscular effort, that of the ciliary muscle. In middle age, the lens gradually loses elasticity, so that, in spite of contraction of the ciliary muscle, it may remain too flattened to afford a good focus on the retina for a near object; this condition, which makes near objects difficult to see clearly, is known as *presbyopia*.

Certain other abnormalities of vision have nothing particularly to do with the ability of the lens to adjust itself for near and far vision. The cornea, the first refracting medium that the light strikes as it enters the eye, may have slight irregularities in its curve; this accounts for the indistinctness of vision known as *astigmatism*. Moreover, the eyeball may have grown out of proportion to its refracting system, to a point beyond which the lens can adjust by changes in its shape. Thus, if the eyeball is too long for its refracting system, objects will be brought to a focus in front of rather than on the retina, whereas if it is too short, the focus will be behind the retina. Either condition, obviously, results in poor vision. Too little refracting power for the length of the eyeball, resulting in a focus point behind the retina, is known as or *hyperopia* or *hypermetropia*, or farsightedness; distance vision is the best here, because less refracting power is needed for distant objects. Too great refractive power for the length of the eyeball, with the result that the focus lies in front of the retina, is *myopia* or near-sightedness; here vision is better for close objects, where greater refractive power is needed anyway.

NOSE AND PARANASAL SINUSES

The development and some general anatomic features of the nose are mentioned in the discussion of the respiratory system (see Chap. 9) The paranasal sinuses are mentioned in the description of the skull (see Chap. 31).

External Nose

The external nose sometimes is compared to a three-sided pyramid (and its skeleton is sometimes referred to as the "nasal pyramid"). The smallest side of the pyramid faces downward and surrounds the nares before it becomes continuous with the upper lip; the other two sides are the sides of the nose. The margin along which these two sides meet is the **dorsum nasi.** This extends from the **root** of the nose, the part continuous with the forehead, to the apex or tip. The flared lower part of the side of the nose is the **ala** (wing). The external openings of the nose are the **nares** (nostrils). They are separated from each other by the lower border of the **nasal septum.**

Over the movable alae and tip of the nose, the skin is tightly attached to the supporting cartilage, but over the rest of the nose it is movable on the underlying skeleton. The blood supply, from both angular and dorsal nasal vessels, and its innervation, mostly from the ophthalmic nerve, are described in connection with the face (see Chap. 31).

The **skeleton of the external nose** (Fig. 33-28) is contributed to laterally by the frontal processes of the maxillas and superiorly by the nasal part of the frontal bone. Articulating with both of these, and completing the bony part of the skeleton, are the two small **nasal bones.** The remainder of the skeleton of the external nose is cartilaginous.

Articulating with the nasal and maxillary bones are the **lateral nasal cartilages,** often referred to as the upper cartilages. In their upper parts, these cartilages are continuous with each other through the **septal cartilage,** which passes backward and downward from them to articulate with the bony septum of the nose. They and the septal cartilage actually are a single piece of cartilage, although named as if they were separate. In their lower parts, the lateral nasal cartilages are separated from each other by a cleft in which the septal cartilage appears on the dorsum of the nose. The septal cartilage extends farther downward toward the apex of the nose than do the lateral nasal cartilages. Below the lateral nasal and septal cartilages are the **greater alar cartilages** (often referred to as the lower nasal cartilages). These are separate cartilages, and each one has a relatively large lateral crus that supports the ala (and overlaps the lower border of the lateral nasal cartilage) and a smaller medial crus that lies close to its fellow of the opposite side and forms a lower part of the nasal septum. In the angle between the lateral nasal

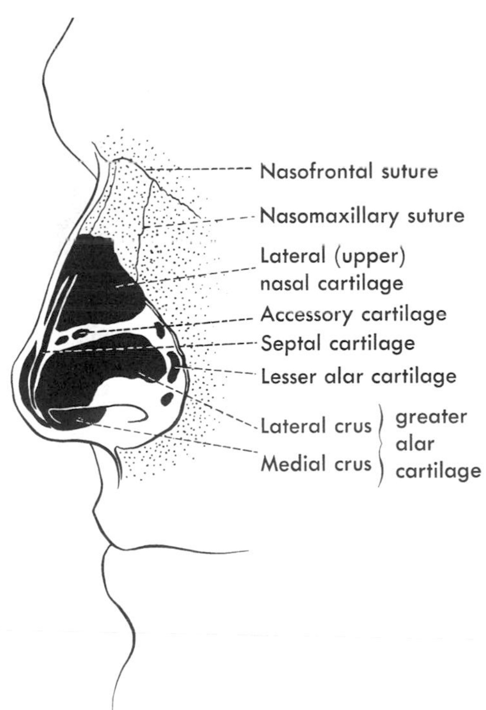

FIGURE *33-28.*
The nasal cartilages, somewhat spread apart.

cartilage, the lateral crus of the greater alar cartilage, and the septal cartilage, there commonly are one or more small **accessory nasal** (sesamoid) **cartilages.** Posterior to the lateral nasal cartilage and the lateral crus of the major alar cartilage, there are usually several **lesser alar cartilages.** These various cartilages are united by dense connective tissue, and this tissue, with fat added, forms a part of the ala.

Nasal Cavity

Each nasal cavity is narrow above and wider below, and the two cavities are separated from each other by the nasal septum. Each cavity begins at the **naris** and extends back to the **choana,** the opening into the pharynx. The first part of the cavity is the **vestibule** (see Fig. 33-30), the lower part of which is lined with skin and provided with hairs. The vestibule is bounded laterally by the greater alar cartilage, and its upper limit, the *limen nasi,* is a crescentic infolding of the lateral wall at the lower border of the lateral nasal cartilage; the medial wall of the vestibule, formed by the nasal septum, has no marking to delimit it from the remainder of the nasal cavity.

The entire medial and lateral nasal walls posterior to the vestibule, except in the uppermost narrow part of the nasal cavity, are covered by a thick glandular and vascular mucous membrane and constitute the **respiratory region** (warming and humidifying the inspired air). In the narrow roof of the nose, extending downward a little on the medial and lateral sides, is the thinner mucous membrane of the **olfactory region** in which the olfactory nerves arise. The mucous membrane of the respiratory region is provided with cilia that have in general a beat backward toward the choanae to carry mucus into the throat where it can be swallowed. The mucous membrane of the conchae (see Fig. 33-30) is particularly vascular, presenting a so-called *cavernous plexus* that resembles erectile tissue. Because of its vascularity, the nasal mucous membrane easily becomes swollen, and when this is combined with increased secretion of mucus a "stopped-up nose" results. Most nose drops contain some epinephrine-like substance that decreases the secretion of mucus and produces vasoconstriction of the arterioles, thus relieving the nasal congestion.

Nasal Septum

The nasal septum presents little in the way of markings and can be studied in part to advantage in a dried skull. As seen through the piriform apertures, the large posterior part of the septum is bony. The upper part of the bony septum is formed by the **perpendicular plate of the ethmoid bone** (Fig. 33-29). Its lower part is formed by the **vomer,** with some contribution from the nasal crests of the maxillary and palatine bones. Most of the remainder of the septum, the anterior and lower part, is cartilaginous and is formed chiefly by the septal cartilage.

The **septal cartilage** has a tongue-and-groove articulation with the edges of the bony septum. Alongside its lower edge is a small cartilage, the **vomeronasal cartilage;** this is connected with a little blind pouch from the nasal cavity, the **vomeronasal organ,** that extends backward between the two cartilages. The septal cartilage does not reach the distal part of the nasal septum; this is formed by the medial crura of the two greater alar cartilages and, therefore, is a double wall. The two medial crura are not closely bound together, and the groove between them can be felt distinctly at the tip of the nose. They are bound to the lower edge of the septal cartilage by a sufficient amount of connective tissue to allow them to be freely movable, and the part of the septum that they form is known as the mobile part.

The nasal septum is covered by mucous membrane, of which an upper posterior part, just below the cribriform plate of the ethmoid, is olfactory. The vomeronasal organ, rudimentary and not always

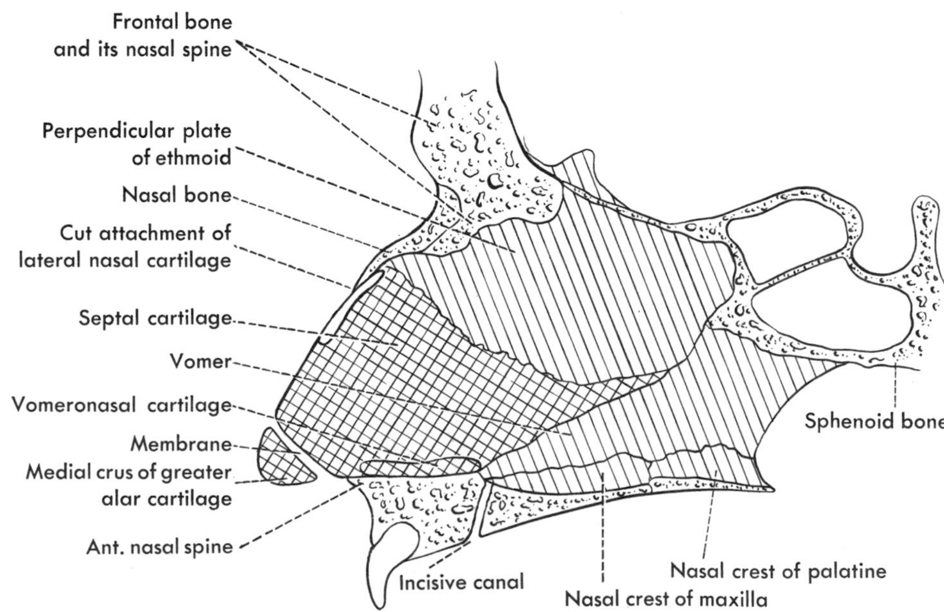

FIGURE *33-29.*
Components of the nasal septum. Cartilage is *crosshatched*.

discernible in humans, is in some mammals large and lined by olfactory epithelium.

Frequently, the nasal septum is deviated to one side or the other and, in conjunction with deviation, may present spurs that project still farther into one nasal cavity. A deviated septum and spur may come in contact with the projecting conchae from the lateral nasal wall, resulting in partial occlusion of the nasal cavity or in discomfort as a result of the contact.

The **nerves and vessels** of the nasal septum are branches of those that also supply the lateral nasal wall and are described in a following section.

Lateral Nasal Wall

The lateral nasal wall presents a number of features deserving study (Figs. 33-30 and 33-31). Most prominent are the **conchae** (also called "turbinates"), curved shelves of bone covered by mucosa that project from the lateral nasal wall and greatly increase the respiratory surface of the nose. They are named inferior, middle, and superior nasal conchae, according to their position. The **inferior concha** is the longest, with the middle being almost as long although it does not come quite as far forward. The **superior concha** is much smaller, only about half the length of the middle concha, and lies above the posterior half of this concha. Above the back end of the superior concha there may be an inconspicuous bulge, the supreme concha. The air passageways deep to the conchae are known as the inferior, middle, and superior **nasal meatuses,** respectively.

Only a few other markings on the lateral wall of the nose can be seen until the conchae are reflected. At the anterior border of the middle concha, a depressed area, the *atrium of the middle meatus,* leads upward into the middle meatus. Anterior to and above the atrium is a variably sized projection, the *agger nasi,* that contains one or more ethmoid air cells. Anterior to and above this is a slight groove, the **olfactory sulcus,** that leads upward to the olfactory region of the nose. Relatively little air normally flows over the sulcus or the agger nasi to the uppermost part of the nose during quiet respiration, so that, when one wants to smell the inspired air better, one sniffs to set up air currents that will carry the air to the olfactory region.

At the uppermost posterior part of the nose, the nasal cavity is bounded posteriorly by a part of the body of the sphenoid bone known as the **sphenoid concha** (this does not at all resemble the nasal conchae). The sphenoid sinus opens through the sphenoid concha; the part of the nasal cavity here is known as the **sphenoethmoidal recess.** The part of the nasal cavity behind the middle and inferior conchae is the **nasopharyngeal meatus;** it ends at the choana where the nasal cavity opens into the nasal part of the pharynx.

The superior and middle nasal conchae are parts of the **ethmoid labyrinth,** the paired parts of the ethmoid bones that form much of the lateral walls of the nasal cavities and medial walls of the orbits. In the bases of the bones and the ethmoid labyrinth, are the air cavities or ethmoid cells that together constitute the ethmoid or **ethmoidal sinus** (see Fig. 33-37). Some of the ethmoid cells open into the superior meatus, and sometimes one or more may open above the superior concha. Other ethmoid cells open under cover of the middle concha. After the middle concha is removed by cutting it close to its base (see Fig. 33-31), the openings of some of these cells and additional modeling of the labyrinth can be observed. A rounded bulge projecting downward and forward below the root of attachment of the middle concha is the **ethmoid bulla,** formed by ethmoid air cells that open into the middle meatus. It varies in size with the size and number of the cells present. Anterior to and below it and projecting upward toward it is a thin process, the **uncinate process.** The gap between the bulla and the uncinate process

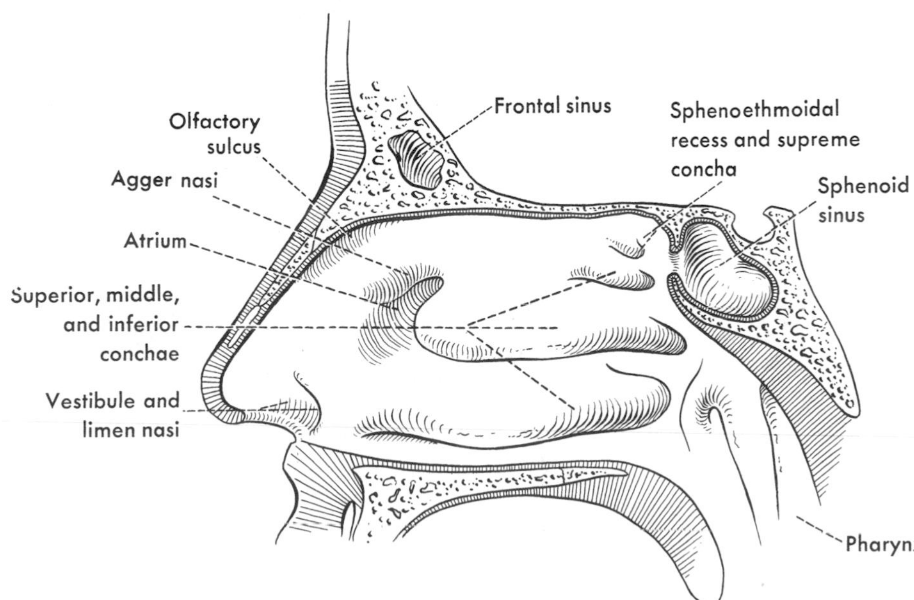

FIGURE *33-30.*
The lateral nasal wall.

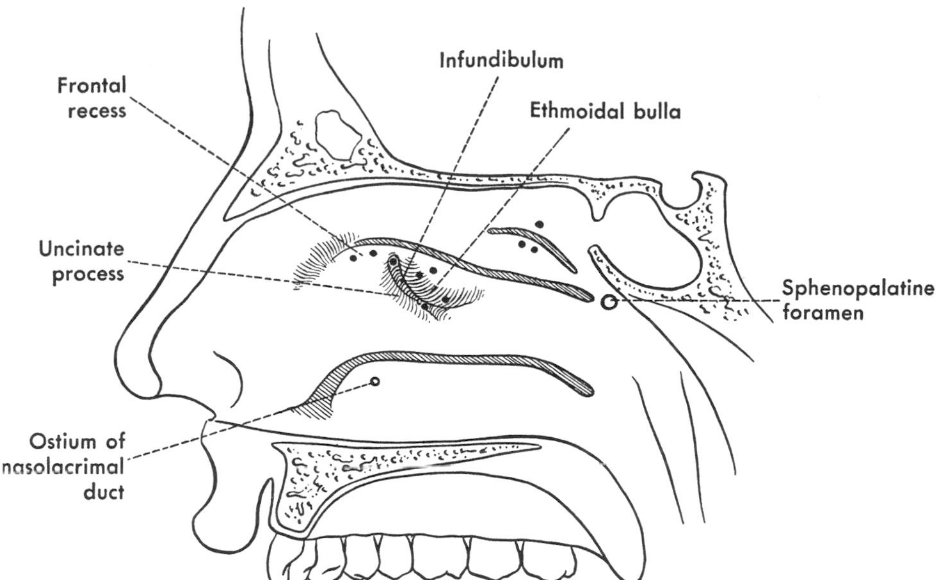

FIGURE *33-31.*
The lateral nasal wall after removal of the conchae; their cut bases are represented by appropriate *shaded areas.* The *unlabeled black dots* are openings of ethmoid cells.

is the **semilunar hiatus,** which leads downward and forward into a curved channel, the **ethmoid infundibulum,** lying lateral to the uncinate process. The maxillary sinus usually opens into the infundibulum under cover of the uncinate process. At its anterior and upper end, the infundibulum expands and regularly receives the openings of ethmoid cells (which may also open into the middle meatus in front of the infundibulum). Often, the infundibulum also receives the opening of the frontal sinus.

The only opening under cover of the inferior concha is that of the **nasolacrimal duct.** The exact position of this opening varies, but it usually is fairly high under the curved anterior end of the concha. The opening also varies in size and shape; it frequently is partly covered by a fold of mucous membrane, the lacrimal fold.

Nerves and Vessels

The nerves and blood vessels of the nasal cavity are fairly simple, although difficult to demonstrate on the average cadaver. The general areas of distribution of various nerves to the lateral nasal wall are shown in Figure 33-32.

The **olfactory nerves,** concerned with smell only, arise from cells in the uppermost part of the nasal mucosa, largely that over the superior concha and a similar area on the septum. The central processes of these cells form the delicate filaments that constitute the olfactory nerve. These penetrate the cribriform plate and end in the overlying olfactory bulb.

The largest nerves and blood vessels of the nasal cavity enter it through the sphenopalatine foramen, in the lateral nasal wall just behind the posterior end of the middle nasal concha. It connects the nasal cavity and the pterygopalatine fossa. In the pterygopalatine fossa are the maxillary nerve, the pterygopalatine ganglion, and branches of the maxillary artery. Sensory fibers from the maxillary nerve combine with postganglionic parasympathetic fibers from the pterygopalatine ganglion and with sympathetic fibers that have reached the ganglion from the deep petrosal nerve to form lateral and medial posterior superior nasal branches (Figs. 33-33 and 33-34). The lateral branches turn forward after traversing the sphenopalatine foramen, and the medial branches cross the body of the sphenoid bone to reach the septum.

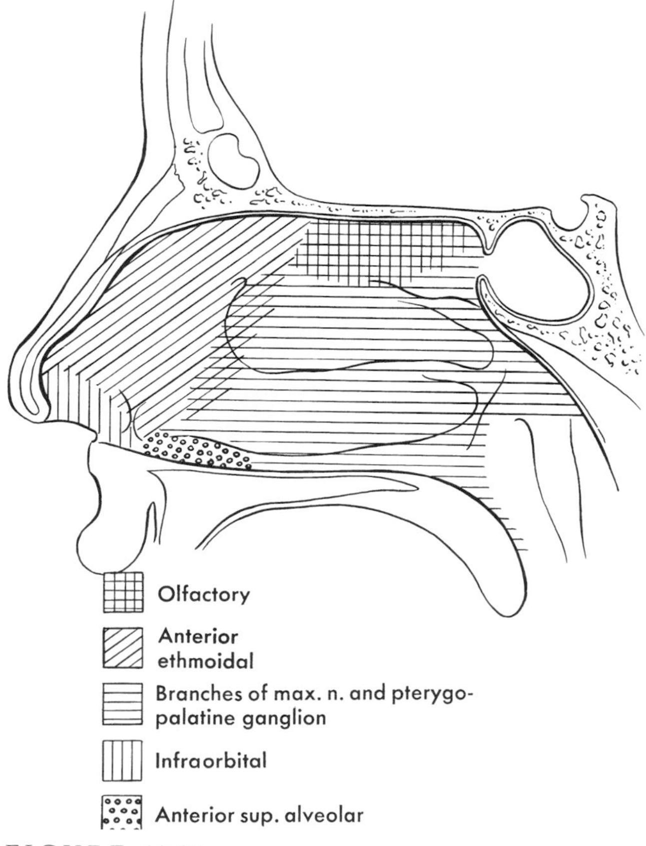

FIGURE *33-32.*
Distribution of nerves to the lateral nasal wall.

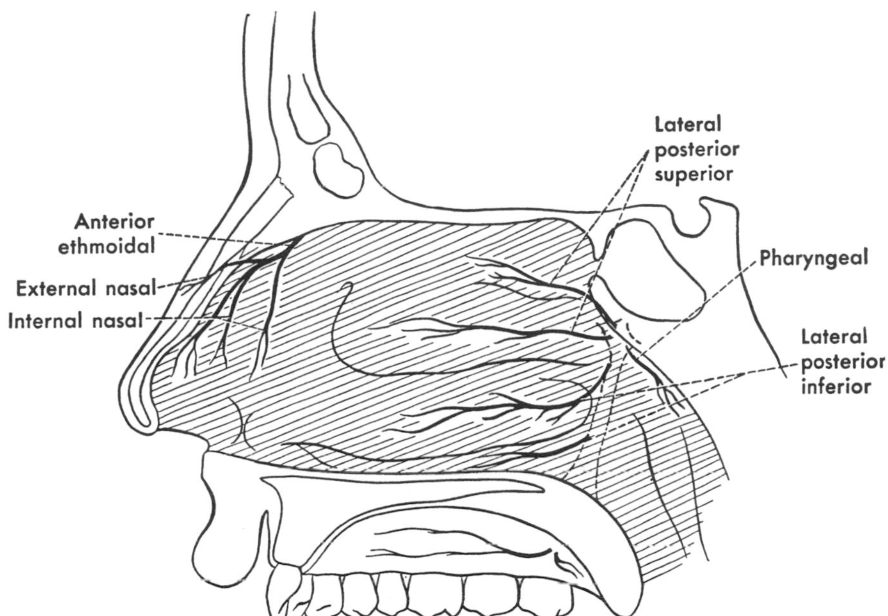

FIGURE *33-33.*
Nerves of the respiratory part of the lateral nasal wall.

One of the latter, the **nasopalatine,** continues downward and forward on the septum, eventually passes through an incisive canal between the nasal cavity and the mouth, and ends by innervating mucosa of the hard palate just behind the incisor teeth. The other posterior nerves of the nasal cavity, the **lateral posterior inferior nasals,** are distributed to the posterior parts of the middle and inferior meatuses and the inferior concha. They descend from the maxillary nerve and the pterygopalatine ganglion as part of the greater palatine nerve, then leave it to penetrate the lateral nasal wall.

The anterior part of the nasal cavity is innervated largely through the *ophthalmic nerve,* although twigs from the maxillary nerve supply parts of the vestibule and of the inferior meatus. Above, the innervation is through the **anterior ethmoidal nerve,** a branch of the nasociliary. It enters the nasal cavity through a slit in its roof on the side of the crista galli and, besides giving twigs to the anterior ethmoidal cells and to the frontal sinus, distributes internal lateral and medial nasal branches to the anterior parts of the nasal cavity. The external nasal branch continues downward and forward to leave the nasal cavity between the nasal bone and the lateral nasal cartilage and supply skin of the dorsum of the nose.

The **arteries** of the nose (Fig. 33-35) run in general with the larger nerves. The *sphenopalatine artery,* a branch of the maxillary, enters the nasal cavity through the sphenopalatine foramen with the posterior superior

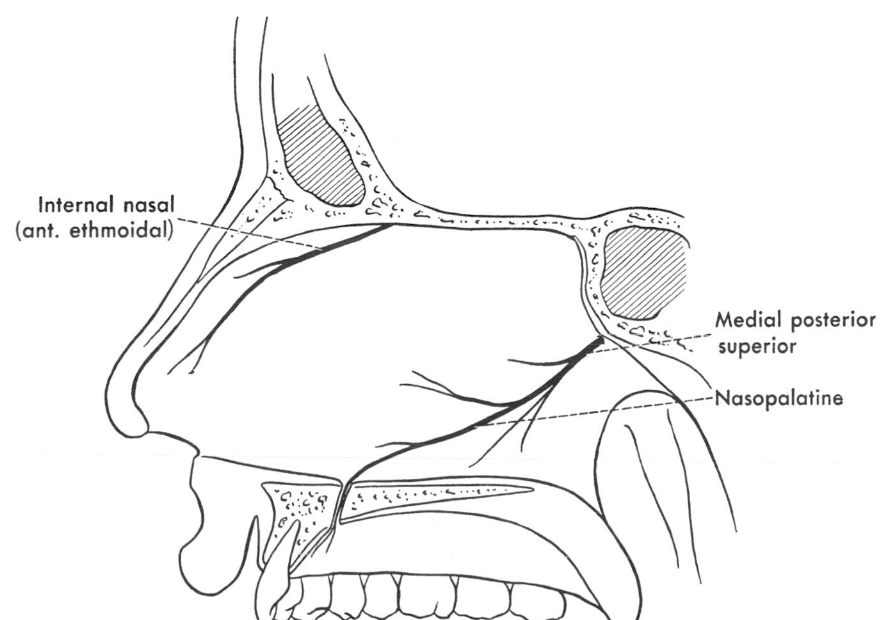

FIGURE *33-34.*
Nerves of the respiratory part of the nasal septum.

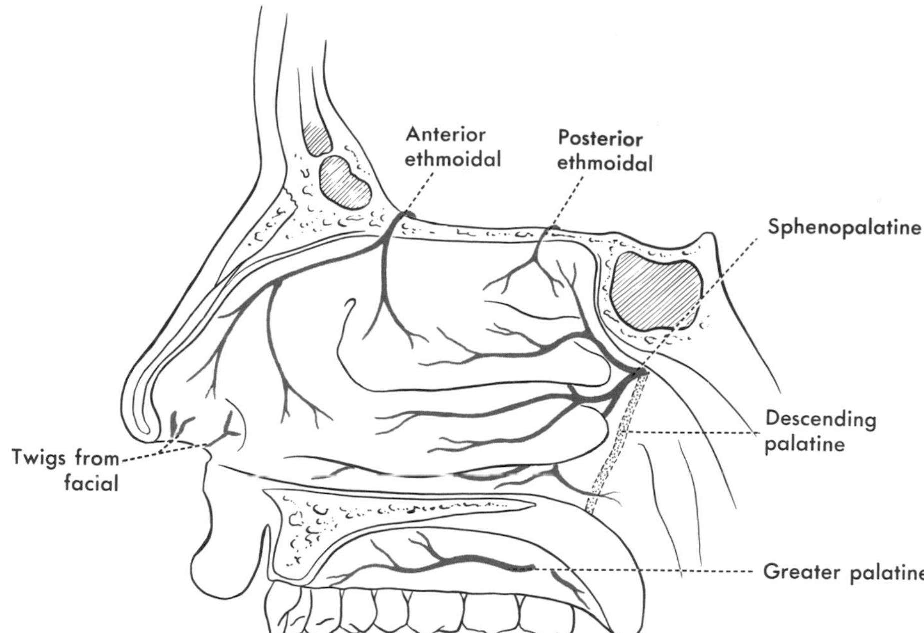

FIGURE 33-35.
Arteries of the lateral nasal wall.

nasal nerves and divides into *lateral* and *septal* (medial) *posterior nasal arteries.* In addition, the posterior and anterior ethmoidal branches of the ophthalmic artery enter the nasal cavity through its roof, alongside the cribriform plate, and divide into medial and lateral branches that are distributed to an upper but particularly an anterior part of the nasal cavity. Finally, the *superior labial artery* (from the facial) usually sends a branch into the nasal cavity along the septum, and the *greater palatine artery* (from the maxillary) sends a branch upward through an incisive canal to reach an anterior lower part of the nasal septum. Here there are rather broad anastomoses between the major arteries of the nose, and this area often is involved when there is nosebleed.

More serious bleeding from the nose may arise from the large vessels, just after they have entered the nasal cavity. Bleeding close to the back end of the middle concha, from the sphenopalatine artery, often can be checked by packs placed in this position. The sphenopalatine artery can be ligated if the severity of the bleeding warrants it, or the external carotid artery can be ligated in the neck, to decrease the amount of blood delivered to the sphenopalatine. Bleeding from the roof of the nasal cavity originates from one of the ethmoidal arteries. Severe bleeding from these arteries has been halted by ligating them intraorbitally.

Most of the **lymphatics** of the nasal cavity join those of the pharynx.

Paranasal Sinuses

The paranasal sinuses (Figs. 33-36 through 33-38) are diverticula of the nasal cavity, which grow from this cavity into neighboring bones and replace the diploë there. Of the four sinuses, the frontal, the maxillary, and the sphenoid are typically large and paired, but the ethmoid sinus of each side consists of a varying number of smaller air-filled cavities known as the ethmoid cells.

The **frontal sinuses** lie in the frontal bone, as their name implies. They vary much in size; one may be considerably larger than the other and grow beyond the midline, overlapping or pushing to one side the sinus of the other side. Usually a frontal sinus has both a perpendicular and a horizontal extension (see Fig. 33-38), so that it lies in both the squama and the orbital part of the frontal bone. Sometimes anterior ethmoid cells protrude markedly into it. The frontal sinus opens beneath the front end of the middle concha, either into the ethmoid infundibulum or anterior to or above this groove in a region known to clinicians as the frontal recess.

The ethmoid cells that collectively form the **ethmoid sinus** vary in number; there may be as few as 3 or as many as 18. *The anterior ethmoid cells,* which tend to be more numerous but also usually are smaller than the middle and posterior ones, open into the middle meatus, either into the ethmoid infundibulum or the frontal recess. Some of these cells are closely related developmentally to the frontal sinus, and it is one of these that may bulge into that sinus. The *middle ethmoid cells* (also known as bullar cells because they form the ethmoid bulla) average about three in number, as compared with an average of five or six for the anterior cells. They also open into the middle meatus, either on the surface of the bulla or immediately above it beneath the attached edge of the middle concha. (Many clinicians include the middle cells with the anterior ones, describing as anterior cells all those that open into the middle meatus.) The *posterior ethmoid cells* are reported to vary from none to six; they typically open into the superior meatus, but occasionally one or more open above the superior concha.

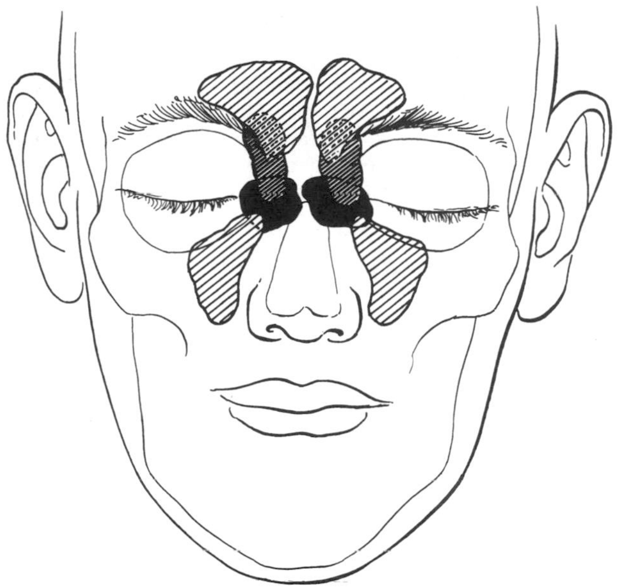

FIGURE 33-36.
Diagram of the paranasal sinuses: The frontal and maxillary sinuses are *shaded by widely spaced lines*, the ethmoid sinuses are *shaded by closely spaced ones*, and the sphenoid sinuses are *black*. (Wakefield EG. Clinical diagnosis. New York: Appleton, 1955.)

Sometimes a posterior ethmoid cell bulges into the sphenoid sinus, or sometimes it becomes intimately related to the optic canal, growing partly or even entirely around the canal so that the optic nerve is separated from the mucosa of the air cell by only a thin lamina of bone. Total blindness of an eye has been reported from careless exploration of such a posterior ethmoid cell.

The **maxillary sinus** lies in the prominence of the cheek, where its roof, lateral wall, and floor are composed primarily of the maxillary bone; and its medial wall is the lateral nasal wall. Its opening is high on its medial wall, usually into the infundibulum where it may be hidden by the uncinate process, but sometimes far enough posteriorly to be into the middle meatus itself and, therefore, more approachable for irrigation when there is infection. Accessory openings into the middle meatus are fairly common.

The **sphenoid sinuses** are placed close together in the body of the sphenoid bone; therefore, the hypophysis, lying in the sella turcica, is above them. On each side are the carotid artery, cavernous sinus, and ophthalmic and maxillary branches of the trigeminal nerve; the nerve of the pterygoid canal runs through the anterior part of the floor. In addition, if a sinus extends forward and upward sufficiently, it becomes closely related to the optic canal. The two sinuses vary much in size and rarely are symmetric; the bony septum between them usually is deviated to one side or the other. Each sphenoid sinus opens through its anterior wall, some distance above its floor, into the sphenoethmoidal recess of the nasal cavity.

From the positions of their openings, it is obvious that, of the large paranasal sinuses, only the frontal sinus has gravity drainage in the erect posture; the maxillary and sphenoid sinuses never do, and the openings of ethmoid cells vary so much that there is no good position for gravity drainage of all of them. Gravity drainage from the maxillary sinuses is best when one is lying on the side opposite the affected sinus. Similarly, best gravity drainage from the sphenoid sinuses can be secured when one lies face down. However, all the paranasal sinuses are provided with *ciliated epithelium,* and the beat of this cilia is toward the normal ostium; thus, under normal circumstances the secretions are carried to the ostia and discharged into the nose. In sinusitis, the ciliary action is not sufficient to empty the sinuses, the ostia of which often are partly or completely closed by swelling of the mucous membrane; hence, lavage of the sinuses and shrinkage of the membrane to allow them to become once again

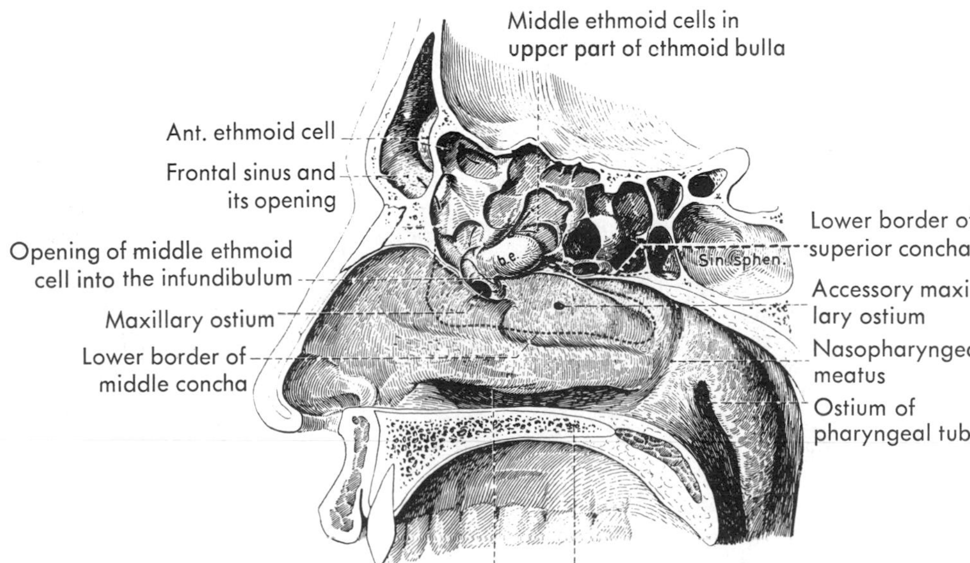

FIGURE 33-37.
The ethmoid air cells, together constituting the ethmoid sinus: *b.e.* is the ethmoid bulla; *Sin. sphen.* is the sphenoid sinus. The posterior ethmoid cells are here more *heavily shaded* than are the anterior and middle ones. "Pharyngeal tube" is an older name for the auditory tube. (Corning HK. Lehrbuch der topographischen Anatomie fur Studierende Und Artze. Munich: JF Bergmann, 1923.)

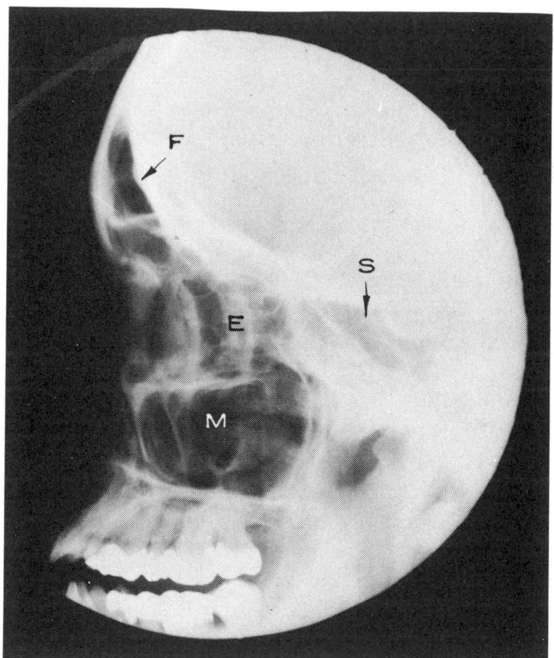

FIGURE *33-38.*
A lateral view of the paranasal sinuses. (Courtesy of Dr. D. G. Pugh)

aerated may be necessary to relieve the condition. Accessory openings for drainage are sometimes made surgically.

The ethmoid cells begin to develop during fetal life, and it is because of this earlier development that they may occupy positions where they bulge into the later-developing frontal and sphenoid sinuses. The frontal and sphenoid sinuses are represented only by rudimentary diverticula at birth; the maxillary sinus is present, but small, at birth. The maxillary, frontal, and sphenoid sinuses develop fairly rapidly during the first 7 to 8 years of life, but the maxillary sinuses do not reach their full development until after the second or permanent dentition has been acquired, and the frontal ones do not reach theirs until after puberty. The invasion of the frontal and maxillary bones by the sinuses apparently is an important cause of the change in features occurring between babyhood and puberty.

The **blood and nerve supply** of the sphenoid, ethmoid, and frontal sinuses is largely from the nerves and vessels that supply the nose—the posterior superior nasal vessels and nerves; the posterior ethmoidal artery and nerve (when this is present) to the sphenoid sinus and more posteriorly lying ethmoid cells; and anterior ethmoidal arteries and nerves to anteriorly lying ethmoid cells and the frontal sinus. The supraorbital artery and nerve are the chief supply to the frontal sinus and also may supply anterior ethmoid cells. The innervation and blood supply to the maxillary sinus is from twigs that leave the posterior superior alveolar and infraorbital nerves and arteries as they run in the wall of the maxillary sinus in close relationship to the mucosa.

RECOMMENDED READINGS

Aykut M, Gümüsburun E, Müderrïs S, Adigüzel E. The secondary nasal middle concha. Surg Radiol Anat 1994; 16: 307.

Basmajian JV, DeLuca CJ. Extraocular muscles and muscles of middle ear. In: Muscles alive: their functions revealed by electromyography. 5th ed. Baltimore: Williams & Wilkins, 1985.

Beard C, Quickert MH. Anatomy of the orbit. Birmingham: Aesculapius, 1988.

Beatie JC, Stilwell DL Jr. Innervation of the eye. Anat Rec 1961; 141: 45.

Blanton PL, Biggs NL. Eighteen hundred years of controversy: the paranasal sinuses. Am J Anat 1969; 124: 135.

Brémond-Gignac DS, Deplus S, Cussenot O, Lassau J-P. Anatomic study of the orbital septum. Surg Radiol Anat 1994; 16: 121.

Caparosa RJ, Klassen D. Congenital anomalies of the stapes and facial nerve. Arch Otolaryngol 1966; 83: 420.

Christensen K. The innervation of the nasal mucosa, with special reference to its afferent supply. Ann Otol Rhinol Laryngol 1934; 43: 1066.

Crowe SJ, Hughson W, Witting EG. Function of the tensor tympani muscle: an experimental study. Arch Otolaryngol 1931; 14: 575.

Davis H. Biophysics and physiology of the inner ear. Physiol Rev 1957; 37: 1.

Dohlman G. Investigations in the function of the semicircular canals. Acta Otolaryngol 1944; 51: 211.

Duckert LG. Anatomy of the skull base, temporal bone, external ear, and middle ear. In: Cummings CW, ed. Otolaryngology—head and neck surgery. 2nd ed, vol 4. St Louis: Mosby-Year Book, 1993: 2483.

Fine BS, Tousimis AJ. The structure of the vitreous body and the suspensory ligaments of the lens. Arch Ophthalmol 1961; 65: 95.

Graney DO, Rice DH. Anatomy of the paranasal sinuses. In: Cummings CW, ed. Otolaryngology—head and neck surgery. 2nd ed. vol 1. St Louis: Mosby-Year Book, 1993: 901.

Graney DO, Baker SR. Anatomy of the nose. In: Cummings CW, ed. Otolaryngology—head and neck surgery. 2nd ed. vol 1. St Louis: Mosby-Year Book, 1993: 627.

Graves GO, Edwards LF. The eustachian tube: a review of its descriptive microscopic, topographic and clinical anatomy. Arch Otolaryngol 1944; 39: 359.

Guild SR. The circulation of the endolymph. Am J Anat 1944; 39: 359.

Hillen B, ed. Paranasal sinuses and anterior skull base [computer software program]. New York: Elsevier Science, 1994.

Hollinshead WH. Anatomy for surgeons; vol 1, the head and neck. 3rd ed. Philadelphia: Harper & Row, 1982.

House WF. Surgical exposure of the internal auditory canal and its contents through the middle cranial fossa. Laryngoscope 1961; 71: 1363.

Jakobiec FA. Ocular anatomy, embryology and teratology. Philadelphia: Harper & Row, 1982.

Johnson RW. Anatomy for ophthalmic anaesthesia. Br J Anaesth 1995; 75: 80.

Kullmann GL, Dyck PJ, Cody DTR. Anatomy of the mastoid portion of the facial nerve. Arch Otolaryngol 1971; 93: 29.

Lang J. Clinical anatomy of the nose, nasal cavity and paranasal sinuses. Stuttgart: Thieme, 1989.

Manson PN, Lazarus RB, Morgan R, Iliff N. Pathways of sympathetic innervation to the superior and inferior (Müller's) tarsal muscles. Plast Reconstr Surg 1986; 78: 33.

Pait TG, Zeal A, Harris FS, Paullus WS, Rhoton AL Jr. Microsurgical anatomy and dissection of the temporal bone. Surg Neurol 1977; 8: 363.

Philippou M, Stenger GM, Goumas PD, Hillen B, Huizing EH. Cross-sectional anatomy of the nose and paranasal sinuses. Rhinology 1990; 28: 221.

Proctor B. Surgical anatomy of the ear and temporal bone. New York: Thieme, 1989.

Robert Y, Rocourt N, Gaillandre L, Lemaitre L, Francke JP. Serial anatomy of the auditory tube: correlation to CT and MR imaging. Surg Radiol Anat 1994; 16: 63.

Vogt-Hohenlinde CH. Topographical anatomy for sinus surgery. Acta Otolaryngol Stockh 1991; suppl: 484.

Watson C, Vijayan N, The sympathetic innervation of the eyes and face: a clinicoanatomic review. Clin Anat 1995; 8: 262.

Hollinshead's Textbook of Anatomy, by Cornelius Rosse and Penelope Gaddum-Rosse.
Lippincott-Raven Publishers, Philadelphia, © 1997.

CHAPTER 34

Pharynx and Larynx

PHARYNX

The pharynx is the continuation of the digestive cavity from the mouth, but also receives in its upper part the posterior openings of the nasal cavities, the choanae. That part above the level of the soft palate is the **pars nasalis** (nasal pharynx); that between the level of the soft palate and the entrance into the larynx is the **pars oralis;** and the part posterior to the larynx down to the beginning of the esophagus is the **laryngeal part** (see Fig. 34-4). Because of the openings of the nose, mouth, and larynx into the pharynx, the musculature of the pharyngeal wall is largely lateral and posterior; even below the opening from the mouth, there is no anterior muscular wall to the pharynx, for the back part of the tongue at first provides this wall, and below this and the laryngeal opening, the posterior wall of the larynx is the anterior pharyngeal wall.

A certain amount of loose connective tissue lies between the two pterygoid muscles and the lateral wall of the pharynx, and this is described as forming the **lateral pharyngeal fascial space.** This space is bounded above by the base of the skull and below by the attachment of the cervical fascia to the hyoid bone, submandibular gland, and mandible (see Fig. 31-32). Anteriorly, however, it becomes continuous with the potential spaces above and below the mylohyoid muscles ("submandibular space"), and posteriorly, it is continuous with the retropharyngeal space.

The **retropharyngeal space** is the loose connective tissue between the pharynx and the vertebral column. It is the uppermost part of the retrovisceral space as that extends upward to the base of the skull, and really, therefore, should not be separately named.

Exterior of the Pharynx

The external surface of the pharynx consists of voluntary muscle covered by a thin **buccopharyngeal fascia** continuous with that on the outer surface of the buccinator muscle. It can best be examined after the posterior part of the occipital bone and the vertebral column have been separated from the pharynx, so that it can be seen from behind as well as laterally. In close relation posterolaterally are the 9th, 10th, and 11th cranial nerves as they emerge through the jugular foramen; just behind these is the upper end of the internal jugular vein as it leaves the jugular fossa; crossing behind the structures from the jugular foramen and running downward, laterally, and forward is the hypoglossal nerve; and anteromedial to them is the upper end of the internal carotid artery as this enters the back end of the carotid canal.

The **blood supply** of the upper part of the pharynx is from the **ascending pharyngeal artery,** which runs upward along the posterolateral wall, and from small descending branches of the palatine arteries; twigs from the superior and inferior thyroid arteries supply the lower part (Fig. 34-1) The **veins** form a *pharyngeal plexus* on the posterior surface of the pharynx. This plexus drains laterally at irregular intervals into the pterygoid plexus, the superior and inferior thyroid veins, and often by separate pharyngeal veins that enter the lower end of the facial vein or the internal jugular close to this ending. Postero-

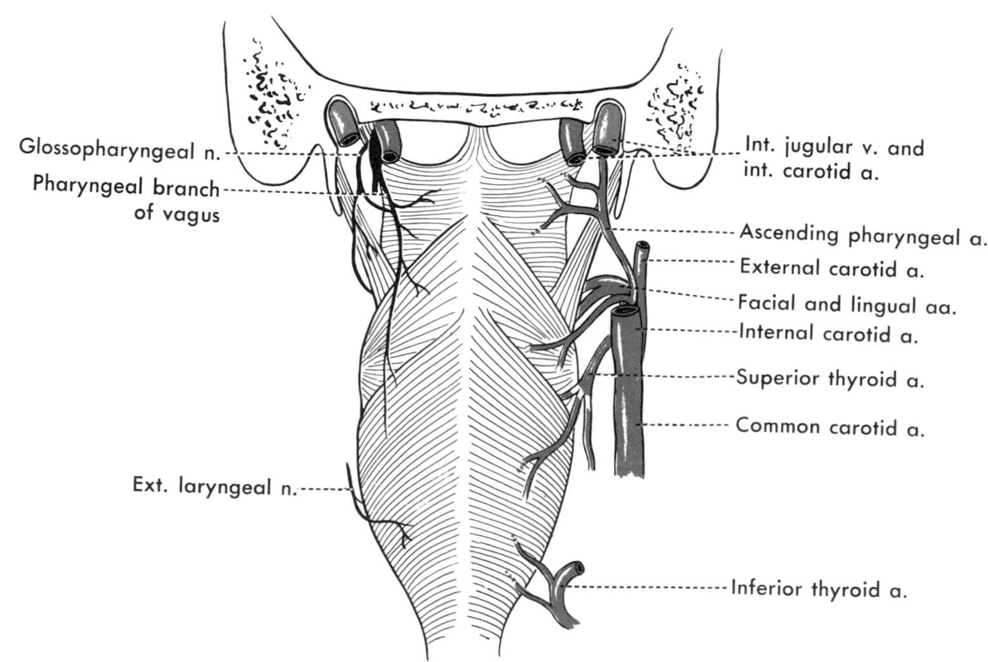

FIGURE *34-1.*
Nerves and arteries of the pharynx.

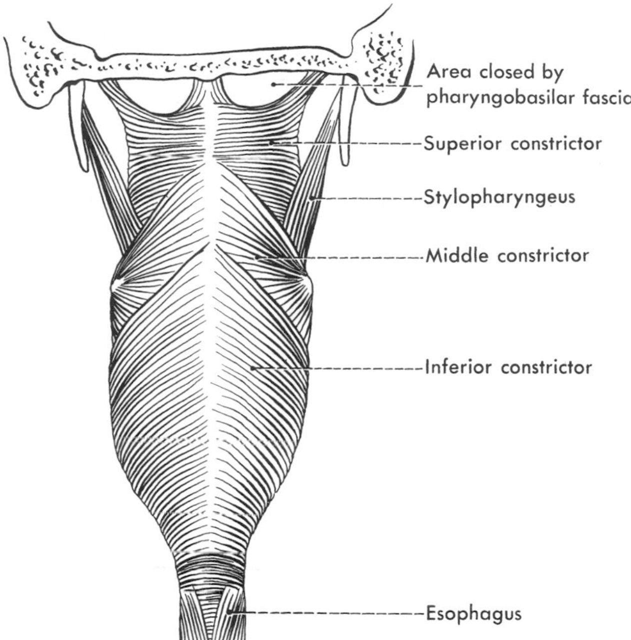

FIGURE *34-2.*
The pharyngeal muscles seen from behind.

laterally on the pharyngeal wall, not much above the level of the carotid bifurcation, there usually is a large **retropharyngeal lymph node;** there also may be smaller nodes present. These receive most of the lymphatic drainage of the pharynx, the nasal cavity, and a posterior part of the tongue.

The **nerve supply** to the pharynx is from the *pharyngeal plexus,* formed by the union of the pharyngeal branches of the glossopharyngeal and vagus nerves. The vagal contribution to the pharyngeal plexus supplies all the muscles of the pharynx except the stylopharyngeus and most of those of the soft palate (tensor veli palatini excepted), but the lowermost muscle of the pharynx, the inferior constrictor, may receive a twig from another branch of the vagus (external laryngeal nerve) that goes primarily to the larynx. It usually is stated that the glossopharyngeal contribution to the pharyngeal plexus is sensory to all the pharynx between the levels of the opening of the auditory tube and the larynx, but the nerve may not reach as high as the auditory tube, leaving much of the pars nasalis to be supplied by the fifth nerve; the vagus nerve apparently may supply sensation to more than the laryngeal part of the pharynx.

The four paired **muscles of the pharynx** visible from the outside (Figs. 34-2 and 34-3) are rather simply arranged. There are three constrictors, each overlapping the one above, and there is a more longitudinally arranged muscle, the stylopharyngeus, that runs downward and disappears between the superior and middle constrictors. The muscle fibers of each pair of pharyngeal constrictors meet in the posterior midline to form a *pharyngeal raphe.*

The **superior constrictor** is a broad muscle, the upper part of which does not completely cover the wall of the pharynx. It has a free upper edge that originates from the posterior border of the medial pterygoid plate, runs posteriorly and somewhat downward, and then loops up to meet the similar component from the other side. The two parts are then attached above by a midline band to the pharyngeal tubercle of the occipital bone. The gap above the muscle on each side is traversed by the auditory tube, but otherwise it is sealed by a heavy **pharyngobasilar fascia** attached above to the base of the skull and to the cartilaginous portion of the auditory tube and anteriorly to the posterior border of the medial pterygoid plate. The pharyngobasilar fascia supports the mucous membrane of most of the nasal part of the pharynx, but becomes

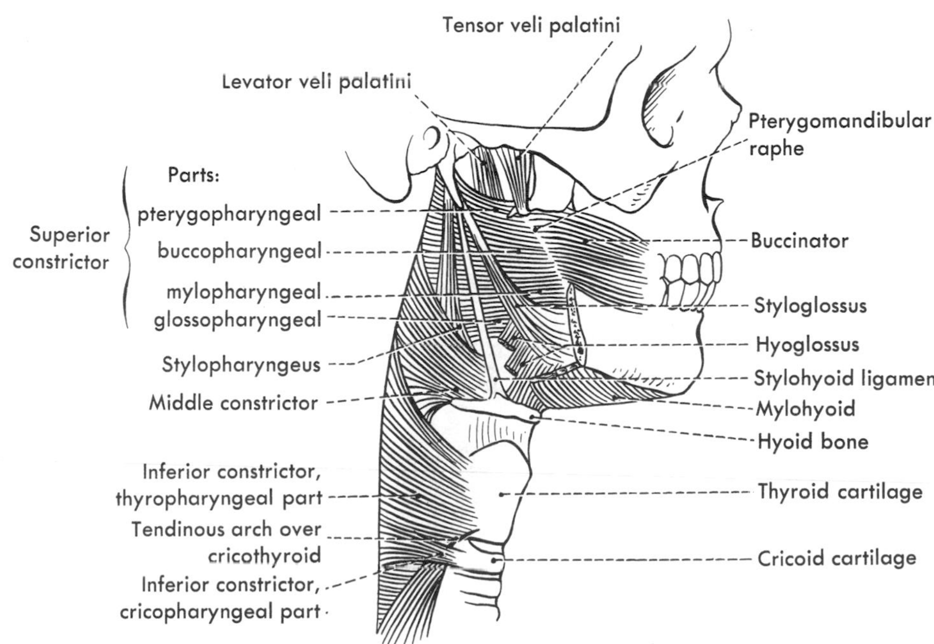

FIGURE *34-3.*
Lateral view of the pharyngeal muscles.

much thinner below, at about the level of the soft palate. Two muscles of the palate lie adjacent to it, and when the fascia is removed, the gap above the superior constrictor is largely hidden by these (see Fig. 34-3).

In addition to its origin from the medial pterygoid plate, the superior constrictor arises also from the *pterygomandibular raphe,* which extends downward from the hamulus of the plate to the mandible and gives origin anteriorly to the buccinator muscle in the cheek. Below this, it takes origin from the mylohyoid line of the mandible, and below this, from the lateral surface of the muscles of the tongue. Four parts corresponding to these four origins are named (see Fig. 34-3), but these terms are seldom used. The lower part of the superior constrictor is covered posteriorly by the middle constrictor, but anterolaterally, there is a gap between the two through which the stylopharyngeus muscle passes.

The **middle constrictor** arises from both the greater and lesser horns of the hyoid bone and from the lower part of the stylohyoid ligament above the lesser horn. From this relatively narrow origin, it spreads out in a fan-shaped manner so that its upper fibers overlap the superior constrictor posteriorly, and its lower fibers are, in turn, overlapped by the inferior constrictor.

The **inferior constrictor** arises from both thyroid and cricoid cartilages. The fibers of thyroid origin run backward, the upper ones, especially, running upward at the same time, to insert into the pharyngeal raphe and overlap the middle constrictor. The lowest fibers of thyroid origin have only a little upward direction, and the uppermost fibers of cricoid origin run still less upward. The lower fibers run almost directly transversely and blend below with the circular fibers of the esophagus, which are exposed here.

The cricopharyngeal part of the inferior constrictor, often called the **cricopharyngeus muscle,** is of considerable importance. In contrast with the other pharyngeal constrictor fibers, it maintains a tonic contraction until swallowing is started and thus serves as the sphincter between the pharynx and the esophagus. This normally prevents regurgitation to the laryngeal level of material passing retrogradely from the stomach into the esophagus, unless there is active vomiting. Also, spasm of the more transverse fibers of the muscle may be a cause of obstruction here and allow the development of a diverticulum (usually called a hypopharyngeal diverticulum). Such diverticula are directed downward and may become very large sacs that interfere with the nutrition of the individual and must be treated surgically.

The **stylopharyngeus muscle** arises from the medial side of the styloid process and passes downward and medially between the external and internal carotid arteries. It enters the pharynx through the gap between the superior and middle constrictors and spreads out on the inner surface of the latter to blend with it and insert in part on the upper and posterior borders of the thyroid cartilage.

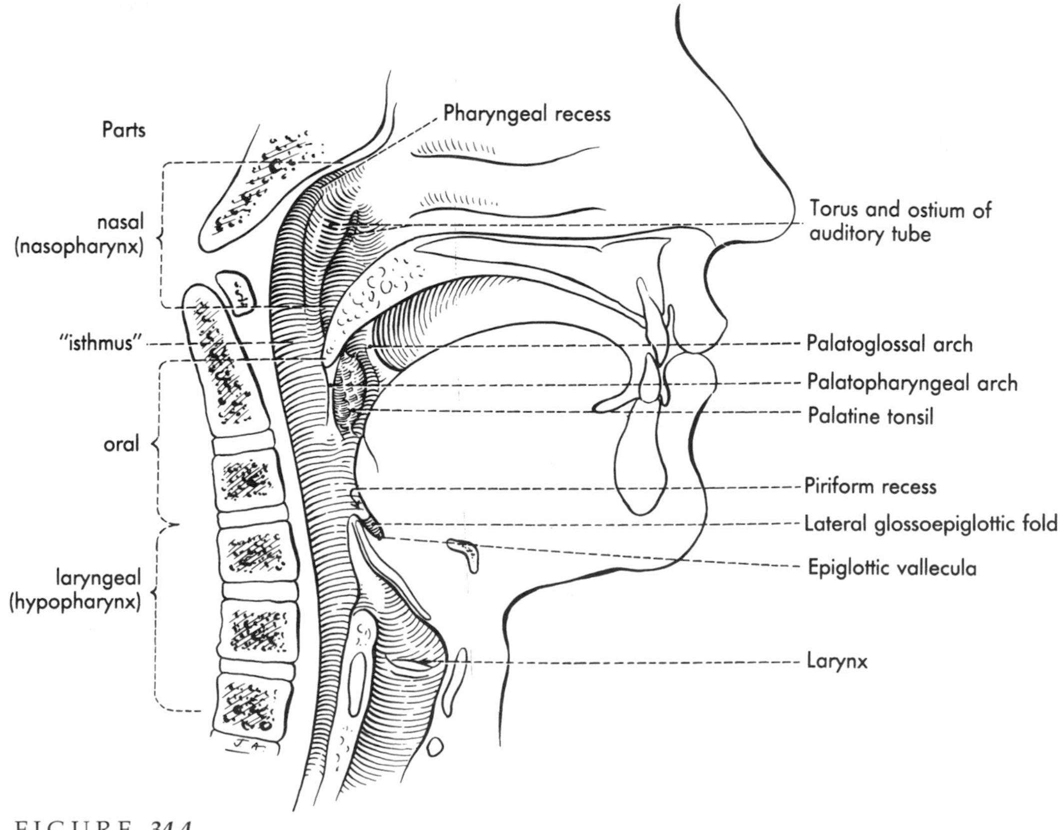

FIGURE *34.4.*
Interior of the pharynx.

The stylopharyngeus is the only muscle innervated by the *glossopharyngeal nerve.* This nerve runs downward medial to the stylopharyngeus and then turns forward toward the tongue around the posterior border and outer surface of the muscle, giving off its lone motor branch at about this point. The stylopharyngeus helps to raise the pharynx, but paralysis of it has no noticeable effect on swallowing.

Interior of the Pharynx

Of the parts of the cavity of the pharynx (Fig. 34-4) the nasal part often is called nasopharynx and the laryngeal part, the hypopharynx.

Nasal Part

The nasal part of the pharynx has a roof and lateral and posterior walls. There is, essentially, no anterior wall, because choanae open here. The roof, called the **fornix,** consists of mucous membrane closely applied to the basal portions of the sphenoid and occipital bones. The lateral and posterior walls consist of the superior constrictors, the pharyngobasilar fascia that lines their internal surfaces, and the mucosa.

The soft palate forms the floor of the anterior part of the nasal pharynx and is the only really mobile wall of this part of the pharynx; thus, the nasal pharynx remains constantly open. On its lateral wall, above the soft palate, is the **pharyngeal ostium of the auditory tube,** the tube to the middle ear cavity.

Above and posterior to the ostium is an elevation, the **torus tubarius,** or tubal torus, produced by the cartilage of the tube. Proceeding down from the torus is a slight fold, the **salpingopharyngeal fold** (*salpinx* meaning tube). Behind the torus and the salpingopharyngeal fold is a slit-like lateral projection of the pharynx, the **pharyngeal recess.** A slight **salpingopalatine fold** runs from the anterior border of the torus tubarius toward the palate. Below the torus tubarius, in front of the salpingopharyngeal fold, another fold or bulge, the **torus levatorius,** or levator torus, is formed by the levator veli palatini and is especially evident when the muscle contracts.

The opening of the nasopharynx behind the soft palate into the oral pharynx is usually called the **pharyngeal isthmus.** At this level the nasal part of the pharynx can be completely closed off from the oral part, for the soft palate can be pulled backward and upward by the levator veli palatini to meet the posterior wall. The meeting of soft palate and posterior pharyngeal wall is necessary for proper phonation, especially of consonants, and also is necessary if fluid swallowed under pressure is to be kept from running into the nose (for instance, one can drink bending over, or standing on one's head, because of the complete closure here).

In the posterior part of the roof and the upper part of the posterior wall of the nasal part of the pharynx is an accumulation of lymphoid tissue that may be prominent in children but that becomes indistinct or disappears by adulthood; this is the **pharyngeal tonsil.** Similar accumulations of lymphoid tissue in children are associated with the posterior lip of the ostium of the auditory tube and are called the **tubal tonsil.** When the pharyngeal and tubal tonsils are enlarged, they are referred to as **adenoids.** These may cause difficulty in nasal breathing because of obstruction of the nasal pharynx, and if the ostium of the tube is occluded, there may be hearing loss because of gradual absorption of the air in the middle ear cavity.

Oral Part

The oral part of the pharynx opens above, behind the soft palate, into the nasal part. It receives anteriorly the opening from the mouth, and below this it is bordered by the posterior part of the dorsum of the tongue. Behind the tongue, the oral part of the pharynx extends laterally and posteriorly downward to the upwardly projecting epiglottis, a portion of the larynx, to become continuous with the laryngeal part.

The **fauces** (meaning throat), the lateral boundaries of the *faucial isthmus,* or the opening of the mouth into the pharynx, deserves special attention. Each consists of two folds ("pillars of the fauces") between which the palatine tonsil, usually known simply as "the tonsil," lies (Fig. 34-5 and also see Fig. 31-24). The anterior fold, the **palatoglossal arch,** curves downward and forward from the soft palate to the tongue. The posterior fold, the **palatopharyngeal arch,** extends downward from the posterolateral border of the soft palate along the wall of the pharynx. Each arch contains a muscle, similarly named—that is, palatoglossus and palatopharyngeus muscles. Between these two arches is the somewhat almond-shaped mass of lymphoid tissue that constitutes the palatine tonsil and that largely fills the space between the folds, the **tonsillar fossa.** The roof and floor of the faucial isthmus, which are not well defined, are the soft palate and the dorsum of the tongue.

A fold of mucous membrane, the **semilunar fold,** extends between the palatoglossal and palatopharyngeal arches across the upper part of the tonsil, and between it and the tonsil is a slit, the **supratonsillar fossa.** A second fold, the *triangular fold,*

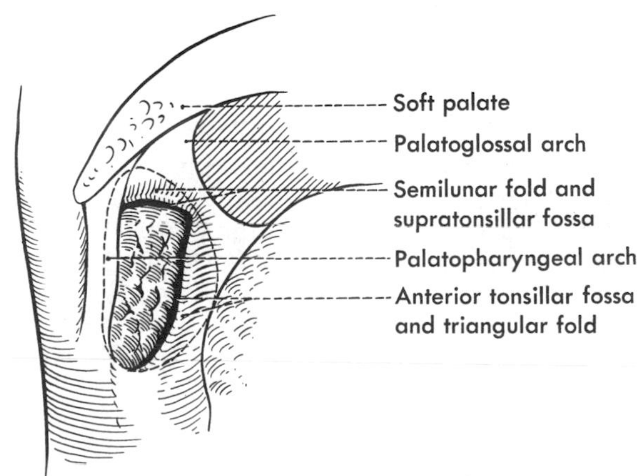

FIGURE 34-5.
The palatine tonsil and its relations.

projects backward from the palatoglossal arch and either may be fused to the tonsil or may leave a slit that usually is called the anterior tonsillar fossa.

The **palatine tonsil** varies considerably in size and shape, for it may bulge markedly between the folds or may be flat and almost hidden in the tonsillar fossa. It often extends into the soft palate deep to the semilunar fold. Its surface is covered with epithelium that has pits, the *tonsillar crypts,* passing into the lymphoid substance. Between it and the superior pharyngeal constrictor, which forms most of its muscular bed, is the pharyngobasilar fascia; the part adjacent to the tonsil sends septa into it and often is described as the *tonsillar capsule.* Loose connective tissue between the "capsule" and the superior constrictor muscle forms a line of cleavage that facilitates removal of the tonsil.

The largest **artery** of the tonsil, the *tonsillar branch of the facial,* enters its lower pole. The ascending pharyngeal, lingual, descending palatine, and ascending palatine branch of the facial are also usually described as having small tonsillar branches. The **glossopharyngeal nerve** runs forward to the tongue medial to the hyoglossus muscle after passing across the gap between the superior and middle pharyngeal constrictors close to the lower pole of the tonsil. Because of this relation, edema about the nerve may result from tonsillectomy, and some patients complain of temporary loss of taste following this operation. The nerve gives off a tonsillar branch that, along with branches of the ninth from the pharyngeal plexus, supplies the region of the tonsil.

Below the fauces, the pharynx is bounded anteriorly by the posterior part of the dorsum of the tongue. This, in addition to presenting the vallate taste buds, also has an accumulation of lymphoid tissue beneath its mucosa. This lymphoid tissue on the pharyngeal surface of the tongue constitutes the **lingual tonsil** and may be sufficiently enlarged to need removal when other tonsillar tissue is removed.

It may be noted that the pharyngeal tonsils posteriorly and above, the palatine tonsils laterally, and the lingual tonsil anteriorly and below form an oblique ring of lymphoid tissue around the pharynx. This apparently has the function of tending to halt infection at this level, but when it becomes enlarged as a result of disease, it is no longer of use as a defense mechanism, and its enlargement may cause obstruction.

The **epiglottis,** behind the tongue, is united to that structure by a midline and two lateral folds, the **median** and the **lateral glossoepiglottic folds,** respectively. The paired depressions between the median and lateral glossoepiglottic folds are the **epiglottic valleculae** (see both Figs. 31-37 and 34-4).

Laryngeal Part

The laryngeal part of the pharynx, continuous with the oral part at the level of the upper border of the epiglottis, is wide above, but narrows rapidly below at the level of the cricoid cartilage of the larynx (Fig. 34-6) to become continuous with the esophagus at the lower border of the cartilage. The anterior wall of this part of the pharynx is the larynx: above is the posterior surface of the epiglottis; below the opening into the larynx are certain muscles of the larynx and the lamina (expanded posterior part) of the cricoid cartilage, covered posteriorly by pharyngeal mucous membrane.

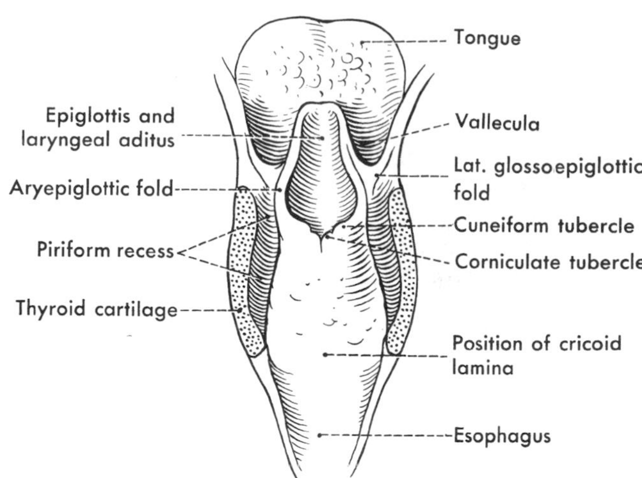

FIGURE *34-6.*
The larynx from behind, after removal of the posterior pharyngeal wall.

The pharynx also extends lateral to the larynx, being separated from that by the **aryepiglottic folds** that run from the upper posterior border of the larynx to the sides of the epiglottis. These lateral extensions are the **piriform recesses** (also called sinuses). As the pharynx narrows at the cricoid level, the piriform recesses are obliterated; thus, they are blind forward extensions of the pharynx.

Because each epiglottic vallecula is a shallow basin, an object such as a safety pin that is thought to have been swallowed or inspired may sometimes lodge in it, or such an object may lodge in a piriform recess. Both the valleculae and the recesses, therefore, usually are examined for objects thought to be inhaled, before a child is subjected to bronchoscopy.

Swallowing (deglutition) is a complex act typically involving contraction of the pharyngeal constrictors and the esophagus from above downward. As the bolus is passed into the oral part of the pharynx, the soft palate is raised to come in contact with the posterior pharyngeal wall, and the pharynx as a whole is raised by the action of its longitudinal muscle. Contraction of the superior pharyngeal constrictor passes the bolus into the region of the relaxed middle constrictor which, in turn, contracts, followed by the inferior constrictor. The cricopharyngeal part of the inferior constrictor ("cricoesophageal sphincter") relaxes as swallowing is started, and a descending contraction of the esophagus passes the bolus into the stomach. The larynx is protected partly by contraction of its sphincteric muscles and partly because the food or liquid tends to pass to the sides of the epiglottis, rather than directly over the laryngeal aditus.

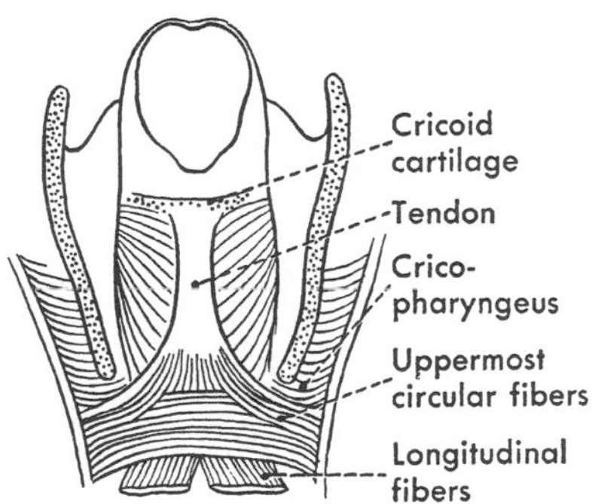

FIGURE 34-7.
Attachment of the esophagus to the larynx.

Attachment of the Esophagus

The mucosa of the esophagus is continuous with that of the pharynx at the lower border of the cricoid cartilage, but the musculature of the two structures is continuous only posteriorly. Here the longitudinal (external) layer of esophageal muscle separates into two bands that diverge anteriorly around the sides of the esophagus, thereby exposing the inner circular muscle posteriorly (see Fig. 34-2). After all the longitudinal muscle is concentrated in the anterior esophageal wall, the two bands unite to form a **cricoesophageal tendon** that is attached to the posterior surface of the cricoid lamina (Fig. 34-7). The posteriorly exposed circular fibers at the upper end of the esophagus blend with the lowest fibers of the inferior pharyngeal constrictor (cricopharyngeal part); anteriorly, however, the fibers largely encircle the esophagus, but a few uppermost ones join the sides of the cricoesophageal tendon. Because the inferior constrictor attaches to the sides of the cricoid cartilage, this leaves a small gap laterally between the lower edge of the cricopharyngeal part of the inferior constrictor and the esophageal muscle. The inferior laryngeal nerve and vessels enter the larynx here (see Fig. 34-20).

Palate

The palate separates the nose from the mouth and partially separates the nasal and oral parts of the pharynx. Its major anterior part, the **hard palate,** consists of the bony palate with a covering of mucosa and numerous mucous glands.

Development. The palate is formed by two palatine (lateral palatine) processes that develop from the maxilla and fuse with each other in the midline and with the fused medial nasal or medial palatine processes (also called the premaxillary or primary palate) anteriorly (Fig. 34-8). Failure of the nasal process to develop or to fuse with one or both lateral processes, or failure of the lateral processes to fuse, produces **cleft palate.** Associated with cleft palate, or sometimes occurring alone, there may be a **cleft upper lip.** Whether the cleft is bilateral, unilateral, or a large midline defect, it often has been called harelip. (Hares and rabbits normally have a cleft upper lip, but their cleft is a midline one. The abnormal cleft in a human is rarely in the midline, occurring more commonly along the line of fusion between medial nasal and palatine processes.) Clefts that involve the posterior part of the palate interfere with swallowing and with phonation. Orthodontists, plastic surgeons, and speech specialists often work together as a team in determining at what age an operation should be done to produce maximum benefit.

The **soft palate** (palatinum molle) is attached anteriorly to the hard palate and blends laterally with the pharynx. Its posteroinferior part, the **velum palatini** (a term used also to mean the entire soft palate), is more in the coronal than the horizontal plane, and from its free edge, a nipplelike projection, the **uvula,** hangs down. The soft palate is mainly muscular in structure (Fig. 34-9), but numerous mucous glands lie between the mucosa and the muscles. With the exception of the tensor veli palatini, the muscles are innervated through the vagus nerve, by way of the pharyngeal plexus; the tensor is innervated by a branch from the mandibular nerve.

Muscles

The **levator veli palatini** (see Fig. 34-3) arises from the inferior surface of the petrous portion of the temporal bone and from a part of the medial surface of the cartilaginous portion of the auditory tube, just inside the attachment of the pharyngobasilar fascia to the tube and the temporal bone. It runs obliquely downward and medially into the posterior part of the soft palate to become continuous with the muscle of the opposite side. As it passes to the palate below the ostium of the auditory tube, it is responsible for the *levator torus,* which may be obvious only when the muscle contracts. The insertion end of this muscle forms much of the bulk of the soft palate.

The **tensor veli palatini** (see Figs. 34-3 and 34-9) lies lateral and in part anterior to the levator. It arises from the scaphoid fossa (at the base of the medial pterygoid process), the spine of the sphenoid bone, and the lateral sur-

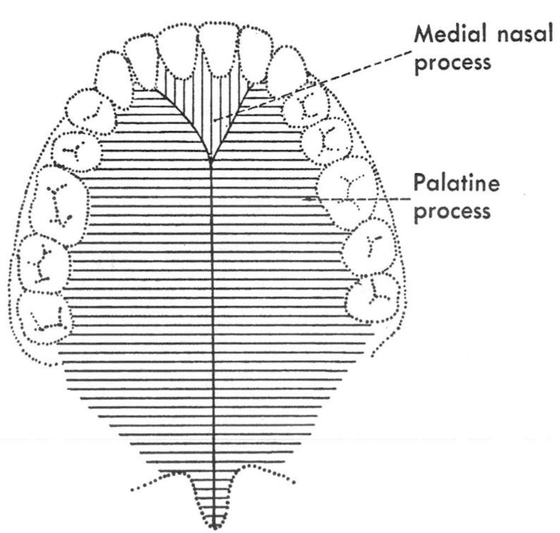

FIGURE 34-8.
Elements entering into the formation of the palate and anterior alveolar region.

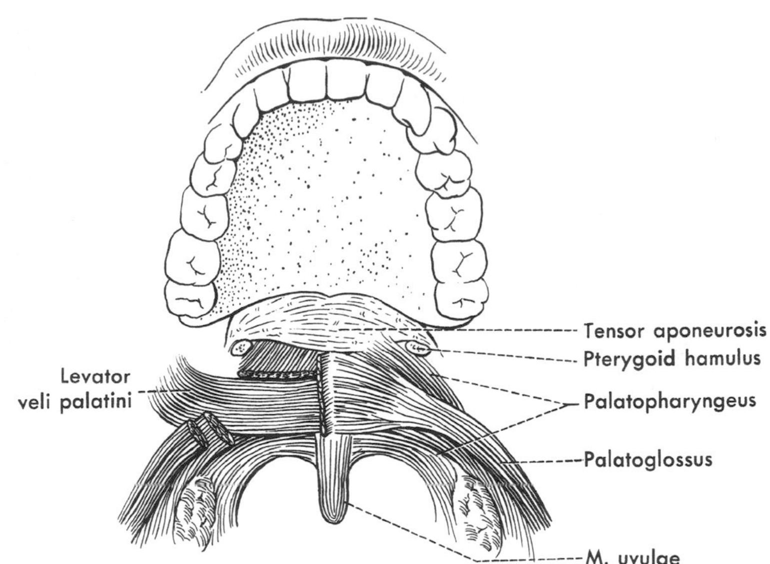

FIGURE 34-9.
Muscles of the soft palate.

face of the cartilaginous portion of the auditory tube (outside the pharyngobasilar fascia, which separates it from the levator) and extends vertically downward lateral to the medial pterygoid process. Its posterior border runs forward, but its anterior border runs straight down, so that at the level of the pterygoid hamulus, it has become narrow. Here it gives rise to a tendon that runs medially below the pterygoid hamulus and spreads out as the more aponeurotic anterior part of the soft palate. Anteriorly, the aponeurosis is attached to the posterior edge and lower surface of the bony palate, and it helps give origin to muscles of the soft palate. Although it is related to the medial pterygoid plate, therefore deep in the infratemporal fossa, the tensor receives its nerve supply from the mandibular nerve, which lies in the infratemporal fossa lateral to the muscle.

These two muscles have different actions on the soft palate. The levator veli palatini raises the soft palate and in so doing also pulls it backward so as to make it approach the posterior wall of the pharynx. The tensor veli palatini, by reason of the sharp turn that it makes around the pterygoid hamulus, cannot raise the soft palate but, rather, pulls laterally and, therefore, tenses it. Both muscles have been said to open the auditory tube (as in yawning, to allow air to enter the middle ear cavity), but the role of the levator in this process is less certain than that of the tensor.

The **musculus uvulae** arises by paired slips from the posterior border of the hard palate just on each side of the midline, and from the palatine aponeurosis behind the hard palate. The slips run backward on each side of the midline into the uvula, blending as they do so.

The **palatoglossus** is a thin sheet of muscle that begins on the lower surface of the soft palate where it is continuous with its fellow of the opposite side. It runs laterally, downward, and forward in front of the tonsil, forming the palatoglossal arch, and inserts into the dorsum and side of the tongue.

The **palatopharyngeus** is attached to the posterior border of the hard palate and to the aponeurotic layer of the soft palate and, in part, is continuous with its fellow of the opposite side. It is split into a superior (posterior) and an inferior (anterior) layer, between which lie the musculus uvulae and the palatine part of the levator. At the lateral border of the palate, the two layers blend and descend internal to the superior pharyngeal constrictor. Some of the anterior fibers form a part of the bed of the tonsil, and some of the posterior ones form the palatopharyngeal arch. The posterior fibers are joined by the small **salpingopharyngeus muscle,** a muscle of the pharynx that takes origin from the pharyngeal end of the auditory tube and raises the salpingopharyngeal fold in the posterolateral wall of the pharynx. The muscle fibers of the two palatopharyngeal muscles then spread toward the posterior midline. They end by attaching, in part, into the thyroid cartilage, but largely into the pharyngobasilar fascia.

The palatopharyngeus muscle is a levator of the pharynx. The salpingopharyngeus also is potentially a pharyngeal levator, but typically is a tiny muscle and may be lacking; it is of no real importance. The palatopharyngeus and the palatoglossus can both depress the palate, and when they do so, they narrow the faucial isthmus.

Nerves and Vessels

The chief nerves and vessels of the palate descend through greater and lesser palatine canals that open above into the pterygopalatine fossa and below by a major and usually two minor palatine foramina on the lower surface of the hard palate. The nerves descending in the canals are listed as branches of the pterygopalatine ganglion. Actually, the fibers composing them are largely from the maxillary, but as these fibers pass the pterygopalatine ganglion, they probably are joined by some postganglionic parasympathetic fibers from it, sympathetic fibers from the internal carotid plexus, and sensory

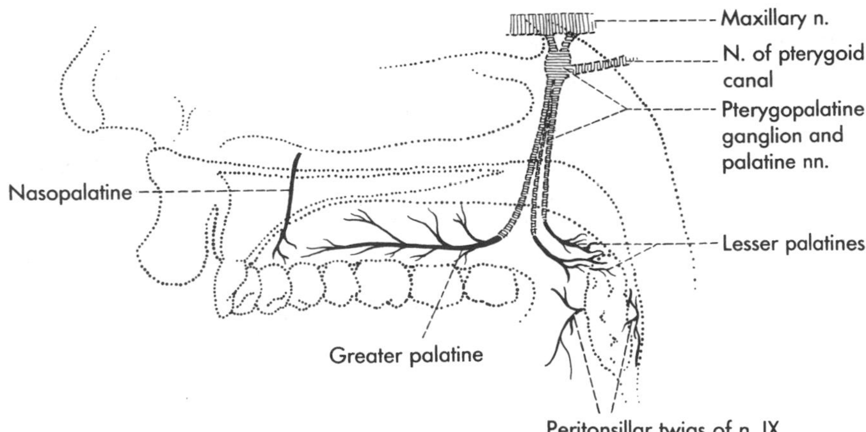

FIGURE *34-10.*
The palatine nerves.

fibers from the facial nerve, the last two brought to the ganglion by the nerve of the pterygoid canal. As the palatine nerves run downward through the palatine canals, they give off posterior inferior nasal branches to the lateral nasal wall and usually emerge on the palate as three nerves (Fig. 34-10).

The **greater palatine nerve,** the largest, emerges from the greater palatine foramen and turns forward to supply the hard palate and the inner surface of the gums of the teeth as far forward as the canine tooth. A small area immediately behind the incisor teeth is supplied by the **nasopalatine nerve,** which descends through an incisive canal from the nose. The **lesser palatine nerves,** emerging through lesser palatine foramina, supply the soft palate and the upper tonsillar region. It presumably is one of these nerves that contains sensory fibers from the facial nerve to a posterior part of the soft palate.

The **descending palatine artery,** derived from the terminal portion of the maxillary artery in the pterygopalatine fossa, is a short trunk that gives off lesser palatine arteries and continues as the **greater palatine artery.** The latter runs, with the nerve of the same name, through the greater palatine canal and emerges at the greater palatine foramen to run forward on the hard palate with the nerve. Instead of stopping short of the incisor teeth, it sends a terminal branch through an incisive canal to reach a lower part of the nasal septum. The **lesser palatine arteries** descend with the lesser palatine nerves to supply the soft palate and the upper tonsillar region. The small **ascending palatine branch** of the facial artery runs over the upper border of the superior constrictor and along the levator veli palatini to anastomose with them.

LARYNX

The larynx, part of the respiratory system, opens posteriorly and above into the pharynx; inferiorly, it is continued by the trachea. Although it is supported by cartilages, its aperture can be varied, for it is provided with muscles that can bring folds together, as in holding the breath or in vocalizing (in which the vocal folds are close together and set in vibration by the expired air), or separate them, as when one gasps for breath.

Laryngeal Skeleton

The major cartilages of the larynx are the thyroid, cricoid, arytenoid, and epiglottic (Figs. 34-11 and 34-12). The largest of these is the **thyroid cartilage,** which forms the laryngeal prominence in the neck. The thyroid cartilage, as its name (shield-shaped) indicates, does not extend around the larynx. It consists of *right and left laminae* that meet in the anterior midline. Projecting upward from the posterior border of each lamina is a *superior cornu,* and projecting downward is an *inferior cornu*. The upper border and superior cornua of the thyroid cartilage are united to the hyoid bone above by the *thyrohyoid membrane,* the thickened lateral edges of which are called the **thyrohyoid ligaments**. The thickened midline part is called the median thyrohyoid ligament. Each side of the thyrohyoid membrane presents, posterolaterally, an aper-

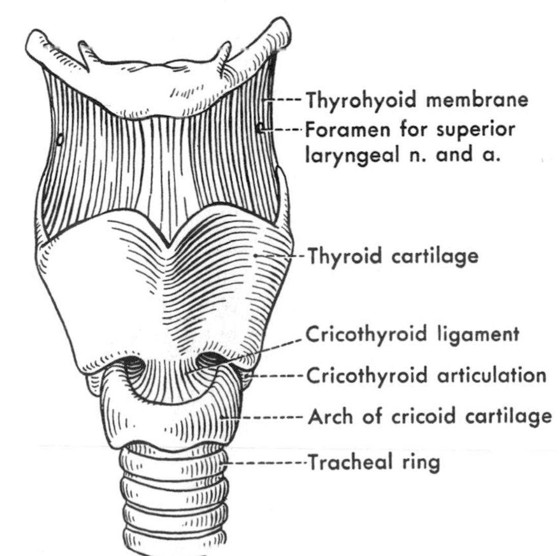

FIGURE *34-11.*
Cartilages of the larynx, anterior view.

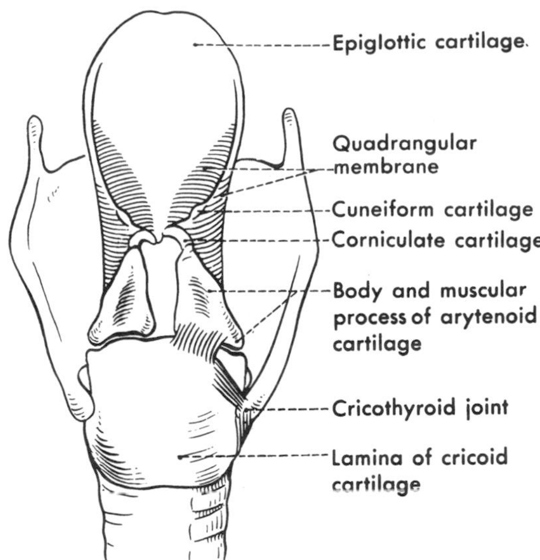

FIGURE *34-12.*
Cartilages of the larynx, posterior view.

ture through which the superior laryngeal nerve (internal branch) and vessels enter the larynx. The thyroid cartilage articulates below, through its inferior horns, with the cricoid cartilage and, besides these synovial articulations, is attached to this same cartilage by the **cricothyroid ligament.**

Only a part of the **cricoid cartilage** can be seen anteriorly; this is mostly its *arch,* united above to the thyroid cartilage by the *cricothyroid ligament* (in the anterior midline) and below to the uppermost ring of the trachea by a *cricotracheal ligament*. Posteriorly, the cricoid cartilage expands to form a *lamina*, on the sides of which are the cricothyroid synovial articulations.

Articulating with the upper lateral borders of the cricoid lamina are the **arytenoid cartilages.** These are particularly important because they are movable upon the cricoid cartilage and have the *vocal folds* attached to them. Each arytenoid cartilage somewhat resembles a three-sided pyramid. The base presents a synovial articular surface on which the arytenoid cartilage can slide laterally and medially, forward and backward, or rotate upon the cricoid cartilage. Projecting laterally from the base is a short blunt *muscular process* (two important muscles insert upon it); projecting anteriorly is a thinner process, the *vocal process*, to which the vocal cords and folds are attached. The posterior surface of the arytenoid cartilage is somewhat concave and gives attachment to a muscle that runs between the two cartilages; the medial surface is small, faces the medial surface of the other cartilage, and is covered by mucous membrane of the larynx; and the anterolateral surface, the largest, gives attachment to thin muscles that line the larynx and also has a large group of mucous glands between it and the mucous membrane. The apex of the cartilage is surmounted by a slender curved **corniculate cartilage** that is directed posteromedially, but does not move independently of the arytenoid cartilage. Its upper end raises the mucosa to produce a small *corniculate tubercle.*

Extending upward, laterally, and forward from the upper part of each arytenoid cartilage and from its surmounting corniculate cartilage to the lateral border of the epiglottic cartilage, there is, in the intact condition, a fold of mucous membrane, the **aryepiglottic fold,** supported by a thin lamina of connective tissue, the **quadrangular membrane** (Fig. 34-12). This membrane separates the piriform recess from the entrance into the larynx, and in its free border a little above and anterior to the corniculate tubercle, there may be a small **cuneiform cartilage** that produces a *cuneiform tubercle* (Fig. 34-13).

The **epiglottic cartilage** is a thin, unpaired cartilage supporting the epiglottis, which projects upward in the pharynx behind the tongue. The cartilage is broad above, but narrows below to a thin stalk or *petiolus.* The upper part of its anterior surface, clothed with mucous membrane, borders the epiglottic valleculae posteriorly. Its posterior surface, also clothed with mucous membrane, forms the anterior wall of the laryngeal vestibule, the first part of the larynx. Below the valleculae, the anterior surface of the epiglottic cartilage is attached to the posterior surface of the hyoid bone by a *hypoepiglottic ligament*, and the petiolus is attached to the posterior surface of the thyroid cartilage by a *thyroepiglottic ligament*. From the edges of the epiglottis, the *aryepiglottic folds*, already mentioned, extend downward to the corniculate and arytenoid cartilages.

Interior of the Larynx

In a hemisection of the larynx (see Fig. 34-13), the general anatomy of its walls can be studied; however, relatively little of the cavity can be seen from above (Fig. 34-14). The aditus or entrance is bounded above by the superior border of the epiglottis, laterally by the aryepiglottic folds, and inferiorly and posteriorly by the interarytenoid fold (enclosing the arytenoideus muscles). The cavity of the larynx is divided into three parts: the **vestibule,** extend-

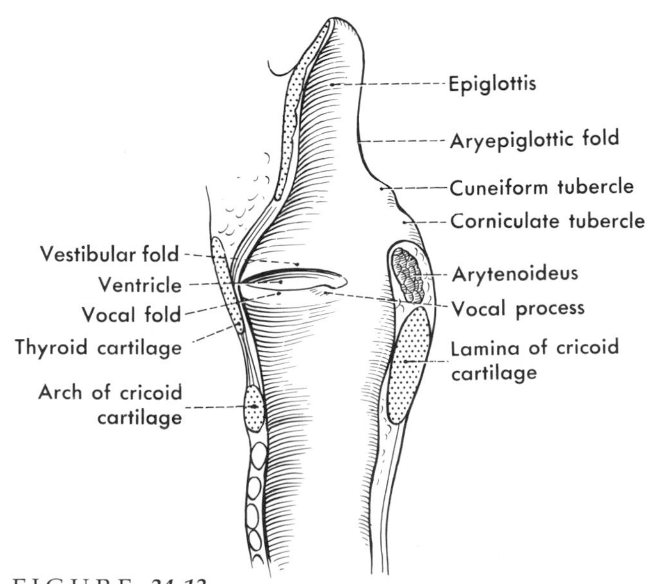

FIGURE *34-13.*
Interior of the larynx.

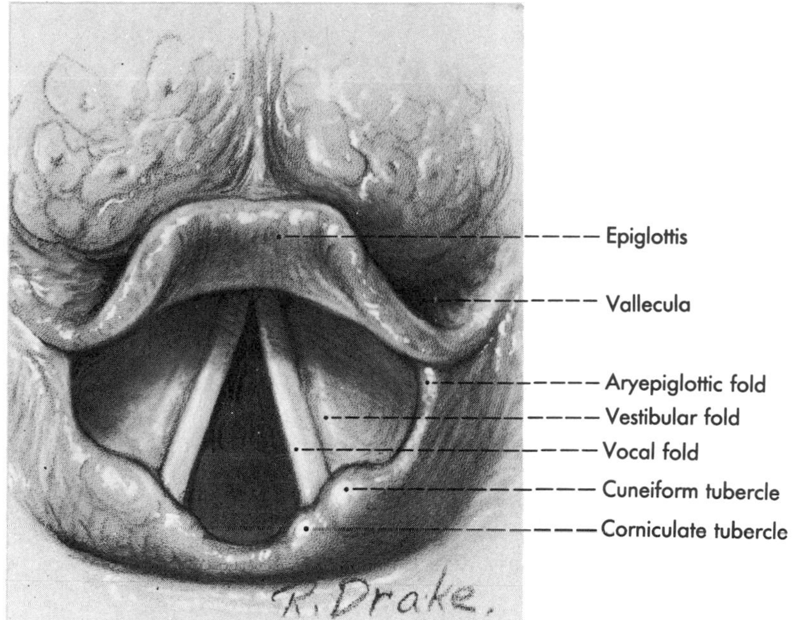

FIGURE 34-14.
View of the larynx from above with the vocal cords abducted.

ing from the aditus to the vestibular folds, prominent transverse folds of mucous membrane; the **ventricle,** lying between the vestibular and vocal folds; and the **infraglottic** (subglottic) **cavity,** lying below the vocal folds and extending downward to the lower border of the cricoid cartilage. The **glottis** consists of the vocal folds and the slit between these.

The bulky **vestibular folds** extend transversely on either side of the larynx and enclose between them a slit, the **rima vestibuli.** Underlying these folds are muscle fibers that can, by their contraction, bring the folds together, and it is this apposition of folds that is essential to holding the breath against pressure in the thoracic cavity when one is, for instance, exerting strain as in lifting a weight.

The **laryngeal ventricles,** lateral expansions of the laryngeal cavity between the vestibular folds and the sharper-edged vocal folds, undercut somewhat the vestibular folds, thereby helping these to resist the pressure of outgoing air when they are brought together. Toward the anterior end of the laryngeal ventricle there is a small blind sac protruding upward, the **laryngeal saccule.**

Rarely, the laryngeal saccule is congenitally enlarged and protrudes out through the thyrohyoid membrane to lie deep to the strap muscles of the neck (as it normally does in certain monkeys). It can also be enlarged by frequent increases in thoracic pressure. Thus, its enlargement can be considered an occupational hazard for such persons as glassblowers.

The **vocal folds** below the ventricles project medially and somewhat upward. Because of their direction, they are readily pushed aside by expired air (this occurs in phonation), but they tend to resist inspiration of air when they are together. The slit between the two vocal folds is the **rima glottidis.** The anterior part of each fold is formed by the vocal ligament (these border the pars intermembranacea of the rima). The posterior part of each fold is formed by the vocal process of the arytenoid cartilage and borders the pars intercartilaginea.

The membranous vocal folds, commonly called the vocal cords, are formed by thickened, upwardly projecting edges of a fibroelastic membrane, the **conus elasticus,** that lies between the laryngeal muscles and the mucous membrane (Fig. 34-15). The conus elasticus arises below from the entire upper border of the arch of the cricoid cartilage; the cricothyroid ligament, visible externally, is the thickened anterior part of the conus. Its upper borders, the **vocal ligaments,** are attached posteriorly to the vocal processes of the two arytenoid cartilages; anteriorly they are attached almost together to the posterior surface of the thyroid cartilage (Fig. 34-16). Apposition of the two vocal folds is necessary for normal phonation, for this allows the setting up of vibrations by them as the air passes between them. Similarly, their abduction is necessary to widen the passageway and allow the utmost in respiratory activity. Because their anterior ends are attached to the thyroid cartilage, it is their posterior ends that are moved apart or brought together by movements of the arytenoid cartilages.

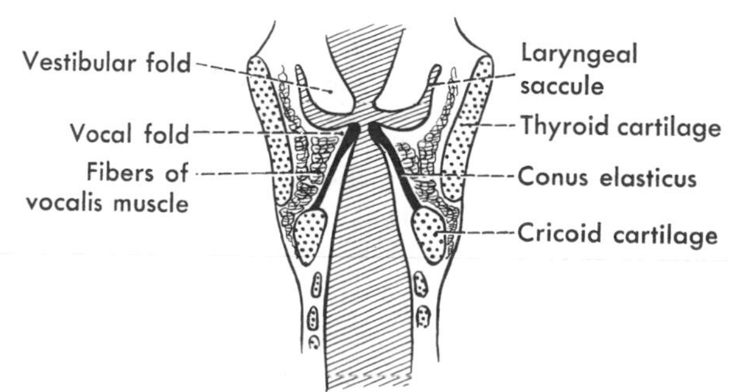

FIGURE 34-15.
Diagram of the conus elasticus.

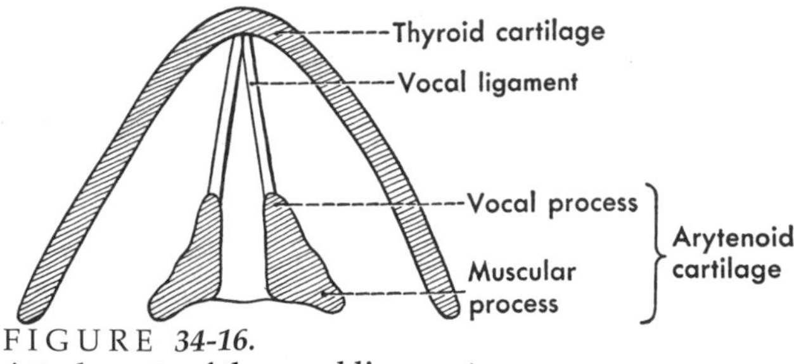

FIGURE *34-16.*
Attachments of the vocal ligaments.

The **infraglottic portion** of the larynx presents nothing of particular importance. It is wider anteroposteriorly than laterally. It narrows anteroposteriorly as it is traced downward toward the trachea, and its narrower lateral dimension widens. Anteriorly, the mucosa of the infraglottic portion of the larynx rests against a lower part of the thyroid cartilage, the cricothyroid ligament, and the arch of the cricoid cartilage. Posteriorly, it rests against the anterior surface of the lamina of the cricoid cartilage. At the lower border of the cricoid cartilage, the larynx is continuous with the trachea.

Elastic and Epithelial Layers

The larynx is lined by a fibroelastic membrane. The mucosa of the larynx is closely attached to the inner surface of this membrane, and many of the muscles are closely attached to the outer surface. The heaviest part of the fibroelastic membrane is the lowest part, or *conus elasticus,* ending above in the vocal ligaments, and the part above is the *quadrangular membrane.* This is particularly thin over the ventricles, but thickens in the vestibular folds to form vestibular ligaments. Above this, it runs upward and forward from the arytenoid and corniculate cartilages to the sides of the epiglottic cartilage, thus supporting the aryepiglottic folds.

The vocal ligaments are covered by stratified squamous epithelium, as is most of the wall of the vestibule, but columnar ciliated epithelium, similar to that of the trachea, is present in the laryngeal ventricle and below the glottis.

Muscles

The muscles listed as laryngeal ones are confined to the larynx and are divisible into two general groups: one group, composed of the aryepiglotticus, the thyroepiglotticus, the thyroarytenoideus, and the oblique arytenoideus, is primarily concerned with protection of the larynx and is sphincteric in action on the laryngeal aditus and vestibule; the other group, composed of the cricothyroideus, the cricoarytenoideus, the vocalis, and the transverse arytenoideus, is concerned with adjustments of the larynx and vocal cords during phonation and respiration. The larynx as a whole is also acted on by the infrahyoid muscles and indeed by all muscles attaching to the hyoid bone, because it moves with the hyoid bone.

The laryngeal muscles are innervated by the vagus nerves (the fibers reaching these nerves through the so-called cranial rootlets and internal ramus of the accessory nerve). The cricothyroid muscle the only external muscle of the larynx, is the only one innervated by the superior laryngeal nerve (which is otherwise only sensory and secretory to the larynx). The remaining muscles are innervated through the recurrent laryngeal branch of the vagus, which enters the larynx from below.

The **cricothyroid muscle** (see Fig. 34-20) arises from the arch of the cricoid cartilage and runs upward and backward, fanning out as it does so, to insert on the lower border and lower medial surface of the thyroid cartilage. The two muscles cover the lateral part of the cricothyroid ligament. When they act together, they tilt the cricoid cartilage on the thyroid. In consequence, they lengthen the distance between the posterior surface of the thyroid cartilage and the vocal processes of the arytenoid cartilages and thus lengthen the vocal cords (Fig. 34-17). Furthermore, because, in the relaxed condition, the vocal cords are bowed, this movement also tends to straighten the vocal cords and thus bring them closer to the midline.

The **external branch of the superior laryngeal nerve** descends on the lateral pharyngeal wall just deep to the superior thyroid artery to reach the cricothyroid muscle and innervate it.

After the pharyngeal mucosa has been removed from the posterior and lateral surfaces of the cricoid and arytenoid cartilages, and a lateral part of the thyroid cartilage has been cut away, most of the remaining muscles of the larynx can be seen (Fig. 34-18). The posterior surface of the lamina of the cricoid cartilage is largely covered on each side by the two **posterior cricoarytenoideus muscles,** which arise from the lamina. The fibers of each muscle converge to an insertion on the muscular process of the arytenoid cartilage. By their contraction, these muscles pull the muscular processes of the arytenoid cartilages medially and backward (Fig. 34-19A), thus producing a rotation of the arytenoid cartilages at the cricoarytenoid joints and swinging the vocal processes laterally. At the same time, they pull the arytenoid cartilages downward on the obliquely sloping cricoarytenoid joints, so that the two cartilages slide away from each other. Thus, both intercartilaginous and intermembranous parts of the rima glottidis are widened; indeed, the posterior cricoary-

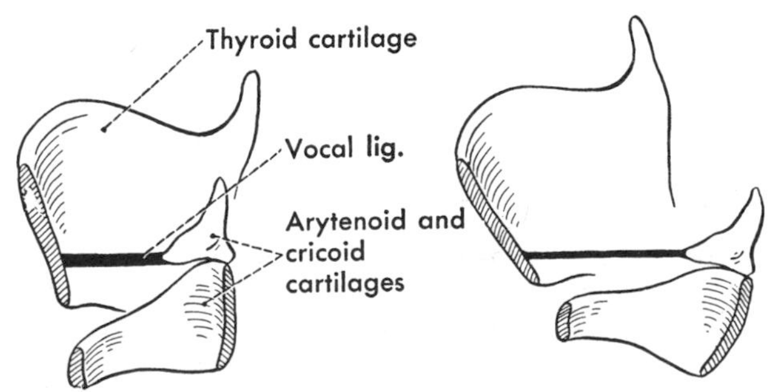

FIGURE *34-17.*
Action of the cricothyroid in lengthening and thinning the vocal cord by tilting the cricoid and thyroid cartilages on each other.

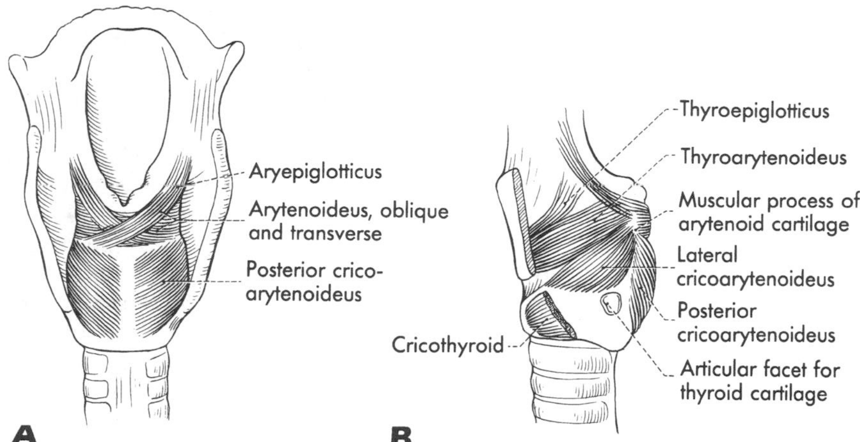

FIGURE *34-18.*
Muscles of the larynx in (A) posterior view, and (B) lateral view, after removal of the thyroid cartilage.

tenoid muscles are the only effective abductors of the vocal cords; therefore, they are particularly important in the preservation of an airway at the rima glottidis.

The **lateral cricoarytenoideus** is smaller than the posterior one. It arises from the upper border of the posterior part of the arch of the cricoid and runs upward and backward to insert on the muscular process of the arytenoid cartilage. It pulls the muscular process of the arytenoid cartilage forward and laterally (see Fig. 34-19B), rotating and sliding the arytenoid cartilage so that it and its vocal process are brought closer to the midline; thus, the lateral cricoarytenoidei are adductors of the vocal cords.

The **transverse arytenoideus** is an unpaired muscle that stretches between the posterior surfaces of the two arytenoid cartilages, uniting them below the interarytenoid notch. It draws the two cartilages together when it contracts, thereby tending to close the rima glottidis.

Posterior to the heavy transverse fibers of the transverse arytenoideus are two slender bands, the **oblique arytenoidei,** that arise from the muscular processes of the two arytenoid cartilages. The fibers swing upward across the midline, crossing those of the other side, to reach the apex of the arytenoid cartilage, where many of them insert. The remainder, joined by other fibers arising here from the arytenoid cartilage, extend upward in the aryepiglottic folds and form the **aryepiglottic muscle.** The oblique arytenoids and the aryepiglottic muscles together constitute a sphincter of the laryngeal aditus. By their contraction, they help prevent solids and liquids from entering the vestibule.

On the side of the larynx, deep to the thyroid cartilage, is a thin lamina of muscle, best developed at the level of the ventricular fold, that is the **thyroarytenoideus muscle.** This arises from the inner surface of the lower part of the thyroid cartilage close to the angle formed by the two laminae. It runs backward and somewhat upward to an insertion on the lateral border of the arytenoid cartilage. It is a sphincter of the vestibule, drawing the arytenoid cartilages closer to the thyroid cartilage and approximating the vestibular folds.

Associated with the upper border of the thyroarytenoideus muscle are other fibers, the **thyroepiglotticus,** that arise in common with the thyroarytenoideus, but leave it to sweep upward into the aryepiglottic fold. Here, they blend with the aryepiglotticus and insert in part into the quadrangular membrane and, in part, into the epiglottic cartilage. The thyroepiglotticus is a part of the sphincteric mechanism of aditus and vestibule.

The **vocalis muscle** is closely associated with the conus elasticus and the vocal ligament (see Fig. 34-15). It lies largely below and deep to the thyroarytenoideus. It is thicker than the thyroarytenoideus and somewhat triangular in cross section. It arises from the inferior part of the angle between the two laminae of the thyroid cartilage and runs backward to an insertion on the lateral surface of the vocal process and the adjacent anterolateral surface of the arytenoid cartilage, but between these two extremes, it is usually said to be attached along the entire length of the vocal ligament or the conus elasticus below the ligament (the details of its insertion are not agreed on). By its contraction, the vocalis muscle would tend to shorten the vocal cord if it acted alone; however, it probably acts when the length of the cord already is fixed by the cricothyroid muscle. By varying the degree of its contraction, it varies the tension of the vocal fold, and it also can hold a posterior part of the fold firmly against the other

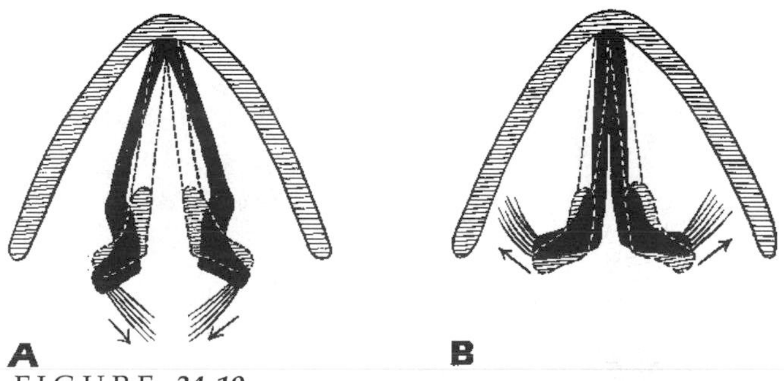

FIGURE *34-19.*
(A) The action of the posterior cricoarytenoid in adducting the vocal cord; (B) the action of the lateral cricoarytenoid in adducting the cord. The final position of the vocal cord and arytenoid cartilage is in *black,* and the starting position is in *outline.*

fold, allowing air to escape only between anterior parts of the folds. Exactly how it does the latter is not agreed on. It has been said variously to pull the conus elasticus upward so that the vocal folds are brought together over a greater area than that provided by their thin edges and to do the opposite, either abducting slightly a variable anterior segment of the cord or so pulling the cord forward that an anterior part of the two adducted cords is more easily separated by the air stream than is the posterior part.

Nerves and Vessels

The nerves and arteries of the larynx consist of the superior and inferior laryngeal nerves and arteries (Fig. 34-20).

The **superior laryngeal nerve,** a branch from the lower end of the inferior ganglion of the vagus, descends anterior to the vagus nerve in the upper part of the neck and, at about the level of the hyoid bone, comes in fairly close relation to the superior thyroid artery, lying just deep to that. Usually, above the level of the hyoid bone, the nerve divides into external and internal branches. The **external branch** descends behind the larynx on the inferior constrictor and with the superior thyroid artery until it curves forward below the thyroid cartilage to end in the cricothyroid muscle, frequently giving off a branch into the inferior constrictor before it does so.

The **internal branch** of the superior laryngeal nerve curves forward below the hyoid bone and accompanies the superior laryngeal artery, a branch of the superior thyroid, in a course across the posterior part of the thyrohyoid membrane. Soon, however, nerve and artery penetrate the membrane and run in the wall or floor of the piriform recess (where the nerve can be anesthetized). The nerve breaks up into branches, most of which penetrate the thyroarytenoideus muscle to be distributed both upward and downward to the mucosal surface of the larynx, largely above the vocal folds (and also to the piriform recess, the epiglottic vallecula, and a small posterior part of the dorsum of the tongue). One or more branches of the superior laryngeal nerve descend to reach the mucous membrane on the pharyngeal surface of the larynx and penetrate the transverse arytenoideus muscle to reach the interior of the larynx. One of these descending branches often anastomoses with the inferior laryngeal nerve.

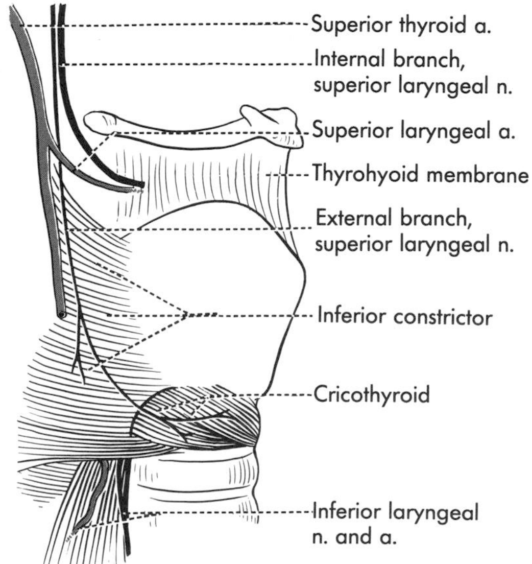

FIGURE *34-20.*
Nerves and arteries to the larynx.

The **inferior laryngeal nerve** is the terminal part of the recurrent laryngeal, a branch of the vagus. The courses of the recurrent nerves in the neck are described in Chapter 30. Each nerve enters the larynx just posterior to the cricothyroid articulation in the lateral gap between the lower edge of the inferior pharyngeal constrictor and the esophagus. Fairly often before it enters the larynx, but if not before then after it has entered, the inferior laryngeal nerve divides into two or more branches. The muscular distribution of the branches is variable, but if there are only two, the **posterior branch** is likely to be distributed to the posterior cricoarytenoid and the transverse and oblique arytenoidei muscles, and the **anterior branch** to the remaining internal muscles of the larynx. Twigs also supply the laryngeal mucosa below the vocal folds. Any of the branches may communicate with the internal laryngeal nerve.

The **inferior laryngeal artery** is a small branch of the inferior thyroid artery that accompanies the inferior laryngeal nerve into the larynx. It anastomoses there with the larger **superior laryngeal artery,** from the superior thyroid, and the two supply the larynx and adjacent portions of the pharynx. The laryngeal arteries are accompanied by laryngeal veins. The **superior laryngeal vein** typically joins the superior thyroid vein and through this empties into the internal jugular. The **inferior laryngeal vein** joins the inferior thyroid vein of its side or anastomosing channels between the thyroid veins across the front of the trachea.

The **lymphatics** of the larynx drain along the vessels and, therefore, both upward and downward. Some of them end in very small lymph nodes that lie on the thyrohyoid membrane and cricotracheal ligament, or on the upper end of the trachea, but these, in turn, drain to the deep cervical nodes, so that all the drainage of the larynx ends here.

Some Functional Aspects

The functions of the individual muscles of the larynx have already been noted, and functional aspects of the larynx as a whole can be fairly briefly summarized. The vestibule of the larynx is particularly sensitive to foreign objects, so that when these come in contact with its epithelium, violent coughing ensues to expel them. This involves first a marked abduction of the vocal cords, brought about particularly by the posterior cricoarytenoid muscles, to enlarge the airway as much as possible and allow a gasp for breath; then a closure of the larynx, primarily brought about by the vestibular folds and, therefore, by the thyroarytenoideus muscle; and when this closure is suddenly released following increase in pressure in the thorax, the air erupts as a cough.

In quiet inspiration, the vocal cords are slightly abducted and somewhat curved, and the arytenoid cartilages also are apart, so that there is a fair-sized slit at the rima glottidis. During forced inspiration, the rima glottidis is widened as much as possible which means that the arytenoid cartilages are pulled laterally and the vocal processes rotated laterally by the posterior cricoarytenoid muscles. During phonation, except for the lowest tones, the vocal cords become straight and move together to meet in the midline. This apparently is brought about by the action of several muscles simultaneously. The cricothyroids adduct and lengthen the vocal cord and fold because they tilt the thyroid and cricoid cartilages upon each other; the lateral cricoarytenoids adduct the vocal cords by swinging the vocal processes together; and the vocalis muscles apparently act differentially on the vocal folds so that a variable anterior segment vibrates.

Although it commonly is the escape of air between anterior segments of the two vocal folds that produces the vibrations that then are modified by the tongue, lips, palate, and so forth, to produce speech, other vibrating mechanisms can be used. For instance, the vestibular folds can be used for vocalization, although the voice then is more hoarse than usual. Also, after the larynx has been removed, as it may have to be for carcinoma, a patient may produce a certain amount of intelligible sound by learning to govern the escape of swallowed air from the stomach and the esophagus.

It perhaps cannot be claimed that the mechanism of vocalization is completely understood, but it seems clear that, under normal circumstances, control of tone (pitch) is brought about by variations in the length of the vibrating segments of the vocal folds. It is the anterior ends of the vocal folds that vibrate for the highest tones, and as progressively lower tones are produced, longer and longer anterior segments of the folds vibrate. Men generally have both longer and heavier vocal folds than women, and this is why the male voice is deeper. The muscles that particularly affect the length of the vocal folds and of their vibratory portions are the cricothyroideus, which lengthens the fold as a whole, and the vocalis, which apparently governs the length of the vibratory portion of the fold. Along with changes in the vibratory portions of the folds, the larynx as a whole also is raised or lowered—raised for high tones, lowered for low tones—so that the pharynx, a part of the resonating chamber above the larynx, is altered in length for different tones, somewhat as organ pipes of different lengths are used for the production of different tones. Insofar as the vocal cords themselves are concerned, it seems clear that changes in pitch are not produced simply by altering the tenseness of the vocal ligaments, as was once believed. The tenseness of the vocal folds is controlled by the vocalis muscles, not by stretch of the vocal ligaments, so that these muscles control both the tenseness and the mass of the vibrating segments of the vocal folds and are responsible for the fine variations in pitch of which the human larynx is capable.

Because the inferior laryngeal nerve innervates all the muscles of the larynx except the cricothyroid, and therefore all the muscles concerned with active movement of the vocal cords, paralysis of that nerve produces paralysis of the vocal cord on its side. A cord so paralyzed is at first bowed outward and can be neither abducted nor adducted. Because the normal vocal cord cannot meet it, the voice is poor (but in longer-standing paralysis, described below, a paralyzed cord may gradually move toward the midline, with consequent improvement of the voice to a point where it seems normal). Paralysis of the left nerve may occur as a result of a lesion in the mediastinum, for this nerve turns upward around the arch of the aorta, or either nerve may be interrupted in the neck. Each nerve is closely related to the posterior aspect of the thyroid gland just before it enters the larynx, and below that crosses the inferior thyroid artery (it may run behind the artery, between its branches, or in front of it); great care, therefore, must be taken to avoid injuring the nerves during thyroidectomy.

In bilateral paralysis of the vocal cords, the voice is almost lost, for the cords cannot be moved together. Often, however, bilaterally paralyzed cords gradually become less bowed and, therefore, move toward each other, as a result of the pull of the unparalyzed cricothyroid muscles. The voice improves as adduction increases, but as the cords cannot be abducted, the airway is simultaneously narrowed. The narrowing may be so severe that operative intervention, usually involving removal of the arytenoid cartilage, is necessary.

If a superior laryngeal nerve or its external branch is interrupted (as they may be in securing the superior thyroid artery in a thyroidectomy), the cricothyroid muscle cannot lengthen the vocal cord. Although such a cord will move as readily to the midline as will its mate on the unaffected side, it is not as straight and tense, for the vocalis muscle is not as effective in acting on the cord as a whole as is the cricothyroid. Consequently, because of the lack of tenseness of one cord, there is a tendency to hoarseness and easy tiring of the voice.

Variations in the position and tenseness of the vocal folds after nerve injury are impossible to quantitate by laryngoscopy, so clinicians commonly classify vocal cords simply as bowed or straight and as movable or immovable.

RECOMMENDED READINGS

Basmajian JV, DeLuca CJ. Mouth, pharynx, and larynx. In: Muscles alive: their functions revealed by electromyography. 5th ed. Baltimore: Williams & Wilkins, 1985.

Curtin HD. Separation of the masticator space from parapharyngeal space. Radiology 1987; 163: 195.

Dorrance GM, Bransfield JW. Studies in the anatomy and repair of cleft palate. Surg Gynecol Obstet 1947; 84: 878.

Eckel HE, Sittel C, Zorowka P, Jerke A. Dimensions of the laryngeal framework in adults. Surg Radiol Anat 1994; 16: 31.

Fink BR. Tensor mechanisms of the vocal folds. Ann Otol Rhinol Laryngol 1962; 71: 591.

Fink BR. The human larynx: a functional study. New York: Raven Press, 1975.

Graney DO, Flint PW. Anatomy of the larynx/hypopharynx. In: Cummings CW, ed. Otolaryngology—head and neck surgery. 2nd ed, vol 3. St Louis: Mosby-Year Book, 1993: 1693.

Graney DO, Petruzzelli GY, Myers EN. Anatomy of the oral cavity/oropharynx/nasopharynx. In: Cummings CW, ed. Otolaryngology—head and neck surgery. 2nd ed. vol 2. St Louis: Mosby-Year Book, 1993: 1101.

Hollinshead WH. Anatomy for surgeons: vol 1, the head and neck. 3rd ed. Philadelphia: Harper & Row, 1982.

Lam KH, Wong J. The preepiglottic and paraglottic spaces in relation to spread of carcinoma of the larynx. Am J Otolaryngol 1983; 4: 81.

Lemere F. Innervation of the larynx: I. Innervation of laryngeal muscles. Am J Anat 1932; 51: 417.

Mitchinson AGH, Yoffey JM. Changes in the vocal folds in humming low and high notes: a radiographic study. J Anat 1948; 82: 88.

Morrison LF. Recurrent laryngeal nerve paralysis: a revised conception based on the dissection of one hundred cadavers. Ann Otol Rhinol Laryngol 1952; 61: 567.

Murtagh JA. The respiratory function of the larynx: some observations in the laryngeal innervation. Ann Otol Rhinol Laryngol 1945; 54: 102.

Pressman JJ, Dowdy A, Libby R, Fields M. Further studies upon the submucosal compartments and lymphatics of the larynx by the injection of dyes and radioisotopes. Ann Otol Rhinol Laryngol 1956; 65: 963.

Ramsey GH, Watson JS, Gramiak R, et al. Cinefluorographic analysis of the mechanism of swallowing. Radiology 1955; 64: 498.

Raven RW. Pouches of the pharynx and oesophagus: with special reference to the embryological and morphological aspects. Br J Surg 1933; 21: 235.

Rich AR. The innervation of the tensor veli palatini and levator veli palatini muscles. Bull Johns Hopkins Hosp 1920; 31: 305.

Reidenbach MM. The cricoarytenoid ligament: its morphology and possible implications for vocal cord movements. Surg Radiol Anat 1995; 17: 301.

Rueger RS. The superior laryngeal nerve and the interarytenoid muscle in humans: an anatomical study. Laryngoscope 1972; 82: 2008.

Sellars IE, Keen EN The anatomy and movements of the cricoarytenoid joint. Laryngoscope 1978; 88: 667.

Stockwell M, Lozanoff S, Lang SA, Nyssen J. Superior laryngeal nerve block: an anatomical study. Clin Anat 1995; 8: 89.

Van Alyea, OE. Ethmoid labyrinth: anatomic study, with consideration of the clinical significance of its structural characteristics. Arch Otolaryngol 1939; 29: 881.

Glossary of Some Synonyms and Eponyms

This relatively short list includes BNA and other terms that are in fairly common use but differ considerably from the NA and, therefore, need definition. With the occasional exception of useful terms that the NA omits entirely, the continued use of these terms should be avoided, but the student will encounter them and needs to understand them. Eponyms, such as those listed here and numerous others, should be discouraged, because they are often vague, do not necessarily indicate the person who first described the structure, and are totally nondescriptive.

Alcock's canal: pudendal canal
Ansa hypoglossi: ansa cervicalis
Antrum: maxillary sinus
  tympanic: mastoid antrum
Appendage, auricular: auricle (of heart)
Arches, lumbocostal: arcuate ligaments
  volar arterial: palmar arterial arches
Artery, auditory, internal: labyrinthine
  buccinator: buccal
  coronary of stomach: left gastric, *or* left and right gastrics
  dental: alveolar
  descending, of heart: interventricular
  digital, volar: palmar digital
  dorsal interosseous, of forearm: posterior interosseous
  frontal: supratrochlear
  genicular, supreme: descending genicular
  hemorrhoidal: rectal
  hypogastric: internal iliac
  innominate: brachiocephalic
  interosseous, dorsal and volar: posterior and anterior interosseous
  of ligamentum teres femoris: a. of the ligament of the femoral head
  mammary, internal: internal thoracic
  maxillary, external: facial

Artery
  internal: maxillary
  metacarpal, volar: palmar metacarpal
  spermatic, internal: testicular *or* ovarian
  transverse scapular: suprascapular
  vesiculodeferential: a. of ductus deferens
Auditory: acoustic
Auerbach's plexus and ganglia: myenteric portion of the enteric nerve plexus
Bartholin's duct: major sublingual duct
  gland: greater vestibular gland
Bell's muscle: lateral edges of the trigonal muscle of the urinary bladder
Bigelow, "Y" ligament of: iliofemoral ligament
Bochdalek's gap: lumbocostal trigone
Bone, astragalus: talus
  cuneiform, first, second, and third: medial, intermediate, and lateral cuneiforms
  innominate: os coxae
  malar: zygomatic
  multangular, greater and lesser: trapezium and trapezoid
  navicular, of hand: scaphoid
  scaphoid, of foot: navicular
  turbinate: nasal concha
Botallo's duct and ligament: ductus arteriosus and ligamentum arteriosum
Broca's convolution: posterior end of left inferior frontal gyrus
Buck's fascia: deep penile fascia
Burn's space: suprasternal fascial space
Calot, triangle of: cystohepatic triangle; *see* Triangle
Camper's fascia: fatty part of superficial fascia (tela subcutanea) on lower abdomen
Canal, pterygopalatine: palatine canals
  of Schlemm: sinus venosus sclerae
  semicircular, membranous: semicircular duct
  subsartorial: adductor canal
Canthi (canthus): the palpebral commissures, or angles at which the eyelids meet

Cartilage, lower nasal: greater alar
sesamoid, nasal: accessory
upper nasal: lateral
Chain, sympathetic: sympathetic trunk
Chopart's joint: transverse tarsal joint
Cisterna magna: cerebellomedullary cistern
Cloquet's septum; node: femoral septum; lymph node at the femoral ring
Colles' fascia: superficial perineal fascia (membranous, deep to the tela subcutanea)
Cooper's ligaments: a) pectineal ligament, b) suspensory ligaments of breast
Corpus cavernosum urethrae: corpus spongiosum penis
Cortex, of cerebral hemisphere: pallium
Corti, ganglion and organ of: spiral ganglion and spiral organ of ear
Cowper's glands: bulbourethral glands
Cuvier, duct of: common cardinal vein
Denonvillier's fascia: rectovesical septum (peritoneoperineal membrane)
Dorsal: posterior, usually, except in hand
Douglas, cavity or pouch of: rectouterine excavation or pouch
fold of: rectouterine fold
line or fold of: arcuate line of sheath of rectus abdominis
Duct, submaxillary: submandibular duct
Eminence, iliopectineal: iliopubic eminence
Eustachian tube: auditory tube
valve: valve of inferior vena cava
Fallopian aqueduct or canal: facial canal
foramen: hiatus of canal of greater petrosal nerve
tube: uterine tube
Fascia bulbi: vagina bulbi
lumbodorsal: thoracolumbar
renal: fibrous portion of the adipose renal capsule
Sibson's: suprapleural membrane
Fenestra ovalis: fenestra vestibuli
rotunda: fenestra cochleae
Filum terminale, internal: filum terminale (of cord)
external: filum of the spinal dura mater
Fissure, of cerebral pallium: sulcus
pterygopalatine: pterygomaxillary fissure
sphenoidal: superior orbital fissure
sphenoidal, inferior, *or* **sphenomaxillary:** inferior orbital fissure
Flexure, hepatic: right colic
lienal: left colic
Fold, ileocecal, inferior: ileocecal
superior: vascular fold of cecum
malleolar: mallear
ventricular: vestibular
Foramen, optic: optic canal
Fossa, antecubital: cubital
navicularis: vestibular fossa
ovalis femoris: saphenous hiatus
Fourchette: frenulum of labia minora
Foveae, inguinal and supravesical: inguinal and supravesical fossae
Frankenhauser's ganglion: uterovaginal nerve plexus
Gärtner's duct: longitudinal duct of epoöphoron, remains of mesonephric duct in female.
Galen, vein of: great cerebral vein
Ganglion, cervical, inferior: unfortunately not included in the NA. This is the lowest cervical sympathetic ganglion, frequently but not always fused with the first thoracic to form the cervicothoracic or stellate ganglion
jugular: superior, of vagus
nodose: inferior, of vagus
petrous: inferior, of glossopharyngeal
semilunar: trigeminal
sphenopalatine: pterygopalatine
submaxillary: submandibular
Gasserian ganglion: trigeminal ganglion
Genu, external, of facial nerve: geniculum
Gerota's capsule or fascia: renal fascia; *see* Fascia
Gimbernat's ligament: lacunar ligament
Gland, adrenal: suprarenal
lymph: lymph node
submaxillary: submandibular
Glaserian fissure: petrotympanic fissure
Glisson's capsule: perivascular fibrous capsule of liver
Groove, bicipital, of humerus: intertubercular groove
Gyrus, fusiform: medial occipitotemporal gyrus
hippocampal: parahippocampal gyrus
Hasner, fold or valve of: lacrimal fold
Haversian canals: central canal of osteon
Heister, spiral valve of: spiral fold of cystic duct
Henle's ligament: part of conjoint tendon
Hensen's duct: ductus reuniens
Hering, nerve of: Carotid sinus branch of cranial nerve IX
Herophilus, torcular of: confluence of the (cranial venous) sinuses
Hesselbach's ligament: interfoveolar ligament
triangle: inguinal triangle
Hiatus, of facial canal: of canal of greater petrosal nerve
Highmore, antrum of: maxillary sinus
His, bundle of: atrioventricular bundle
Horner's muscle: pars lacriminalis of orbicularis oculi
Houston's valves or folds: transverse rectal folds
Humphrey, ligament of: anterior meniscofemoral ligament
Hunter's canal: adductor canal
Inscription, tendinous: tendinous intersection
Ischiadic: sciatic
Jacobson's cartilage, organ: vomeronasal cartilage and organ
nerve: tympanic branch, cranial nerve IX
Labbé, vein of: inferior anastomotic vein of cerebrum
Labrum, glenoid (of hip): acetabular labrum
Lacertus fibrosus: bicipital aponeurosis
Lamina papyracea: orbital lamina of ethmoid bone
Langer's lines: cleavage lines of skin
Ligament, cruciate crural: inferior extensor retinaculum of ankle
dorsal carpal: extensor retinaculum at wrist
iliopectineal: iliopectineal arch

laciniate: flexor retinaculum at ankle
periodontal: same as periodontal membrane
supensory of eyeball: thickened lower part of bulbar sheath
transverse carpal: flexor retinaculum at wrist
transverse crural: superior extensor retinaculum of leg and ankle
umbilical, lateral: medial umbilical ligament.
Ligamentum teres (of femur): ligament of the head of the femur
Line, pectinate or mucocutaneous: a line connecting the anal valves at the bases of the anal columns
Linea semicircularis: arcuate line of sheath of rectus abdominis
Lister's tubercle: dorsal radial tubercle; *see* Tubercle
Littré, glands of: urethral glands
Lockwood's ligament: thickened lower part of the bulbar sheath
Louis (Ludovici), angle of: sternal angle
Luschka's body or glomus: coccygeal body
foramina: lateral apertures of fourth ventricle
Mackenrodt's ligament: cardinal (lateral cervical) ligament of uterus
Magendie, foramen of: median aperture of fourth ventricle
Marshall, ligament or fold of: fold of the left superior vena cava in the pericardial sac
vein of: oblique vein of left atrium
Mayo, vein of: prepyloric vein
Meatus, urethral: external urethral ostium in male
Meckel's cartilage: the cartilage of the first branchial arch
cave: trigeminal cavum, the subarachnoid space around cranial nerve V as it lies in the middle cranial fossa
diverticulum: ileal diverticulum, a persistent proximal part of the vitellointestinal duct
ganglion: pterygopalatine, *sometimes* submandibular ganglion
Meibomian glands: tarsal glands
Membrane, basilar (of ear): lamina basilaris
periodontal: the dental term for the periodontium; in dentistry, periodontium includes also the surrounding bone and the gums
Monro, foramina of: interventricular foramina
Morgagni, appendix of hydatid of: appendix testis *or* vesicular appendix of epoöphoron
columns of: anal columns
foramen of: a) foramen cecum linguae, b) sternocostal triangle; *see* Triangle
fossa of: fossa navicularis urethrae
sinus of: a) laryngeal ventricle, b) anal sinus, c) space between superior constrictor and base of skull, d) pharyngeal recess
Morison, pouch or space of: hepatorenal recess
Müller's duct: paramesonephric duct
muscle: any of four bits of smooth muscle related to orbit, but most commonly the superior tarsal muscle
Muscle, bulbocavernosus: bulbospongiosus
caninus: levator anguli oris
compressor naris: transverse part of nasalis
dilator naris: alar part of nasalis
flexor digitorum sublimis: flexor digitorum superficialis
quadratus labii inferioris: depressor labii inferioris
quadratus labii superioris: zygomaticus minor levator labii superioris, *and* levator labii superioris alaeque nasi
thyroarytenoideus externus: thyroarytenoideus
internus: vocalis
triangularis: depressor anguli oris
Nerve, acoustic: vestibulocochlear
anterior thoracic: pectoral nerves
buccinator: buccal branch of trigeminal nerve
cutaneous colli: transversus colli
dorsal, in forearm: posterior
hemorrhoidal: rectal
of Hering: carotid sinus nerve
petrosal, superficial, greater and lesser: greater and lesser petrosals
statoacoustic: vestibulocochlear
vidian: nerve of pterygoid canal
volar: in forearm, anterior; in hand, palmar
Nuck, canal of: persistent processus vaginalis in female
Oddi, sphincter of: sphincter of hepatopancreatic ampulla
Olive, inferior: olive
Os, external: uterine ostium
Otoliths: statoconia
Pacchionian bodies or granulations: arachnoidal granulations
Passavant, fold or ridge of: a fold developing on the posterior pharyngeal wall to help close the nasopharynx
Petit, triangle of: lumbar triangle
Plexus, hypogastric: pelvic plexus
Portio major, of trigeminal nerve: sensory root
minor, of trigeminal nerve: motor root
Pouches, perineal: perineal spaces
Poupart's ligament: inguinal ligament
Process, odontoid: dens of axis
Purkinje fibers: modified muscle fibers of the conduction system of the heart
Ranvier, nodes of: constrictions of the myelin of nerve fibers
Rathke's pouch: hypophyseal, craniobuccal, *or* neurobuccal pouch, from which the anterior lobe of the hypophysis develops
Reil, island of: insula of cerebral hemisphere
Reissner's membrane: vestibular membrane
Retzius, cave of: retropubic space
veins of: retroperitoneal veins connecting portal and caval systems
Riolan, arc of: usually an anastomosis between the left and middle colic arteries at the base of the mesocolon
Rivinus, ducts of: lesser sublingual ducts
Rolandic fissure: central sulcus of cerebral hemisphere
Rosenmöller, fossa of: pharyngeal recess
Rosenthal, vein of: basal vein of cerebrum

Sac, lesser: omental bursa
Santorini, cartilage of: corniculate cartilage
  duct of: accessory pancreatic duct
Sappey's veins: small veins in the falciform ligament
Scala media: cochlear duct
Scarpa's fascia: membranous part of superficial fascia of lower abdomen
  ganglion: vestibular ganglion
  triangle: femoral triangle
Schlemm, canal of: sinus venosus sclerae
Sibson's fascia: suprapleural membrane
Sinus, piriform: piriform recess
  rectal: anal sinus
Skene's ducts or glands: paraurethral ducts or glands
Spieghel's (spigelian) line: semilunar line of abdomen
  lobe: caudate lobe of liver
Stensen, canal of: incisive canal
  duct of: parotid duct
Sylvian aqueduct: cerebral aqueduct
  fissure: lateral sulcus of cerebral hemisphere
Tables, of skull: laminae
Tenon's capsule or fascia: the fascial sheath of the eyeball
Thebesian valve: valve of coronary sinus
  veins: least cardiac veins
Treitz, muscle or ligament of: suspensory muscle of duodenum
Treves, bloodless fold of: ileocecal fold
Triangle, cystohepatic: triangle between cystic duct, common hepatic duct, and liver
sternocostal: triangle between sternal and costal origins of diaphragm, transmitting superior epigastric vessels
Trolard, vein of: superior anastomotic vein of cerebrum
Tuberosity, bicipital: radial
  of humerus: tubercle
Tunnel, carpal: carpal canal
Turbinate: concha
Urethra, anterior: spongy, or spongy and membranous, part of male urethra
  posterior: prostatic, or prostatic and membranous, part of male urethra
Uvea, or uveal tract: the choroid, ciliary body, and iris of the eyeball
Valsalva, sinus of: aortic sinus
Vas deferens: ductus deferens
Vasa efferentia testis: ductuli efferentes
Vater, ampulla of: hepatopancreatic ampulla
Vein, coronary: usually left gastric
  facial, anterior: facial **common:** lower end of facial vein after it is joined by retromandibular vein
   posterior: retromandibular
  hemorrhoidal: rectal
  hypogastric: internal iliac
  innominate: brachiocephalic
  maxillary, internal: maxillary
  pyloric: usually right gastric, sometimes prepyloric vein
Verumontanum: colliculus seminalis
Vidian canal, nerve: pterygoid canal, nerve of pterygoid canal
Volar: in forearm, anterior; in hand, palmar
Waldeyer's ring: lymphatic ring in the pharynx
Wharton's duct: submandibular duct
Willis, circle of: circulus arteriosus cerebri
Window: *see* Fenestra
Winslow, foramen of: epiploic foramen
Wirsung, duct of: pancreatic (chief) duct
Wolffian body and duct: mesonephros and mesonephric duct
Wormian bones: sutural bones of skull
Wrisberg, cartilage of: cuneiform cartilage
  ganglion of: a cardiac ganglion
  ligament of: posterior meniscofemoral ligament
Zinn, annulus of: annulus tendineus communis
Zuckerkandl, organs of: groups of chromaffin cells on the aorta near origin of inferior mesenteric artery

Index

PLEASE NOTE: Anatomical terms are found under the type of structure, printed in **BOLDFACE CAPITALS**. For example, to find *femoral artery* look under **ARTERY(IES)**. Page numbers in boldface type indicate more substantive information on that subject. Figures and tables are identified by "f" or "t" after the page number.

E

H

N

O

U

V